Code of
Medical Ethics

of the American Medical Association

Council on Ethical and Judicial Affairs
Current Opinions with Annotations

2012–2013 Edition

Annotations prepared by the
Southern Illinois University Schools of Medicine and Law

AMA
AMERICAN
MEDICAL
ASSOCIATION

Contents

Preface ix

History xi

Guide to Use of Annotations xiii

Principles of Medical Ethics

Preamble xv

Principles of Medical Ethics, with annotations xvi

Principles of Medical Ethics I xx

Principles of Medical Ethics II. xxvi

Principles of Medical Ethics III xxxiii

Principles of Medical Ethics IV xxxvii

Principles of Medical Ethics V lvi

Principles of Medical Ethics VI lix

Principles of Medical Ethics VII. lxviii

Principles of Medical Ethics VIII lxxi

Principles of Medical Ethics IX lxxvi

1.00 Introduction

1.01   Terminology 1

1.02   The Relation of Law and Ethics 1

2.00 Opinions on Social Policy Issues

2.01   Abortion 5

2.015   Mandatory Parental Consent to Abortion 6

2.02   Physicians' Obligations in Preventing, Identifying, and Treating Violence and Abuse   8

2.03   Allocation of Limited Medical Resources 11

2.035   Futile Care 16

2.037   Medical Futility in End-of-Life Care 18

2.04   Artificial Insemination by Known Donor 20

2.05   Artificial Insemination by Anonymous Donor 22

2.055   Ethical Conduct in Assisted Reproductive Technology 23

2.06   Capital Punishment 24

2.065   Court-Initiated Medical Treatments in Criminal Cases 34

2.067   Torture 35

2.068   Physician Participation in Interrogation 37

2.07   Clinical Investigation 38

2.071   Subject Selection for Clinical Trials 42

2.075   The Use of Placebo Controls in Clinical Trials 43

2.076   Surgical "Placebo" Controls 44

2.077   Ethical Considerations in International Research 45

2.078   Guidelines to Prevent Malevolent Use of Biomedical Research 46

2.079   Safeguards in the Use of DNA Databanks in Genomic Research 47

2.08	Commercial Use of Human Tissue	48
2.09	Costs	50
2.095	The Provision of Adequate Health Care	52
2.10	Fetal Research Guidelines	53
2.105	Patenting Human Genes	54
2.11	Gene Therapy	56
2.12	Genetic Counseling	57
2.13	Genetic Engineering	59
2.131	Disclosure of Familial Risk in Genetic Testing	59
2.132	Genetic Testing by Employers	60
2.135	Insurance Companies and Genetic Information	63
2.136	Genetic Information and the Criminal Justice System	63
2.137	Ethical Issues in Carrier Screening of Genetic Disorders	64
2.138	Genetic Testing of Children	65
2.139	Multiplex Genetic Testing	66
2.14	In Vitro Fertilization	67
2.141	Frozen Pre-embryos	68
2.145	Pre-embryo Splitting	70
2.146	Research With Stem Cells	70
2.147	Cloning to Produce Children	72
2.15	Transplantation of Organs From Living Donors	73
2.151	Cadaveric Organ Donation: Encouraging the Study of Motivation	76
2.152	Solicitation of the Public for Directed Donation of Organs for Transplantation	77
2.155	Presumed Consent and Mandated Choice for Organs From Deceased Donors	78
2.157	Organ Donation After Cardiac Death	80
2.16	Organ Transplantation Guidelines	81
2.161	Medical Applications of Fetal Tissue Transplantation	83
2.162	Anencephalic Neonates as Organ Donors	83
2.165	Umbilical Cord Blood Banking	85
2.169	The Ethical Implications of Xenotransplantation	86
2.17	Quality of Life	87
2.18	Surrogate Mothers	90
2.19	Unnecessary Medical Services	91
2.191	Advance Care Planning	92
2.20	Withholding or Withdrawing Life-Sustaining Medical Treatment	93
2.201	Sedation to Unconsciousness in End-of-Life Care	113
2.21	Euthanasia	114
2.211	Physician-Assisted Suicide	117
2.215	Treatment Decisions for Seriously Ill Newborns	126
2.22	Do-Not-Resuscitate Orders	128
2.225	Optimal Use of Orders Not-to-Intervene and Advance Directives	131
2.23	HIV Testing	133
2.24	Impaired Drivers and Their Physicians	135
2.25	The Use of Quarantine and Isolation as Public Health Interventions	136
2.30	Information From Unethical Experiments	138
2.40	Radio-Frequency ID Devices in Humans	139

3.00 Opinions on Interprofessional Relations

3.01	Nonscientific Practitioners	140
3.02	Nurses	143
3.03	Allied Health Professionals	143
3.04	Referral of Patients	144
3.041	Chiropractic	145
3.05	Physician Employment by a Nonphysician Supervisee	146
3.06	Sports Medicine	146
3.08	Sexual Harassment and Exploitation Between Medical Supervisors and Trainees	147
3.09	Medical Students Performing Procedures on Fellow Students	148

4.00 Opinions on Hospital Relations

4.01	Admission Fee	149
4.02	Assessments, Compulsory	149
4.03	Billing for Housestaff and Student Services	149
4.04	Economic Incentives and Levels of Care	150
4.05	Organized Medical Staff	151
4.06	Physician-Hospital Contractual Relations	151
4.07	Staff Privileges	151

5.00 Opinions on Confidentiality, Advertising, and Communications Media Relations

5.01	Advertising and Managed Care Organizations	153
5.015	Direct-to-Consumer Advertisements of Prescription Drugs	154
5.02	Advertising and Publicity	155
5.025	Physician Advisory or Referral Services by Telecommunication	159
5.026	The Use of Electronic Mail	159
5.027	Use of Health-Related Online Sites	161
5.04	Communications Media: Standards of Professional Responsibility	162
5.045	Filming Patients in Health Care Settings	163
5.046	Filming Patients for the Education of Health Professionals	165
5.05	Confidentiality	166
5.051	Confidentiality of Medical Information Postmortem	184
5.055	Confidential Care for Minors	185
5.059	Privacy in the Context of Health Care	187
5.0591	Patient Privacy and Outside Observers to the Clinical Encounter	188
5.06	Confidentiality: Attorney-Physician Relation	188
5.07	Confidentiality: Computers	189
5.075	Confidentiality: Disclosure of Records to Data Collection Companies	193
5.08	Confidentiality: Insurance Company Representative	194
5.09	Confidentiality: Industry-Employed Physicians and Independent Medical Examiners	195
5.10	A Physician's Role Following a Breach of Electronic Health Information	197

6.00 Opinions on Fees and Charges

6.01	Contingent Physician Fees	199
6.02	Fee Splitting	201

6.021   Financial Incentives to Patients for Referrals 203
6.03   Fee Splitting: Referrals to Health Care Facilities 203
6.05   Fees for Medical Services 204
6.07   Insurance Form Completion Charges 204
6.08   Interest Charges and Finance Charges 205
6.09   Laboratory Bill 206
6.10   Services Provided by Multiple Physicians 206
6.11   Competition 206
6.12   Forgiveness or Waiver of Insurance Copayments 207
6.13   Professional Courtesy 208

7.00   Opinions on Physician Records

7.01   Records of Physicians: Availability of Information to Other Physicians 209
7.02   Records of Physicians: Information and Patients 210
7.025   Records of Physicians: Access by Nontreating Medical Staff 212
7.03   Records of Physicians Upon Retirement or Departure From a Group 212
7.04   Sale of a Medical Practice 214
7.05   Retention of Medical Records 215

8.00   Opinions on Practice Matters

8.01   Appointment Charges 217
8.02   Ethical Guidelines for Physicians in Administrative or
        Other Nonclinical Roles 217
8.021   Ethical Obligations of Medical Directors 218
8.03   Conflicts of Interest: Guidelines 219
8.031   Conflicts of Interest: Biomedical Research 224
8.0315   Managing Conflicts of Interest in the Conduct of Clinical Trials 226
8.0321   Physicians' Self-referral 228
8.04   Consultation 233
8.041   Second Opinions 234
8.043   Ethical Implications of Surgical Comanagement 235
8.045   Direct-to-Consumer Diagnostic Imaging Tests 236
8.047   Industry Representatives in Clinical Settings 237
8.05   Contractual Relationships 237
8.0501   Professionalism and Contractual Relations 241
8.051   Conflicts of Interest Under Capitation 241
8.052   Negotiating Discounts for Specialty Care 243
8.053   Restrictions on Disclosure in Health Care Plan Contracts 243
8.054   Financial Incentives and the Practice of Medicine 244
8.055   Retainer Practices 246
8.056   Physician Pay-for-Performance Programs 248
8.06   Prescribing and Dispensing Drugs and Devices 249
8.061   Gifts to Physicians From Industry 252
8.062   Sale of Non–Health-Related Goods From Physicians' Offices 266
8.063   Sale of Health-Related Products From Physicians' Offices 266
8.07   Expedited Partner Therapy 268
8.08   Informed Consent 269
8.081   Surrogate Decision Making 277
8.082   Withholding Information From Patients 279

8.083	Placebo Use in Clinical Practice	280
8.085	Waiver of Informed Consent for Research in Emergency Situations	281
8.087	Medical Student Involvement in Patient Care	282
8.088	Resident Physicians' Involvement in Patient Care	282
8.09	Laboratory Services	283
8.095	Reporting Clinical Test Results: General Guidelines	284
8.10	Lien Laws	285
8.11	Neglect of Patient	285
8.115	Termination of the Physician-Patient Relationship	288
8.12	Patient Information	290
8.121	Ethical Responsibility to Study and Prevent Error and Harm	293
8.13	Managed Care	295
8.132	Referral of Patients: Disclosure of Limitations	303
8.135	Cost Containment Involving Prescription Drugs in Health Care Plans	305
8.14	Sexual Misconduct in the Practice of Medicine	307
8.145	Sexual or Romantic Relations Between Physicians and Key Third-Parties	312
8.15	Substance Abuse	313
8.16	Substitution of Surgeon Without Patient's Knowledge or Consent	313
8.17	Use of Restraints	315
8.18	Informing Families of a Patient's Death	316
8.181	Performing Procedures on the Newly Deceased for Training Purposes	316
8.19	Self-treatment or Treatment of Immediate Family Members	317
8.191	Peers as Patients	318
8.20	Invalid Medical Treatment	319
8.21	Use of Chaperones During Physical Exams	319

9.00 Opinions on Professional Rights and Responsibilities

9.01	Accreditation	321
9.011	Continuing Medical Education	321
9.0115	Financial Relationships With Industry in Continuing Medical Education	323
9.012	Physicians' Political Communications With Patients and Their Families	325
9.02	Restrictive Covenants and the Practice of Medicine	325
9.021	Covenants Not-to-Compete for Physicians-in-Training	331
9.025	Advocacy for Change in Law and Policy	331
9.03	Civil Rights and Professional Responsibility	332
9.0305	Physician Health and Wellness	333
9.031	Reporting Impaired, Incompetent, or Unethical Colleagues	333
9.032	Reporting Adverse Drug or Device Events	335
9.035	Gender Discrimination in the Medical Profession	336
9.037	Signing Bonuses to Attract Graduates of US Medical Schools	337
9.04	Discipline and Medicine	337
9.045	Physicians With Disruptive Behavior	339
9.05	Due Process	340
9.055	Disputes Between Medical Supervisors and Trainees	341
9.06	Free Choice	342
9.065	Caring for the Poor	346
9.0651	Financial Barriers to Health Care Access	348
9.067	Physician Obligation in Disaster Preparedness and Response	349

9.07	Medical Testimony	350
9.08	New Medical Procedures	354
9.09	Patent for Surgical or Diagnostic Instrument	356
9.095	The Use of Patents and Other Means to Limit Availability of Medical Procedures.	357
9.10	Peer Review	360
9.11	Ethics Committees in Health Care Institutions	360
9.115	Ethics Consultations.	362
9.12	Patient-Physician Relationship: Respect for Law and Human Rights.	363
9.121	Racial and Ethnic Health Care Disparities	366
9.122	Gender Disparities in Health Care	368
9.123	Disrespect and Derogatory Conduct in the Patient-Physician Relationship	370
9.124	Professionalism in the Use of Social Media.	371
9.13	Physicians and Infectious Diseases	372
9.131	HIV-Infected Patients and Physicians	373
9.132	Health Care Fraud and Abuse.	380
9.133	Routine Universal Immunization of Physicians for Vaccine-Preventable Diseases	380
9.14	Quality.	381

10.00 Opinions on the Patient-Physician Relationship

10.01	Fundamental Elements of the Patient-Physician Relationship	382
10.015	The Patient-Physician Relationship	390
10.016	Pediatric Decision-Making	395
10.017	Gifts From Patients	396
10.018	Physician Participation in Soliciting Contributions From Patients.	396
10.02	Patient Responsibilities	397
10.03	Patient-Physician Relationship in the Context of Work-Related and Independent Medical Examinations	400
10.05	Potential Patients	401

Appendix

American Medical Association: Relevant Bylaws.	403
Preface to the Rules of the Council on Ethical and Judicial Affairs	413
General Rules of the Council on Ethical and Judicial Affairs	414
Rules for Review of Membership	418
Rules of the Council on Ethical and Judicial Affairs in Original Jurisdiction Cases.	421

Table of Cases	424
Table of Articles	433
Index to Opinions	483

Preface

The *Code of Medical Ethics: Current Opinions with Annotations* represents the Council on Ethical and Judicial Affairs' application of the American Medical Association's (AMA) Principles of Medical Ethics to more than 200 ethical issues in medicine. This edition, which includes the Principles of Medical Ethics most recently revised in 2001 and Opinions issued through 2011, replaces all previous editions.

The nine Principles of Medical Ethics are the primary component of the Code. They describe the core ethical principles of the medical profession. A single Principle should not be read in isolation from others; the overall intent of the nine Principles, read together, guides physicians' behavior.

The AMA House of Delegates has the authority to establish the Principles of Medical Ethics. However, the Council on Ethical and Judicial Affairs is responsible for determining the Association's positions on ethical issues through its interpretations of the Principles, which are expressed in the Opinions. Each Opinion is followed by one or more roman numerals to identify the Principle(s) from which the Opinion is derived.

Most Opinions are explained by background reports, which provide a detailed analysis of the salient ethical considerations, as well as the rationale behind the Council's recommendations. These reports are referenced at the end of Opinions as appropriate and made available separately (www.ama-assn.org/go/cejareports).

Finally, each Opinion is followed by a list of annotations reflecting citations to the Opinion in judicial rulings and the medical, ethical, and legal literature (as described in more detail in the Guide to Use of Annotations).

The Code of Medical Ethics is published every two years. New Opinions are issued at the Annual and/or Interim meetings of the AMA's House of Delegates and are available through the Council's online version of the Code page (www.ama-assn.org/go/code) and the AMA's online policy database, PolicyFinder (www.ama-assn.org/go/policyfinder). The Council on Ethical and Judicial Affairs encourages comments and suggestions for future editions of this publication.

Council on Ethical and Judicial Affairs

2010-2011

John "Jack" W. McMahon, Sr, MD
CHAIR

Sharon P. Douglas, MD
VICE CHAIR

Stephen L. Brotherton, MD

Ronald J. Clearfield, MD, FACR

Susan Dorr Goold, MD, MHSA

H. Rex Greene, MD

Julia Halsey

Patrick McCormick, MD

Kavita Shah, MD, MBE

2011-2012

Sharon P. Douglas, MD
CHAIR

H. Rex Greene, MD
VICE CHAIR

Dennis S. Agliano, MD, FACS

Stephen L. Brotherton, MD

Ronald J. Clearfield, MD, FACR

Susan Dorr Goold, MD, MHSA

Patrick McCormick, MD

Kavita Shah, MD, MBE

Leon Vorobeichik

Audiey C. Kao, MD, PhD, Vice President, Ethics Group

Bette Crigger, PhD, Council Secretary

Valarie Blake, JD, MA, Senior Research Associate

Danielle Hahn, MS, Research Associate

Thomas Wagner, Council Coordinator

James L. Madara, MD, Executive Vice President/Chief Executive Officer

Modena Wilson, MD, MPH, Senior Vice President, Professional Standards

History

The Oath of Hippocrates, a brief statement of principles, has come down through history as a living statement of ideals to be cherished by the physician. This Oath was conceived some time during the period of Grecian greatness, probably in the fifth century BC. It protected rights of the patient and appealed to the inner and finer instincts of the physician without imposing sanctions or penalties on him or her. Other civilizations subsequently developed written principles, but the Oath of Hippocrates (Christianized in the tenth or eleventh century AD to eliminate reference to pagan gods) has remained in Western civilization as an expression of ideal conduct for the physician.

The most significant contribution to Western medical ethical history subsequent to Hippocrates was made by Thomas Percival, an English physician, philosopher, and writer. In 1803, he published his Code of Medical Ethics. His personality, his interest in sociological matters, and his close association with the Manchester Infirmary led to the preparation of a scheme of professional conduct relative to hospitals and other charities from which he drafted the code that bears his name.

At the first official meeting of the American Medical Association (AMA) at Philadelphia in 1847, the two principal items of business were the establishment of a code of ethics and the creation of minimum requirements for medical education and training. Although the Medical Society of the State of New York and the Medico-Chirurgical Society of Baltimore had formal written codes of medical ethics prior to this time, it is clear the AMA's first adopted Code of Ethics was based on Percival's Code.

In general, the language and concepts of the original Code drafted by Isaac Hays, MD, and John Bell, MD, and adopted by the Association in 1847 remained the same throughout the years. There were revisions, of course, which reflected the temper of the times and the eternal quest to express basic concepts with clarity. Major revisions did occur in 1903, 1912, 1947, and 1994.

In December 1955, an attempt was made to distinguish medical ethics from matters of etiquette. A draft of a two-part code seeking to accomplish this was submitted to the House of Delegates at that time but was not accepted. This proposal was, in effect, a separation of then existing statements found in the Principles into two categories. Little or no change was made in the language of the 48 sections of the Principles.

Subsequently, in June 1956, a seemingly radical proposal was submitted to the House of Delegates for consideration. This proposal, a short version of the Principles, was discussed at the December 1956 session of the House after wide publication and broad consideration among members of the medical profession. It was postponed for final consideration until the June 1957 meeting of the House of Delegates, when the short version was adopted.

The format of the Principles adopted in June 1957 is a change from the format of the Principles promulgated by Percival in 1803 and accepted by the Association in 1847. Ten short sections, preceded by a preamble, succinctly express the fundamental concepts embodied in the present (1955) Principles, according to the report of the Council on Constitution and Bylaws. That Council assured the House of Delegates in its June 1957 report that "every basic principle has been preserved; on the other hand, as much as possible of the prolixity and ambiguity which in the past obstructed ready explanation, practical codification and particular selection of basic concepts has been eliminated."

In 1977, the Judicial Council recommended to the House of Delegates that the AMA Principles of Medical Ethics be revised to clarify and update the language, to eliminate reference to gender, and to seek a proper and reasonable balance between professional standards and contemporary legal standards in our changing society. Given the desire of the Judicial Council for a new version of the Principles to be widely accepted and accurately understood, in 1978 the Judicial Council recommended that a special committee of the House be appointed to consider such a revision. This was done in 1980, and the House of Delegates adopted the revision of the AMA Principles of Medical Ethics at its Annual Meeting in June 1980. In June 2001, the House adopted further revisions, adding two new Principles.

In June 1985, the Judicial Council became the Council on Ethical and Judicial Affairs.

Guide to Use of Annotations

Over the years, the American Medical Association (AMA) Principles of Medical Ethics and the Code of Medical Ethics of the Council on Ethical and Judicial Affairs have emerged as an important source of guidance for responsible professional medical behavior, as well as the primary compendium of medical professional value statements in the United States.

The Opinions included in this volume are derived from two sources. The Council may issue Opinions directly at any time, usually during the Annual and Interim meetings of the AMA House of Delegates. Other Opinions are derived from the conclusions or recommendations of longer reports of the Council that are available from the AMA. Many of the Reports from which Opinions are derived are also published in peer-reviewed medical journals.

In this volume, an Opinion that is derived from a longer Report is followed by a citation to that Report and, if applicable, to a peer-reviewed medical journal. Opinions that are issued directly rather than derived from Reports are followed by information giving the date of issuance or most recent revision. For some of the older Opinions, however, this information is not available.

The impact of the Principles and Opinions has been significant. In this regard, attorneys and judges have shown an increasing willingness to look to the Principles and Opinions as a predicate for legal advocacy and decision-making in matters of health care law and litigation.

Against this backdrop of increasing reliance on the Principles and Opinions, these annotations have been prepared. They are designed to provide a research and reference tool for practitioners, scholars, jurists, and others who seek ready access to the Principles and Opinions in their work.

The annotations include summaries of all reported court decisions and selected state attorney general opinions that make substantive reference to the Principles or Opinions. Additionally, the annotations summarize selected articles from the medical, legal, and ethical literature.

These materials were gathered on the basis of carefully structured searches of a variety of computerized databases. Annotations are inclusive through December 2011.

The annotations have been prepared to maximize their usefulness as reference and research tools. After a brief synopsis of the facts and legal issues, each case annotation focuses on the court's reference to the Principle(s) or Opinion(s) and the role it played in the decision. In addition to the particular source referred to by the court, case annotations include, where necessary, a cross-reference to the relevant provision(s) of the present version of the Principles and Opinions.

Journal annotations provide a general summary of the subject article, along with an indication of the specific Principle(s) or Opinion(s) referenced therein. Again, a cross-reference feature is included. For convenience, consistent terminology is used in the journal annotations. When an author generally refers to the Principle or Opinion, the term references is used. When a Principle or Opinion is cited, this term is used. Finally, if an author directly quotes from a Principle or an Opinion, then the annotation so indicates.

With respect to both case and journal annotations, specific page references are provided to identify where the Principle(s) or Opinion(s) are discussed. This feature is intended to facilitate efficient use of these annotations. A Table of Cases and a Table of Articles also have been compiled to further enhance the usefulness of this compendium.

It is important to recognize that the Principles and Opinions have a long and evolving history. Many of the annotations included herein refer to older versions of the Principles and Opinions, some of which have been eliminated or substantially amended, revised, or updated. Nonetheless, these annotations may be valuable to the user. Efforts were made to identify the most appropriate provisions of the present Principles and Opinions to which to assign case and journal annotations. However, in some instances the correspondence is not exact and the user will need to review carefully the particular case or article under consideration with respect to the user's specific interests.

The annotators would like to express appreciation to Melanie Basham, Keleigh Biggins, John Castronova, Frank Choi, Michelle Dillon, Charles Ellington, Elizabeth Foster, Roberto Hernandez, Jean Kirchner, Elizabeth Lingle, Alisha Logan, Laura McMullen, Michele Miller, Thomas Morrow, Holly Noyes, Jo Powers, Nicholas Schroer, David Slade, Susan Tedrick, Elizabeth Valencia, Laura Wardwell, and Christopher White, who provided valuable research, editing, and other assistance on this project. Finally, we owe a special debt of thanks to Pamela Graham, Bonnie Miller, and Susan Williams of the Southern Illinois University School of Law, and Sarah Peters of the Southern Illinois University School of Medicine, who handled the difficult task of entry of annotations into the database with skill and enthusiasm.

This project was supported by a contract from the AMA.

Annotators

Ross D. Silverman, JD, MPH
Southern Illinois University
School of Medicine
Department of Medical Humanities

Frank G. Houdek, JD, MLS
Associate Dean
Southern Illinois University
School of Law

W. Eugene Basanta, JD, LLM
Southern Illinois University
School of Law
Center for Health Law and Policy

Connie Poole, AMLS
Southern Illinois University
School of Medicine
Department of Information and
Communication Sciences

March 2012

American Medical Association
Principles of Medical Ethics

Preamble

The medical profession has long subscribed to a body of ethical statements developed primarily for the benefit of the patient. As a member of this profession, a physician must recognize responsibility to patients first and foremost, as well as to society, to other health professionals, and to self. The following Principles adopted by the American Medical Association are not laws, but standards of conduct which define the essentials of honorable behavior for the physician.

   I. A physician shall be dedicated to providing competent medical care, with compassion and respect for human dignity and rights.

  II. A physician shall uphold the standards of professionalism, be honest in all professional interactions, and strive to report physicians deficient in character or competence, or engaging in fraud or deception, to appropriate entities.

  III. A physician shall respect the law and also recognize a responsibility to seek changes in those requirements which are contrary to the best interests of the patient.

  IV. A physician shall respect the rights of patients, colleagues, and other health professionals, and shall safeguard patient confidences and privacy within the constraints of the law.

  V. A physician shall continue to study, apply, and advance scientific knowledge, maintain a commitment to medical education, make relevant information available to patients, colleagues, and the public, obtain consultation, and use the talents of other health professionals when indicated.

  VI. A physician shall, in the provision of appropriate patient care, except in emergencies, be free to choose whom to serve, with whom to associate, and the environment in which to provide medical care.

  VII. A physician shall recognize a responsibility to participate in activities contributing to the improvement of the community and the betterment of public health.

  VIII. A physician shall, while caring for a patient, regard responsibility to the patient as paramount.

  IX. A physician shall support access to medical care for all people.

Adopted June 1957; revised June 1980; revised June 2001.

American Medical Association
Principles of Medical Ethics

Preamble

The medical profession has long subscribed to a body of ethical statements developed primarily for the benefit of the patient. As a member of this profession, a physician must recognize responsibility to patients first and foremost, as well as to society, to other health professionals, and to self. The following Principles adopted by the American Medical Association are not laws, but standards of conduct which define the essentials of honorable behavior for the physician.

Haw. 1995 After physician was convicted of attempted first-degree sexual abuse and kidnapping, the civil court affirmed the Board of Medical Examiner's decision to suspend him from practicing medicine for one year. In challenging Board's action, physician argued, among other things, that convictions were not related to his qualifications, functions, or duties as a physician. The court disagreed with all of physician's points of error on appeal. In considering physician's claim that convictions were not related to his duties as a physician, the court referred to the Preamble as reflecting a duty to the public generally. *Loui v. Board of Medical Examiners, 78 Haw. 21, 889 P.2d 705, 714.*

Ind. 1991 Plaintiff sued physician for injuries caused by physician's patient as the result of medication administered by the physician. Weighing (1) the relationship between the parties, (2) the reasonable foreseeability of harm to the injured party, and (3) public policy, the court held that a physician generally owes no duty to unknown third parties who may be injured by the physician's treatment of a patient. Concurring opinion quoted the Preamble which mandates that a physician "recognize responsibility . . . to society" arguing that there is no absolute immunity to third-party suits. *Webb v. Jarvis, 575 N.E.2d 992, 998.*

N.J. 1979 In wrongful death action against a psychiatrist whose patient murdered plaintiff's decedent, the court concluded, in accord with Principle 9 (1957) [now Principle IV], that a psychiatrist may owe a duty to warn potential victims of possible danger from psychiatrist's patient despite the general emphasis on confidentiality. The court also noted the Preamble and Principles 1 and 3 (1957) [now revised Preamble, Principle I and Opinion 5.05] in discussing the psychiatrist-patient relationship. *McIntosh v. Milano, 168 N.J. Super. 466, 403 A.2d 500, 510, 512-13.*

Journal 2011 Discusses the development of lethal autonomous robots, as well as issues raised by this new military technology. Concludes discussion on the advancement and acceptance of lethal autonomous robots is needed on the national and international levels in order to successfully manage advancements in robotic technology. Cites Preamble and Principles I and VI. Allenby, Arkin, Barrett, Borenstein, Gaudet, Kittrie, Lin, Lucas, Marchant, O'Meara, & Silberman, *International Governance of Autonomous Military Robots*, 12 Colum. Sci. & Tech. L. Rev. 272, 291 (2011).

Journal 2010 Analyzes factors contributing to the emergence of medical repatriation and evaluates whether this practice comports with current legal and ethical standards. Proposes changes to federal regulations that govern hospitals and clarifications to medical ethical standards. Quotes the Preamble and Principles I, II, III, IV, V, VI, VII, VIII, and IX. Zoellner, *Medical Repatriation:*

Examining the Legal and Ethical Implications of an Emerging Practice, 32 Wash. U. J. L. & Pol'y 515, 530-532 (2010).

Journal 2009 Examines the ethical guidelines regarding physicians' participation in interrogations and statutory approaches aimed at eliminating such physician involvement. Concludes that to maintain the integrity of the medical profession, physician involvement in interrogations must be precluded by legislative action. Quotes Preamble and Opinions 2.067 and 2.068. Cites Opinions 2.06 and 2.068; Bahnassi, *Keeping Doctors Out of the Interrogation Room: A New Ethical Obligation That Requires the Backing of the Law,* 19 Health Matrix 447, 449-51, 461, 464, 465-67, 469-70, 474-75 (2009).

Journal 2009 Explores the Supreme Court's *Baze v. Rees* decision and the three-drug protocol for lethal injection. Discusses the necessity of judicial intervention to improve lethal injection protocols. Concludes courts should carefully consider their approach to challenges to lethal injection as an opportunity to prevent violation of Eighth Amendment rights. Quotes Preamble and Opinion 1.02. Cites Opinion 2.06. Berger, *Lethal Injection and the Problem of Constitutional Remedies,* 27 Yale L. & Pol'y Rev. 259, 319, 320 (2009).

Journal 2009 Discusses the essential role of professionals in the community and the conflicting moral obligations facing professionals. Concludes the legal profession's insistence that priority be given exclusively to the client's interests prevents it from successfully addressing ethical problems. Cites Preamble and Principle VII. Greenstein, *Against Professionalism,* 22 Geo. J. Legal Ethics 327, 349 (2009).

Journal 2009 Explores the nature of the physician-patient relationship and the impact of increased availability of medical information on patient autonomy and physician responsibility to exercise independent judgment. Concludes physicians must treat patients in accordance with their fiduciary obligation to use their own judgment when confronted with a patient demanding unnecessary medical services. Quotes Preamble, Principles I and VIII, and Opinions 2.035, 8.03, and 10.015. Hafemeister, *The Fiduciary Obligation of Physicians to "Just Say No" If an "Informed" Patient Demands Services That Are Not Medically Indicated,* 39 Seton Hall L. Rev. 335, 372, 373, 374 (2009).

Journal 2009 Discusses the right of health care professionals to refuse to provide health care services to lesbian, gay, or bisexual (LGB) individuals, because of moral or religious objections, and its impact on access to health care services, including assisted reproduction and elder health care services, for such patients. Concludes physicians should adhere to professional ethical standards to promote LGB patients' autonomy and equal access to care. Quotes Preamble. Cites Opinion 10.05. Reibman, *The Patient Wanted the Doctor to Treat Her in the Closet, but the Janitor Wouldn't Open the Door: Healthcare Provider Rights of Refusal Versus LGB Rights to Reproductive and Elder Healthcare,* 28 Temp. J. Sci. Tech. & Envtl. L. 65, 90-91 (2009).

Journal 2009 Discusses the tension between duties of confidentiality and to protect third parties owed by mental health professionals to their patients and the public. Analyzes current Illinois law regarding these duties. Argues because Illinois law causes confusion regarding a professional's duty to disclose, inappropriately restricts the protected class, and leads to unnecessary breaches of confidentiality, clarification is necessary. Quotes Preamble and Opinion 5.05. Wood, *Protective Privilege versus Public Peril: How Illinois Has Failed to Balance Patient Confidentiality With the Mental Health Professional's Duty to Protect the Public,* 29 N. Ill. U. L. Rev. 571, 581, 598 (2009).

Journal 2008 Discusses issues arising from the increase in retail clinics and their impact on patients. Concludes the growth of retail clinics should be established on the same principles as traditional clinics to maximize their benefits to patients and to the health care community. Quotes Preamble. Hsu, *Legal Issues Concerning Retail Clinics,* 20 Health Law 13, 22 (June 2008).

Journal 2008 Examines the ethical reasons why physicians choose to provide treatment in disaster situations, even at great risk to themselves. Concludes that individual values play a substantial role in such decision making. Quotes Preamble, Opinion 9.131, and Ch. III, Art. 1, Sec. 1 (1847) [now Opinions 2.25 and 9.067]. Iserson, Heine, Larkin, Moskop, Baruch, & Aswegan, *Fight or Flight: The Ethics of Emergency Physician Disaster Response,* 51 Annals of Emergency Med. 345, 346-47 (2008).

Journal 2007 Compares the role of conscience clauses in various professions. Concludes that conscience clauses in the area of health care must not impede access to care. Quotes Preamble and Principles V, VI, and VIII. Chudoba, *Conscience in America: The Slippery Slope of Mixing Morality With Medicine,* 36 Sw. U. L. Rev. 85, 86, 103, 104, 105 (2007).

Journal 2007 Addresses physician liability for an extramarital affair with a patient's spouse. Concludes that such an affair should be regarded as a breach of a fiduciary duty. Quotes Preamble, Principles I, II, and VIII, and Opinions 8.145, 9.04, 9.123, and 10.015. Demaine, *"Playing Doctor" With the Patient's Spouse: Alternative Conceptions of Health Professional Liability,* 14 Va. J. Soc. Pol'y & L. 308, 325, 330-31, 331-32 (2007).

Journal 2007 Compares laws of client abandonment with those of patient abandonment by physicians. Concludes that physicians should be required to show good cause to justify abandonment. Quotes Ch. II, Art. I, Sec. 5 (1903) [now Preamble]. References Opinion 8.115. LeBlanc, *Abandoning Patients and Clients: Where Medicine Can Learn From Law,* 1 Charleston L. Rev. 237, 237-38, 256 (2007).

Journal 2007 Analyzes scientific, ethical, and legal issues raised in the exhumation and genetic analysis of historical figures. Concludes that biohistorical review boards should be created to generate guidelines for such research. Quotes Preamble and Opinion 2.08. Cites Opinions 2.079, 2.105, 5.05, 5.051, 5.075, 8.03, 8.031, 9.095, and 9.10. Paradise & Andrews, *Tales From the Crypt: Scientific, Ethical, and Legal Considerations for Biohistorical Analysis of Deceased Historical Figures,* 26 Temp. J. Sci. Tech. & Envtl. L. 223, 287-88 (2007).

Journal 2007 Examines how the subject of medical ethics is taught in US medical schools. Concludes that ethics should be broadly integrated into the curriculum throughout medical school. Quotes Preamble. Rooksby, *Ethics Education in Medical Schools: Problems, Practices, and Possibilities,* 10 Quinnipiac Health L. J. 181, 205 (2007).

Journal 2006 Examines the legal and public health issues raised by increased rates of hepatitis C in prison populations. Concludes that reform is needed to provide adequate health care to prisoners and that courts have the power to require such care under the Eighth Amendment. Quotes Preamble, Principles VII, VIII, and IX, and Opinion 10.015. Brunsden, *Hepatitis C in Prisons: Evolving Toward Decency Through Adequate Medical Care and Public Health Reform,* 54 UCLA L. Rev. 465, 500 (2006).

Journal 2006 Considers the interaction of laws, rules, and guidelines in the area of health law. Suggests that the legislature should revise current laws to reflect local variability in practice. Quotes Preamble and Principles VII and IX. Heimer, *Responsibility in Health Care: Spanning the Boundary Between Law and Medicine,* 41 Wake Forest L. Rev. 465, 498 (2006).

Journal 2006 Examines a mental health professional's competing duties of confidentiality and reporting a patient's threats of violence. Suggests new legislation should clarify duty to report a threat. Quotes Preamble and Principles III, IV, and VIII. Cites Opinion 5.05. Mossman, *Critique of Pure Risk Assessment or, Kant Meets Tarasoff,* 75 U. Cin. L. Rev. 523, 579 (2006).

Journal 2006 Addresses the problem of disruptive dialysis patients. Concludes that the dialysis care system must change to prevent dismissal of these patients. Quotes Preamble. Smetanka, *Who Will Protect the "Disruptive" Dialysis Patient?* 32 Am. J. L. & Med. 53, 89 (2006).

Journal 2004 Discusses the "no-harm" doctrine as a long-held legal and moral principle. Concludes that this doctrine protects personal liberties and shields citizens from harmful religious or secular action. Quotes Preamble. Hamilton, *Religious Institutions, the No-Harm Doctrine, and the Public Good,* 2004 B.Y.U. L. Rev. 1099, 1175, 1176 (2004).

Journal 2004 Analyzes various issues relating to the role of mental health professionals in capital punishment in light of Albert Bandura's model of "mechanisms of moral disengagement." Concludes that facilitating participation of mental health professionals in executions creates conflicts with the humanistic norms of the profession. Quotes Preamble and Opinions 1.01, 1.02, 2.06, 2.067, 2.20, 2.21, 2.211, and 8.14. Judges, *The Role of Mental Health Professionals in Capital Punishment: An Exercise in Moral Disengagement,* 41 Hous. L. Rev. 515, 562, 568, 569, 570, 571-72, 581, 586, 588, 598 (2004).

Journal 2003 Examines policy options for integration of traditional and modern medicine. Concludes that solid cross-sectoral linkages between different traditions can stabilize an integrated health care system. Quotes Preamble and Principle V. Holliday, *Traditional Medicines in Modern Societies: An Exploration of Integrationist Options Through East Asian Experience,* 28 J. Med. & Phil. 373, 387 (2003).

Journal 2003 Considers conflicts of interest and potential liability that a team physician faces when treating an injured athlete. Concludes that an athlete's health should be the team physician's primary concern in making treatment decisions. References Principles I and II. Landis, *The Team Physician: An Analysis of the Causes of Action, Conflicts, Defenses and Improvements*, 1 DePaul J. Sports L. & Contemp. Probs. 139, 144 (2003).

Journal 2002 Explores the implications of withholding medical treatment when abortion results in a live birth. Concludes that, in these situations, abortive parents and physicians should not solely decide the child's best interest. Quotes Preamble, Principles I and III, and Opinions 2.035, 2.20, and 2.215. Casagrande, *Children Not Meant to Be: Protecting the Interests of the Child When Abortion Results in Live Birth*, 6 Quinnipiac Health L. J. 19, 44, 45, 47-48 (2002).

Journal 2002 Considers the dilemma of informed consent in the context of prescribing psychotropic medication to patients with mental illness and mental retardation. Recognizes the need for substituted decision-making in certain situations. Concludes that legislation would help address this issue. Quotes Preamble, Principles I, III, IV, VIII, and IX, and Opinion 8.08. O'Sullivan & Borcherding, *Informed Consent for Medication in Persons With Mental Retardation and Mental Illness*, 12 Health Matrix 63, 75, 86, 87, 88 (2002).

Journal 2002 Discusses legal and medical policies that protect confidentiality in the physician-patient relationship. Concludes that reducing the current level of privacy protection would jeopardize health care. Quotes Preamble and Opinions 2.136, 5.05, and 10.01. References Principles VIII and IX. Sciarrino, *Ferguson v. City of Charleston: "The Doctor Will See You Now, Be Sure to Bring Your Privacy Rights in With You!"* 12 Temp. Pol. & Civ. Rts. L. Rev. 197, 213, 215, 220, 221, 222 (2002).

Journal 2000 Examines the increased prominence of medical ethics in light of various changes in medicine and society. Concludes with observations regarding how "preventive ethics" can enhance patient care. Quotes Preamble. Nandi, *Ethical Aspects of Clinical Practice*, 135 Arch. Surg. 22, 23 (2000).

Journal 2000 Examines current laws prohibiting discrimination in the context of access to health care, placing emphasis on people with HIV/AIDS. Considers the implications of *Bragdon v. Abbott*. Concludes that everyone should be entitled to health care in the absence of an acceptable justification for its denial. Quotes Preamble, Principle VI, and Opinion 9.131. Shepherd, *HIV, the ADA, and the Duty to Treat*, 37 Hous. L. Rev. 1055, 1061, 1083-84 (2000).

Journal 1999 Asserts that patient autonomy is closely linked to patient-physician discourse. Proposes a constitutional framework for evaluating how governmental regulations may interfere with such discourse. Concludes by emphasizing the importance of protecting the quality of physician-patient discourse. Quotes Preamble and Opinion 8.03. Gatter, *Protecting Patient-Doctor Discourse: Informed Consent and Deliberative Autonomy*, 78 Or. L. Rev. 941, 956 (1999).

Journal 1998 Argues that the doctrine of informed consent should not be abandoned. Explains why informed consent is needed. Suggests that even if physicians cannot determine patients' best interests, they can determine patients' reasonable interests. Quotes Preamble. White & Zimbelman, *Abandoning Informed Consent: An Idea Whose Time Has Not Yet Come*, 23 J. Med. Phil. 477, 496 (1998).

Journal 1997 Examines noncompetition clauses in the medical field. Reviews policy concerns and historical and common-law analyses of agreements not to compete. Posits that the more commercialized the medical profession becomes, the more noncompetition clauses infringe upon the physician-patient relationship and patients' rights. Quotes Opinions 9.02 and 9.06. Cites Preamble and Opinion 6.11. Comment, *Noncompetition Clauses in Physician Employment Contracts in Oregon*, 76 Or. L. Rev. 195, 204-06 (1997).

Journal 1997 Considers principles of confidentiality in the physician-patient relationship. Notes the current trend emphasizing public reporting obligations of physicians to protect members of society. Emphasizes need for balance between patient rights and societal interests. Quotes Principle IV and Opinion 5.05. References Preamble. Jozefowicz, *The Case Against Having Professional Privilege in the Physician-Patient Relationship*, 16 Med. & L. 385, 386-87, 391 (1997).

Journal 1997 Discusses the need for balance between business ethics and medical ethics in the context of managed care. Explores two models for integrating ethics and managed care. Proposes the adoption of a collective responsibility model to improve quality of care. Quotes Principles I, II, III, IV, and V. Cites Preamble. References Opinion 8.13. Regan, *Regulating the Business of Medicine: Models for Integrating Ethics and Managed Care*, 30 Colum. J. L. & Soc. Probs. 635, 651, 656, 657 (1997).

Journal 1996 Considers the impact of gag clauses on the physician-patient relationship. Undertakes an extensive legal, ethical, and policy analysis. Concludes that gag clauses are violative of legal and ethical principles. Quotes Principles II, V, and VI, and Fundamental Elements (1). Cites Preamble. Martin & Bjerknes, *The Legal and Ethical Implications of Gag Clauses in Physician Contracts*, XXII Am. J. Law & Med. 433, 465-66 (1996).

Journal 1996 Considers prearraignment forensic evaluations. Notes the prohibition against use of such evaluations. Examines underlying ethical precepts. Observes that principles of beneficence are misapplied to forensic psychiatry in this context. Advocates a new ethical framework. Quotes Preamble. References Principle IV and Opinion 5.05. Ornish, Mills, & Ornish, *Prearraignment Forensic Evaluations: Toward a New Policy*, 24 Bull. Am. Acad. Psychiatry Law 453, 454, 469 (1996).

Journal 1995 Examines the metaphor of physicians as fiduciaries. Considers how the law holds physicians accountable in this regard. Quotes Preamble. Cites Opinion 8.03 (1986) [now Opinion 8.032]. Rodwin, *Strains in the Fiduciary Metaphor: Divided Physician Loyalties and Obligations in a Changing Health Care System*, XXI Am. J. Law & Med. 241, 246, 250 (1995).

Journal 1994 Reviews the evolution of the physician-patient relationship, with attention to patient autonomy. Examines the changing health care delivery environment. Quotes Preamble, Principles I, II, III, IV, V, and VI, Fundamental Elements (1) and (2), and Opinions 1.02 and 8.07 (1981) [now Opinion 8.08]. Cites Opinion 1.01. Szczygiel, *Beyond Informed Consent*, 21 Ohio N. U. L. Rev. 171, 217, 218, 220, 225, 226, 256 (1994).

Journal 1993 Discusses ethical issues that may arise in the context of caring for the critically ill. Emphasizes the need for organization of patient care when multiple providers are involved. Quotes Preamble. Bruening, Andrew, & Smith, *Concurrent Care: An Ethical Issue for Family Physicians*, 36 J. Fam. Practice 606, 607 (1993).

Journal 1991 Examines the informed consent doctrine and how it was broadened in *Moore v. Regents of the University of California*. Concludes that, in California, under Moore, a physician must disclose to patients any economic or research interest he or she might have in the patient's medical treatment. Quotes Preamble. Guise, *Expansion of the Scope of Disclosure Required Under the Informed Consent Doctrine: Moore v. The Regents of the University of California*, 28 San Diego L. Rev. 455, 462 (1991).

Journal 1990 Discusses the moral dilemma in deciding whether to withdraw artificial nutrition and hydration from a patient and the appropriate role of the judiciary. Concludes that judicial decisions do not represent the moral viewpoint of society and that moral pronouncements should not be made in the courtroom. Quotes Preamble, Principles I, II, III, IV, V, VI, and VII, and Opinion 2.20. Peccarelli, *A Moral Dilemma: The Role of Judicial Intervention in Withholding or Withdrawing Nutrition and Hydration*, 23 John Marshall L. Rev. 537, 539, 540, 541 (1990).

I. A physician shall be dedicated to providing competent medical care, with compassion and respect for human dignity and rights.

10th Cir. 2001 Plaintiffs, former employees of a public medical center, brought suit against medical director under 42 USC § 1983, based upon medical director's racially and sexually harassing actions and statements. The district court awarded compensatory and punitive damages against the medical director. Affirming the award of damages, the court quoted Principles I and IV and concluded that the medical director's behavior impacted not only plaintiffs, but the overall public health. *Nieto v. Kapoor*, 268 F.3d 1208, 1223 n. 12.

D. Kan. 1995 Plaintiff, an occupational medicine physician, alleged that defendant, medical group, wrongfully discharged him in violation of public policy and in breach of the implied covenant of good faith and fair dealing. Defendant complained that plaintiff consistently granted excess time off to patients. Even though defendant warned plaintiff that he would be terminated if he continued this practice, plaintiff refused to comply stating that he was ethically obligated to serve the best interests of his patients. Plaintiff claimed that to place the defendant's interests above his legal and ethical duties to his patients would violate public policy as set out by statute and the Principles of Medical Ethics, with apparent reference to Principle I. Since plaintiff failed to show that defendant's practice caused harm to patients or deviated from accepted standards, the court disregarded plaintiff's public policy exception to the employment-at-will doctrine and granted defendant's motion for summary judgment. *Aiken v. Business & Indus. Health Group*, 886 F. Supp. 1565, 1571.

N.J. 1979 In wrongful death action against a psychiatrist whose patient murdered plaintiff's decedent, the court concluded, in accord with Principle 9 (1957) [now Principle IV], that a psychiatrist may owe a duty to warn potential victims of possible danger from psychiatrist's patient despite the general emphasis on confidentiality. The court also noted the Preamble and Principles 1 and 3 (1957) [now revised Preamble, Principle I, and Opinion 5.05] in discussing the psychiatrist-patient relationship. *McIntosh v. Milano, 168 N.J. Super. 466, 403 A.2d 500, 510, 512-13.*

Ohio 2009 Physician appealed from a judgment affirming an order of the State Medical Board that permanently revoked appellant's certificate to practice medicine. The Board found that appellant's sexual contact with patients violated Ohio statutes governing physician conduct and the Code of Ethics of the AMA, citing Principles I, II, IV, and VIII. The Court of Appeals held that Ohio state law allows the Board to revoke a physician's certificate if it finds that the person violated any provision of the Code of Ethics of the AMA. *D'Souza v. State Med. Bd. of Ohio, 2009 WL 5108774, 6.*

Ohio 2000 Hospital sought court order permitting administration of antipsychotic medication to an involuntarily committed mentally ill patient without consent. The court said that forced medication is permitted in certain instances, including where medical personnel determine that patients present an imminent risk of harm to themselves or others. Quoting Principle I, the court found that placing such authority in a physician's hands is appropriate. Because the treating physician testified the patient did not pose a risk, the court ruled forced medication could not be required on this basis. *Steele v. Hamilton County Cmty. Mental Health Bd., 90 Ohio St. 3d 176, 736 N.E.2d 10, 18.*

Ohio 1991 State medical board revoked license of physician who had consensual sexual relations with his patient. The court upheld the board's ruling that this violated Principles I, II, and IV. Dissenting judge, citing AMA Council on Ethical and Judicial Affairs, Sexual Misconduct in the Practice of Medicine, 266 JAMA 2741 [now Opinion 8.14], argued that until 1991, the AMA did not clearly deem sexual contact with a patient unethical. *Pons v. Ohio State Medical Bd., 66 Ohio St. 3d 619, 623, 625, 614 N.E.2d 748, 752, 753.*

Ohio App. 2005 The Ohio State Medical Board permanently revoked the license of the appellant, a psychiatrist, for having inappropriate physical and sexual contact with a female patient. The trial court affirmed the Board's ruling, and the appellant appealed. The Board claimed that the appellant's relationship with his patient violated the AMA's Code of Medical Ethics citing Principles I, II, and IV. The appellate court affirmed stating that permanent revocation of the appellant's license was not excessive and was not a violation of due process as the Board may revoke the appellant's license if treatment did not meet minimal standards of care and violated any provision of the AMA's Code of Medical Ethics. *Schechter v. Ohio State Med. Bd., 2005 WL 1869733, 9.*

Ohio App. 1999 Physician appealed trial court's affirmation of state medical board's decision to suspend his medical license because the physician engaged in sexual relationships with mothers of his pediatric patients. On appeal the physician claimed that he was denied due process because physicians were not adequately notified that having sexual relations with parents of pediatric patients was unethical. The physician also claimed that the board had not presented adequate evidence that AMA Principles I and IV extend to the parents of pediatric patients. The court quoted Principles I and IV, and stated that medical experts who testified were of the opinion that having sexual relationships with parents of pediatric patients constituted ethical violations. *Gladieux v. Ohio State Medical Board, 1999 WL 770959, *2, *4.*

Journal 2011 Discusses the development of lethal autonomous robots, as well as issues raised by this new military technology. Concludes discussion on the advancement and acceptance of lethal autonomous robots is needed on the national and international levels in order to successfully manage advancements in robotic technology. Cites Preamble and Principles I and VI. Allenby, Arkin, Barrett, Borenstein, Gaudet, Kittrie, Lin, Lucas, Marchant, O'Meara, & Silberman, *International Governance of Autonomous Military Robots, 12 Colum. Sci. & Tech. L. Rev. 272, 291 (2011).*

Journal 2011 Discusses compassion in the medical field and a proposed change to New Zealand law creating a patient's right to be treated with compassion. Concludes in order to eliminate the need for compassion legislation, physicians should have more education on suffering and patient values, and regulators should inform health care providers about what constitutes inappropriate behavior by setting standards of conduct. Quotes Principle I. Paterson, *Can We Mandate Compassion?* 41*Hastings Center Rep.* 20, 21 (Mar.-Apr. 2011).

Journal 2011 Argues that regulation of physicians' off-label use of prescription medications is necessary to prevent harm to both the patient and to society via unnecessary increases in health care spending. Concludes the state should intervene in the physician-patient relationship when physicians prescribe medicine off-label that is not justified by high-quality evidence of safety and efficacy. Quotes Principles I and V. Rosoff & Coleman, *The Case for Legal Regulation of Physicians' Off-Label Prescribing*, 86 *Notre Dame L. Rev.* 649, 675 (2011).

Journal 2010 Argues the medicalization of the concepts of "health" and "harm" has led to a simplistic use of evidence to answer complicated ethical questions, such as the permissibility of the reduction of twins to a singleton. Concludes empirical evidence cannot be a substitute for ethical deliberation. References Principle I. McClimans, *Elective Twin Reductions: Evidence and Ethics*, 24 *Bioethics* 295, 297 (2010).

Journal 2010 Analyzes factors contributing to the emergence of medical repatriation and evaluates whether this practice comports with current legal and ethical standards. Proposes changes to federal regulations that govern hospitals and clarifications to medical ethical standards. Quotes the Preamble and Principles I, II, III, IV, V, VI, VII, VIII, and IX. Zoellner, *Medical Repatriation: Examining the Legal and Ethical Implications of an Emerging Practice*, 32 *Wash. U. J. L. & Pol'y* 515, 530-532 (2010).

Journal 2009 Explores emerging issues in conflict management systems design (CMSD). Concludes as the practice of CMSD in the organizational context continues to expand, practitioners should openly discuss the emerging issues of the field. References Principles I, II, V, and VIII. Costantino, *Second Generation Organizational Conflict Management Systems Design: A Practitioner's Perspective on Emerging Issues*, 14 *Harv. Negot. L. Rev.* 81, 95 (2009).

Journal 2009 Discusses tobacco use in psychiatric institutions and its impact on the health and behavior of patients. Concludes legislative action should be taken to remove tobacco from psychiatric institutions to provide patients with the health and safety benefits of smoke-free facilities. Quotes Principles I and III. Hackett, *Smoke-Free State Psychiatric Facility Grounds: Is Legislation Necessary and Appropriate to Remove Tobacco From These Treatment Settings?* 53 *N. Y. L. Sch. L. Rev.* 99, 122-23 (2009).

Journal 2009 Discusses whether or not patients have a right to pain management. Concludes that no physician duty is established by law or ethics to provide pain management outside the traditional physician-patient relationship. Cites Principles I, II, IV, and VIII. Hall & Boswell, *Ethics, Law, and Pain Management as a Patient Right*, 12 *Pain Physician* 499, 500 (2009).

Journal 2009 Examines the advent of a consumerist model of providing health care services to patients. Concludes that patients as consumers cannot, by themselves, achieve the desired policy goals of containing health care costs and optimizing care quality because the demands on patients and health care providers are too numerous. Cites Principle I. Hall & Schneider, *When Patients Say No (To Save Money): An Essay on the Tectonics of Health Law*, 41 *Conn. L. Rev.* 743, 770 (2009).

Journal 2009 Explores the nature of the physician-patient relationship and the impact of increased availability of medical information on patient autonomy and physician responsibility to exercise independent judgment. Concludes physicians must treat patients in accordance with their fiduciary obligation to use their own judgment when confronted with a patient demanding unnecessary medical services. Quotes Preamble, Principles I and VIII, and Opinions 2.035, 8.03, and 10.015. Hafemeister, *The Fiduciary Obligation of Physicians to "Just Say No" if an "Informed" Patient Demands Services That Are Not Medically Indicated*, 39 *Seton Hall L. Rev.* 335, 372, 373, 374 (2009).

Journal 2008 Explores the legal, ethical, and policy implications of concierge medicine. Argues physicians engaged in concierge care must strive to meet ethical and legal standards, and take care to communicate clearly with patients about services and fees. Quotes Opinion 8.055. Cites Principles II and VI and Opinion 8.055. Portman & Romanow, *Concierge Medicine: Legal Issues, Ethical Dilemmas, and Policy Challenges*, 1 *J. Health & Life Sci. L.* 1, 4, 28-29 (2008).

Journal 2008 Examines the development of bioethics and environmental ethics, as well as laws promoting the role of bioethicists in decision making. Concludes environmental ethicists must convince legislatures of the role of environmental ethics in order to have a greater impact on decision making. Quotes Principles I, II, III, IV, V, VI, VII, VIII, and IX. Robertson, *Seeking a Seat at the Table: Has Law Left Environmental Ethics Behind as It Embraces Bioethics?* 32 Wm. & Mary Envtl. L. & Pol'y Rev. 273, 307 (2008).

Journal 2008 Explores the fiduciary relationship between physicians and patients, professional and ethical obligations of both physicians and lawyers, and the implications for conflict resolution in health care. Concludes physicians must put patient interests above their own and lawyers must work to discern clients' best interests and support client welfare. Quotes Principle VIII and Opinions 8.12 and 10.015. Cites Principles I and II and Opinions 10.01 and 10.015. Scott, *Doctors as Advocates, Lawyers as Healers*, 29 Hamline J. Pub. L. Pol'y, 331, 340-41, 347, 371 (2008).

Journal 2007 Addresses physician liability for an extramarital affair with a patient's spouse. Concludes that such an affair should be regarded as a breach of a fiduciary duty. Quotes Preamble, Principles I, II, and VIII, and Opinions 8.145, 9.04, 9.123, and 10.015. Demaine, *"Playing Doctor" With the Patient's Spouse: Alternative Conceptions of Health Professional Liability*, 14 Va. J. Soc. Pol'y & L. 308, 325, 330-31, 331-32 (2007).

Journal 2007 Discusses the evolution of informed consent doctrine. Concludes that, in context of research, informed consent exceptions should be substantially narrowed. Quotes Ch. I, Art. I, Sec. 4 (May 1847) [now Opinion 8.082] and Ch. I, Art. I, Sec. 1 (May 1847) [now Principles I and VIII]. References Opinions 2.08 and 8.08. Grimm, *Informed Consent for All! No Exceptions*, 37 N. M. L. Rev. 39, 39, 61 (2007).

Journal 2007 Highlights inconsistencies in applying judicial deference to medical ethics. Concludes that courts should afford greater deference to established medical ethics standards. Quotes Principle I and Opinion 2.06 and Ch. II, Art. I, Sec. 3 (May 1847) [now Opinion 5.02]. Cites Opinions 4.01 and 7.05. Lerman, *Second Opinion: Inconsistent Deference to Medical Ethics in Death Penalty Jurisprudence*, 95 Geo. L. J. 1941, 1945, 1974-75, 1976, 1977 (2007).

Journal 2007 Argues that issuance of apologies from physicians who commit medical errors will diminish the number of malpractice suits brought. Concludes that patients desire apologies in the case of medical errors and are less likely to sue when they are given. Cites Principles I, II, III, and IV and Opinion 8.12. Tabler, *Should Physicians Apologize for Medical Errors?* 19 Health Lawyer 23, 23 (Jan. 2007).

Journal 2006 Examines ethical dilemmas physicians may face as providers of pay-for-performance medical care. Concludes that this strategy offers a benefit to patients as long as physicians uphold stringent ethical standards and work together to ensure optimum patient care. Cites Principles I, V, VIII, and IX and Opinions 2.035, 2.095, 6.01, 8.021, 8.03, 8.0501, 8.053, 8.054, and 8.121. Bostick, Sade & McMahon, *Report of the Council on Ethical and Judicial Affairs: Physician Pay-For-Performance Programs*, 3 Ind. Health L. Rev. 429, 430, 431, 432-33, 434, 435, 436 (2006).

Journal 2006 Explores conscience clause legislation relating to the dispensing of oral contraceptives. Concludes that such legislation must balance the interests of the patient and the health care provider. Cites Principles I, II, III, IV, V, VI, VII, VIII, and IX. Collins, *Conscience Clauses and Oral Contraceptives: Conscientious Objection or Calculated Obstruction?* 15 Ann. Health L. 37, 54 (2006).

Journal 2006 Discusses mentally incompetent inmates and capital punishment. Proposes that, to be permissible, involuntary medication of death-row inmates must represent the best medically appropriate treatment. Quotes Principles I, III, and VIII and Opinion 2.06. Gabos, *The Perils of Singleton v. Norris: Ethics and Beyond*, 32 Am. J. L. & Med. 117, 118, 125-26, 127 (2006).

Journal 2005 Considers the legal and ethical implications of tracking dementia patients with global positioning system (GPS) technology. Concludes that GPS tracking may infringe on fundamental rights of privacy, autonomy, and human dignity and that the only justification for tracking is to prevent harm to the individual being tracked. References Principle I. Eltis, *Predicating Dignity on Autonomy? The Need for Further Inquiry Into the Ethics of Tagging and Tracking Dementia Patients With GPS Technology*, 13 Elder L. J. 387, 403 (2005).

Journal 2005 Examines issues surrounding tort reform proposals. Concludes that more can be done to correct the current tort system before moving toward a "one size fits all" approach. Quotes Principles I, II, III, IV, V, VI, VII, VIII, and IX. Messerly & Warwick, *Nowhere to Turn: A Glance at the Facts Behind the Supposed Need for Tort "Reform,"* 28 Hamline L. Rev. 489, 506 (2005).

Journal 2003 Considers the legal, medical, and ethical issues of physician-patient confidentiality in disclosure of paternity. Concludes that a balancing test should be applied to making determinations regarding disclosure of paternity. Quotes Principles I, IV, and V and Opinions 1.02, 5.055, and 10.01. Cites Principle II and Opinion 5.05. Richards & Wolf, *Medical Confidentiality and Disclosure of Paternity*, 48 S. D. L. Rev. 409, 411, 412, 413 (2003).

Journal 2002 Explores the implications of withholding medical treatment when abortion results in a live birth. Concludes that, in these situations, abortive parents and physicians should not solely decide the child's best interest. Quotes Preamble, Principles I and III, and Opinions 2.035, 2.20, and 2.215. Casagrande, *Children Not Meant to Be: Protecting the Interests of the Child When Abortion Results in Live Birth*, 6 Quinnipiac Health L. J. 19, 44, 45, 47-48 (2002).

Journal 2002 Analyzes the expanded use of the Civil False Claims Act in prosecuting health care fraud. Concludes that, in enforcing the law, government must balance its promises to beneficiaries, health care providers, and the public. Quotes Principles I, II, and IV. Krause, *"Promises to Keep": Health Care Providers and the Civil False Claims Act*, 23 Cardozo L. Rev. 1363, 1365 (2002).

Journal 2002 Considers the dilemma of informed consent in the context of prescribing psychotropic medication to patients with mental illness and mental retardation. Recognizes the need for substituted decision-making in certain situations. Concludes that legislation would help address this issue. Quotes Preamble, Principles I, III, IV, VIII, and IX, and Opinion 8.08. O'Sullivan & Borcherding, *Informed Consent for Medication in Persons With Mental Retardation and Mental Illness*, 12 Health Matrix 63, 75, 86, 87, 88 (2002).

Journal 2002 Examines the origin and dynamics of the scope-of-practice laws governing health care providers. Concludes that the current system is not working and offers recommendations for change. Quotes Principles I and II. Safriet, *Closing the Gap Between Can and May in Health-Care Providers' Scopes of Practice: A Primer for Policymakers*, 19 Yale J. on Reg. 301, 311 (2002).

Journal 2001 Discusses the physician unionization debate with emphasis on the perspective of physicians. Concludes that physicians' arguments against managed care articulate a moral claim in favor of collective bargaining rights. Quotes Principle I. Fine, *Exploitation of the Elite: A Case for Physician Unionization*, 45 St. Louis L. J. 207, 207 (2001).

Journal 2000 Examines the AMA Code of Ethics. Explores historical developments. Concludes that professional ethical principles meaningfully affect the conduct of physicians and make a difference to the patients and the public they serve. Cites Principle I. Baker & Emanuel, *The Efficacy of Professional Ethics: The AMA Code of Ethics in Historical and Current Perspective*, 30 Hastings Center Rep. S13, S14 (July/Aug. 2000).

Journal 2000 Considers the rules governing expert testimony. Explores professional ethical standards affecting expert witnesses and concludes that codes of ethics have not succeeded in eliminating biased expert testimony. Recommends creation of an organization to assist courts in obtaining reliable expert witness testimony. Quotes Principle III and Opinion 6.01. Cites Principles I, II, and V and Opinions 1.02 and 9.07. Murphy, *Expert Witnesses at Trial: Where Are the Ethics?* 14 Geo. J. Legal Ethics 217, 231-32 (2000).

Journal 1999 Analyzes the federal rules of evidence from a feminist perspective. Proposes a new "apology" evidence rule to serve as an exception to the general rule that statements by party opponents are admissible during trial. Suggests that physicians who commit medical errors may ease patients' anger by apologizing. The new evidence rule would permit physicians to be more forthcoming in this regard. Quotes Principles I and II. Orenstein, *Apology Excepted: Incorporating a Feminist Analysis Into Evidence Policy Where You Would Least Expect It*, 28 S.W. U. L. Rev. 221, 264 (1999).

Journal 1998 Explores the impact of managed care on the health care system. Discusses legal and ethical conflicts that have arisen and emphasizes the need to balance the interests of patients with the integrity of the system. Quotes Principle I. Field, *New Ethical Relationships Under Health Care's New Structure: The Need for a New Paradigm*, 43 Vill. L. Rev. 467, 468 (1998).

Journal 1998 Discusses managed care and the expansion of physicians' duties under such programs. Focuses on the current legal standard of care for physicians. Proposes that physicians who are mandated by managed care organizations to provide services performed by specialists be held to the same standard of care as other physicians who are required to deliver those services. Quotes Principle I. Friedland, *Managed Care and the Expanding Scope of Primary Care Physicians'*

Duties: A Proposal to Redefine Explicitly the Standard of Care, 26 J. Law Med. & Ethics 100, 104 (1998).

Journal 1998 Examines the US Supreme Court's decision in *Zinermon v. Burch* in relation to other Supreme Court decisions regarding the role of the courts in mental health treatment determinations. Argues that the government must strike a balance between the duty to care for the mentally ill and the duty to respect individual liberty. Provides approaches legislatures could adopt regarding mental health issues. References Principles I and III. Nidich, *Zinermon v. Burch and Voluntary Admissions to Public Hospitals: A Common Sense Proposal for Compromise, 25 N. Ky. L. Rev. 699, 710 (1998).*

Journal 1997 Discusses the practice of physician deselection by managed care organizations. Suggests that deselection harms the physician-patient relationship and creates a conflict of interest. Argues that solutions to deselection should consider effects on the patient rather than on the physician. Quotes Principle III. Cites Principle I and Opinions 8.05 and 8.13. Liner, *Physician Deselection: The Dynamics of a New Threat to the Physician-Patient Relationship, 23 Am. J. Law & Med. 511, 513, 527 (1997).*

Journal 1997 Discusses the need for balance between business ethics and medical ethics in the context of managed care. Explores two models for integrating ethics and managed care. Proposes the adoption of a collective responsibility model to improve quality of care. Quotes Principles I, II, III, IV, and V. Cites Preamble. References Opinion 8.13. Regan, *Regulating the Business of Medicine: Models for Integrating Ethics and Managed Care, 30 Colum. J. L. & Soc. Probs. 635, 651, 656, 657 (1997).*

Journal 1996 Discusses the trend toward conserving resources expended on health care by withholding services absent a showing of necessity. Claims that the high standard of care physicians owe patients is jeopardized by medical treatment decisions based on coverage concerns. Concludes that the legal structure regarding health care plans should be changed. Quotes Preamble, Principles I, II, III, IV, V, VI, and VII and Opinion 2.03. Hirshfeld & Thomason, *Medical Necessity Determinations: The Need for a New Legal Structure, 6 Health Matrix 3, 8-9 (1996).*

Journal 1995 Examines the rights of health care professionals to refuse to participate in patient care on the basis of conscientious objection. Suggests steps that health care facilities may take when dealing with health care professionals who object to participating in patient care. Quotes Principles I and VI and Opinions 1.02, 2.035, and 9.055. Dellinger & Vickery, *When Staff Object to Participating in Care, 28 J. Health & Hospital Law 269, 272, 276 (1995).*

Journal 1994 Considers whether an exception should be made to physician-patient confidentiality that would allow a physician to reveal parental medical history to a child. Concludes that such an exception would not completely erode physician-patient confidentiality. Quotes Principle IV, Fundamental Elements (4), and Opinion 5.05. Cites Principle I and Fundamental Elements (1). Friedland, *Physician-Patient Confidentiality: Time to Re-examine a Venerable Concept in Light of Contemporary Society and Advances in Medicine, 15 J. Legal Med. 249, 257, 264, 276 (1994).*

Journal 1994 Argues that physician aid-in-dying should be protected by the US Constitution and that patients should have a federal cause of action to challenge prohibitive state statutes. Considers how such a cause of action might affect public policy. Quotes Principles I and III. References Opinion 2.06. Note, *Toward a More Perfect Union: A Federal Cause of Action for Physician Aid-in-Dying, 27 U. Mich. J. L. Ref. 521, 538 (1994).*

Journal 1994 Reviews the evolution of the physician-patient relationship, with attention to patient autonomy. Examines the changing health care delivery environment. Quotes Preamble, Principles I, II, III, IV, V, and VI, Fundamental Elements (1) and (2), and Opinions 1.02 and 8.07 (1981) [now Opinion 8.08]. Cites Opinion 1.01. Szczygiel, *Beyond Informed Consent, 21 Ohio N. U. L. Rev. 171, 217, 218, 220, 225, 226, 256 (1994).*

Journal 1993 Discusses physicians' duty to disclose to patients medical treatment alternatives that are not readily available. Proposes that based on the historical development and legal requirements of the informed consent doctrine, physicians should be required to inform patients of nonreadily available alternatives or face liability for breach of such obligation. Quotes Principles I, II, III, IV, and V and Opinion 8.08. Note, *Informed Choice: Physicians' Duty to Disclose Nonreadily Available Alternatives, 43 Case W. Res. L. Rev. 491, 491, 498-99, 508, 509 (1993).*

Journal 1990 Discusses the moral dilemma in deciding whether to withdraw artificial nutrition and hydration from a patient and the appropriate role of the judiciary. Concludes that judicial decisions do not represent the moral viewpoint of society and that moral pronouncements should not be made in the courtroom. Quotes Preamble, Principles I, II, III, IV, V, VI, and VII, and Opinion 2.20. Peccarelli, *A Moral Dilemma: The Role of Judicial Intervention in Withholding or Withdrawing Nutrition and Hydration*, 23 John Marshall L. Rev. 537, 539, 540, 541 (1990).

Journal 1986 Observes that the AMA policy on capital punishment expressly forbids psychiatrists from making determinations of competency for execution. Compares the psychiatrist's determination of competency for execution to the behavior of Nazi physicians, and condemns as inherently dishonest any therapy not grounded in the patient's best interests. References Principle I and Opinion 2.06. Sargent, *Treating the Condemned to Death*, 16 Hastings Center Rep. 5, 5 (Dec. 1986).

II. A physician shall uphold the standards of professionalism, be honest in all professional interactions, and strive to report physicians deficient in character or competence, or engaging in fraud or deception, to appropriate entities.

E.D. Mo. 2007 Defendant-physician's husband, also a physician, suffered brain damage during surgery, yet continued to practice medicine. Following a patient death, plaintiff brought a wrongful death action against the physician and a separate action against his wife for negligent failure to report her husband's impairment. The court found that the wife, although a physician, had no duty to warn of her husband's "dangerous propensities." Plaintiff cited Principle II's ethical requirement to report a fellow physician's deficiencies in competence. However, the court noted that the defendant was not a member of the AMA and that Missouri law does not impose such a duty. *Phelps v. DeMello*, 2007 WL 1063567, 3.

Cal. App. 2004 Trial court sustained a demur to the appellants' first amended complaint. The appellate court quoted Principles II and V in concluding the coroner's practice of hiring a pathologist who had a close working relationship with a company which treats individuals whose death the pathologist may be required to investigate was a questionable policy due to the pathologist's wide discretion. The appellate court, however, affirmed the trial court's decision that appellants had not stated any viable claims. *Miller v. Rupf*, 2004 WL 2092015, 11 n. 9.

Cal. App. 1956 Physician-petitioner sought mandamus against local medical association whose bylaws provided for the expulsion of any member who violated the Principles. Petitioner had been expelled under the provision for alleged violation of Principles Ch. III, Art IV, Sec.4 (1947) [now Opinions 9.04 and 9.07] for making disparaging statements regarding another physician in a report used in judicial proceedings. In holding that application of the provision to petitioner was contrary to public policy, the court noted that the physician's statements had been made at the request of a civil litigant and enjoyed a statutory testimonial privilege. Further, the court found that the AMA's right to formulate ethical principles did not extend to defining the duties of witnesses. Expulsion was also based on petitioner's critical comments about other physicians overheard by their patients in violation of Principles Ch. III, Art. IV, Sec.1 (1947) [now Principle II and Opinion 9.04]. The court found application of this Principle under the circumstances reasonable and not contrary to public policy. *Bernstein v. Alameda-Contra Costa Medical Ass'n*, 139 Cal. App. 2d 241, 293 P.2d 862, 863, 863 nn.1, 2 865 nn.4, 6, 866, 866 n.8, 867.

Fla. App. 1995 The court considered the issue of the effect of § 455.241(2) of the Florida Statutes on right of defense in a medical malpractice action to engage in ex parte communications with plaintiff's nonparty treating physician. The court held that a 1988 amendment to § 455.241(2) negated the applicability of the statute to medical malpractice cases. The dissent, citing *Petrillo v. Syntex Laboratories, Inc.*, 148 Ill. App. 3d 581, 499 N.E.2d 952 (1986), quoted Principles II and IV and Opinions 5.05, 5.06, and 5.08 as strong public policy support for its position that ex parte communications should be barred altogether. *Castillo-Plaza v. Green*, 655 So. 2d 197, 206 n.4.

Ill. App. 1986 Defense attorney in product liability suit was held in contempt of court for conducting ex parte discussions with plaintiff-patient's treating physician without patient's consent and contrary to authorized methods of discovery. The court held that the strong public policy favoring physician-patient confidentiality articulated in Principles II and IV and Opinions 5.05, 5.06, 5.07, and 5.08 justified a rule against such ex parte discussions. Further, the court held that the public has the right to rely on physicians to faithfully execute their ethical obligations. *Petrillo v. Syntex Laboratories, Inc.*, 148 Ill. App. 3d 581, 499 N.E.2d 952, 957, 958, 959.

Ky. App. 1978 Plaintiff-physician attempted to enjoin defendant medical society from expelling him for actions contrary to a variety of Principles, the most relevant to his alleged unethical behavior being Principle 4 (1957) [now Principles II and III]. After reviewing the procedures followed by the medical society in considering the evidence pertaining to the charges, the court affirmed judgment dismissing the action, concluding that plaintiff was not deprived of due process. *Kirk v. Jefferson County Medical Soc'y, 577 S.W.2d 419, 421.*

Md. App. 2007 The Maryland State Board of Physicians suspended the medical license of physician-appellant upon finding he lied to a peer review committee and left an anesthetized patient unattended. The circuit court affirmed suspension and the physician appealed. Quoting Principle II to support finding a breach of the physician's duty of honesty, the court ruled there was a reasonable factual and legal basis for the Board's decision. *Cornfeld v. State Board of Physicians, 174 Md. App. 456, 921 A.2d 893,906-07.*

Md. App. 1993 State Board of Physician Quality Assurance received a complaint that psychiatrist was having a romantic relationship with a former patient. When, as part of its investigation, the Board subpoenaed psychiatrist's records, patient raised the constitutional right to privacy. The court held that the state's interest in investigating possible disciplinary action against psychiatrist outweighed patient's constitutional right to privacy. The court cited Principle II as a potential basis to justify the Board's investigation of possible unprofessional conduct by physician. *Dr. K. v. State Board of Physician Quality Assur., 98 Md. App. 103, 632 A.2d 453, 456, cert. denied, 334 Md. 18, 637 A.2d 1191 (1994), and cert. denied, 115 S. Ct. 75, 130 L. Ed. 29 (1994).*

Mass. 1955 Plaintiff-physician was charged under state licensing statute by defendant-board with conspiracy and fee-splitting. Both parties sought a declaratory judgment as to whether the defendant-board had jurisdiction to determine plaintiff's guilt or innocence. In holding that the board was qualified to determine if plaintiff's actions constituted gross misconduct under the statute, the court referred to Principles Ch.I, Secs.1 and 6 (1947) [now Principle II and Opinion 6.02] delineating, in part, limitations on payment for medical services. These provisions, the court said, reflected the medical profession's understanding of its peculiar obligations. *Forziati v. Board of Registration in Medicine, 333 Mass. 125, 128 N.E.2d 789, 791.*

Mich. App. 2007 Plaintiff-physician had privileges at defendant-hospital. After a decline in referrals, plaintiff sued the hospital and two physicians for tortious interference with a business relationship and civil conspiracy. Plaintiff attempted to establish illegitimate business practices on the part of defendants by showing that a defendant-physician was not qualified to handle the cases referred to him. With apparent reference to Principle II, plaintiff claimed that this defendant improperly held himself out to have expertise in the field of gynecologic oncology. The court found the honesty requirement in Principle II to be too vague to support any of the claims brought by the plaintiff and affirmed summary judgment for defendants. *Boike v. McLaren Health Care Corp., 2007 WL 1932029, 4.*

Mich. App. 1968 Physician was properly dismissed from hospital staff for violating Principle 4 (1957) [now Principle II and Opinion 9.11] when on numerous occasions physician vilified other physicians, swore and screamed in the hospital, and quarreled with staff and hospital visitors. *Anderson v. Board of Trustees of Caro Community Hosp., 10 Mich. App. 348, 159 N.W.2d 347, 348-50.*

Minn. 1970 Defendant-physician appealed order to answer interrogatories, claiming that a medical malpractice plaintiff is prohibited from compelling expert testimony from a defendant to prove a charge of malpractice without calling other medical witnesses. In holding that a defendant could be compelled to provide expert medical opinion in response to interrogatories, the court quoted Principle 1 (1957) [now Principle II and Opinion 8.12] for the proposition that physicians owe a duty of disclosure to their patients. *Anderson v. Florence, 288 Minn. 351, 181 N.W.2d 873, 880, 880 n.7.*

N.Y. Sup. 1965 Physician sued publishing company to bar insertion of advertisement for baby and child care products in physician's book, seeking declaration that book contract was void to the extent that it allowed inclusion of such an advertisement. Physician asserted that the advertisement was contrary to public policy, citing Opinions and Reports of the Judicial Council Sec. 5, Para. 29 (1965) [now Opinion 5.02] which stated that a doctor should not lend his name to any product. In rejecting the physician's claim, the court was willing to give careful consideration to the Association's view but concluded that it did not, in itself, constitute an expression of public policy. *Spock v. Pocket Books, Inc., 48 Misc. 2d 812, 266 N.Y.S.2d 77, 79.*

Ohio 2009 Physician appealed from a judgment affirming an order of the state medical board that permanently revoked appellant's certificate to practice medicine. The board found that appellant's sexual contact with patients violated Ohio statutes governing physician conduct and the code of ethics of the AMA, citing Principles I, II, IV, and VIII. The Court of Appeals held that Ohio state law allows the board to revoke a physician's certificate if it finds that the person violated any provision of the code of ethics of the AMA. *D'Souza v. State Med. Bd. of Ohio,* 2009 WL 5108774, 6.

Ohio 1991 State medical board revoked license of physician who had consensual sexual relations with his patient. The court upheld the board's ruling that this violated Principles I, II, and IV. Dissenting judge, citing AMA Council on Ethical and Judicial Affairs, Sexual Misconduct in the Practice of Medicine, 266 JAMA 2741 [now Opinion 8.14], argued that until 1991, the AMA did not clearly deem sexual contact with a patient unethical. *Pons v. Ohio State Medical Bd.,* 66 Ohio St. 3d 619, 623, 625, 614 N.E.2d 748, 752, 753.

Ohio 1980 A physician, charged with violating the state medical licensing statute by distributing controlled substances without a proper license and writing prescriptions for narcotics in the name of one person when they were intended for another, challenged the state medical board's decision to suspend his license and place him on two years' probation. Under the statute, a physician could be disciplined for various activities including violation of any provision of a code of ethics of a national professional organization such as the AMA. The board found in part that the physician's actions violated Principles 4 and 7 (1957) [now Principles II and III and Opinions 8.06 and 9.04]. The trial court reversed, holding that the board had insufficient evidence for its decision, and the court of appeals affirmed. On appeal, the supreme court held that expert testimony was not required at a hearing before a medical licensing board because they were experts and could determine for themselves whether the Principles had been violated. *Arlen v. State,* 61 Ohio St. 2d 168, 399 N.E.2d 1251, 1252, 1253-54.

Ohio App. 2005 The Ohio State Medical Board permanently revoked the license of the appellant, a psychiatrist, for having inappropriate physical and sexual contact with a female patient. The trial court affirmed the board's ruling, and the appellant appealed. The board claimed that the appellant's relationship with his patient violated the AMA's Code of Medical Ethics citing Principles I, II, and IV. The appellate court affirmed stating that permanent revocation of the appellant's license was not excessive and was not a violation of due process as the board may revoke the appellant's license if treatment did not meet minimal standards of care and violated any provision of the AMA's Code of Medical Ethics. *Schechter v. Ohio State Med. Bd.,* 2005 WL 1869733, 9.

Journal 2010 Analyzes factors contributing to the emergence of medical repatriation and evaluates whether this practice comports with current legal and ethical standards. Proposes changes to federal regulations that govern hospitals and clarifications to medical ethical standards. Quotes the Preamble and Principles I, II, III, IV, V, VI, VII, VIII, and IX. Zoellner, *Medical Repatriation: Examining the Legal and Ethical Implications of an Emerging Practice,* 32 Wash. U. J. L. & Pol'y 515, 530-532 (2010).

Journal 2009 Explores emerging issues in conflict management systems design (CMSD). Concludes as the practice of CMSD in the organizational context continues to expand, practitioners should openly discuss the emerging issues of the field. References Principles I, II, V, and VIII. Costantino, *Second Generation Organizational Conflict Management Systems Design: A Practitioner's Perspective on Emerging Issues,* 14 Harv. Negot. L. Rev. 81, 95 (2009).

Journal 2009 Discusses the interaction between statutes and case law governing the medical field and the core principles of medical professionalism. Concludes the legal framework of medical professionalism does not encompass all the elements required of a medical professional. Quotes Principles II, III, IV, V, VI, VII, and VIII. Fichter, *The Law of Doctoring: A Study of the Codification of Medical Professionalism,* 19 Health Matrix 317, 338, 339, 340, 343, 351 (2009).

Journal 2009 Discusses whether or not patients have a right to pain management. Concludes that no physician duty is established by law or ethics to provide pain management outside the traditional physician-patient relationship. Cites Principles I, II, IV, and VIII. Hall & Boswell, *Ethics, Law, and Pain Management as a Patient Right,* 12 Pain Physician 499, 500 (2009).

Journal 2008 Discusses procedural guidelines for treating HIV-positive patients seeking cosmetic surgery for lipodystrophy syndrome. Concludes that this patient group is increasing in number, and that physicians could risk violating legal and ethical rules by refusing to provide treatment.

Quotes Principle II and Opinion 9.131. Davison, Reisman, Pellegrino, Larson, Dermody, & Hutchison, *Perioperative Guidelines for Elective Surgery in the Human Immunodeficiency Virus–Positive Patient*, 121 Plastic and Reconstructive Surgery 1831, 1838 (2008).

Journal 2008 Explores the legal, ethical, and policy implications of concierge medicine. Argues physicians engaged in concierge care must strive to meet ethical and legal standards, and take care to communicate clearly with patients about services and fees. Quotes Opinion 8.055. Cites Principles II and VI and Opinion 8.055. Portman & Romanow, *Concierge Medicine: Legal Issues, Ethical Dilemmas, and Policy Challenges*, 1 J. Health & Life Sci. L. 1, 4, 28-29 (2008).

Journal 2008 Examines the development of bioethics and environmental ethics, as well as laws promoting the role of bioethicists in decision making. Concludes environmental ethicists must convince legislatures of the role of environmental ethics in order to have a greater impact on decision making. Quotes Principles I, II, III, IV, V, VI, VII, VIII, and IX. Robertson, *Seeking a Seat at the Table: Has Law Left Environmental Ethics Behind as It Embraces Bioethics?* 32 Wm. & Mary Envtl. L. & Pol'y Rev. 273, 307 (2008).

Journal 2008 Explores the fiduciary relationship between physicians and patients, professional and ethical obligations of both physicians and lawyers, and the implications for conflict resolution in health care. Concludes physicians must put patient interests above their own and lawyers must work to discern clients' best interests and support client welfare. Quotes Principle VIII and Opinions 8.12 and 10.015. Cites Principles I and II and Opinions 10.01 and 10.015. Scott, *Doctors as Advocates, Lawyers as Healers*, 29 Hamline J. Pub. L. Pol'y, 331, 340-41, 347, 371 (2008).

Journal 2007 Addresses physician liability for an extramarital affair with a patient's spouse. Concludes that such an affair should be regarded as a breach of a fiduciary duty. Quotes Preamble, Principles I, II, and VIII, and Opinions 8.145, 9.04, 9.123, and 10.015. Demaine, *"Playing Doctor" With the Patient's Spouse: Alternative Conceptions of Health Professional Liability*, 14 Va. J. Soc. Pol'y & L. 308, 325, 330-31, 331-32 (2007).

Journal 2007 Argues that issuance of apologies from physicians who commit medical errors will diminish the number of malpractice suits brought. Concludes that patients desire apologies in the case of medical errors and are less likely to sue when they are given. Cites Principles I, II, III, and IV and Opinion 8.12. Tabler, *Should Physicians Apologize for Medical Errors?* 19 Health Lawyer 23, 23 (Jan. 2007).

Journal 2007 Discusses military policies on the ethical treatment of enemy combatants. Concludes that military medical personnel should adhere to the ethical standards of their profession at all times. References Principle II. Xenakis, *How Should We Respond? Seton Hall University School of Law Guantanamo Teach-In*, 37 Seton Hall L. Rev. 703, 709 (2007).

Journal 2006 Evaluates the constitutionality of federal faith-based initiative programs. Concludes that such programs violate the First Amendment under the combined Lemon and Zelman test. Cites Principles II and VIII. Boden, *Compassion Inaction: Why President Bush's Faith-Based Initiatives Violate the Establishment Clause*, 29 Seattle U. L. Rev. 991, 1023 (2006).

Journal 2006 Explores conscience clause legislation relating to the dispensing of oral contraceptives. Concludes that such legislation must balance the interests of the patient and the health care provider. Cites Principles I, II, III, IV, V, VI, VII, VIII, and IX. Collins, *Conscience Clauses and Oral Contraceptives: Conscientious Objection or Calculated Obstruction?* 15 Ann. Health L. 37, 54 (2006).

Journal 2006 Examines physician criminal activity and subsequent disciplinary actions by state licensing boards. Concludes that licensing boards should impose greater penalties on physicians convicted of crimes. Quotes Principles II and III. Jung, Lurie, & Wolfe, *U.S. Physicians Disciplined for Criminal Activity*, 16 Health Matrix 335, 335 (2006).

Journal 2006 Reviews Supreme Court decisions on protection of a public employee's freedom of speech. Concludes that the law should provide constitutional protection when an employee's speech is critical of his or her public employer. Quotes Principle II. Note, *Leading Cases–Public Employee Speech*, 120 Harv. L. Rev. 125, 282 (2006).

Journal 2005 Argues that disciplining physicians who give questionable expert testimony in medical malpractice cases may reduce insurance premiums for physicians. Concludes that state regulation of medical expert testimony is vital to tort liability reform. Cites Principle II. Gomez, *Silencing the Hired Guns: Ensuring Honesty in Medical Expert Testimony Through State Legislation*, 26 J. Legal Med. 385, 399 (2005).

Journal 2005 Examines issues surrounding tort reform proposals. Concludes that more can be done to correct the current tort system before moving toward a "one size fits all" approach. Quotes Principles I, II, III, IV, V, VI, VII, VIII, and IX. Messerly & Warwick, *Nowhere to Turn: A Glance at the Facts Behind the Supposed Need for Tort "Reform,"* 28 Hamline L. Rev. 489, 506 (2005).

Journal 2003 Considers conflicts of interest and potential liability that a team physician faces when treating an injured athlete. Concludes that an athlete's health should be the team physician's primary concern in making treatment decisions. References Principles I and II. Landis, *The Team Physician: An Analysis of the Causes of Action, Conflicts, Defenses and Improvements,* 1 DePaul J. Sports L. & Contemp. Probs. 139, 144 (2003).

Journal 2003 Examines social norms, using public choice theory, to determine how certain groups in society use these norms to benefit their members. Concludes that the benefits provided by social norms may dissipate depending on various considerations. Quotes Principles II and VIII. Miller, *Norms and Interests,* 32 Hofstra L. Rev. 637, 650, 670 (2003).

Journal 2003 Considers the legal, medical, and ethical issues of physician-patient confidentiality in disclosure of paternity. Concludes that a balancing test should be applied to making determinations regarding disclosure of paternity. Quotes Principles I, IV, and V and Opinions 1.02, 5.055, and 10.01. Cites Principle II and Opinion 5.05. Richards & Wolf, *Medical Confidentiality and Disclosure of Paternity,* 48 S. D. L. Rev. 409, 411, 412, 413 (2003).

Journal 2003 Uses public policy arguments to support a preponderance standard for medical license revocations in situations involving false testimony by a medical expert witness. Concludes that medical licensing boards can more effectively protect the public by using a preponderance standard. Quotes Principles II, III, and IV and Opinions 1.02 and 9.07. Widmer, *South Dakota Should Follow Public Policy and Switch to the Preponderance Standard for Medical License Revocation After In Re the Medical License of Dr. Reuben Setliff, M.D.,* 48 S. D. L. Rev. 388, 396-97, 402 (2003).

Journal 2002 Discusses therapeutic jurisprudence and the importance of trust in the structure of health care law. Concludes that understanding trust provides tools to formulate responses to new ethical, legal, and policy challenges. Quotes Principle Ch. I, Art. I, Sec. 4 (1847) [now Principle II and Opinion 8.12]. Hall, *Law, Medicine, and Trust,* 55 Stan. L. Rev. 463, 471 (2002).

Journal 2002 Analyzes the expanded use of the Civil False Claims Act in prosecuting health care fraud. Concludes that, in enforcing the law, government must balance its promises to beneficiaries, health care providers, and the public. Quotes Principles I, II, and IV. Krause, *"Promises to Keep": Health Care Providers and the Civil False Claims Act,* 23 Cardozo L. Rev. 1363, 1365 (2002).

Journal 2002 Explores the development and current status of collective bargaining and unionization in the medical profession. Concludes that, because collective bargaining traditionally addresses conditions of employment, a focus on patient care will be difficult to ensure. References Principle II. Levy, *Collective Bargaining in the Elite Professions–Doctors' Application of the Labor Law Model to Negotiations With Health Plan Providers,* 13 U. Fla. J. L. & Pub. Pol'y. 269, 277 (2002).

Journal 2002 Examines the origin and dynamics of the scope-of-practice laws governing health care providers. Concludes that the current system is not working and offers recommendations for change. Quotes Principles I and II. Safriet, *Closing the Gap Between Can and May in Health-Care Providers' Scopes of Practice: A Primer for Policymakers,* 19 Yale J. on Reg. 301, 311 (2002).

Journal 2002 Considers the case of *Ferguson v. City of Charleston.* Concludes that the Supreme Court's rationale in that case reflects insights from feminist legal theory. Quotes Opinion 10.01. Cites Principles II and IV. Taslitz, *A Feminist Fourth Amendment?: Consent, Care, Privacy, and Social Meaning in Ferguson v. City of Charleston,* 9 Duke J. Gender L. & Pol'y 1, 18, 19 (2002).

Journal 2001 Discusses whether or not the medical profession needs a policy on honesty. Reviews ethical codes and concludes they fail to offer physicians with meaningful guidance about what constitutes "the truth" and when and how to disclose it. Quotes Principle II and Opinions 8.12 and 10.01. DeVita, *Honestly, Do We Need a Policy on Truth?* 11 Kennedy Inst. Ethics J. 157, 158 (2001).

Journal 2001 Compares and contrasts certain ethical positions articulated by the legal and medical professions. Concludes that both professions generally agree on ethical principles, but sometimes differ in the manner of implementation. Quotes Principle II. Cites Opinion 5.02. Needell, *Legal Ethics in Medicine: Are Medical Ethics Different From Legal Ethics?* 14 St. Thomas L. Rev. 31, 35, 50 (2001).

Journal 2000 Considers whether government regulators should allow managed care organizations to cover the costs of alternative treatments. Concludes that legislation should be more attentive to its consumer protection role. Quotes Principle II. Boozang, *Is the Alternative Medicine? Managed Care Apparently Thinks So,* 32 Conn. L. Rev. 567, 606 (2000).

Journal 2000 Considers the rules governing expert testimony. Explores professional ethical standards affecting expert witnesses and concludes that codes of ethics have not succeeded in eliminating biased expert testimony. Recommends creation of an organization to assist courts in obtaining reliable expert witness testimony. Quotes Principle III and Opinion 6.01. Cites Principles I, II, and V and Opinions 1.02 and 9.07. Murphy, *Expert Witnesses at Trial: Where Are the Ethics?* 14 Geo. J. Legal Ethics 217, 231-32 (2000).

Journal 2000 Discusses traditional medical ethics and the physician's duty to benefit patients. Concludes that in the twenty-first century, physicians will no longer be expected to determine on their own what will benefit their patients. Quotes Principle II and Opinion 8.08. Veatch, *Doctor Does Not Know Best: Why in the New Century Physicians Must Stop Trying to Benefit Patients,* 25 J. Med. & Phil. 701, 710, 711 (2000).

Journal 1999 Provides examples in which psychiatrists might use deception in their practice. Explains the motivations for such conduct and raises questions about possible blameworthiness for such conduct. Quotes Principles II and III. Haroun & Morris, *Weaving a Tangled Web: The Deceptions of Psychiatrists,* 10 J. Contemp. Leg. Issues 227, 235 (1999).

Journal 1999 Examines fraud and abuse throughout government health care programs, with emphasis on enforcement and available sanctions. Concludes that consideration of strategies for revising enforcement protocols is advisable. Quotes Principle II. Jost & Davies, *The Empire Strikes Back: A Critique of the Backlash Against Fraud and Abuse Enforcement,* 51 Ala. L. Rev. 239, 240 (1999).

Journal 1999 Describes historical and present views regarding medical diagnosis. Discusses pressures physicians face that may affect the diagnostic process. Suggests that legal institutions can reduce these pressures, which will enhance the physician-patient therapeutic relationship. Quotes Principle II and Opinion 9.07. Noah, *Pigeonholing Illness: Medical Diagnosis as a Legal Construct,* 50 Hastings L. J. 241, 301, 302 (1999).

Journal 1999 Analyzes the federal rules of evidence from a feminist perspective. Proposes a new "apology" evidence rule to serve as an exception to the general rule that statements by party opponents are admissible during trial. Suggests that physicians who commit medical errors may ease patients' anger by apologizing. The new evidence rule would permit physicians to be more forthcoming in this regard. Quotes Principles I and II. Orenstein, *Apology Excepted: Incorporating a Feminist Analysis Into Evidence Policy Where You Would Least Expect It,* 28 S.W. U. L. Rev. 221, 264 (1999).

Journal 1999 Evaluates changes in direct-to-consumer advertising of prescription pharmaceuticals. Discusses FDA regulation of this type of advertising. Recognizes the important role of the FDA in this context. Quotes Principles II and III. Terzian, *Direct-to-Consumer Prescription Drug Advertising,* 25 Am. J. Law & Med. 149, 165 (1999).

Journal 1998 Discusses gag provisions in physicians' contracts with managed care organizations. Examines effects of gag rules on physicians. Explores state legislation and proposed federal legislation pertaining to gag provisions. Cites Principle II. Munoz, Nichols, Okata, Pitt, & Seager, *The Two Faces of Gag Provisions: Patients and Physicians in a Bind,* 17 Yale L. & Pol'y Rev. 249, 258 (1998).

Journal 1997 Reports on a study of physician attitudes regarding expert witnesses. Notes that a majority of physicians believe that medical expert testimony should be subject to peer review and, when appropriate, medical licensing board discipline. Quotes Principles II and VI and Opinion 9.07. Eitel, Hegeman, & Evans, *Medicine on Trial: Physicians' Attitudes About Expert Medical Witnesses,* 18 J. Legal Med. 345, 355, 358 (1997).

Journal 1997 Discusses physician frustration with managed care plans caused by gag clauses and cost-containment mechanisms. Reviews the development of managed care organizations and federal attempts at limiting the use of gag clauses. Concludes that gag clauses are inherently flawed and compromise quality health care. Quotes Principles II and V, Fundamental Elements (1), and Opinion 8.13. Note, *Physicians, Bound and Gagged: Federal Attempts to Combat Managed Care's Use of Gag Clauses, 21 Seton Hall Legis. J. 567, 601-02 (1997).*

Journal 1997 Discusses the need for balance between business ethics and medical ethics in the context of managed care. Explores two models for integrating ethics and managed care. Proposes the adoption of a collective responsibility model to improve quality of care. Quotes Principles I, II, III, IV, and V. Cites Preamble. References Opinion 8.13. Regan, *Regulating the Business of Medicine: Models for Integrating Ethics and Managed Care, 30 Colum. J. L. & Soc. Probs. 635, 651, 656, 657 (1997).*

Journal 1996 Discusses the trend toward conserving resources expended on health care by withholding services absent a showing of necessity. Claims that the high standard of care physicians owe patients is jeopardized by medical treatment decisions based on coverage concerns. Concludes that the legal structure regarding health care plans should be changed. Quotes Preamble, Principles I, II, III, IV, V, VI, and VII, and Opinion 2.03. Hirshfeld & Thomason, *Medical Necessity Determinations: The Need for a New Legal Structure, 6 Health Matrix 3, 8-9 (1996).*

Journal 1996 Considers the impact of gag clauses on the physician-patient relationship. Undertakes an extensive legal, ethical, and policy analysis. Concludes that gag clauses are violative of legal and ethical principles. Quotes Principles II, V, and VI and Fundamental Elements (1). Cites Preamble. Martin & Bjerknes, *The Legal and Ethical Implications of Gag Clauses in Physician Contracts, XXII Am. J. Law & Med. 433, 465-66 (1996).*

Journal 1996 Examines the issue of attorney-client sexual relationships and the ethical problems inherent in such conduct. Recommends promulgation of a rule regulating such relationships. Quotes Principle II. Myers, Sonenshein, & Hofstein, *To Regulate or Not To Regulate Attorney-Client Sex? The Ethical Question in Pennsylvania, 69 Temp. L. Rev. 741, 780 (1996).*

Journal 1996 Discusses the ethical implications of sexual misconduct in the medical field. Examines the current civil and criminal tools used to curb physician-patient misconduct. Notes the inadequacy of physician reporting. Proposes a statutory approach to discipline physicians who abuse their fiduciary duties. Quotes Principle II. References Opinion 8.14. Note, *Sexual Conduct Within the Physician-Patient Relationship: A Statutory Framework for Disciplining This Breach of Fiduciary Duty, 1 Widener L. Symp. J. 501, 507 (1996).*

Journal 1994 Compares Texas law with Illinois law on the issue of ex parte communications between defense counsel and the patient/plaintiff's physician in civil litigation. Argues that preservation of the physician-patient relationship requires prohibition of such contact. Quotes Principles II and IV and Opinion 5.05. Comment, *From the Land of Lincoln a Healing Rule: Proposed Texas Rule of Civil Procedure Prohibiting Ex Parte Contact Between Defense Counsel and a Plaintiff's Treating Physician, 25 Tex. Tech L. Rev. 1081, 1081, 1082 (1994).*

Journal 1994 Reviews the evolution of the physician-patient relationship, with attention to patient autonomy. Examines the changing health care delivery environment. Quotes Preamble, Principles I, II, III, IV, V, and VI, Fundamental Elements (1) and (2), and Opinions 1.02 and 8.07 (1981) [now Opinion 8.08]. Cites Opinion 1.01. Szczygiel, *Beyond Informed Consent, 21 Ohio N. U. L. Rev. 171, 217, 218, 220, 225, 226, 256 (1994).*

Journal 1993 Discusses physicians' duty to disclose to patients medical treatment alternatives that are not readily available. Proposes that based on the historical development and legal requirements of the informed consent doctrine, physicians should be required to inform patients of non–readily available alternatives or face liability for breach of such obligation. Quotes Principles I, II, III, IV, and V and Opinion 8.08. Note, *Informed Choice: Physicians' Duty to Disclose Nonreadily Available Alternatives, 43 Case W. Res. L. Rev. 491, 491, 498-99, 508, 509 (1993).*

Journal 1993 Discusses the problems physicians may encounter by exposing an errant colleague, such as harm to the reporting physician's reputation and the fear of litigation. States that problems involving physician competency and unethical behavior should be investigated, and that physicians should take personal responsibility for reporting problems they observe. References

Principle II and Opinions 8.14 and 9.031. Morreim, *Am I My Brother's Warden? Responding to the Unethical or Incompetent Colleague*, 23 Hastings Center Rep. 19, 23 (May/June 1993).

Journal 1993 Explores problems associated with parental requests to withhold diagnoses from children. Discusses the physician's conflict between a duty to respect parents' wishes and a duty to tell children the truth. Quotes Principle II. Sigman, Kraut, & La Puma, *Disclosure of a Diagnosis to Children and Adolescents When Parents Object*, 147 Am. J. Diseases Children 764, 766 (1993).

Journal 1991 Examines the issues surrounding judicial use of professional ethics codes in private litigation. Concludes that judges should more extensively use professional ethics codes to define public policy, standards of care, and legal causes of action. Quotes Principle II and Opinion 2.19. Note, *Professional Ethics Codes in Court: Redefining the Social Contract Between the Public and the Professions*, 25 Georgia L. Rev. 1327, 1335, 1351 (1991).

Journal 1990 Examines the extent to which forensic psychiatrists are consulted in medical malpractice cases. Considers the appropriate standard of care, particularly for psychiatric malpractice cases, and the problems associated with its determination. References Principles II and IV. Modlin, *Forensic Psychiatry and Malpractice*, 18 Bull. Am. Acad. Psychiatry Law 153, 161 (1990).

Journal 1990 Discusses the moral dilemma in deciding whether to withdraw artificial nutrition and hydration from a patient and the appropriate role of the judiciary. Concludes that judicial decisions do not represent the moral viewpoint of society and that moral pronouncements should not be made in the courtroom. Quotes Preamble, Principles I, II, III, IV, V, VI, and VII, and Opinion 2.20. Peccarelli, *A Moral Dilemma: The Role of Judicial Intervention in Withholding or Withdrawing Nutrition and Hydration*, 23 John Marshall L. Rev. 537, 539, 540, 541 (1990).

Journal 1989 Discusses the history of the physician-patient privilege up through changes implemented under the Ohio Tort Reform Act of 1987. Aspects of the physician-patient privilege that are most significantly affected by this Tort Reform Act are highlighted, with recommendations for further refinement of the privilege in Ohio. Quotes Principles II and IV and Opinion 5.05. Note, *The Ohio Physician-Patient Privilege: Modified, Revised, and Defined*, 49 Ohio St. L. J. 1147, 1167 (1989).

Journal 1985 Initially describes how existing doctrines protect the value of autonomy in the context of the physician-patient relationship, then examines various problems in the current protective scheme. Concludes by recommending the creation of an independent articulable protected interest in patient autonomy. Quotes Principles II and IV. Cites Opinions 4.04 (1984) [now Opinions 8.03 and 8.032] and 6.03 (1984) [now Opinion 6.02]. Shultz, *From Informed Consent to Patient Choice: A New Protected Interest*, 95 Yale L. J. 219, 275 (1985).

III. A physician shall respect the law and also recognize a responsibility to seek changes in those requirements which are contrary to the best interests of the patient.

Ariz. 1965 Physician appealed denial of medical license which was based on alleged violations of local medical society rules and Principles 3, 5, and 10 (1957) [now Principles III and VII and Opinions 3.01, 8.11, and 9.06]. Alleged violations included treating a patient without first obtaining a prior treating physician's permission, inadequate patient care, performing operations without hospital privileges, and signing the medical record of a deceased patient who had been treated by interns. The court held that the evidence failed to show any clear violation of the Principles and that a local medical society had no right to prescribe a code of ethics for state licensing purposes. *Arizona State Bd. of Medical Examiners v. Clark*, 97 Ariz. 205, 398 P.2d 908, 914-15, 915 n.3.

Ky. App. 1978 Plaintiff-physician attempted to enjoin defendant medical society from expelling him for actions contrary to a variety of Principles, the most relevant to his alleged unethical behavior being Principle 4 (1957) [now Principles II and III]. After reviewing the procedures followed by the medical society in considering the evidence pertaining to the charges, the court affirmed judgment dismissing the action, concluding that plaintiff was not deprived of due process. *Kirk v. Jefferson County Medical Soc'y*, 577 S.W.2d 419, 421.

Ohio 1980 A physician, charged with violating the state medical licensing statute by distributing controlled substances without a proper license and writing prescriptions for narcotics in the name of one person when they were intended for another, challenged the state medical board's decision to suspend his license and place him on two years' probation. Under the statute, a physician could be disciplined for various activities including violation of any provision of a code of ethics of a national professional organization such as the AMA. The board found in part that the physician's actions violated Principles 4 and 7 (1957) [now Principles II and III and Opinions 8.06 and 9.04]. The trial court reversed, holding that the board had insufficient evidence for its decision, and the court of appeals affirmed. On appeal, the Supreme Court held that expert testimony was not required at a hearing before a medical licensing board because they were experts and could determine for themselves whether the Principles had been violated. *Arlen v. State, 61 Ohio St. 2d 168, 399 N.E.2d 1251, 1252, 1253-54.*

Journal 2011 Proposes fundamental reforms to the medical liability system based on the development of clinical practice guidelines by private, for-profit firms that in turn would bear the liability cost for providers who buy or license, and then follow the firm's prescribed guidelines. Quotes Principle III. Avraham, *Private Regulation, 34 Harv. J. L. & Pub. Pol'y 543, 614-15 (2011).*

Journal 2011 Reviews the use and current regulation of medical marijuana to alleviate pain in terminally ill patients. Focusing on patient autonomy, concludes that patients should have access to medical marijuana in controlled doses under controlled conditions. Quotes Principle III and Opinions 10.01, 10.015, and 10.02. References Principle VIII. Pfeifer, *Smoking Gun: The Moral and Legal Struggle for Medical Marijuana, 27 Touro L. Rev. 339, 340-41, 345-346 (2011).*

Journal 2010 Analyzes factors contributing to the emergence of medical repatriation and evaluates whether this practice comports with current legal and ethical standards. Proposes changes to federal regulations that govern hospitals and clarifications to medical ethical standards. Quotes the Preamble and Principles I, II, III, IV, V, VI, VII, VIII, and IX. Zoellner, *Medical Repatriation: Examining the Legal and Ethical Implications of an Emerging Practice, 32 Wash. U. J. L. & Pol'y 515, 530-532 (2010).*

Journal 2009 Discusses the interaction between statutes and case law governing the medical field and the core principles of medical professionalism. Concludes the legal framework of medical professionalism does not encompass all the elements required of a medical professional. Quotes Principles II, III, IV, V, VI, VII, and VIII. Fichter, *The Law of Doctoring: A Study of the Codification of Medical Professionalism, 19 Health Matrix 317, 338, 339, 340, 343, 351 (2009).*

Journal 2009 Discusses tobacco use in psychiatric institutions and its impact on the health and behavior of patients. Concludes legislative action should be taken to remove tobacco from psychiatric institutions to provide patients with the health and safety benefits of smoke-free facilities. Quotes Principles I and III. Hackett, *Smoke-Free State Psychiatric Facility Grounds: Is Legislation Necessary and Appropriate to Remove Tobacco From These Treatment Settings? 53 N. Y. L. Sch. L. Rev. 99, 122-23 (2009).*

Journal 2009 Explores the jurisprudential foundation of the fiduciary duty physicians owe their patients and discusses the failure of physicians to disclose to patients errors and other emergent medical risks. Concludes law should recognize the physician's duty to disclose such risks by enforcing a cause of action for breach of that duty. Quotes Principles III and VIII and Opinions 8.12, 10.015, and 10.02. References Opinion 8.12. Hafemeister, *Lean on Me: A Physician's Fiduciary Duty to Disclose an Emergent Medical Risk to the Patient, 86 Wash. U. L. Rev. 1167, 1172-1173, 1178, 1182, 1185, 1188, 1209 (2009).*

Journal 2008 Examines the development of bioethics and environmental ethics, as well as laws promoting the role of bioethicists in decision making. Concludes environmental ethicists must convince legislatures of the role of environmental ethics in order to have a greater impact on decision making. Quotes Principles I, II, III, IV, V, VI, VII, VIII, and IX. Robertson, *Seeking a Seat at the Table: Has Law Left Environmental Ethics Behind as It Embraces Bioethics? 32 Wm. & Mary Envtl. L. & Pol'y Rev. 273, 307 (2008).*

Journal 2007 Argues that issuance of apologies from physicians who commit medical errors will diminish the number of malpractice suits brought. Concludes that patients desire apologies in the case of medical errors and are less likely to sue when they are given. Cites Principles I, II, III, and IV and Opinion 8.12. Tabler, *Should Physicians Apologize for Medical Errors? 19 Health Lawyer 23, 25 (Jan. 2007).*

Journal 2007 Examines relative vs absolute rights to confidentiality for military detainees considering the utilitarian need to protect the public at large. Concludes that evolving standards may favor individual rights to confidentiality, even from a utilitarian perspective. Quotes Opinions 1.02 and 5.05. References Principle III. Wynia, *Breaching Confidentiality to Protect the Public: Evolving Standards of Medical Confidentiality for Military Detainees, 7 Am. J. Bioethics 1, 2 (Aug. 2007).*

Journal 2006 Explores conscience clause legislation relating to the dispensing of oral contraceptives. Concludes that such legislation must balance the interests of the patient and the health care provider. Cites Principles I, II, III, IV, V, VI, VII, VIII and IX. Collins, *Conscience Clauses and Oral Contraceptives: Conscientious Objection or Calculated Obstruction? 15 Ann. Health L. 37, 54 (2006).*

Journal 2006 Discusses mentally incompetent inmates and capital punishment. Proposes that, to be permissible, involuntary medication of death-row inmates must represent the best medically appropriate treatment. Quotes Principles I, III, and VIII, and Opinion 2.06. Gabos, *The Perils of Singleton v. Norris: Ethics and Beyond, 32 Am. J. L. & Med. 117, 118, 125-26, 127 (2006).*

Journal 2006 Examines physician criminal activity and subsequent disciplinary actions by state licensing boards. Concludes that licensing boards should impose greater penalties on physicians convicted of crimes. Quotes Principles II and III. Jung, Lurie, & Wolfe, *U.S. Physicians Disciplined for Criminal Activity, 16 Health Matrix 335, 335 (2006).*

Journal 2006 Examines a mental health professional's competing duties of confidentiality and reporting a patient's threats of violence. Suggests new legislation should clarify duty to report a threat. Quotes Preamble and Principles III, IV, and VIII. Cites Opinion 5.05. Mossman, *Critique of Pure Risk Assessment or, Kant Meets Tarasoff, 75 U. Cin. L. Rev. 523, 579 (2006).*

Journal 2005 Examines issues surrounding tort reform proposals. Concludes that more can be done to correct the current tort system before moving toward a "one size fits all" approach. Quotes Principles I, II, III, IV, V, VI, VII, VIII, and IX. Messerly & Warwick, *Nowhere to Turn: A Glance at the Facts Behind the Supposed Need for Tort "Reform," 28 Hamline L. Rev. 489, 506 (2005).*

Journal 2005 Argues that medicating a criminal defendant to restore competency is ethical, even in capital cases. Concludes that principles justifying administration of punishment in the legal system give rise to an ethical imperative for physicians to provide competence-restoring medical therapy. Quotes Principle III and Opinion 2.06. Mossman, *Is Prosecution "Medically Appropriate?" 31 New Eng. J. on Crim. & Civ. Confinement 15, 53-54, 59 (2005).*

Journal 2003 Uses public policy arguments to support a preponderance standard for medical license revocations in situations involving false testimony by a medical expert witness. Concludes that medical licensing boards can more effectively protect the public by using a preponderance standard. Quotes Principles II, III, and IV and Opinions 1.02 and 9.07. Widmer, *South Dakota Should Follow Public Policy and Switch to the Preponderance Standard for Medical License Revocation After In Re the Medical License of Dr. Reuben Setliff, M.D., 48 S. D. L. Rev. 388, 396-97, 402 (2003).*

Journal 2002 Explores the implications of withholding medical treatment when abortion results in a live birth. Concludes that, in these situations, abortive parents and physicians should not solely decide the child's best interest. Quotes Preamble, Principles I and III, and Opinions 2.035, 2.20, and 2.215. Casagrande, *Children Not Meant to Be: Protecting the Interests of the Child When Abortion Results in Live Birth, 6 Quinnipiac Health L. J. 19, 44, 45, 47-48 (2002).*

Journal 2002 Advocates in favor of disclosure of information regarding a physician's clinical experience when obtaining informed consent. Concludes that the physician's experience is material and patients who inquire should be given this information. Quotes Principle Ch. I, Art. I, Sec. 4 (1847) [now Principle II and Opinion 8.12]. Iheukwumere, *Doctor, Are You Experienced? The Relevance of Disclosure of Physician Experience to a Valid Informed Consent, 18 J. Contemp. Health L. & Pol'y 373, 376-77 (2002).*

Journal 2002 Considers the dilemma of informed consent in the context of prescribing psychotropic medication to patients with mental illness and mental retardation. Recognizes the need for substituted decision-making in certain situations. Concludes that legislation would help address this issue. Quotes Preamble, Principles I, III, IV, VIII, and IX, and Opinion 8.08. O'Sullivan & Borcherding, *Informed Consent for Medication in Persons With Mental Retardation and Mental Illness, 12 Health Matrix 63, 75, 86, 87, 88 (2002).*

Journal 2001 Considers whether or not it is ethical for physicians to prescribe, and pharmacists to dispense, syringes for use by injection drug users. Concludes that ethical considerations suggest such actions are permissible but not obligatory. Quotes Principle III and Opinion 1.02. References Opinion 5.05. Lazzarini, *An Analysis of Ethical Issues in Prescribing and Dispensing Syringes to Injection Drug Users*, 11 Health Matrix 85, 107, 119 (2001).

Journal 2000 Considers the rules governing expert testimony. Explores professional ethical standards affecting expert witnesses and concludes that codes of ethics have not succeeded in eliminating biased expert testimony. Recommends creation of an organization to assist courts in obtaining reliable expert witness testimony. Quotes Principle III and Opinion 6.01. Cites Principles I, II, and V and Opinions 1.02 and 9.07. Murphy, *Expert Witnesses at Trial: Where Are the Ethics?* 14 Geo. J. Legal Ethics 217, 231-32 (2000).

Journal 1999 States that current First Amendment opinions do not give clear guidelines on professional speech. Describes the US Supreme Court's approach to commercial speech. Examines Supreme Court opinions and points out similarities between the Court's stance on commercial and professional speech. Cites Principle III. Halberstam, *Commercial Speech, Professional Speech, and the Constitutional Status of Social Institutions*, 147 U. Pa. L. Rev. 771, 857 (1999).

Journal 1999 Provides examples in which psychiatrists might use deception in their practice. Explains the motivations for such conduct and raises questions about possible blameworthiness for such conduct. Quotes Principles II and III. Haroun & Morris, *Weaving a Tangled Web: The Deceptions of Psychiatrists*, 10 J. Contemp. Leg. Issues 227, 235 (1999).

Journal 1999 Evaluates changes in direct-to-consumer advertising of prescription pharmaceuticals. Discusses Food and Drug Administration (FDA) regulation of this type of advertising. Recognizes the important role of the FDA in this context. Quotes Principles II and III. Terzian, *Direct-to-Consumer Prescription Drug Advertising*, 25 Am. J. Law & Med. 149, 165 (1999).

Journal 1998 Examines the US Supreme Court's decision in *Zinermon v. Burch* in relation to other Supreme Court decisions regarding the role of the courts in mental health treatment determinations. Argues that the government must strike a balance between the duty to care for the mentally ill and the duty to respect individual liberty. Provides approaches legislatures could adopt regarding mental health issues. References Principles I and III. Nidich, *Zinermon v. Burch and Voluntary Admissions to Public Hospitals: A Common Sense Proposal for Compromise*, 25 N. Ky. L. Rev. 699, 710 (1998).

Journal 1997 Discusses the practice of physician deselection by managed care organizations. Suggests that deselection harms the physician-patient relationship and creates a conflict of interest. Argues that solutions to deselection should consider effects on the patient rather than on the physician. Quotes Principle III. Cites Principle I and Opinions 8.05 and 8.13. Liner, *Physician Deselection: The Dynamics of a New Threat to the Physician-Patient Relationship*, 23 Am. J. Law & Med. 511, 513, 527 (1997).

Journal 1997 Discusses the need for balance between business ethics and medical ethics in the context of managed care. Explores two models for integrating ethics and managed care. Proposes the adoption of a collective responsibility model to improve quality of care. Quotes Principles I, II, III, IV, and V. Cites Preamble. References Opinion 8.13. Regan, *Regulating the Business of Medicine: Models for Integrating Ethics and Managed Care*, 30 Colum. J. L. & Soc. Probs. 635, 651, 656, 657 (1997).

Journal 1996 Discusses the trend toward conserving resources expended on health care by withholding services absent a showing of necessity. Claims that the high standard of care physicians owe patients is jeopardized by medical treatment decisions based on coverage concerns. Concludes that the legal structure regarding health care plans should be changed. Quotes Preamble, Principles I, II, III, IV, V, VI, and VII, and Opinion 2.03. Hirshfeld & Thomason, *Medical Necessity Determinations: The Need for a New Legal Structure*, 6 Health Matrix 3, 8-9 (1996).

Journal 1995 Offers relevant historical perspectives and provides comprehensive ethical and legal discussion of physician-assisted suicide and euthanasia. Highlights important legislative developments, including the Oregon Death with Dignity Act, and analyzes significant judicial opinions. Quotes Principles III, IV, and VI and Opinions 2.21 and 9.12. Cites Opinions 2.20 and 8.11. Stone & Winslade, *Physician-Assisted Suicide and Euthanasia in the United States: Legal and Ethical Observations*, 16 J. Legal Med. 481, 483, 490, 497, 498, 499 (1995).

Journal 1994 Explores the ethical issues involved in a multidisciplinary team working with children in legal proceedings. Focuses on the relationships between professionals and the conflicts that arise regarding disclosure of confidential information and forced disclosure of nonprivileged information. Quotes Principles III and IV, Fundamental Elements (4), and Opinions 1.02 (1992) and 5.07 (1992) [now Opinion 5.05]. Cites Opinion 2.02. Glynn, *Multidisciplinary Representation of Children: Conflicts Over Disclosures of Client Communications, 27 J. Marshall L. Rev. 617, 625, 626, 630-32, 637, 639, 643 (1994).*

Journal 1994 Argues that physician aid-in-dying should be protected by the US Constitution and that patients should have a federal cause of action to challenge prohibitive state statutes. Considers how such a cause of action might affect public policy. Quotes Principles I and III. References Opinion 2.06. Note, *Toward a More Perfect Union: A Federal Cause of Action for Physician Aid-In-Dying, 27 U. Mich. J. L. Ref. 521, 538 (1994).*

Journal 1994 Reviews the evolution of the physician-patient relationship, with attention to patient autonomy. Examines the changing health care delivery environment. Quotes Preamble, Principles I, II, III, IV, V, and VI, Fundamental Elements (1) and (2), and Opinions 1.02 and 8.07 (1981) [now Opinion 8.08]. Cites Opinion 1.01. Szczygiel, *Beyond Informed Consent, 21 Ohio N. U. L. Rev. 171, 217, 218, 220, 225, 226, 256 (1994).*

Journal 1993 Discusses physicians' duty to disclose to patients medical treatment alternatives that are not readily available. Proposes that based on the historical development and legal requirements of the informed consent doctrine, physicians should be required to inform patients of non–readily available alternatives or face liability for breach of such obligation. Quotes Principles I, II, III, IV, and V and Opinion 8.08. Note, *Informed Choice: Physicians' Duty to Disclose Nonreadily Available Alternatives, 43 Case W. Res. L. Rev. 491, 491, 498-99, 508, 509 (1993).*

Journal 1991 Examines the wisdom and likely results of medicalizing psychoactive drugs of abuse. Concludes that although many physicians would consider prescribing psychoactive drugs of abuse for drug abusers in order to end dependence, few would be willing to prescribe such drugs for recreational purposes. Quotes Principle III. Levine, *Medicalization of Psychoactive Substance Use and the Doctor-Patient Relationship, 69 Milbank Quarterly 623, 624 (1991).*

Journal 1990 Discusses the moral dilemma in deciding whether to withdraw artificial nutrition and hydration from a patient and the appropriate role of the judiciary. Concludes that judicial decisions do not represent the moral viewpoint of society and that moral pronouncements should not be made in the courtroom. Quotes Preamble, Principles I, II, III, IV, V, VI, and VII, and Opinion 2.20. Peccarelli, *A Moral Dilemma: The Role of Judicial Intervention in Withholding or Withdrawing Nutrition and Hydration, 23 John Marshall L. Rev. 537, 539, 540, 541 (1990).*

IV.   A physician shall respect the rights of patients, colleagues, and other health professionals, and shall safeguard patient confidences and privacy within the constraints of the law.

10th Cir. 2001 Plaintiffs, former employees of a public medical center, brought suit against medical director under 42 USC § 1983, based upon medical director's racially and sexually harassing actions and statements. The district court awarded compensatory and punitive damages against the medical director. Affirming the award of damages, the court quoted Principles I and IV and concluded that the medical director's behavior impacted not only plaintiffs, but the overall public health. *Nieto v. Kapoor, 268 F.3d 1208, 1223 n. 12.*

D. Kan. 1991 With apparent reliance on Principle IV and Opinion 5.05, plaintiff claimed that other than in discovery or judicial proceedings, the physician-patient privilege is absolute and precludes ex parte communications with defense counsel. While recognizing the confidential nature of the physician-patient relationship, the court held that the ethical standards promulgated by the AMA are not binding law and that, where a litigant-patient has placed his or her medical status in issue, the physician is released from the constraints imposed by the physician-patient relationship for the purposes of the litigation. *Bryant v. Hilst, 136 F.R.D. 487, 490.*

E.D. La. 2005 Plaintiff filed a motion to modify the district court's order requiring five days' notice to opposing counsel before interviewing plaintiff's prescribing physician. The court quoted Opinion 5.05 and cited Principle IV when discussing the physician-patient relationship and the physician's duty to protect confidences revealed by a patient. The court granted the plaintiff's motion and modified the order to ensure that defendants were faced with the same restrictions as the plaintiff and that plaintiff could conduct ex parte interviews with physicians not named as defendants. *In re Vioxx Products Liability Litigation, 230 F.R.D. 473, 476 n. 17.*

N.D. Ohio 1965 Plaintiff-patient alleged that the defendant-malpractice insurer induced physician to reveal confidential information about plaintiff on pretext that plaintiff filed a malpractice suit. In denying defendant's motion for reconsideration of the court's earlier opinion, the court confirmed its holding that actions of a third party inducing a physician to divulge confidential information may result in liability to the patient. In so holding, the court quoted (with incorrect citation to Ch. II, Sec.1) Principles Ch. I, Sec.2 (1912), [now Principle IV and Opinion 5.08], to emphasize the medical profession's established views regarding confidentiality. *Hammonds v. Aetna Casualty & Sur. Co., 243 F. Supp. 793, 803.*

M.D. Pa. 1987 Plaintiff in a medical malpractice action sought to preclude his treating physicians from serving as defendant's expert witnesses at trial. The court held that defense counsel's failure to provide prior notice of ex parte communication with plaintiff's treating physicians barred their use as defense experts. Referring to *Petrillo v. Syntex Laboratories, Inc.,* 148 Ill. App. 3d 581, 499 N.E.2d 952 (1986), the court noted that the court there favorably cited Principle IV and Opinions 5.05, 5.06, and 5.07 (1984) in support of a public policy protecting confidentiality between physician and patient and against ex parte discussion. *Manion v. N.P.W. Medical Ctr. of N.E. Pa., Inc., 676 F.Supp. 585, 591.*

Ala. 1973 Physician revealed patient information to the patient's employer, contrary to instructions of patient. Patient sued for breach of fiduciary duty. Citing Principle 9 (1957) [now Principle IV and Opinion 5.05], as well as cases from other states, the court held that even in the absence of a testimonial privilege statute, as a matter of public policy, a physician has a fiduciary duty not to make extrajudicial disclosures of patient information acquired in the course of treatment unless the public interest or the private interest of the patient demands otherwise. In holding that the physician had breached his contract with patient, the court found the Principles together with state licensing requirements sufficient to establish the public policy of confidentiality. *Horne v. Patton, 291 Ala. 701, 287 So. 2d 824, 829, 832.*

Alaska 1977 Physician–school board member failed to fully comply with state's conflict of interest law by refusing to reveal the names of patients from whom he had received over $100 in income. The physician claimed a legal privilege or ethical duty not to disclose the information under Principle 9 (1957) [now Principle IV and Opinion 5.05] and, alternatively, that the conflict of interest law unconstitutionally invaded a patient's right to privacy. The court held that disclosure was not barred by a legal privilege or ethical mandate, but that the conflict of interest law unconstitutionally invaded patient privacy due to the absence of protective regulations. In ruling on the ethical duty issue, the court noted that under Alaska law, a physician's license may be revoked for violating the Principles. However, the court found this licensing provision irrelevant to the privileged relationship exception in the conflict of interest law. The court found that otherwise the privilege exception in the statute could be changed by the AMA, a private organization, simply by amending the Principles. *Falcon v. Alaska Pub. Offices Comm'n, 570 P.2d 469, 474 n.13.*

Ariz. App. 1992 Employer argued that workers' compensation statute abrogated the physician-patient privilege statute, permitting ex parte communications with employee's treating physician. Recognizing that a physician is ethically bound to protect the confidentiality of privileged information pursuant to Principle IV, yet lacks the legal training to distinguish between privileged and unprivileged information, the court held that a claimant has the right to insist that his attorney be present when his employer interviews the employee's physician. *Salt River Project v. Industrial Comm'n, 1992 Ariz. App. LEXIS 323, 129 Ariz. Adv. Rep. 39.*

Ariz. App. 1989 In a medical malpractice action, defense counsel interviewed several of plaintiff's treating physicians ex parte and notified plaintiff of this in preparation for a medical liability review panel hearing. Plaintiff moved to bar all testimony by those physicians and to disqualify defense counsel from representing defendants. The appellate court noted a physician's obligation of confidentiality pursuant to Principle IV and Opinion 5.05 and held that defense counsel in a medical malpractice action may not engage in nonconsensual ex parte communications with plaintiff's treating physicians. *Duquette v. Superior Court, 161 Ariz. 269, 778 P.2d 634, 641.*

Cal. 1976 Parents sued psychotherapists to recover for murder of daughter by psychiatric patient, alleging that failure to warn victim of patient's violent threat was a proximate cause of her death. In considering whether such a revelation would have been a violation of professional ethics, the Court noted that Principle 9 (1957) [now Principle IV and Opinion 5.05] recognized that the confidential nature of a physician-patient communication must yield when disclosure is necessary to protect an individual or community as a whole. The court concluded that, in the circumstances of this case, disclosure would not have violated medical ethics and held that psychotherapists are under a duty to warn when they determine or should determine that a patient poses a serious danger of violence to someone else. *Tarasoff v. Regents of Univ. of Cal.*, 17 Cal.3d 425, 551 P.2d 334, 347, 131 Cal. Rptr. 14, 27.

Cal. 1970 Psychiatrist-witness in civil assault case applied for writ of habeas corpus after being held in contempt of court for refusing to produce patient's psychiatric records. Patient, plaintiff in the assault action, neither expressly claimed nor waived the statutory psychotherapist-patient privilege. The court held that the litigant-patient exception to the statutory psychotherapist-patient privilege does not unconstitutionally infringe rights of privacy of either psychotherapists or their patients. The court noted that in such a context a psychiatrist does not violate Principle 9 (1957) [now Principle IV and Opinion 5.05] since the Principle allows for legally compelled disclosure. *In re Lifschutz*, 2 Cal. 3d 415, 467 P.2d 557, 565-66 n.9, 85 Cal. Rptr. 829, 837-38 n.9.

Cal. App. 1982 Defendant was convicted of lewd act with a child and child molestation or annoyance, after licensed clinical psychologist reported defendant's admission of sexual conduct to authorities. The court held that the psychologist's testimony was properly admitted since a statute requiring the reporting of actual or suspected child abuse expressly made the psychotherapist-patient privilege inapplicable. The court quoted Principle 9 (1957) [now Principle IV and Opinions 2.02 and 5.05] in concluding the disclosure was not a breach of professional ethics. *People v. Stritzinger*, 137 Cal. App. 3d 126, 186 Cal. Rptr. 750, 752 rev'd, 34 Cal.3d 505, 668 P.2d 738, 194 Cal. Rptr. 431 (1983).

Colo. 1989 Spouse of police officer killed by released psychiatric patient sued state mental hospital and psychiatrist for negligence. Patient had blamed police for his misfortunes during repeated involuntary commitments for paranoid schizophrenia, and psychiatrist knew that patient would have access to a gun after release. The court held that a psychiatrist owed a duty of care in determining whether patient had propensity for violence and posed unreasonable risk of serious bodily harm to others. In so holding, the court cited Principle 9 (1957) [now Principle IV and Opinion 5.05], in support of the view that there are situations in which the need to protect an individual or the community from the threat of harm from a patient may outweigh the strong policy in favor of nondisclosure of patient confidences. *Perreira v. State*, 768 P.2d 1198, 1210 n.7.

Del. Super. 1993 Plaintiff-patient brought action for invasion of privacy, breach of confidentiality, and breach of implied contract against defendants, a physician and nurse. Plaintiff alleged that defendant-nurse, without plaintiff's consent, informed plaintiff's mother and grandmother that she was pregnant. Plaintiff also alleged that defendant-physician was liable for the nurse's conduct based on respondeat superior. The defendants questioned whether plaintiff had stated a cause of action and, if so, whether the cause should be treated as a medical malpractice action. Quoting Principle IV and noting that the legislature and the courts had recognized the duty of confidentiality, the court held that plaintiff had a cause of action for breach of confidentiality. *Martin v. Baehler*, 1993 WL 258843, 3.

D.C. App. 2005 Appellant widow filed suit against appellee hospital for negligence in relation to her husband's suicide after his release from hospital. The district court granted appellee's motion for summary judgment, finding that patient suicide occurring six hours after release was not foreseeable. The appellate court affirmed. In the dissenting opinion, Principle IV is quoted to support the position that the hospital, although the information was confidential, should have told appellant of her husband's suicidal tendencies because of the risk he posed to himself. *Garby v. George Washington University Hosp.*, 886 A.2d 510, 526.

D.C. App. 1985 Patient sued plastic surgeon for breach of confidential physician-patient relationship following surgeon's use of before and after photographs of her plastic surgery in a department store presentation. In considering whether such a breach was an actionable tort, the court made reference to an earlier case quoting Principles Ch. II, Sec. 2 (1947) [erroneously cited in the earlier case as Ch. II, Sec. 1 (1943)] [now Principle IV and Opinion 5.05] as evidence of the strong public policy which exists in favor of maintaining a patient's confidences. *Vassiliades v. Garfinckel's, Brooks Bros.*, 492 A.2d 580, 590, 591.

Fla. App. 1995 The court considered the issue of the effect of § 455.241(2) of the Florida Statutes on right of defense in a medical malpractice action to engage in ex parte communications with plaintiff's nonparty treating physician. The court held that a 1988 amendment to § 455.241(2) negated the applicability of the statute to medical malpractice cases. The dissent, citing *Petrillo v. Syntex Laboratories, Inc.*, 148 Ill. App. 3d 581, 499 N.E.2d 952 (1986), quoted Principles II and IV and Opinions 5.05, 5.06, and 5.08 as strong public policy support for its position that ex parte communications should be barred altogether. *Castillo-Plaza v. Green*, 655 So. 2d 197, 206 n.4.

Ill. 1997 Trial court held various statutory sections, including those permitting unlimited disclosure of a patient's medical records, unconstitutional. On appeal, state Supreme Court affirmed. Regarding provisions mandating consent to the disclosure of medical records, the court noted, with reference to Principle IV and Opinion 5.05, the crucial importance of confidentiality in the physician-patient relationship. *Best v. Taylor Machine Works*, 179 Ill. 2d 367, 689 N.E. 2d 1057, 1099.

Ill. 1997 Plaintiffs brought action for medical malpractice and loss of consortium against physicians. Defendants sought the release of medical information according to a statute providing for unlimited access to a plaintiff's medical records. The trial court found this provision unconstitutional as a violation of separation of powers and of patients' privacy rights. On appeal, the court agreed that the statute violated separation of powers. Further, with apparent reference to Principle IV, the court noted the ethical duty of physicians to maintain patient confidentiality. The court, in turn, held that the statute violated the right to privacy, as patients hold confidentiality of personal medical information to be an integral part of privacy interests. *Kunkel v. Walton*, 179 Ill. 2d 519, 689 N.E. 2d 1047, 1055.

Ill. App. 1987 In appeal of malpractice action, an issue was whether expert testimony of plaintiff's treating physician, based upon discussions with the defense counsel without patient's consent, was admissible. The court held that ex parte communications between a plaintiff's treating physician and legal adversary violated public policy. In determining the existence of such a policy favoring the sanctity of the doctor-patient relationship, the court noted *Petrillo v. Syntex Laboratories Inc.*, 148 Ill. App. 3d 581, 499 N.E.2d 952 (1st Dist. 1986) and its reference to the Principles and Opinions, namely Principle IV and Opinion 5.05 (1984), which establish an ethical obligation to keep physician-patient communications confidential, generally requiring a patient's consent before information is released. *Yates v. El-Deiry*, 160 Ill. App. 3d 198, 513 N.E.2d 519, 522.

Ill. App. 1986 Defense attorney in product liability suit was held in contempt of court for conducting ex parte discussions with plaintiff-patient's treating physician without patient's consent and contrary to authorized methods of discovery. The court held that the strong public policy favoring physician-patient confidentiality articulated in Principles II and IV and Opinions 5.05, 5.06, 5.07, and 5.08 (1984) justified a rule against such ex parte discussions. Further, the court held that the public has the right to rely on physicians to faithfully execute their ethical obligations. *Petrillo v. Syntex Laboratories, Inc.*, 148 Ill. App. 3d 581, 499 N.E.2d 952, 957, 958, 959 cert. denied, 483 US 1007 (1987).

Ill. App. 1979 Patient filed suit against physician for breach of contract and breach of confidential relationship after physician's employee disclosed patient's name to police. Patient alleged that implied contract arose out of a statutory physician-patient privilege, and provisions of the Canons of Medical Ethics, with apparent reference to Principle 9 (1957) [now Principle IV and Opinion 5.05]. The court held that disclosure of patient's name alone by a physician or the physician's agents is insufficient to state a cause of action in contract and does not violate the physician-patient privilege. *Geisberger v. Willuhn*, 72 Ill. App. 3d 435, 390 N.E.2d 945, 946, 948.

Ind. App. 1996 A patient filed suit against a mental health counseling center for disclosing to a third party death threats made by the patient during therapy. The patient claimed this was a breach of the standard of care owed to her. The trial court found that the counseling center was not statutorily prohibited from disclosing death threats the patient made. On appeal, the court affirmed the decision. It noted, with apparent reference to Principle IV and Opinion 5.05, that physicians may disclose confidential information to ensure the safety of the public or of individuals. In clarifying its holding, the court observed that while free and frank communication should be promoted to aid proper diagnosis and treatment, public policy supports disclosure of confidential information when appropriate. *Rocca v. Southern Hills Counseling Center, Inc.*, 671 N.E. 2d 913, 916.

Me. 1999 Physician appealed decision of the Board of Licensure in Medicine imposing a civil penalty for his failure to release medical records to patient's physicians. Physician argued that the Board did not specify the ethical standards that his conduct violated. The court vacated the Board's decision on the grounds that the physician was denied the opportunity to refute evidence of a violation of professional standards or to develop a defense predicated on those standards. The Board, in defense of its decision, presented Opinions 7.01 and 7.02 to the court. The court, in vacating the decision, pointed out that the hearing record did not demonstrate which Opinions the Board applied. Furthermore, the court, quoting Principle IV, stated that the physician had a responsibility to protect the patient's medical records. *Balian v. Board of Licensure in Medicine, 722 A.2d 364, 368.*

Md. App. 2007 In an espionage case, a psychiatrist was engaged to evaluate defendant's competency. Defendant disclosed confidential information which the psychiatrist later disclosed to defendant's wife and the media. Defendant and his wife filed a complaint for breach of confidentiality with the State Board of Physicians which revoked the psychiatrist's medical license. On appeal, the psychiatrist denied any unprofessional conduct. The court, quoting Principle IV, found the psychiatrist's behavior was unethical and unprofessional. With apparent reference to Opinion 5.05, the psychiatrist argued there was an exception to the duty of confidentiality when disclosure would protect the "community interest." The court found no such "community interest" exception. *Salerian v. Maryland State Board of Physicians, 176 Md. App. 231, 932 A.2d 1225, 1235-36, 1241-42.*

Md. Att'y Gen. 1989 Except as required by statute, physicians are not legally obligated to report that an adult has been sexually assaulted. Quoting Principle IV regarding the safeguarding of patient confidences within the constraints of the law, the opinion concludes that a physician must consider the confidential nature of the physician-patient relationship when deciding whether to report that a patient has been sexually assaulted. *Maryland Att'y Gen. Op. No. 89-022.*

Md. Att'y Gen. 1986 State attorney general opined that statute authorized physicians to report to the Motor Vehicle Administration patients with certain disorders that would impair their ability to drive. The opinion cites Principle IV in support of the conclusion that, where required by law, a physician's disclosure of patient information is proper. *Maryland Att'y Gen. Op. No. 86-030 71 Op. Att'y. Gen. 407, 410.*

Md. Att'y Gen. 1977 Opinion addresses the obligation of a psychiatrist to report child abuse information obtained from a parent-patient. Referring to state statutes and to Principle 9 (1957) [now Principle IV and Opinions 2.02 and 5.05], the opinion concludes that the question of whether to disclose suspected child abuse is a matter left to the individual psychiatrist's professional and moral judgment. *Maryland Att'y. Gen. Opinion, 62 Op. Att'y Gen. 157, 160.*

Mass. 1989 Physician appealed after being disciplined for discussing anticipated deposition testimony with malpractice defendant's attorney one day prior to scheduled deposition. The court, referring to Principle IV, noted that the AMA's ethical standards did not specifically address situation presented. After weighing the fact that physician had specifically asked attorney whether discussion was appropriate, the court held that the physician's behavior did not constitute gross misconduct and thus he could not be disciplined under licensing statute. *Hellman v. Board of Registration in Medicine, 404 Mass. 800, 537 N.E.2d 150, 153 n.4.*

Mass. 1984 Employee sued employer for libel and invasion of privacy following disclosure of medical facts about employee to other employees. In part, claim involved disclosure of opinion about employee's mental state to his supervisor by physician retained by employer. Citing Principle 9 (1957) [now Principle IV and Opinions 5.05 and 5.09], the court held that a physician retained by an employer may disclose to the employer information concerning an employee if receipt of the information is reasonably necessary to serve a substantial and valid business interest of the employer. *Bratt v. Intn'l Business Mach. Corp., 392 Mass. 508, 467 N.E.2d 126, 137 n.23.*

Minn. 1976 Plaintiff-patient in malpractice action appealed trial court's order to provide authorization for private, informal interview between defense counsel and patient's treating physician. In holding that formal pretrial discovery provided the exclusive procedure by which defendant could obtain medical testimony, the court noted, without deciding the issue, that a physician who discloses confidential patient information in a private interview may be subject to tort liability for breach of patient's right to privacy or professional discipline for unprofessional conduct, citing Principle 9 (1957) [now Principle IV and Opinion 5.05]. *Wenninger v. Muesing, 240 N.W.2d 333, 337 n.3.*

Mo. 1998 Defendant convicted of first-degree murder claimed that a physician's testimony at trial violated Principle IV and the statutory physician-patient privilege because the physician contacted the press, provided interviews about his examination of defendant, and testified for the prosecution to rebut defendant's posttraumatic stress disorder defense. The court stated that the defendent waived any privilege and that it was not its place to enforce professional ethical standards. *State v. Johnson, 968 S.W.2d 123, 131.*

Mo. 1993 Patient sued physicians alleging a breach of fiduciary duty of confidentiality for participating in an unauthorized ex parte discussion with defendant's attorney. While recognizing this duty, the court held that, where the plaintiff's medical condition is in issue, this constitutes a waiver of both the testimonial privilege and the physician's fiduciary duty in so far as the information is related to the medical issues. Quoting Opinion 5.05 and citing Principle IV, the court stated that courts may apply ethical principles to frame the specific limits of the legal duty of confidentiality. *Brandt v. Medical Defense Assoc., 856 S.W.2d 667, 671 n.1.*

Mo. 1989 In a personal injury suit, plaintiff challenged trial court's authority to compel plaintiff to authorize ex parte meetings between defendant insurance company and plaintiff's treating physician. Applying a balancing test between preserving the physician-patient confidential and fiduciary relationship, the physician-patient testimonal privilege, and the quest for truth in civil litigation, the court held that such information could be obtained through the methods of formal discovery. The court quoted Principle IV and Opinion 5.05 (1984) as statements of the policy underlying medical confidentiality and a basis for a patient's affirmative right to rely on the confidential nature of disclosures to a treating physician. *State ex. rel. Woytus v. Ryan, 776 S.W.2d 389, 392-93.*

Mo. App. 1985 In a prohibition proceeding arising from a medical malpractice action, defense attorneys sought order compelling plaintiff to authorize a private interview between defense attorneys and physician who treated plaintiff for injuries allegedly caused by defendant-physician. The appellate court, after discussing Principle IV and Opinion 5.05 (1984), held that the defense attorneys had the right to seek an ex parte interview with the treating physician, subject to the willingness of the physician to grant the interview. Furthermore, the court noted that Opinion 5.05 prevents a physician from revealing a patient's confidences only where there is a lack of consent from the patient and found that consent did exist here in the form of a medical authorization executed by plaintiff during pendency of the malpractice action. *State ex rel. Stufflebam v. Appelquist, 694 S.W.2d 882, 886, 888 n.7, overruled by State ex. rel. Woytus v. Ryan, 776 S.W.2d 389 (Mo. 1989).*

N.J. 1985 Plaintiff provided authorization for release of decedent's medical records from former treating physicians but refused to consent to depositions or interviews between defense counsel and physicians. The court noted physicians' ethical duty to avoid unauthorized disclosure, as stated in Principle 9 (1957) [now Principle IV and Opinion 5.05], but recognized that a patient's right to confidentiality was not absolute. After balancing the competing interests involved, the court held that defense counsel had a right to seek ex parte interviews of decedent's other treating physicians regarding litigation matters, provided procedural safeguards were met including clear statements that participation in such an interview is voluntary on the part of a physician. *Stempler v. Speidell, 100 N.J. 368, 495 A.2d 857, 860, cert. denied, 483 US 1007 (1987).*

N.J. 1979 In wrongful death action against a psychiatrist whose patient murdered plaintiff's decedent, the court concluded, in accord with Principle 9 (1957) [now Principle IV], that a psychiatrist may owe a duty to warn potential victims of possible danger from psychiatrist's patient despite the general emphasis on confidentiality. The court also noted the Preamble and Principles 1 and 3 (1957) [now revised Preamble, Principle I, and Opinion 5.05] in discussing the psychiatrist-patient relationship. *McIntosh v. Milano, 168 N.J. Super. 466, 403 A.2d 500, 510, 512-13.*

N.J. 1962 Parents sued pediatrician for unauthorized disclosure to life insurer of deceased infant's congenital heart defect. The court quoted Principle 9 (1957) [now Principle IV and Opinion 5.05] as an articulation of a physician's legal duty to his or her patient subject to exceptions of compelling social or patient interests. The court held that the parents had lost their limited right to nondisclosure by filing an insurance claim. *Hague v. Williams, 37 N.J. 328, 181 A.2d 345, 347.*

N.J. Super. 2002 Patient brought suit against physician for releasing her medical records to opposing counsel in a divorce action without her authorization or consent. The lower court dismissed the complaint for failure to state a claim and ruled the records were discoverable. The New Jersey Superior Court reversed holding that the patient had a cause of action against both the physician and opposing counsel. Quotes Principle IV. *Crescenzo v. Crane, 350 N.J. Super. 531, 796 A.2d 283, 290.*

N.J. Super. 1991 Physician's estate sued hospital alleging that it violated state law against discrimination by restricting the physician's surgery privileges and requiring him to inform patients of his HIV-infected status before performing invasive procedures. The defendant hospital was also alleged to have breached its duty to maintain confidentiality of his seropositive diagnosis. The court held that the hospital had not discriminated against the physician since the hospital had relied on ethical and professional standards, including a report of the Council on Ethical and Judicial Affairs of the AMA dealing with the issue of AIDS [now Opinions 9.13 and 9.131]. However, the hospital was held to have breached its fiduciary duty to maintain the confidentiality of the physician's medical records. Referring to *McIntosh v. Milano,* 168 N.J. Super. 466, 403 A.2d 500 (1979) which had quoted AMA Principles of Medical Ethics sec. 9 (1957) [now Principle IV and Opinion 5.05] in applying the "duty to warn" exception, the court noted that the disclosure in this case went far beyond the medical personnel directly involved in the treatment of the physician and those patients entitled to informed consent. *Estate of Behringer v. Medical Ctr., 249 N.J. Super. 597, 614, 633, 592 A.2d 1251, 1259, 1268.*

N.J. Super. 1988 Several portions of state department of corrections regulations concerning exceptions to privileged communications between psychologist and inmates were invalidated by appellate court because they permitted disclosure of confidences that did not present clear and imminent danger to the inmate or others, or failed to identify any intended victim. Court made general reference (with erroneous quotation) to Principle 9 (1957) [now Principle IV and Opinion 5.05]. *In re Rules Adoption, 224 N.J. Super. 252, 540 A.2d 212, 215.*

N.J. Super. 1987 Defendant in a personal injury suit sought to offer testimony from plaintiff's treating physician regarding plaintiff's prognosis. The court denied plaintiff's motion to exclude that evidence, despite the ethical obligation of physicians to uphold patients' communications as confidential under Principle 9 (1957) [now Principle IV and Opinion 5.05]. The court's decision was based on New Jersey case law permitting disclosure of a patient's medical condition to someone having a legitimate interest where the physical condition of the patient is made an element of a claim. *Kurdek v. West Orange Bd. of Educ., 222 N.J. Super. 218, 536 A.2d 332, 335.*

N.J. Super. 1967 In a suit for separate maintenance, communications between plaintiff-wife and her psychiatrist were not protected from disclosure during depositions, despite Principle 9 (1957) [now Principle IV and Opinion 5.05] which prohibited physicians from disclosing patient confidences except where necessary to protect the welfare of the individual or of the community. The court concluded that the patient had only a limited right of nondisclosure, subject to exceptions created by supervening interest of society and that the institution of litigation by the patient constituted a vitiation of that right. *Ritt v. Ritt, 98 N.J. Super. 590, 238 A.2d 196, 199 rev'd, 52 N.J. 177, 244 A.2d 497 (1968).*

N.Y. Sup. 2000 Physician brought wrongful discharge claim against corporate employer. The physician alleged she was discharged because she refused to reveal confidential medical information regarding employees. With apparent reference to Principle IV and Opinions 5.05 and 5.09, the affidavit filed by the physician claimed she had an ethical and legal duty to protect patient confidentiality. The court found termination of an employee at will based upon such grounds is sufficient to state a cause of action for breach of contract. The court ruled that obligations of good faith and fair dealing may be implied in a contract for the employment of a physician and that no physician should be placed in the position of choosing between retaining employment and violating ethical standards. *Horn v. New York Times, 186 Misc. 2d 469, 719 N.Y.S. 2d 471, 474.*

N.Y. Sup. 1977 Plaintiff, a psychiatric patient, sued her psychiatrist and the psychiatrist's spouse for violating several state statutes and her privacy rights by publishing a book about the intimate details of plaintiff's psychotherapy. The court found for plaintiff, basing its decision in part upon Principle 9 (1957) [now Principle IV and Opinion 5.05] which requires a physician to uphold the confidences of a patient. *Doe v. Roe, 93 Misc. 2d 201, 400 N.Y.S.2d 668, 674.*

N.Y. Surr. 1977 In a discovery proceeding, respondent-psychiatrist, who had treated some patients of deceased psychiatrist subsequent to his death, allegedly misappropriated decedent's patient records. Estate petitioned court for return of records and damages for injury to value of decedent's practice. Respondent sought dismissal of claim arguing that estate could not sell patient records. The court rejected respondent's request. In so ruling, the court noted that under Principle 9 (1957) [now Principle IV and Opinion 5.05] prohibiting physicians from revealing patient confidences, various guidelines had been issued regarding sale of a medical practice [now Opinion 7.04]. Whether respondent's actions had interfered with the estate's efforts to dispose of decedent's practice in keeping with these guidelines presented the court with factual issues for later resolution. *Estate of Finkle, 90 Misc. 2d 550, 395 N.Y.S.2d 343, 346.*

N.C. 1990 Plaintiff in a malpractice case was granted an order prohibiting ex parte conferences between defendant's attorney and nonparty treating physicians. The court noted that both the Principles of Medical Ethics and Current Opinions affirm the physician's duty to protect patient confidentiality, in apparent reference to Principle IV and Opinion 5.05. In consideration of (1) the patient's right to privacy, (2) physician-patient confidentiality, (3) the adequacy of formal discovery procedures, and (4) the dilemma in which nonparty treating physicians are placed by ex parte conferences, the court held that an attorney may not interview a patient's nonparty treating physicians privately without express authorization. *Crist v. Moffatt, 326 N.C. 326, 333, 389 S.E.2d 41, 46.*

Ohio 2009 Physician appealed from a judgment affirming an order of the state medical board that permanently revoked appellant's certificate to practice medicine. The board found that appellant's sexual contact with patients violated Ohio statutes governing physician conduct and the AMA's Code of Medical Ethics, citing Principles I, II, IV, and VIII. The Court of Appeals held that Ohio state law allows the board to revoke a physician's certificate if it finds that the person violated any provision of the AMA's Code of Medical Ethics. *D'Souza v. State Med. Bd. of Ohio, 2009 WL 5108774, 6.*

Ohio 1999 Patients brought a class action suit against hospital on grounds that the hospital disclosed patients' confidential medical information to the hospital's law firm, in order to determine whether the patients were eligible for government benefits to pay for unpaid hospital bills. The trial court granted defendants' motion for summary judgment. On appeal, the court held that a physician or a hospital can be held liable for unauthorized out-of-court disclosure of patients' confidential information. In addition, the court found that an independent tort exists for unauthorized, unprivileged disclosure of patients' private medical information to a third party. The court cited Principle 9 (1957) [now Principle IV and Opinion 5.05], noting that courts have looked to such sources in providing a cause of action for breach of patient confidentiality. *Biddle v. Warren General Hospital, 86 Ohio St. 3d 395, 715 N.E.2d 518, 523.*

Ohio 1997 Estates of victims who were killed by their mentally ill son brought suit against son's psychotherapist for failing to disclose potential for violence. Son had been institutionalized and treated for schizophrenia. After release, he continued to take medication and see a psychotherapist. Despite parents' objections and attempts to have him involuntarily recommitted, psychotherapist reduced his medication and continued to recommend outpatient treatment. The court held that the psychotherapist had a duty to exercise reasonable care to control the son so as to prevent him from causing harm to his family. The court expressed concern for safeguarding the confidentiality of psychotherapeutic communications but noted that Principle 9 (1957) [now Principle IV and Opinion 5.05] has long allowed breaches of confidence when it becomes necessary to protect the welfare of the individual or the community. *Estates of Morgan v. Fairfield Family Counseling Center, 77 Ohio St. 3d 284, 303, 673 N.E.2d 1311, 1326.*

Ohio 1991 State medical board revoked license of physician who had consensual sexual relations with his patient. The court upheld the board's ruling that this violated Principles I, II, and IV. Dissenting judge, citing AMA Council on Ethical and Judicial Affairs, Sexual Misconduct in the Practice of Medicine, 266 JAMA 2741 [now Opinion 8.14], argued that until 1991, the AMA did not clearly deem sexual contact with a patient unethical. *Pons v. Ohio State Medical Bd., 66 Ohio St. 3d 619, 623, 625, 614 N.E.2d 748, 752, 753.*

Ohio 1988 Administrator sued psychiatrist for wrongful death after recently discharged patient killed her infant daughter. In determining whether a professional judgment rule should be adopted in the malpractice standard of care where the prediction of violent behavior is involved, the court referred favorably to Principle 9 (1957) [now Principle IV and Opinion 5.05] which allows breaches of patient confidences when necessary to protect potential victims. *Littleton v. Good Samaritan Hosp., 39 Ohio St. 3d 86, 529 N.E.2d 449, 459 n.19.*

Ohio App. 2005 The Ohio State Medical Board permanently revoked the license of the appellant, a psychiatrist, for having inappropriate physical and sexual contact with a female patient. The trial court affirmed the board's ruling, and the appellant appealed. The board claimed that the appellant's relationship with his patient violated the AMA's Code of Medical Ethics citing Principles I, II, and IV. The appellate court affirmed stating that permanent revocation of the appellant's license was not excessive and was not a violation of due process as the board may revoke the appellant's license if treatment did not meet minimal standards of care and violated any provision of the AMA's Code of Medical Ethics. *Schechter v. Ohio State Med. Bd., 2005 WL 1869733, 9.*

Ohio App. 1999 Physician appealed trial court's affirmation of state medical board's decision to suspend his medical license because the physician engaged in sexual relationships with mothers of his pediatric patients. On appeal, the physician claimed that he was denied due process because physicians were not adequately notified that having sexual relations with parents of pediatric patients was unethical. The physician also claimed that the board had not presented adequate evidence that AMA's Code of Medical Ethics, Principles I and IV extend to the parents of pediatric patients. The court quoted Principles I and IV, and stated that medical experts who testified were of the opinion that having sexual relationships with parents of pediatric patients constituted ethical violations. *Gladieux v. Ohio State Medical Board, 1999 WL 770959, *2, *4.*

Okla. 1988 In response to a police request, physician reported patient treated for a penile bite. Patient sued physician for negligence after information furnished by physician led to patient's arrest and conviction for rape. Patient alleged a tortious breach of the physician-patient confidential relationship, breach of contract, violation of licensing statute, and breach of Principle 9 (1957) [now Principle IV and Opinion 5.05]. The court reasoned that the benefit of the divulgence inured to the public at large and thus fell within the public policy exception to the testimonial privilege, created no liability in tort or contract, and was not a breach of medical ethics under the licensing statute or the Principles. *Bryson v. Tillinghast, 749 P.2d 110, 113, 114.*

Pa. 1973 Plaintiff in personal injury suit resulting from auto accident claimed that trial court should have allowed showing on cross-examination that defendant's expert medical witness, who had treated plaintiff, violated Principle 9 (1957) [now Principle IV and Opinion 5.05] by ex parte communications with defense counsel, in order to impeach his medical testimony. The court held that any connection between an alleged breach of medical ethics and the credibility of a physician on the witness stand was tenuous. Therefore, the trial court's decision barring further inquiry in this regard was proper. *Downey v. Weston, 451 Pa. 259, 301 A.2d 635, 638.*

Pa. Super. 1988 Plaintiff-patient sued her physician for breach of confidentiality when physician conferred with defense counsel in plaintiff's malpractice suit against the hospital (physician's employer). In its majority opinion, the court cited Principle IV, commenting that it gave very little guidance to physicians but nonetheless was not violated by the physician. The court also noted Opinion 5.07 (1986) finding that the plaintiff's suit minimized her expectations of confidentiality. The dissent, however, interpreted these same provisions, along with Opinion 5.05 (1986), as protecting plaintiff's expectations of confidentiality. *Moses v. McWilliams, 379 Pa. Super. 150, 549 A.2d 950, 956, 962 (dissent), appeal denied, 521 Pa. 630, 558 A.2d 532 (1989).*

S.C. 2003 Worker's Compensation Commission ordered injured employee's attorney to stop obstructing ex parte contacts between rehabilitative nurse hired by employer and treating physicians regarding employee's medical condition. The South Carolina Supreme Court reversed and held that the Worker's Compensation Act did not authorize such ex parte communication. Quotes Principle IV. *Brown v. Bi-Lo, Inc, 354 S.C. 436, 581 S.E.2d 836, 840, n. 5.*

S.C. App. 1997 Patient sued physician for breaching duty of confidentiality after physician divulged patient's emotional health status in a letter which was introduced during patient's divorce proceeding. The trial court dismissed the action for failure to state a cause of action, finding state law did not support a duty of confidentiality. The appeals court reversed. In part, it found a basis for such an action in medical and ethical principles, with apparent reference to Principle IV. Absent a compelling public interest in disclosure, confidences must be preserved. The court remanded to consider whether the disclosure was essential to the best interests of the patient or others. *McCormick v. England, 328 S.C. 627, 494 S.E. 2d 431, 435.*

Tenn. App. 1994 Plaintiff sought damages for wrongful death from defendant-surgeon. Defendant requested that the court require plaintiff to sign a form authorizing release of medical records and information to defense counsel. Trial court denied defendant's motion noting, with apparent reference to Principle IV and Opinion 5.05, that confidential relationship exists between physician and patient. Appellate court affirmed although it did not reach the ethical issue of the propriety of disclosures by a physician. *Wright v. Wasudev, 1994 Tenn. App. LEXIS 657.*

Utah Att'y Gen. 1978 A physician who, acting in good faith, discloses confidential information to proper authorities concerning a patient's unfitness to drive is not liable for doing so. Reference is made to Principle 9 (1957) [now Principle IV and Opinion 5.05] to support propriety of such disclosure where the public interest is involved. *Utah Att'y Gen. Op. No. 77-294.*

Wash. 1988 Personal representative brought wrongful death action against decedent's physicians. At issue was whether defense counsel in a personal injury action may communicate ex parte with plaintiff's treating physician where plaintiff has waived the physician-patient relationship. In holding that defense counsel may not engage in ex parte communication, and is limited to formal discovery methods, the court cited Principle IV and Opinion 5.05 (1986) with approval, reasoning that the mere threat of disclosure of private conversations between a physician and defense counsel would chill the physician-patient relationship and hinder further treatment. *Loudon v. Mhyre, 110 Wash. 2d 675, 756 P.2d 138, 141, 141 n.3.*

Wash. App. 2000 Patient sued a physician under medical malpractice statute, seeking damages for emotional distress resulting from the physician's disclosure of confidential information to the patient's ex-husband. Trial court granted the defendant's motion for summary judgment. On appeal, the court held that a tort action did exist under the statute for damages resulting from the unauthorized disclosure of confidential information related to health care obtained within the physician-patient relationship. The court quoted Principle IV, stating that the accepted standard of care includes a duty to maintain confidentiality with respect to patient information. *Berger v. Sonneland, 101 Wash. App. 141, 1 P.3d 1187, 1192.*

W. Va. 1993 Plaintiff, in a malpractice action, sought a writ of prohibition to prevent the enforcement of a trial court order allowing ex parte interviews. The court, in granting the writ, held that any benefit from ex parte interviews that occurs is minimal compared to the danger that they will undermine the confidential nature of the physician-patient relationship. Quoting Principles of Medical Ethics Ch. II, sec. 1 (1943) [now Principle IV and Opinion 5.05], the court noted that the medical profession is well aware of the importance of patient confidentiality. *State ex. rel. Kitzmiller v. Henning, 437 S.E.2d 452, 454.*

W. Va. 1988 Patient-wife sued psychiatrist who disclosed subpoenaed confidential information to her husband's attorney in divorce proceedings. The court held that a tort action lies when confidential communications regarding mental health patients are released, except under limited circumstances such as a binding court order. The court, however, declined to recognize an enforceable contractual right to confidentiality, although it noted that some states have recognized such a right based upon Principle IV. *Allen v. Smith, 368 S.E.2d 924, 928.*

Wis. 1995 In medical malpractice suit, the court held that (1) subject to restrictions, defense counsel may engage in ex parte communications with plaintiff's treating physician if the communications do not involve disclosure of confidential information; (2) outside a judicial proceeding, defendant-physician may communicate ex parte with plaintiff's treating physician subject to a physician's duty of confidentiality; and (3) if defense counsel elicits confidential information from a treating physician during ex parte communications, the appropriate sanction is within the discretion of the court. The court expressly overruled *State ex rel. Klieger v. Alby,* 125 Wis. 2d 468, 373 N.W.2d 57 (Ct. App. 1985) and the cases applying it. The majority and concurring opinions referred to Principle IV and Opinion 5.05. *Steinberg v. Jensen, 194 Wis. 2d 440, 534 N.W.2d 361, 370, 377.*

Wis. App. 1994 In medical malpractice suit, defense counsel engaged in ex parte communications with plaintiff's consulting physicians. Plaintiff amended her complaint seeking punitive damages for breach of confidentiality. The court concluded that the rule of *State ex rel. Klieger v. Alby,* 125 Wis. 2d 468, 373 N.W.2d 57 (Ct. App. 1985), which prohibits ex parte communications that have the potential to breach physician-patient confidentiality, was violated and sanctions were required. The court referred to *Petrillo v. Syntax Labs., Inc.,* 148 Ill. App. 3d 581, 499 N.E.2d 952 (1986) and its use of Principle IV and Opinion 5.05. *Steinberg v. Jensen, 186 Wis. 2d 237, 519 N.W.2d 753, 761 n.9, rev'd, 194 Wis. 2d 440, 534 N.W.2d 361 (1995).*

Wis. Att'y Gen. 1987 Physicians may report cases of suspected child abuse or neglect when a patient discloses that he or she has abused a child in some manner. Where report is made in good faith, physicians are immune from any civil or criminal liability. Passing reference is made to Principle 9 (1957) [now Principle IV and Opinions 2.02 and 5.05] in support of this position. *Wisconsin Att'y Gen. Op. 10-87 (Mar. 16, 1987) (LEXIS, States library, Wis. file).*

Journal 2010 Examines published resources within the medical and legal fields that focus on confidentiality and evaluates those resources to determine if they help clarify confidentiality issues. Further, discusses differences between these professions that may be hindrances when serving the same patient or client. Concludes that, while both professions guard against disclosure of patient/client communications, they also allow for disclosure in certain instances such as imminent death, harm, or injury. References Principle IV and cites Opinions 2.02, 2.23, 2.24, and 5.05. Johns, *Multidisciplinary Practice and Ethics Part II—Lawyers, Doctors, and Confidentiality*, 6 *NAELA J*. 55, 57-65, 68 (2010).

Journal 2010 Discusses the effects of using deidentified health information on privacy and considers the dangers of nonconsensual use of health information. Concludes deidentification of health information is a necessary though insufficient protection of privacy, and further research and regulations should be developed to demonstrate respect for individuals without unduly burdening research. Quotes Principle IV and Opinions 5.05 and 7.025. Rothstein, *Is Deidentification Sufficient to Protect Health Privacy in Research?* 10 *Am. J. Bioethics* 3, 5 (Sept. 2010).

Journal 2010 Analyzes factors contributing to the emergence of medical repatriation and evaluates whether this practice comports with current legal and ethical standards. Proposes changes to federal regulations that govern hospitals and clarifications to medical ethical standards. Quotes the Preamble and Principles I, II, III, IV, V, VI, VII, VIII, and IX. Zoellner, *Medical Repatriation: Examining the Legal and Ethical Implications of an Emerging Practice*, 32 *Wash. U. J. L. & Pol'y* 515, 530-532 (2010).

Journal 2009 Explores the history of the debate over when lawyers may or must disclose client confidences. Concludes a lawyer's duty to keep client confidences involves a philosophical question of the lawyer's role in society. Quotes Principle 9 (1957) [now Principle IV]. Ariens, *"Playing Chicken": An Instant History of the Battle Over Exceptions to Client Confidences*, 33 *J. Legal Prof*. 239, 255 (2009).

Journal 2009 Discusses the interaction between statutes and case law governing the medical field and the core principles of medical professionalism. Concludes the legal framework of medical professionalism does not encompass all the elements required of a medical professional. Quotes Principles II, III, IV, V, VI, VII, and VIII. Fichter, *The Law of Doctoring: A Study of the Codification of Medical Professionalism*, 19 *Health Matrix* 317, 338, 339, 340, 343, 351 (2009).

Journal 2009 Discusses whether or not patients have a right to pain management. Concludes that no physician duty is established by law or ethics to provide pain management outside the traditional physician-patient relationship. Cites Principles I, II, IV, and VIII. Hall & Boswell, *Ethics, Law, and Pain Management as a Patient Right*, 12 *Pain Physician* 499, 500 (2009).

Journal 2009 Discusses the judicial standard for reviewing physician noncompete covenants. Concludes courts should apply a strict standard to such covenants, rather than declare the covenants per se invalid. Quotes Principles IV and VII, Principles of Medical Ethics §5 (1957) [now Principle VI], Code of Medical Ethics Ch. II, Art. I §3 (1847) [now Opinion 5.02], Opinion 9.02, and Code of Medical Ethics Ch. II, Art. I §4 (1847) [now Opinion 9.09]. Cites Opinions 8.041, 8.115, 9.02, 9.06, 9.065, 9.067, 10.01, and 10.015. Koons, *Physician Employee Non-Compete Agreements on the Examining Table: The Need to Better Protect Patients' and the Public's Interests in Indiana*, 6 *Ind. Health L. Rev*. 253, 272-77, 280-81 (2009).

Journal 2009 Examines genetic discrimination, the Genetic Information Nondiscrimination Act, and the social fairness ideas behind its categorical protections for genetic information. Concludes genetic antidiscrimination acts based on broad categorical protections may be misguided. Cites Code of Ethics of the AMA § 8 (1848) [now Principle IV]. Morrow, *Insuring Fairness: The Popular Creation of Genetic Antidiscrimination*, 98 *Geo. L. J*. 215, 237 (2009).

Journal 2009 Examines a new Internal Revenue Service program for "whistleblower awards" given to informants who identify noncompliant taxpayers. Concludes that while whistleblowers may be useful for discovering noncompliance, Congress should prohibit awards given to those who breach confidential relationships. Quotes Principle IV. Morse, *Whistleblowers and Tax Enforcement: Using Inside Information to Close the "Tax Gap,"* 24 *Akron Tax J*. 1, 33 (2009).

Journal 2009 Examines Health Information Portability and Accountability Act (HIPAA) and the common law doctrine of informed consent with respect to electronic health record programs and the duty to obtain informed consent before allowing use of electronic health record services. Concludes that in order to protect individual privacy, electronic health record service providers should obtain informed consent before allowing their users to post their medical histories. Cites Principle IV. Prasse, *Hippocrates Would Roll Over in His Grave: An Examination of Why Internet Health Care Programs Should Obtain Informed Consent From Their Users, 42 Creighton L. Rev. 733, 746 (2009).*

Journal 2009 Explores the process of an attorney advising a client to seek mental health treatment and how that recommendation impacts the attorney-client relationship. Concludes attorneys must be willing to advise clients to seek treatment if appropriate. Quotes Principle IV. Suzuki, *When Something Is Not Quite Right: Considerations for Advising a Client to Seek Mental Health Treatment, 6 Hastings Race & Poverty L. J. 209, 250 (2009).*

Journal 2008 Discusses ex parte interviews with a treating physician in discovery before and after the HIPAA Privacy Rule and the issues facing physicians contacted for such interviews. Concludes courts and attorneys should work together to allow for efficient discovery while protecting physicians. Quotes Principles IV and VIII and Opinions 5.05 and 10.01. Burnette & Morning, *HIPAA and Ex Parte Interviews—the Beginning of the End? 1 J. Health & Life Sci. L. 73, 100-01 (2008).*

Journal 2008 Argues a general physician-patient privilege is needed in West Virginia and outlines the manner in which the privilege could be adopted. Concludes that the privilege will allow physicians to maintain their fiduciary role, foster open communication between patient and physician, and encourage patients to freely seek medical treatment. Quotes Principle IV and Opinion 5.05. Johnson, *"I Will Not Divulge": How to Resolve the "Mass of Legal Confusion" Surrounding the Physician-Patient Relationship in West Virginia, 110 W. Va. L. Rev. 1231, 1247 (2008).*

Journal 2008 Examines the pattern of school shootings perpetuated by mentally unstable individuals, focusing on the shooter at Virginia Tech and the failings of the mental health system in that situation. Concludes schools and universities should implement new policies to protect the privacy of mental health records while ensuring a safe learning environment for all students. Quotes Principle IV. Muñoz, *Privacy at the Cost of Public Safety: Reevaluating Mental Health Laws in the Wake of the Virginia Tech Shootings, 18 S. Cal. Interdisc. L. J. 161, 172 (2008).*

Journal 2008 Examines the development of bioethics and environmental ethics, as well as laws promoting the role of bioethicists in decision making. Concludes environmental ethicists must convince legislatures of the role of environmental ethics in order to have a greater impact on decision making. Quotes Principles I, II, III, IV, V, VI, VII, VIII, and IX. Robertson, *Seeking a Seat at the Table: Has Law Left Environmental Ethics Behind as it Embraces Bioethics? 32 Wm. & Mary Envtl. L. & Pol'y Rev. 273, 307 (2008).*

Journal 2007 Reviews American Bar Association (ABA) Model Rule of Professional Conduct 3.6, governing the speech of attorneys while involved in trials, and analyzes how it applies distinctly to speech directed at judges, prosecutors, and the court system. Concludes that Rule 3.6 affords more protection to judges than to prosecutors or the court system. Quotes Principle IV. Hinkie, *Free Speech and Rule 3.6: How the Object of Attorney Speech Affects the Right to Make Public Criticism, 20 Geo. J. Legal Ethics 695, 695 (2007).*

Journal 2007 Discusses confidentiality privileges under the law. Concludes that the short story, "Mr. Prinzo's Breakthrough," is a valuable tool for teaching students about exceptions to confidentiality privileges. Quotes Principle IV. Moore, *Mr. Prinzo's Breakthrough and the Limits of Confidentiality, 51 St. Louis L. J. 1059, 1064 (2007).*

Journal 2007 Argues that issuance of apologies from physicians who commit medical errors will diminish the number of malpractice suits brought. Concludes that patients desire apologies in the case of medical errors and are less likely to sue when they are given. Cites Principles I, II, III, and IV and Opinion 8.12. Tabler, *Should Physicians Apologize for Medical Errors? 19 Health Lawyer 23, 23 (Jan. 2007).*

Journal 2006 Analyzes cases where a patient's right to refuse care conflicts with the physician's obligation to protect that patient's well-being. Concludes health care providers should seek a compromise that best promotes both patient autonomy and well-being. Quotes Principle IV and Ch. I, Art. II, Sec. 6 (May 1847) [now Opinion 10.01]. Carrese, *Refusal of Care: Patients' Well-being and Physicians' Ethical Obligations, 296 JAMA 691, 692, 693 (2006).*

Journal 2006 Explores conscience clause legislation relating to the dispensing of oral contraceptives. Concludes that such legislation must balance the interests of the patient and the health care provider. Cites Principles I, II, III, IV, V, VI, VII, VIII, and IX. Collins, *Conscience Clauses and Oral Contraceptives: Conscientious Objection or Calculated Obstruction?* 15 Ann. Health L. 37, 54 (2006).

Journal 2006 Analyzes the ethical and legal problems of confidentiality which arise in the context of genetic testing. Concludes that the disclosure of a patient's genetic disease to others is only allowable when the patient is a minor and the family has a right to know. Quotes Principle IV and references Principle 9 (1957) [now Principle IV and Opinion 5.05]. Denbo, *What Your Genes Know Affects Them: Should Patient Confidentiality Prevent Disclosure of Genetic Test Results to a Patient's Biological Relatives?* 43 Am. Bus. L. J. 561, 572, 577 (2006).

Journal 2006 Evaluates the influence that Justice Blackmun's experience at the Mayo Clinic had on his opinions related to medicine. Concludes that Blackmun's experience had less of an impact on his opinions than is traditionally assumed. Quotes Principle 9 (1957) [now Principle IV and Opinion 5.05]. Hunter, *Justice Blackmun, Abortion, and the Myth of Medical Independence,* 72 Brooklyn L. Rev. 147, 190-91 (2006).

Journal 2006 Examines a mental health professional's competing duties of confidentiality and reporting a patient's threats of violence. Suggests new legislation should clarify duty to report a threat. Quotes Preamble and Principles III, IV, and VIII. Cites Opinion 5.05. Mossman, *Critique of Pure Risk Assessment or, Kant Meets Tarasoff,* 75 U. Cin. L. Rev. 523, 579 (2006).

Journal 2006 Analyzes the privacy risks associated with introducing a system of electronic medical records. Concludes that cost and confidentiality concerns mandate that security must be built into the initial system. Cites Ch. I, Art. I, Sec. 2 (May 1847) [now Principle IV and Opinion 5.05]. Rothstein & Talbott, *Compelled Disclosure of Health Information: Protecting Against the Greatest Potential Threat to Privacy,* 295 JAMA 2882, 2883 (2006).

Journal 2006 Examines situations where physician-patient confidentiality may be breached to prevent violations of human rights. Suggests that new laws should be enacted to specify when a physician may testify about a violation of human rights. Quotes Principle IV and Opinion 5.05. Weissbrodt & Wilson, *Piercing the Confidentiality Veil: Physician Testimony in International Criminal Trials Against Perpetrators of Torture,* 15 Minn. J. Int'l L. 43, 68, 68-69 (2006).

Journal 2005 Discusses the current "market approach" regarding who controls personal genetic information. Concludes that, consistent with principles of individualism, American citizens should have the right to their own genetic information. Quotes Principle IV. Cole, *Authentic Democracy: Endowing Citizens With a Human Right in Their Genetic Information,* 33 Hofstra L. Rev. 1241, 1251 (2005).

Journal 2005 Examines issues surrounding tort reform proposals. Concludes that more can be done to correct the current tort system before moving toward a "one size fits all" approach. Quotes Principles I, II, III, IV, V, VI, VII, VIII, and IX. Messerly & Warwick, *Nowhere to Turn: A Glance at the Facts Behind the Supposed Need for Tort "Reform,"* 28 Hamline L. Rev. 489, 506 (2005).

Journal 2004 Argues that courts should put safeguards in place to protect the confidential relationship between at-risk children and health care professionals. Concludes that such protection may limit disclosure of private information in court proceedings, enhance the dignity of minors, and facilitate their well-being. Quotes Principle IV. Katner, *Confidentiality and Juvenile Mental Health Records in Dependency Proceedings,* 12 Wm. & Mary Bill of Rts. J. 511, 529 (2004).

Journal 2004 Argues that the privacy model rather than the property model is the most appropriate way to protect an individual's interest in genetic information. Concludes that privacy interests must nevertheless be balanced against other societal factors. References Principle IV and Opinion 5.05. Suter, *Disentangling Privacy From Property: Toward a Deeper Understanding of Genetic Privacy,* 72 Geo. Wash. L. Rev. 737, 787 (2004).

Journal 2003 Considers the legal, medical, and ethical issues of physician-patient confidentiality in disclosure of paternity. Concludes that a balancing test should be applied to making determinations regarding disclosure of paternity. Quotes Principles I, IV, and V and Opinions 1.02, 5.055, and 10.01. Cites Principle II and Opinion 5.05. Richards & Wolf, *Medical Confidentiality and Disclosure of Paternity,* 48 S. D. L. Rev. 409, 411, 412, 413 (2003).

Journal 2003 Uses public policy arguments to support a preponderance standard for medical license revocations in situations involving false testimony by a medical expert witness.

Concludes that medical licensing boards can more effectively protect the public by using a preponderance standard. Quotes Principles II, III, and IV and Opinions 1.02 and 9.07. Widmer, *South Dakota Should Follow Public Policy and Switch to the Preponderance Standard for Medical License Revocation After In Re the Medical License of Dr. Reuben Setliff, M.D., 48 S. D. L. Rev. 388, 396-97, 402 (2003).*

Journal 2002 Analyzes the expanded use of the Civil False Claims Act in prosecuting health care fraud. Concludes that, in enforcing the law, government must balance its promises to beneficiaries, health care providers, and the public. Quotes Principles I, II, and IV. Krause, *"Promises to Keep": Health Care Providers and the Civil False Claims Act, 23 Cardozo L. Rev. 1363, 1365 (2002).*

Journal 2002 Considers the dilemma of informed consent in the context of prescribing psychotropic medication to patients with mental illness and mental retardation. Recognizes the need for substituted decision-making in certain situations. Concludes that legislation would help address this issue. Quotes Preamble, Principles I, III, IV, VIII, and IX, and Opinion 8.08. O'Sullivan & Borcherding, *Informed Consent for Medication in Persons With Mental Retardation and Mental Illness, 12 Health Matrix 63, 75, 86, 87, 88 (2002).*

Journal 2002 Considers the ethical and legal issues regarding breach of confidentiality in situations where a patient is pregnant and uses teratogenic substances. Concludes that a breach of confidentiality causes damage to the physician-patient relationship. Quotes Principle IV and Opinion 10.01. Plambeck, *Divided Loyalties: Legal and Bioethical Considerations of Physician–Pregnant Patient Confidentiality and Prenatal Drug Abuse, 23 J. Legal Med. 1, 8, 25 (2002).*

Journal 2002 Analyzes the role of prognostication in physician-patient communication. Concludes that the patient-physician model of shared decision-making offers the best hope for reestablishing prognostication. Quotes Principles Ch. I, Art. I, Sec. 2 and 4 (1846) [now Principle IV and Opinions 8.12 and 10.01]. Cites Opinion 8.08. Rich, *Prognostication in Clinical Medicine: Prophecy or Professional Responsibility? 23 J. Legal Med. 297, 299, 318, 327 (2002).*

Journal 2002 Considers the case of *Ferguson v. City of Charleston.* Concludes that the Supreme Court's rationale in that case reflects insights from feminist legal theory. Quotes Opinion 10.01. Cites Principles II and IV. Taslitz, *A Feminist Fourth Amendment?: Consent, Care, Privacy, and Social Meaning in Ferguson v. City of Charleston, 9 Duke J. Gender L. & Pol'y 1, 18, 19 (2002).*

Journal 2001 Discusses issues surrounding the privacy of genetic information. Considers the social, ethical, and legal responses to problems that arise in this context. Concludes with a unique view of privacy that would protect the right of individuals not to know genetic information about themselves. Quotes Principle IV and Opinion 10.01. Laurie, *Challenging Medical-Legal Norms: The Role of Autonomy, Confidentiality, and Privacy in Protecting Individual and Familial Group Rights in Genetic Information, 22 J. Legal Med. 1, 24 (2001).*

Journal 2001 Considers ethical aspects of physician conflicts of interest in the context of human subjects research. Focuses on conflicts that are associated with clinical trials of new drugs and devices. Concludes by discussing the impact of these conflicts of interest on trust in the physician-patient relationship. References Principle IV and Opinion 8.032. Miller, *Trusting Doctors: Tricky Business When It Comes to Clinical Research, 81 B. U. L. Rev. 423, 427-28 (2001).*

Journal 2001 Considers conflicts of interest in clinical research and other types of medical practice. Compares the way in which physicians and lawyers address conflicts of interest in professional practice. Concludes that physicians are unaware of the need to create a meaningful conflict-of-interest doctrine for medical practice. Quotes Preamble, Principle IV, and Opinions 2.07, 8.03, 8.031, and 10.01. Moore, *What Doctors Can Learn From Lawyers About Conflicts of Interest, 81 B. U. L. Rev. 445, 447, 449-50 (2001).*

Journal 2001 Discusses linkages between governmental regulation of medical privacy and reduced medical error. Concludes that protection of patient privacy and the reduction of medical error will be important aspects of health care reform and will spur structural changes in health care delivery that will positively affect evolution of medical malpractice law. Quotes Principle IV. Terry, *An eHealth Diptych: The Impact of Privacy Regulation on Medical Error and Malpractice Litigation, 27 Am. J. L. & Med. 361, 402 (2001).*

Journal 2000 Discusses the development and history of the ethical doctrine of informed consent. Examines the current state of the law in Pennsylvania and concludes it does not adequately fulfill the goals of ethical and legal doctrines. Quotes Principle IV and Opinion 10.01. References

Opinion 8.08. Warren, *Pennsylvania Medical Informed Consent Law: A Call to Protect Patient Autonomy Rights by Abandoning the Battery Approach*, 38 Duq. L. Rev. 917, 925 (2000).

Journal 1999 Examines reporting of AIDS and HIV under Texas law. Discusses limitations on a physician's ability to warn potentially at-risk third parties. Concludes that Texas law should be changed to place a duty upon physicians to notify at-risk third parties of a patient's HIV-positive status. Quotes Principle IV and Opinion 10.01. Acosta, *The Texas Communicable Disease Prevention and Control Act: Are We Offering Enough Protection to Those Who Need It Most?* 36 Hous. L. Rev. 1819, 1822, 1830, 1831 (1999).

Journal 1999 Discusses whether a physician has the duty to disclose cancer-related gene mutations to a patient's children. Reviews current legislation regarding disclosure of genetic information. Argues that the potential for harm outweighs imposition of a duty to disclose. Quotes Principle IV. Brownrigg, *Mother Still Knows Best: Cancer-Related Gene Mutations, Familial Privacy, and a Physician's Duty to Warn*, 26 Fordham Urb. L. J. 247 (1999).

Journal 1999 Discusses the use of expert witnesses. Points out that, although some professions have a code of ethics, there is not a single source that defines professional ethics for expert witnesses. Argues that ethical and professional standards for expert witnesses must be defined. Cites Principle IV. Lubet, *Expert Witnesses: Ethics and Professionalism*, 12 Geo. J. Legal Ethics 465, 466 (1999).

Journal 1999 Discusses the practice of male circumcision in the US. Examines situations where the state may intervene in parental decision-making affecting minor children. Argues that males should be afforded the same protection as females in statutes prohibiting the mutilation of genital organs. Quotes Principle IV. Povenmire, *Do Parents Have the Legal Authority to Consent to the Surgical Amputation of Normal, Healthy Tissue From Their Infant Children?: The Practice of Circumcision in the United States*, 7 Am. U. J. Gender Soc. Pol. & L. 87, 96 (1999).

Journal 1999 Discusses the need for physicians to advocate on behalf of patients' rights in the context of health care delivery. Evaluates the nature and scope of the physician's role as advocate, noting that physicians cannot be expected to engage in attorney-like advocacy. Quotes Principles IV and VI, Fundamental Elements (2), (4), and (6) [now Opinion 10.01], Patient Responsibilities 5 [now Opinion 10.02], and Opinions 2.03, 2.07, 2.09, 2.16, 2.19, 3.06, 4.01, 4.04, 6.01, 7.02, 8.02, 8.03, 8.13, 8.132, 9.06, 9.07, and 9.131. Cites Opinions 5.05, 5.09, 7.01, 8.135, and 9.02. Sage, *Physicians as Advocates*, 35 Hous. L. Rev. 1529, 1537, 1541, 1542, 1552-53, 1554, 1556, 1557, 1559, 1561-62, 1564, 1571, 1574, 1576, 1580 (1999).

Journal 1999 Discusses the Department of Health and Human Services recommendations for federal legislation regarding confidentiality of health information. Points out that the recommendations include an exception for law enforcement access to medical records. Argues that such an exception must be narrow and clearly defined. Quotes Principle IV. Van Der Goes, *Opportunity Lost: Why and How to Improve the HHS-Proposed Legislation Governing Law Enforcement Access to Medical Records*, 147 U. Pa. L. Rev. 1009, 1063 (1999).

Journal 1999 Explores Model Rules of Professional Conduct focusing on the attorney-client relationship. Compares confidentiality provisions in the Model Rules with the rules of confidentiality governing the medical profession. Observes that existing confidentiality rules are incomplete and ambiguous. Concludes that one remedy is to embrace a discretionary confidentiality rule. Quotes Opinion 5.05. Cites Principle IV and Opinion 5.07. Zer-Gutman, *Revising the Ethical Rules of Attorney-Client Confidentiality: Towards a New Discretionary Rule*, 45 Loy. L. Rev. 669, 683-84, 699, 709, 718 (1999).

Journal 1998 Discusses issues of privacy arising out of collection and dissemination of genetic information about specific individuals. Emphasizes the need for privacy and confidentiality in this context. Suggests that future public policy should accommodate this need. Quotes Principle IV. Balint, *Issues of Privacy and Confidentiality in the New Genetics*, 9 Alb. L. J. Sci. & Tech. 27, 32 (1998).

Journal 1998 Recommends the passage of Ohio's proposed bill that would recognize an accountant-client privilege. Describes current recognized privileges, including the physician-patient privilege. Quotes Principle IV. Canning, *Privileged Communications in Ohio and What's New on the Horizon: Ohio House Bill 52 Accountant-Client Privilege*, 31 Akron L. Rev. 505, 550 (1998).

Journal 1998 Suggests that professional ethics correspond well to many governmental areas. Argues that the professional rules are more difficult for politically appointed attorneys. Indicates that ethical questions for government-appointed attorneys are often resolved through personal ethics rather than professional codes. Cites Principle IV. Lund, *The President as Client and the Ethics of the President's Lawyers*, 61 L. & Contemp. Probs. 65, 68 (1998).

Journal 1998 Discusses issues of patient consent regarding disclosure of medical information. Points out that recent changes in the health care system have presented medical record privacy concerns. Discloses findings of a study regarding hospital consent forms and calls for more research to be conducted. Cites Principle IV and Opinion 5.05. Merz, Sankar, & Yoo, *Hospital Consent for Disclosure of Medical Records*, 26 J. Law Med. & Ethics 241, 248 (1998).

Journal 1998 Examines the transition from paper medical records to electronic medical records. Identifies issues of confidentiality and privacy that arise as a result of the move to electronic medical records. Concludes that federal protection is needed to safeguard personal medical information. Quotes Principle IV and Opinions 5.07 and 5.075. Cites Opinion 8.061. Tsai, *Cheaper and Better: The Congressional Administrative Simplification Mandate Facilitates the Transition to Electronic Medical Records*, 19 J. Legal Med. 549, 570, 581 (1998).

Journal 1998 Explores the increased use and benefits of telemedicine. Points out that there is inadequate protection of privacy rights regarding electronic medical information. Concludes that federal law does not uniformly address medical record privacy and that Missouri law lacks adequate specificity. Quotes Principle IV. References Opinion 5.05. Young, *Telemedicine: Patient Privacy Rights of Electronic Medical Records*, 66 UMKC L. Rev. 921, 926 (1998).

Journal 1997 Discusses the Massachusetts statute that prohibits disclosure of a person's HIV status without obtaining informed consent. Suggests that legislation should be enacted mandating reporting of HIV to the department of public health. Quotes Principle IV. Agnello, *Advocating for a Change in the Massachusetts HIV Statute: Putting an End to Physician Uncertainty*, 2 J. Trial App. Advoc. 105, 107 (1997).

Journal 1997 Discusses the need for health care providers to have accurate medical information to treat patients effectively. Explains the benefits of computerized patient medical records and the privacy and confidentiality concerns raised. Concludes that patient privacy needs to be assured to improve service. Quotes Principle IV. Cuzmanes & Orlando, *Automation of Medical Records: The Electronic Superhighway and Its Ramifications for Health Care Providers*, 6 J. Pharmacy & L. 19, 27 (1997).

Journal 1997 Discusses principles of autonomy in the physician-patient relationship. Notes that rights to privacy and confidentiality are grounded in patient autonomy. Concludes that patients may be harmed when privacy rights are breached. Quotes Principle IV. Doyal, *Human Need and the Right of Patients to Privacy*, 14 J. Contemp. Health L. & Pol'y 1, 3 (1997).

Journal 1997 Considers principles of confidentiality in the physician-patient relationship. Notes the current trend emphasizing public reporting obligations of physicians to protect members of society. Emphasizes need for balance between patient rights and societal interests. Quotes Principle IV and Opinion 5.05. References Preamble. Jozefowicz, *The Case Against Having Professional Privilege in the Physician-Patient Relationship*, 16 Med. & L. 385, 386-87, 391 (1997).

Journal 1997 Suggests that ex parte conferences between treating physicians and opposing counsel undermine the physician-patient relationship. Notes that there are no significant benefits within the fact-finding process that justify the conflicts of interest created. Concludes that ex parte conferences are unnecessary. Quotes Principle IV and Opinion 5.05. Kassel, *Counterpoint . . . Defense Counsel's Ex Parte Communication with Plaintiff's Doctors: A Bad One-Sided Deal*, 9 S. C. Law. 42, 43 (Sept./Oct. 1997).

Journal 1997 Discusses the need for balance between business ethics and medical ethics in the context of managed care. Explores two models for integrating ethics and managed care. Proposes the adoption of a collective responsibility model to improve quality of care. Quotes Principles I, II, III, IV, and V. Cites Preamble. References Opinion 8.13. Regan, *Regulating the Business of Medicine: Models for Integrating Ethics and Managed Care*, 30 Colum. J. L. & Soc. Probs. 635, 651, 656, 657 (1997).

Journal 1997 Explores confidentiality problems that arise as a result of new health information systems. Examines legal aspects of medical records confidentiality. Advocates legislation at the national level to protect privacy of personal health information. Cites Principles of Medical

Ethics § 9 (1957) [now Principle IV]. Turkington, *Medical Record Confidentiality Law, Scientific Research, and Data Collection in the Information Age, 25 J. Law Med. & Ethics 113, 126 (1997).*

Journal 1996 Explores whether patients have a duty to disclose their HIV status to treating physicians. Suggests that recognizing such a duty may subject patients to a lower standard of care and provide a disincentive to be tested. Concludes that courts should not impose a duty to disclose on patients. Quotes Principle 9 (1957) [now Principle IV] and Opinion 9.131. DeNatale & Parrish, *Health Care Workers' Ability to Recover in Tort for Transmission or Fear of Transmission of HIV From a Patient, 36 Santa Clara L. Rev. 751, 782-83, 787 (1996).*

Journal 1996 Discusses the trend toward conserving resources expended on health care by withholding services absent a showing of necessity. Claims that the high standard of care physicians owe patients is jeopardized by medical treatment decisions based on coverage concerns. Concludes that the legal structure regarding health care plans should be changed. Quotes Preamble, Principles I, II, III, IV, V, VI, and VII, and Opinion 2.03. Hirshfeld & Thomason, *Medical Necessity Determinations: The Need for a New Legal Structure, 6 Health Matrix 3, 8-9 (1996).*

Journal 1996 Discusses sexual abuse litigation in which accusers have recovered memories of molestation in psychotherapy sessions. Observes that to successfully defend against such claims, it is necessary for the accused to have access to the clinical record. Posits that confidentiality problems can be eliminated with in camera record inspections. References Principle IV and Opinion 5.05. Loftus, Paddock, & Guernsey, *Patient-Psychotherapist Privilege: Access to Clinical Records in the Tangled Web of Repressed Memory Litigation, 30 U. Rich L. Rev. 109, 127 (1996).*

Journal 1996 Reviews two Washington State Supreme Court decisions in which subsequent treating physicians testified against their patients and on behalf of defendant physicians in malpractice litigation. Observes that these decisions erode the physician-patient privilege. Posits that the decisions are inconsistent with current medical ethics and proposes a statutory enactment as a solution. Quotes Opinion 5.05. Cites Principle 9 (1957) [now Principle IV]. Oppenheim, *Physicians as Experts Against Their Own Patients? What Happened to the Privilege? 63 Def. Couns. J. 254, 257, 261 (1996).*

Journal 1996 Considers prearraignment forensic evaluations. Notes the prohibition against use of such evaluations. Examines underlying ethical precepts. Observes that principles of beneficence are misapplied to forensic psychiatry in this context. Advocates a new ethical framework. Quotes Preamble. References Principle IV and Opinion 5.05. Ornish, Mills, & Ornish, *Prearraignment Forensic Evaluations: Toward a New Policy, 24 Bull. Am. Acad. Psychiatry Law 453, 454, 469 (1996).*

Journal 1996 Examines the psychiatrist-patient duty of confidentiality. Notes that Principles of Medical Ethics prohibit the disclosure of patient confidences and medical records. Observes that exceptions to this prohibition exist when required by law or to protect the community. Quotes Principle 9 (1957) [now Principle IV and Opinion 5.05]. Sadoff, *Ethical Obligations for the Psychiatrist: Confidentiality, Privilege, and Privacy in Psychiatric Treatment, 29 Loy. L.A. L. Rev. 1709, 1710, 1711 (1996).*

Journal 1996 Examines the theories courts have used when evaluating claims for emotional distress damages arising from HIV misdiagnosis. Observes that the physical injury requirement is outdated but notes that alternatives may give rise to potentially unlimited liability. Concludes that physicians should be afforded good faith immunity from suits. Quotes Principle 9 (1957) [now Principle IV]. Schmid, *Protecting the Physician in HIV Misdiagnosis Cases, 46 Duke L. J. 431, 458 (1996).*

Journal 1995 Discusses the belief of health care providers that they have an ethical obligation to warn the partners of HIV-positive patients. Examines both the scope of a Massachusetts statute that prevents providers from releasing HIV test results of patients and possible defenses that providers may assert. Quotes Principle IV and Opinion 5.05. Friedland, *HIV Confidentiality and the Right to Warn—The Health Care Provider's Dilemma, 80 Mass. L. Rev. 3, 4 (March 1995).*

Journal 1995 Examines federal legislative proposals intended to protect confidentiality of computerized medical records. Concludes that proposed legislation will significantly undermine confidentiality. Cites Opinion 5.07. References Principle IV. Hoge, *Proposed Federal Legislation Jeopardizes Patient Privacy, 23 Bull. Am. Acad. Psychiatry Law 495, 498, 500 (1995).*

Journal 1995 Offers relevant historical perspectives and provides comprehensive ethical and legal discussion of physician-assisted suicide and euthanasia. Highlights important legislative developments, including the Oregon Death with Dignity Act, and analyzes significant judicial opinions. Quotes Principles III, IV, and VI and Opinions 2.21 and 9.12. Cites Opinions 2.20 and 8.11. Stone & Winslade, *Physician-Assisted Suicide and Euthanasia in the United States: Legal and Ethical Observations*, 16 J. Legal Med. 481, 483, 490, 497, 498, 499 (1995).

Journal 1994 Compares Texas law with Illinois law on the issue of ex parte communications between defense counsel and the patient/plaintiff's physician in civil litigation. Argues that preservation of the physician-patient relationship requires prohibition of such contact. Quotes Principles II and IV and Opinion 5.05. Comment, *From the Land of Lincoln a Healing Rule: Proposed Texas Rule of Civil Procedure Prohibiting Ex Parte Contact Between Defense Counsel and a Plaintiff's Treating Physician*, 25 Tex. Tech L. Rev. 1081, 1081, 1082 (1994).

Journal 1994 Considers whether an exception should be made to physician-patient confidentiality that would allow a physician to reveal parental medical history to a child. Concludes that such an exception would not completely erode physician-patient confidentiality. Quotes Principle IV, Fundamental Elements (4), and Opinion 5.05. Cites Principle I and Fundamental Elements (1). Friedland, *Physician-Patient Confidentiality: Time to Re-examine a Venerable Concept in Light of Contemporary Society and Advances in Medicine*, 15 J. Legal Med. 249, 257, 264, 276 (1994).

Journal 1994 Explores the ethical issues involved in a multidisciplinary team working with children in legal proceedings. Focuses on the relationships between professionals and the conflicts that arise regarding disclosure of confidential information and forced disclosure of nonprivileged information. Quotes Principles III and IV, Fundamental Elements (4), and Opinions 1.02 (1992) and 5.07 (1992) [now Opinion 5.05]. Cites Opinion 2.02. Glynn, *Multidisciplinary Representation of Children: Conflicts Over Disclosures of Client Communications*, 27 J. Marshall L. Rev. 617, 625, 626, 630-32, 637, 639, 643 (1994).

Journal 1994 Discusses physician-patient confidentiality and the exception that permits breach of a patient's confidence if required by law. Argues that this is always a legitimate exception to the confidentiality rule. Quotes Principle IV and Fundamental Elements (4). McConnell, *Confidentiality and the Law*, 20 J. Med. Ethics 47, 47 (1994).

Journal 1994 Reviews the evolution of the physician-patient relationship, with attention to patient autonomy. Examines the changing health care delivery environment. Quotes Preamble, Principles I, II, III, IV, V, and VI, Fundamental Elements (1) and (2), and Opinions 1.02 and 8.07 (1981) [now Opinion 8.08]. Cites Opinion 1.01. Szczygiel, *Beyond Informed Consent*, 21 Ohio N. U. L. Rev. 171, 217, 218, 220, 225, 226, 256 (1994).

Journal 1994 Discusses the importance of confidentiality in the physician-patient relationship and under what circumstances patient information may be released. Examines unique considerations that apply when a physician provides medical care to a minor or an HIV-infected individual. Quotes Principle IV and Fundamental Elements (4). Weiner & Wettstein, *Confidentiality of Patient-Related Information*, 112 Arch. Ophthalmology 1032, 1033 (1994).

Journal 1993 Discusses family privacy rights and considers the meaning of justice, self-respect, and the fundamental principles of physician ethics. Concludes that physicians have an ethical duty to intervene in domestic violence so long as such intervention does not breach confidentiality or violate patient autonomy. Quotes Principle IV and Opinion 5.05. References Opinions 8.14 and 9.131. Jecker, *Privacy Beliefs and the Violent Family: Extending the Ethical Argument for Physician Intervention*, 269 JAMA 776, 778, 779 (1993).

Journal 1993 Discusses physicians' duty to disclose to patients medical treatment alternatives that are not readily available. Proposes that based on the historical development and legal requirements of the informed consent doctrine, physicians should be required to inform patients of non–readily available alternatives or face liability for breach of such obligation. Quotes Principles I, II, III, IV, and V and Opinion 8.08. Note, *Informed Choice: Physicians' Duty to Disclose Nonreadily Available Alternatives*, 43 Case W. Res. L. Rev. 491, 491, 498-99, 508, 509 (1993).

Journal 1993 Explores the idea of reverse informed consent, which would impose a duty on patients to inform health care professionals of their infectious status. Concludes that such a duty is justified. Quotes Principles IV and VI and Opinions 8.11 and 9.131. Oddi, *Reverse Informed Consent: The Unreasonably Dangerous Patient*, 46 V and. L. Rev. 1417, 1449, 1463, 1465, 1479 (1993).

Journal 1993 Discusses the issues surrounding the confidentiality of electronic and computerized medical records. Concludes that any legal standard addressing this problem should balance the need to protect patient confidentiality with the practical constraints, such as cost and accessibility limiting ideal security. References Principle IV and Opinion 5.07. Waller & Fulton, *The Electronic Chart; Keeping It Confidential and Secure, 26 J. Health & Hosp. L. 104, 105 (April 1993).*

Journal 1992 Discusses legal issues in the context of disclosing health information in adoptions. Presents the arguments for and against disclosure, including the traditional view favoring non-disclosure. References Principle IV. Blair, *Lifting the Genealogical Veil: The Blueprint for Legislative Reform of the Disclosure of Health-Related Information in Adoption, 70 No. Carolina L. Rev. 681, 692 (1992).*

Journal 1991 Discusses the case of *Crist v. Moffat,* which prohibits ex parte communications with a plaintiff's treating physician in North Carolina. Examines the physician-patient privilege and looks at various jurisdictions that permit and forbid ex parte communications. Quotes Principle IV and Opinion 5.06. Comment, *Shielding the Plaintiff and Physician: The Prohibition of Ex Parte Contacts With a Plaintiff's Treating Physician, 13 Campbell L. Rev. 233, 243, 248 (1991).*

Journal 1990 Examines the relationship between professional ethics and professional autonomy, perceived problems of health care rationing under a prospective payment vs a fee-for-service system, and the relationship between professional ethics and the problem of rationing. Concludes that rationing is inevitable, forcing important ethical questions to be addressed. Quotes Principles IV and VI. Agich, *Rationing and Professional Autonomy, 18 Law Med. & Health Care 77, 79, 82 (1990).*

Journal 1990 Examines the extent to which forensic psychiatrists are consulted in medical malpractice cases. Considers the appropriate standard of care, particularly for psychiatric malpractice cases, and the problems associated with its determination. References Principles II and IV. Modlin, *Forensic Psychiatry and Malpractice, 18 Bull. Am. Acad. Psychiatry Law 153, 161 (1990).*

Journal 1990 Discusses the moral dilemma in deciding whether to withdraw artificial nutrition and hydration from a patient and the appropriate role of the judiciary. Concludes that judicial decisions do not represent the moral viewpoint of society and that moral pronouncements should not be made in the courtroom. Quotes Preamble, Principles I, II, III, IV, V, VI, and VII, and Opinion 2.20. Peccarelli, *A Moral Dilemma: The Role of Judicial Intervention in Withholding or Withdrawing Nutrition and Hydration, 23 John Marshall L. Rev. 537, 539, 540, 541 (1990).*

Journal 1990 Presents current issues, policies, legislation, and judicial decisions regarding impaired physicians. Concludes by proposing enhanced confidentiality requirements in disciplinary proceedings and nationwide adoption of a uniform law in this area. Quotes Opinion 4.07. References Principle IV. Walzer, *Impaired Physicians: An Overview and Update of the Legal Issues, 11 J. Legal Med. 131, 174, 192 (1990).*

Journal 1989 Discusses the history of the physician-patient privilege up through changes implemented under the Ohio Tort Reform Act of 1987. Aspects of the physician-patient privilege that are most significantly affected by this Tort Reform Act are highlighted, with recommendations for further refinement of the privilege in Ohio. Quotes Principles II and IV and Opinion 5.05. Note, *The Ohio Physician-Patient Privilege: Modified, Revised, and Defined, 49 Ohio St. L. J. 1147, 1167 (1989).*

Journal 1985 Initially describes how existing doctrines protect the value of autonomy in the context of the physician-patient relationship, then examines various problems in the current protective scheme. Concludes by recommending the creation of an independent articulable protected interest in patient autonomy. Quotes Principles II and IV. Cites Opinions 4.04 (1984) [now Opinions 8.03 and 8.032] and 6.03 (1984) [now Opinion 6.02]. Shultz, *From Informed Consent to Patient Choice: A New Protected Interest, 95 Yale L. J. 219, 275 (1985).*

Journal 1983 Examines the evolution and impact of decisions in *Tarasoff v. Regents of the University of California,* 131 Cal. Rptr. 14 (Cal. 1976) and *McIntosh v. Milano,* 403 A.2d 500 (N.J. Super. 1979) which established a duty on the part of a physician or psychotherapist to warn third parties foreseeably endangered by a patient. In establishing such a duty, the courts endeavored to balance the physician's duty to warn endangered third parties with the duty to maintain confidentiality within the physician-patient relationship. Quotes Principle IV. Roth & Levin, *Dilemma of Tarasoff: Must Physicians Protect the Public or Their Patients? 11 Law Med. & Health Care 104, 106 (1983).*

Journal 1981 Observes that a reevaluation of medicine and the medical profession is occurring on at least three levels: theoretical, educational, and professional. Notes that physicians are facing various challenges to the exercise of many of their societal functions and emphasizes that physicians view law and the medical profession as the source most responsible for these challenges. Quotes Principle IV. Schwartz & Gibson, *Defining the Role of the Physician: Medical Education, Tradition, and the Legal Process*, 18 Houston L. Rev. 779, 791 (1981).

V. A physician shall continue to study, apply, and advance scientific knowledge, maintain a commitment to medical education, make relevant information available to patients, colleagues, and the public, obtain consultation, and use the talents of other health professionals when indicated.

S.D. Ind. 1992 Drug manufacturer sought protective order to prevent disclosure of patients' and physicians' names from adverse drug reaction reports. Plaintiff, quoting Principle V which requires that physicians "make relevant information available to . . . the public," argued that requiring the disclosure of physicians' names would not deter physicians from reporting adverse drug reactions. The court held that the Principle notwithstanding, disclosure of physicians' names would seriously undermine the FDA's voluntary reporting system. *In re Eli Lilly & Co.*, 142 F.R.D. 454, 458.

D.S.C. 1968 Military dependent sued government physicians under Federal Tort Claims Act where child with acute abdominal pain was twice referred to naval hospital with diagnosis of possible appendicitis and twice sent home without treatment, eventually suffering ruptured appendix and serious complications. In finding for the plaintiff, the court quoted Principle 8 (1957) [now Principle V and Opinion 8.04] in considering whether the physicians had a duty to seek consultation in such a situation. *Steeves v. United States*, 294 F. Supp. 446, 454.

Cal. App. 2004 Trial court sustained a demur to the appellants' first amended complaint. The appellate court quoted Principles II and V in concluding the coroner's practice of hiring a pathologist who had a close working relationship with a company which treats individuals whose death the pathologist may be required to investigate was a questionable policy due to the pathologist's wide discretion. The appellate court, however, affirmed the trial court's decision that appellants had not stated any viable claims. *Miller v. Rupf*, 2004 WL 2092015, 11 n. 9.

Minn. 1999 Plaintiffs sought declaratory relief against hospital for its refusal to grant plaintiffs access to peer review materials. The trial court granted the defendant's motion for summary judgment. On appeal the Minnesota Supreme Court held that physicians' private right to access a hospital's peer review materials did not outweigh public interest in quality health care. The court stated that quality care could be jeopardized if physicians had access to peer review material. The court also cited Principle V, stating that physicians have an ethical duty to participate in the peer review process. *Amaral v. Saint Cloud Hospital*, 598 N.W.2d 379, 388.

Tex. 1993 Estate of man who committed suicide after taking drug filed suit against manufacturer and sought adverse reaction or drug experience reports submitted to the FDA. These reports are voluntarily submitted by physicians and other health care providers and, according to 21 CFR § 314.430(e)(4)(ii), the FDA must keep the identity of the reporters and the patients confidential. Noting the public interest in the voluntary reporting system and that the trial court had ordered disclosure of confidential information without applying the standard of relevance and need, the court denied disclosure of the reporters' identities. Quoting Principle V, the dissent declared that the decision adversely affected public health and safety by leaving drug manufacturers free to conceal important information. *Eli Lilly & Co. v. Marshall*, 850 S.W.2d 155, 163.

Journal 2011 Examines ethical reasons for excluding medical methods from patent protection and discusses whether they are appropriate. Compares the treatment of medical methods under the Japanese patent system with laws in Europe and the US. Concludes the ethical issues surrounding Japan's patent system should be viewed from the standpoint of whether the patent system can be socially justified and would lead to industrial development. Quotes Principle 2 (1957) [now Principle V]. Liu & Sato, *Patent Protection of Medical Methods—Focusing on Ethical Issues*, 20 Pac. Rim. L. & Pol'y J. 125, 135 (2011).

Journal 2011 Argues that regulation of physicians' off-label use of prescription medications is necessary to prevent harm to both the patient and to society via unnecessary increases in health care spending. Concludes the state should intervene in the physician-patient relationship when physicians prescribe medicine off-label that is not justified by high-quality evidence of safety and efficacy. Quotes Principles I and V. Rosoff & Coleman, *The Case for Legal Regulation of Physicians' Off-Label Prescribing, 86 Notre Dame L. Rev. 649, 675 (2011).*

Journal 2010 Analyzes factors contributing to the emergence of medical repatriation and evaluates whether this practice comports with current legal and ethical standards. Proposes changes to federal regulations that govern hospitals and clarifications to medical ethical standards. Quotes the Preamble and Principles I, II, III, IV, V, VI, VII, VIII, and IX. Zoellner, *Medical Repatriation: Examining the Legal and Ethical Implications of an Emerging Practice, 32 Wash. U. J. L. & Pol'y 515, 530-532 (2010).*

Journal 2009 Explores emerging issues in conflict management systems design (CMSD). Concludes as the practice of CMSD in the organizational context continues to expand, practitioners should openly discuss the emerging issues of the field. References Principles I, II, V, and VIII. Costantino, *Second Generation Organizational Conflict Management Systems Design: A Practitioner's Perspective on Emerging Issues, 14 Harv. Negot. L. Rev. 81, 95 (2009).*

Journal 2009 Discusses the interaction between statutes and case law governing the medical field and the core principles of medical professionalism. Concludes the legal framework of medical professionalism does not encompass all the elements required of a medical professional. Quotes Principles II, III, IV, V, VI, VII, and VIII. Fichter, *The Law of Doctoring: A Study of the Codification of Medical Professionalism, 19 Health Matrix 317, 338, 339, 340, 343, 351 (2009).*

Journal 2008 Considers whether certain medical and surgical procedures should be removed from the scope of patentability. Concludes "pure" medical and surgical techniques should not be patentable while granting medical process patents for other procedures. Quotes Principle V and Opinion 9.08. Peschel, *Revisiting the Compromise of 35 USC § 287(c), 16 Tex. Intell. Prop. L. J. 299, 315 (2008).*

Journal 2008 Examines the development of bioethics and environmental ethics, as well as laws promoting the role of bioethicists in decision making. Concludes environmental ethicists must convince legislatures of the role of environmental ethics in order to have a greater impact on decision making. Quotes Principles I, II, III, IV, V, VI, VII, VIII, and IX. Robertson, *Seeking a Seat at the Table: Has Law Left Environmental Ethics Behind as It Embraces Bioethics? 32 Wm. & Mary Envtl. L. & Pol'y Rev. 273, 307 (2008).*

Journal 2007 Compares the role of conscience clauses in various professions. Concludes that conscience clauses in the area of health care must not impede access to care. Quotes Preamble and Principles V, VI, and VIII. Chudoba, *Conscience in America: The Slippery Slope of Mixing Morality With Medicine, 36 Sw. U. L. Rev. 85, 86, 103, 104, 105 (2007).*

Journal 2007 Examines ethical issues raised by advances in computed tomography (CT) imaging technology. Concludes that widespread cooperation and patient advocacy are needed to ensure ethical use of CT. Quotes Principle v. Wann, Nassef, Jeffrey, Messer, Wilke, Duerinckx, Blankenship, Rosenberg, & Dembo, *Ethical Considerations in CT Angiography, 23 Int. J. Cardiovasc. Imaging 379, 384 (2007).*

Journal 2006 Examines ethical dilemmas physicians may face as providers of pay-for-performance medical care. Concludes that this strategy offers a benefit to patients as long as physicians uphold stringent ethical standards and work together to ensure optimum patient care. Cites Principles I, V, VIII, and IX and Opinions 2.035, 2.095, 6.01, 8.021, 8.03, 8.0501, 8.053, 8.054, and 8.121. Bostick, Sade, & McMahon, *Report of the Council on Ethical and Judicial Affairs: Physician Pay-for-Performance Programs, 3 Ind. Health L. Rev. 429, 430, 431, 432-33, 434, 435, 436 (2006).*

Journal 2006 Explores conscience clause legislation relating to the dispensing of oral contraceptives. Concludes that such legislation must balance the interests of the patient and the health care provider. Cites Principles I, II, III, IV, V, VI, VII, VIII, and IX. Collins, *Conscience Clauses and Oral Contraceptives: Conscientious Objection or Calculated Obstruction? 15 Ann. Health L. 37, 54 (2006).*

Journal 2005 Examines issues surrounding tort reform proposals. Concludes that more can be done to correct the current tort system before moving toward a "one size fits all" approach. Quotes Principles I, II, III, IV, V, VI, VII, VIII, and IX. Messerly & Warwick, *Nowhere to Turn: A Glance at the Facts Behind the Supposed Need for Tort "Reform," 28 Hamline L. Rev. 489, 506 (2005).*

Journal 2004 Discusses the need for a greater understanding of and openness to religious values by the professions. Concludes that, although such openness is important, problems may arise when professional values and religious values clash. Quotes Opinion 5.05. References Principle V. Sullivan, *Naked Fitzies and Iron Cages: Individual Values, Professional Virtues, and the Struggle for Public Space*, 78 Tul. L. Rev. 1687, 1702, 1703 (2004).

Journal 2003 Examines policy options for integration of traditional and modern medicine. Concludes that solid cross-sectoral linkages between different traditions can stabilize an integrated health care system. Quotes Preamble and Principle V. Holliday, *Traditional Medicines in Modern Societies: An Exploration of Integrationist Options Through East Asian Experience*, 28 J. Med. & Phil. 373, 387 (2003).

Journal 2003 Considers the legal, medical, and ethical issues of physician-patient confidentiality in disclosure of paternity. Concludes that a balancing test should be applied to making determinations regarding disclosure of paternity. Quotes Principles I, IV, and V and Opinions 1.02, 5.055, and 10.01. Cites Principle II and Opinion 5.05. Richards & Wolf, *Medical Confidentiality and Disclosure of Paternity*, 48 S. D. L. Rev. 409, 411, 412, 413 (2003).

Journal 2002 Reviews how changes in the health care delivery system underscore the importance of information in patient empowerment. Concludes that patients should use information to take charge of their health care. Quotes Principle V and Opinion 10.02. Cites Opinion 10.01. Kane, *Information Is the Key to Patient Empowerment*, 11 Annals Health L. 25, 29-30, 44 (2002).

Journal 2002 Evaluates pain management treatment for prisoners. Concludes that withholding treatment for, or failing to adequately treat, pain violates the Eighth Amendment. Quotes Principle V and Opinion 2.20. McGrath, *Raising the "Civilized Minimum" of Pain Amelioration for Prisoners to Avoid Cruel and Unusual Punishment*, 54 Rutgers L. Rev. 649, 657, 660 (2002).

Journal 2002 Evaluates the application of biomedical knowledge in clinical practice. Concludes that serious inadequacies exist in the current practice of evidence-based medicine. Quotes Principle V and Opinion 9.08. References Opinion 9.095. Noah, *Medicine's Epistemology: Mapping the Haphazard Diffusion of Knowledge in the Biomedical Community*, 44 Ariz. L. Rev. 373, 404, 447, 448 (2002).

Journal 2000 Discusses patent law and policy. Examines whether or not those who practice medicine should be excused from patent laws because of the conflict that medical procedure patents create with respect to the practice of medicine. Concludes that Congress should repeal section 287(c) of the Patent Act. Quotes Principle V and Opinions 9.08 and 9.09. Cites Opinion 8.03. References Opinion 10.01. Ho, *Patents, Patients, and Public Policy: An Incomplete Intersection at 35 USC § 287(c)*, 33 U.C. Davis L. Rev. 601, 603, 623, 624, 625, 631 (2000).

Journal 2000 Considers the rules governing expert testimony. Explores professional ethical standards affecting expert witnesses and concludes that codes of ethics have not succeeded in eliminating biased expert testimony. Recommends creation of an organization to assist courts in obtaining reliable expert witness testimony. Quotes Principle III and Opinion 6.01. Cites Principles I, II, and V and Opinions 1.02 and 9.07. Murphy, *Expert Witnesses at Trial: Where Are the Ethics?* 14 Geo. J. Legal Ethics 217, 231-32 (2000).

Journal 2000 Describes possible solutions designed to improve postapproval regulation of prescription drugs so that fewer patients will suffer from adverse drug reactions. Concludes that the FDA along with physicians and clinical researchers should rethink the existing approach to monitoring of unexpected side effects. Quotes Principle V and Opinion 9.032. Cites Opinion 5.05. Noah, *Adverse Drug Reactions: Harnessing Experimental Data to Promote Patient Welfare*, 49 Cath. U. L. Rev. 449, 477, 497-98 (2000).

Journal 2000 Evaluates the regulatory framework governing prescription drugs. Considers problems faced by elderly patients when taking FDA-approved medications. Concludes that in order to optimize patient safety, the existing regulatory system must undergo important structural changes. Quotes Principle V and Opinion 9.032. Noah & Brushwood, *Adverse Drug Reactions in Elderly Patients: Alternative Approaches to Postmarket Surveillance*, 33 J. Health L. 383, 400, 445 (2000).

Journal 1997 Discusses physician frustration with managed care plans caused by gag clauses and cost-containment mechanisms. Reviews the development of managed care organizations and federal attempts at limiting the use of gag clauses. Concludes that gag clauses are inherently flawed and compromise quality health care. Quotes Principles II and V, Fundamental Elements (1), and

Opinion 8.13. Note, *Physicians, Bound and Gagged: Federal Attempts to Combat Managed Care's Use of Gag Clauses,* 21 *Seton Hall Legis. J.* 567, 601-02 (1997).

Journal 1997 Discusses the need for balance between business ethics and medical ethics in the context of managed care. Explores two models for integrating ethics and managed care. Proposes the adoption of a collective responsibility model to improve quality of care. Quotes Principles I, II, III, IV, and V. Cites Preamble. References Opinion 8.13. Regan, *Regulating the Business of Medicine: Models for Integrating Ethics and Managed Care,* 30 *Colum. J. L. & Soc. Probs.* 635, 651, 656, 657 (1997).

Journal 1996 Discusses the trend toward conserving resources expended on health care by withholding services absent a showing of necessity. Claims that the high standard of care physicians owe patients is jeopardized by medical treatment decisions based on coverage concerns. Concludes that the legal structure regarding health care plans should be changed. Quotes Preamble, Principles I, II, III, IV, V, VI, and VII, and Opinion 2.03. Hirshfeld & Thomason, *Medical Necessity Determinations: The Need for a New Legal Structure,* 6 *Health Matrix* 3, 8-9 (1996).

Journal 1996 Considers the impact of gag clauses on the physician-patient relationship. Undertakes an extensive legal, ethical, and policy analysis. Concludes that gag clauses are violative of legal and ethical principles. Quotes Principles II, V, and VI and Fundamental Elements (1). Cites Preamble. Martin & Bjerknes, *The Legal and Ethical Implications of Gag Clauses in Physician Contracts,* XXII *Am. J. Law & Med.* 433, 465-66 (1996).

Journal 1994 Reviews the evolution of the physician-patient relationship, with attention to patient autonomy. Examines the changing health care delivery environment. Quotes Preamble, Principles I, II, III, IV, V, and VI, Fundamental Elements (1) and (2), and Opinions 1.02 and 8.07 (1981) [now Opinion 8.08]. Cites Opinion 1.01. Szczygiel, *Beyond Informed Consent,* 21 *Ohio N. U. L. Rev.* 171, 217, 218, 220, 225, 226, 256 (1994).

Journal 1993 Discusses physicians' duty to disclose to patients medical treatment alternatives that are not readily available. Proposes that based on the historical development and legal requirements of the informed consent doctrine, physicians should be required to inform patients of nonreadily available alternatives or face liability for breach of such obligation. Quotes Principles I, II, III, IV, and V and Opinion 8.08. Note, *Informed Choice: Physicians' Duty to Disclose Nonreadily Available Alternatives,* 43 *Case W. Res. L. Rev.* 491, 491, 498-99, 508, 509 (1993).

Journal 1990 Discusses the moral dilemma in deciding whether to withdraw artificial nutrition and hydration from a patient and the appropriate role of the judiciary. Concludes that judicial decisions do not represent the moral viewpoint of society and that moral pronouncements should not be made in the courtroom. Quotes Preamble, Principles I, II, III, IV, V, VI, and VII, and Opinion 2.20. Peccarelli, *A Moral Dilemma: The Role of Judicial Intervention in Withholding or Withdrawing Nutrition and Hydration,* 23 *John Marshall L. Rev.* 537, 539, 540, 541 (1990).

VI. A physician shall, in the provision of appropriate patient care, except in emergencies, be free to choose whom to serve, with whom to associate, and the environment in which to provide medical care.

2d Cir. 1980 Appeal by hospital of National Labor Relations Board order to employ two part-time staff physicians on a full-time basis and to consider their applications for permanent admitting privileges. Physicians had joined picket line in sympathy with striking union employees without giving advance notice and were allegedly denied full-time positions in retaliation. The court held that support of the strike was activity protected by the National Labor Relations Act but that the physicians lost protection when they told patients the facility was unable to provide adequate care, in careless disregard of the truth. Further, the court noted that the failure to give notice before striking raised ethical questions under Principle 5 (1957) [now Principle VII]. *Montefiore Hosp. & Medical Ctr. v. NLRB,* 621 F.2d 510, 516.

4th Cir. 1984 Prisoner sued private physician under 42 USC § 1983 for failure to provide medical treatment in violation of his Eighth Amendment rights. The court held that the exercise of the physician's medical judgment did not constitute action under color of state law. While not specifically referring to Principle VI (1980), the court cited the Principles for the general proposition that the physician-patient relationship is independent of state administrative supervision. This concept is apparently embodied in Principle VI. *Calvert v. Sharp, 748 F.2d 861, 863, cert. denied, 471 US 1132 (1975).*

6th Cir. 1989 Plaintiff, a chiropractic association, alleged that the AMA and several other professional associations violated antitrust law by conspiring to contain and ultimately eliminate the practice of chiropractic. The court provided a historical overview of the AMA's gradual, but incomplete, recognition of chiropractors and limited licensed practitioners referring specifically to Principle 3 (1957) as well as to the Opinions and Reports of the Judicial Council Sec. 3, Para. 8 (1969) and to the Opinions and Reports 3.60 and 3.70 (1977) [now Principle VI and Opinions 3.01 and 3.04]. Based on its reading of these Principles and Opinions, the court reversed the trial court's grant of summary judgment to the AMA because there remained a material issue of fact of whether it had continued to illegally boycott chiropractic. *Chiropractic Coop. Ass'n v. AMA, 867 F.2d 270, 272-75.*

W.D. Ark. 1989 Physician sued hospital alleging that it had acted in bad faith when it terminated his employment for failure to accept responsibility for "medical" as opposed to "surgical" patients. Plaintiff argued that the incorporation of the AMA's Principles of Medical Ethics into the hospital's by-laws gave him the right to choose which patients to serve, in apparent reference to Principle VI. While recognizing this right, the court held that the hospital had a corresponding right to consider such a refusal in its employment decisions. *Maxey v. United States, 1989 US Dist. LEXIS 5827.*

N.D. Ga. 1981 Decedent's widow brought wrongful death action against hospital, treating physician, and physician supervising a group of emergency room physicians who had independent contracts with the hospital. Plaintiff claimed the supervising physician was vicariously liable in damages to her under the doctrine of respondeat superior. The court noted that the traditional control test used to identify agency relationships is ineffective in the context of physician-hospital relationships because physicians are bound by Principle 6 (1957) [now most closely embodied by the independent judgment aspects of Principle VI] which requires physicians to practice medicine according to their independent professional judgment. *Stewart v. Midani, 525 F. Supp. 843, 848-49.*

E.D. Mich. 1986 Plaintiff-chiropractors claimed violation of the Sherman Antitrust Act alleging that the AMA conspired with others to injure them professionally and financially. In support of their claim, plaintiffs cited Principle 3 (1957) and the Opinions and Reports of the Judicial Council Sec.3, Para. 8 (1969) [now Principle VI and Opinions 3.01 and 3.04]. The court, noting the 1977 change in the AMA's position regarding chiropractic reflected in the Opinions and Reports of the Judicial Council 3.60 and 3.70 (1977) [now Opinion 3.04], held that plaintiffs failed to demonstrate evidence of an overt act by the AMA within the statutory limitations period. Summary judgment entered for AMA. *Chiropractic Coop. Ass'n v. AMA, 1986-2 Trade Cas. (CCH) & 67,294, aff'd in part and rev'd in part, 867 F.2d 270 (6th Cir. 1989).*

E.D. Mich. 1985 In an antitrust case brought by plaintiff-chiropractic association against the AMA, plaintiffs presented the court with a motion in limine asking that the court strike defendant's affirmative defense of a good faith concern with public health and patient care. Plaintiffs argued that the defense was unprecedented, in conflict with existing law, and dramatically wrong. Plaintiffs referred to Principle 3 (1957) [now Principle VI and Opinions 3.01 and 3.04] as the source of the AMA's antitrust violations. The court denied plaintiffs' motion to strike, stating that under the rule of reason test, the AMA had the right to present evidence that its actions furthered the public interest and patient care. *Chiropractic Coop. Ass'n v. AMA, 617 F. Supp. 264, 266, aff'd in part and rev'd in part, 867 F.2d 270 (6th Cir. 1989).*

D.N.M. 1987 In an antitrust action against major health insurance provider and state medical society, group of chiropractors alleged that a conspiracy existed in which the insurer refused to provide health cost reimbursement coverage for chiropractic services. Plaintiffs urged court to apply a per se analysis, rather than the rule of reason analysis, to determine the legality of defendants' restrictive practices. The court declined to apply the per se test. In part, court's conclusion was based on view that concerns of defendant-physicians about relationship with chiropractors because of ethical restrictions imposed by Principle 3 (1957) [now Principle VI and Opinions 3.01 and 3.04] deserved more consideration than the per se test would afford. *Johnson v. Blue Cross/Blue Shield, 677 F. Supp. 1112, 1118.*

D. Vt. 1986 Prisoner sued prison officials and private physician under section 42 USC § 1983, claiming cruel and unusual punishment in violation of his constitutional rights after physician allegedly frightened the prisoner while he was physically restrained, performed a colonoscopy with the examining room door open to a main hallway, and allowed guards to participate in the exam. The court held that although state law required the provision of medical care to inmates, the ethical canons upon which the physician-patient relationship was based were not derived from state law and the physician's actions did not constitute state action. In so holding, the court relied on *Calvert v. Sharpe*, 748 F.2d 861 (4th cir. 1984) which cites generally to the Principles for the proposition that the physician-patient relationship is independent of state supervision. Principle VI reflects this concept. *Nash v. Wennar, 645 F.Supp. 238, 242.*

Ariz. 1984 Mother sued hospital and physicians after minor son was transferred to another facility for solely financial reasons although emergency surgical care was medically indicated. In holding that the hospital's transfer policy pre-empted further care by the physicians and that the record revealed no physician negligence, the court stated that generally the standard of care for physicians is determined by what is usually done by members of the profession. The court then cited Principle VI, apparently for the proposition that in emergency situations there may be an ethical, rather than legal, obligation to provide care. *Thompson v. Sun City Community Hosp., Inc., 141 Ariz. 597, 688 P.2d 605, 612 n.7.*

Ariz. App. 2009 Outpatient treatment center, which was not owned by a licensed physician or other licensed medical professional, sued automobile insurer for refusal to reimburse injured persons treated by the center. The court quoted Principle VI and discussed the changes made to the Principle to comply with federal antitrust law. The court explained that Principle VI permits physicians to practice in a variety of business structures consistent with the lack of any restriction as to corporate ownership of an outpatient treatment center. The appeals court held that the center was legally licensed. *Midtown Medical Group, Inc. v. State Farm Mutual Automobile Insurance Co., 220 Ariz. 341, 206 P.3d 790, 797-98. .*

Ariz. App. 1980 Malpractice suit against a paid on-call physician for refusal to treat decedent resulting in delay in treatment. The court quoted Principle 5 (1957) [now Principle VI and Opinion 8.11] as establishing an ethical duty to provide emergency care. However, court distinguished any such ethical obligation from its holding that physician had a contractual duty to treat emergency patients to the best of his ability. *Hiser v. Randolph, 126 Ariz. 608, 617 P.2d 774, 776 n.1, 777, 778.*

Cal. App. 2003 Patient and her husband sued medical clinic for terminating care after the patient filed malpractice claims against two clinic physicians. Clinic's policy required termination of all medical care for patients and their families in such a situation. Appeals court upheld summary judgment for the clinic on several claims, but denied summary judgment on claims for interference with contractual relations, negligent infliction of emotional distress, and breach of fiduciary duty. Quotes Principles VI and VIII. *Scripps Clinic v. Superior Court, 108 Cal. App.4th 917, 134 Cal. Rptr. 2d 101, 117.*

Cal. App. 1978 Surviving spouse sued physicians who were on emergency surgical call panel for malpractice where patient died during surgery. Although defendants claimed immunity under state Good Samaritan statute, the court held the statute inapplicable since the legislative purpose was to encourage physicians to render care on an irregular basis to unattended persons discovered by chance at the scene of an emergency. In so holding, the court noted that Principle 5 (1957) [now Principle VI and Opinions 8.11 and 9.06] imposed an ethical duty to render emergency medical care. *Colby v. Schwartz, 78 Cal. App. 3d 885, 144 Cal. Rptr. 624, 627 n.2.*

Ky. App. 1989 Malpractice suit was initiated against physician for failure to treat plaintiff's brother where defendant had repeatedly rebuffed plaintiff's request for emergency assistance and told him to get in line or sign in. Plaintiff removed his brother to another hospital where he subsequently died of heart attack. Plaintiff argued that defendant was under a duty to treat based upon, inter alia, the AMA Code of Ethics [apparently Principle VI and Opinion 8.11]. The court rejected the argument, finding that a breach of ethical standards may establish grounds for professional discipline, but not a civil cause of action, and held that defendant was under no legal duty to treat. *Noble v. Sartori, 1989 Ky. App. LEXIS 67.*

Minn. 2005 Respondents, providers of massage services, physical therapy, and chiropractic care, attempted to recover benefits from automobile insurers. The trial court dismissed respondents' complaint because it found they violated the corporate practice of medicine doctrine. The appellate court later reversed. The Minnesota Supreme Court affirmed in part and reversed in part. In a separate opinion, concurring in part and dissenting in part, three justices quoting Principle VI would have overruled *Granger v. Adson*, 190 Minn. 23, 250 N.W. 722 (1933) to the extent that it made the corporate practice of medicine doctrine part of Minnesota common law, and found that a ban on the corporate practice of medicine is no longer sound public policy. *Isles Wellness, Inc. v. Progressive N. Ins. Co., 703 N.W.2d 513, 528.*

N.J. Super. 1994 Plaintiff-physician alleged that nursing home violated public policy when it terminated his at-will employment in retaliation for his refusal to see and treat patients in excess of his original workload. With apparent reference to Principle VI, physician argued that caring for excessive numbers of patients violated his ethical responsibilities and public policy. The court held that even though physician's objections to nursing home's practices may have supported a reasonable belief that public policy was violated, there was insufficient evidence that objections contributed to termination. *Fineman v. New Jersey Dept. of Human Servs., 272 N.J. Super. 606, 640 A.2d 1161, 1163, 1166, 1169-70, cert. denied, 138 N.J. 267, 649 A.2d 1287 (1994).*

N.J. Super. 1960 Plaintiff, a graduate of a school of osteopathy and licensed to practice medicine and surgery in New Jersey, sought to compel the defendant medical society to admit him to full membership. Defendant claimed as an affirmative defense that to admit plaintiff would violate Principle 3 (1957) [now Principle VI and Opinion 3.01] because plaintiff possessed a degree in osteopathy rather than an M.D. The court noted that the defendant society had virtually monopolistic control of medical practice in the state and that exclusion from membership caused substantial injury. In view of this, the court ordered the defendant society to admit plaintiff to its membership. To bar membership of a licensed graduate of an approved school of osteopathy would, the court held, violate public policy. *Falcone v. Middlesex County Medical Soc'y, 62 N.J. Super. 184, 162 A.2d 324, 328-29, aff'd, 34 N.J. 582, 170 A.2d 791 (1961).*

N.Y. Sup. 1993 Defendant was charged with violating state statute imposing criminal sanction on a physician who refuses to treat a person seeking emergency medical care. Defendant sought dismissal of the charge challenging the constitutionality of the statute and arguing that [it requires mens rea.] The court denied defendant's motion for dismissal, concluding that the statute was constitutional and that the legislature clearly imposed strict liability. The court quoted Principle VI in support of its strict liability conclusion. *People v. Anyakora, 162 Misc. 2d 47, 616 N.Y.S.2d 149, 155.*

Ohio App. 1991 Medical corporation sought an injunction to enforce a covenant not to compete against defendant-physician. The lower court granted summary judgment based on a referee's report which concluded that under Principle VI and Opinions 6.11, 9.02, and 9.06 (1989), restrictive covenants were per se unenforceable as a matter of public policy. While recognizing a strong public interest in allowing open access to health care, the appellate court in reversing held that Opinion 9.02, which applied specifically to restrictive covenants, only "discouraged" such covenants. *Ohio Urology, Inc. v. Poll, 72 Ohio. App. 446, 450, 451, 594 N.E.2d 1027, 1030, 1031.*

Wash. 1951 Plaintiff, a charitable, not-for-profit medical corporation, offered prepaid health care services to members and their families. Suit was filed against county medical society and others for damages and injunction for defendants' alleged efforts to monopolize prepaid medical care in area and unlawfully restrain competition by plaintiff and its physicians. Defendants alleged as affirmative defense that their efforts were designed to curb unethical prepaid contract practice by plaintiff. Court examined at length AMA's position regarding contract practice including Principles Ch. III, Art. VI, Secs. 3 and 4 (1947) [now Principle VI and Opinions 8.05 and 9.06] concluding nothing in plaintiff's practice violated the AMA's ethical guidelines. Further, quoting Principles Ch. III, Art. III, Sec.1 (1947) [now Opinion 8.04] dealing with consultations, court noted that defendants' efforts impeded plaintiff's physicians from obtaining consultations. Court concluded that defendants' actions constituted unlawful, monopolistic behavior and issued an injunction, although it declined to award damages. *Group Health Coop. v. King County Medical Soc'y, 39 Wash. 2d 586, 237 P.2d 737, 744, 750-51, 759-60.*

Wash. App. 1984 Plaintiff-pathologist sued his corporate employer and one of its subsidiaries for breach of his employment contract; defendants counterclaimed, alleging that plaintiff had tortiously interfered with defendants' business relationships. Plaintiff had discouraged the transfer of laboratory specimens for analysis at a distant lab because he allegedly believed that to do so would be a violation of medical ethics, particularly Principle 6 (1957) [now Principle VI]. In finding for plaintiff, the court acknowledged that a physician was bound to uphold duly prescribed medical ethical principles despite his employment status, especially where such a principle coincided with a public policy favoring acts that tend to prevent a deterioration of the quality of medical care. *Wood v. Upjohn Co., No. 6093-1-II (Sept. 4, 1984) (LEXIS, States library, Wash. file).*

Journal 2011 Discusses the development of lethal autonomous robots, as well as issues raised by this new military technology. Concludes discussion on the advancement and acceptance of lethal autonomous robots is needed on the national and international levels in order to successfully manage advancements in robotic technology. Cites Preamble and Principles I and VI. Allenby, Arkin, Barrett, Borenstein, Gaudet, Kittrie, Lin, Lucas, Marchant, O'Meara, & Silberman, *International Governance of Autonomous Military Robots, 12 Colum. Sci. & Tech. L. Rev. 272, 291 (2011)*.

Journal 2011 Examines barriers to seeking services for communication impairments perceived by lesbian, gay, bisexual, and transgender (LGBT) people. Concludes assumptions of heterosexuality are perceived as prejudices by LGBT patients and impair the delivery of speech pathologist or audiologist services. References Principle VI. Kelly & Robinson, *Disclosure of Membership in the Lesbian, Gay, Bisexual, and Transgender Community by Individuals With Communication Impairments: A Preliminary Web-Based Survey, 20 Am. J. Speech-Language Pathology 86, 90 (2011)*.

Journal 2010 Discusses the inadequacy of sexual minority health care education in medical school curricula and the disparities that exist in medical access for sexual minorities. Concludes medical schools should reevaluate their curricula to improve student understanding of sexual minority health care. Quotes Principle VI. Kolder & Julian, *Teaching About Sexual Minorities: An Iowa Experience, 1 Proc. Obstetrics Gynecology 1, 1 (April 2010, Article 10)*.

Journal 2010 Analyzes factors contributing to the emergence of medical repatriation and evaluates whether this practice comports with current legal and ethical standards. Proposes changes to federal regulations that govern hospitals and clarifications to medical ethical standards. Quotes the Preamble and Principles I, II, III, IV, V, VI, VII, VIII, and IX. Zoellner, *Medical Repatriation: Examining the Legal and Ethical Implications of an Emerging Practice, 32 Wash. U. J. L. & Pol'y 515, 530-532 (2010)*.

Journal 2009 Examines the role of physicians during natural and man-made disasters. Concludes hospitals must make plans to define disaster response procedures that shift responsibility for survival from the physician to the community. Quotes Code of Ethics, Ch. III, Art. I §1 (1847) [now Opinion 9.067], Principle 5 (1957) [now Principle VI], Principle VI, and Opinions 2.23, 9.067, and 9.131. Cites Opinions 9.06, 9.067, and 9.12. Ahronheim, *Service by Health Care Providers in a Public Health Emergency: The Physician's Duty and the Law, 12 J. Health Care L. & Pol'y 195, 209-11, 215, 225 (2009)*.

Journal 2009 Discusses the interaction between statutes and case law governing the medical field and the core principles of medical professionalism. Concludes the legal framework of medical professionalism does not encompass all the elements required of a medical professional. Quotes Principles II, III, IV, V, VI, VII, and VIII. Fichter, *The Law of Doctoring: A Study of the Codification of Medical Professionalism, 19 Health Matrix 317, 338, 339, 340, 343, 351 (2009)*.

Journal 2009 Discusses the judicial standard for reviewing physician noncompete covenants. Concludes courts should apply a strict standard to such covenants, rather than declare the covenants per se invalid. Quotes Principles IV and VII, Principles of Medical Ethics §5 (1957) [now Principle VI], Code of Medical Ethics Ch. II, Art. I §3 (1847) [now Opinion 5.02], Opinion 9.02, and Code of Medical Ethics Ch. II, Art. I §4 (1847) [now Opinion 9.09]. Cites Opinions 8.041, 8.115, 9.02, 9.06, 9.065, 9.067, 10.01, and 10.015. Koons, *Physician Employee Non-Compete Agreements on the Examining Table: The Need to Better Protect Patients' and the Public's Interests in Indiana, 6 Ind. Health L. Rev. 253, 272-77, 280-81 (2009)*.

Journal 2008 Discusses the ethics of physicians offering diagnoses reached through observation of signs in a person who has not approached them for medical advice. Concludes that diagnosis of a nonpatient may be ethical based on considerations of relationship, urgency, risk of harm, and accuracy. Quotes Principle VI. Mitchell, *The Ethics of Passer-By Diagnosis, 371 Lancet 85, 87 (2008)*.

Journal 2008 Explores the legal, ethical, and policy implications of concierge medicine. Argues physicians engaged in concierge care must strive to meet ethical and legal standards, and take care to communicate clearly with patients about services and fees. Quotes Opinion 8.055. Cites Principles II and VI and Opinion 8.055. Portman & Romanow, *Concierge Medicine: Legal Issues, Ethical Dilemmas, and Policy Challenges, 1 J. Health & Life Sci. L. 1, 4, 28-29 (2008)*.

Journal 2008 Examines the development of bioethics and environmental ethics, as well as laws promoting the role of bioethicists in decision making. Concludes environmental ethicists must convince legislatures of the role of environmental ethics in order to have a greater impact on decision making. Quotes Principles I, II, III, IV, V, VI, VII, VIII, and IX. Robertson, *Seeking a Seat at the Table: Has Law Left Environmental Ethics Behind as It Embraces Bioethics?* 32 Wm. & Mary Envtl. L. & Pol'y Rev. 273, 307 (2008).

Journal 2008 Examines the benefits and costs of adopting a tort duty to affirmatively aid and the implications of a criminal law duty to aid. Concludes the absence in American tort and criminal law of an affirmative duty to aid is appropriate despite its contradiction of social and moral values. Quotes Principle VI. Scordato, *Understanding the Absence of a Duty to Reasonably Rescue in American Tort Law,* 82 Tul. L. Rev. 1447, 1486 (2008).

Journal 2007 Compares the role of conscience clauses in various professions. Concludes that conscience clauses in the area of health care must not impede access to care. Quotes Preamble and Principles V, VI, and VIII. Chudoba, *Conscience in America: The Slippery Slope of Mixing Morality With Medicine,* 36 Sw. U. L. Rev. 85, 86, 103, 104, 105 (2007).

Journal 2007 Considers how a physician should treat a patient who has suffered a bad outcome from care provided via "medical tourism." Concludes that the ethical response is to provide care for the patient as for any other. Quotes Principle VI. Jones & McCullough, *What to Do When a Patient's International Medical Care Goes South,* 46 J. of Vascular Surgery 1077, 1078 (2007).

Journal 2007 Questions whether it is ethical for a physician to provide medical care to a family member. Concludes that providing such care becomes increasingly problematic as the likelihood of complications increases. Quotes Principle VI and Opinion 8.19. Oberheu, Jones, & Sade, *A Surgeon Operates on His Son: Wisdom or Hubris?* 84 Ann. Thorac. Surg. 723, 725, 726 (2007).

Journal 2006 Explores the legal and ethical issues surrounding concierge medicine. Concludes that concierge medicine is best restricted to a small class of wealthy individuals. Quotes Principle IX and Opinion 8.055. Cites Principle VI and Opinions 8.055, 8.11, 8.115, 9.065, and 10.05. Carnahan, *Law, Medicine, and Wealth: Does Concierge Medicine Promote Health Care Choice, or is it a Barrier to Access?* 17 Stan. L. & Pol'y Rev. 121, 149-50, 151, 152, 153-54 (2006).

Journal 2006 Explores conscience clause legislation relating to the dispensing of oral contraceptives. Concludes that such legislation must balance the interests of the patient and the health care provider. Cites Principles I, II, III, IV, V, VI, VII, VIII, and IX. Collins, *Conscience Clauses and Oral Contraceptives: Conscientious Objection or Calculated Obstruction?* 15 Ann. Health L. 37, 54 (2006).

Journal 2005 Examines issues surrounding tort reform proposals. Concludes that more can be done to correct the current tort system before moving toward a "one size fits all" approach. Quotes Principles I, II, III, IV, V, VI, VII, VIII, and IX. Messerly & Warwick, *Nowhere to Turn: A Glance at the Facts Behind the Supposed Need for Tort "Reform,"* 28 Hamline L. Rev. 489, 506 (2005).

Journal 2003 Discusses whether compassion represents an adequate ethical response when an individual is suffering. Concludes that compassion may not have a proper role in social or legal decision-making because of its potential to ignore those who are in need. Quotes Principle VI. Shepherd, *Face to Face: A Call for Radical Responsibility in Place of Compassion,* 77 St. John's L. Rev. 445, 472 (2003).

Journal 2001 Discusses the prohibition on nonlawyer ownership of legal service providers. Considers how ethical rules and standards governing physicians have been directed toward preserving independent judgment. Concludes that ethical conflicts created by abandoning the prohibition on nonlawyer ownership of legal service providers may be managed by following the medical ethics model. Quotes Principle VI and Opinions 2.03, 2.09, 8.02, 8.021, 8.03, 8.05, 8.051, 8.054, 8.13, and 8.132. Harris & Foran, *The Ethics of Middle-Class Access to Legal Services and What We Can Learn From the Medical Profession's Shift to a Corporate Paradigm,* 70 Fordham L. Rev. 775, 817, 821, 822, 823, 824 (2001).

Journal 2000 Examines the ethical, social, and moral dilemmas faced by gays and lesbians who desire to have genetically related children. Discusses assisted reproductive technologies most commonly used by gays and lesbians. Explores the barriers associated with access to reproductive technologies by these individuals. Quotes Principle VI. DeLair, *Ethical, Moral, Economic and Legal Barriers to Assisted Reproductive Technologies Employed by Gay Men and Lesbian Women,* 4 DePaul J. Health Care L. 147, 150 (2000).

Journal 2000 Discusses and evaluates different systems for addressing consumer concerns about managed health care. Asserts that current legal systems for identifying and resolving consumer concerns are not understood by most consumers and are not accessible by many, especially the uninsured. Concludes that several immediate steps are realistic for moving toward reform. Cites Principle VI. References Opinions 8.13 and 9.065. Kinney, *Tapping and Resolving Consumer Concerns About Health Care, 26 Am. J. Law & Med. 335, 337, 375 (2000).*

Journal 2000 Discusses managed care in terms of problems, responses, and accomplishments. Demonstrates how a physician union's collective bargaining process can benefit patients and physicians in addressing problems with managed care. Concludes that barriers preventing such unions should be removed. Quotes Principles VI and VII and Opinion 10.01. Rugg, *An Old Solution to a New Problem: Physician Unions Take the Edge Off Managed Care, 34 Colum. J. L. & Soc. Probs. 1, 41 (2000).*

Journal 2000 Examines current laws prohibiting discrimination in the context of access to health care, placing emphasis on people with HIV/AIDS. Considers the implications of *Bragdon v. Abbott.* Concludes that everyone should be entitled to health care in the absence of an acceptable justification for its denial. Quotes Preamble, Principle VI, and Opinion 9.131. Shepherd, *HIV, the ADA, and the Duty to Treat, 37 Hous. L. Rev. 1055, 1061, 1083-84 (2000).*

Journal 1999 Discusses potential conflicts between a criminal defense attorney's religious beliefs and representation of the client. Explores theories that would allow an attorney to put religious beliefs over the client's interest. Offers analogies within the physician-patient relationship. Concludes that a defense attorney is bound by duty and must set aside conflicting religious beliefs. Quotes Principle VI and Opinions 8.11, 9.06, and 9.12. Reza, *Religion and the Public Defender, 26 Fordham Urb. L. J. 1051, 1062, 1063 (1999).*

Journal 1999 Discusses the need for physicians to advocate on behalf of patients' rights in the context of health care delivery. Evaluates the nature and scope of the physician's role as advocate, noting that physicians cannot be expected to engage in attorney-like advocacy. Quotes Principles IV and VI, Fundamental Elements (2), (4), and (6) [now Opinion 10.01], Patient Responsibilities 5 [now Opinion 10.02], and Opinions 2.03, 2.07, 2.09, 2.16, 2.19, 3.06, 4.01, 4.04, 6.01, 7.02, 8.02, 8.03, 8.13, 8.132, 9.06, 9.07, and 9.131. Cites Opinions 5.05, 5.09, 7.01, 8.135, and 9.02. Sage, *Physicians as Advocates, 35 Hous. L. Rev. 1529, 1537, 1541, 1542, 1552-53, 1554, 1556, 1557, 1559, 1561-62, 1564, 1571, 1574, 1576, 1580 (1999).*

Journal 1999 Discusses whether health care professionals have the right to refuse to treat patients under common law and federal statutes and regulations. Explores the impact of the Americans with Disabilities Act and the US Supreme Court decision in *Bragdon v. Abbott* on the duties of health care professionals in the context of providing treatment to HIV-positive patients. Quotes Principle VI and Opinions 2.23 and 9.131. White, *Health Care Professionals and Treatment of HIV-Positive Patients, 20 J. Legal Med. 67, 86 (1999).*

Journal 1998 Discusses the development and existence of the corporate practice of medicine doctrine. Points out that the doctrine is inconsistent with recent changes in the health care system. Suggests that the ban on corporate practice should be eliminated. Cites Principle VI. Freiman, *The Abandonment of the Antiquated Corporate Practice of Medicine Doctrine: Injecting a Dose of Efficiency Into the Modern Health Care Environment, 47 Emory L. J. 697, 712 (1998).*

Journal 1998 Focuses on conflicts of interest and pressures physicians face when treating professional athletes. Discusses case law regarding team physician liability. Concludes that team physicians and their attorneys need to be aware of conflicts of interest that may arise from treatment of professional athletes. Quotes Principle VI (1957) [now most closely embodied by the independent judgment aspects of Principle VI]. Polsky, *Winning Medicine: Professional Sports Team Doctors' Conflicts of Interest, 14 J. Contemp. Health L. & Pol'y 503, 505 (1998).*

Journal 1997 Reports on a study of physician attitudes regarding expert witnesses. Notes that a majority of physicians believe that medical expert testimony should be subject to peer review and, when appropriate, medical licensing board discipline. Quotes Principles II and VI and Opinion 9.07. Eitel, Hegeman, & Evans, *Medicine on Trial: Physicians' Attitudes About Expert Medical Witnesses, 18 J. Legal Med. 345, 355, 358 (1997).*

Journal 1997 Analyzes the prohibition against employment agreements between corporations and licensed physicians. Discusses the origins and development of the corporate practice of medicine doctrine. Proposes that state legislatures should adopt doctrinal modifications to aid in the movement toward managed care. Quotes Principle VI. Mars, *The Corporate Practice of Medicine: A Call for Action,* 7 Health Matrix 241, 267 (1997).

Journal 1996 Discusses the trend toward conserving resources expended on health care by withholding services absent a showing of necessity. Claims that the high standard of care physicians owe patients is jeopardized by medical treatment decisions based on coverage concerns. Concludes that the legal structure regarding health care plans should be changed. Quotes Preamble, Principles I, II, III, IV, V, VI, and VII, and Opinion 2.03. Hirshfeld & Thomason, *Medical Necessity Determinations: The Need for a New Legal Structure,* 6 Health Matrix 3, 8-9 (1996).

Journal 1996 Considers the impact of gag clauses on the physician-patient relationship. Undertakes an extensive legal, ethical, and policy analysis. Concludes that gag clauses are violative of legal and ethical principles. Quotes Principles II, V, and VI and Fundamental Elements (1). Cites Preamble. Martin & Bjerknes, *The Legal and Ethical Implications of Gag Clauses in Physician Contracts,* XXII Am. J. Law & Med. 433, 465-66 (1996).

Journal 1996 Discusses commercialization of the medical industry. Addresses ethical and policy considerations that form the basis for the corporate practice of medicine doctrine. Observes that the doctrine is now outdated. Quotes Principle VI. Parker, *Corporate Practice of Medicine: Last Stand or Final Downfall?* 29 J. Health & Hosp. L. 160, 167, 173 (1996).

Journal 1996 Examines the recent trend in health care laws and ethics to focus on the alleviation of suffering. Expresses concern that such a focus may result in the valuation of one life over another. Emphasizes the need to evaluate multiple, diverse responses to suffering. Quotes Principle VI. References Opinion 2.162. Shepherd, *Sophie's Choices: Medical and Legal Responses to Suffering,* 72 Notre Dame L. Rev. 103, 106, 133 (1996).

Journal 1995 Examines the rights of health care professionals to refuse to participate in patient care on the basis of conscientious objection. Suggests steps that health care facilities may take when dealing with health care professionals who object to participating in patient care. Quotes Principles I and VI and Opinions 1.02, 2.035, and 9.055. Dellinger & Vickery, *When Staff Object to Participating in Care,* 28 J. Health & Hospital Law 269, 272, 276 (1995).

Journal 1995 Offers relevant historical perspectives and provides comprehensive ethical and legal discussion of physician-assisted suicide and euthanasia. Highlights important legislative developments, including the Oregon Death with Dignity Act, and analyzes significant judicial opinions. Quotes Principles III, IV, and VI and Opinions 2.21 and 9.12. Cites Opinions 2.20 and 8.11. Stone & Winslade, *Physician-Assisted Suicide and Euthanasia in the United States: Legal and Ethical Observations,* 16 J. Legal Med. 481, 483, 490, 497, 498, 499 (1995).

Journal 1995 Examines the history of Medicaid physician reimbursement and physician participation. Concludes that states should facilitate tie-ins among Medicaid patients and privately insured patients rather than raising physician fees. Cites Principle VI. Watson, *Medicaid Physician Participation: Patients, Poverty, and Physician Self-interest,* XXI Am. J. Law & Med. 191, 218 (1995).

Journal 1994 Analyzes the corporate practice of medicine doctrine. Asserts that viability of the doctrine is questionable in the modern health care industry. Quotes Principle VI. Dowell, *The Corporate Practice of Medicine Prohibition: A Dinosaur Awaiting Extinction,* 27 J. Health & Hospital Law 369, 370 (1994).

Journal 1994 Explores how the Americans with Disabilities Act has created, through federal civil rights mechanisms, a legal duty to treat HIV-infected patients. Discusses previous attempts to create a professional obligation to treat patients with AIDS. Quotes Principle VI and Opinion 9.131. Cites Opinion 9.12. Halevy & Brody, *Acquired Immunodeficiency Syndrome and the Americans with Disabilities Act: A Legal Duty to Treat,* 96 Am. J. Med. 282, 283, 284 (1994).

Journal 1994 Reviews the evolution of the physician-patient relationship, with attention to patient autonomy. Examines the changing health care delivery environment. Quotes Preamble, Principles I, II, III, IV, V, and VI, Fundamental Elements (1) and (2), and Opinions 1.02 and 8.07 (1981) [now Opinion 8.08]. Cites Opinion 1.01. Szczygiel, *Beyond Informed Consent,* 21 Ohio N. U. L. Rev. 171, 217, 218, 220, 225, 226, 256 (1994).

Journal 1993 Explores the traditional view that lawyers have unfettered discretion to select clients and New York's antidiscrimination disciplinary rule, statutes, and case law. Concludes that the legal profession should prohibit invidious or improper discrimination. Quotes Principle VI and Opinions 9.12 and 9.131. Begg, *Revoking the Lawyers' License to Discriminate in New York: The Demise of a Traditional Professional Prerogative*, 7 Geo. J. Legal Ethics 275, 298, 299 (1993).

Journal 1993 Addresses both patient rights under California consent and confidentiality laws relating to AIDS and prohibitions on unreasonable searches and seizures under the US Constitution. Concludes that any health care worker who can document an exposure to blood or body fluids should have the option of compelling a nonconsenting patient to be tested for HIV. Quotes Principle VI and Opinion 9.131. Comment, *Nonconsensual HIV Testing in the Health Care Setting: The Case for Extending the Occupational Protections of California Proposition 96 to Health Care Workers*, 26 Loy. L. A. L. Rev. 1251, 1269 (1993).

Journal 1993 Discusses physicians' duty to disclose to patients medical treatment alternatives that are not readily available. Proposes that based on the historical development and legal requirements of the informed consent doctrine, physicians should be required to inform patients of non–readily available alternatives or face liability for breach of such obligation. Quotes Principles I, II, III, IV, and V and Opinion 8.08. Note, *Informed Choice: Physicians' Duty to Disclose Nonreadily Available Alternatives*, 43 Case W. Res. L. Rev. 491, 491, 498-99, 508, 509 (1993).

Journal 1993 Explores the idea of reverse informed consent, which would impose a duty on patients to inform health care professionals of their infectious status. Concludes that such a duty is justified. Quotes Principles IV and VI and Opinions 8.11 and 9.131. Oddi, *Reverse Informed Consent: The Unreasonably Dangerous Patient*, 46 Vand. L. Rev. 1417, 1449, 1463, 1465, 1479 (1993).

Journal 1992 Discusses the plight of undocumented aliens and their need for access to medical care. Considers existing systems for providing such care, as well as barriers to the receipt of medical attention. Cites Principles VI and VII. Loue, *Access to Health Care and the Undocumented Alien*, 13 J. Legal Med. 271, 291 (1992).

Journal 1991 Considers whether physicians have an obligation to provide medical care to HIV-infected patients. Examines various sources for such a duty, including a moral obligation not to discriminate and a social responsibility to provide access to health care. Quotes Opinion 9.131. Cites Principle VI. Daniels, *Duty to Treat or Right to Refuse?* 21 Hastings Center Rep. 36, 37, 42 (March/April 1991).

Journal 1991 Discusses the problem of noncompliant patients and whether a physician may deny treatment to these individuals. Concludes that physicians are not relieved of their duty to treat noncompliant patients, especially because these patients may not be able to adequately control their behavior. Cites Principle VI and Opinion 9.12. Orentlicher, *Denying Treatment to the Noncompliant Patient*, 265 JAMA 1579, 1581 (1991).

Journal 1990 Examines the relationship between professional ethics and professional autonomy, perceived problems of health care rationing under a prospective payment vs a fee-for-service system, and the relationship between professional ethics and the problem of rationing. Concludes that rationing is inevitable, forcing important ethical questions to be addressed. Quotes Principles IV and VI. Agich, *Rationing and Professional Autonomy*, 18 Law Med. & Health Care 77, 79, 82 (1990).

Journal 1990 Considers the propriety of HIV testing for hospital patients prior to nonemergency surgery. Concludes that testing of patients should be permitted so long as it is not done with the intent, nor the effect, of discriminating against individual patients. Quotes Principle VI and Opinion 9.131. Naccasha, *The Permissibility of Routine AIDS Testing in the Health Care Context*, 5 Notre Dame J. L. Ethics & Pub. Pol'y, 223, 241 (1990).

Journal 1990 Discusses a physician's duty to treat AIDS patients. Concludes that there is a weak basis for imposing an ethical duty to treat, but suggests that a legal duty may be fashioned. Quotes Principle V (1980) [now Principle VII]. Note, *Ethics and AIDS: A Summary of the Law and a Critical Analysis of the Individual Physician's Ethical Duty to Treat*, XVI Am. J. Law & Med. 249, 262 (1990).

Journal 1990 Discusses the moral dilemma in deciding whether to withdraw artificial nutrition and hydration from a patient and the appropriate role of the judiciary. Concludes that judicial decisions do not represent the moral viewpoint of society and that moral pronouncements should not be made in the courtroom. Quotes Preamble, Principles I, II, III, IV, V, VI, and VII and

Opinion 2.20. Peccarelli, *A Moral Dilemma: The Role of Judicial Intervention in Withholding or Withdrawing Nutrition and Hydration*, 23 John Marshall L. Rev. 537, 539, 540, 541 (1990).

Journal 1989 Discusses the legal and ethical challenges that AIDS poses for health care providers. Proposes that health care providers actively participate in preventing HIV infection, providing care for HIV-infected individuals, and fighting AIDS and its associated stigma. Quotes Principle VI and Opinion 9.131. Forrester, *AIDS: The Responsibility to Care*, 34 Vill. L. Rev. 799, 811 (1989).

Journal 1989 Discusses common law developments in the 1960s and 1970s that established a duty to provide emergency care and treatment. Observes that the common law met with only limited success in this regard and concludes that the Consolidated Omnibus Budget Reconciliation Act of 1985 offers the greatest likelihood for creating a nationally enforceable legal duty to provide emergency care. Quotes Principle VI. Rothenberg, *Who Cares? The Evolution of the Legal Duty to Provide Emergency Care*, 26 Houston L. Rev. 21, 22 (1989).

Journal 1988 Noting that safety precautions have been recommended by Centers for Disease Control and Prevention (CDC) and Occupational Safety and Health Administration (OSHA), observes that, despite these measures, if health care providers believe that a risk of contagion exists when caring for HIV-seropositive patients, they may take steps to limit exposure by reducing care. Against this background, it is suggested that policies be developed to help ensure that the threat of AIDS does not limit access to care for such patients. Quotes Principle 5 (1980) [sic] [now Principle VI]. Brennan, *Ensuring Adequate Health Care for the Sick: The Challenge of the Acquired Immunodeficiency Syndrome as an Occupational Disease*, 1988 Duke L. J. 29, 47.

Journal 1988 Discusses the question of whether health professionals are obligated to subject themselves to the risks that attend treating patients with communicable diseases, particularly AIDS. Examines the ethical pronouncements and codes of the nursing and medical professions in this respect, noting that the most recent statements of professional values imply the existence of an obligation to treat HIV-infectious patients. Quotes Opinion 8.10 (1986) [now Opinion 8.11] and Principle VI. Cites Opinion 9.11 (1986) [now Opinion 9.12]. Freedman, *Health Professions, Codes, and the Right to Refuse to Treat HIV-Infectious Patients*, 18 Hastings Center Rep. 20 (Supp.), 23, 24 (April/May 1988).

Journal 1986 Examines common law and statutory law applicable to patient dumping, and emphasizes the antidumping provisions of Consolidated Omnibus Budget Reconciliation Act (COBRA). Weaknesses in this federal legislative scheme are highlighted, and recommendations for strengthening the statute and maximizing access to emergency medical care are offered. Quotes Principle VI and Opinion 8.10 (1986) [now Opinion 8.11]. Note, *Preventing Patient Dumping: Sharpening the COBRA's Fangs*, 61 N. Y. U. L. Rev. 1186, 1189-90 (1986).

VII. A physician shall recognize a responsibility to participate in activities contributing to the improvement of the community and the betterment of public health.

Ariz. 1965 Physician appealed denial of medical license which was based on alleged violations of local medical society rules and Principles 3, 5, and 10 (1957) [now Principles III and VII and Opinions 3.01, 8.11, and 9.06]. Alleged violations included treating a patient without first obtaining a prior treating physician's permission, inadequate patient care, performing operations without hospital privileges, and signing the medical record of a deceased patient who had been treated by interns. The court held that the evidence failed to show any clear violation of the Principles and that a local medical society had no right to prescribe a code of ethics for state licensing purposes. *Arizona State Bd. of Medical Examiners v. Clark*, 97 Ariz. 205, 398 P.2d 908, 914-15, 915 n.3.

Journal 2010 Examines the physicians' "Right of Conscience" (ROC) and professional integrity within the context of the patient-physician relationship. Discusses the evolution of the patient-physician relationship and the legal transition of empowering patient autonomy. Concludes physicians should be allowed limited ROC to prevent marginalization of physicians' morals and values while ultimately strengthening the patient-physician relationship. Quotes Principle VII. Gold, *Physicians' "Right of Conscience"—Beyond Politics*, 38 J. L. Med & Ethics, 134, 138 (2010).

Journal 2010 Analyzes factors contributing to the emergence of medical repatriation and evaluates whether this practice comports with current legal and ethical standards. Proposes changes to federal regulations that govern hospitals and clarifications to medical ethical standards. Quotes the Preamble and Principles I, II, III, IV, V, VI, VII, VIII, and IX. Zoellner, *Medical Repatriation: Examining the Legal and Ethical Implications of an Emerging Practice, 32 Wash. U. J. L. & Pol'y 515, 530-532 (2010)*.

Journal 2009 Discusses the interaction between statutes and case law governing the medical field and the core principles of medical professionalism. Concludes the legal framework of medical professionalism does not encompass all the elements required of a medical professional. Quotes Principles II, III, IV, V, VI, VII, and VIII. Fichter, *The Law of Doctoring: A Study of the Codification of Medical Professionalism, 19 Health Matrix 317, 338, 339, 340, 343, 351 (2009)*.

Journal 2009 Discusses the essential role of professionals in the community and the conflicting moral obligations facing professionals. Concludes the legal profession's insistence that priority be given exclusively to the client's interests prevents it from successfully addressing ethical problems. Cites Preamble and Principle VII. Greenstein, *Against Professionalism, 22 Geo. J. Legal Ethics 327, 349 (2009)*.

Journal 2009 Discusses the judicial standard for reviewing physician noncompete covenants. Concludes courts should apply a strict standard to such covenants, rather than declare the covenants per se invalid. Quotes Principles IV and VII, Principles of Medical Ethics §5 (1957) [now Principle VI], Code of Medical Ethics Ch. II, Art. I §3 (1847) [now Opinion 5.02], Opinion 9.02, and Code of Medical Ethics Ch. II, Art. I §4 (1847) [now Opinion 9.09]. Cites Opinions 8.041, 8.115, 9.02, 9.06, 9.065, 9.067, 10.01, and 10.015. Koons, *Physician Employee Non-Compete Agreements on the Examining Table: The Need to Better Protect Patients' and the Public's Interests in Indiana, 6 Ind. Health L. Rev. 253, 272-77, 280-81 (2009)*.

Journal 2008 Examines the development of bioethics and environmental ethics, as well as laws promoting the role of bioethicists in decision making. Concludes environmental ethicists must convince legislatures of the role of environmental ethics in order to have a greater impact on decision making. Quotes Principles I, II, III, IV, V, VI, VII, VIII, and IX. Robertson, *Seeking a Seat at the Table: Has Law Left Environmental Ethics Behind as it Embraces Bioethics? 32 Wm. & Mary Envtl. L. & Pol'y Rev. 273, 307 (2008)*.

Journal 2008 Argues that as a matter of public health, physicians must control antibiotic administration to combat antibiotic resistance. Concludes that despite limited incentives for antibiotic conservation, physicians must acknowledge their important role in mitigating the public health threat of antibiotic resistance. Quotes Principles VII and VIII and Opinions 2.09 and 10.015. Cites Opinion 2.03. Saver, *In Tepid Defense of Population Health: Physicians and Antibiotic Resistance, 34 Am. J. L. & Med. 431, 457 (2008)*.

Journal 2008 Questions why pediatricians are not more involved in community activities. Concludes that greater community involvement might boost morale in the profession. Quotes Principle VII. Wilson, *Dwindling Community Involvement: A Sign of Professional Failure to Thrive? 162 Arch. Pediatr. Adolesc. Med. 695, 695 (2008)*.

Journal 2007 Examines physicians' duty to treat victims of highly infectious diseases during an epidemic. Concludes that no clear duty exists, and that if physicians are compelled to provide care by law they must be afforded sufficient due process to protect their property interests in their medical licenses. Quotes Ch. III, Art. I, Sec. I (May 1847) [now Opinions 2.25 and 9.067] and Opinion 9.131. References Principle 10 (1957) [now Principle VII]. Schwartz, *Doubtful Duty: Physicians' Legal Obligation to Treat During an Epidemic, 60 Stan. L. Rev. 657, 662, 663 (2007)*.

Journal 2006 Examines the legal and public health issues raised by increased rates of hepatitis C in prison populations. Concludes that reform is needed to provide adequate health care to prisoners and that courts have the power to require such care under the Eighth Amendment. Quotes Preamble, Principles VII, VIII, and IX, and Opinion 10.015. Brunsden, *Hepatitis C in Prisons: Evolving Toward Decency Through Adequate Medical Care and Public Health Reform, 54 UCLA L. Rev. 465, 500 (2006)*.

Journal 2006 Explores conscience clause legislation relating to the dispensing of oral contraceptives. Concludes that such legislation must balance the interests of the patient and the health care provider. Cites Principles I, II, III, IV, V, VI, VII, VIII, and IX. Collins, *Conscience Clauses and Oral Contraceptives: Conscientious Objection or Calculated Obstruction? 15 Ann. Health L. 37, 54 (2006)*.

Journal 2006 Considers the interaction of laws, rules, and guidelines in the area of health law. Suggests that the legislature should revise current laws to reflect local variability in practice. Quotes Preamble and Principles VII and IX. Heimer, *Responsibility in Health Care: Spanning the Boundary Between Law and Medicine, 41 Wake Forest L. Rev. 465, 498 (2006).*

Journal 2006 Examines methods of teaching law students about social justice. Concludes that a change in teaching methods would encourage students to place a higher value on furthering social justice. Quotes Principle VII. Rand, *An Interdisciplinary Search for Help Through Social Work's Empowerment Approach, 13 Clinical L. Rev. 459, 477 (2006).*

Journal 2005 Examines issues surrounding tort reform proposals. Concludes that more can be done to correct the current tort system before moving toward a "one size fits all" approach. Quotes Principles I, II, III, IV, V, VI, VII, VIII, and IX. Messerly & Warwick, *Nowhere to Turn: A Glance at the Facts Behind the Supposed Need for Tort "Reform," 28 Hamline L. Rev. 489, 506 (2005).*

Journal 2005 Examines the practice of "boutique medicine" and considers legal and ethical implications. Concludes that boutique medical services would be ethical only if physicians used retainer money from their boutique clients to augment health care costs of the poor. Quotes Principles VII and IX and Opinion 8.055. Russano, *Is Boutique Medicine a New Threat to American Health Care or a Logical Way of Revitalizing the Doctor-Patient Relationship? 17 Wash. U. J. L. & Pol'y 313, 331, 332 (2005).*

Journal 2005 Discusses ethical, legal, and policy issues associated with treatment and research involving patients who are in a persistent vegetative or minimally conscious state. Concludes that patients in these states are at risk for therapeutic failures until physicians can more accurately determine which patients will benefit from treatment and accurately convey such information to families or surrogates. Quotes Principles VII and IX and Opinions 8.031, 8.0315, 9.065, 10.01, and 10.015. Tovino & Winslade, *A Primer on the Law and Ethics of Treatment, Research, and Public Policy in the Context of Severe Traumatic Brain Injury, 14 Ann. Health L. 1, 18, 38, 39, 40, 41 (2005).*

Journal 2004 Argues that the corporate practice of medicine doctrine is no longer practical in today's health care system. Concludes that federal legislation must be enacted to align the states on the issue and to ensure that physicians may practice in a way that benefits patients and the health care system. Quotes Principle VI. Huberfeld, *Be Not Afraid of Change: Time to Eliminate the Corporate Practice of Medicine Doctrine, 14 Health Matrix 243, 256 (2004).*

Journal 2003 Discusses conflicts of interest caused when managed care organizations provide financial incentives to physicians. Concludes that the focus of managed care is not well-suited for the doctor-patient relationship. Quotes Opinion 8.03. Cites Principle VII. References Opinion 8.051. Hall, *Bargaining With Hippocrates: Managed Care and the Doctor-Patient Relationship, 54 SC L. Rev. 689, 696, 735 (2003).*

Journal 2003 Considers a legislative plan allowing voluntary, consensual organ donation by condemned prisoners. Concludes that, in view of the current organ shortage, the benefits of such a plan outweigh the concerns. Quotes Principle VII and Opinion 2.06. Perales, *Rethinking the Prohibition of Death Row Prisoners as Organ Donors: A Possible Lifeline to Those on Organ Donor Waiting Lists, 34 St. Mary's L. J. 687, 721, 725 (2003).*

Journal 2001 Examines international ethical guidelines for psychiatrists. Observes that many psychiatrists are unaware of the relevant guidelines. Concludes that information about these guidelines should be more widely disseminated with a goal of increased compliance. Quotes Principle VII. Martens, *Necessity of Adapting Psychiatric Treatment to Relevant Ethical Guidelines, 20 Med. Law 393, 394 (2001).*

Journal 2000 Discusses managed care in terms of problems, responses, and accomplishments. Demonstrates how a physician union's collective bargaining process can benefit patients and physicians in addressing problems with managed care. Concludes that barriers preventing such unions should be removed. Quotes Principles VI and VII and Opinion 10.01. Rugg, *An Old Solution to a New Problem: Physician Unions Take the Edge Off Managed Care, 34 Colum. J. L. & Soc. Probs. 1, 41 (2000).*

Journal 1996 Discusses the trend toward conserving resources expended on health care by withholding services absent a showing of necessity. Claims that the high standard of care physicians owe patients is jeopardized by medical treatment decisions based on coverage concerns.

Concludes that the legal structure regarding health care plans should be changed. Quotes Preamble, Principles I, II, III, IV, V, VI, and VII, and Opinion 2.03. Hirshfeld & Thomason, *Medical Necessity Determinations: The Need for a New Legal Structure, 6 Health Matrix 3, 8-9 (1996).*

Journal 1996 Proposes an alternative method of capital punishment to allow for organ donation by executed prisoners. Provides justifications for this proposal. Concludes that physicians should be able to ethically participate in this process. Quotes Principle VII. Cites Opinion 2.06. References Opinion 2.162 (1994) [subsequently amended]. Patton, *A Call for Common Sense: Organ Donation and the Executed Prisoner, 3 Va. J. Soc. Pol'y & L. 387, 404, 405, 407-10 (1996).*

Journal 1995 Explores the debates and commentaries regarding patenting medical instruments and processes. Concludes that current patent law fails to address the ethical concerns of physicians and their patients. Quotes Principles of Medical Ethics §10 (1971) [now Principle VII] and Principle §2 (1971) [now Opinion 9.095] and Opinions 9.08 and 9.09. Reisman, *Physicians and Surgeons as Inventors: Reconciling Medical Process Patents and Medical Ethics, 10 High Tech. L. J. 355, 356, 368-70, 385 (1995).*

Journal 1992 Discusses the problem of discrimination based on HIV status, particularly among women and children. Examines medical and public health issues involving HIV. Cites Principle VII. References Opinion 9.131. Gittler & Rennart, *HIV Infection Among Women and Children and Antidiscrimination Laws: An Overview, 77 Iowa L. Rev. 1313, 1363 (1992).*

Journal 1992 Discusses the plight of undocumented aliens and their need for access to medical care. Considers existing systems for providing such care, as well as barriers to the receipt of medical attention. Cites Principles VI and VII. Loue, *Access to Health Care and the Undocumented Alien, 13 J. Legal Med. 271, 291 (1992).*

Journal 1990 Discusses the moral dilemma in deciding whether to withdraw artificial nutrition and hydration from a patient and the appropriate role of the judiciary. Concludes that judicial decisions do not represent the moral viewpoint of society and that moral pronouncements should not be made in the courtroom. Quotes Preamble, Principles I, II, III, IV, V, VI, and VII, and Opinion 2.20. Peccarelli, *A Moral Dilemma: The Role of Judicial Intervention in Withholding or Withdrawing Nutrition and Hydration, 23 John Marshall L. Rev. 537, 539, 540, 541 (1990).*

VIII.   A physician shall, while caring for a patient, regard responsibility to the patient as paramount.

Cal. App. 2003 Patient and her husband sued medical clinic for terminating care after the patient filed malpractice claims against two clinic physicians. Clinic's policy required termination of all medical care for patients and their families in such a situation. Appeals court upheld summary judgment for the clinic on several claims, but denied summary judgment on claims for interference with contractual relations, negligent infliction of emotional distress, and breach of fiduciary duty. Quotes Principles VI and VIII. *Scripps Clinic v. Superior Court, 108 Cal. App.4th 917, 134 Cal. Rptr. 2d 101, 117.*

Ohio 2009 Physician appealed from a judgment affirming an order of the state medical board that permanently revoked appellant's certificate to practice medicine. The board found that appellant's sexual contact with patients violated Ohio statutes governing physician conduct and the AMA's Code of Medical Ethics, citing Principles I, II, IV, and VIII. The Court of Appeals held that Ohio state law allows the board to revoke a physician's certificate if it finds that the person violated any provision of the Code of Ethics of the AMA. *D'Souza v. State Med. Bd. of Ohio, 2009 WL 5108774, 6.*

Journal 2011 Examines the way in which the actuary delivers services in the context of the pension funding crises that exist in the United States. Concludes by offering proposals for self-regulatory mechanisms to address the practices within the profession that have been identified as factors that contributed to the crisis in pension funding. Cites Principle VIII. Gunz & Jennings, *A Proactive Proposal for Self-regulation of the Actuarial Profession: A Means of Avoiding the Audit Profession's Post-Enron Regulatory Fate, 48 Am. Bus. L.J. 641, 654 (2011).*

Journal 2011 Reviews the responsible conduct of research (RCR) domains of publication practices and authorship, conflicts of interest, and research misconduct. Concludes that because the accuracy, completeness, and value of the scientific record impact the health of society, scientists are obligated to use the highest possible standards of research conduct. Quotes Principle VIII and Opinion 8.031. Horner & Minifie, *Research Ethics III: Publication Practices and Authorship, Conflicts of Interest, and Research Misconduct*, 54 J. Speech, Language, & Hearing Res. S346, S351, S352 (2011).

Journal 2011 Reviews the use and current regulation of medical marijuana to alleviate pain in terminally ill patients. Focusing on patient autonomy, concludes that patients should have access to medical marijuana in controlled doses under controlled conditions. Quotes Principle III and Opinions 10.01, 10.015, and 10.02. References Principle VIII. Pfeifer, *Smoking Gun: The Moral and Legal Struggle for Medical Marijuana*, 27 Touro L. Rev. 339, 340-41, 345-346 (2011).

Journal 2010 Examines the growth and regulation of donor-assisted reproduction. Concludes reform is needed to permit children to access genetic and health information, with the goal of increasing the safety of donor-assisted reproduction while maintaining donor anonymity. Quotes Principle VIII. Luetkemeyer, *Who's Guarding the Henhouse and What Are They Doing With the Eggs (and Sperm)? A Call for Increased Regulation of Gamete Donation and Long-term Tracking of Donor Gametes*, 3 St. Louis U. J. Health L. & Pol'y 397, 414 (2010).

Journal 2010 Analyzes factors contributing to the emergence of medical repatriation and evaluates whether this practice comports with current legal and ethical standards. Proposes changes to federal regulations that govern hospitals and clarifications to medical ethical standards. Quotes the Preamble and Principles I, II, III, IV, V, VI, VII, VIII, and IX. Zoellner, *Medical Repatriation: Examining the Legal and Ethical Implications of an Emerging Practice*, 32 Wash. U. J. L. & Pol'y 515, 530-532 (2010).

Journal 2009 Explores emerging issues in conflict management systems design (CMSD). Concludes as the practice of CMSD in the organizational context continues to expand, practitioners should openly discuss the emerging issues of the field. References Principles I, II, V, and VIII. Costantino, *Second Generation Organizational Conflict Management Systems Design: A Practitioner's Perspective on Emerging Issues*, 14 Harv. Negot. L. Rev. 81, 95 (2009).

Journal 2009 Examines therapeutic uses of cannabis and the legal and social controversies surrounding its legalization. Concludes changes in the regulation of medical cannabis are necessary to better care for patients and better utilize resources that are currently directed toward the war on drugs. Quotes Principle VIII and Opinion 2.17. DiFonzo, *The End of the Red Queen's Race: Medical Marijuana in the New Century*, 27 Quinnipiac L. Rev. 673, 736, 737 (2009).

Journal 2009 Discusses the interaction between statutes and case law governing the medical field and the core principles of medical professionalism. Concludes the legal framework of medical professionalism does not encompass all the elements required of a medical professional. Quotes Principles II, III, IV, V, VI, VII, and VIII. Fichter, *The Law of Doctoring: A Study of the Codification of Medical Professionalism*, 19 Health Matrix 317, 338, 339, 340, 343, 351 (2009).

Journal 2009 Discusses the importance of trust in the physician-patient and in the attorney-client relationship. Notes the lack of an appropriate remedy for breaches of fiduciary duties. Concludes there should be a statutory remedy for breaches of trust in the professional relationship. Quotes Principle VIII. Forell & Sortun, *The Tort of Betrayal of Trust*, 42 U. Mich. J. L. Reform, 557, 603 (2009).

Journal 2009 Explores the jurisprudential foundation of the fiduciary duty physicians owe their patients and discusses the failure of physicians to disclose to patients errors and other emergent medical risks. Concludes law should recognize the physician's duty to disclose such risks by enforcing a cause of action for breach of that duty. Quotes Principles III and VIII and Opinions 8.12, 10.015, and 10.02. References Opinion 8.12. Hafemeister, *Lean on Me: A Physician's Fiduciary Duty to Disclose an Emergent Medical Risk to the Patient*, 86 Wash. U. L. Rev. 1167, 1172-1173, 1178, 1182, 1185, 1188, 1209 (2009).

Journal 2009 Explores the nature of the physician-patient relationship and the impact of increased availability of medical information on patient autonomy and physician responsibility to exercise independent judgment. Concludes physicians must treat patients in accordance with their fiduciary obligation to use their own judgment when confronted with a patient demanding unnecessary medical services. Quotes Preamble, Principles I and VIII, and Opinions 2.035, 8.03, and 10.015. Hafemeister, *The Fiduciary Obligation of Physicians to "Just Say No" if an "Informed" Patient Demands Services That Are Not Medically Indicated*, 39 Seton Hall L. Rev. 335, 372, 373, 374 (2009).

Journal 2009 Discusses whether or not patients have a right to pain management. Concludes that no physician duty is established by law or ethics to provide pain management outside the traditional physician-patient relationship. Cites Principles I, II, IV, and VIII. Hall & Boswell, *Ethics, Law, and Pain Management as a Patient Right*, 12 Pain Physician 499, 500 (2009).

Journal 2008 Discusses ex parte interviews with a treating physician in discovery before and after the HIPAA Privacy Rule and the issues facing physicians contacted for such interviews. Concludes courts and attorneys should work together to allow for efficient discovery while protecting physicians. Quotes Principles IV and VIII and Opinions 5.05 and 10.01. Burnette & Morning, HIPAA *and Ex Parte Interviews—The Beginning of the End?* 1 J. Health & Life Sci. L. 73, 100-01 (2008).

Journal 2008 Discusses legal and ethical considerations in making organ transplants available to qualified incarcerated individuals at public expense. Concludes legal and ethical norms suggest organ transplants should be made available to prisoners and new policies should be established to provide necessary transplant services. Apparent reference to Principle VIII. McKinney, Winslade, & Stone, *Offender Organ Transplants: Law, Ethics, Economics, and Health Policy*, 9 Hous. J. Health L. & Pol'y 39, 62 (2008).

Journal 2008 Discusses covenants not to compete and Kentucky cases dealing with physician noncompetition agreements. Concludes Kentucky should enact legislation permitting reasonable noncompetition agreements ancillary to sale of practice contracts to increase patient choice of physician. Quotes Principle VIII and Opinion 9.02. Naiser, *Physician Noncompetition Agreements in Kentucky: The Past Discounting of Public Interests and a Proposed Solution*, 47 U. Louisville L. Rev. 195, 195, 200 (2008).

Journal 2008 Examines the development of bioethics and environmental ethics, as well as laws promoting the role of bioethicists in decision making. Concludes environmental ethicists must convince legislatures of the role of environmental ethics in order to have a greater impact on decision making. Quotes Principles I, II, III, IV, V, VI, VII, VIII, and IX. Robertson, *Seeking a Seat at the Table: Has Law Left Environmental Ethics Behind as It Embraces Bioethics?* 32 Wm. & Mary Envtl. L. & Pol'y Rev. 273, 307 (2008).

Journal 2008 Examines ethical issues related to broadcasting cardiothoracic surgeries for educational and media purposes. Concludes that seven ethical guidelines should be followed to ensure patient safety. Quotes Principle VIII and Opinion 8.121. Sade, *Broadcast of Surgical Procedures as a Teaching Instrument in Cardiothoracic Surgery*, 86 Ann. Thorac. Surg. 357, 359 (2008).

Journal 2008 Argues that as a matter of public health, physicians must control antibiotic administration to combat antibiotic resistance. Concludes that despite limited incentives for antibiotic conservation, physicians must acknowledge their important role in mitigating the public health threat of antibiotic resistance. Quotes Principles VII and VIII and Opinions 2.09 and 10.015. Cites Opinion 2.03. Saver, *In Tepid Defense of Population Health: Physicians and Antibiotic Resistance*, 34 Am. J. L. & Med. 431, 457 (2008).

Journal 2008 Explores the fiduciary relationship between physicians and patients, professional and ethical obligations of both physicians and lawyers, and the implications for conflict resolution in health care. Concludes physicians must put patient interests above their own and lawyers must work to discern clients' best interests and support client welfare. Quotes Principle VIII and Opinions 8.12 and 10.015. Cites Principles I and II and Opinions 10.01 and 10.015. Scott, *Doctors as Advocates, Lawyers as Healers*, 29 Hamline J. Pub. L. Pol'y, 331, 340-41, 347, 371 (2008).

Journal 2007 Compares the role of conscience clauses in various professions. Concludes that conscience clauses in the area of health care must not impede access to care. Quotes Preamble and Principles V, VI, and VIII. Chudoba, *Conscience in America: The Slippery Slope of Mixing Morality With Medicine*, 36 Sw. U. L. Rev. 85, 86, 103, 104, 105 (2007).

Journal 2007 Addresses physician liability for an extramarital affair with a patient's spouse. Concludes that such an affair should be regarded as a breach of a fiduciary duty. Quotes Preamble, Principles I, II, and VIII, and Opinions 8.145, 9.04, 9.123, and 10.015. Demaine, *"Playing Doctor" With the Patient's Spouse: Alternative Conceptions of Health Professional Liability*, 14 Va. J. Soc. Pol'y & L. 308, 325, 330-31, 331-32 (2007).

Journal 2007 Discusses the evolution of informed consent doctrine. Concludes that, in context of research, informed consent exceptions should be substantially narrowed. Quotes Ch. I, Art. I, Sec. 4 (May 1847) [now Opinion 8.082] and Ch. I, Art. I, Sec. 1 (May 1847) [now Principles I and

VIII]. References Opinions 2.08 and 8.08. Grimm, *Informed Consent for All! No Exceptions, 37 N. M. L. Rev. 39, 39, 61 (2007).*

Journal 2007 Analyzes drafters' original intent for the Confrontation Clause as well as the contemporary interpretation under Crawford. Concludes that only statements taken by law enforcement agents should be considered testimonial in nature. Quotes Principle VIII. Harbinson, *Crawford v. Washington and Davis v. Washington's Originalism: Historical Arguments Showing Child Abuse Victims' Statements to Physicians Are Nontestimonial and Admissible as an Exception to the Confrontation Clause, 58 Mercer L. Rev. 569, 617 (2007).*

Journal 2007 Evaluates the added cost of extrarenal findings in CT imaging of kidney donors. Concludes that because incidental findings arise in 28% of cases, pertinent ethical issues should be considered. References Principle VIII. Maizlin, Barnard, Gourlayz, & Brown, *Economic and Ethical Impact of Extrarenal Findings on Potential Living Kidney Donor Assessment with Computed Tomography Angiography, 20 Transplant Int'l. 338, 341 (2007).*

Journal 2006 Evaluates the constitutionality of federal faith-based initiative programs. Concludes that such programs violate the First Amendment under the combined Lemon and Zelman test. Cites Principles II and VIII. Boden, *Compassion Inaction: Why President Bush's Faith-Based Initiatives Violate the Establishment Clause, 29 Seattle U. L. Rev. 991, 1023 (2006).*

Journal 2006 Examines ethical dilemmas physicians may face as providers of pay-for-performance medical care. Concludes that this strategy offers a benefit to patients as long as physicians uphold stringent ethical standards and work together to ensure optimum patient care. Cites Principles I, V, VIII, and IX and Opinions 2.035, 2.095, 6.01, 8.021, 8.03, 8.0501, 8.053, 8.054, and 8.121. Bostick, Sade, & McMahon, *Report of the Council on Ethical and Judicial Affairs: Physician Pay-for-Performance Programs, 3 Ind. Health L. Rev. 429, 430, 431, 432-33, 434, 435, 436 (2006).*

Journal 2006 Examines the legal and public health issues raised by increased rates of Hepatitis C in prison populations. Concludes that reform is needed to provide adequate health care to prisoners and that courts have the power to require such care under the Eighth Amendment. Quotes Preamble, Principles VII, VIII, and IX, and Opinion 10.015. Brunsden, *Hepatitis C in Prisons: Evolving Toward Decency Through Adequate Medical Care and Public Health Reform, 54 UCLA L. Rev. 465, 500 (2006).*

Journal 2006 Explores conscience clause legislation relating to the dispensing of oral contraceptives. Concludes that such legislation must balance the interests of the patient and the health care provider. Cites Principles I, II, III, IV, V, VI, VII, VIII, and IX. Collins, *Conscience Clauses and Oral Contraceptives: Conscientious Objection or Calculated Obstruction? 15 Ann. Health L. 37, 54 (2006).*

Journal 2006 Discusses mentally incompetent inmates and capital punishment. Proposes that, to be permissible, involuntary medication of death-row inmates must represent the best medically appropriate treatment. Quotes Principles I, III, and VIII and Opinion 2.06. Gabos, *The Perils of Singleton v. Norris: Ethics and Beyond, 32 Am. J. L. & Med. 117, 118, 125-26, 127 (2006).*

Journal 2006 Examines the practice of law firms employing their own in-house counsel. Concludes there will likely be an increase in firms that retain in-house counsel to represent them. Quotes Principle VIII. Gorman, *Empirical Studies of the Legal Profession: What Do We Know About Lawyers' Lives?: Explaining the Spread of Law Firm In-House Counsel Positions: A Response to Professor Chambliss. 84 N. C. L. Rev. 1577, 1585.*

Journal 2006 Discusses the prevalence and cause of physicians' failure to provide proper care. Concludes that patients should be able to sue their physicians for breach of fiduciary duty. Quotes Principle VIII and Opinion 8.03. Mehlman, *Dishonest Medical Mistakes, 59 Vand. L. Rev. 1137, 1144 (2006).*

Journal 2006 Examines a mental health professional's competing duties of confidentiality and reporting a patient's threats of violence. Suggests new legislation should clarify duty to report a threat. Quotes Preamble and Principles III, IV, and VIII. Cites Opinion 5.05. Mossman, *Critique of Pure Risk Assessment or, Kant Meets Tarasoff, 75 U. Cin. L. Rev. 523, 579 (2006).*

Journal 2006 Examines the constitutionality of conscience clauses under the Fourteenth Amendment. Concludes that state involvement through the enactment of such clauses may violate the Fourteenth Amendment. Cites Principle VIII. Rozenek, *Whose Conscience Is It Anyway? The State's Role in Conscience Clause Creation and the Denial of Contraception, 40 Suffolk U. L. Rev. 215, 220 (2006).*

Journal 2006 Reviews conflicts which arise when a physician must choose between violating a law and adhering to an ethical principle. Concludes the physician must consider the needs of the patient and acknowledges that there are cases where violating a law may be justified. Quotes Principle VIII and Opinion 1.02. Schwartz, *The Ethical Health Lawyer: When Doing the Right Thing Means Breaking the Law: What Is the Role of the Health Lawyer? 34 J. L. Med. & Ethics 624,* 625, 626 (2006).

Journal 2005 Discusses physician responses to the medical malpractice liability crisis. Concludes that certain responses may violate ethical obligations that physicians owe to their patients and to society as a whole. Cites Opinions 9.025 and 10.015. References Principle VIII. Kachalia, Choudhry, & Studdert, *Physician Responses to the Malpractice Crisis: From Defense to Offense, 33 J. L. Med. & Ethics 416, 419, 421, 424 (2005).*

Journal 2005 Argues that the Eighth Circuit's ruling in *Singleton v. Norris* failed to consider the ethical standards of the medical community. Concludes that, as a result, physicians may be placed in an untenable position regarding treatment of mentally ill death-row inmates. Quotes Principle VIII and Opinions 1.02 and 2.06. Lloyd, *Primum Non Nocere: Singleton v. Norris and the Ethical Dilemma of Medicating the Condemned, 58 Ark. L. Rev. 225, 232, 233 (2005).*

Journal 2005 Examines issues surrounding tort reform proposals. Concludes that more can be done to correct the current tort system before moving toward a "one size fits all" approach. Quotes Principles I, II, III, IV, V, VI, VII, VIII, and IX. Messerly & Warwick, *Nowhere to Turn: A Glance at the Facts Behind the Supposed Need for Tort "Reform," 28 Hamline L. Rev. 489,* 506 (2005).

Journal 2005 Argues that in *Aetna v. Davila/Cigna v. Calad,* the Supreme Court missed an opportunity to overturn unjust ERISA policies. Concludes that the principle of complete ERISA preemption as articulated in these consolidated cases is unsatisfactory because it violates the separation of powers doctrine. Quotes Principle VIII. Cites Opinions 8.054, 8.13, 8.135, 9.123, 10.01, and 10.015. Nelson, *AETNA v. DAVILA/CIGNA v. CALAD: A Missed Opportunity, 31 Wm. Mitchell L. Rev. 843, 847, 849, 850, 880 (2005).*

Journal 2004 Examines the requirements of the Privacy Rule regarding use and disclosure of a patient's identifiable health information in the context of research. Concludes that the Rule's burdensome administrative requirements may discourage research and thus outweigh any benefits for research subject autonomy. Quotes Principle VIII and Opinions 5.051, 8.031, and 10.015. Tovino, *The Use and Disclosure of Protected Health Information for Research Under the HIPAA Privacy Rule: Unrealized Patient Autonomy and Burdensome Government Regulation, 49 S. D. L. Rev. 447, 496, 502 (2004).*

Journal 2003 Examines social norms, using public choice theory, to determine how certain groups in society use these norms to benefit their members. Concludes that the benefits provided by social norms may dissipate depending on various considerations. Quotes Principles II and VIII. Miller, *Norms and Interests, 32 Hofstra L. Rev. 637, 650, 670 (2003).*

Journal 2002 Examines how managed care has adversely affected information disclosure in the physician-patient relationship. Concludes that, unless courts expand applicability of principles of informed consent, patient self-determination and autonomy will continue to be undermined. Quotes Principle VIII and Opinions 8.03, 8.053, 8.054, and 8.08. Morris, *Dissing Disclosure: Just What the Doctor Ordered, 44 Ariz. L. Rev. 313, 344, 349, 362, 363, 366 (2002).*

Journal 2002 Considers the dilemma of informed consent in the context of prescribing psychotropic medication to patients with mental illness and mental retardation. Recognizes the need for substituted decision-making in certain situations. Concludes that legislation would help address this issue. Quotes Preamble, Principles I, III, IV, VIII, and IX, and Opinion 8.08. O'Sullivan & Borcherding, *Informed Consent for Medication in Persons With Mental Retardation and Mental Illness, 12 Health Matrix 63, 75, 86, 87, 88 (2002)*

Journal 2002 Discusses legal and medical policies that protect confidentiality in the physician-patient relationship. Concludes that reducing the current level of privacy protection would jeopardize health care. Quotes Preamble and Opinions 2.136, 5.05, and 10.01. References Principles VIII and IX. Sciarrino, *Ferguson v. City of Charleston: "The Doctor Will See You Now, Be Sure to Bring Your Privacy Rights in With You!" 12 Temp. Pol. & Civ. Rts. L. Rev. 197, 213, 215,* 220, 221, 222 (2002).

IX. A physician shall support access to medical care for all people.

Journal 2011 Argues the medical profession has no commitment to political advocacy because civic virtues are outside the professional realm, civic participation is not necessary for civic virtue, and because the medical profession should not mandate any political stance for its members. Concludes the medical profession should be dedicated to competent and ethical professional work rather than require political advocacy. Quotes Principle IX. Huddle, *Medical Professionalism and Medical Education Should Not Involve Commitments to Political Advocacy*, 86 Acad. Med. 378, 379 (2011).

Journal 2010 Analyzes factors contributing to the emergence of medical repatriation and evaluates whether this practice comports with current legal and ethical standards. Proposes changes to federal regulations that govern hospitals and clarifications to medical ethical standards. Quotes the Preamble and Principles I, II, III, IV, V, VI, VII, VIII, and IX. Zoellner, *Medical Repatriation: Examining the Legal and Ethical Implications of an Emerging Practice*, 32 Wash. U. J. L. & Pol'y 515, 530-532 (2010).

Journal 2008 Examines the development of bioethics and environmental ethics, as well as laws promoting the role of bioethicists in decision making. Concludes environmental ethicists must convince legislatures of the role of environmental ethics in order to have a greater impact on decision making. Quotes Principles I, II, III, IV, V, VI, VII, VIII, and IX. Robertson, *Seeking a Seat at the Table: Has Law Left Environmental Ethics Behind as It Embraces Bioethics?* 32 Wm. & Mary Envtl. L. & Pol'y Rev. 273, 307 (2008).

Journal 2006 Examines ethical dilemmas physicians may face as providers of pay-for-performance medical care. Concludes that this strategy offers a benefit to patients as long as physicians uphold stringent ethical standards and work together to ensure optimum patient care. Cites Principles I, V, VIII, and IX and Opinions 2.035, 2.095, 6.01, 8.021, 8.03, 8.0501, 8.053, 8.054, and 8.121. Bostick, Sade, & McMahon, *Report of the Council on Ethical and Judicial Affairs: Physician Pay-For-Performance Programs*, 3 Ind. Health L. Rev. 429, 430, 431, 432-33, 434, 435, 436 (2006).

Journal 2006 Examines the legal and public health issues raised by increased rates of Hepatitis C in prison populations. Concludes that reform is needed to provide adequate health care to prisoners and that courts have the power to require such care under the Eighth Amendment. Quotes Preamble, Principles VII, VIII, and IX, and Opinion 10.015. Brunsden, *Hepatitis C in Prisons: Evolving Toward Decency Through Adequate Medical Care and Public Health Reform*, 54 UCLA L. Rev. 465, 500 (2006).

Journal 2006 Explores the legal and ethical issues surrounding concierge medicine. Concludes that concierge medicine is best restricted to a small class of wealthy individuals. Quotes Principle IX and Opinion 8.055. Cites Principle VI and Opinions 8.055, 8.11, 8.115, 9.065, and 10.05. Carnahan, *Law, Medicine, and Wealth: Does Concierge Medicine Promote Health Care Choice, or Is It a Barrier to Access?* 17 Stan. L. & Pol'y Rev. 121, 149-50, 151, 152, 153-54 (2006).

Journal 2006 Explores conscience clause legislation relating to the dispensing of oral contraceptives. Concludes that such legislation must balance the interests of the patient and the health care provider. Cites Principles I, II, III, IV, V, VI, VII, VIII, and IX. Collins, *Conscience Clauses and Oral Contraceptives: Conscientious Objection or Calculated Obstruction?* 15 Ann. Health L. 37, 54 (2006).

Journal 2006 Considers the interaction of laws, rules, and guidelines in the area of health law. Suggests that the legislature should revise current laws to reflect local variability in practice. Quotes Preamble and Principles VII and IX. Heimer, *Responsibility in Health Care: Spanning the Boundary Between Law and Medicine*, 41 Wake Forest L. Rev. 465, 498 (2006).

Journal 2006 Discusses the role of EMTALA in mandating care for the uninsured. Concludes EMTALA is inadequate and Congress should take steps toward establishing a program for universal health care. Quotes Principle IX and Ch. II, Art. V, Sec. 9 (May 1847) [now Opinion 9.065] and Ch. III, Art. I, Sec. 3 (May 1847) [now Opinion 9.065]. Hermer, *The Scapegoat: EMTALA and Emergency Department Overcrowding*, 14 J. L. & Pol'y 695, 713-14 (2006).

Journal 2005 Discusses legal and ethical problems associated with patient surcharges. Concludes that surcharges are necessary to combat rising malpractice insurance premiums and a declining payment environment. Cites Principle IX and Opinion 6.12. Landfair, *Transforming Physicians Into Business Savvy Entrepreneurs: Patient Surcharges Charge Onto the Scene of Physician Reimbursement*, 43 Duq. L. Rev. 257, 268, 269 (2005).

Journal 2005 Examines issues surrounding tort reform proposals. Concludes that more can be done to correct the current tort system before moving toward a "one size fits all" approach. Quotes Principles I, II, III, IV, V, VI, VII, VIII, and IX. Messerly & Warwick, *Nowhere to Turn: A Glance at the Facts Behind the Supposed Need for Tort "Reform,"* 28 Hamline L. Rev. 489, 506 (2005).

Journal 2005 Examines the practice of "boutique medicine" and considers legal and ethical implications. Concludes that boutique medical services would be ethical only if physicians used retainer money from their boutique clients to augment health care costs of the poor. Quotes Principles VII and IX and Opinion 8.055. Russano, *Is Boutique Medicine a New Threat to American Health Care or a Logical Way of Revitalizing the Doctor-Patient Relationship?* 17 Wash. U. J. L. & Pol'y 313, 331, 332 (2005).

Journal 2005 Discusses ethical, legal, and policy issues associated with treatment and research involving patients who are in a persistent vegetative or minimally conscious state. Concludes that patients in these states are at risk for therapeutic failures until physicians can more accurately determine which patients will benefit from treatment and accurately convey such information to families or surrogates. Quotes Principles VII and IX and Opinions 8.031, 8.0315, 9.065, 10.01, and 10.015. Tovino & Winslade, *A Primer on the Law and Ethics of Treatment, Research, and Public Policy in the Context of Severe Traumatic Brain Injury,* 14 Ann. Health L. 1, 18, 38, 39, 40, 41 (2005).

Journal 2002 Considers the dilemma of informed consent in the context of prescribing psychotropic medication to patients with mental illness and mental retardation. Recognizes the need for substituted decision-making in certain situations. Concludes that legislation would help address this issue. Quotes Preamble, Principles I, III, IV, VIII, and IX, and Opinion 8.08. O'Sullivan & Borcherding, *Informed Consent for Medication in Persons With Mental Retardation and Mental Illness,* 12 Health Matrix 63, 75, 86, 87, 88 (2002).

Journal 2002 Discusses legal and medical policies that protect confidentiality in the physician-patient relationship. Concludes that reducing the current level of privacy protection would jeopardize health care. Quotes Preamble and Opinions 2.136, 5.05, and 10.01. References Principles VIII and IX. Sciarrino, *Ferguson v. City of Charleston: "The Doctor Will See You Now, Be Sure to Bring Your Privacy Rights in With You!"* 12 Temp. Pol. & Civ. Rts. L. Rev. 197, 213, 215, 220, 221, 222 (2002).

Adopted June 1957; revised June 1980; revised June 2001.

Introduction

1.00

1.01 **Terminology**

The term "ethical" is used in opinions of the Council on Ethical and Judicial Affairs to refer to matters involving (1) moral principles or practices and (2) matters of social policy involving issues of morality in the practice of medicine. The term "unethical" is used to refer to professional conduct which fails to conform to these moral standards or policies.

Many of the Council's opinions lay out specific duties and obligations for physicians. Violation of these principles and opinions represents unethical conduct and may justify disciplinary action such as censure, suspension, or expulsion from medical society membership. (II)

Issued prior to April 1977. Updated June 1994 and June 1996.

Journal 2011 Critiques Kristen Shotwell's article *Secretly Falling in Love: America's Love Affair With Controlling the Hearts and Minds of Public School Teachers* which argues that a teacher's private conduct should not be subject to closer scrutiny than other members of the community. Concludes that a teacher's adverse notoriety for private conduct should remain a factor in terms of teacher retention. Cites Opinion 1.01. DeMitchell, *Immorality, Teacher Private Conduct, and Adverse Notoriety: A Needed Recalculation of Nexus? 40 J. L & Educ. 327, 336 (2011).*

Journal 2008 Questions what entity should be responsible for critically evaluating chiropractors. Concludes that chiropractic should be a self-regulated profession. Quotes Introduction (1847) [now Opinions 1.01 and 1.02]. References Ch. II, Art. I, Sec. 3 (1847) [now Opinion 5.02] and Ch. II, Art. IV, Sec. 1 (May 1847) [now Opinion 3.01]. Johnson, *Keeping a Critical Eye on Chiropractic, 31 J. of Manipulative and Physiological Therapeutics 559, 559 (2008).*

Journal 2004 Analyzes various issues relating to the role of mental health professionals in capital punishment in light of Albert Bandura's model of "mechanisms of moral disengagement." Concludes that facilitating participation of mental health professionals in executions creates conflicts with the humanistic norms of the profession. Quotes Preamble and Opinions 1.01, 1.02, 2.06, 2.067, 2.20, 2.21, 2.211, and 8.14. Judges, *The Role of Mental Health Professionals in Capital Punishment: An Exercise in Moral Disengagement, 41 Hous. L. Rev. 515, 562, 568, 569, 570, 571-72, 581, 586, 588, 598 (2004).*

Journal 1994 Discusses the role of professional societies in establishing ethical guidelines for physicians in the context of using medical innovations and new technologies. Observes that these standards must be supplemented by additional external measures or incentives in order to be most effective. Cites Opinions 1.01, 1.02, 8.061, 9.04, and 9.131. Orentlicher, *The Influence of a Professional Organization on Physician Behavior, 57 Alb. L. Rev. 583, 592, 593, 594, 595, 596 (1994).*

Journal 1994 Reviews the evolution of the physician-patient relationship, with attention to patient autonomy. Examines the changing health care delivery environment. Quotes Preamble, Principles I, II, III, IV, V, and VI, Fundamental Elements (1) and (2), and Opinions 1.02 and 8.07 (1981) [now Opinion 8.08]. Cites Opinion 1.01. Szczygiel, *Beyond Informed Consent, 21 Ohio N. U. L. Rev. 171, 217, 218, 220, 225, 226, 256 (1994).*

1.02 **The Relation of Law and Ethics**

The following statements are intended to clarify the relationship between law and ethics.

Ethical values and legal principles are usually closely related, but ethical obligations typically exceed legal duties. In some cases, the law mandates unethical conduct. In general, when physicians believe a law is unjust, they should work to change the law. In exceptional circumstances of unjust laws, ethical responsibilities should supersede legal obligations.

The fact that a physician charged with allegedly illegal conduct is acquitted or exonerated in civil or criminal proceedings does not necessarily mean that the physician acted ethically. (III)

Issued prior to April 1977. Updated June 1994.

Journal 2011 Explores whether legal professionals, in their practice, take responsibility for legal outcomes. Examines different approaches including a "dissociative paradigm" requiring legal professionals to separate personal views from legal reasoning and an "ownership principle" directing that legal professionals not set aside personal conscience in providing legal services. Concludes by recommending that legal professionals follow the ownership principle over the dissociation paradigm regarding legal outcomes. Quotes Opinion 1.02. Khan, *Taking Ownership of Legal Outcomes: An Argument Against Dissociation Paradigm and Analytical Gaming*, 55 St. Louis U. L.J. 887, 911 (2011).

Journal 2010 Explores dilemmas arising when military mental health providers encounter conflicts between a professional ethical obligation and a federal statute. Concludes ethical-legal conflict in military practice may be managed by recognizing when a true conflict exists, possessing adequate knowledge of the professional ethical code and the relevant federal laws, developing a process for ethical decision making, and maintaining a commitment to the professional code of ethics. Quotes Opinion 1.02. Johnson, Grasso, & Maslowski, *Conflicts Between Ethics and Law for Military Mental Health Providers*, 175 Mil. Med. 548, 549 (2010).

Journal 2009 Explores the Supreme Court's *Baze v. Rees* decision and the three-drug protocol for lethal injection. Discusses the necessity of judicial intervention to improve lethal injection protocols. Concludes courts should carefully consider their approach to challenges to lethal injection as an opportunity to prevent violation of Eighth Amendment rights. Quotes Preamble and Opinion 1.02. Cites Opinion 2.06. Berger, *Lethal Injection and the Problem of Constitutional Remedies*, 27 Yale L. & Pol'y Rev. 259, 319, 320 (2009).

Journal 2009 Examines physician violation of both business-related and patient care–related laws. Concludes lawmakers should lend thoughtful consideration to physicians' complaints that at times adherence to a particular law constrains appropriate patient care. Quotes Opinion 1.02. Hoffmann, *Physicians Who Break the Law*, 53 St. Louis U. L. J. 1049, 1065 (2009).

Journal 2008 Questions what entity should be responsible for critically evaluating chiropractors. Concludes that chiropractic should be a self-regulated profession. Quotes Introduction (1847) [now Opinions 1.01 and 1.02]. References Ch. II, Art. I, Sec. 3 (1847) [now Opinion 5.02] and Ch. II, Art. IV, Sec. 1 (May 1847) [now Opinion 3.01]. Johnson, *Keeping a Critical Eye on Chiropractic*, 31 J. of Manipulative and Physiological Therapeutics 559, 559 (2008).

Journal 2007 Examines relative vs absolute rights to confidentiality for military detainees considering the utilitarian need to protect the public at large. Concludes that evolving standards may favor individual rights to confidentiality, even from a utilitarian perspective. Quotes Opinions 1.02 and 5.05. References Principle III. Wynia, *Breaching Confidentiality to Protect the Public: Evolving Standards of Medical Confidentiality for Military Detainees*, 7 Am. J. Bioethics, 1, 2 (Aug. 2007).

Journal 2006 Reviews conflicts which arise when a physician must choose between violating a law and adhering to an ethical principle. Concludes the physician must consider the needs of the patient and acknowledges that there are cases where violating a law may be justified. Quotes Principle VIII and Opinion 1.02. Schwartz, *The Ethical Health Lawyer: When Doing the Right Thing Means Breaking the Law: What Is the Role of the Health Lawyer?* 34 J. L. Med. & Ethics 624, 625, 626 (2006).

Journal 2005 Discusses ongoing violations of professional codes of ethics by US military medical personnel. Proposes that medical licensing boards should monitor and discipline all such breaches. Quotes Opinion 1.02. Philip, Conant, & Heilig, *Participation of Health Care Personnel in Torture and Interrogation*, 353 New Eng. J. Med. 1634, 1634 (2005).

Journal 2005 Argues that the Eighth Circuit's ruling in *Singleton v. Norris* failed to consider the ethical standards of the medical community. Concludes that, as a result, physicians may be placed in an untenable position regarding treatment of mentally ill death-row inmates. Quotes Principle VIII and Opinions 1.02 and 2.06. Lloyd, *Primum Non Nocere: Singleton v. Norris and the Ethical Dilemma of Medicating the Condemned*, 58 Ark. L. Rev. 225, 232, 233 (2005).

Journal 2005 Examines ethical guidelines for health personnel created by the Department of Defense in response to recent allegations of abuse and torture by US forces. Concludes that the guidelines allow physicians to participate in interrogation practices that contravene international ethical principles. Cites Opinion 1.02. References Opinion 2.067. Rubenstein, Pross, Davidoff, & Iacopino, *Coercive US Interrogation Policies: A Challenge to Medical Ethics*, 294 JAMA 1544 (2005).

Journal 2004 Analyzes various issues relating to the role of mental health professionals in capital punishment in light of Albert Bandura's model of "mechanisms of moral disengagement." Concludes that facilitating participation of mental health professionals in executions creates conflicts with the humanistic norms of the profession. Quotes Preamble and Opinions 1.01, 1.02, 2.06, 2.067, 2.20, 2.21, 2.211, and 8.14. Judges, *The Role of Mental Health Professionals in Capital Punishment: An Exercise in Moral Disengagement*, 41 Hous. L. Rev. 515, 562, 568, 569, 570, 571-72, 581, 586, 588, 598 (2004).

Journal 2003 Considers the legal, medical, and ethical issues of physician-patient confidentiality in disclosure of paternity. Concludes that a balancing test should be applied to making determinations regarding disclosure of paternity. Quotes Principles I, IV, and V and Opinions 1.02, 5.055, and 10.01. Cites Principle II and Opinion 5.05. Richards & Wolf, *Medical Confidentiality and Disclosure of Paternity*, 48 S. D. L. Rev. 409, 411, 412, 413 (2003).

Journal 2003 Uses public policy arguments to support a preponderance standard for medical license revocations in situations involving false testimony by a medical expert witness. Concludes that medical licensing boards can more effectively protect the public by using a preponderance standard. Quotes Principles II, III, and IV and Opinions 1.02 and 9.07. Widmer, *South Dakota Should Follow Public Policy and Switch to the Preponderance Standard for Medical License Revocation After In Re the Medical License of Dr. Reuben Setliff, M.D.*, 48 S. D. L. Rev. 388, 396-97, 402 (2003).

Journal 2002 Discusses issues regarding regulation of elderly drivers. Concludes that mandating physicians to report unfit elderly patients will protect the public and help resolve ethical and legal dilemmas. Quotes Opinions 1.02, 2.24, 5.05, and 10.01. Kane, *Driving Into the Sunset: A Proposal for Mandatory Reporting to the DMV by Physicians Treating Unsafe Elderly Drivers*, 25 U. Haw. L. Rev. 59, 59, 61, 62, 67, 69, 82, 83 (2002).

Journal 2001 Considers whether or not it is ethical for physicians to prescribe, and pharmacists to dispense, syringes for use by injection drug users. Concludes that ethical considerations suggest such actions are permissible but not obligatory. Quotes Principle III and Opinion 1.02. References Opinion 5.05. Lazzarini, *An Analysis of Ethical Issues in Prescribing and Dispensing Syringes to Injection Drug Users*, 11 Health Matrix 85, 107, 119 (2001).

Journal 2001 Explores utilization of the Gannett Principles to develop uniform ethical and legal standards in journalism. Concludes that these principles are an inevitable and useful response to legal realities. Quotes Opinion 1.02. Storey, *Does Ethics Make Good Law? A Case Study*, 19 Cardozo Arts & Ent. L. J. 467, 470 (2001).

Journal 2000 Considers the rules governing expert testimony. Explores professional ethical standards affecting expert witnesses and concludes that codes of ethics have not succeeded in eliminating biased expert testimony. Recommends creation of an organization to assist courts in obtaining reliable expert witness testimony. Quotes Principle III and Opinion 6.01. Cites Principles I, II, and V and Opinions 1.02 and 9.07. Murphy, *Expert Witnesses at Trial: Where Are the Ethics?* 14 Geo. J. Legal Ethics 217, 231-32 (2000).

Journal 1995 Examines the rights of health care professionals to refuse to participate in patient care on the basis of conscientious objection. Suggests steps that health care facilities may take when dealing with health care professionals who object to participating in patient care. Quotes Principles I and VI and Opinions 1.02, 2.035, and 9.055. Dellinger & Vickery, *When Staff Object to Participating in Care*, 28 J. Health & Hospital Law 269, 272, 276 (1995).

Journal 1994 Explores the ethical issues involved in a multidisciplinary team working with children in legal proceedings. Focuses on the relationships between professionals and the conflicts that arise regarding disclosure of confidential information and forced disclosure of nonprivileged information. Quotes Principles III and IV, Fundamental Elements (4), and Opinion 1.02 (1992) and 5.07 (1992) [now Opinion 5.05]. Cites Opinion 2.02. Glynn, *Multidisciplinary Representation of Children: Conflicts Over Disclosures of Client Communications, 27 J. Marshall L. Rev. 617, 625, 626, 630-32, 637, 639, 643 (1994).*

Journal 1994 Discusses the role of professional societies in establishing ethical guidelines for physicians in the context of using medical innovations and new technologies. Observes that these standards must be supplemented by additional external measures or incentives in order to be most effective. Cites Opinions 1.01, 1.02, 8.061, 9.04, and 9.131. Orentlicher, *The Influence of a Professional Organization on Physician Behavior, 57 Alb. L. Rev. 583, 592, 593, 594, 595, 596 (1994).*

Journal 1994 Reviews the evolution of the physician-patient relationship, with attention to patient autonomy. Examines the changing health care delivery environment. Quotes Preamble, Principles I, II, III, IV, V, and VI, Fundamental Elements (1) and (2), and Opinions 1.02 and 8.07 (1981) [now Opinion 8.08]. Cites Opinion 1.01. Szczygiel, *Beyond Informed Consent, 21 Ohio N. U. L. Rev. 171, 217, 218, 220, 225, 226, 256 (1994).*

Journal 1992 Argues that legal ethics and state laws governing attorney conduct are in conflict. Concludes that legal ethics continue to play a prominent role because states are "weakly committed" to regulation of the profession. Cites Opinion 1.02. Koniak, *The Law Between the Bar and the State, 70 No. Carolina L. Rev. 1389, 1396 (1992).*

Journal 1991 Explores ethical problems unique to the field of forensic psychiatry. Presents the results of a survey of members of the American Academy of Psychiatry and the Law (AAPL), asking their opinions regarding proposed ethical guidelines. Quotes Opinions 1.02 and 5.09. Weinstock, Leong, & Silva, *Opinions by AAPL Forensic Psychiatrists on Controversial Ethical Guidelines: A Survey, 19 Bull. Am. Acad. Psychiatry Law 237, 238 (1991).*

2.00 **Opinions on Social Policy Issues**

2.01 **Abortion**

The Principles of Medical Ethics of the AMA do not prohibit a physician from performing an abortion in accordance with good medical practice and under circumstances that do not violate the law. (III, IV)

Issued prior to April 1977.

U.S. 1973 Pregnant woman and physician sought declaratory relief and injunction against Texas criminal abortion statute. In holding that the constitutional right of privacy includes a woman's decision whether to terminate a pregnancy prior to viability, the Court reviewed the medical and legal history of abortion, including the AMA's lobbying efforts in support of criminal abortion statutes (1859, 1871), its opposition to induced abortion except when threat to life or health of mother exists (1967), its statement that lobbying efforts were consistent with the Principles of Medical Ethics (1957), and the Preamble, Sec. 10 (1971) [now Opinion 2.01], which stated that a physician was not prohibited from performing an abortion in accordance with good medical practice and consistent with local law. *Roe v. Wade, 410 U.S. 113, 144 n.39.*

Journal 2010 Discusses issues arising from the enactment of legislation by North Dakota involving a minor's reproductive rights. Explores ethical principles that govern physician's actions within the context of reproductive health. Concludes that, while a patient's expectation of confidentiality with a physician is critical, competing values come into play when the patient is a minor and parental involvement may be important. Provides practical guidance to address issues in this context. Quotes Opinions 2.01, 2.015, 5.055, 8.08, 8.115, 9.12, 10.01, 10.015, and 10.05. Cites Opinions 5.05, 5.055, 8.08, 8.11, 8.115, 9.12, and 10.05. Haas, *"Doctor, I'm Pregnant and Fifteen—I Can't Tell My Parents—Please Help Me": Minor Consent, Reproductive Rights, and Ethical Principles for Physicians, 86 N.D. L. Rev. 63, 70, 73, 75-78, 82, 84, 86-88, (2010).*

Journal 2005 Discusses Wisconsin Act 110. Concludes the Act was unnecessary, and that if an infant does survive an abortion, the decision of whether treatment should be administered must be left to the physician. Quotes Opinion 2.01. Frishman, *Wisconsin Act 110: When an Infant Survives an Abortion, 20 Wis. Women's L. J. 101, 117 (2005).*

Journal 2005 Examines the legal and ethical aspects of physician participation in capital punishment. Concludes that federal and state laws addressing this practice must be amended to harmonize the law with applicable principles of medical ethics. Quotes Opinion 2.06. Cites Opinion 2.21. References Opinion 2.01. Levy, *Conflict of Duty: Capital Punishment Regulations and AMA Medical Ethics, 26 J. Legal Med. 261, 268, 269, 270, 273 (2005).*

Journal 2004 Asks whether pharmacists should be protected from civil liability when they refuse to dispense birth control medication based on their moral convictions. Concludes that moral beliefs of health care providers should not get in the way of patient care. Cites Opinion 2.01. Cantor & Baum, *The Limits of Conscientious Objection—May Pharmacists Refuse to Fill Prescriptions for Emergency Contraception? 351 New Eng. J. Med. 2008, 2012 (2004).*

Journal 2000 Examines physician value neutrality (PVN). Defines PVN as providing a foundation to suggest physicians must keep their values—religious, political, or otherwise—out of the patient-physician relationship. Concludes it is not clear how values can be removed from the patient-physician relationship without removing the very thing PVN supporters are trying to protect, the intrinsic value of persons. References Opinions 2.01, 2.02, 8.032, 8.05, 8.08, and 8.132. Beckwith & Peppin, *Physician Value Neutrality: A Critique, 28 J. L. Med. & Ethics 67, 72-73 (2000).*

Journal 1995 Examines four essential principles of bioethics—patient autonomy, nonmalefi-cence, beneficence, and justice—and describes their application in clinical settings according to bioethical norms and AMA opinions. Concludes that such an approach promotes compassionate medical caregiving and that laws should reflect these values. Quotes Opinions 2.01 and 8.18. References Opinion 2.211. Cohen, *Toward a Bioethics of Compassion*, 28 Ind. L. Rev. 667, 673, 681-82, 683 (1995).

2.015 Mandatory Parental Consent to Abortion

Physicians should ascertain the law in their state on parental involvement to ensure that their procedures are consistent with their legal obligations.

Physicians should strongly encourage minors to discuss their pregnancy with their parents. Physicians should explain how parental involvement can be help-ful and that parents are generally very understanding and supportive. If a minor expresses concerns about parental involvement, the physician should ensure that the minor's reluctance is not based on any misperceptions about the likely consequences of parental involvement.

Physicians should not feel or be compelled to require minors to involve their parents before deciding whether to undergo an abortion. The patient, even an adolescent, generally must decide whether, on balance, parental involvement is advisable. Accordingly, minors should ultimately be allowed to decide whether parental involvement is appropriate. Physicians should explain under what circumstances (eg, life-threatening emergency) the minor's confidentiality will need to be abrogated.

Physicians should try to ensure that minor patients have made an informed decision after giving careful consideration to the issues involved. They should encourage their minor patients to consult alternative sources if parents are not going to be involved in the abortion decision. Minors should be urged to seek the advice and counsel of those adults in whom they have confidence, includ-ing professional counselors, relatives, friends, teachers, or the clergy. (III, IV)

Issued June 1994 based on the report "Mandatory Parental Consent to Abortion," adopted June 1992 (JAMA. 1993;269:82-86).

6th Cir. 1999 Plaintiff challenged state law requiring minors to appeal, within 24 hours, a denied petition to bypass parental consent to obtain an abortion. The court stated that the 24-hour appeal requirement did not unduly burden the minor's ability to obtain an abortion. The dissent cited Opinion 2.015, to support its view that the 24-hour appeal requirement imposed an undue burden by jeopardizing the minor's ability to obtain an abortion. *Memphis Planned Parenthood v. Sundquist*, 175 F.3d 456, 473.

8th Cir. 1995 Court held several provisions of the South Dakota abortion law unconstitutional, including parental notice provision. In ruling that parental notice requirement, which lacked a bypass provision, unduly burdened liberty interests of some minors, the court cited AMA Council on Ethical and Judicial Affairs, Mandatory Parental Consent to Abortion, 269 JAMA 82 (1993) [now Opinion 2.015]. *Planned Parenthood v. Miller*, 63 F.3d 1452, 1462.

Mass. 1997 Plaintiffs brought suit seeking a declaration that statute prohibiting, with certain exceptions, a pregnant unmarried minor from obtaining an abortion unless either both parents consent or a judge authorizes the procedure, is unconstitutional. The court concluded that the statute did not facially violate due process or equal protection and was thus constitutional. However, the court struck down the provision requiring both parents' consent as lacking suffi-cient justification to overcome the minor's constitutional right to choose. The court cited AMA Council on Ethical and Judicial Affairs, Mandatory Parental Consent to Abortion, 269 JAMA 82 (1993) [now Opinion 2.015]. *Planned Parenthood League of Massachusetts, Inc. v. Attorney General*, 424 Mass. 586, 596, 608, 677 N.E.2d 101, 107, 114.

N.J. 2000 Prior to the effective date of the Parental Notification for Abortion Act, the plaintiffs sought a declaratory judgment and preliminary injunction precluding the enforcement of the Act. The trial court dismissed the challenge, but the state Supreme Court struck down the statute. The state, in support of the Act, argued that it was passed to facilitate and foster familial communications. The court rejected this as a legitimate governmental interest, noting that the Act applies to many young women who are justified in not telling their parents about their abortion decisions. The court quoted AMA Council on Ethics and Judicial Affairs, Mandatory Parental Consent to Abortion, 269 JAMA 82 (1983) [now Opinion 2.015] in support of this argument. *Planned Parenthood of Central New Jersey v. Farmer*, 165 N.J. 609, 762 A.2d 620, 640.

Journal 2010 Discusses issues arising from the enactment of legislation by North Dakota involving a minor's reproductive rights. Explores ethical principles that govern physician's actions within the context of reproductive health. Concludes that, while a patient's expectation of confidentiality with a physician is critical, competing values come into play when the patient is a minor and parental involvement may be important. Provides practical guidance to address issues in this context. Quotes Opinions 2.01, 2.015, 5.055, 8.08, 8.115, 9.12, 10.01, 10.015, and 10.05. Cites Opinions 5.05, 5.055, 8.08, 8.11, 8.115, 9.12, and 10.05. Haas, *"Doctor, I'm Pregnant and Fifteen—I Can't Tell My Parents—Please Help Me": Minor Consent, Reproductive Rights, and Ethical Principles for Physicians*, 86 N.D. L. Rev. 63, 70, 73, 75-78, 82, 84, 86-88, (2010).

Journal 2003 Uses the medical self-consent rights of minors to challenge the legal assumption that teens lack decisional capacity for abortions. Concludes with discussion of an empirical study that supports this challenge. References Opinion 2.015. Ehrlich, *Grounded in the Reality of Their Lives: Listening to Teens Who Make the Abortion Decision Without Involving Their Parents*, 18 Berkeley Women's L. J. 61, 72, 84-85, 175-76 (2003).

Journal 2003 Explores conflict in the legal treatment of minors in situations involving reproductive decision-making and the commission of crimes. Concludes that different approaches are justified. References Opinion 2.015. Ehrlich, *Shifting Boundaries: Abortion, Criminal Culpability and the Indeterminate Legal Status of Adolescents*, 18 Wis. Women's L. J. 77, 105 (2003).

Journal 2002 Argues attorneys should be appointed to represent minors in judicial bypass proceedings. Concludes that appointing a guardian ad litem raises ethical and constitutional problems. References Opinion 2.015. Graybill, *Assisting Minors Seeking Abortions in Judicial Bypass Proceedings: A Guardian Ad Litem Is No Substitute for an Attorney*, 55 Vand. L. Rev. 581, 583 (2002).

Journal 2002 Examines how Alabama juvenile courts are handling petitions for waiver of parental consent for abortion. Concludes the courts are not correctly handling these matters, thus adversely affecting the rights of pregnant minors. References Opinion 2.015. Silverstein & Speitel, *"Honey, I Have No Idea": Court Readiness to Handle Petitions to Waive Parental Consent for Abortion*, 88 Iowa L. Rev. 75, 116, 117 (2002).

Journal 2001 Considers proposed state legislation requiring a minor to notify a parent when she intends to obtain an abortion. Concludes that notification serves the minor's best interests. References Opinion 2.015. Collett, *Protecting Our Daughters: The Need for the Vermont Parental Notification Law*, 26 Vt. L. Rev. 101, 106-07 (2001).

Journal 2000 Explores issues associated with mandatory parental consent to abortion laws. Examines the failure of the US Supreme Court to consider medical decision-making by minors when evaluating the constitutionality of such laws. References Opinion 2.015. Ehrlich, *Minors as Medical Decision Makers: The Pretextual Reasoning of the Court in the Abortion Cases*, 7 Mich. J. Gender & L. 65, 91 (2000).

Journal 1999 Discusses minors' rights to an abortion. Examines parental notification requirements and procedures to bypass parental notification laws. Argues that minors should be afforded the same rights in seeking an abortion as adult women. References Opinion 2.015. Katz, *The Pregnant Child's Right to Self-determination*, 62 Alb. L. Rev. 1119, 1142 (1999).

Journal 1998 Discusses parental consent laws pertaining to minors seeking abortions. Examines *Roe v. Wade* and the federal constitutional challenge to the Massachusetts parental consent law. States that the purpose of parental involvement laws is to limit abortion rights, rather than to promote family discourse. References Opinion 2.015. Ehrlich, *Journey Through the Courts: Minors, Abortion and the Quest for Reproductive Fairness*, 10 Yale J. L. & Feminism 1, 19 (1998).

Journal 1997 Addresses the issue of teenage pregnancy. Examines governmental actions that have made it more difficult for teenagers to receive abortions. Suggests that parental consent and judicial bypass provisions are an infringement on their reproductive freedom. Advocates lawyer participation in abortion reform. References Opinion 2.015. Schiff, *The Lawyer's Role in Restoring Adolescents' Abortion Rights*, 44 Fed. Law. 60, 62 (May 1997).

Journal 1996 Reviews Supreme Court decisions that address parental involvement in the abortion decisions of mature minors. Suggests that the Court's position on parental involvement should be reevaluated. Posits that many young women are mature enough to make their own pregnancy decisions. References Opinion 2.015. O'Shaughnessy, *The Worst of Both Worlds?: Parental Involvement Requirements and the Privacy Rights of Mature Minors*, 57 Ohio St. L. J. 1731, 1764-65 (1996).

2.02   The previous Opinion 2.02, "Abuse of Spouses, Children, Elderly Persons, and Others at Risk," issued December 1982, was replaced by the current Opinion 2.02, "Physicians' Obligations in Preventing, Identifying, and Treating Violence and Abuse."

2.02   Physicians' Obligations in Preventing, Identifying, and Treating Violence and Abuse

Interpersonal violence and abuse were once thought to primarily affect specific high-risk patient populations, but it is now understood that all patients may be at risk. The complexity of the issues arising in this area requires three distinct sets of guidelines for physicians. The following guidelines address assessment, prevention, and reporting of interpersonal violence and abuse.

(1) When seeking to identify and diagnose past or current experiences with violence and abuse, physicians should adhere to the following guidelines:

    (a) Physicians should routinely inquire about physical, sexual, and psychological abuse as part of the medical history. Physicians should also consider abuse as a factor in the presentation of medical complaints because patients' experiences with interpersonal violence or abuse may adversely affect their health status or ability to adhere to medical recommendations.

    (b) Physicians should familiarize themselves with the detection of violence or abuse, the community and health care resources available to abused or vulnerable persons, and the legal requirements for reporting violence or abuse.

    (c) Physicians should not be influenced in the diagnosis and management of abuse by such misconceptions as the beliefs that abuse is a rare occurrence, does not occur in "normal" families, is a private problem best resolved without outside interference, or is caused by the victim's own actions.

(2) The following guidelines are intended to guide physicians' efforts to address acts of violence and abuse:

    (a) Physicians must treat the immediate symptoms and sequelae of violence and abuse, while also providing ongoing care for patients so as to address any long-term health consequences that may arise as the result of exposure.

    (b) Physicians should be familiar with current information about cultural variations in response to abuse, public health measures that are effective in preventing violence and abuse, and how to work cooperatively with relevant community services. Physicians should help in developing educational resources for identifying and caring for victims. Comprehensive training in matters pertaining to violence and abuse should be required in medical school curricula and in postgraduate training programs.

(c) Physicians should also provide leadership in raising awareness regarding the need to assess and identify signs of abuse. By establishing guidelines and institutional policies it may be possible to reduce the volume of abuse cases that go unidentified, and consequently, help to ensure that all patients receive the benefit of appropriate assessment regardless of their age, gender, ethnicity, or social circumstances. The establishment of appropriate mechanisms should also direct physicians to external community or private resources that might be available to aid patients.

(d) Physicians should support research in the prevention of violence and abuse and seek collaboration with relevant public health authorities and community organizations.

(3) Physicians should comply with the following guidelines when reporting evidence of violence or abuse:

(a) Physicians should familiarize themselves with any relevant reporting requirements within the jurisdiction in which they practice.

(b) When a jurisdiction mandates reporting suspicion of violence and abuse, physicians should comply. However, physicians should only disclose minimal information in order to safeguard patients' privacy. Moreover, if available evidence suggests that mandatory reporting requirements are not in the best interests of patients, physicians should advocate for changes in such laws.

(c) In jurisdictions where reporting suspected violence and abuse is not legally mandated, physicians should discuss the issue sensitively with the patient by first suggesting the possibility of abuse, followed by describing available safety mechanisms. Reporting when not required by law requires the informed consent of the patient. However, exceptions can be made if a physician reasonably believes that a patient's refusal to authorize reporting is coerced and therefore does not constitute a valid informed treatment decision. (I, III)

Issued June 2008 based on the report "Physicians' Obligations in Preventing, Identifying, and Treating Violence and Abuse," adopted November 2007.

Cal. App. 1982 Defendant was convicted of lewd act with a child and child molestation or annoyance, after licensed clinical psychologist reported defendant's admission of sexual conduct to authorities. The court held that the psychologist's testimony was properly admitted since a statute requiring the reporting of actual or suspected child abuse expressly made the psychotherapist-patient privilege inapplicable. The court quoted Principle 9 (1957) [now Principle IV and Opinions 2.02 and 5.05] in concluding the disclosure was not a breach of professional ethics. *People v. Stritzinger, 137 Cal. App. 3d 126, 186 Cal. Rptr. 750, 752 rev'd 34 Cal. 3d 505, 668 p.2d 738, 194 Cal. Rptr. 431 (1983).*

Md. Att'y Gen. 1977 Opinion addresses the obligation of a psychiatrist to report child abuse information obtained from a parent-patient. Referring to state statutes and to Principle 9 (1957) [now Principle IV and Opinions 2.02 and 5.05] the opinion concludes that the question of whether to disclose suspected child abuse is a matter left to the individual psychiatrist's professional and moral judgment. *Maryland Att'y. Gen. Opinion, 62 Op. Att'y Gen. Md. 157, 160.*

Wis. Att'y Gen. 1987 Physicians may report cases of suspected child abuse or neglect when a patient discloses that he or she has abused a child in some manner. Where report is made in good faith, physicians are immune from any civil or criminal liability. Passing reference is made to Principle 9 (1957) [now Principle IV and Opinions 2.02 and 5.05] in support of this position. *Wisconsin Att'y Gen. Op. 10-87 (March 16, 1987) (LEXIS, States library, Wis. file).*

Journal 2010 Discusses futility disputes where a patient's surrogate wishes to prolong treatment that the physician deems medically ineffective, and the current lack of legal remedies to resolve them. Concludes that states need to establish fair, impartial, and patient-centered methods of resolving futility disputes including independent medical boards that would operate under procedural and substantive regulations. Quotes Opinions 2.02 and 2.035. References Opinions 2.17 and 2.20. Bassel, *Order at the End of Life: Establishing a Clear and Fair Mechanism for the Resolution of Futility Disputes,* 63 Vand. L. Rev. 491, 494, 523 (2010).

Journal 2010 Examines published resources within the medical and legal fields that focus on confidentiality and evaluates those resources to determine if they help clarify confidentiality issues. Further, discusses differences between these professions that may be hindrances when serving the same patient or client. Concludes that, while both professions guard against disclosure of patient/client communications, they also allow for disclosure in certain instances such as imminent death, harm, or injury. References Principle IV and cites Opinions 2.02, 2.23, 2.24, and 5.05. Johns, *Multidisciplinary Practice and Ethics Part II—Lawyers, Doctors, and Confidentiality,* 6 NAELA J. 55, 57-65, 68 (2010).

Journal 2009 Examines the influence of HIV/AIDS on intimate partner violence and the current legal response to this violence. Concludes courts and legislatures must recognize the relationship between HIV/AIDS and domestic violence and take steps to allow victims to tell their stories in court. Cites Opinion 2.02. Stoever, *Stories Absent From the Courtroom: Responding to Domestic Violence in the Context of HIV and AIDS,* 87 N. C. L. Rev. 1157, 1226 (2009).

Journal 2008 Discusses the effect of *Crawford* and *Davis* on out-of-court statements made to medical personnel and the application of the Sixth Amendment Confrontation Clause to such statements. Concludes courts, when making a confrontation determination, must consider the intent of the declarant and the circumstances that influence the content of the declarant's statement. Quotes Opinion 9.07. Cites Opinion 2.02. Gordon, *Is There an Accuser in the House?: Evaluating Statements Made to Physicians and Other Medical Personnel in the Wake of Crawford v. Washington and Davis v. Washington,* 38 N. M. L. Rev. 529, 529 (2008).

Journal 2000 Examines physician value neutrality (PVN). Defines PVN as providing a foundation to suggest physicians must keep their values—religious, political, or otherwise—out of the patient-physician relationship. Concludes it is not clear how values can be removed from the patient-physician relationship without removing the very thing PVN supporters are trying to protect, the intrinsic value of persons. References Opinions 2.01, 2.02, 8.032, 8.05, 8.08, and 8.132. Beckwith & Peppin, *Physician Value Neutrality: A Critique,* 28 J. L. Med. & Ethics 67, 72-73 (2000).

Journal 2000 Examines public policies and medical practices intended to protect victims of domestic violence. Explores the possibility of liability for failure to act by health care professionals. Concludes that states need to develop public policy initiatives to address this and other related issues. References Opinion 2.02. Brown-Cranstoun, *Kringen v. Boslough and Saint Vincent Hospital: A New Trend for Healthcare Professionals Who Treat Victims of Domestic Violence?* 33 J. Health L. 629, 649, 650 (2000).

Journal 2000 Discusses the physical health consequences of psychological intimate partner violence (IPV). Concludes that clinicians should screen for psychological, physical, and sexual IPV in order to minimize physical health consequences. References Opinion 2.02. Coker, Smith, Bethea, King, & McKeown, *Physical Health Consequences of Physical and Psychological Intimate Partner Violence,* 9 Arch. Fam. Med. 451, 456, 457 (2000).

Journal 2000 Describes the epidemiology of intimate partner violence. Explores medical, legal, and law enforcement responses to intimate partner violence. Urges further research relating to medical and legal issues associated with intimate partner violence as well as additional training of attorneys, health care providers, judges, and law enforcement personnel. References Opinion 2.02. Loue, *Intimate Partner Violence: Bridging the Gap Between Law and Science,* 21 J. Legal Med. 1, 18 (2000).

Journal 2000 Examines public reporting statutes and introduces the provisions of the Violence Against Women Act (VAWA). Compares VAWA and public reporting laws. Concludes that VAWA is superior legislation because it requires women to initiate their own claims against abusers. References Opinion 2.02. Vital, *Mandatory Reporting Statutes and the Violence Against Women Act: An Analytical Comparison, 10 Geo. Mason U. Civ. Rts. L. J. 171, 189 (2000).*

Journal 1999 Discusses the basis for holding professionals liable for failing to report abuse. Explains reasons why professionals should be held liable in tort when they fail to report abuse. Argues that imposing such liability will increase early detection and deter future abuse. References Opinion 2.02. Jones, *Kentucky Tort Liability for Failure to Report Family Violence, 26 N. Ky. L. Rev. 43, 58 (1999).*

Journal 1998 Emphasizes that physicians need to be aware of the signs of domestic violence. Points out that, because many victims seek medical treatment, physicians are in a key position to identify domestic violence. Argues that Florida should follow other states' examples and adopt a mandatory reporting act. References Opinion 2.02. Makar, *Domestic Violence: Why the Florida Legislature Must Do More to Protect the "Silent" Victims, 72 Fla. Bar J. 10, 16 (Nov. 1998).*

Journal 1998 Discusses proposed legislation in New York that would mandate physician reporting of domestic violence. Argues that mandatory reporting harms patients by threatening the physician-patient relationship. Suggests that victims of domestic violence may be less likely to seek treatment or will be hesitant to speak freely with their physicians if reporting is mandatory. Cites Opinion 2.02. McFarlane, *Mandatory Reporting of Domestic Violence: An Inappropriate Response for New York Health Care Professionals, 17 Buff. Pub. Int. L. J. 1, 29 (1998).*

Journal 1998 Points out that most victims of elder abuse are socially isolated and thus few incidents of elder abuse are reported to authorities. Argues that current protections against elder abuse are inadequate. Suggests that the legal system and health professionals can make a difference in reducing elder abuse. Quotes Opinion 5.05. References Opinion 2.02. Moskowitz, *Saving Granny From the Wolf: Elder Abuse and Neglect—The Legal Framework, 31 Conn. L. Rev. 77, 116, 120, 121, 122 (1998).*

Journal 1997 Considers the best interests of children who are victims of domestic abuse. Advocates a rebuttable presumption against granting custody to a perpetrator. Concludes that courts should be educated about domestic violence. References Opinion 2.02. Comment, *Protecting Children Exposed to Domestic Violence in Contested Custody and Visitation Litigation, 6 B. U. Pub. Int. L. J. 501, 502, 505 (1997).*

Journal 1997 Reviews the historical treatment of domestic violence in tort law. Explores the difficulties victims of domestic violence suffer in pursuing traditional forms of relief. Considers this issue in the context of divorce proceedings. Offers practical guidance for achieving justice. References Opinion 2.02. Dalton, *Domestic Violence, Domestic Torts and Divorce: Constraints and Possibilities, 31 New. Eng. L. Rev. 319, 354 (1997).*

Journal 1996 Considers means of combating spousal abuse problems. Suggests various schemes of liability to increase aid to victims and reporting of problems. Observes that physicians may play an important role in eliminating spousal abuse. Concludes that imposition of civil liability on physicians for failure to report abuse will help remedy problems. References Opinion 2.02. Jones, *Battered Spouses' Damage Actions Against Non-Reporting Physicians, 45 DePaul L. Rev. 191 (1996).*

Journal 1994 Explores the ethical issues involved in a multidisciplinary team working with children in legal proceedings. Focuses on the relationships between professionals and the conflicts that arise regarding disclosure of confidential information and forced disclosure of nonprivileged information. Quotes Principles III and IV, Fundamental Elements (4), and Opinions 1.02 (1992) and 5.07 (1992) [now Opinion 5.05]. Cites Opinion 2.02. Glynn, *Multidisciplinary Representation of Children: Conflicts Over Disclosures of Client Communications, 27 J. Marshall L. Rev. 617, 625, 626, 630-32, 637, 639, 643 (1994).*

2.03 Allocation of Limited Medical Resources

A physician has a duty to do all that he or she can for the benefit of the individual patient. Policies for allocating limited resources have the potential to limit the ability of physicians to fulfill this obligation to patients. Physicians

have a responsibility to participate and to contribute their professional expertise in order to safeguard the interests of patients in decisions made at the
societal level regarding the allocation or rationing of health resources.

Decisions regarding the allocation of limited medical resources among
patients should consider only ethically appropriate criteria relating to medical
need. These criteria include likelihood of benefit, urgency of need, change in
quality of life, duration of benefit, and, in some cases, the amount of resources
required for successful treatment. In general, only very substantial differences
among patients are ethically relevant; the greater the disparities, the more
justified the use of these criteria becomes. In making quality-of-life judgments,
patients should first be prioritized so that death or extremely poor outcomes
are avoided; then, patients should be prioritized according to change in quality of life, but only when there are very substantial differences among patients.
Nonmedical criteria, such as ability to pay, age, social worth, perceived obstacles to treatment, patient contribution to illness, or past use of resources, should
not be considered.

Allocation decisions should respect the individuality of patients and the
particulars of individual cases as much as possible. When very substantial differences do not exist among potential recipients of treatment on the basis of
the appropriate criteria defined above, a "first-come-first-served" approach or
some other equal opportunity mechanism should be employed to make final
allocation decisions. Though there are several ethically acceptable strategies for implementing these criteria, no single strategy is ethically mandated.
Acceptable approaches include a three-tiered system, a minimal threshold
approach, and a weighted formula. Decision-making mechanisms should be
objective, flexible, and consistent to ensure that all patients are treated equally.

The treating physician must remain a patient advocate and therefore should
not make allocation decisions. Patients denied access to resources have the
right to be informed of the reasoning behind the decision. The allocation
procedures of institutions controlling scarce resources should be disclosed to
the public as well as subject to regular peer review from the medical profession.
(I, VII)

Issued March 1981. Updated June 1994 based on the report "Ethical Considerations in the
Allocation of Organs and Other Scarce Medical Resources Among Patients," adopted June 1993
(*Arch Intern Med.* 1995;155:29-40).

Journal 2010 Examines recent health care reform proposals and their failure to address many
issues, including health disparities. Concludes that access to health care should be treated as a
human right to reform the health care system to harmonize with core values. Cites Opinion 2.03.
McClellan, *Health Disparities, Health Care Reform, Morality, and the Law: "Keep Your Government
Hands Off of My Medicare,"* 82 Temp. L. Rev 1141, 1151, 1154-55 (2010).

Journal 2010 Addresses whether health care workers should receive priority in treatment during an influenza epidemic. Using distributive justice principles and practical considerations,
concludes that health care workers should not get priority treatment in such an epidemic and
that medical utility should be the sole criterion in determining any treatment priority. Quotes
Opinion 2.03. Cites Opinion 9.067. Rothstein, *Should Health Care Providers Get Treatment
Priority in an Influenza Pandemic?* 38 J. L. Med. & Ethics 412, 413, 415 (2010).

Journal 2009 Proposes a novel method of predicting risk of liver transplant for any donor/
recipient pair. Concludes that considering the age of the donor, together with the sickness
of the recipient, provides the best prediction of outcome. Cites Opinion 2.03. Halldorson,

Bakthavatsalam, Fix, Reyes, & Perkins, *D-MELD, a Simple Predictor of Post Liver Transplant Mortality for Optimization of Donor/Recipient Matching, 9 Am. J. of Transplantation 318, 324 (2009).*

Journal 2008 Argues that as a matter of public health, physicians must control antibiotic administration to combat antibiotic resistance. Concludes that despite limited incentives for antibiotic conservation, physicians must acknowledge their important role in mitigating the public health threat of antibiotic resistance. Quotes Principles VII and VIII and Opinions 2.09 and 10.015. Cites Opinion 2.03. Saver, *In Tepid Defense of Population Health: Physicians and Antibiotic Resistance, 34 Am. J. L. & Med. 431, 457 (2008).*

Journal 2006 Examines the public reaction to the Terri Schiavo case. Concludes that public fears were misplaced and that all persons benefited from the decision. Quotes Opinions 2.03, 2.035, and 2.17. Cites Opinion 2.22. Cerminara, *Musings on the Need to Convince Some People With Disabilities That End-of-Life Decision-Making Advocates Are Not Out to Get Them, 37 Loy. U. Chi. L. J. 343, 347 (2006).*

Journal 2006 Reviews policy surrounding medical futility in the US and UK. Concludes that communication and collaboration with patients and their families is the best solution for addressing decisions about futile care. Quotes Opinion 2.035. Cites Opinion 2.03. Rowland, *Communicating Past the Conflict: Solving the Medical Futility Controversy With Process-Based Approaches, 14 U. Miami Int'l & Comp. L. Rev. 271, 278-79 (2006).*

Journal 2003 Discusses the practice of gainsharing and argues that providing physicians and hospitals with certain financial incentives to reduce health costs may be of value in health care reform. Concludes with suggestions for how best to proceed in this difficult context. Quotes Opinions 2.03, 2.09, 4.04, and 8.03. References Opinion 8.13. Saver, *Squandering the Gain: Gainsharing and the Continuing Dilemma of Physician Financial Incentives, 98 Nw. U. L. Rev. 145, 219, 221, 222 (2003).*

Journal 2002 Examines whether managed care organizations should be obligated to disclose physician financial incentives that may limit patient care. Concludes that mandatory disclosure is in the best interest of patients and physicians. Quotes Opinions 2.03 and 8.13. Talesh, *Breaking the Learned Helplessness of Patients: Why MCOs Should Be Required to Disclose Financial Incentives, 26 Law & Psychol. Rev. 49, 60-61, 63 (2002).*

Journal 2001 Examines issues relating to health care cost containment. Concludes that, if physicians are to meet the goals assigned to them in a cost-constrained health care system, then professional standards must be reevaluated and modified to afford meaningful guidance for clinical decision-making in the face of health care spending controls. Quotes Opinions 2.03, 2.09, 2.095, 8.032, and 9.04. Cites Opinions 8.02, 8.021, 8.051, and 8.13. Agrawal, *Resuscitating Professionalism: Self-regulation in the Medical Marketplace, 66 Mo. L. Rev. 341, 354, 355, 360, 361, 378, 388 (2001).*

Journal 2001 Discusses the prohibition on nonlawyer ownership of legal service providers. Considers how ethical rules and standards governing physicians have been directed toward preserving independent judgment. Concludes that ethical conflicts created by abandoning the prohibition on nonlawyer ownership of legal service providers may be managed by following the medical ethics model. Quotes Principle VI and Opinions 2.03, 2.09, 8.02, 8.021, 8.03, 8.05, 8.051, 8.054, 8.13, and 8.132. Harris & Foran, *The Ethics of Middle-Class Access to Legal Services and What We Can Learn From the Medical Profession's Shift to a Corporate Paradigm, 70 Fordham L. Rev. 775, 817, 821, 822, 823, 824 (2001).*

Journal 2000 Considers how social and political values shape normative understandings of health and disease. Concludes that the challenge for developing universal canonical accounts of health and disease arises out of moral diversity. Quotes Opinion 2.03. Cherry, *Polymorphic Medical Ontologies: Fashioning Concepts of Disease, 25 J. Med. & Phil. 519, 532 (2000).*

Journal 1999 Analyzes federal regulations regarding allocation of organs for transplantation. Explores the political background and controversy surrounding allocation of human organs. Cites Opinion 2.03. McMullen, *Equitable Allocation of Human Organs: An Examination of the New Federal Regulation, 20 J. Legal Med. 405, 412 (1999).*

Journal 1999 Points out that several states do not allow patients to designate their physicians as health care proxies. Observes that such restrictions inhibit patient autonomy. Provides justification in support of permitting appointments of physicians as proxies. Cites Opinion 2.03. Rai,

Siegler, & Lantos, *The Physician as a Health Care Proxy*, 29 Hastings Center Rep. 14, 19 (Sep./ Oct. 1999).

Journal 1999 Discusses the need for physicians to advocate on behalf of patients' rights in the context of health care delivery. Evaluates the nature and scope of the physician's role as advocate, noting that physicians cannot be expected to engage in attorney-like advocacy. Quotes Principles IV and VI, Fundamental Elements (2), (4), and (6) [now Opinion 10.01], Patient Responsibilities 5 [now Opinion 10.02], and Opinions 2.03, 2.07, 2.09, 2.16, 2.19, 3.06, 4.01, 4.04, 6.01, 7.02, 8.02, 8.03, 8.13, 8.132, 9.06, 9.07, and 9.131. Cites Opinions 5.05, 5.09, 7.01, 8.135, and 9.02. Sage, *Physicians as Advocates*, 35 Hous. L. Rev. 1529, 1537, 1541, 1542, 1552-53, 1554, 1556, 1557, 1559, 1561-62, 1564, 1571, 1574, 1576, 1580 (1999).

Journal 1999 Explores the impact managed care organizations have had on health care. Explains that patients may not understand restrictions and incentives imposed by their managed care organizations when entering the program. Argues that such information should be disclosed at various times during the period of plan coverage. Cites Opinions 2.03, 8.03, 8.032, 8.051, 8.13, and 8.132. Wolf, *Toward a Systemic Theory of Informed Consent in Managed Care*, 35 Hous. L. Rev. 1631, 1641, 1658, 1661, 1662, 1679 (1999).

Journal 1998 Discusses the physician's fiduciary duty to the patient. Explores the expansion of the "honest services" mail fraud statute to prosecute undisclosed fiduciary breaches. Concludes that the mail fraud statute may be used to prosecute physicians who fail to disclose financial incentives to their patients. Quotes Opinion 8.03. Cites Opinions 2.03 and 8.07 [now Opinion 8.06]. Jones, *Primum Non Nocere: The Expanding "Honest Services" Mail Fraud Statute and the Physician-Patient Fiduciary Relationship*, 51 Vand. L. Rev. 139, 161, 164 (1998).

Journal 1997 Posits that cost-containment schemes in managed care systems have eroded the fiduciary duty physicians owe patients. Notes that MCOs are prohibiting patients from trusting and relying on physicians. Concludes that patients must seek quality assurance from sources other than their physicians. Quotes Opinions 2.03, 2.09, and 8.13. Jacobi, *Patients at a Loss: Protecting Health Care Consumers Through Data Driven Quality Assurance*, 45 U. Kan. L. Rev. 705, 720, 721, 759 (1997).

Journal 1996 Examines the role of physicians in managed health care. Posits that the new system of managed care is beneficial because it combines high performance with affordable outcomes. Concludes that outcome-based payment systems, with tort reform, will maximize results. Quotes Opinion 2.03 (1984) [subsequently amended]. Furrow, *Incentivizing Medical Practice: What (if Anything) Happens to Professionalism?* 1 Widener L. Symp. J. 1, 9 (1996).

Journal 1996 Discusses the trend toward conserving resources expended on health care by withholding services absent a showing of necessity. Claims that the high standard of care physicians owe patients is jeopardized by medical treatment decisions based on coverage concerns. Concludes that the legal structure regarding health care plans should be changed. Quotes Preamble, Principles I, II, III, IV, V, VI, and VII, and Opinion 2.03. Hirshfeld & Thomason, *Medical Necessity Determinations: The Need for a New Legal Structure*, 6 Health Matrix 3, 8-9 (1996).

Journal 1996 Considers whether the Oregon Health Plan discriminates on the basis of race by excluding coverage for obesity which disproportionately affects African American women. Discusses discrimination in federally funded health care programs and the purpose of Title VI. Quotes Opinion 2.03. Jurevic, *Disparate Impact Under Title VI: Discrimination, By Any Other Name, Will Still Have the Same Impact*, 15 St. Louis U. Pub. L. Rev. 237, 253 (1996).

Journal 1996 Discusses conflicts of interest between health care professionals and patients created by managed health care and the drive toward reduction of costs. Suggests that a multidisciplinary group of health professionals could act as patient advocates to help protect their interests. Quotes Opinion 2.03. Mehlman, *Medical Advocates: A Call for a New Profession*, 1 Widener L. Symp. J. 299, 314 (1996).

Journal 1996 Considers the change from traditional medical care systems to managed care, noting the conflicts of interest this creates between physicians' ethical obligations and financial concerns. Discusses these issues in the context of managed behavioral health care. Suggests community-based care and social supports as a solution. Quotes Opinions 2.03 and 4.04. Petrila, *Ethics, Money, and the Problem of Coercion in Managed Behavioral Health Care*, 40 St. Louis U. L. J. 359, 377 (1996).

Journal 1994 Considers how greater patient autonomy has led to situations in which medical care may be viewed as futile. Suggests that the law has intruded too far into this area of medicine. Quotes Opinion 2.035. Cites Opinions 2.03, 2.095, 2.17, 2.19, 2.20, and 2.22. Cultice, *Medical Futility: When Is Enough, Enough? 27 J. Health & Hosp. Law 225, 230, 256 (1994).*

Journal 1994 Discusses the practice of physician rationing and how the principles of beneficence and autonomy are consistent with the practice. Explores the objection to using financial incentives, commonly adopted by health maintenance organizations (HMOs), to promote rationing and concludes that rationing should be allowed in some circumstances. Quotes Opinion 2.03. Hall, *Rationing Health Care at the Bedside, 69 N. Y. U. L. Rev. 693, 704 (1994).*

Journal 1994 Observes that health care reform proposals present significant challenges to the role and ethics of attending physicians. Emphasizes that reform proposals must set forth the role envisioned for physicians and must articulate an acceptable ethical framework within which physicians may fulfill that role. Quotes Opinions 4.04, 9.121, and 9.122. Cites Opinions 2.03, 2.09, 5.01, and 8.03. Wolf, *Health Care Reform and the Future of Physician Ethics, 24 Hastings Center Rep. 28, 32, 40 (March/April 1994).*

Journal 1992 Discusses two California cases focusing on the liability of physicians and third-party payers when medically necessary care is denied. Concludes that physicians also may be obligated to advocate patient interests in attempting to secure payment from third parties when appropriate. Quotes Opinion 2.03. Comment, *Who's in Charge: The Doctor or the Dollar? Assessing the Relative Liability of Third Party Payors and Doctors After Wickline and Wilson, 18 J. Contemp. L. 285, 301, 302 (1992).*

Journal 1992 Examines the major health care rationing issues facing the US including increasing costs and decreasing access. Concludes that the standard of care should not be changed and that rationing should be a separate enterprise undertaken pursuant to explicit criteria. Quotes Opinions 2.03, 2.09, and 4.04. Hirshfeld, *Should Ethical and Legal Standards for Physicians Be Changed to Accommodate New Models for Rationing Health Care? 140 Univ. Pa. L. Rev. 1809, 1816 (1992).*

Journal 1991 Focuses on the denial of insurance benefits for experimental medical procedures, and explains the de novo review process under ERISA. Concludes that there is need for a structure that will permit greater objectivity in the context of data collection as well as judicial determination. Cites Opinions 2.03 and 2.09. Note, *Denial of Coverage for "Experimental" Medical Procedures: The Problem of De Novo Review Under ERISA, 79 Kentucky L. J. 801, 824 (1990-91).*

Journal 1990 Discusses economic considerations in clinical decision-making, with emphasis on the standard of care. Concludes that organized medicine has made valuable contributions through development of practice parameters that offer guidance in the exercise of clinical judgment. Cites Opinions 2.03 and 2.09. Hirshfeld, *Economic Considerations in Treatment Decisions and the Standard of Care in Medical Malpractice Litigation, 264 JAMA 2004, 2007 (1990).*

Journal 1990 Discusses efforts of third-party payers to control health care expenditures for beneficiaries. Concludes that financial incentives to limit care and other cost-control techniques should be disclosed and that the rationale for such disclosure is compelling. Quotes Opinions 2.03, 2.09, and 8.03. Cites Opinions 2.19, 4.04, and 4.06. Hirshfeld, *Should Third Party Payors of Health Care Services Disclose Cost Control Mechanisms to Potential Beneficiaries? 14 Seton Hall Legis. J. 115, 130, 131, 144, 145, 146 (1990).*

Journal 1988 Discusses various circumstances that have led to proposals for the rationing of health care by hospitals and other providers in order to contain health care costs. Because of the impact such proposals may have on older persons, focus is placed on the Age Discrimination Act of 1975 and its likely effect on the use of age as a criterion for rationing in the context of heart transplantation. Quotes Opinion 2.02 (1982) [now Opinion 2.03]. Silver, *From Baby Doe to Grandpa Doe: The Impact of the Federal Age Discrimination Act on the Hidden Rationing of Medical Care, 37 Catholic Univ. L. Rev. 993, 1013 (1988).*

Journal 1985 Notes that considerations of cost and availability of advanced medical technology raise troublesome ethical and legal issues. In addressing these issues, examines potential mechanisms for rationing expensive lifesaving medical treatment, concluding that the cost of rationing probably exceeds the benefits. Quotes Opinion 2.02 (1982) [now Opinion 2.03]. Mehlman, *Rationing Expensive Lifesaving Medical Treatments, 1985 Wisconsin L. Rev. 239, 250, 260 (1985).*

2.035 Futile Care

Physicians are not ethically obligated to deliver care that, in their best professional judgment, will not have a reasonable chance of benefiting their patients. Patients should not be given treatments simply because they demand them. Denial of treatment should be justified by reliance on openly stated ethical principles and acceptable standards of care, as defined in Opinion 2.03, "Allocation of Limited Medical Resources," and Opinion 2.095, "The Provision of Adequate Health Care," not on the concept of "futility," which cannot be meaningfully defined. (I, IV)

Issued June 1994.

Journal 2010 Discusses futility disputes where a patient's surrogate wishes to prolong treatment that the physician deems medically ineffective, and the current lack of legal remedies to resolve them. Concludes that states need to establish fair, impartial, and patient-centered methods of resolving futility disputes including independent medical boards that would operate under procedural and substantive regulations. Quotes Opinions 2.02 and 2.035. References Opinions 2.17 and 2.20. Bassel, *Order at the End of Life: Establishing a Clear and Fair Mechanism for the Resolution of Futility Disputes,* 63 Vand. L. Rev. 491, 494, 523 (2010).

Journal 2009 Examines criteria defining when renal dialysis becomes futile. Concludes that uniform guidelines should be adopted defining when medical care is futile and should be withheld. Cites Opinion 2.035. Fink, *Time to Stop Dialyzing the Dead (and Treating Other Patients Too Aggressively, Too),* 38 Dialysis & Transplantation 184, 185 (May 2009, 1, 1).

Journal 2009 Explores the nature of the physician-patient relationship and the impact of increased availability of medical information on patient autonomy and physician responsibility to exercise independent judgment. Concludes physicians must treat patients in accordance with their fiduciary obligation to use their own judgment when confronted with a patient demanding unnecessary medical services. Quotes Preamble, Principles I and VIII, and Opinions 2.035, 8.03, and 10.015. Hafemeister, *The Fiduciary Obligation of Physicians to "Just Say No" if an "Informed" Patient Demands Services That Are Not Medically Indicated,* 39 Seton Hall L. Rev. 335, 372, 373, 374 (2009).

Journal 2008 Discusses medical options when the physician can do nothing further to cure the patient and examines the Texas Advance Directives Act, a medical futility statute. Concludes conflicts may be reduced if physician-patient communication is initiated when treatment begins rather than when further treatment becomes futile. Cites the Texas medical futility process as an example for providing physicians a mechanism for resolving conflicts with patients. Quotes Opinions 2.035, 2.037, and 2.20. Dahm, *Medical Futility and the Texas Medical Futility Statute: A Model to Follow or One to Avoid?* 20 Health Law 25, 26 (Aug. 2008).

Journal 2007 Argues that it is unethical for a physician to withhold CPR without seeking consent of the patient. Concludes that standards for withholding care should be agreed upon by society and passed into law. Cites Opinion 2.035. Manthous, *Counterpoint: Is It Ethical to Order "Do Not Resuscitate" Without Patient Consent?* 132 Chest 751, 753 (2007).

Journal 2007 Compares US and international policy on end-of-life decision making. Concludes that interests of patient autonomy should be balanced with family interests and advocates a comprehensive "best interest" model. Quotes Opinion 2.037. Cites Opinions 2.035 and 2.20. Rode, *End-of-Life Decision Making for Patients in Persistent Vegetative States: A Comparative Analysis,* 30 Hastings Int'l & Comp. L. Rev. 477, 499, 500 (2007).

Journal 2007 Discusses patients' right to refuse medical treatment and the corresponding duties of health care professionals. Concludes that detailed, carefully prepared advance directives are necessary to fulfill patients' wishes. Quotes Ch. II (1940) [now Opinions 8.08 and 8.082] and Opinions 2.035, 2.037, 2.20, 2.225, 8.081, and 10.015. Cites Opinions 9.11 and 9.115. Stamatakis, *Beyond Advance Directives: Personal Autonomy and the Right to Refuse Life-Sustaining Medical Treatment,* 47 N. H. B. J. 20, 29-30 (2007).

Journal 2006 Examines ethical dilemmas physicians may face as providers of pay-for-performance medical care. Concludes that this strategy offers a benefit to patients as long as physicians uphold stringent ethical standards and work together to ensure optimum patient care. Cites Principles I, V, VIII, and IX and Opinions 2.035, 2.095, 6.01, 8.021, 8.03, 8.0501, 8.053, 8.054, and 8.121. Bostick, Sade, & McMahon, *Report of the Council on Ethical and Judicial Affairs: Physician Pay-For-Performance Programs, 3 Ind. Health L. Rev. 429, 430, 431, 432-33, 434, 435, 436 (2006).*

Journal 2006 Examines the public reaction to the Terri Schiavo case. Concludes that public fears were misplaced and that all persons benefited from the decision. Quotes Opinions 2.03, 2.035, and 2.17. Cites Opinion 2.22. Cerminara, *Musings on the Need to Convince Some People With Disabilities That End-of-Life Decision-Making Advocates Are Not Out to Get Them, 37 Loy. U. Chi. L. J. 343, 347 (2006).*

Journal 2006 Reviews policy surrounding medical futility in the US and UK. Concludes that communication and collaboration with patients and their families is the best solution for addressing decisions about futile care. Quotes Opinion 2.035. Cites Opinion 2.03. Rowland, *Communicating Past the Conflict: Solving the Medical Futility Controversy With Process-Based Approaches, 14 U. Miami Int'l & Comp. L. Rev. 271, 278-79 (2006).*

Journal 2006 Discusses the ethical controversy surrounding physician-assisted suicide. Concludes that natural law and individual autonomy are important considerations in the ethical debate. Quotes Opinion 2.211. Cites Opinion 2.035. Wong, *Whose Life Is It Anyway? 5 Cardozo Pub. L. Pol'y & Ethics J. 233, 271-72 (2006).*

Journal 2005 Examines ethical rules governing various forms of alternative dispute resolution. Concludes that a unique set of guidelines is needed for negotiation which encourages greater disclosure, communication, and trust between parties. References Opinion 2.035. Bordone, *Fitting the Ethics to the Forum: A Proposal for Process-Enabling Ethical Codes, 21 Ohio St. J. on Disp. Resol. 1, 35 (2005).*

Journal 2005 Discusses the evidentiary standards utilized to permit withdrawal of life-sustaining treatment by substitute decision-makers when patients are in a persistent vegetative state. Concludes that a futility rationale for making end-of-life decisions may represent the best approach in these situations. Quotes Opinion 2.035. Cites Opinion 2.20. Mareiniss, *A Comparison of Cruzan and Schiavo: The Burden of Proof, Due Process, and Autonomy in the Persistently Vegetative Patient, 26 J. Legal Med. 233, 248, 250 (2005).*

Journal 2004 Discusses a physician's conflict of interest in making end-of-life decisions when there is pressure to maximize ICU profits. Concludes that formal guidelines are needed to ensure that proper life-ending decisions are made in the ICU. Quotes Opinion 2.035. Fleming, *Healthcare Access: Conflicts of Interest Presented by Managed Care ICU Bedside Rationing and Their Impact on Minorities and Women, 5 Geo. J. Gender & L. 663, 667 (2004).*

Journal 2004 Examines conflicts that arise when a hospice may be obligated to resuscitate a patient who has not executed an advance directive regarding CPR. Concludes that the Patient Self-Determination Act must be amended to allow hospice providers to administer CPR in only a limited number of circumstances. References Opinions 2.035 and 2.22. Rutkow, *Dying to Live: The Effect of the Patient Self-Determination Act on Hospice Care, 7 N. Y. U. J. Legis. & Pub. Pol'y 393, 413, 430 (2004).*

Journal 2004 Discusses the law in Tennessee regarding surrogate decision-making. Concludes that recent legislation passed in Tennessee will assist those who care for incapacitated patients. Cites Opinions 2.035, 8.081, and 8.115. Wampler, *To Be or Not to Be in Tennessee: Deciding Surrogate Issues, 34 U. Mem. L. Rev. 333, 365 (2004).*

Journal 2002 Explores the implications of withholding medical treatment when abortion results in a live birth. Concludes that, in these situations, abortive parents and physicians should not solely decide the child's best interest. Quotes Preamble, Principles I and III, and Opinions 2.035, 2.20, and 2.215. Casagrande, *Children Not Meant to Be: Protecting the Interests of the Child When Abortion Results in Live Birth, 6 Quinnipiac Health L. J. 19, 44, 45, 47-48 (2002).*

Journal 2002 Discusses the precautions lawyers must take when advising clients about living wills. Concludes clients must be reminded that medical advances or changes in circumstances may affect their living wills. Quotes Opinion 2.035. Kruse, *A Call for New Perspectives for Living Wills (You Might Like It Here), 37 Real Prop., Prob. & Tr. J. 545, 550 (2002).*

Journal 2001 Observes that many aspects of managed care have increased the tensions between patients and their health care providers. Notes that patient dissatisfaction is on the rise for other reasons as well. Concludes that Congress should take a comprehensive legislative approach in addressing these issues. Quotes Opinion 2.17. Cites Opinion 2.035. References Opinions 2.037 and 2.22. Sanematsu, *Taking a Broader View of Treatment Disputes Beyond Managed Care: Are Recent Legislative Efforts the Cure?* 48 UCLA L. Rev. 1245, 1258, 1284 (2001).

Journal 2000 Considers whether or not age is a sufficient justification to limit or deny access to health care. Concludes that the use of advance care directives, further research, and educational programs can help physicians address this ethical challenge. Quotes Opinion 2.035. Tadd & Bayer, *Commentary: Medical Decision Making Based on Chronological Age—Cause for Concern*, 11 J. Clinical Ethics 328, 330 (2000).

Journal 1998 Explains when a surrogate is required to make health care decisions. Discusses limitations of a surrogate's authority. Emphasizes that the health care provider must recognize that ultimate decision-making regarding care first belongs to the patient, and then to the surrogate. Quotes Opinion 2.035. Cites Opinion 8.11. References Opinion 2.22. O'Neill, *Surrogate Health Care Decisions for Adults in Illinois—Answers to the Legal Questions That Health Care Providers Face on a Daily Basis*, 29 Loy. Univ. Chi. L. J. 411, 445, 448 (1998).

Journal 1997 Examines case law pertaining to medical futility disputes. Reviews hospital policies regarding futility and notes a variety of definitions and guidelines. Concludes that, absent a clear consensus, physicians should not act solely to decide questions of futility. References Opinions 2.035 and 2.22. Johnson, Gibbons, Goldner, Wiener, & Eton, *Legal and Institutional Policy Responses to Medical Futility*, 30 J. Health & Hosp. L. 21, 26, 31, 35, 36 (1997).

Journal 1995 Considers how the judiciary, legislatures, and provider institutions balance the values of patients and their physicians. Recommends that physicians and hospitals promulgate written policies outlining their preferred treatment parameters in any given circumstance. Quotes Opinion 2.035. Daar, *Medical Futility and Implications for Physician Autonomy*, XXI Am. J. Law & Med. 221, 234 (1995).

Journal 1995 Examines the rights of health care professionals to refuse to participate in patient care on the basis of conscientious objection. Suggests steps that health care facilities may take when dealing with health care professionals who object to participating in patient care. Quotes Principles I and VI and Opinions 1.02, 2.035, and 9.055. Dellinger & Vickery, *When Staff Object to Participating in Care*, 28 J. Health & Hospital Law 269, 272, 276 (1995).

Journal 1994 Considers how greater patient autonomy has led to situations in which medical care may be viewed as futile. Suggests that the law has intruded too far into this area of medicine. Quotes Opinion 2.035. Cites Opinions 2.03, 2.095, 2.17, 2.19, 2.20, and 2.22. Cultice, *Medical Futility: When Is Enough, Enough?* 27 J. Health & Hosp. Law 225, 230, 256 (1994).

2.037 Medical Futility in End-of-Life Care

When further intervention to prolong the life of a patient becomes futile, physicians have an obligation to shift the intent of care toward comfort and closure. However, there are necessary value judgments involved in coming to the assessment of futility. These judgments must give consideration to patient or proxy assessments of worthwhile outcome. They should also take into account the physician or other provider's perception of intent in treatment, which should not be to prolong the dying process without benefit to the patient or to others with legitimate interests. They may also take into account community and institutional standards, which in turn may have used physiological or functional outcome measures.

Nevertheless, conflicts between the parties may persist in determining what is futility in the particular instance. This may interrupt satisfactory decision-making and adversely affect patient care, family satisfaction, and physician–clinical team functioning. To assist in fair and satisfactory decision-making about what constitutes futile intervention:

(1) All health care institutions, whether large or small, should adopt a policy on medical futility; and

(2) Policies on medical futility should follow a due process approach. The following seven steps should be included in such a due process approach to declaring futility in specific cases:

   (a) Earnest attempts should be made in advance to deliberate over and negotiate prior understandings between patient, proxy, and physician on what constitutes futile care for the patient, and what falls within acceptable limits for the physician, family, and possibly also the institution.

   (b) Joint decision-making should occur between patient or proxy and physician to the maximum extent possible.

   (c) Attempts should be made to negotiate disagreements if they arise, and to reach resolution within all parties' acceptable limits, with the assistance of consultants as appropriate.

   (d) Involvement of an institutional committee such as the ethics committee should be requested if disagreements are irresolvable.

   (e) If the institutional review supports the patient's position and the physician remains unpersuaded, transfer of care to another physician within the institution may be arranged.

   (f) If the process supports the physician's position and the patient/proxy remains unpersuaded, transfer to another institution may be sought and, if done, should be supported by the transferring and receiving institutions.

   (g) If transfer is not possible, the intervention need not be offered. (I, V)

Issued June 1997 based on the report "Medical Futility in End-of-Life Care," adopted December 1996 (JAMA. 1999;281:937-941).

Journal 2008 Discusses medical options when the physician can do nothing further to cure the patient and examines the Texas Advance Directives Act, a medical futility statute. Concludes conflicts may be reduced if physician-patient communication is initiated when treatment begins rather than when further treatment becomes futile. Cites the Texas medical futility process as an example for providing physicians a mechanism for resolving conflicts with patients. Quotes Opinions 2.035, 2.037, and 2.20. Dahm, *Medical Futility and the Texas Medical Futility Statute: A Model to Follow or One to Avoid? 20 Health Law 25, 26 (Aug. 2008).*

Journal 2007 Compares US and international policy on end-of-life decision making. Concludes that interests of patient autonomy should be balanced with family interests and advocates a comprehensive "best interest" model. Quotes Opinion 2.037. Cites Opinions 2.035 and 2.20. Rode, *End-of-Life Decision Making for Patients in Persistent Vegetative States: A Comparative Analysis, 30 Hastings Int'l & Comp. L. Rev. 477, 499, 500 (2007).*

Journal 2007 Discusses patients' right to refuse medical treatment and the corresponding duties of health care professionals. Concludes that detailed, carefully prepared advance directives are necessary to fulfill patients' wishes. Quotes Ch. II (1940) [now Opinions 8.08 and 8.082] and Opinions 2.035, 2.037, 2.20, 2.225, 8.081, and 10.015. Cites Opinions 9.11 and 9.115. Stamatakis, *Beyond Advance Directives: Personal Autonomy and Their Right to Refuse Life-Sustaining Medical Treatment, 47 N. H. B. J. 20, 29-30 (2007).*

Journal 2006 Examines US and UK terminal illness jurisprudence. Proposes new legislation should be drafted to allow for palliative care when curative treatments are no longer appropriate. Cites Opinions 2.037 and 9.115. Feldhammer, *Medical Torture: End of Life Decision-Making in the United Kingdom and United States, 14 Cardozo J. Int'l & Comp. L. 511, 514-15, 532 (2006).*

Journal 2006 Reviews Texas statutory policies related to the handling of cases of medical futility. Concludes that effective communication is the best means of resolving a conflict over treatment and that statutory guidelines are best used as a last resort. Cites Opinion 2.037. Halevy & McGuire, *The History, Successes and Controversies of the Texas "Futility" Policy, 43 Houston Lawyer 38, 39 (2006).*

Journal 2006 Discusses decision-making authority in cases of medical futility. Concludes that unilateral decision-making by the health care provider poses numerous ethical and legal problems. Quotes Opinion 2.037. Kwiecinski, *To Be or Not to Be, Should Doctors Decide? Ethical and Legal Aspects of Medical Futility Policies*, 7 Marq. Elder's Advisor 313, 323-24 (2006).

Journal 2002 Critiques Daniel Callahan's theory of rationing health resources according to age. Concludes age should not be a controlling factor in end-of-life decision-making. References Opinion 2.037. Cohen-Almagor, *A Critique of Callahan's Utilitarian Approach to Resource Allocation in Health Care*, 17 Issues L. & Med. 247, 261 (2002).

Journal 2002 Analyzes ethical positions on futility in light of the California Uniform Health Care Decisions Act. Concludes the Act provides only a preliminary framework and considers AMA guidelines on medical futility in offering suggestions for change. Quotes Opinion 2.037. Ferguson, *Ethical Postures of Futility and California's Uniform Health Care Decisions Act*, 75 S. Cal. L. Rev. 1217, 1252-53 (2002).

Journal 2001 Observes that many aspects of managed care have increased the tensions between patients and their health care providers. Notes that patient dissatisfaction is on the rise for other reasons as well. Concludes that Congress should take a comprehensive legislative approach in addressing these issues. Quotes Opinion 2.17. Cites Opinion 2.035. References Opinions 2.037 and 2.22. Sanematsu, *Taking a Broader View of Treatment Disputes Beyond Managed Care: Are Recent Legislative Efforts the Cure?* 48 UCLA L. Rev. 1245, 1258, 1284 (2001).

Journal 2000 Discusses the rise and fall of the futility movement. Focuses on attempts to define and develop a process for resolving futility disputes. Concludes that the decision-making dilemma surrounding treatments of minimal benefit still exists and that talking to patients and families should be viewed as the primary method by which physicians may address this problem. References Opinion 2.037. Helft, Siegler, & Lantos, *The Rise and Fall of the Futility Movement*, 343 New Eng. J. Med. 293, 294 (2000).

Journal 2000 Evaluates documentation of decision-making in the treatment of hospitalized elderly trauma patients who died. Considers the frequency of withdrawal of therapy and who made the decisions. Concludes that further research is needed regarding methods to resolve disputes involving futility and withdrawal of therapy. References Opinion 2.037. Trunkey, Cahn, Lenfesty, & Mullins, *Management of the Geriatric Trauma Patient at Risk of Death: Therapy Withdrawal Decision Making*, 135 Arch. Surg. 34, 35 (2000).

Journal 2000 Discusses medical futility and offers a case-based assessment of circumstances under which continued use of treatment may exceed the boundaries of reasonableness. Suggests a procedural approach for making decisions on a case-by-case basis. References Opinion 2.037. Truog, *Futility in Pediatrics: From Case to Policy*, 11 J. Clinical Ethics 136, 139, 141 (2000).

2.04   The previous Opinion 2.04, "Artificial Insemination by Known Donor," issued prior to April 1977, was replaced by the current Opinion 2.04, "Artificial Insemination by Known Donor."

2.04   Artificial Insemination by Known Donor

Any individual or couple contemplating artificial insemination by husband, partner, or other known donor should be counseled about the full range of infectious and genetic diseases for which the donor or recipient can be screened, including communicable disease agents and diseases. Full medical history disclosure and appropriate diagnostic screening should be recommended to the donor and recipient but are not required.

Informed consent for artificial insemination should include disclosure of risks, benefits, and likely success rate of the method proposed and potential alternative methods. Individuals should receive information about screening, costs, and procedures for confidentiality, when applicable. The prospective parents or parent should be informed of the laws regarding the rights of children conceived by artificial insemination, as well as the laws regarding parental rights and obligations.

Sex selection of sperm for the purposes of avoiding a sex-linked inheritable disease is appropriate. However, physicians should not participate in sex selection for reasons of gender preference. Physicians should encourage a prospective parent or parents to consider the value of both sexes.

If semen is frozen and the donor dies before it is used, the frozen semen should not be used or donated for purposes other than those originally intended by the donor. If the donor left no instructions, it is reasonable to allow the remaining partner to use the semen for artificial insemination but not to donate it to someone else. However, the donor should be advised of such a policy at the time of donation and be given an opportunity to override it. (I, V)

Issued June 1993; updated December 2004.

Colo. 1989 State statute prohibiting a sperm donor from asserting his parental status was held to be inapplicable where known donor and unmarried recipient agreed that the donor would have parental rights. Concurring opinion argued that the statute bars any nonhusband donor, regardless of relationship to the recipient, from asserting parental rights. However, the concurring opinion found the statute inapplicable because its provision requiring "supervision" by a physician had not been met. In apparent reference to the standards set out under Opinions 2.04 and 2.05, the concurring opinion said that "supervision" should at the least require an examination to determine whether there are any health risks to the recipient as a result of the procedure and to protect the child from hereditary disease. *In re R.C., 775 P.2d 27, 37 n.3.*

Journal 2010. Addresses issues involving posthumous conception. Concludes that an estate fiduciary does not have absolute discretion to make decisions regarding the disposition of a decedent's reproductive matter. Cites Opinion 2.04. Cooper & Harper, *Life After Death: The Authority of Estate Fiduciaries to Dispose of Decedents' Reproductive Matter, 26 Touro L. Rev. 649, 658 (2010).*

Journal 2009 Discusses advancements in assisted reproductive technology and the law concerning posthumous conception. Concludes the Model Act Concerning Assisted Reproductive Technology should be used as a basis for legislation to regulate the use of assisted reproductive technology for posthumous conception. Cites Opinion 2.04. O'Brien, *The Momentum of Posthumous Conception: A Model Act, 25 J. Contemp. Health L. & Pol'y 332, 363 (2009).*

Journal 2004 Explores whether a child born through postmortem conception (PMC) can claim an inheritance from a deceased father. Concludes that, under common law rules, a PMC child generally will not be able to inherit; however, the final outcome may be affected by available extrinsic evidence. Quotes Opinion 2.04. Knaplund, *Postmortem Conception and a Father's Last Will, 46 Ariz. L. Rev. 91, 96 (2004).*

Journal 1987 Examines various ethical issues surrounding surrogate motherhood, artificial insemination, in vitro fertilization, and embryonic/fetal research. Reports on the positions of four ethics groups: the Warnock Committee of Inquiry into Human Fertilization and Embryology; the AMA's Council on Ethical and Judicial Affairs; the Ethics Committee of the American Fertility Society; and the Ethics Committee of the American College of Obstetricians and Gynecologists. References Opinions 2.04, 2.05, and 2.13 (1986) [now Opinion 2.14]. Quotes Opinion 2.18. Rosner, Cassell, Friedland, Landolt, Loeb, Numann, Ora, Risemberg, & Sordillo, *Ethical Considerations of Reproductive Technologies, 87 N. Y. State J. Med. 398, 399-400 (1987).*

2.05   The previous Opinion 2.05, "Artificial Insemination by Donor," issued 1983, was replaced by the current Opinion 2.05, "Artificial Insemination by Anonymous Donor."

2.05 Artificial Insemination by Anonymous Donor

Thorough medical histories must be taken of all candidates for anonymous semen donation. All potential donors must also be screened for infectious or inheritable diseases which could adversely affect the recipient or the resultant child. Frozen semen should be used for artificial insemination because it enables the donor to be tested for communicable disease agents and diseases at the time of donation, and again after an interval before the original semen is used, thus increasing the likelihood that the semen is free of blood-borne pathogens. Physicians should rely on the guidelines formulated by relevant professional organizations, such as the American Society of Reproductive Medicine, the Centers for Disease Control and Prevention, and the Food and Drug Administration, in determining which disorders to screen for and which procedures to use in screening. Physicians should maintain a permanent record which includes both identifying and nonidentifying health and genetic screening information. Other than exceptional situations where identifying information may be required, physicians should release only nonidentifying health-related information in order to preserve the confidentiality of the semen donor.

Physicians should maintain permanent records of donors to fulfill the following obligations: (1) to exclude individuals from the donor pool who test positive for infectious or inheritable diseases, (2) to limit the number of pregnancies resulting from a single donor source so as to avoid future consanguineous marriages or reproduction, (3) to notify donors of screening results which indicate the presence of an infectious or inheritable disease, and (4) to notify donors if a child born through artificial insemination has a disorder which may have been transmitted by the donor.

Informed consent for artificial insemination should include disclosure of risks, benefits, likely success rate of the method proposed and potential alternative methods, and costs. Both recipients and donors should be informed of the reasons for screening and confidentiality. They should also know the extent of access to nonidentifying and identifying information about the donor. Participants should be advised to consider the legal ramifications, if any, of artificial insemination by anonymous donor.

The consent of the husband is ethically appropriate if he is to become the legal father of the resultant child from artificial insemination by anonymous donor. Anonymous donors cannot assume the rights or responsibilities of parenthood for children born through therapeutic donor insemination, nor should they be required to assume them.

In the case of single women or women who are part of a homosexual couple, it is not unethical to provide artificial insemination as a reproductive option.

Sex selection of sperm for the purposes of avoiding a sex-linked inheritable disease is appropriate. However, physicians should not participate in sex selection of sperm for reasons of gender preference. Physicians should encourage a prospective parent or parents to consider the value of both sexes.

In general, it is inappropriate to offer compensation to donors to encourage donation over and above reimbursement for time and actual expenses. (I, V)

Issued June 1993; updated December 2004.

Colo. 1989 State statute prohibiting a sperm donor from asserting his parental status was held to be inapplicable where known donor and unmarried recipient agreed that the donor would have parental rights. Concurring opinion argued that the statute bars any nonhusband donor, regardless of relationship to the recipient, from asserting parental rights. However, the concurring opinion found the statute inapplicable because its provision requiring "supervision" by a physician had not been met. In apparent reference to the standards set out under Opinions 2.04 and 2.05, the concurring opinion said that "supervision" should at the least require an examination to determine whether there are any health risks to the recipient as a result of the procedure and to protect the child from hereditary disease. *In re R.C., 775 P.2d 27, 37 n.3.*

Journal 2006 Examines protection and regulation of sperm donor genetic information. Concludes that children born as a result of artificial insemination should have a legal right to both medical and genetic information about the donor. References 2.05. D'Orazio, *Half of the Family Tree: A Call For Access to a Full Genetic History for Children Born by Artificial Insemination, 2 J. Health & Biomedical L. 249, 256 (2006).*

Journal 1987 Examines various ethical issues surrounding surrogate motherhood, artificial insemination, in vitro fertilization, and embryonic/fetal research. Reports on the positions of four ethics groups: the Warnock Committee of Inquiry into Human Fertilization and Embryology; the AMA's Council on Ethical and Judicial Affairs; the Ethics Committee of the American Fertility Society; and the Ethics Committee of the American College of Obstetricians and Gynecologists. References Opinions 2.04, 2.05, and 2.13 (1986) [now Opinion 2.14]. Quotes Opinion 2.18. Rosner, Cassell, Friedland, Landolt, Loeb, Numann, Ora, Risemberg, & Sordillo, *Ethical Considerations of Reproductive Technologies, 87 N. Y. State J. Med. 398, 399-400 (1987).*

2.055 Ethical Conduct in Assisted Reproductive Technology

The following guidelines are intended to emphasize the value of existing standards to ensure ethical practices in assisted reproductive technology (ART):

(1) The medical profession's development of technical and ethical guidelines for ART should continue. Education of the profession and patients should be pursued through widely disseminated information. Such material should include information on clinic-specific success rates.

(2) Fertility laboratories not currently participating in a credible professional accreditation program are encouraged to do so. Professional self-regulation is also encouraged through signed pledges to meet established ethical standards and to comply with laboratory accreditation efforts. Physicians who become aware of unethical practices must report such conduct to the appropriate body. Physicians also should be willing to provide expert testimony when needed. Specialty societies should discuss the development of mechanisms for disciplinary action, such as revocation of membership, for members who fail to comply with ethical standards.

(3) Patients should be fully informed about all aspects of ART applicable to their particular clinical profile. A well-researched, validated informed consent instrument would be useful for the benefit of patients and professionals. Payment based on clinical outcome is unacceptable.

(4) Physicians and clinicians practicing ART should use accurate descriptors of available services, success rates, and fee structure and payment obligations in promotional materials.

If legislation on regulation of ART laboratories, advertising practices, or related issues is adopted, it should include adequate financial resources to ensure the intended action can be implemented. Improved legislative protection may be needed to protect physicians and their professional organizations when they provide testimony on unethical conduct of colleagues. (I, V)

Issued December 1998 based on the report "Issues of Ethical Conduct in Assisted Reproductive Technology," adopted June 1996.

Journal 2010 Describes how physicians act as bankers in financing fertility treatments for patients and how this significantly contributes to medical debt and bankruptcies. Proposes regulations which would address these issues within fertility markets. Quotes Opinion 6.08. Cites Opinion 2.055. Hawkins, *Doctors as Bankers: Evidence From Fertility Markets*, 84 Tul. L. Rev. 841, 848, 874 (2010).

Journal 2009 Discusses the costs parents, children, and society incur as a result of multiple gestation pregnancies. Concludes the US should adopt increased regulation similar to that prevalent in European countries to address these costs. Quotes Opinion 2.055. Velikonja, *The Costs of Multiple Gestation Pregnancies in Assisted Reproduction*, 32 Harv. J. L. & Gender 463, 484 (2009).

Journal 2005 Examines legal controversies triggered by advances in technology, using in vitro fertilization as an example. Concludes that no single legislative solution is capable of dealing with the many problems associated with changes in technology. Cites Opinions 2.055 and 2.141. Moses, *Understanding Legal Responses to Technological Change: The Example of In Vitro Fertilization*, 6 Minn. J. L. Sci. & Tech. 505, 543, 615 (2005).

2.06 Capital Punishment

An individual's opinion on capital punishment is the personal moral decision of the individual. A physician, as a member of a profession dedicated to preserving life when there is hope of doing so, should not be a participant in a legally authorized execution. Physician participation in execution is defined generally as actions which would fall into one or more of the following categories: (1) an action which would directly cause the death of the condemned; (2) an action which would assist, supervise, or contribute to the ability of another individual to directly cause the death of the condemned; (3) an action which could automatically cause an execution to be carried out on a condemned prisoner.

Physician participation in an execution includes, but is not limited to, the following actions: prescribing or administering tranquilizers and other psychotropic agents and medications that are part of the execution procedure; monitoring vital signs on site or remotely (including monitoring electrocardiograms); attending or observing an execution as a physician; and rendering of technical advice regarding execution.

In the case where the method of execution is lethal injection, the following actions by the physician would also constitute physician participation in execution: selecting injection sites; starting intravenous lines as a port for a lethal injection device; prescribing, preparing, administering, or supervising injection drugs or their doses or types; inspecting, testing, or maintaining lethal injection devices; and consulting with or supervising lethal injection personnel.

The following actions do not constitute physician participation in execution: (1) testifying as to medical history and diagnoses or mental state as they relate to competence to stand trial, testifying as to relevant medical evidence during trial, testifying as to medical aspects of aggravating or mitigating circumstances during the penalty phase of a capital case, or testifying as to medical diagnoses as they relate to the legal assessment of competence for execution; (2) certifying death, provided that the condemned has been declared dead by another person; (3) witnessing an execution in a totally nonprofessional capacity; (4) witnessing an execution at the specific voluntary request of the condemned person, provided that the physician observes the execution in a nonprofessional capacity; and (5) relieving the acute suffering of a condemned person while awaiting execution, including providing tranquilizers at the specific voluntary request of the condemned person to help relieve pain or anxiety in anticipation of the execution.

Physicians should not determine legal competence to be executed. A physician's medical opinion should be merely one aspect of the information taken into account by a legal decision maker such as a judge or hearing officer. When a condemned prisoner has been declared incompetent to be executed, physicians should not treat the prisoner for the purpose of restoring competence unless a commutation order is issued before treatment begins. The task of re-evaluating the prisoner should be performed by an independent physician examiner. If the incompetent prisoner is undergoing extreme suffering as a result of psychosis or any other illness, medical intervention intended to mitigate the level of suffering is ethically permissible. No physician should be compelled to participate in the process of establishing a prisoner's competence or be involved with treatment of an incompetent, condemned prisoner if such activity is contrary to the physician's personal beliefs. Under those circumstances, physicians should be permitted to transfer care of the prisoner to another physician.

Organ donation by condemned prisoners is permissible only if (1) the decision to donate was made before the prisoner's conviction, (2) the donated tissue is harvested after the prisoner has been pronounced dead and the body removed from the death chamber, and (3) physicians do not provide advice on modifying the method of execution for any individual to facilitate donation. (I)

Issued July 1980. Updated June 1994 based on the report "Physician Participation in Capital Punishment," adopted December 1992 (JAMA. 1993;270:365-368); updated June 1996 based on the report "Physician Participation in Capital Punishment: Evaluations of Prisoner Competence to Be Executed; Treatment to Restore Competence to Be Executed," adopted in June 1995; updated December 1999; and updated June 2000 based on the report "Defining Physician Participation in State Executions," adopted June 1998.

U.S. 2008 Affirmed Kentucky Supreme Court decision that Kentucky's lethal injections protocol does not violate the Eighth Amendment's ban on cruel and unusual punishment. Alito, J., concurring, cited Opinion 2.06 and recognized (1) the ethical rules of the profession prohibiting physician participation in lethal injection executions and (2) that a modification of a lethal injection protocol is not "feasible" or "readily available" if it would require participation by persons whose professional ethics impede participation. *Baze v. Rees, 553 U.S. 35, 64 (2008) (Alito, J., concurring).*

6th Cir. 2009 Death row inmate intervened in action brought challenging Ohio's lethal injection protocol. Inmate argued the state's new one-drug protocol was inadequate regarding the competency, training, and supervision of execution personnel. In rejecting the argument that physicians should be required to oversee execution, the court noted Ohio statute permitting revocation of a physician's license for a violation of the Code of Ethics of the AMA. The court cited Opinion 2.06 prohibiting physician participation in executions. *Cooey v. Strickland, 589 F.3d 210, 227.*

6th Cir. 2007 A death row inmate challenged the method of execution under the Eighth Amendment. State officials moved to dismiss the complaint as untimely. The district court denied the motion. The Court of Appeals held that the state two-year statute of limitations applied and that, although the discovery rule extended the limitations period to the date when information about the execution procedure was available, plaintiff's claim was still untimely. The dissent argued that information about the execution procedure available to plaintiff was misleading. For example, the available information stated that a physician pronounces death. Quoting

Opinion 2.06, the dissent noted this could constitute unethical conduct by a physician. *Cooey v. Strickland, 479 F.3d 412, 428.*

8th Cir. 2003 Prisoner convicted of capital felony murder was involuntarily medicated after a review panel held he was a danger to himself and others. Thereafter, the state set an execution date for prisoner because he was competent due to the medication. The Court of Appeals, en banc, affirmed lower court's denial of the prisoner's habeus corpus petition. Court found state had a duty to medicate the prisoner and that Eighth Amendment is not violated when a prisoner on death row regains competency as a result of involuntary medication. Dissenting judges, with apparent reference to Opinion 2.06, noted that the ethical standards of the AMA prohibit physicians from assisting in executions. *Singleton v. Norris, 319 F.3d 1018, 1036.*

D.D.C. 2001 District court found that the government was permitted to treat the defendant involuntarily with antipsychotic medication in order to render him nondangerous and mentally competent to stand trial. The court in making its decision that a pretrial detainee is not afforded the same prohibition against involuntary medication as a convicted defendant waiting to be executed apparently relied on Opinion 2.06. *United States v. Weston, 134 F. Supp. 2d 115, 126-27.*

E.D. Ky. 2007 Plaintiff, a death-row inmate, challenged the constitutionality of the state's method of execution. The state's execution protocol stipulated that if an IV could not be properly inserted, a request to postpone the execution should be made to the governor. Plaintiff sought to depose the state's governor (who was a physician) to determine what his response would be in such a situation and argued that because the governor was also a physician, he might issue medical advice. The court found this question irrelevant to the constitutional issue. Additionally, the court noted that, under the state's law, physicians must abide by the AMA Code of Medical Ethics and that Opinion 2.06 expressly prohibits supervising an execution. *Moore v. Rees, 2007 WL 1035013, 6.*

La. 1992 State's attempt to circumvent prohibition against execution of insane prisoners by forcibly medicating prisoner was held to be a violation of the prisoner's right to privacy and constituted cruel and unusual punishment. Noting that a physician's administration of medication in order to facilitate the prisoner's execution is contrary to the AMA's ethical code, in apparent reference to Opinion 2.06, the court held that involuntary administration of medication is not medical treatment but constitutes a part of capital punishment. *State v. Perry, 610 So. 2d 746, 753.*

N.C. 2009 Department of corrections and prison warden brought action against state medical board to enjoin board from taking any disciplinary action against physicians for participating in executions. The court cited the board's position statement prohibiting physician participation in executions, quoting Opinion 2.06. The court held the position statement was an invalid exercise of board's statutory powers. *North Carolina Department of Corrections v. North Carolina Medical Board, 363 N.C. 189, 675 S.E.2d 641, 644-65.*

S.C. 1993 State sought to reverse order vacating death sentence and imposing life imprisonment. The court stated that the critical issue inherent in the state's contention of error was whether the state could forcibly medicate a prisoner solely to make prisoner competent enough to execute. Citing Opinion 2.06, the court held that the AMA's position reinforces the prohibition against the state's use of medication solely to facilitate an insane prisoner's execution. *Singleton v. State, 437 S.E. 2d 53, 61.*

Tenn. App. 2004 Appeal from a district court order finding that Tennessee's three-drug lethal injection procedure does not constitute "cruel and unusual" punishment under the US or Tennessee constitutions or violate state professional practice statutes. The Court of Appeals of Tennessee, citing Opinion 2.06, concluded that the state legislature likely anticipated that licensed health care professionals would not participate in executions because such participation violates professional ethics codes. *Abdur'Rahman v. Bredesen, 2004 WL 2246227, n. 45.*

Va. Att'y Gen. 1994 Attorney General responded in the negative when asked whether a physician employed by the department of corrections may be disciplined by the board of medicine for participating in the execution of a prisoner where "participating" was defined as "attending or observing an execution, for making a determination that death has occurred, for issuing a certificate of death, or for performing any other function that applicable state statutes lawfully require to be performed by a physician in connection with an execution." Citing Opinion 2.06, the Attorney General noted that such ethical opinions are not legally conclusive and that if they conflict with a state statute, the statute controls. *Va. Att'y Gen. Op., 1994 Va. AG LEXIS 12.*

Journal 2011 Argues physicians should have the choice to participate in lethal injection executions. Concludes that although executions may proceed without physician involvement and the integrity and ethics of the medical profession must be protected, because executions performed without a physician have been mishandled, physician involvement is needed. Quotes Opinion 2.211. References Opinion 2.06. Nelson & Ashby, *Rethinking the Ethics of Physician Participation in Lethal Injection Execution, 41 Hastings Center Rep., 28, 29, 35 (May-June 2011).*

Journal 2010 Examines recent constitutional challenges to new guidelines for execution by lethal injection in Missouri under the Eighth Amendment's cruel and unusual punishment provisions. Concludes that, while the new Missouri guidelines were upheld as constitutional, legal challenges to the death penalty and lethal injections will continue. Cites Opinion 2.06. Maerz, *Death of the Challenge to Lethal Injection? Missouri's Protocol Deemed Constitutional Yet Again, 75 Mo. L. Rev. 1323, 1340-41 (2010).*

Journal 2010. Addresses whether states may forcibly administer antipsychotic drugs to insane death row inmates to restore their competence for execution. Concludes that execution after forcible medication with antipsychotic drugs violates both the Eighth and Fourteenth Amendments. Cites Opinion 2.06. Sewall, *Pushing Execution Over the Constitutional Line: Forcible Medication of Condemned Inmates and the Eighth and Fourteenth Amendments, 51 B.C. L. Rev. 1279, 1301 (2010).*

Journal 2010 Examines ethical implications of physician involvement in assessments of competence for execution. Concludes forensic psychiatrists should participate in such assessments to prevent executions of those lacking requisite competence. References Opinion 2.06. Weinstock, Leong, & Silva, *Competence to Be Executed: an Ethical Analysis Post Panetti, 28 Behav. Sci. Law 690, 691 (2010).*

Journal 2010 Discusses the right of prison inmates to refuse psychotropic medications and the evolution of medical, ethical, and legal guidelines for physicians in dealing with death row inmates. Concludes physicians need to strictly adhere to the medical-ethical guidelines that are in place regarding death row inmates. Quotes Opinion 2.06. Zonana, *Physicians Must Honor Refusal of Treatment to Restore Competency by Non-Dangerous Inmates on Death Row, 38 J. L. Med. & Ethics 764, 766 (2010).*

Journal 2009 Examines opinions in *Baze v. Rees* from the US Supreme Court discussing the constitutionality of execution by lethal injection. Concludes the Supreme Court did not answer the medical ethics questions regarding lethal injection and urges physicians to remove themselves from the lethal injection procedure entirely. References Opinion 2.06. Annas, *Toxic Tinkering—Lethal-Injection Execution and the Constitution, 359 New Engl. J. Med. 1512, 1512 (2009).*

Journal 2009 Examines the ethical guidelines regarding physicians' participation in interrogations and statutory approaches aimed at eliminating such physician involvement. Concludes that to maintain the integrity of the medical profession, physician involvement in interrogations must be precluded by legislative action. Quotes Preamble and Opinions 2.067 and 2.068. Cites Opinions 2.06 and 2.068. Bahnassi, *Keeping Doctors Out of the Interrogation Room: A New Ethical Obligation That Requires the Backing of the Law, 19 Health Matrix 447, 449-51, 461, 464, 465-67, 469-70, 474-75 (2009).*

Journal 2009 Explores the Supreme Court's *Baze v. Rees* decision and the three-drug protocol for lethal injection. Discusses the necessity of judicial intervention to improve lethal injection protocols. Concludes courts should carefully consider their approach to challenges to lethal injection as an opportunity to prevent violation of Eighth Amendment rights. Quotes Preamble and Opinion 1.02. Cites Opinion 2.06. Berger, *Lethal Injection and the Problem of Constitutional Remedies, 27 Yale L. & Pol'y Rev. 259, 319, 320 (2009).*

Journal 2009 Examines the history of the anti–death penalty movement and analyzes recent Supreme Court decisions and their implications for protection of Eighth Amendment rights. Concludes America ultimately will abolish the death penalty as a violation of international law, consistent with its standing on other forms of cruel and degrading punishments. Cites Opinion 2.06. Bessler, *Revisiting Beccaria's Vision: The Enlightenment, America's Death Penalty, and the Abolition Movement, 4 NW J. L. & Soc. Pol'y 195, 299 (2009).*

Journal 2009 Examines historical and modern methods of execution and discusses the plurality, concurring, and dissenting opinions in *Baze v. Rees.* Concludes scientific testing and medical evidence should be used to conduct a thorough pain analysis of lethal injection to ensure the protocol comports with the Eighth Amendment. Quotes Opinion 2.06. Butler, *Baze v. Rees: Lethal Injection as a Constitutional Method of Execution*, 86 *Denv. U. L. Rev.* 509, 530 (2009).

Journal 2009 Discusses the development of the lethal injection method of execution and the lack of a constitutional standard for reviewing method-of-execution challenges. Concludes that states should strengthen their execution protocols in order to increase the likelihood of overcoming constitutional challenges. References Opinion 2.06. Heilman, *Contemplating "Cruel and Unusual": A Critical Analysis of Baze v. Rees in the Context of the Supreme Court's Eighth Amendment "Proportionality" Jurisprudence*, 58 *Am. U. L. Rev.* 633, 652 (2009).

Journal 2009 Argues that the trichemical combination used in lethal injection carries with it great risk of a needlessly painful execution. Concludes use of this execution method is inconsistent with the Eighth Amendment's Cruel and Unusual Punishment Clause. References Opinion 2.06. Hughes, *The Tri-Chemical Cocktail: Serene Brutality*, 72 *Alb. L. Rev.* 527, 540 (2009).

Journal 2009 Discusses US Supreme Court decisions shaping the law concerning capital punishment. Concludes that the October 2007 term produced opinions displaying conflicting views on the death penalty, but ultimately was important for those seeking to abolish the death penalty. Quotes Opinion 2.06. Klein, *An Analysis of the Death Penalty Jurisprudence of the October 2007 Supreme Court Term*, 25 *Touro L. Rev.* 625, 630 (2009).

Journal 2009 Describes death penalty cases in California wherein prosecutorial misconduct led to a reversal of either the sentence or the conviction. Concludes such misconduct is a systemic problem in California and clear distinctions are needed to help prosecutors avoid misconduct as they try death penalty cases. Cites Opinion 2.06. Minsker, *Prosecutorial Misconduct in Death Penalty Cases*, 45 *Cal. W. L. Rev.* 373, 400 (2009).

Journal 2009 Examines the element of pain present in lethal injection with respect to the Eighth Amendment prohibition on cruel and unusual punishment. Concludes use of the drug Pavulon causes paralysis and severe pain when administered and constitutes cruel and unusual punishment. Argues further that use of Pavulon in human executions should be eliminated. Quotes Opinion 2.06. Tapocsi, *Three Steps to Death: The Use of the Drug Pavulon in the Lethal Injection Protocol Utilized Today Violates the Eighth Amendment's Protection Against Cruel and Unusual Punishment*, 35 *Ohio N. U. L. Rev.* 425, 440 (2009).

Journal 2008 Discusses whether drug-induced competence warrants a finding of sanity in capital punishment cases, thereby qualifying an inmate for execution. Argues the practice of medicating mentally ill inmates to allow for their execution contradicts society's ethical and moral values and poses a question of constitutionality that should be addressed by the courts. Cites Opinion 2.06. Barua, *"Synthetic Sanity": A Way Around the Eighth Amendment?* 44 *Crim. Law Bulletin* 561, 574 (2008).

Journal 2008 Argues pain and punishment are inseparable components of the American justice system. Concludes lethal injection must include an element of pain and calls for renewed efforts to establish capital punishment protocols that conform to societal goals. Cites Opinion 2.06. Blecker, *Killing Them Softly: Meditations on a Painful Punishment of Death*, 35 *Fordham Urb. L. J.* 969, 988 (2008).

Journal 2008 Analyzes the constitutionality of the three-drug lethal injection protocol and legal challenges to this method of execution. Concludes that because lethal injection is a complex and flawed procedure, the legislature should carefully evaluate current execution techniques to ensure humane punishment. Quotes Opinion 2.06. Gaitan, *Challenges Facing Society in the Implementation of the Death Penalty*, 35 *Fordham Urb. L. J.* 763, 767 (2008).

Journal 2008 Considers physician involvement in executions and the resulting ethical complications. Concludes the presence of physicians at executions compromises the physician's duties to society and to the medical profession. Quotes Opinion 2.06. Groner, *The Hippocratic Paradox: The Role of the Medical Profession in Capital Punishment in the United States*, 35 *Fordham Urb. L. J.* 883, 903-04 (2008).

Journal 2008 Discusses disciplinary safe harbor policies as a device for allowing physician participation in executions and examines several justifications relied upon by legislatures for such participation. Concludes the legal justifications of safe harbors are weak, that they may lead to a loss of confidence in the medical profession, and, if so, should not be adopted. Quotes Opinion 2.06. Sawicki, *Doctors, Discipline, and the Death Penalty: Professional Implications of Safe Harbor Policies*, 27 *Yale L. & Pol'y Rev.* 107, 121 (2008).

Journal 2007 Examines the role of the medical profession in participating in state sanctioned lethal injection. Concludes that any participation is unethical because it causes harm and undermines trust. Cites Opinion 2.06. References Opinions 2.211 and 9.02. Black & Sade, *Lethal Injection and Physicians: State Law vs Medical Ethics,* 298 JAMA 2779, 2780, 2781 (2007).

Journal 2007 Examines flaws in lethal injection protocols across states. Concludes that a collaborative effort between legal and medical professionals is needed to revise protocols to meet basic constitutional requirements. Quotes Opinion 2.06. Denno, *The Lethal Injection Quandary: How Medicine Has Dismantled Death,* 76 Fordham L. Rev. 49, 80-81 (2007).

Journal 2007 Discusses challenges to the constitutionality of lethal injection made pursuant to 42 USC § 1983. Concludes that the Supreme Court must rule on the constitutionality of lethal injection to stem a flood of litigation in the lower federal courts. Quotes Opinion 2.06. Greer, *Legal Injection: The Supreme Court Enters the Lethal Injection Debate: Hill v. McDonough, 126 S. Ct. 2096 (2006),* 30 Harv. J. L. & Pub. Pol'y 767, 774 (2007).

Journal 2007 Analyzes the impact of recent death penalty cases. Concludes that, in similar cases, the manner of execution may be challenged under 42 USC § 1983 and that a denial of the right to counsel of choice may result in an overturned conviction. Quotes Opinion 2.06. Klein, *Death Penalty and Right to Counsel Decisions in the October 2005 Term,* 22 Touro L. Rev. 1003, 1012 (2007).

Journal 2007 Examines the constitutionality of lethal injection protocols. Concludes that current protocols are unconstitutional under the Eighth Amendment and suggests that, at minimum, the legislature should conduct a thorough investigation into humane methods of execution. Quotes Opinion 2.06. Kreitzberg & Richter, *But Can It Be Fixed? A Look at Constitutional Challenges to Lethal Injection Executions,* 47 Santa Clara L. Rev. 445, 448, 449, 499, 502 (2007).

Journal 2007 Highlights inconsistencies in applying judicial deference to medical ethics. Concludes that courts should afford greater deference to established medical ethics standards. Quotes Principle I and Opinions 2.06 and Ch. II, Art. I, Sec. 3 (May 1847) [now Opinion 5.02]. Cites Opinions 4.01 and 7.05. Lerman, *Second Opinion: Inconsistent Deference to Medical Ethics in Death Penalty Jurisprudence,* 95 Geo. L. J. 1941, 1945, 1974-75, 1976, 1977 (2007).

Journal 2007 Examines the potential for error in lethal injection procedures. Concludes that such procedures must be changed to ensure a painless execution and should cease to require participation of medical professionals. Quotes Opinion 2.06. Mottor, *Morales and Taylor: The Future of Lethal Injection,* 6 Appalachian J. L. 287, 300-01 (2007).

Journal 2007 Argues that there is a public right to know the identity of state executioners. Concludes that the state must be able to prove the qualification of the executioner, and that this is best accomplished by revealing their identity. Quotes Opinion 2.06. Roko, *Executioner Identities: Toward Recognizing a Right to Know Who Is Hiding Beneath the Hood,* 75 Fordham L. Rev. 2791, 2799 (2007).

Journal 2006 Discusses the ethical issue of incompetent inmates who face capital punishment. Formally recommends that all states adopt policy against execution of incompetent defendants. References Opinion 2.06. American Bar Association Task Force on Mental Disability and the Death Penalty (Igasaki, et al), *Recommendation and Report on the Death Penalty and Persons With Mental Disabilities,* 30 Mental & Physical Disability L. Rep. 668, 676 (2006).

Journal 2006 Evaluates legal and ethical challenges to the use of the drug Pavulon in lethal injection executions. Concludes Pavulon should not be used because of the risk of cruel and unusual punishment. Cites Opinion 2.06. Ewart, *Use of the Drug Pavulon In Lethal Injections: Cruel and Unusual?* 14 Wm. & Mary Bill of Rts. J. 1159, 1182 (2006).

Journal 2006 Discusses mentally incompetent inmates and capital punishment. Proposes that, to be permissible, involuntary medication of death-row inmates must represent the best medically appropriate treatment. Quotes Principles I, III, and VIII and Opinion 2.06. Gabos, *The Perils of Singleton v. Norris: Ethics and Beyond,* 32 Am. J. L. & Med. 117, 118, 125-26, 127 (2006).

Journal 2006 Examines conflicts between physicians' personal and professional ethical obligations. Concludes that courts should give greater deference to professional moral guidelines. Quotes Opinion 2.06. Gottlieb, *Executions and Torture: The Consequences of Overriding Professional Ethics,* 6 Yale J. Health Pol'y, L. & Ethics 351, 366, 367 (2006).

Journal 2006 Examines the probability that lethal injection results in unnecessary suffering. Concludes that legislators should ban the practice until this can be disproven. Quotes Opinion

2.06. Wong, *Lethal Injection Protocols: The Failure of Litigation to Stop Suffering and the Case for Legislative Reform*, 25 Temp. J. Sci. Tech. & Envtl. L. 263, 282 (2006).

Journal 2005 Examines various justifications for postponing the execution of mentally ill prisoners on death row. Concludes that mistakes in postconviction adjudication should be minimized and that prisoners who lack genuine understanding of the nature of or purpose for their punishment should not be executed. References Opinion 2.06. Bonnie, *Mentally Ill Prisoners on Death Row: Unsolved Puzzles for Courts and Legislatures*, 54 Cath. U. L. Rev. 1169, 1175 (2005).

Journal 2005 Discusses the case of *Singleton v. Norris*. Concludes that a psychiatrist should not withhold necessary and appropriate treatment of a psychotic death-row inmate, even if it might restore competency for execution. Quotes Opinion 2.06. Cantor, *Of Pills and Needles: Involuntarily Medicating the Psychotic Inmate When Execution Looms*, 2 Ind. Health L. Rev. 119, 154, 156, 164 (2005).

Journal 2005 Considers legal issues raised by forcible medication of an inmate to restore competence prior to court-ordered execution. Concludes that the best solution is to delay execution until the inmate regains competency and it is no longer necessary to medicate. References Opinion 2.06. Kimbler, *Psychotic Journeys of the Green Mile*, 22 T. M. Cooley L. Rev. 27, 48 (2005).

Journal 2005 Examines the legal and ethical aspects of physician participation in capital punishment. Concludes that federal and state laws addressing this practice must be amended to harmonize the law with applicable principles of medical ethics. Quotes Opinion 2.06. Cites Opinion 2.21. References Opinion 2.01. Levy, *Conflict of Duty: Capital Punishment Regulations and AMA Medical Ethics*, 26 J. Legal Med. 261, 268, 269, 270, 273 (2005).

Journal 2005 Argues that the Eighth Circuit's ruling in *Singleton v. Norris* failed to consider the ethical standards of the medical community. Concludes that, as a result, physicians may be placed in an untenable position regarding treatment of mentally ill death-row inmates. Quotes Principle VIII and Opinions 1.02 and 2.06. Lloyd, *Primum Non Nocere: Singleton v. Norris and the Ethical Dilemma of Medicating the Condemned*, 58 Ark. L. Rev. 225, 232, 233 (2005).

Journal 2005 Argues that medicating a criminal defendant to restore competency is ethical, even in capital cases. Concludes that principles justifying administration of punishment in the legal system give rise to an ethical imperative for physicians to provide competence-restoring medical therapy. Quotes Principle III and Opinion 2.06. Mossman, *Is Prosecution "Medically Appropriate"?* 31 New Eng. J. on Crim. & Civ. Confinement 15, 53-54, 59 (2005).

Journal 2004 Discusses the history of restoring competency to execute and the Supreme Court's decision not to grant certiorari in *Singleton v. Norris*. Concludes that the Court must grant certiorari in a medicate-to-execute case and establish guidelines in this area. Quotes Opinion 2.06. Campbell, *Sell, Singleton, and Forcible Medication—Running Roughshod Over Liberty*, 35 U. Tol. L. Rev. 691, 716 (2004).

Journal 2004 Evaluates the constitutionality of involuntarily medicating mentally ill patients to restore competency for execution. Concludes that this practice should be held unconstitutional. Cites Opinion 2.06. References Opinion 2.065. Hensl, *Restored to Health to Be Put to Death: Reconciling the Legal and Ethical Dilemmas of Medicating to Execute in Singleton v. Norris*, 49 Vill. L. Rev. 291, 324 (2004).

Journal 2004 Analyzes various issues relating to the role of mental health professionals in capital punishment in light of Albert Bandura's model of "mechanisms of moral disengagement." Concludes that facilitating participation of mental health professionals in executions creates conflicts with the humanistic norms of the profession. Quotes Preamble and Opinions 1.01, 1.02, 2.06, 2.067, 2.20, 2.21, 2.211, and 8.14. Judges, *The Role of Mental Health Professionals in Capital Punishment: An Exercise in Moral Disengagement*, 41 Hous. L. Rev. 515, 562, 568, 569, 570, 571-72, 581, 586, 588, 598 (2004).

Journal 2004 Argues the existence of an international *jus cogens* norm against implementation of the death penalty. Concludes that this norm has developed in international law and may lead to abolition of the death penalty. Quotes Opinion 2.06. Sawyer, *The Death Penalty Is Dead Wrong: Jus Cogens Norms and the Evolving Standard of Decency*, 22 Penn. St. Int'l L. Rev. 459, 477 (2004).

Journal 2004 Analyzes the moral and ethical conflicts that are created by requiring health care professionals to involuntarily medicate death-row inmates to restore competency for execution.

Concludes that it is cruel and unusual punishment to execute individuals who are forcibly medicated for this purpose. Quotes Opinion 2.06. Shaivitz, *Medicate-to-Execute: Current Trends in Death Penalty Jurisprudence and the Perils of Dual Loyalty,* 7 J. Health Care L. & Pol'y 149, 167, 168 (2004).

Journal 2003 Examines the manner in which psychiatrists participate in the criminal justice system. Concludes that, in some situations, this participation may violate principles of medical ethics. Cites Opinions 2.06 and 8.08. Dolin, *A Healer or an Executioner? The Proper Role of a Psychiatrist in a Criminal Justice System,* 17 J. L. & Health 169, 206, 213-14 (2003).

Journal 2003 Discusses the inconsistent governmental regulation of drugs used in physician-assisted suicide (PAS) and lethal injections. Concludes that the FDA should regulate drugs used in lethal injections in the same manner it has attempted to regulate drugs used in PAS. Quotes Opinions 2.06 and 2.211. Miller, *A Death by Any Other Name: The Federal Government's Inconsistent Treatment of Drugs Used in Lethal Injections and Physician-Assisted Suicide,* 17 J. L. & Health 217, 234-35 (2003).

Journal 2003 Considers a legislative plan allowing voluntary, consensual organ donation by condemned prisoners. Concludes that, in view of the current organ shortage, the benefits of such a plan outweigh the concerns. Quotes Principle VII and Opinion 2.06. Perales, *Rethinking the Prohibition of Death Row Prisoners as Organ Donors: A Possible Lifeline to Those on Organ Donor Waiting Lists,* 34 St. Mary's L. J. 687, 721, 725 (2003).

Journal 2003 Discusses history of the death penalty in Colorado. Concludes that the trend is moving toward its abolition. Quotes Opinion 2.06. Radelet, *Capital Punishment in Colorado: 1859-1972,* 74 U. Colo. L. Rev. 885, 940 (2003).

Journal 2002 Addresses the problems arising out of legislative changes in methods of execution. Focuses on the change from electrocution to lethal injection. Concludes that, despite changes, executions are not necessarily more humane. Quotes Opinion 2.06. Denno, *When Legislatures Delegate Death: The Troubling Paradox Behind State Uses of Electrocution and Lethal Injection and What It Says About Us,* 63 Ohio St. L. J. 63, 112-13 (2002).

Journal 2002 Examines the standard for determining competency to be executed as applied to mentally ill death-row inmates. Favors commuting their sentences. Concludes a new standard that comports with the Eighth Amendment should be adopted. Quotes Opinion 2.06. Horstman, *Commuting Death Sentences of the Insane: A Solution for a Better, More Compassionate Society,* 36 U. S. F. L. Rev. 823, 848 (2002).

Journal 2002 Analyzes Arizona case law and other relevant law regarding medical treatment of individuals who are not competent to be executed. Concludes that the law should address this difficult problem in a more uniform manner. Cites Opinion 2.06. Levitt & Ryan, *Not Competent to Be Executed: Dilemmas Faced by Psychiatrists and Attorneys,* 23 Am. J. Forensic Psych. 39, 47 (July 2002).

Journal 2002 Examines medical professionalism. Considers how changes in health care give rise to physician frustration, which has served as an anchor for the Charter on Medical Professionalism. Quotes Opinion 2.06. Miles, *On a New Charter to Defend Medical Professionalism: Whose Profession Is It Anyway?* 32 Hastings Center Rep. 46, 47 (May/June 2002).

Journal 2001 Discusses the ethical, legal, and policy arguments affecting physician participation in capital punishment. Examines the tension created by conflicting state death penalty laws and medical practice acts. Concludes that an active role for physicians in lethal injection should be supported in an effort to reduce mishaps that may occur during executions. Quotes Opinion 2.06. Baum, *"To Comfort Always": Physician Participation in Executions,* 5 N. Y. U. J. Legis. & Pub. Pol'y 47, 56-57 (2001).

Journal 2001 Addresses the issue of whether death-row prisoners may be compelled to take psychotropic medications to render them mentally competent to be executed. Considers whether physicians should be required to violate principles of medical ethics in order to treat death-row inmates for this purpose. Quotes Opinion 2.06. Daugherty, *"Synthetic Sanity": The Ethics and Legality of Using Psychotropic Medications to Render Death Row Inmates Competent for Execution,* 17 J. Contemp. H. L. & Pol'y 715, 730 (2001).

Journal 2001 Discusses policies that consider physician participation in capital punishment to be unethical. Observes that such policies are without merit. Argues that such policies attempt to override the will of the people, their elected representatives, and the administration of justice.

Concludes that these policies should be rescinded by state and national medical associations. Quotes Opinion 2.06. Keyes, *The Choice of Participation by Physicians in Capital Punishment*, 22 *Whittier L. Rev.* 809, 810-11, 838 (2001).

Journal 2000 Explores physicians' views regarding involvement in capital punishment. Concludes that, despite medical society policies, a majority of physicians believe participation in capital punishment is acceptable in certain circumstances. Quotes Opinion 2.06. Farber, Davis, Weiner, Jordan, Boyer, & Ubel, *Physicians' Attitudes About Involvement in Lethal Injection for Capital Punishment*, 160 *Arch. Intern. Med.* 2912, 2912 (2000).

Journal 2000 Explores issues and concerns associated with capital punishment. Discusses the controversy surrounding ways that physicians participate in capital punishment in this country. Concludes that capital punishment is not needed and cannot be fairly administered. Quotes Opinion 2.06. Martin, *Tessie Hutchinson and the American System of Capital Punishment*, 59 *Md. L. Rev.* 553, 565 (2000).

Journal 2000 Explores the history and legal rationale behind the prohibition against executing the insane. Considers relevant case law addressing the forced medication issue, especially as it relates to death-row inmates. Concludes the ultimate question should focus on what is in the prisoner's best interest. Cites Opinion 2.06. Miller-Rice, *The "Insane" Contradiction of Singleton v. Norris: Forced Medication in a Death Row Inmate's Medical Interest Which Happens to Facilitate His Execution*, 22 *U. Ark. Little Rock L. Rev.* 659, 673 (2000).

Journal 2000 Explores the debate regarding physician-assisted suicide. Concludes that autonomy should be respected and that an individual's wishes for assisted suicide should be honored, unless the individual is misinformed or legally incompetent. Quotes Opinion 2.211. References Opinion 2.06. Urofsky, *Justifying Assisted Suicide: Comments on the Ongoing Debate*, 14 *Notre Dame J. L. Ethics & Pub. Pol'y* 893, 918, 923 (2000).

Journal 1999 Discusses the Uniform Declaration of Death Act and the dead-donor rule. Provides ethical justifications for sustaining current policies on non–heart-beating organ donation. Cites Opinions 2.06 and 2.162. DuBois, *Non–Heart-Beating Organ Donation: A Defense of the Required Determination of Death*, 27 *J. Law Med. & Ethics* 126, 128 (1999).

Journal 1998 Describes a survey regarding physician-assisted suicide given to members of the Group for the Advancement of Psychiatry. Discusses the results of the survey, noting that most surveyed psychiatrists oppose assisting patients to die. Cites Opinions 2.06 and 2.20. Kramer, Gruenberg, & Fidler, *Psychiatrists' Attitudes Toward Physician-Assisted Suicide: A Survey*, 19 *Am. J. Forensic Psychiatry* 81, 87, 90 (1998).

Journal 1998 Explains that a determination of mental capacity to consent must be made when a person requests physician-assisted suicide in a jurisdiction where such practice is legal. Explores the potential for liability in the context of making such a determination. Argues that standards regarding determination of mental capacity must be established by case law or legislation. Cites Opinion 2.211. References Opinion 2.06. Lipschitz, *Psychiatry and Consent for Physician-Assisted Suicide*, 19 *Am. J. Forensic Psychiatry* 91, 103, 104 (1998).

Journal 1997 Explores the Eighth Amendment prohibition against cruel and unusual punishment in the context of capital punishment. Discusses widely used methods of execution. Suggests that execution methods may be unconstitutionally excessive. Concludes the death penalty should not be imposed until methods are more humane. Quotes Opinion 2.06. Denno, *Getting to Death: Are Executions Constitutional?* 82 *Iowa L. Rev.* 319, 385-86 (1997).

Journal 1997 Describes capital punishment in the US. Considers ethical and moral issues implicated by physician participation. Opines that executions constitute harm and that physician participation contravenes professional ethical obligations. Quotes Opinion 2.06. Michalos, *Medical Ethics and the Executing Process in the United States of America*, 16 *Med. & Law* 125, 131, 133 (1997).

Journal 1996 Examines how execution practices affect crime deterrence. Explores trend toward private and more humane executions. Discusses similarity between lethal injection and medical procedures. Concludes that deterrence is not served by current execution practices and should not be advanced as support for the death penalty. Cites Opinion 2.06. Abernethy, *The Methodology of Death: Reexamining the Deterrence Rationale*, 27 *Colum. Hum. Rts. L. Rev.* 379, 410-11 (1996).

Journal 1996 Examines the death penalty statute in New York. Discusses statutory provisions and notes it is unethical for medical personnel to assist with executions. Concludes that the death penalty statute fails to deter crime and may be unconstitutional. Quotes Opinion 2.06. Acker, *When the Cheering Stopped: An Overview and Analysis of New York's Death Penalty Legislation*, 17 Pace L. Rev. 41, 221-22 (1996).

Journal 1996 Discusses the current shortage of available organs for transplant patients. Suggests several new methods for increasing the supply. Includes among these suggestions a proposal that inmates sentenced to death should be allowed to donate organs. Quotes Opinion 2.06. Coleman, *Brother, Can You Spare a Liver? Five Ways to Increase Organ Donation*, 31 Val. U. L. Rev. 1, 30, 31 (1996).

Journal 1996 Discusses the involvement of psychiatrists in capital punishment. Posits that physicians should not aid legal executions. Expresses support for the ethical resolutions of psychiatric and medical associations regarding this issue. Quotes Opinion 2.06. Freedman & Halpern, *The Erosion of Ethics and Morality in Medicine: Physician Participation in Legal Executions in the United States*, 41 N. Y. L. Sch. L. Rev. 169, 174 (1996).

Journal 1996 Proposes an alternative method of capital punishment to allow for organ donation by executed prisoners. Provides justifications for this proposal. Concludes that physicians should be able to ethically participate in this process. Quotes Principle VII. Cites Opinion 2.06. References Opinion 2.162 (1994) [subsequently amended]. Patton, *A Call for Common Sense: Organ Donation and the Executed Prisoner*, 3 Va. J. Soc. Pol'y & L. 387, 404, 405, 407-10 (1996).

Journal 1996 Considers physician participation in execution of capital offenders. Observes that this practice is unethical and contrary to the physician's role as a healer. Concludes that physicians should not participate in any aspect of executions. Quotes Opinion 2.06. Schoenholtz, Freedman, & Halpern, *The Legal Abuse of Physicians in Deaths in the United States: The Erosion of Ethics and Morality in Medicine*, 42 Wayne L. Rev. 1505, 1542 (1996).

Journal 1996 Discusses the role psychiatrists play in capital punishment. Notes that the ethical prohibition against physician participation in the process creates complications for psychiatrists. References Opinion 2.06. Zwirn, *Professionalism, Mental Disability, and the Death Penalty*, 41 N. Y. L. Sch. L. Rev. 163, 165 (1996).

Journal 1995 Summarizes the US Supreme Court's capital punishment jurisprudence. Explores the history and methodology of the New York Court of Appeals' constitutional adjudication of capital punishment issues and examines constitutional challenges to the death penalty in other states. Quotes Opinion 2.06. Falk & Cary, *Death-Defying Feats: State Constitutional Challenges to New York's Death Penalty*, 4 J. L. & Pol'y 161, 233, 234 (1995).

Journal 1995 Explores the relevance of historical account of capital punishment in New York to the contemporary debate regarding televised executions. Concludes that increased publicity may give both the public and the condemned more power over how executions are conducted. Cites Opinion 2.06. Madow, *Forbidden Spectacle: Executions, the Public and the Press in Nineteenth Century New York*, 43 Buff. L. Rev. 461, 475 (1995).

Journal 1994 Argues that assisted suicide is not an implicit right under the Fourteenth Amendment's liberty guarantee. Suggests that giving physicians the authority to determine the appropriateness of assisted suicide furthers no legitimate state interest. Cites Opinion 2.06. References Opinion 2.211. Marzen, *Out, Out Brief Candle: Constitutionally Prescribed Suicide for the Terminally Ill*, 21 Hastings Const. L. Q. 799, 821 (1994).

Journal 1994 Argues that physician aid-in-dying should be protected by the US Constitution and that patients should have a federal cause of action to challenge prohibitive state statutes. Considers how such a cause of action might affect public policy. Quotes Principles I and III. References Opinion 2.06. Note, *Toward a More Perfect Union: A Federal Cause of Action for Physician Aid-In-Dying*, 27 U. Mich. J. L. Ref. 521, 538 (1994).

Journal 1993 Considers whether criminal penalties should be imposed on a physician who assists in the suicide of a competent, nonterminal patient who requested such assistance. Presents the arguments for and against active euthanasia, with emphasis on the "slippery slope" argument. References Opinions 2.06 and 2.20. Persels, *Forcing the Issue of Physician-Assisted Suicide: Impact of the Kevorkian Case on the Euthanasia Debate*, 14 J. Legal Med. 93, 115 (1993).

Journal 1993 Explores the extent to which physicians may participate in capital punishment. Explains the policy behind prohibiting physicians from taking part in executions. Cites Opinion

2.06. Truog & Brennan, *Participation of Physicians in Capital Punishment, 329 New Eng. J. Med.* 1346 (1993).

Journal 1991 Considers ethical issues raised by the case of *Perry v. Louisiana,* where the state attempted to treat an insane death-row inmate in order to render him fit for execution. Explores various ethical questions involving mentally ill defendants/inmates and proposes increased discussion and reform of ethical guidelines. Quotes Opinion 2.06. Note, *Perry v. Louisiana: Medical Ethics on Death Row—Is Judicial Intervention Warranted? 4 Georgetown J. Legal Ethics 707,* 714 (1991).

Journal 1987 Concludes that a policy or practice of active voluntary euthanasia is not desirable, linking a moral prohibition against active voluntary euthanasia to the moral prohibition against physicians actively participating in capital punishment. In place of any practice of active voluntary euthanasia, recommends increased use of hospices, greater emphasis on training physicians to care for the dying patient, and further research aimed at producing symptomatic relief in dying patients. Cites Opinions 2.06, 8.10 (1986) [now Opinion 8.11], and 9.06. Shewmon, *Active Voluntary Euthanasia: A Needless Pandora's Box, 3 Issues in Law and Med. 219, 220, 222,* 243 (1987).

Journal 1987 Focuses on the decision of the US Supreme Court in *Ford v. Wainwright,* wherein the Court ruled that the Eighth Amendment forbids the execution of a condemned inmate who has become insane. Noting that physicians should not ethically participate in a legally authorized execution, except to make a determination or certification of death, concludes that participation by mental health professionals in assessing competency for execution is incompatible with the general ethics of the profession. Cites Opinion 2.06. Wallace, *Incompetency for Execution: The Supreme Court Challenges the Ethical Standards of the Mental Health Professions,* 8 J. Legal Med. 265, 267 (1987).

Journal 1986 Observes that the AMA policy on capital punishment expressly forbids psychiatrists from making determinations of competency for execution. Compares the psychiatrist's determination of competency for execution to the behavior of Nazi physicians, and condemns as inherently dishonest any therapy not grounded in the patient's best interests. References Principle I and Opinion 2.06. Sargent, *Treating the Condemned to Death, 16 Hastings Center Rep.* 5, 5 (Dec. 1986).

Journal 1983 Focuses on the medical-ethical dilemma inherent in the application of medical technology to bring about death and observes that medical professional organizations have done little to solve the dilemma. Concludes that there is a need for federal legislation preempting the multiplicity of state-sanctioned methods to reduce the potential of abuse of civil and human rights. References 1980 AMA Policy Statement [now Opinion 2.06]. Finks, *Lethal Injection: An Uneasy Alliance of Law and Medicine, 4 J. Legal Med. 383, 392, 394 (1983).*

2.065 Court-Initiated Medical Treatments in Criminal Cases

Physicians can ethically participate in court-initiated medical treatments only if the procedure being mandated is therapeutically efficacious and is therefore undoubtedly not a form of punishment or solely a mechanism of social control. While a court has the authority to identify criminal behavior, a court does not have the ability to make a medical diagnosis or to determine the type of treatment that will be administered. In accordance with ethical practice, physicians should treat patients based on sound medical diagnoses, not court-defined behaviors. This is particularly important where the treatment involves inpatient therapy, surgical intervention, or pharmacological treatment. In these cases, diagnosis can be made initially by the physician who will do the treatment, but must then be confirmed by an independent physician or a panel of physicians not responsible to the state. A second opinion is not necessary in cases of court-ordered counseling or referrals for psychiatric evaluations.

A recognized, authoritative medical body, such as a national specialty society, should pre-establish scientifically valid treatments for medically determined diagnoses. Such pre-established acceptable treatments should then be applied on a case-by-case basis.

The physician who will perform the treatment must be able to conclude, in good conscience and to the best of his or her professional judgment, that the informed consent was given voluntarily to the extent possible, recognizing the element of coercion that is inevitably present. In cases involving inpatient therapy, surgical intervention, or pharmacological treatment, an independent physician or a panel of physicians not responsible to the state should confirm that the informed consent was given in accordance with these guidelines. (I, III)

Issued December 1998 based on the report "Court-Initiated Medical Treatment in Criminal Cases," adopted June 1998.

Wis. Sup. 2010 State petitioned for involuntary administration of psychotropic medication for defendant who was in custody after acquittal due to mental illness. Defendant argued that Wisconsin statute allowing for such treatment unconstitutionally violated his due process rights. The majority quotes Opinions 2.065 and 2.19 in finding the Wisconsin statute in question facially valid on procedural due process grounds. *State v. Wood, 323 Wis. 2d 321, 780 N.W.2d 63, 82-83.*

Journal 2011 Discusses the doctrine of informed consent and the influence of physician groups on the dissemination of information to patients. Concludes the doctrine of informed consent should be expanded by the courts, rather than continuing to allow professional societies to dictate provider guidelines for obtaining informed consent. Quotes Opinions 8.08, 10.01, and 10.015. References Opinion 2.065. Ginsberg, *Informed Consent: No Longer Just What the Doctor Ordered? The "Contributions" of Medical Associations and Courts to a More Patient Friendly Doctrine, 15 Mich. St. J. Med. & Law 17, 23, 24, 25, 26, 46 (2011).*

Journal 2008 Examines various types of neuroscience-based techniques used to prevent criminal behavior and the problems associated with such interventions. Concludes any treatments utilizing neuroscience in an effort to mitigate criminal behavior must be proven safe and effective prior to implementation. Quotes Opinion 2.065. Greely, *Neuroscience and Criminal Justice: Not Responsibility but Treatment, 56 U. Kan. L. Rev. 1103, 1131 (2008).*

Journal 2006 Examines the practice of chemically castrating repeat sex offenders. Concludes that chemical castration is cruel and unusual punishment which violates the Eighth Amendment. Cites Opinion 2.065. Stinneford, *Incapacitation Through Maiming: Chemical Castration, The Eighth Amendment, and the Denial of Human Dignity, 3 U. St. Thomas L. J. 559, 576 (2006).*

Journal 2004 Evaluates the constitutionality of involuntarily medicating mentally ill patients to restore competency for execution. Concludes that this practice should be held unconstitutional. Cites Opinion 2.06. References Opinion 2.065. Hensl, *Restored to Health to Be Put to Death: Reconciling the Legal and Ethical Dilemmas of Medicating to Execute in Singleton v. Norris, 49 Vill. L. Rev. 291, 324 (2004).*

2.067 Torture

Torture refers to the deliberate, systematic, or wanton administration of cruel, inhumane, and degrading treatments or punishments during imprisonment or detainment.

Physicians must oppose and must not participate in torture for any reason. Participation in torture includes, but is not limited to, providing or withholding any services, substances, or knowledge to facilitate the practice of torture. Physicians must not be present when torture is used or threatened.

Physicians may treat prisoners or detainees if doing so is in their best interest, but physicians should not treat individuals to verify their health so that torture can begin or continue. Physicians who treat torture victims should not be persecuted. Physicians should help provide support for victims of torture and, whenever possible, strive to change situations in which torture is practiced or the potential for torture is great. (I, III)

Issued December 1999.

W.D. Mich. 2006 Plaintiffs, state prisoners, filed a class action alleging that inadequate medical care violated the Eighth Amendment. Quoting Opinion 2.067, plaintiff's medical expert testified that prison conditions should be classified as torture and that it was unethical for any physician to support or fail to oppose such conditions. Upon further findings of inadequate care, the court held the practices violated the Eighth Amendment, granted a preliminary injunction, and ordered other relief. *Hadix v. Caruso, 461 F.Supp. 2d 574, 581, 596.*

Journal 2011 Examines the participation of medical personnel in torture of Guantanamo detainees and violations of international and domestic law that occurred as a result. Concludes that the government should take certain steps to address such violations, including civil remedies for victims of torture. Cites Opinions 2.067 and 2.068. Brennan, *Torture of Guantanamo Detainees With the Complicity of Medical Health Personnel: The Case for Accountability and Providing a Forum for Redress for These International Wrongs, 45 U.S.F. L. Rev. 1005, 1045 (2011).*

Journal 2009 Examines the ethical guidelines regarding physicians' participation in interrogations and statutory approaches aimed at eliminating such physician involvement. Concludes that to maintain the integrity of the medical profession, physician involvement in interrogations must be precluded by legislative action. Quotes Preamble and Opinions 2.067 and 2.068. Cites Opinions 2.06 and 2.068, Bahnassi, *Keeping Doctors Out of the Interrogation Room: A New Ethical Obligation That Requires the Backing of the Law, 19 Health Matrix 447, 449-51, 461, 464, 465-67, 469-70, 474-75 (2009).*

Journal 2009 Proposes revisions to the Declaration of Tokyo regarding physician participation in the practice of torture. Concludes that physicians have a duty to be proactive in preventing torture. Cites Opinion 2.067. References Opinion 2.068. Miles & Freedman, *Medical Ethics and Torture: Revising the Declaration of Tokyo, 373 Lancet 344, 344-45 (2009).*

Journal 2007 Discusses physician involvement in abuse of enemy combatants detained by the US. Concludes that the AMA will continue to advocate for ethical treatment of detainees. Cites Opinions 2.067 and 2.068. Langston, *Ethical Treatment of Military Detainees, 370 Lancet 1999, 1999 (2007).*

Journal 2007 Discusses the responsibilities of health care professionals compelled by the US government to participate in torture and other unethical practices against detainees. Concludes that health care professionals must adhere to the Geneva Conventions and uphold the ethical practice of medicine. Quotes Opinion 2.067. Rubenstein, *First, Do No Harm: Health Professionals and Guantanamo, 37 Seton Hall L. Rev. 733, 738 (2007).*

Journal 2006 Examines conflicting loyalties of military medical personnel, which lead to militarily sanctioned human rights abuses. Concludes that immediate reform is necessary to prevent abuses and proposes an increase in education, supervision, and sanctioning. Quotes Opinion 2.067. Clark, *Medical Ethics at Guantanamo Bay and Abu Ghraib: The Problem of Dual Loyalty, 34 J. L. Med. & Ethics 570, 573 (2006).*

Journal 2006 Reviews the policy of the US government regarding the use of torture. Concludes that all forms of torture must be prohibited. Quotes Opinion 2.067. Goldstone, *Symposium: "Torture and the War on Terror": Combating Terrorism: Zero Tolerance for Torture, 37 Case W. Res. J. Int'l L. 343, 346 (2006).*

Journal 2005 Examines ethical guidelines for health personnel created by the Department of Defense in response to recent allegations of abuse and torture by US forces. Concludes that the guidelines allow physicians to participate in interrogation practices that contravene international ethical principles. Cites Opinion 1.02. References Opinion 2.067. Rubenstein, Pross, Davidoff, & Iacopino, *Coercive US Interrogation Policies: A Challenge to Medical Ethics, 294 JAMA 1544 (2005).*

Journal 2004 Analyzes various issues relating to the role of mental health professionals in capital punishment in light of Albert Bandura's model of "mechanisms of moral disengagement."

Concludes that facilitating participation of mental health professionals in executions creates conflicts with the humanistic norms of the profession. Quotes Preamble and Opinions 1.01, 1.02, 2.06, 2.067, 2.20, 2.21, 2.211, and 8.14. Judges, *The Role of Mental Health Professionals in Capital Punishment: An Exercise in Moral Disengagement, 41 Hous. L. Rev. 515, 562, 568, 569, 570, 571-72, 581, 586, 588, 598 (2004).*

2.068 Physician Participation in Interrogation

Interrogation is defined as questioning related to law enforcement or to military and national security intelligence gathering, designed to prevent harm or danger to individuals, the public, or national security. Interrogations are distinct from questioning used by physicians to assess the physical or mental condition of an individual. To be appropriate, interrogations must avoid the use of coercion—that is, threatening or causing harm through physical injury or mental suffering. In this Opinion, "detainee" is defined as a criminal suspect, prisoner of war, or any other individual who is being held involuntarily.

Physicians who engage in any activity that relies on their medical knowledge and skills must continue to uphold principles of medical ethics. Questions about the propriety of physician participation in interrogations and in the development of interrogation strategies may be addressed by balancing obligations to individuals with obligations to protect third parties and the public. The further removed the physician is from direct involvement with a detainee, the more justifiable is a role serving the public interest. Applying this general approach, physician involvement with interrogations during law enforcement or intelligence gathering should be guided by the following:

(1) Physicians may perform physical and mental assessments of detainees to determine the need for and to provide medical care. When so doing, physicians must disclose to the detainee the extent to which others have access to information included in medical records. Treatment must never be conditional on a patient's participation in an interrogation.

(2) Physicians must neither conduct nor directly participate in an interrogation, because a role as physician-interrogator undermines the physician's role as healer and thereby erodes trust in the individual physician-interrogator and in the medical profession.

(3) Physicians must not monitor interrogations with the intention of intervening in the process, because this constitutes direct participation in interrogation.

(4) Physicians may participate in developing effective interrogation strategies for general training purposes. These strategies must not threaten or cause physical injury or mental suffering and must be humane and respect the rights of individuals.

(5) When physicians have reason to believe that interrogations are coercive, they must report their observations to the appropriate authorities. If authorities are aware of coercive interrogations but have not intervened, physicians are ethically obligated to report the offenses to independent authorities that have the power to investigate or adjudicate such allegations. (I, III, VII, VIII)

Issued November 2006 based on the report "Physician Participation in Interrogation," adopted June 2006.

Journal 2011 Examines the participation of medical personnel in torture of Guantanamo detainees and violations of international and domestic law that occurred as a result. Concludes that the government should take certain steps to address such violations, including civil remedies for victims of torture. Cites Opinions 2.067 and 2.068. Brennan, *Torture of Guantanamo Detainees With the Complicity of Medical Health Personnel: The Case for Accountability and Providing a Forum for Redress for These International Wrongs*, 45 U.S.F. L. Rev. 1005, 1045 (2011).

Journal 2009 Examines the ethical guidelines regarding physicians' participation in interrogations and statutory approaches aimed at eliminating such physician involvement. Concludes that to maintain the integrity of the medical profession, physician involvement in interrogations must be precluded by legislative action. Quotes Preamble and Opinions 2.067 and 2.068. Cites Opinions 2.06 and 2.068, Bahnassi, *Keeping Doctors Out of the Interrogation Room: A New Ethical Obligation that Requires the Backing of the Law*, 19 Health Matrix 447, 449-51, 461, 464, 465-67, 469-70, 474-75 (2009).

Journal 2009 Asserts that military psychiatrists should not participate in interrogations. Concludes that the US military should revise its policies to conform to the ethical standards of the medical profession. Cites Opinion 2.068. Heyman, *Military Medical Ethics*, 395 New Eng. J. Med. 2728, 2729 (2009).

Journal 2009 Proposes revisions to the Declaration of Tokyo regarding physician participation in the practice of torture. Concludes that physicians have a duty to be proactive in preventing torture. Cites Opinion 2.067. References Opinion 2.068. Miles & Freedman, *Medical Ethics and Torture: Revising the Declaration of Tokyo*, 373 Lancet 344, 344-45 (2009).

Journal 2007 Discusses physician involvement in abuse of enemy combatants detained by the US. Concludes that the AMA will continue to advocate for ethical treatment of detainees. Cites Opinions 2.067 and 2.068. Langston, *Ethical Treatment of Military Detainees*, 370 Lancet 1999, 1999 (2007).

Journal 2007 Considers how health care professionals should respond to interrogation and detention policies used in Guantanamo Bay. Concludes that while individuals face pressure to comply with military orders, they should adhere to principles of medical ethics. Quotes Opinion 2.068. Marks, *Doctors as Pawns? Law and Medical Ethics at Guantanamo Bay*, 37 Seton Hall L. Rev. 711, 725 (2007).

Journal 2007 Describes ethical issues surrounding physician participation in the interrogation of military detainees. Concludes medical professionals are required to put the well-being of the detainee ahead of other "dual-loyalty" considerations. Quotes Opinion 2.068. Miles, *Medical Ethics and the Interrogation of Guantanamo 063*, 7 Am. J. Bioethics 5, 9 (April 2007).

Journal 2006 Analyzes liability of the US government and private contractors for acts of torture committed at Abu Ghraib. Concludes that human rights law should be further developed to provide for liability analogous to tort law. References Opinion 2.068. Garfield, *Bridging a Gap in Human Rights Law: Prisoner of War Abuse as "War Tort,"* 37 Geo. J. Int'l L. 725, 743 (2006).

2.07 Clinical Investigation

The following guidelines are intended to aid physicians in fulfilling their ethical responsibilities when they engage in the clinical investigation of new drugs and procedures:

(1) A physician may participate in clinical investigation only to the extent that those activities are a part of a systematic program competently designed, under accepted standards of scientific research, to produce data which are scientifically valid and significant.

(2) In conducting clinical investigation, the investigator should demonstrate the same concern and caution for the welfare, safety, and comfort of the person involved as is required of a physician who is furnishing medical care to a patient independent of any clinical investigation.

(3) Minors or mentally incompetent persons may be used as subjects in clinical investigation only if:

(a) The nature of the investigation is such that mentally competent adults would not be suitable subjects.

(b) Consent, in writing, is given by a legally authorized representative of the subject under circumstances in which informed and prudent adults would reasonably be expected to volunteer themselves or their children as subjects.

(4) In clinical investigation primarily for treatment:

(a) The physician must recognize that the patient-physician relationship exists and that professional judgment and skill must be exercised in the best interest of the patient.

(b) Voluntary written consent must be obtained from the patient, or from the patient's legally authorized representative if the patient lacks the capacity to consent, following: (i) disclosure that the physician intends to use an investigational drug or experimental procedure; (ii) a reasonable explanation of the nature of the drug or procedure to be used, risks to be expected, and possible therapeutic benefits; (iii) an offer to answer any inquiries concerning the drug or procedure; and (iv) a disclosure of alternative drugs or procedures that may be available. Physicians should be completely objective in discussing the details of the drug or procedure to be employed, the pain and discomfort that may be anticipated, known risks and possible hazards, the quality of life to be expected, and particularly the alternatives. Especially, physicians should not use persuasion to obtain consent which otherwise might not be forthcoming, nor should expectations be encouraged beyond those which the circumstances reasonably and realistically justify.

(i) In exceptional circumstances, where the experimental treatment is the only potential treatment for the patient and full disclosure of information concerning the nature of the drug or experimental procedure or risks would pose such a serious psychological threat of detriment to the patient as to be medically contraindicated, such information may be withheld from the patient. In these circumstances, such information should be disclosed to a responsible relative or friend of the patient where possible.

(ii) Ordinarily, consent should be in writing, except where the physician deems it necessary to rely upon consent in other than written form because of the physical or emotional state of the patient.

(5) In clinical investigation primarily for the accumulation of scientific knowledge:

(a) Adequate safeguards must be provided for the welfare, safety, and comfort of the subject. It is fundamental social policy that the advancement of scientific knowledge must always be secondary to primary concern for the individual.

(b) Consent, in writing, should be obtained from the subject, or from a legally authorized representative if the subject lacks the capacity to consent, following: (i) disclosure of the fact that an investigational drug or procedure is to be used, (ii) a reasonable explanation of the nature of the procedure to be used and risks to be expected, and (iii) an offer to answer any inquiries concerning the drug or procedure.

(6) No person may be used as a subject in clinical investigation against his or her will.

(7) The overuse of institutionalized persons in research is an unfair distribution of research risks. Participation is coercive and not voluntary if the participant is subjected to powerful incentives and persuasion.

(8) The ultimate responsibility for the ethical conduct of science resides within the institution (academic, industrial, public, or private) which conducts scientific research and with the individual scientist. Research institutions should assure that rigorous scientific standards are upheld by each of their faculty, staff, and students and should extend these standards to all reports, publications, and databases produced by the institution. All medical schools and biomedical research institutions should implement guidelines for a review process for dealing with allegations of fraud. These guidelines should ensure that (a) the process used to resolve allegations of fraud does not damage science, (b) all parties are treated fairly and justly with a sensitivity to reputations and vulnerabilities, (c) the highest degree of confidentiality is maintained, (d) the integrity of the process is maintained by an avoidance of real or apparent conflicts of interest, (e) resolution of charges is expeditious, (f) accurate and detailed documentation is kept throughout the process, and (g) responsibilities to all involved individuals, the public, research sponsors, the scientific literature, and the scientific community are met after resolution of charges. Academic institutions must be capable of, and committed to, implementing effective procedures for examining allegations of scientific fraud. No system of external monitoring should replace the efforts of an institution to set its own standards which fulfill its responsibility for the proper conduct of science and the training of scientists.

(9) With the approval of the patient or the patient's lawful representative, physicians should cooperate with the press and media to ensure that medical news concerning the progress of clinical investigation or the patient's condition is available more promptly and more accurately than would be possible without their assistance. On the other hand, the Council does not approve of practices designed to create fanfare, sensationalism to attract media attention, and unwarranted expressions of optimism because of short-term progress, even though longer range prognosis is known from the beginning to be precarious. With the approval of the patient or the patient's family, the Council, however, encourages the objective disclosure to the press and media of pertinent information. If at all possible, the identity of the patient should remain confidential if the patient or the patient's family so desires. The situation should not be used for the commercial ends of participating physicians or the institutions involved. (I, III, V)

Issued prior to April 1977. Updated June 1994 and June 1998.

N.J. 1980 Physician employed to do research sued pharmaceutical company for wrongful discharge claiming that as an employee at will she had a cause of action for termination following her refusal to continue research she viewed as medically unethical. The court held that an employee has a cause of action when discharged contrary to a clearly mandated public policy. However, the court affirmed summary judgment because human testing was not imminent and because plaintiff failed to demonstrate the existence of a clear public policy based upon any statements of medical ethics to support her refusal to continue work on controversial drug. The dissent argued that the Opinions and Reports of the Judicial Council 5.03 and 5.18 (1979) [now Opinion 2.07] and other medical ethical statements did provide a clear expression of public policy and that plaintiff's failure to specifically cite them was merely a technical defect, and not fatal. *Pierce v. Ortho Pharmaceutical Corp., 84 N. J. 58, 417 A.2d 505, 516, 518.*

Wyo. 2000 Physician sought judicial review of board of medicine's disciplinary order. Among its holdings, the board found the physician's participation in a patient case study using testing and treatment procedures of no proven medical efficacy was unprofessional conduct contrary to recognized standards of medical ethics. The board quoted and relied on Opinion 2.07. The Supreme Court reversed the board's decision for failure to provide expert testimony regarding whether the physician's conduct was contrary to the standards set out in Opinion 2.07. *Painter v. Abels, 998 P.2d 931, 935, 939.*

Journal 2010 Discusses the shortfalls and inadequacies of current informed consent protocols in the context of sham surgery-controlled trials. Concludes that investigating institutions should strengthen their informed consent protocols in this area. Cites Opinions 2.07 and 2.076. Bertram, *How Current Informed Consent Protocols Flunk the Sham Surgery Test: A New Frontier in Medicine and Ethics, 14 Quinnipiac Health L. J. 131, 133, 161-162 (2010).*

Journal 2007 Reviews recent essays on the regulation of biomedical research and laws governing conflicts of interest. Concludes that all aspects of research are financially driven and that civil liability is a strong deterrent to unethical practice. Quotes Opinion 2.07. Bergin, *Book Review: Law and Ethics in Biomedical Research: Regulation, Conflict of Interest, and Liability, 23 Windsor Rev. Legal & Soc. Issues 117, 122 (2007).*

Journal 2005 Proposes a therapeutic approach to be used by insurers in making decisions and communicating with patients about coverage for last-chance therapies. Concludes that an approach based upon conflict management rather than dispute resolution is better equipped to treat insureds as individuals. Cites Opinion 2.07. Cerminara, *Dealing With Dying: How Insurers Can Help Patients Seeking Last-Chance Therapies (Even When the Answer is "NO"), 15 Health Matrix 285, 293-94 (2005).*

Journal 2005 Examines potential legal issues that physician investigators face in conducting placebo-controlled trials. Concludes that physician investigators who harm patients by giving them a placebo may be subject to liability. Quotes Opinion 2.07. Glass & Waring, *The Physician/Investigator's Obligation to Patients Participating in Research: The Case of Placebo Controlled Trials, 33 J. L. Med. & Ethics, 575, 576 (2005).*

Journal 2002 Challenges the general use of special informed consent disclosure rules in experimental therapy. Discusses the lack of a bright-line distinction between standard and experimental interventions. Concludes that focus should be placed on the distinctiveness of experimentation. Quotes Opinion 2.07. References Opinion 9.032. Noah, *Informed Consent and the Elusive Dichotomy Between Standard and Experimental Therapy, 28 Am. J. L. & Med. 361, 394, 395 (2002).*

Journal 2001 Considers conflicts of interest in clinical research and other types of medical practice. Compares the way in which doctors and lawyers address conflicts of interest in professional practice. Concludes that physicians are unaware of the need to create a meaningful conflict-of-interest doctrine for medical practice. Quotes Preamble, Principle IV, and Opinions 2.07, 8.03, 8.031, and 10.01. Moore, *What Doctors Can Learn From Lawyers About Conflicts of Interest, 81 B. U. L. Rev. 445, 447, 449-50 (2001).*

Journal 1999 Explores the duty to disclose genetic test results in research and clinical settings. Characterizes the legal duty to disclose. Concludes with guidelines regarding ways that medical researchers can reduce the potential for liability in this context. Quotes Opinion 2.07. Furman, *Genetic Test Results and the Duty to Disclose: Can Medical Researchers Control Liability? 23 Seattle Univ. L. R. 391, 408-09 (1999).*

Journal 1999 Discusses the need for physicians to advocate on behalf of patients' rights in the context of health care delivery. Evaluates the nature and scope of the physician's role as advocate, noting that physicians cannot be expected to engage in attorney-like advocacy. Quotes Principles IV and VI, Fundamental Elements (2), (4), and (6) [now Opinion 10.01], Patient

Responsibilities 5 [now Opinion 10.02], and Opinions 2.03, 2.07, 2.09, 2.16, 2.19, 3.06, 4.01, 4.04, 6.01, 7.02, 8.02, 8.03, 8.13, 8.132, 9.06, 9.07, and 9.131. Cites Opinions 5.05, 5.09, 7.01, 8.135, and 9.02. Sage, *Physicians as Advocates, 35 Hous. L. Rev. 1529, 1537, 1541, 1542, 1552-53, 1554, 1556, 1557, 1559, 1561-62, 1564, 1571, 1574, 1576, 1580 (1999).*

Journal 1998 Discusses conflicts of interest in the physician-patient relationship arising out of use of financial incentives by managed care organizations. Considers how such conflicts are dealt with in the attorney-client relationship. Suggests that a financial incentive should be legally denounced if it unreasonably interferes with a physician's duty to properly care for and treat patients. Quotes Preamble, Fundamental Elements (1) [now Opinion 10.01], and Opinions 4.04, 5.01, 8.03, 8.13, and 9.06. Cites Fundamental Elements (4) [now Opinion 10.01] and Opinions 2.07, 2.08, and 2.132. Hall, *Third-Party Payor Conflicts of Interest in Managed Care: A Proposal for Regulation Based on the Model Rules of Professional Conduct, 29 Seton Hall L. Rev. 95, 96, 107, 108, 109, 110, 111, 112, 134, 135, 136 (1998).*

Journal 1998 Discusses the use of mentally impaired individuals as research subjects. Argues that a common set of rules needs to be promulgated to protect the decisionally impaired from certain risks of human research. Quotes Opinion 2.07. Sundram, *In Harm's Way: Research Subjects Who Are Decisionally Impaired, 1 J. Health Care L. & Pol'y 36, 43-44 (1998).*

Journal 1997 Considers emergency room research informed consent standards. Reviews new federal regulations and related moral and ethical concerns. Concludes that regulations will require a case-by-case approach to balancing competing interests between research and ethics. References Opinion 2.07. Brody, *New Perspectives on Emergency Room Research, 27 Hastings Center Rep. 7, 9 (Jan./Feb. 1997).*

Journal 1997 Considers informed consent and the principle of self-determination. Analyzes the tradition of informed consent in medical research, with emphasis on international considerations. Concludes that research subjects need better protection. Cites Opinion 2.07. Note, *The Informed-Consent Policy of the International Conference on Harmonization of Technical Requirements for Registrations of Pharmaceuticals for Human Use: Knowledge Is the Best Medicine, 30 Cornell Int'l L. J. 203, 209 (1997).*

Journal 1993 Considers the legitimacy of neonatal HIV screening studies conducted without parental notice or consent. Asserts that such testing is morally and legally questionable. Quotes Opinion 2.07. Isaacman & Miller, *Neonatal HIV Seroprevalence Studies, 14 J. Legal Med. 413, 428 (1993).*

Journal 1989 Discusses various social control mechanisms that have an impact upon biomedical research. Emphasis is placed upon a comparison of the effectiveness of intra- and extraprofessional methods of control. References Opinion 2.07. Benson, *The Social Control of Human Biomedical Research: An Overview and Review of the Literature, 29 Soc. Sci. Med. 1, 3 (1989).*

2.071 Subject Selection for Clinical Trials

Ethical considerations in clinical research have traditionally focused on protecting research subjects. These protections may be especially important for those from socioeconomically diasdavantaged populations who may be more vulnerable to coercive pressures. The benefits from altruism that result from participation in research, particularly for severely chronically ill persons, may justify equitable consideration of historically disadvantaged populations such as the poor. With these considerations in mind, the following guidelines are offered:

(1) Although the burdens of research should not fall disproportionately on socioeconomically disadvantaged populations, neither should such populations be categorically excluded, or discouraged, from research protocols.

(2) Inclusion and exclusion criteria for a clinical study should be based on sound scientific principles. Conversely, participants in a clinical trial should be drawn from the qualifying population in the general geographic area of the trial without regard to race, ethnicity, economic status, or gender.

If a subject's primary care physician determines that the subject received a clear medical benefit from the experimental intervention which is now moving toward marketing approval and chooses to seek authorization from the Food and Drug Administration (FDA) for continued use of the investigational therapy during the time period between the end of the protocol and the availability of the drug on the market, the investigator should work with the primary care physician, the product sponsor, and the FDA to allow continued availability of the product. (I, V, VII)

Issued June 1998 based on the report "Subject Selection for Clinical Trials," adopted December 1997 (*IRB*. 1998;20(2-3):12-15).

Journal 2004 Evaluates weaknesses in institutional review board (IRB) protection of human subjects. Concludes that one vehicle for enhancing human subjects protection is to hold IRBs legally accountable for negligent conduct. Cites Opinions 2.071, 2.075, and 8.0315. Noah, *Bioethical Malpractice: Risk and Responsibility in Human Research, 7 J. Health Care L. & Pol'y 175, 183, 235 (2004).*

2.075 The Use of Placebo Controls in Clinical Trials

Placebo controls are an important part of medicine's commitment to ensuring that the safety and efficacy of new drugs are sufficiently established. Used appropriately, placebo controls can safely provide valuable data and should continue to be considered in the design of clinical trials. The existence of an accepted therapy does not necessarily preclude the use of such controls; however, physician-investigators should adhere to the following guidelines to ensure that the interests of patients who participate in clinical trials are protected.

(1) Investigators must be extremely thorough in obtaining informed consent from patients. To the extent that research is dependent upon the willingness of patients to accept a level of risk, their understanding of the potential harms involved must be a top priority of any clinical investigation. The possibility presented in some studies that patients often do not fully understand the research protocol and therefore truly cannot give informed consent demonstrates a need to heighten the efforts of researchers to impress upon their subjects the nature of clinical research and the risks involved. Patients are capable of making decisions when presented with sufficient information, and it is the responsibility of the institutional review board (IRB) and the individual investigators involved to ensure that each subject has been adequately informed and has given voluntary consent. Each patient must also be made aware that he or she can terminate his or her participation in a study at any time.

(2) Informed consent cannot be invoked to justify an inappropriate trial design. IRBs as well as investigators have an obligation to evaluate each study protocol to determine whether a placebo control is necessary and whether an alternative study design with another type of control would be sufficient for the purposes of research. Protocols that involve conditions causing death or irreversible damage cannot ethically employ a placebo control if alternative treatment would prevent or slow the illness progression. When studying illnesses characterized by severe or painful symptoms, investigators should thoroughly explore alternatives to the use

of placebo controls. In general, the more severe the consequences and symptoms of the illness under study, the more difficult it will be to justify the use of a placebo control when alternative therapy exists. Consequently, there will almost certainly be conditions for which placebo controls cannot be justified. Similarly, the use of a placebo control will more easily be justified as the severity and number of negative side effects of standard therapy increase.

(3) Researchers and IRBs should continue to minimize the amount of time patients are given placebo. The rationale provided by investigators for the length of study will give IRBs the opportunity to ensure that patients are given placebo therapy for as short a time as possible to provide verifiable results. Additionally, the interim data analysis and monitoring currently in practice will allow researchers to terminate the study because of either positive or negative results, thus protecting patients from remaining on placebo unnecessarily. (I, V)

Issued June 1997 based on the report "Ethical Use of Placebo Controls in Clinical Trials," adopted June 1996.

Journal 2004 Evaluates weaknesses in institutional review board (IRB) protection of human subjects. Concludes that one vehicle for enhancing human subjects protection is to hold IRBs legally accountable for negligent conduct. Cites Opinions 2.071, 2.075, and 8.0315. Noah, *Bioethical Malpractice: Risk and Responsibility in Human Research, 7 J. Health Care L. & Pol'y 175, 183, 235 (2004).*

Journal 2003 Provides an update on the Declaration of Helsinki and the FDA's position on placebo-controlled medical research. Concludes that the FDA should reconsider its position in light of the principles articulated in the Declaration. Quotes Opinion 2.075. Michels & Rothman, *Update on Unethical Use of Placebos in Randomised Trials, 17 Bioethics 188, 200 (2003)*

Journal 2001 Reviews federal regulations and discusses challenges associated with developing guidelines relating to the use of placebos. Concludes that the use of placebo controls in human subjects research must be carefully regulated. Quotes Opinion 2.075. Hoffman, *The Use of Placebos in Clinical Trials: Responsible Research or Unethical Practice? 33 Conn. L. Rev. 449, 454-55, 496 (2001).*

2.076 Surgical "Placebo" Controls

The term surgical "placebo" controls refers to the control arm of a research study where subjects undergo surgical procedures that have the appearance of therapeutic interventions, but during which the essential therapeutic maneuver is omitted.

The appropriateness of a surgical placebo control should be evaluated on the basis of guidelines provided in Opinion 2.07, "Clinical Investigation," as well as the following requirements:

(1) Surgical placebo controls should be used only when no other trial design will yield the requisite data.

(2) Particular attention must be paid to the informed consent process when enrolling subjects in trials that use surgical placebo controls. Careful explanation of the risks of the operations must be disclosed, along with a description of the differences between the trial arms emphasizing the essential procedure that will or will not be performed. Additional safeguards around the informed consent process may be appropriate such as

using a neutral third party to provide information and get consent, or using consent monitors to oversee the consent process.

(3) The use of surgical placebo controls may be justified when an existing, accepted surgical procedure is being tested for efficacy. It is not justified when testing the effectiveness of an innovative surgical technique that represents only a minor modification of an existing, accepted surgical procedure.

(4) When a new surgical procedure is developed with the prospect of treating a condition for which no known surgical therapy exists, using surgical placebo controls may be justified, but must be evaluated in light of whether the current standard of care includes a nonsurgical treatment and the benefits, risks, and side effects of that treatment.

   (a) If forgoing standard treatment would result in significant injury and the standard treatment is efficacious and acceptable to the patient (in terms of side effects, personal beliefs, etc), then it must be offered as part of the study design.

   (b) When the standard treatment is not fully efficacious, or not acceptable to the patient, surgical placebo controls may be used and the standard treatment forgone, but additional safeguards must be put in place around the informed consent process. (I, V)

Issued December 2000 based on the report "Surgical Placebo Controls," adopted June 2000 (*Ann Surg.* 2002;235:303-307). Updated June 2003.

Journal 2010 Discusses the shortfalls and inadequacies of current informed consent protocols in the context of sham surgery-controlled trials. Concludes that investigating institutions should strengthen their informed consent protocols in this area. Cites Opinions 2.07 and 2.076. Bertram, *How Current Informed Consent Protocols Flunk the Sham Surgery Test: A New Frontier in Medicine and Ethics*, 14 Quinnipiac Health L. J. 131, 133, 161-162 (2010).

2.077   Ethical Considerations in International Research

Physicians, either in their role as investigators or as decision-makers involved in the deliberations related to the funding or the review of research, hold an ethical obligation to ensure the protection of research participants. When the research is to be conducted in countries with differing cultural traditions, health care systems, and ethical standards, and in particular in countries with developing economies and with limited health care resources, US physicians should respect the following guidelines:

(1) First and foremost, physicians involved in clinical research that will be carried out internationally should be satisfied that a proposed research design has been developed according to a sound scientific design. Therefore, investigators must ascertain that there is genuine uncertainty within the clinical community about the comparative merits of the experimental treatment and the one to be offered as a control in the population among which the study is to be undertaken. In some instances, a three-pronged protocol, which offers the standard treatment in use in the US, a treatment that meets a level of care that is attainable and sustainable by the host country, and a placebo (see Opinion 2.076, "Surgical 'Placebo' Controls"), may be the best method to evaluate the safety and efficacy of a treatment in a given population. When US investigators participate in international

research they must obtain approval for such protocols from US institutional review boards (IRBs).

(2) IRBs, which are responsible for ensuring the protection of research participants, must determine that risks have been minimized and that the protocol's ratio of risks to benefits is favorable to participants. In evaluating the risks and benefits that a protocol presents to a population, IRBs should obtain relevant input from representatives from the host country and from the research population. It is also appropriate for IRBs to consider the harm that is likely to result from forgoing the research.

(3) Also, IRBs are required to protect the welfare of individual participants. This can best be achieved by assuring that a suitable informed consent process is in place. Therefore, IRBs should ensure that individual potential participants will be informed of the nature of the research endeavor and that their voluntary consent will be sought. IRBs should recognize that, in some instances, information will be meaningful only if it is communicated in ways that are consistent with local customs.

(4) Overall, to ensure that the research does not exploit the population from which participants are recruited, IRBs should ensure that the research corresponds to a medical need in the region where it is undertaken. Furthermore, they should foster research with the potential for lasting benefits, especially when it is undertaken among populations that are severely deficient in health care resources. This can be achieved by facilitating the development of a health care infrastructure that will be of use during and beyond the conduct of the research. Additionally, physicians conducting studies must encourage research sponsors to continue to provide beneficial study interventions to all study participants at the conclusion of the study. (I, IV, VII, VIII, IX)

Issued December 2001 based on the report "Ethical Considerations in International Research," adopted June 2001.

2.078 Guidelines to Prevent Malevolent Use of Biomedical Research

Physicians who engage in biomedical research are bound by the ethical obligations of the medical profession and also are required to meet responsibilities of the scientific community. Beyond their commitment to the advancement of scientific knowledge and the betterment of public health, physician-researchers must strive to maintain public trust in the profession through their commitment to public welfare and safety, as demonstrated through individual responsibility, commitment to peer review, and transparency in the design, execution, and reporting of research.

Biomedical research may generate knowledge with potential for both beneficial and harmful application. Before participating in research, physician-researchers should assess foreseeable ramifications of their research in an effort to balance the promise of benefit from biomedical innovation against potential harms from corrupt application of the findings.

In exceptional cases, assessment of the balance of future harms and benefits of research may preclude participation in the research, for instance, when the goals of research are antithetical to the foundations of the medical profession, as with the development of biological or chemical weapons. Properly designed biomedical research to develop defenses against such weapons is ethical.

The potential harms associated with some research may warrant regulatory oversight. Physician-researchers have a responsibility not only to adhere to standards for research, but also to lend their expertise to the development of safeguards and oversight mechanisms, both nationally and internationally. Oversight mechanisms should balance the need to advance science with the risk of malevolent application.

After research has been conducted, consideration should be given to the risk of unrestricted dissemination of the results. Only under rare circumstances should findings be withheld, and then only to the extent required to reasonably protect against dangerous misuse.

These ethical principles should be part of the education and training of all physicians involved in biomedical research.

Issued December 2004 based on the report "Guidelines to Prevent Malevolent Use of Biomedical Research," adopted June 2004.

2.079 Safeguards in the Use of DNA Databanks in Genomic Research

The following safeguards should be applied to the use of databases for the purpose of population-based genomic research:

(1) Physicians who participate as investigators in genomic research should have adequate training in genomic research and related ethical issues so as to be able to discuss these issues with patients and/or potential research subjects.

(2) If research is to be conducted within a defined subset of the general population, that is, an identifiable community, then investigators should consult with the community to design a study that will minimize harm not only for individual subjects, but also for the community. When substantial opposition to the research is expressed within the community, investigators should not conduct the study. When the community supports a proposal, investigators nevertheless should obtain individual consent in the usual manner. The same procedure should be followed whether the investigators intend to collect new samples and data or whether they wish to use previously archived data sets.

(3) When obtaining the informed consent of individuals to participate in genomic research, standard informed consent requirements apply (see Opinion 2.07, "Clinical Investigation"). In addition:

(a) Special emphasis should be placed on disclosing the specific standards of privacy contained in the study: whether the material will be coded (ie, encrypted so that only the investigator can trace materials back to specific individuals) or be completely deidentified (ie, stripped of identifiers).

(b) If data are to be coded, subjects should be told whether they can expect to be contacted in the future to share in findings or to consider participating in additional research, which may relate to the current protocol or extend to other research purposes.

(c) Individuals should always be free to refuse the use of their biological materials in research, without penalty.

(d) Disclosure should include information about whether investigators or subjects stand to gain financially from research findings (see Opinion 2.08, "Commercial Use of Human Tissue"). Such disclosure should refer to the possible conflicts of interest of the investigators (see Opinion 8.0315, "Managing Conflicts of Interest in the Conduct of Clinical Trials").

(e) Subjects should be informed of when, if ever, and how archived information and samples will be discarded.

(4) To strengthen the protection of confidentiality, genomic research should not be conducted using information and samples that identify the individuals from whom they were obtained (ie, by name or Social Security number). Furthermore, to protect subsets of the population from such harms as stigmatization and discrimination, demographic information not required for the study's purposes should be coded. (I, IV, V, VII)

Issued June 2002 based on the report "The Use of DNA Databanks in Genomic Research: The Imperative of Informed Consent," adopted December 2001 (*Genetics in Medicine*, 2004;6(6): 526-529).

Journal 2011 Discusses scientific and technological advancements in genetic research and the controversy surrounding patenting human genomic material. Concludes that although patent protection should be provided, modifications to the current system are necessary to ensure that genetic sequencing information is available to researchers to further advancement in health care. Cites Council on Ethical and Judicial Affairs Report 2-I-97 [now Opinion 2.105] and Report 4-I-01 [now Opinion 2.079]. Ratcliffe, *The Ethics of Genetic Patenting and the Subsequent Implications on the Future of Health Care*, 27 Touro L. Rev. 435, 438-39, 449 (2011).

Journal 2007 Analyzes scientific, ethical, and legal issues raised in the exhumation and genetic analysis of historical figures. Concludes that biohistorical review boards should be created to generate guidelines for such research. Quotes Preamble and Opinion 2.08. Cites Opinions 2.079, 2.105, 5.05, 5.051, 5.075, 8.03, 8.031, 9.095, and 9.10. Paradise & Andrews, *Tales From the Crypt: Scientific, Ethical, and Legal Considerations for Biohistorical Analysis of Deceased Historical Figures*, 26 Temp. J. Sci. Tech. & Envtl. L. 223, 287-88 (2007).

2.08 The previous Opinion 2.08, "Clinical Investigation: Replacement of Vital Humans Organs," issued July 1986, was deleted in 1994 and combined with Opinion 2.07, "Clinical Investigation."

2.08 Commercial Use of Human Tissue

The rapid growth of the biotechnology industry has resulted in the commercial availability of numerous therapeutic and other products developed from human tissue. Physicians contemplating the commercial use of human tissue should abide by the following guidelines:

(1) Informed consent must be obtained from patients for the use of organs or tissues in clinical research.

(2) Potential commercial applications must be disclosed to the patient before a profit is realized on products developed from biological materials.

(3) Human tissue and its products may not be used for commercial purposes without the informed consent of the patient who provided the original cellular material.

(4) Profits from the commercial use of human tissue and its products may be shared with patients, in accordance with lawful contractual agreements.

(5) The diagnostic and therapeutic alternatives offered to patients by their physicians should conform to standards of good medical practice and should not be influenced in any way by the commercial potential of the patient's tissue. (II, V)

Issued June 1994 based on the report "Who Should Profit From the Economic Value of Human Tissue? An Ethical Analysis," adopted June 1990.

S.D. Fla. 2003 Donors of tissue samples sought equitable and injunctive relief against a physician-researcher and affiliated hospitals doing research on Canavan disease. The researcher used the donations to obtain a gene patent and the hospitals restricted any activity related to the patent. District court dismissed all counts except the unjust enrichment claim. Court quoted Opinion 2.08 with respect to disclosure to patients of possible commercial application of research. *Greenberg v. Miami Children's Hospital Research Institute, Inc.*, 264 F. Supp. 2d 1064, 1070-71, n. 2.

Journal 2009 Discusses legislative changes and the increase in patentable material that led to the commercialization of scientific research. Concludes a mandatory disclosure regimen is necessary to preserve the interests of researchers and tissue donors in scientific research. Quotes Opinion 2.08. Overgaard, *Balancing the Interests of Researchers and Donors in the Commercial Scientific Research Marketplace*, 74 Brook. L. Rev. 1473, 1501, 1506 (2009).

Journal 2007 Discusses the evolution of informed consent doctrine. Concludes that, in context of research, informed consent exceptions should be substantially narrowed. Quotes Ch. I, Art. I, Sec. 4 (May 1847) [now Opinion 8.082] and Ch. I, Art. I, Sec. 1 (May 1847) [now Principles I and VIII]. References Opinions 2.08 and 8.08. Grimm, *Informed Consent for All! No Exceptions*, 37 N. M. L. Rev. 39, 39, 61 (2007).

Journal 2007 Analyzes scientific, ethical, and legal issues raised in the exhumation and genetic analysis of historical figures. Concludes that biohistorical review boards should be created to generate guidelines for such research. Quotes Preamble and Opinion 2.08. Cites Opinions 2.079, 2.105, 5.05, 5.051, 5.075, 8.03, 8.031, 9.095, and 9.10. Paradise & Andrews, *Tales From the Crypt: Scientific, Ethical, and Legal Considerations for Biohistorical Analysis of Deceased Historical Figures*, 26 Temp. J. Sci. Tech. & Envtl. L. 223, 287-88 (2007).

Journal 2006 Explores whether patients have a property interest in their own tissue. Concludes that courts must carefully consider evolving thought about interests of patients in their tissue samples. Cites Opinion 2.08. Andrews, *Two Perspectives: Rights of Donors: Who Owns Your Body? A Patient's Perspective on Washington University v. Catalona*, 34 J. L. Med. & Ethics 398, 404 (2006).

Journal 2006 Evaluates unjust enrichment claims against those patenting human genetic material. Concludes that opponents of the practice of patenting genetic material may bring such claims. Cites Opinion 2.08. Greenfield, *Greenberg v. Miami Children's Hospital: Unjust Enrichment and the Patenting of Human Genetic Material*, 15 Ann. Health L. 213, 248 (2006).

Journal 2005 Examines financial, ethical, moral, and legal issues surrounding the use of tissue samples stored in biobanks. Concludes that a fiduciary duty should exist between health care providers and researchers who have established biobanks and individuals submitting tissue samples. Quotes Opinion 2.08. Andrews, *Harnessing the Benefits of Biobanks*, 33 J. L. Med. & Ethics 22, 25 (2005).

Journal 2004 Urges that Congress pass legislation authorizing the sale of human tissue for research purposes, but holding liable any researcher who wrongfully uses such tissue. Concludes this legislation would balance the interests of research subjects with those of the biotechnology industry. Cites Opinion 2.08. Gitter, *Ownership of Human Tissue: A Proposal for Federal Recognition of Human Research Participants' Property Rights in Their Biological Material*, 61 Wash. & Lee L. Rev. 257, 334 (2004).

Journal 2002 Examines various concerns regarding gene patents and discusses other policy alternatives. Concludes that policymakers are exploring alternatives to ensure that gene patents will benefit society. Quotes Opinion 2.08. Cites Opinion 9.095. Andrews, *The Gene Patent Dilemma: Balancing Commercial Incentives With Health Needs*, 2 Hous. J. Health L. & Pol'y 65, 74, 104 (2002).

Journal 1998 Discusses conflicts of interest in the physician-patient relationship arising out of use of financial incentives by managed care organizations. Considers how such conflicts are dealt with in the attorney-client relationship. Suggests that a financial incentive should be legally denounced if it unreasonably interferes with a physician's duty to properly care for and treat patients. Quotes Preamble, Fundamental Elements (1) [now Opinion 10.01], and Opinions 4.04, 5.01, 8.03, 8.13, and 9.06. Cites Fundamental Elements (4) [now Opinion 10.01] and Opinions 2.07, 2.08, and 2.132. Hall, *Third-Party Payor Conflicts of Interest in Managed Care: A Proposal for Regulation Based on the Model Rules of Professional Conduct,* 29 Seton Hall L. Rev. 95, 96, 107, 108, 109, 110, 111, 112, 134, 135, 136 (1998).

2.09 Costs

While physicians should be conscious of costs and not provide or prescribe unnecessary medical services, concern for the quality of care the patient receives should be the physician's first consideration. This does not preclude the physician, individually or through medical or other organizations, from participating in policy-making with respect to social and economic issues affecting health care. (I, VII)

Issued March 1981. Updated June 1994, June 1998, and December 2003.

Journal 2011 Examines the Patient Protection and Affordable Care Act and its impact on patient access to physician services. Also considers the possibility that physicians might be required to provide services to all patients as a condition to practice. Concludes that regulations that try to conscript physician services would be practically ineffective, legally dubious, and unwise public policy. Quotes Opinion 9.06 and 10.015. Cites Opinion 2.09. Kapp, *Conscripted Physician Services and the Public's Health,* 39 J. L. Med. & Ethics 414, 414, 418 (2011).

Journal 2009 Discusses methods of allocation and rationing of health care resources in an effort to curb health care costs and how these methods impact the elderly. Concludes that in order to make the greatest use of the available resources, an equitable policy regarding elder health care must be adopted and adhered to. Quotes Opinion 2.09. Smith, *The Elderly and Health Care Rationing,* 7 Pierce L. Rev. 171, 181 (2009).

Journal 2008 Argues that as a matter of public health, physicians must control antibiotic administration to combat antibiotic resistance. Concludes that despite limited incentives for antibiotic conservation, physicians must acknowledge their important role in mitigating the public health threat of antibiotic resistance. Quotes Principles VII and VIII and Opinions 2.09 and 10.015. Cites Opinion 2.03. Saver, *In Tepid Defense of Population Health: Physicians and Antibiotic Resistance,* 34 Am. J. L. & Med. 431, 457 (2008).

Journal 2003 Discusses the practice of gainsharing and argues that providing physicians and hospitals with certain financial incentives to reduce health costs may be of value in health care reform. Concludes with suggestions for how best to proceed in this difficult context. Quotes Opinions 2.03, 2.09, 4.04, and 8.03. References Opinion 8.13. Saver, *Squandering the Gain: Gainsharing and the Continuing Dilemma of Physician Financial Incentives,* 98 Nw. U. L. Rev. 145, 219, 221, 222 (2003).

Journal 2001 Examines issues relating to health care cost containment. Concludes that, if physicians are to meet the goals assigned to them in a cost-constrained health care system, then professional standards must be reevaluated and modified to afford meaningful guidance for clinical decision-making in the face of health care spending controls. Quotes Opinions 2.03, 2.09, 2.095, 8.032, and 9.04. Cites Opinions 8.02, 8.021, 8.051, and 8.13. Agrawal, *Resuscitating Professionalism: Self-regulation in the Medical Marketplace,* 66 Mo. L. Rev. 341, 354, 355, 360, 361, 378, 388 (2001).

Journal 2001 Discusses the prohibition on nonlawyer ownership of legal service providers. Considers how ethical rules and standards governing physicians have been directed toward preserving independent judgment. Concludes that ethical conflicts created by abandoning the prohibition on nonlawyer ownership of legal service providers may be managed by following the medical ethics model. Quotes Principle VI and Opinions 2.03, 2.09, 8.02, 8.021, 8.03, 8.05, 8.051, 8.054, 8.13, and 8.132. Harris & Foran, *The Ethics of Middle-Class Access to Legal Services and*

What We Can Learn From the Medical Profession's Shift to a Corporate Paradigm, 70 Fordham L. Rev. 775, 817, 821, 822, 823, 824 (2001).

Journal 1999 Discusses the need for physicians to advocate on behalf of patients' rights in the context of health care delivery. Evaluates the nature and scope of the physician's role as advocate, noting that physicians cannot be expected to engage in attorney-like advocacy. Quotes Principles IV and VI, Fundamental Elements (2), (4), and (6) [now Opinion 10.01], Patient Responsibilities 5 [now Opinion 10.02], and Opinions 2.03, 2.07, 2.09, 2.16, 2.19, 3.06, 4.01, 4.04, 6.01, 7.02, 8.02, 8.03, 8.13, 8.132, 9.06, 9.07, and 9.131. Cites Opinions 5.05, 5.09, 7.01, 8.135, and 9.02. Sage, *Physicians as Advocates, 35 Hous. L. Rev. 1529, 1537, 1541, 1542, 1552-53, 1554, 1556, 1557, 1559, 1561-62, 1564, 1571, 1574, 1576, 1580 (1999).*

Journal 1997 Posits that cost-containment schemes in managed care systems have eroded the fiduciary duty physicians owe patients. Notes that managed care organizations (MCOs) are prohibiting patients from trusting and relying on physicians. Concludes that patients must seek quality assurance from sources other than their physicians. Quotes Opinions 2.03, 2.09, and 8.13. Jacobi, *Patients at a Loss: Protecting Health Care Consumers Through Data Driven Quality Assurance, 45 U. Kan. L. Rev. 705, 720, 721, 759 (1997).*

Journal 1996 Explores changing health care delivery environment and proposes a new approach to medical ethics. Suggests ways to improve the roles of care managers in capitated systems. Advocates disclosure of information to patients regarding coverage limitations and cost-containment policies. Quotes Opinion 2.09. Malinowski, *Capitation, Advances in Medical Technology, and the Advent of a New Era in Medical Ethics, XXII Am. J. Law & Med. 331, 337 (1996).*

Journal 1996 Discusses the health care system as it pertains to the elderly. Observes that age-based rationing decisions create significant value conflicts. Suggests that, in developing national health policy, decisions regarding resource allocation for the elderly must incorporate principles of ethical and moral reasoning. Quotes Opinion 2.09. Smith, *Our Hearts Were Once Young and Gay: Health Care Rationing and the Elderly, 8 U. Fla. J. L. & Pub. Pol'y 1, 21 (1996).*

Journal 1994 Considers how patients with insufficient financial resources place physicians in a conflict-of-interest situation with respect to patient needs and the financial interests of the physician, other patients, and society. Suggests that rules of contract and malpractice law do not provide satisfactory guidelines to resolve these conflicts. Cites Opinions 2.09 and 2.095. Mehlman & Massey, *The Patient-Physician Relationship and the Allocation of Scarce Resources: A Law and Economics Approach, 4 Kennedy Inst. Ethics J. 291, 292 (1994).*

Journal 1994 Observes that health care reform proposals present significant challenges to the role and ethics of attending physicians. Emphasizes that reform proposals must set forth the role envisioned for physicians and must articulate an acceptable ethical framework within which physicians may fulfill that role. Quotes Opinions 4.04, 9.121, and 9.122. Cites Opinions 2.03, 2.09, 5.01, and 8.03. Wolf, *Health Care Reform and the Future of Physician Ethics, 24 Hastings Center Rep. 28, 32, 40 (March/April 1994).*

Journal 1993 Discusses the problem of physicians withholding needed medical treatment from HIV-infected infants. Concludes that current law should be expanded to eliminate this discrimination. Quotes Opinions 2.09, 2.17, 2.20, 2.22, 4.04, and 8.03. Crossley, *Of Diagnoses and Discrimination: Discriminatory Nontreatment of Infants With HIV Infection, 93 Columbia L. Rev. 1581, 1620, 1621 (1993).*

Journal 1993 Defines the physician-patient relationship within the framework of contract, tort, and fiduciary law. Concludes that the law does not require a physician to provide care for the nonpaying patient. Quotes Opinion 2.09. Mehlman, *The Patient-Physician Relationship in an Era of Scarce Resources: Is There a Duty to Treat? 25 Conn. L. Rev. 349 (1993).*

Journal 1992 Examines the major health care rationing issues facing the US including increasing costs and decreasing access. Concludes that the standard of care should not be changed and that rationing should be a separate enterprise undertaken pursuant to explicit criteria. Quotes Opinions 2.03, 2.09, and 4.04. Hirshfeld, *Should Ethical and Legal Standards for Physicians Be Changed to Accommodate New Models for Rationing Health Care? 140 Univ. Pa. L. Rev. 1809, 1816 (1992).*

Journal 1991 Focuses on the denial of insurance benefits for experimental medical procedures. Explains the de novo review process under ERISA. Concludes that there is need for a structure that will permit greater objectivity in the context of data collection as well as judicial determination. Cites Opinions 2.03 and 2.09. Note, *Denial of Coverage for "Experimental" Medical Procedures: The Problem of De Novo Review Under ERISA*, 79 Kentucky L. J. 801, 824 (1990-91).

Journal 1990 Discusses economic considerations in clinical decision-making, with emphasis on the standard of care. Concludes that organized medicine has made valuable contributions through development of practice parameters that offer guidance in the exercise of clinical judgment. Cites Opinions 2.03 and 2.09. Hirshfeld, *Economic Considerations in Treatment Decisions and the Standard of Care in Medical Malpractice Litigation*, 264 JAMA 2004, 2007 (1990).

Journal 1990 Discusses efforts of third-party payers to control health care expenditures for beneficiaries. Concludes that financial incentives to limit care and other cost-control techniques should be disclosed and that the rationale for such disclosure is compelling. Quotes Opinions 2.03, 2.09, and 8.03. Cites Opinions 2.19, 4.04, and 4.06. Hirshfeld, *Should Third Party Payors of Health Care Services Disclose Cost Control Mechanisms to Potential Beneficiaries?* 14 Seton Hall Legis. J. 115, 130, 131, 144, 145, 146 (1990).

2.095 The Provision of Adequate Health Care

Because society has an obligation to make access to an adequate level of health care available to all of its members regardless of ability to pay, physicians should contribute their expertise at a policy-making level to help achieve this goal. In determining whether particular procedures or treatments should be included in the adequate level of health care, the following ethical principles should be considered: (1) degree of benefit (the difference in outcome between treatment and no treatment), (2) likelihood of benefit, (3) duration of benefit, (4) cost, and (5) number of people who will benefit (referring to the fact that a treatment may benefit the patient and others who come into contact with the patient, as with a vaccination or an antimicrobial drug).

Ethical principles require that a just process be used to determine the adequate level of health care. To ensure justice, the process for determining the adequate level of health care should include the following considerations: (1) democratic decision making with broad public input at both the developmental and final approval stages, (2) monitoring for variations in care that cannot be explained on medical grounds with special attention to evidence of discriminatory impact on historically disadvantaged groups, and (3) adjustment of the adequate level over time to ensure continued and broad public acceptance.

Because of the risk that inappropriate biases will influence the content of the basic benefits package, it may be desirable to avoid rigid or precise formulas to define the specific components of the basic benefits package. After applying the five ethical values listed above, it will be possible to designate some kinds of care as either clearly basic or clearly discretionary. However, for care that is not clearly basic or discretionary, seemingly objective formulas may result in choices that are inappropriately biased. For that care, therefore, it may be desirable to give equal consideration (eg, through a process of random selection) to the different kinds of care when deciding which will be included in the basic benefits package. The mechanism for providing an adequate level of health care should ensure that the health care benefits for the poor will not be eroded over time. (VII)

Issued June 1994 based on the report "Ethical Issues in Health System Reform: The Provision of Adequate Health Care," adopted December 1993 (JAMA. 1994;272:1056-1062).

Journal 2011 Analyzes the ability of Medicaid patients to access subspecialty care in Connecticut based on a questionnaire directed towards physicians. Concludes reform in

Medicaid reimbursement, changes in licensing requirements, new rules for participation in Medicaid, and greater regulation of community service could help equalize Medicaid patients' access to subspecialty care. Quotes Opinions 2.095 and 9.065. Grewal, Sofair, Guevara, & Manthous, *Medicaid Patients' Access to Subspecialty Care in Connecticut*, 75 Conn. Med. 489, 490 (2011).

Journal 2006 Examines ethical dilemmas physicians may face as providers of pay-for-performance medical care. Concludes that this strategy offers a benefit to patients as long as physicians uphold stringent ethical standards and work together to ensure optimum patient care. Cites Principles I, V, VIII, and IX and Opinions 2.035, 2.095, 6.01, 8.021, 8.03, 8.0501, 8.053, 8.054, and 8.121. Bostick, Sade, & McMahon, *Report of the Council on Ethical and Judicial Affairs: Physician Pay-for-Performance Programs*, 3 Ind. Health L. Rev. 429, 430, 431, 432-33, 434, 435, 436 (2006).

Journal 2004 Analyzes the constitutions of countries throughout the world, focusing on language that pertains to health care. Concludes that, although a majority of constitutions have such language, this fact is not highly related to each nation's allocation of resources to health and health care. References Opinion 2.095. Kinney & Clark, *Provisions for Health and Health Care in the Constitutions of the Countries of the World*, 37 Cornell Int'l L. J. 285, 289 (2004).

Journal 2001 Examines issues relating to health care cost containment. Concludes that, if physicians are to meet the goals assigned to them in a cost-constrained health care system, then professional standards must be reevaluated and modified to afford meaningful guidance for clinical decision-making in the face of health care spending controls. Quotes Opinions 2.03, 2.09, 2.095, 8.032, and 9.04. Cites Opinions 8.02, 8.021, 8.051, and 8.13. Agrawal, *Resuscitating Professionalism: Self-regulation in the Medical Marketplace*, 66 Mo. L. Rev. 341, 354, 355, 360, 361, 378, 388 (2001).

Journal 1996 Considers challenges to the psychiatrist-patient relationship that are triggered by managed care cost-containment methodologies. Offers guidance to psychiatrists for addressing these challenges. References Opinions 2.095, 8.13, and 8.132. Hoge, *APA Resource Document: I. The Professional Responsibilities of Psychiatrists in Evolving Health Care Systems*, 24 Bull. Am. Acad. Psychiatry Law 393, 405 (1996).

Journal 1994 Considers how greater patient autonomy has led to situations in which medical care may be viewed as futile. Suggests that the law has intruded too far into this area of medicine. Quotes Opinion 2.035. Cites Opinions 2.03, 2.095, 2.17, 2.19, 2.20, and 2.22. Cultice, *Medical Futility: When Is Enough, Enough?* 27 J. Health & Hosp. Law 225, 230, 256 (1994).

Journal 1994 Considers how patients with insufficient financial resources place physicians in a conflict-of-interest situation with respect to patient needs and the financial interests of the physician, other patients, and society. Suggests that rules of contract and malpractice law do not provide satisfactory guidelines to resolve these conflicts. Cites Opinions 2.09 and 2.095. Mehlman & Massey, *The Patient-Physician Relationship and the Allocation of Scarce Resources: A Law and Economics Approach*, 4 Kennedy Inst. Ethics J. 291, 292 (1994).

2.10 Fetal Research Guidelines

The following guidelines are offered as aids to physicians when they are engaged in fetal research:

(1) Physicians may participate in fetal research when their activities are part of a competently designed program, under accepted standards of scientific research, to produce data which are scientifically valid and significant.

(2) If appropriate, properly performed clinical studies on animals and nongravid humans should precede any particular fetal research project.

(3) In fetal research projects, the investigator should demonstrate the same care and concern for the fetus as a physician providing fetal care or treatment in a nonresearch setting.

(4) All valid federal or state legal requirements should be followed.

(5) There should be no monetary payment to obtain any fetal material for fetal research projects.

(6) Competent peer review committees, review boards, or advisory boards should be available, when appropriate, to protect against the possible abuses that could arise in such research.

(7) Research on the so-called dead fetus, macerated fetal material, fetal cells, fetal tissue, or fetal organs should be in accord with state laws on autopsy and state laws on organ transplantation or anatomical gifts.

(8) In fetal research primarily for treatment of the fetus:

    (a) Voluntary and informed consent, in writing, should be given by the gravid woman, acting in the best interest of the fetus.

    (b) Alternative treatment or methods of care, if any, should be carefully evaluated and fully explained. If simpler and safer treatment is available, it should be pursued.

(9) In research primarily for treatment of the gravid female:

    (a) Voluntary and informed consent, in writing, should be given by the patient.

    (b) Alternative treatment or methods of care should be carefully evaluated and fully explained to the patient. If simpler and safer treatment is available, it should be pursued.

    (c) If possible, the risk to the fetus should be the least possible, consistent with the gravid female's need for treatment.

(10) In fetal research involving a fetus in utero, primarily for the accumulation of scientific knowledge:

    (a) Voluntary and informed consent, in writing, should be given by the gravid woman under circumstances in which a prudent and informed adult would reasonably be expected to give such consent.

    (b) The risk to the fetus imposed by the research should be the least possible.

    (c) The purpose of research is the production of data and knowledge which are scientifically significant and which cannot otherwise be obtained.

    (d) In this area of research, it is especially important to emphasize that care and concern for the fetus should be demonstrated. (I, III, V)

Issued March 1980. Updated June 1994.

Journal 1991 Explores arguments for and against fetal tissue transplantation research, including arguments for and against the use of federal funds to support such research. Considers whether the donation model is appropriate for the transfer of fetal tissue, and whether a woman who chooses elective abortion is an appropriate donor. References Opinion 2.10. Childress, *Ethics, Public Policy, and Human Fetal Tissue Transplantation Research*, Vol 1 Kennedy Inst. Ethics J. 93, 116 (June 1991).

Journal 1991 Considers how the use of in vitro fertilization (IVF) has blurred the distinction between medical practice and research. Argues that medical-professional responsibility standards should be used to curtail the creation of life in vitro. Quotes Opinions 2.10 and 2.14. Comment, *Dangerous Relations: Doctors and Extracorporeal Embryos, The Need for New Limits to Medical Inquiry*, 7 J. Contemp. Health L. & Pol'y 307, 309 (1991).

2.105   Patenting Human Genes

A patent grants the holder the right, for a limited amount of time, to prevent others from commercializing his or her inventions. At the same time, the patent system is designed to foster information sharing. Full disclosure of the invention—enabling another trained in the art to replicate it—is necessary to obtain a patent. Patenting is also thought to encourage private investment into research. Arguments have been made that the patenting of human genomic material sets a troubling precedent for the ownership or commodification of human life. DNA sequences, however, are not tantamount to human life, and it is unclear where and whether qualities uniquely human are found in genetic material.

Genetic research holds great potential for achieving new medical therapies. It remains unclear what role patenting will play in ensuring such development. At this time the Council concludes that granting patent protection should not hinder the goal of developing new beneficial technology and offers the following guidelines:

(1) Patents on processes—for example, processes used to isolate and purify gene sequences, genes and proteins, or vehicles of gene therapy—do not raise the same ethical problems as patents on the substances themselves and are thus preferable.

(2) Substance patents on purified proteins present fewer ethical problems than patents on genes or DNA sequences and are thus preferable.

(3) Patent descriptions should be carefully constructed to ensure that the patent holder does not limit the use of a naturally occurring form of the substance in question. This includes patents on proteins, genes, and genetic sequences.

One of the goals of genetic research is to achieve better medical treatments and technologies. Granting patent protection should not hinder this goal. Individuals or entities holding patents on genetic material should not allow patents to languish and should negotiate and structure licensing agreements in such a way as to encourage the development of better medical technology. (V, VII)

Issued June 1998 based on the report "Patenting the Human Genome," adopted December 1997.

Journal 2011 Discusses scientific and technological advancements in genetic research and the controversy surrounding patenting human genomic material. Concludes that although patent protection should be provided, modifications to the current system are necessary to ensure that genetic sequencing information is available to researchers to further advancement in health care. Cites Council on Ethical and Judicial Affairs Report 2-I-97 [now Opinion 2.105] and Report 4-I-01 [now Opinion 2.079]. Ratcliffe, *The Ethics of Genetic Patenting and the Subsequent Implications on the Future of Health Care*, 27 Touro L. Rev. 435, 438-39, 449 (2011).

Journal 2007 Analyzes scientific, ethical, and legal issues raised in the exhumation and genetic analysis of historical figures. Concludes that biohistorical review boards should be created to generate guidelines for such research. Quotes Preamble and Opinion 2.08. Cites Opinions 2.079, 2.105, 5.05, 5.051, 5.075, 8.03, 8.031, 9.095, and 9.10. Paradise & Andrews, *Tales From the Crypt: Scientific, Ethical, and Legal Considerations for Biohistorical Analysis of Deceased Historical Figures*, 26 Temp. J. Sci. Tech. & Envtl. L. 223, 287-88 (2007).

Journal 2001 Examines whether or not DNA patents violate or threaten human dignity. Supports legislation banning patents on the whole human genome. Concludes that only patents that comprise complete commodification of human beings violate human dignity. References Opinion 2.105. Resnik, *DNA Patents and Human Dignity*, 29 J. L. Med. & Ethics 152, 158, 159 (2001).

2.11   Gene Therapy

Gene therapy involves the replacement or modification of a genetic variant to restore or enhance cellular function or to improve the reaction of nongenetic therapies.

Two types of gene therapy have been identified: (1) somatic cell therapy, in which human cells other than germ cells are genetically altered, and (2) germline therapy, in which a replacement gene is integrated into the genome of human gametes or their precursors, resulting in expression of the new gene in the patient's offspring and subsequent generations. The fundamental difference between germline therapy and somatic cell therapy is that germline therapy affects the welfare of subsequent generations and may be associated with increased risk and the potential for unpredictable and irreversible results. Because of the far-reaching implications of germline therapy, it is appropriate to limit genetic intervention to somatic cells at this time.

The goal of both somatic cell and germline therapy is to alleviate human suffering and disease by remedying disorders for which available therapies are not satisfactory. This goal should be pursued only within the ethical tradition of medicine, which gives primacy to the welfare of the patient whose safety and well-being must be vigorously protected. To the extent possible, experience with animal studies must be sufficient to assure the effectiveness and safety of the techniques used and the predictability of the results.

Moreover, genetic manipulation generally should be utilized only for therapeutic purposes. Efforts to enhance "desirable" characteristics through the insertion of a modified or an additional gene, or efforts to "improve" complex human traits—the eugenic development of offspring—are contrary not only to the ethical tradition of medicine, but also to the egalitarian values of our society. Because of the potential for abuse, genetic manipulation to affect non-disease traits may never be acceptable and perhaps should never be pursued. If it is ever allowed, at least three conditions would have to be met before it could be deemed ethically acceptable: (1) there would have to be a clear and meaningful benefit to the person, (2) there would have to be no trade-off with other characteristics or traits, and (3) all citizens would have to have equal access to the genetic technology, irrespective of income or other socioeconomic characteristics. These criteria should be viewed as a minimal, not an exhaustive test of the ethical propriety of non–disease-related genetic intervention. As genetic technology and knowledge of the human genome develop further, additional guidelines may be required.

As gene therapy becomes feasible for a variety of human disorders, there are several practical factors to consider to ensure safe application of this technology in society. First, any gene therapy research should meet the Council's guidelines on clinical investigation (Opinion 2.07, "Clinical Investigation") and investigators must adhere to the standards of medical practice and professional responsibility. The proposed procedure must be fully discussed with the patient, and the written informed consent of the patient or the patient's legal representative must be voluntary. Investigators must be thorough in their attempts to eliminate any unwanted viral agents from the viral vector containing the corrective gene. The potential for adverse effects of the viral delivery system must be disclosed to the patient. The effectiveness of gene therapy must be evaluated fully, including the determination of the natural history of the disease and follow-up examination of subsequent generations. Gene therapy should be pursued only after the availability or effectiveness of other possible therapies is found to be insufficient. These considerations should be reviewed, as appropriate, as procedures and scientific information develop. (I, V)

Issued December 1988. Updated June 1994 based on the report "Prenatal Genetic Screening," adopted December 1992 (*Arch Fam Med.* 1994;3:633-642) and June 1996.

Journal 2006 Explores legal and ethical issues which may arise from prebirth genetic screening and enhancement. Concludes that courts will have to strongly weigh a woman's right to choose abortion against potential ethical problems. Quotes Opinion 2.11. McConnell, *Quality Control: The Implications of Negative Genetic Selection and Pre-Birth Genetic Enhancement, 15 UCLA Women's L. J. 47, 61 (2006).*

Journal 2000 Defines and describes human genetic enhancement. Explores the legal implications of this emerging technology as well as related societal concerns. Quotes Opinion 2.11. References Opinion 2.12. Mehlman, *The Law of Above Averages: Leveling the New Genetic Enhancement Playing Field, 85 Iowa L. Rev. 517, 527-28, 559 (2000).*

Journal 1999 Discusses regulatory concerns regarding genetic technology. Provides ideas on how society might regulate genetic enhancements. Argues that a variety of means of regulation need to be utilized to govern genetic technology. Quotes Opinion 2.11. Cites Opinion 9.065. References Opinion 2.138. Mehlman, *How Will We Regulate Genetic Enhancement? 34 Wake Forest L. Rev. 671, 693-94, 695 (1999).*

2.12 Genetic Counseling

Three primary areas of prenatal genetic testing are (1) screening or evaluating prospective parents for genetic disease before conception to predict the likelihood of conceiving an affected child; (2) analysis of a pre-embryo at the preimplantation stage of artificial reproductive techniques; and (3) in utero testing after conception, such as ultrasonography, amniocentesis, fetoscopy, and chorionic villus sampling, to determine the condition of the fetus. Physicians engaged in genetic counseling are ethically obligated to provide prospective parents with the basis for an informed decision for childbearing. Counseling should include reasons for and against testing as well as discussion of inappropriate uses of genetic testing. Prenatal genetic testing is most appropriate for women or couples whose medical histories or family backgrounds indicate an elevated risk of fetal genetic disorders. Women or couples without an elevated risk of genetic disease may legitimately request prenatal diagnosis, provided they understand and accept the risks involved. When counseling prospective parents, physicians should avoid the imposition of their personal moral values and the substitution of their own moral judgment for that of the prospective parents.

The physician should be aware that where a genetic defect is found in the fetus, prospective parents may request or refuse an abortion. Physicians who consider the legal and ethical requirements applicable to genetic counseling to be in conflict with their moral values and conscience may choose to limit their services to preconception diagnosis and advice or not provide any genetic services. However, the physician who is so disposed is nevertheless obligated to alert prospective parents when a potential genetic problem does exist, so that the parent may decide whether to seek further genetic counseling from another qualified specialist.

Genetic selection refers to the abortion or discard of a fetus or pre-embryo with a genetic abnormality. In general, it is ethically permissible for physicians to participate in genetic selection to prevent, cure, or treat genetic disease. However, selection to avoid a genetic disease may not always be appropriate, depending on factors such as the severity of the disease, the probability of its occurrence, the age at onset, and the time of gestation at which selection would occur. It would not be ethical to engage in selection on the basis of non–disease-related characteristics or traits. (II, IV, V, VI)

Issued June 1983. Updated June 1994 based on the report "Prenatal Genetic Screening," adopted December 1992 (*Arch Fam Med.* 1994;3:633-642).

Journal 2006 Evaluates policies regarding regulation of preimplantation genetic diagnosis. Concludes the US should require a separate license for health care professionals to perform the procedure. Cites Opinion 2.12. Fahrenkrog, *A Comparison of International Regulation of Preimplantation Genetic Diagnosis and a Regulatory Suggestion for the United States,* 15 Transnat'l L. & Contemp. Probs. 757, 759 (2006).

Journal 2006 Discusses the ethical issues surrounding preimplantation genetic diagnosis (PGD) for cancer syndromes. Concludes that patients must be afforded psychosocial support for participation in PGD and that there is ongoing need for professional guidance to physicians on this topic. Quotes Opinion 2.12. Offit, Sagi, & Hurley, *Preimplantation Genetic Diagnosis for Cancer Syndromes: A New Challenge for Preventive Medicine,* 296 JAMA 2727, 2727 (2006).

Journal 2003 Applies professional standards to determine the technology that practitioners should utilize in prenatal diagnosis. Concludes that appropriate uses of prenatal diagnostic methodologies must be articulated by society. Quotes Opinion 2.12. Botkin, *Prenatal Diagnosis and the Selection of Children,* 30 Fla. St. U. L. Rev. 265, 289 (2003).

Journal 2003 Proposes a method to distinguish between good and bad eugenics. Concludes that prenatal testing for Down syndrome, followed by termination of pregnancy, characterizes bad eugenics. References Opinion 2.12. Mahowald, *Aren't We All Eugenicists? Commentary on Paul Lombardo's "Taking Eugenics Seriously,"* 30 Fla. St. U. L. Rev. 219, 234 (2003).

Journal 2003 Considers the medical, ethical, and legal issues associated with using preimplantation genetic diagnosis (PGD) to create a stem cell donor. Concludes by offering important guidelines and limitations in connection with use of PGD. Quotes Opinion 2.12. Wolf, Kahn, & Wagner, *Using Preimplantation Genetic Diagnosis to Create a Stem Cell Donor: Issues, Guidelines & Limits,* 31 J. L. Med. & Ethics 327, 329, 339 (2003).

Journal 2000 Defines and describes human genetic enhancement. Explores the legal implications of this emerging technology as well as related societal concerns. Quotes Opinion 2.11. References Opinion 2.12. Mehlman, *The Law of Above Averages: Leveling the New Genetic Enhancement Playing Field,* 85 Iowa L. Rev. 517, 527-28, 559 (2000).

Journal 1998 Discusses genetic testing to determine hereditary hearing impairment. Explains ways in which genetic counselors can assist people. Points out how presymptomatic diagnosis can help parents and children. References Opinion 2.12. Chen, Mueller, Prasad, Greinwald, Manaligod, Muilenburg, Verhoeven, Van Camp, & Smith, *Presymptomatic Diagnosis of Nonsyndromic Hearing Loss by Genotyping,* 124 Arch. Otolaryngol. Head Neck Surg. 20, 23 (1998).

Journal 1997 Discusses techniques and possibilities for genetic testing. Presents a series of problems designed as a starting point for understanding the conflicts surrounding genetic testing. Reviews the applications of state-of-the-art genetic research. Suggests potential difficulties that testing may cause in society. References Opinion 2.12. Underwood & Cadle, *Genetics, Genetic Testing, and the Specter of Discrimination: A Discussion Using Hypothetical Cases,* 85 Ky. L. J. 665, 684 (1996-97).

2.13 Genetic Engineering

The Federal Recombinant DNA Advisors Committee and the Food and Drug Administration oversee and regulate gene splicing, recombinant DNA research, chemical synthesis of DNA molecules, and other genetic engineering research. However, for genetic engineering technologies that represent a significant departure from familiar practices there should be independent input from the scientific community, organized medicine, industry, the public, and others, in addition to the federal government, to prevent abuse from any sector of society, private or public. Such departures include the use of novel vectors, gene transfer in utero, potential germline modification, and gene transfer to normal volunteers.

If and when gene replacement with normal DNA becomes a practical reality for the treatment of human disorders, the following factors should be considered:

(1) If procedures are performed in a research setting, reference should be made to the Council's guidelines on clinical investigation.

(2) If procedures are performed in a nonresearch setting, adherence to usual and customary standards of medical practice and professional responsibility would be required.

(3) Full discussion of the proposed procedure with the patient would be required. The consent of the patient or the patient's legal representative should be informed, voluntary, and written.

(4) There must be no hazardous or other unwanted virus on the viral DNA containing the replacement or corrective gene.

(5) The inserted DNA must function under normal control within the recipient cell to prevent metabolic damage that could damage tissue and the patient.

(6) The effectiveness of the gene therapy should be evaluated as well as possible. This will include determination of the natural history of the disease and follow-up examination of subsequent generations.

(7) Such procedures should be undertaken in the future only after careful evaluation of the availability and effectiveness of other possible therapy. If simpler and safer treatment is available, it should be pursued.

(8) These considerations should be reviewed, as appropriate, as procedures and scientific information are developed in the future. (I, V, VII)

Issued March 1980. Updated June 1996.

2.131 Disclosure of Familial Risk in Genetic Testing

(1) Physicians have a professional duty to protect the confidentiality of their patients' information, including genetic information.

(2) Pre- and post-test counseling must include implications of genetic information for patients' biological relatives. At the time patients are considering undergoing genetic testing, physicians should discuss with them whether to invite family members to participate in the testing process. Physicians also should identify circumstances under which they would expect patients to notify biological relatives of the availability of information related to risk

of disease. In this regard, physicians should make themselves available to assist patients in communicating with relatives to discuss opportunities for counseling and testing, as appropriate.

(3) Physicians who order genetic tests should have adequate knowledge to interpret information for patients. In the absence of adequate expertise in pre-test and post-test counseling, a physician should refer the patient to an appropriate specialist.

(4) Physicians should encourage genetic education throughout a medical career. (I, IV, V, VIII)

Issued December 2003 based on the report "Disclosure of Familial Risk in Genetic Testing," adopted June 2003 (*Genetic Testing*, 2004;8(3):356-359).

Journal 2007 Examines the legal and ethical considerations surrounding disclosure of *BRCA1/2* genetic testing results to family members. Concludes that genetic providers play a valuable role in facilitating the communication process between family members. Cites Opinion 2.131. DeMarco & McKinnon, *Life After BRCA1/2 Testing: Family Communication and Support Issues*, 27 *Breast Disease 127, 127* (2007).

Journal 2004 Discusses the conflict between a physician's duty to keep genetic information private and potential liability for failure to inform at-risk relatives of the possibility of genetic disorders. Concludes that physicians should encourage patients to share genetic information with at-risk relatives, while abiding by legal and ethical principles. Quotes Opinion 2.131. Offit, Groeger, Turner, Wadsworth, & Weiser, *The "Duty to Warn" a Patient's Family Members About Hereditary Disease Risks*, 292 JAMA 1469, 1471 (2004).

2.132 Genetic Testing by Employers

As a result of the human genome project, physicians will be able to identify a greater number of genetic risks of disease. Among the potential uses of the tests that detect these risks will be screening of potential workers by employers. Employers may want to exclude workers with certain genetic risks from the workplace because these workers may become disabled prematurely, impose higher health care costs, or pose a risk to public safety. In addition, exposure to certain substances in the workplace may increase the likelihood that a disease will develop in the worker with a genetic risk for the disease.

(1) It would generally be inappropriate to exclude workers with genetic risks of disease from the workplace because of their risk. Genetic tests alone do not have sufficient predictive value to be relied upon as a basis for excluding workers. Consequently, use of the tests would result in unfair discrimination against individuals who have positive test results. In addition, there are other ways for employers to serve their legitimate interests. Tests of a worker's actual capacity to meet the demands of the job can be used to ensure future employability and protect the public's safety. Routine monitoring of a worker's exposure can be used to protect workers who have a genetic susceptibility to injury from a substance in the workplace. In addition, employees should be advised of the risks of injury to which they are being exposed.

(2) There may be a role for genetic testing in the exclusion from the workplace of workers who have a genetic susceptibility to injury. At a minimum, several conditions would have to be met:

(a) The disease develops so rapidly that serious and irreversible injury would occur before monitoring of either the worker's exposure to the toxic substance or the worker's health status could be effective in preventing the harm.

(b) The genetic testing is highly accurate, with sufficient sensitivity and specificity to minimize the risk of false-negative and false-positive test results.

(c) Empirical data demonstrate that the genetic abnormality results in an unusually elevated susceptibility to occupational injury.

(d) It would require undue cost to protect susceptible employees by lowering the level of the toxic substance in the workplace. The costs of lowering the level of the substance must be extraordinary relative to the employer's other costs of making the product for which the toxic substance is used. Since genetic testing with exclusion of susceptible employees is the alternative to cleaning up the workplace, the cost of lowering the level of the substance must also be extraordinary relative to the costs of using genetic testing.

(e) Testing must not be performed without the informed consent of the employee or applicant for employment. (IV)

Issued June 1991 based on the report "Genetic Testing by Employers," adopted June 1991 (JAMA. 1991;266:1827-1830).

Journal 2003 Focuses on the controversial use of genetic information in employment and insurance. Concludes that reformers must reexamine the ethical and legal duties of professionals regarding protection of genetic information. References Opinion 2.132. Partlett, *Misuse of Genetic Information: The Common Law and Professionals' Liability*, 42 Washburn L. J. 489, 503 (2003).

Journal 2001 Discusses same-sex marriages in the transgender community. Explores Defense of Marriage Act statutes. Considers whether same-sex transgender marriages can prevail against attacks brought under such statutes. Cites Opinions 2.132, 2.135, 2.137, 5.08, and 5.09. Frye & Meiselman, *Same-Sex Marriages Have Existed Legally in the United States for a Long Time Now*, 64 Alb. L. Rev. 1031, 1053 (2001).

Journal 2001 Examines the distinction between preplacement and postplacement examinations in the workplace. Analyzes the possible dangers that might result if preplacement medical testing is not restricted. Concludes that any such testing must relate to the potential employee's ability to perform assigned job duties. References Opinions 2.132 and 2.139. Hoffman, *Preplacement Examinations and Job-Relatedness: How to Enhance Privacy and Diminish Discrimination in the Workplace*, 49 U. Kan. L. Rev. 517, 534, 535, 556, 565 (2001).

Journal 2000 Explores the benefits and harms of the new era of genomic medicine. Discusses the needs of tissue donors, noting they should be carefully balanced with the needs of the medical research community. Concludes that a multifaceted effort is essential to ensuring trust in the medical community as the benefits of genomic medicine are realized. References Opinion 2.132. Ashburn, Wilson, & Eisenstein, *Human Tissue Research in the Genomic Era of Medicine*, 160 Arch. Intern. Med. 3377, 3378 (2000).

Journal 2000 Examines the effects of genetic information on medical care. Concludes that the existing rules and regulations, which try to protect a patient's absolute control over personal genetic data, should be modified. Suggests that a statutory board might better decide when personal genetic information may be divulged to others. References Opinion 2.132. Bruns & Wolman, *Morality of the Privacy of Genetic Information: Possible Improvements of Procedures*, 19 Med. Law 127, 129 (2000).

Journal 2000 Evaluates transgender legal and political activity in the US. Discusses the International Bill of Gender Rights against the background of the Texas case, *Littleton v. Prange.* Cites Opinions 2.132, 2.135, 2.137, 5.08, and 5.09. Frye, *The International Bill of Gender Rights* *vs. the Cider House Rules: Transgenders Struggle With the Courts Over What Clothing They Are Allowed to Wear on the Job, Which Restroom They Are Allowed to Use on the Job, Their Right to Marry, and the Very Definition of Their Sex, 7 Wm. & Mary J. Women & L. 133, 149 (2000).*

Journal 2000 Explores the legal, ethical, social, and economic considerations associated with use of new genetic techniques in the prediction and diagnosis of Alzheimer disease. Outlines the potential responsibilities and liabilities of physicians in connection with use of these techniques. References Opinions 2.132, 2.139, and 8.032. Kapp, *Physicians' Legal Duties Regarding the Use of Genetic Tests to Predict and Diagnose Alzheimer Disease, 21 J. Legal Med. 445, 456-57, 465-66 (2000).*

Journal 2000 Discusses the adverse effects of predisposition genetic testing on personal and familial relationships as well as insurability and employment opportunities. Concludes that health care providers and policy makers must ensure that individuals who undergo genetic testing have access to proper counseling, appropriate medical resources, and protection from genetic discrimination. References Opinion 2.132. Schneider, *Adverse Impact of Predisposition Testing on Major Life Activities: Lessons From BRCA1/2 Testing, 3 J. Health Care L. & Pol'y 365, 380 (2000).*

Journal 1999 Explains physicians' potential liability as corporate professionals and how that reinforces professional standards. Discusses physicians' pursuit of preventive health and its impact on reducing company liability. References Opinion 2.132. Draper, *Preventive Law by Corporate Professional Team Players: Liability and Responsibility in the Work of Company Doctors, 15 J. Contemp. Health L. & Pol'y. 525, 564 (1999).*

Journal 1999 Argues that current Fourth Amendment jurisprudence needs to be changed. Describes two different theories—an antidiscrimination model and an individual rights model—and applies them to different situations. States that the Fourth Amendment needs to protect personal sovereignty for the sake of the individual and society. References Opinion 2.132. Luna, *Sovereignty and Suspicion, 48 Duke L. J. 787, 884 (1999).*

Journal 1998 Discusses conflicts of interest in the physician-patient relationship arising out of use of financial incentives by managed care organizations. Considers how such conflicts are dealt with in the attorney-client relationship. Suggests that a financial incentive should be legally denounced if it unreasonably interferes with a physician's duty to properly care for and treat patients. Quotes Preamble, Fundamental Elements (1) [now Opinion 10.01], and Opinions 4.04, 5.01, 8.03, 8.13, and 9.06. Cites Fundamental Elements (4) [now Opinion 10.01] and Opinions 2.07, 2.08, and 2.132. Hall, *Third-Party Payor Conflicts of Interest in Managed Care: A Proposal for Regulation Based on the Model Rules of Professional Conduct, 29 Seton Hall L. Rev. 95, 96, 107, 108, 109, 110, 111, 112, 134, 135, 136 (1998).*

Journal 1998 Discusses the use of genetic information by employers. Argues that people may forgo genetic testing for fear that the results will be used by their employers in a discriminatory manner. Concludes that the Minnesota statute prohibiting employers from performing medical tests or obtaining medical information, which is not job-related, is better than other approaches. References Opinion 2.132. Rothstein, Gelb, & Craig, *Protecting Genetic Privacy by Permitting Employer Access Only to Job-Related Employee Medical Information: Analysis of a Unique Minnesota Law, 24 Am. J. Law & Med. 399, 400 (1998).*

Journal 1997 Explores the legality of pre-employment screening techniques. Considers legal reforms that would balance the interests of employers and job applicants. Offers suggestions that would enhance fairness and consistency in this screening process. References Opinion 2.132. Befort, *Pre-Employment Screening and Investigation: Navigating Between a Rock and a Hard Place, 14 Hofstra Lab. L. J. 365, 391 (1997).*

Journal 1997 Explores parents' legal rights to subject their children to genetic testing for untreatable, late-onset disorders or for carrier status. Examines potential negative aspects of genetic testing. Proposes that parents should not have the right to subject their children to such testing. References Opinion 2.132. Holland, *Should Parents Be Permitted to Authorize Genetic Testing for Their Children? 31 Fam. L. Q. 321, 346-47 (1997).*

Journal 1997 Discusses the collection and storage of human tissues. Notes the use of genetic testing by employers. Examines whether those with biomedical experience perceive genetic research as dangerous. Considers problems of privacy and confidentiality raised by genetic technology and the storage of tissues. References Opinion 2.132. Merz, *Psychosocial Risks of Storing and Using Human Tissues in Research, 8 Risk Health Safety & Env't. 235, 236 (1997).*

Journal 1993 Examines how genetic tests to diagnose disease may be useful to private insurance companies in identifying persons for whom coverage will be provided. Concludes that this issue should be considered as part of the national health care reform debate. References Opinion 2.132. Jecker, *Genetic Testing and the Social Responsibility of Private Health Insurance Companies,* 21 J. Law Med. & Ethics 109, 112 (1993).

2.135 Insurance Companies and Genetic Information

Physicians should not participate in genetic testing by health insurance companies to predict a person's predisposition for disease. As a corollary, it may be necessary for physicians to maintain separate files for genetic testing results to ensure that the results are not sent to health insurance companies when requests for copies of patient medical records are fulfilled. Physicians who withhold testing results should inform insurance companies that, when medical records are sent, genetic testing results are not included. This disclosure should occur with all patients, not just those who have undergone genetic testing. (IV)

Issued June 1994 based on the report "Physician Participation in Genetic Testing by Health Insurance Companies," adopted June 1993. Updated June 1996.

Journal 2001 Discusses same-sex marriages in the transgender community. Explores Defense of Marriage Act statutes. Considers whether same-sex transgender marriages can prevail against attacks brought under such statutes. Cites Opinions 2.132, 2.135, 2.137, 5.08, and 5.09. Frye & Meiselman, *Same-Sex Marriages Have Existed Legally in the United States for a Long Time Now,* 64 Alb. L. Rev. 1031, 1053 (2001).

Journal 2000 Evaluates transgender legal and political activity in the US. Discusses the International Bill of Gender Rights against the background of the Texas case, *Littleton v. Prange.* Cites Opinions 2.132, 2.135, 2.137, 5.08, and 5.09. Frye, *The International Bill of Gender Rights vs. the Cider House Rules: Transgenders Struggle With the Courts Over What Clothing They Are Allowed to Wear on the Job, Which Restroom They Are Allowed to Use on the Job, Their Right to Marry, and the Very Definition of Their Sex,* 7 Wm. & Mary J. Women & L. 133, 149 (2000).

2.136 Genetic Information and the Criminal Justice System

The release of genetic information from a physician's records without the consent of the patient constitutes a breach of confidentiality. Opinion 5.05, "Confidentiality," acknowledges that law and overriding social considerations may permit physicians to disclose confidential information in limited circumstances. However, such circumstances present ethical challenges. The following guidelines are intended to aid physicians in considering the ethical basis for the release of genetic information to the criminal justice system:

(1) Physicians should release a patient's genetic information only with the patient's consent or in compliance with a warrant or other order of a court of law. The circumstances in which law enforcement may seek a suspect's genetic information from the suspect's physician depend on whether any specific suspect has been identified and if the suspect is in custody.

    (a) If law enforcement personnel have identified a suspect and the suspect cannot be located to provide a genetic sample, physicians should release clinical genetic information only when a warrant or court order mandates such a release.

    (b) When law enforcement personnel have identified a suspect, and the suspect has been located but refuses to provide a sample or is deceased (but his or her body is available), physicians should not be required to release genetic information as in these circumstances a court can authorize collection of a sample from the suspect or from postmortem tissue.

(c) Searching clinical and research databases of genetic information or extracting and analyzing DNA from clinical or research tissue repositories should not be conducted for the mere possibility that there is a match to a suspect's DNA unless there is a warrant or court order to do so.

(2) When genetic information is provided to the judicial system, physicians should provide the minimum amount of information necessary for the explicit identification procedure being performed. Other elements of the medical record or the results of any genetic testing or genetic diagnosis should not be released without the patient's consent or further warrant or order of the court.

(3) It is unethical for any genetic information obtained from a physician for identification purposes to be used subsequently for other purposes, such as research, unless appropriate ethical guidelines are followed and the informed consent of the individual is obtained (or the legally appropriate surrogate if the individual is incompetent or deceased, in compliance with Opinion 5.051, "Confidentiality of Medical Information Postmortem").

(4) Databases that contain only the genetic identifiers from the specific loci that are typically used for identification purposes do not present the same ethical concerns that are presented by databases which contain genotypic or phenotypic information. Physicians participating in the creation of genetic databases for the exclusive use of the criminal justice system should ensure that the database is not used inappropriately for purposes other than identification.

(5) In general, requiring that the genetic sample be destroyed or returned after the analysis necessary for identification is performed affords protection against inappropriate uses.

(6) When the criminal justice system seeks genetic information for the purposes of identifying a deceased victim, the above relevant guidelines also apply. (III, IV)

Issued June 2001 based on the report "Genetic Information and the Criminal Justice System," adopted June 2000. (*J. Law Med. & Ethics.* 2002;30:88-94).

Journal 2002 Discusses legal and medical policies that protect confidentiality in the physician-patient relationship. Concludes that reducing the current level of privacy protection would jeopardize health care. Quotes Preamble and Opinions 2.136, 5.05, and 10.01. References Principles VIII and IX. Sciarrino, *Ferguson v. City of Charleston: "The Doctor Will See You Now, Be Sure to Bring Your Privacy Rights in With You!" 12 Temp. Pol. & Civ. Rts. L. Rev. 197, 213, 215, 220, 221, 222 (2002)*

2.137   Ethical Issues in Carrier Screening of Genetic Disorders

All carrier testing must be voluntary, and informed consent from screened individuals is required. Confidentiality of results is to be maintained. Results of testing should not be disclosed to third parties without the explicit informed consent of the screened individual. Patients should be informed as to potential uses for the genetic information by third parties, and whether other ways of obtaining the information are available when appropriate.

Carrier testing should be available uniformly among the at-risk population being screened. One legitimate exception to this principle is the limitation of carrier testing to individuals of childbearing age. In pursuit of uniform access, physicians should not limit testing only to patients specifically requesting testing. If testing is offered to some patients, it should be offered to all patients within the same risk category.

The direction of future genetic screening tests should be determined by well-thought-out and well-coordinated social policy. Third parties, including insurance companies and employers, should not be permitted to discriminate against carriers of genetic disorders through policies which have the ultimate effect of influencing decisions about testing and reproduction. (IV, V)

Issued June 1994 based on the report "Ethical Issues in Carrier Screening for Cystic Fibrosis and Other Genetic Disorders," adopted June 1991.

Journal 2007 Evaluates the ethical issues surrounding "neoeugenics." Concludes that, in formulating future policy, societal concerns must be balanced with individual rights to reproductive autonomy. References Opinion 2.137. Suter, *A Brave New World of Designer Babies? 22 Berkeley Tech. L. J. 897, 936-37 (2007).*

Journal 2001 Discusses same-sex marriages in the transgender community. Explores Defense of Marriage Act statutes. Considers whether same-sex transgender marriages can prevail against attacks brought under such statutes. Cites Opinions 2.132, 2.135, 2.137, 5.08, and 5.09. Frye & Meiselman, *Same-Sex Marriages Have Existed Legally in the United States for a Long Time Now, 64 Alb. L. Rev. 1031, 1053 (2001).*

Journal 2000 Evaluates transgender legal and political activity in the US. Discusses the International Bill of Gender Rights against the background of the Texas case, *Littleton v. Prange.* Cites Opinions 2.132, 2.135, 2.137, 5.08, and 5.09. Frye, *The International Bill of Gender Rights vs. the Cider House Rules: Transgenders Struggle With the Courts Over What Clothing They Are Allowed to Wear on the Job, Which Restroom They Are Allowed to Use on the Job, Their Right to Marry, and the Very Definition of Their Sex, 7 Wm. & Mary J. Women & L. 133, 149 (2000).*

2.138 Genetic Testing of Children

Genetic testing of children implicates important concerns about individual autonomy and the interest of the patients. Before testing of children can be performed, there must be some potential benefit from the testing that can reasonably be viewed as outweighing the disadvantages of testing, particularly the harm from abrogating the children's future choice in knowing their genetic status. When there is such a potential benefit, parents should decide whether their children will undergo testing. If parents unreasonably request or refuse testing of their child, the physician should take steps to change or, if necessary, use legal means to override the parents' choice. Applying these principles to specific circumstances yields the following conclusions:

(1) When a child is at risk for a genetic condition for which preventive or other therapeutic measures are available, genetic testing should be offered or, in some cases, required.

(2) When a child is at risk for a genetic condition with pediatric onset for which preventive or other therapeutic measures are not available, parents generally should have discretion to decide about genetic testing.

(3) When a child is at risk for a genetic condition with adult onset for which preventive or other therapeutic measures are not available, genetic testing of children generally should not be undertaken. Families should still be informed of the existence of tests and given the opportunity to discuss the reasons why the tests are generally not offered for children.

(4) Genetic testing for carrier status should be deferred until either the child reaches maturity, the child needs to make reproductive decisions, or, in the case of children too immature to make their own reproductive decisions, reproductive decisions need to be made for the child.

(5) Genetic testing of children for the benefit of a family member should not be performed unless the testing is necessary to prevent substantial harm to the family member.

When a child's genetic status is determined incidentally, the information should be retained by the physician and entered into the patient record. Discussion of the existence of this finding should then be taken up when the child reaches maturity or needs to make reproductive decisions, so that the individual can decide whether to request disclosure of the information. It is important that physicians be consistent in disclosing both positive and negative results in the same way since if physicians raise the existence of the testing results only when the results are positive, individuals will know what the results must be. This information should not be disclosed to third parties. Genetic information should be maintained in a separate portion of the medical record to prevent mistaken disclosure.

When a child is being considered for adoption, the guidelines for genetic testing should be the same as for other children. (IV)

Issued June 1996 based on the report "Testing Children for Genetic Status," adopted June 1995.

Journal 2007 Explores the impact of genetic testing on disability insurance. Concludes that predictive genetic tests should not act to limit access to disability insurance. Cites Opinion 2.138. Wolf & Kahn, *Genetic Testing and the Future of Disability Insurance: Ethics, Law & Policy, 35 J. L. Med. & Ethics 6, 23 (2007).*

Journal 1999 Discusses regulatory concerns regarding genetic technology. Provides ideas on how society might regulate genetic enhancements. Argues that a variety of means of regulation need to be utilized to govern genetic technology. Quotes Opinion 2.11. Cites Opinion 9.065. References Opinion 2.138. Mehlman, *How Will We Regulate Genetic Enhancement? 34 Wake Forest L. Rev. 671, 693-94, 695 (1999).*

Journal 1998 Discusses ramifications of genetic research. Points out that genetic information affects not only the tested individual, but the person's family as well. Suggests that a greater awareness of potential risk will reduce possible hazards stemming from genetic research. Cites Opinion 2.138. Green & Thomas, *DNA: Five Distinguishing Features for Policy Analysis, 11 Harv. J. L. & Tech. 571, 582-83 (1998).*

Journal 1997 Discusses the National Human Genome Research Institute and the activities of the Office of Genome Ethics. Offers an overview and evaluation, with emphasis on bioethical education and counsel that was provided to genetic researchers. References Opinion 2.138. Green, *NHGRI's Intramural Ethics Experiment, 7 Kennedy Inst. of Ethics J. 181, 185, 188 (1997).*

2.139 Multiplex Genetic Testing

Multiplex testing—where tests are offered for several different medical conditions in a single session—presents a series of challenges to adequate communication between the patient and the physician. It increases the total number of marginally indicated or nonindicated tests, thereby bolstering the rate of false results. These results may lead to psychological stress and misinformed life-altering decisions, and may also impact the ability of a physician to obtain informed consent. Multiplex testing and its resultant information may also have widespread societal implications that include discriminatory practices against not only individuals, but also specific ethnic groups that have been designated "at-risk" populations.

Before such tests reach health care providers, clinics, and drugstores, the ethical and social implications of these tests must be well-understood, and careful restrictions and regulations must be established. The following guidelines are offered on the future possibilities of multiplex genetic testing:

(1) Physicians should not routinely order tests for multiple genetic conditions.

(2) Tests for more than one genetic condition should be ordered only when clinically relevant and after the patient has had full counseling and has given informed consent for each test.

(3) Efforts should be made to educate clinicians and society about the uncertainty surrounding genetic testing. (IV, V)

Issued June 1998 based on the report "Multiplex Genetic Testing," adopted December 1996 (*Hastings Center Report*. 1998;28(4):15-21).

Journal 2001 Examines the distinction between preplacement and postplacement examinations in the workplace. Analyzes the possible dangers that might result if preplacement medical testing is not restricted. Concludes that any such testing must relate to the potential employee's ability to perform assigned job duties. References Opinions 2.132 and 2.139. Hoffman, *Preplacement Examinations and Job-Relatedness: How to Enhance Privacy and Diminish Discrimination in the Workplace, 49 U. Kan. L. Rev. 517, 534, 535, 556, 565 (2001).*

Journal 2000 Explores issues relating to genetic privacy and considers how the law should evolve in this context. Identifies contrasting ideological viewpoints regarding the role government should play in regulating public use of personal genetic data. Concludes that because of unregulated information markets, people may be afraid to use genetic technologies. References Opinion 2.139. Fedder, *To Know or Not to Know: Legal Perspectives on Genetic Privacy and Disclosure of an Individual's Genetic Profile, 21 J. Legal Med. 557, 563 (2000).*

Journal 2000 Explores the legal, ethical, social, and economic considerations associated with use of new genetic techniques in the prediction and diagnosis of Alzheimer disease. Outlines the potential responsibilities and liabilities of physicians in connection with use of these techniques. References Opinions 2.132, 2.139, and 8.032. Kapp, *Physicians' Legal Duties Regarding the Use of Genetic Tests to Predict and Diagnose Alzheimer Disease, 21 J. Legal Med. 445, 456-57, 465-66 (2000).*

2.14 In Vitro Fertilization

The technique of in vitro fertilization and embryo transplantation enables certain couples previously incapable of conception to bear a child. It is also useful in the field of research directed toward an understanding of how genetic defects arise and are transmitted and how they might be prevented or treated. Because of serious ethical and moral concerns, however, any fertilized egg that has the potential for human life and that will be implanted in the uterus of a woman should not be subjected to laboratory research.

All fertilized ova not utilized for implantation and that are maintained for research purposes shall be handled with the strictest adherence to the Principles of Medical Ethics, to the guidelines for research and medical practice expressed in the Council's opinion on fetal research, and to the highest standards of medical practice. (I, V, VII)

Issued June 1983.

Journal 2005 Discusses legal and ethical issues in conducting embryonic research in the US. Concludes that failure to pursue such research may be viewed as unethical and that the British experience might offer a model for moving forward in this regard. Cites Opinion 2.14. Clemmens, *Creating Human Embryos for Research: A Scientist's Perspective on Managing the Legal and Ethical Issues, 2 Ind. Health L. Rev. 95, 99 (2005).*

Journal 1991 Considers how the use of in vitro fertilization (IVF) has blurred the distinction between medical practice and research. Argues that medical-professional responsibility standards should be used to curtail the creation of life in vitro. Quotes Opinions 2.10 and 2.14. Comment, *Dangerous Relations: Doctors and Extracorporeal Embryos, The Need for New Limits to Medical Inquiry, 7 J. Contemp. Health L. & Pol'y 307, 309 (1991).*

Journal 1987 Examines various ethical issues surrounding surrogate motherhood, artificial insemination, in vitro fertilization, and embryonic/fetal research. Reports on the positions of four ethics groups: the Warnock Committee of Inquiry Into Human Fertilization and Embryology; the AMA's Council on Ethical and Judicial Affairs; the Ethics Committee of the American Fertility Society; and the Ethics Committee of the American College of Obstetricians and Gynecologists. References Opinions 2.04, 2.05, and 2.13 (1986) [now Opinion 2.14]. Quotes Opinion 2.18. Rosner, Cassell, Friedland, Landolt, Loeb, Numann, Ora, Risemberg, & Sordillo, *Ethical Considerations of Reproductive Technologies, 87 N. Y. State J. Med. 398, 399-400 (1987).*

2.141   Frozen Pre-embryos

The practice of freezing extra pre-embryos harvested during the in vitro fertilization (IVF) process has enhanced the ability of infertile couples to preserve embryos for future implantation. This practice has also posed a number of ethical and legal dilemmas, including questions regarding decision-making authority over the pre-embryos and appropriate uses of pre-embryos.

This country's cultural and legal traditions indicate that the logical persons to exercise control over a frozen pre-embryo are the woman and man who provided the gametes (the ovum and sperm). The gamete providers have a fundamental interest at stake, their potential for procreation. In addition, the gamete providers are the parties most concerned with the interests of a frozen pre-embryo and most likely to protect those interests.

Gamete providers should be able to use the pre-embryos themselves or donate them for use by other parties, but not sell them. In addition, research on pre-embryos should be permitted as long as the pre-embryos are not destined for transfer to a woman for implantation and as long as the research is conducted in accordance with the Council's guidelines on fetal research. Frozen pre-embryos may also be allowed to thaw and deteriorate.

The gamete providers should have an equal say in the use of their pre-embryos and, therefore, the pre-embryos should not be available for use by either provider or changed from their frozen state without the consent of both providers. The man and woman each has contributed half of the pre-embryo's genetic code. In addition, whether a person chooses to become a parent and assume all of the accompanying obligations is a particularly personal and fundamental decision. Even if the individual could be absolved of any parental obligations, he or she may have a strong desire not to have offspring. The absence of a legal duty does not eliminate the moral duty many would feel toward any genetic offspring.

Advance agreements are recommended for deciding the disposition of frozen pre-embryos in the event of divorce or other changes in circumstances. Advance agreements can help ensure that the gamete providers undergo IVF and pre-embryo freezing after a full contemplation of the consequences but should not be mandatory. (I, III, IV, V)

Issued March 1992 based on the report "Frozen Pre-Embryos," adopted December 1989 (*JAMA.* 1990;263:2484-2487). Updated June 1994.

Journal 2006 Discusses the ethical issues surrounding embryonic stem cell research, gamete donation, and embryo adoption. Concludes that conflation of these concepts does not advance solutions in the current climate of abortion politics. Cites Opinion 2.141. Conde, *Embryo Donation: The Government Adopts a Cause*, 13 Wm. & Mary J. Women & L. 273, 288 (2006).

Journal 2005 Examines legal controversies triggered by advances in technology, using in vitro fertilization as an example. Concludes that no single legislative solution is capable of dealing with the many problems associated with changes in technology. Cites Opinions 2.055 and 2.141. Moses, *Understanding Legal Responses to Technological Change: The Example of In Vitro Fertilization*, 6 Minn. J. L. Sci. & Tech. 505, 543, 615 (2005).

Journal 2003 Reviews legal methods for resolving disputes involving disposition of cryopreserved pre-embryos. Concludes that federal legislation is needed to address existing problems. Cites Opinion 2.141. Windsor, *Disposition of Cryopreserved Preembryos After Divorce*, 88 Iowa L. Rev. 1001, 1026 (2003).

Journal 2001 Examines the ethical and legal dilemmas associated with stem cell and fetal tissue research. Discusses current federal law. Concludes that Congress should allow researchers to obtain stem cells from discarded human embryos provided by in vitro fertilization clinics. Cites Opinion 2.141. Casell, *Lengthening the Stem: Allowing Federally Funded Researchers to Derive Human Pluripotent Stem Cells From Embryos*, 34 U. Mich. J. L. Ref. 547, 563 (2001).

Journal 1999 Describes cryopreservation and in vitro fertilization (IVF) procedures. Examines statutory and case law regarding the use of IVF and discusses theories about how frozen preembryos should be discarded. Concludes by suggesting that, in legal disputes, the party opposing implantation ordinarily should prevail. Quotes Opinion 2.141. Fiestal, *A Solomonic Decision: What Will Be the Fate of Frozen Preembryos?* 6 Cardozo Women's L. J. 103, 110 (1999).

Journal 1999 Describes the approaches various courts have taken toward disposition of cryopreserved embryos after dissolution of marriage. Concludes that, while a prior agreement should be binding, various contract defenses may apply where circumstances have substantially changed. References Opinion 2.141. Haut, *Divorce and the Disposition of Frozen Embryos*, 28 Hofstra L. Rev. 493, 519 (1999).

Journal 1998 Addresses the ethical and legal issues regarding storage and disposition of frozen human embryos. Suggests that courts should seek to honor the donors' wishes. Proposes that future legislation should mandate embryo disposition after a certain length of time. Quotes Opinion 2.141. Forster, *The Legal and Ethical Debate Surrounding the Storage and Destruction of Frozen Human Embryos: A Reaction to the Mass Disposal in Britain and the Lack of Law in the United States*, 76 Wash. U. L. Q. 759, 766-67, 770 (1998).

Journal 1998 Discusses legal issues regarding reproductive biotechnology, with emphasis on freezing of eggs and embryos, research involving frozen embryos, and cloning. Argues that legislation should protect society from unacceptable uses of reproductive technology but, at the same time, ensure advancement of technology for the benefit of society. References Opinion 2.141. Godoy, *Where Is Biotechnology Taking the Law? An Overview of Assisted Reproductive Technology, Research on Frozen Embryos and Human Cloning*, 19 J. Juv. L. 357, 363 (1998).

Journal 1990 Considers ways in which the frozen pre-embryo can be legally described and argues that it should not be considered either person or property. Concludes that in vitro fertilization research is valuable to society and proposes research guidelines. References Opinion 2.141. Martin & Lagod, *The Human Preembryo, the Progenitors, and the State: Toward a Dynamic Theory of Status, Rights, and Research Policy*, 5 High Tech. L. J. 257, 304 (1990).

Journal 1990 Considers problems created by frozen pre-embryos that result from in vitro fertilization therapy. Explores problems with disposing of these pre-embryos and how prior agreements between couples have surfaced as a potential solution. References Opinion 2.141. Robertson, *Prior Agreements for Disposition of Frozen Embryos, 51 Ohio St. L. J. 407, 419 (1990).*

2.145 Pre-embryo Splitting

The technique of splitting in vitro fertilized pre-embryos may result in multiple genetically identical siblings.

The procedure of pre-embryo splitting should be available so long as both gamete providers agree. This procedure may greatly increase the chances of conception for an infertile couple or for a couple whose future reproductive capacity will likely be diminished. Pre-embryo splitting also can reduce the number of invasive procedures necessary for egg retrieval and the necessity for hormonal stimulants to generate multiple eggs. The use and disposition of any pre-embryos that are frozen for future use should be consistent with the Council's opinion on frozen pre-embryos (Opinion 2.141, "Frozen Pre-embryos").

The use of frozen pre-embryo identical siblings many years after one child has been born raises new ethical issues. Couples might wait until they can discover the mental and physical characteristics of a child before transferring a genetically identical sibling for implantation, they might sell their frozen pre-embryos based upon the outcome of a genetically identical child, or they might decide to transplant a genetically identical sibling based on the need to harvest the child's tissue.

The Council does not find that these considerations are sufficient to prohibit pre-embryo splitting for the following reasons:

(1) It would take many years to determine the outcome of a child and most families want to complete their childbearing within a shorter time.

(2) The sale of pre-embryos can and should be prohibited.

(3) The small number of couples who might bear identical siblings solely for purposes of harvesting their tissue does not outweigh the benefits which might be derived from pre-embryo splitting. Additionally, it is not evident that a sibling would have negative psychological or emotional consequences from having acted as an organ or tissue donor. Indeed, the child may derive psychological benefits from having saved the life of a sibling.

To the extent possible, discussion of these issues should be had with gamete providers prior to pre-embryo splitting and freezing so as to inform the prospective parents of possible future ethical dilemmas. (I, III, IV, V)

Issued June 1994.

2.146 The previous Opinion 2.146, "Cloing for Biomedical Research," issued December 2003, was replaced by the current Opinion 2.146, "Research With Stem Cells."

2.146 Research With Stem Cells

Human stem cells are widely seen as offering a source of potential treatment for a range of diseases and are thus the subject of much research. Clinical studies have validated the use of adult stem cells in a limited number of therapies, but have yet to confirm the utility of embryonic stem cells.

Physicians who conduct research using stem cells obtained from any source (established tissue, umbilical cord blood, or embryos) must, at a minimum:

(a) adhere to institutional review board (IRB) requirements;

(b) ensure that the research is carried out with appropriate oversight and monitoring;

(c) ensure that the research is carried out with appropriate informed consent. In addition to disclosure of research risks and potential benefits, at minimum, the consent disclosure should address:

(i) for a donor of cells to be used in stem cell research:
(a) the process by which stem cells will be obtained;
(b) what specifically will be done with the stem cells;
(c) whether an immortal cell line will result; and
(d) the primary and anticipated secondary uses of donated embryos and/or derived stem cells, including potential commercial uses.

(ii) for a recipient of stem cells in clinical research:
(a) the types of tissue from which the stem cells derive (eg, established tissue, umbilical cord blood, or embryos); and
(b) unique risks posed by investigational stem cell products (when applicable), such as tumorigenesis, immunological reactions, unpredictable behavior of cells, and unknown long-term health effects.

The professional community as well as the public remain divided about the use of embryonic stem cells for either research or therapeutic purposes. The conflict regarding research with embryonic stem cells centers on the moral status of embryos, a question that divides ethical opinion and that cannot be resolved by medical science. Regardless whether they are obtained from embryos donated by individuals or couples undergoing in vitro fertilization, or from cloned embryos created by somatic cell nuclear transfer (SCNT), use of embryonic stem cells currently requires the destruction of the human embryo from which the stem cells derive.

The pluralism of moral visions that underlies this debate must be respected. Participation in research involving embryonic stem cells requires respect for embryos, research participants, donors, and recipients. Embryonic stem cell research does not violate the ethical standards of the profession. Every physician remains free to decide whether to participate in stem cell research or to use its products. Physicians should continue to be guided by their commitment to the welfare of patients and the advancement of medical science.

Physicians who conduct research using embryonic stem cells should be able to justify greater risks for subjects, and the greater respect due embryos than stem cells from other sources, based on expectations that the research offers substantial promise of contributing significantly to scientific or therapeutic knowledge. (V)

Issued November 2011 based on the report "Amendment to Opinion E-2.146, 'Cloning for Biomedical Research,'" adopted June 2011.

2.147 **Cloning to Produce Children**

Somatic cell nuclear transfer (SCNT) is the process in which the nucleus of a somatic cell of an organism is transferred into an enucleated oocyte. "Cloning to produce children" is the application of SCNT to the creation of a human being that shares all of its nuclear genes with the donor of the human somatic cell.

To clarify the many existing misconceptions about this use of cloning, physicians should help educate the public about the intrinsic limits of cloning to produce children as well as about the current ethical and legal protections that would prevent certain uses of cloned human embryos. These include the following:

(1) Using cloning to produce children as an approach to replicate a person (the donor of the somatic cell) is a concept based on the mistaken notion that one's genotype largely determines one's individuality. A cloned child created via this process would not be identical to the donor of the somatic cell.

(2) Current ethical and legal standards hold that under no circumstances should any use of cloning occur without informed consent from the somatic cell and the oocyte donor(s).

(3) Current ethical and legal standards hold that a child produced from a clone would be entitled to the same rights, freedoms, and protections as every other individual in society. The fact that a human clone's nuclear genes would derive from a single individual rather than two would not change its moral standing.

Physicians have an ethical obligation to consider the harms and benefits of new medical procedures and technologies. Physicians should not participate in cloning to produce children at this time because further investigation and discussion regarding the harms and benefits of this use of cloning are required. Concerns include:

(1) Unknown physical harms introduced by SCNT technology. SCNT has not yet been refined, and its long-term safety has not yet been proven. The risk of producing individuals with genetic anomalies gives rise to an obligation to seek better understanding of—and potential medical therapies for—the unforeseen medical consequences that could stem from cloning to produce children.

(2) Psychosocial harms introduced by cloning, including violations of privacy and autonomy. Cloning to produce children risks limiting, at least psychologically, the seemingly unlimited potential of new human beings and thus creating enormous pressures on the cloned child to live up to expectations based on the life of the somatic cell donor.

(3) The impact of cloning to produce children on familial and societal relations. The family unit may be altered with the introduction of this use of cloning, and more thought is required on a societal level regarding how to construct familial relations.

(4) Potential effects on the gene pool. Like other interventions that can change individuals' reproductive patterns and the resulting genetic characteristics of a population, cloning to produce children has the potential to

be used in a eugenic or discriminatory fashion—practices that are incompatible with the ethical norms of medical practice. Moreover, cloning to produce children could alter irreversibly the gene pool and exacerbate genetic problems that arise from deleterious genetic mutations, resulting in harms to future generations.

Two potentially realistic and possibly appropriate medical uses of cloning to produce children are for assisting individuals or couples to reproduce and for generating tissues when the donor is not harmed or sacrificed. Given the unresolved issues regarding cloning identified above, the medical profession should not undertake cloning to produce children at this time and pursue alternative approaches that raise fewer ethical concerns.

Because SCNT technology is not limited to the United States, physicians should help establish international guidelines governing uses. (V)

Issued December 1999 based on the report "The Ethics of Human Cloning," adopted June 1999. Updated December 2003, based on the report "Cloning for Biomedical Research," adopted June 2003.

Journal 2009 Explores ethical concerns surrounding organ donation from anencephalic infants. Concludes that, by viewing anencephalic infants as having been born into a state of death, an infant's organs may be donated without violating the dead donor rule. Cites Opinion 2.147. References Opinion 2.162. Khan & Lea, *Paging King Solomon: Towards Allowing Organ Donation From Anencephalic Infants*, 6 Ind. Health L. Rev. 17, 38 (2009).

Journal 1999 Discusses arguments against cloning. Points out that, as medical knowledge advances, and physicians can safely undertake this procedure, increasing emphasis will be placed on ethical concerns. Concludes that cloning may benefit infertile couples and single people who want to have children without involving a third party in their procreational activities. References Opinion 2.147. Orentlicher, *Cloning and the Preservation of Family Integrity*, 59 La. L. Rev. 1019, 1022 (1999).

2.15   Opinion 2.15, "Financial Incentives to Living Donors," originally issued June 1984, was replaced by the Opinion 2.15, "Transplantation of Organs From Living Donors," November 2005, which was replaced by the current Opinion 2.15, "Transplantation of Organs From Living Donors," June 2011.

2.15 Transplantation of Organs From Living Donors

Living organ donors are exposed to surgical procedures that pose risks but offer no physical benefits. The medical profession has pursued living donation because the lives and quality of life of patients with end-stage organ failure depend on the availability of transplantable organs and some individuals are willing to donate the needed organs. This practice is consistent with the goals of the profession—treating illness and alleviating suffering—only insofar as the benefits to both donor and recipient outweigh the risks to both.

(1) Because donors are initially healthy and then are exposed to potential harms, they require special safeguards. Accordingly, every donor should be assigned an advocate team that includes a physician. This team is primarily concerned with the well-being of the donor. Though some individuals on the donor advocate team may participate in the care of the recipient, this team ideally should be as independent as possible from those caring for

the recipient. This can help avoid actual or perceived conflicts of interest between donors and recipients.

(a) To determine whether a potential living donor is an appropriate candidate, the advocate team must provide a complete medical evaluation to identify any serious risk to the potential donor's life or health. This includes a psychosocial evaluation of the potential donor to identify disqualifying factors, address specific needs, and explore potential motivations to donate.

(b) Before the potential donor agrees to donate, the advocate team should provide information regarding the donation procedure and its indications, as well as the risks and potential complications to both donor and recipient. Informed consent for donation is distinct from informed consent for the actual surgery to remove the organ.

(i) The potential donor must have decision-making capacity, and the decision to donate must be free from undue pressure. The potential donor must demonstrate adequate understanding of the disclosed information.

(ii) Unemancipated minors and legally incompetent adults ordinarily should not be accepted as living donors because of their inability to fully understand and decide voluntarily. However, in exceptional circumstances, minors with substantial decision-making capability who agree to serve as donors, with the informed consent of their legal guardians, may be considered for donation to recipients with whom they are emotionally connected. Since minors' guardians may be emotionally connected to the organ recipient, when an unemancipated minor agrees to donate, it may be appropriate to seek advice from another adult trusted by the minor or an independent body, such as consultation with an ethics committee, pastoral service, or other counseling resource.

(iii) Potential donors must be informed that they may withdraw from donation at any time before undergoing the operation and that, should this occur, the health care team is committed to protect the potential donor from pressures to reveal the reasons for withdrawal. If the potential donor withdraws, the health care team should report simply that the individual was unsuitable for donation. From the outset, all involved parties must agree that the reasons why any potential donor does not donate will remain confidential for the potential donor's protection. In situations of paired, domino, or chain donation withdrawal must still be permitted. Physicians should make special efforts to present a clear and comprehensive description of the commitment being made by the donor and the implications for other parties to the paired donation during the informed consent process.

(c) Living donation should never be considered if the best medical judgment indicates that transplantation cannot reasonably be expected to yield the intended clinical benefit or achieve agreed-on goals for care for the intended recipient.

(2) Living donors should not receive payment for any of their solid organs. However, donors should be treated fairly; reimbursement for travel, lodging, meals, lost wages, and the medical care associated with donation is ethically appropriate.

(3) The distribution of organs from living donors may take several different forms:

    (a) It is ethically acceptable for donors to designate a recipient, whether a close relative or a known, unrelated recipient.

    (b) Designation of a stranger as the intended recipient is ethical if it produces a net gain of organs in the organ pool without unreasonably disadvantaging others on the waiting list. Variations involve potential donors who respond to public solicitation for organs or who wish to participate in a paired donation or "organ swap" (eg, blood type incompatible donor-recipient pairs Y and Z are recombined to make compatible pairs: donor-Y with recipient-Z and donor-Z with recipient-Y), domino paired donation, and nonsimultaneous extended altruistic donation (also known as chain donation).

    (c) Organs donated by living donors who do not designate a recipient should be allocated according to the algorithm that governs the distribution of deceased donor organs.

(4) Novel variants of living donation call for special attention to protect both donors and recipients:

    (a) Physicians must ensure utmost respect for the privacy and confidentiality of donors and recipients, which may be more difficult when many patients are involved and when donation-transplantation cycles may be extended over time (as in domino or chain donation)

    (b) Physicians should monitor prospective donors and recipients in a proposed nontraditional donation for signs of psychological distress during screening and after the transplant is complete.

    (c) Physicians must protect the donor's right to withdraw in living paired-donations and ensure that the individual is not pressured to donate.

(5) To enhance the safety of living organ donation through better understanding of the harms and benefits associated with living organ donation, physicians should support the development and maintenance of a national database of living donor outcomes, similar to that of deceased donation. (I, V, VII, VIII)

Issued June 2011 based on the report "Amendment to Opinion E-2.15, Amendment to E-2.15, "Transplantation of Organs From Living Donors,'" adopted November 2010.

Journal 2005 Discusses policy issues and moral and ethical dilemmas associated with facial transplant surgery. Concludes that while the government should not stall the progress of biomedical science, facial transplantation practices must be regulated to ensure that progress is consistent with social norms. References Opinion 2.15. Hartman, *Face Value: Challenges of Transplant Technology, 31 Am. J. L. & Med. 7, 25, 31 (2005).*

Journal 2004 Explores the moral and political rationales for current organ acquisition policies. Concludes that, in a secular society, no plausible moral reason exists to ban the sale of organs. Quotes Opinions 2.15 and 2.151. Engelhardt, Jr, *Giving, Selling, and Having Taken: Conflicting Views of Organ Transfer, 1 Ind. Health L. Rev. 29, 33-34 (2004).*

Journal 2004 Examines state laws dealing with a minor's right to consent to medical treatment. Concludes that physicians must be aware of these laws for purposes of compliance, protection against liability, and providing minors the highest level of care. Quotes Opinion 2.015. Vukadinovich, *Minors' Rights to Consent to Treatment: Navigating the Complexity of State Laws*, 37 J. Health L. 667, 689-90 (2004).

Journal 2003 Proposes a moral, communitarian approach to address organ shortages. Concludes the next step should involve a demonstration that the communitarian approach can succeed. Quotes Opinion 2.155. Cites Opinion 2.15. Etzioni, *Organ Donation: A Communitarian Approach*, 13 Kennedy Inst. Ethics J. 1, 3, 4, 16 (March 2003).

Journal 2003 Examines the benefits of paired organ exchanges and proposes a statutory framework for implementation. Concludes this approach supplements the current US organ procurement system without resorting to use of financial incentives. Quotes Opinion 2.15. Morley, *Increasing the Supply of Organs for Transplantation Through Paired Organ Exchanges*, 21 Yale L. & Pol'y Rev. 221, 255 (2003).

Journal 2003 Suggests that financial incentives for organ procurement should be reconsidered. Concludes that the ban on marketing organs should be lifted. References Opinion 2.15. Veatch, *Why Liberals Should Accept Financial Incentives for Organ Procurement*, 13 Kennedy Inst. Ethics J. 19, 34 (March 2003).

Journal 1995 Examines legal and ethical issues surrounding organ transplant procurement practices, with emphasis on a possible commercial system. Concludes that adequate market safeguards need to be developed to protect vulnerable donors and citizens. References Opinions 2.15 and 2.167. Banks, *Legal and Ethical Safeguards: Protection of Society's Most Vulnerable Participants in a Commercialized Organ Transplantation System*, XXI Am. J. Law & Med. 45, 77, 79, 95-96, 103-04 (1995).

2.151 Cadaveric Organ Donation: Encouraging the Study of Motivation

Physicians have an obligation to hold their patients' interests paramount and to support access to medical care (Principles VIII and IX). To discharge these obligations, physicians should participate in efforts to increase organ donation including promotion of voluntary donation. Beyond educational programs, however, physicians should support innovative approaches to encourage organ donation. Such efforts may include encouragement of and, if appropriate, participation in the conduct of ethically designed research studies of financial incentives.

Because the potential benefits and harms of financial incentives for cadaveric organ donation are unknown, physicians have an obligation to study financial incentives. Whether or not they are ethical depends upon the balance of benefits and harms that result from them. Physicians should encourage and support pilot studies, limited to relatively small populations, that investigate the effects of financial incentives for cadaveric organ donation for the purpose of examining and possibly revising current policies in the light of scientific evidence.

Pilot studies of the effects of financial incentives for cadaveric organ donation should be implemented only after certain considerations have been met, including:

(1) Consultation and advice is sought from the population within which the pilot study is to take place.

(2) Objectives and strategies as well as sound scientific design, measurable outcomes, and set time frames are clearly defined in written protocols that are publicly available and approved by appropriate oversight bodies, such as institutional review boards.

(3) Incentives are of moderate value and at the lowest level that can be reasonably expected to increase organ donation.

(4) Payment for an organ from a living donor is not a part of any study.

(5) Financial incentives apply to cadaveric donation only, and must not lead to the purchase of donated organs; the distribution of organs for transplantation should continue to be governed by United Network for Organ Sharing (UNOS), based on ethically appropriate criteria related to medical need. (I, III, V, VII, VIII, IX)

Issued December 2002 based on the report "Cadaveric Organ Donation: Encouraging the Study of Motivation," adopted June 2002 (*Transplantation*. 2003;76(4):748-751).

Journal 2007 Reviews major medical and legal developments in the field of organ transplantation. Concludes that introducing a policy of donor payments would be another major success. References Opinion 2.151. Kaserman, *Fifty Years of Organ Transplants: The Successes and the Failures, 23 Issues L. & Med. 45, 60 (2007).*

Journal 2007 Considers the benefits and risks associated with commodification of organs. Concludes that risks can likely be minimized and that the legal and medical communities should undertake extensive research into the benefits of commodification. References Opinion 2.151. Woan, *Buy Me a Pound of Flesh: China's Sale of Death Row Organs on the Black Market and What Americans Can Learn From It, 47 Santa Clara L. Rev. 413, 439 (2007).*

Journal 2006 Examines federal law governing organ procurement. Suggests that Congress should reconsider its policy banning financial incentives for cadaveric organ donation. References Opinion 2.151. Carlson, *Organ Donation Recovery and Improvement Act: How Congress Missed an Opportunity to Say "Yes" to Financial Incentives for Organ Donation, 23 J. Contemp. Health L. & Pol'y 136, 145 (2006).*

Journal 2006 Examines the problem of organ donor shortage in New York. Concludes that the legislature should establish a financial incentive program of "modest value" to increase the rate of donations. References Opinions 2.151 and 2.16. Flamholz, *A Penny for Your Organs: Revising New York's Policy on Offering Financial Incentives for Organ Donation, 14 J. L. & Pol'y 329, 330, 374 (2006).*

Journal 2004 Explores the moral and political rationales for current organ acquisition policies. Concludes that, in a secular society, no plausible moral reason exists to ban the sale of organs. Quotes Opinions 2.15 and 2.151. Engelhardt, Jr, *Giving, Selling, and Having Taken: Conflicting Views of Organ Transfer, 1 Ind. Health L. Rev. 29, 33-34 (2004).*

Journal 2004 Discusses regulations prohibiting financial incentives for organ donation. Concludes that repealing regulations prohibiting financial incentives for organ donation will lead to the exploitation of the poor. References Opinion 2.151. Hurley, *Cashing in on the Transplant List: An Argument Against Offering Valuable Compensation for the Donation of Organs, 4 J. High Tech. L. 117, 130 (2004).*

2.152 Solicitation of the Public for Directed Donation of Organs for Transplantation

The obligation of physicians to hold their patients' interests paramount and to support access to medical care requires that maximizing the number of medically suitable solid organs for transplantation by ethical means should remain a priority of the medical profession. Donation of organs to specified recipients has been permitted since the beginning of organ transplantation. Although directed donation is permitted under current national policy, solicitation of organs from potential donors who have no preexisting relationship with the recipient is controversial. The following guidelines regarding solicitation of organ donors are offered:

(1) Solicitation of the public for organ donation has unknown effects on the organ supply and on transplant waiting lists. Policies should be based, as far as possible, on facts rather than assumptions, so physicians should support

study of the current system and development of policy based on the results of such studies.

(2) Directed donation policies that produce a net gain of organs in the organ pool and do not unreasonably disadvantage others on the waiting list are ethically acceptable, as long as donors receive no payment beyond reimbursement for travel, lodging, lost wages, and the medical care associated with donation.

(3) The health care team must fully evaluate the medical and psychosocial suitability of all potential donors, regardless of the nature of the relationship between the potential donor and transplant candidate.

A physician should resist pressure to participate in a transplant that he or she believes to be ethically improper and should not pressure others to participate if they refuse on ethical or moral grounds. (VII, VIII, IX)

Issued November 2006 based on the report "Solicitation of the Public for Directed Donation of Organs for Transplantation," adopted June 2006.

2.155   The previous Opinion 2.155, "Mandated Choice and Presumed Consent for Cadaveric Organ Donation," issued June 1994, was replaced by the current Opinion 2.155, "Presumed Consent and Mandated Choice for Organs From Deceased Donors."

2.155 Presumed Consent and Mandated Choice for Organs From Deceased Donors

The supply of organs for transplantation to treat end-stage organ failure is inadequate to meet the clinical need. Therefore, physicians should support the development of policies that will increase the number of organ donors. Two prominent proposals aimed at increasing organ donation would change the approach to consent for deceased donation: mandated choice and presumed consent.

Under a presumed consent model, deceased individuals are presumed to be organ donors unless they indicate their refusal to donate. Such donations would be ethically appropriate only if it could be determined that individuals were aware of the presumption and if effective and easily accessible mechanisms for documenting and honoring refusals to donate were established. Moreover, physicians could proceed with organ procurement only after verifying that there was no documented prior refusal by the decedent and that the family was unaware of any objection to donation by the decedent.

Under a mandated choice model, individuals are required to express their preferences regarding organ donation at the time of performing a state-regulated task. This contrasts with the widespread model of voluntary organ donation under which individuals are afforded an opportunity to indicate their preferences. A mandated choice model would be ethically appropriate only if an individual's choice were made in accordance with the principles of informed consent, which would require a meaningful exchange of information. Physicians could proceed with organ procurement only after verifying that an individual's consent to donation was documented.

It is not known whether implementation of ethically appropriate models of presumed consent or mandated choice for deceased donation would positively or negatively affect the number of organs transplanted. Therefore, physicians should encourage and support properly designed pilot studies, in relatively small populations, that investigate the effects of these policies. Unless there are data that suggest a positive effect on donation, neither presumed consent nor mandated choice for deceased donation should be widely implemented.

In all models, education of individuals to facilitate informed consent is requisite. (I, III, V)

Issued November 2005 based on the report "Presumed Consent for Organ Donation," adopted June 2005.

Journal 2011 Analyzes mandated choice as a method of alleviating the shortage of organs for transplant in the US. Concludes that mandated choice, with appropriate safeguards, is the best option for increasing organ donation in the US. Cites Opinion 2.155. Cotter, *Increasing Consent for Organ Donation: Mandated Choice, Individual Autonomy, and Informed Consent, 21 Health Matrix 599, 606,607 (2011).*

Journal 2007 Argues for a policy allowing tax deductions for expenses associated with organ donation by living donors. Concludes that such a policy would properly compensate donors and reward them for reducing the cost of medical care. References Opinion 2.155. Molen, *Recognizing the Larger Sacrifice: Easing the Burdens Borne by Living Organ Donors Through Federal Tax Deductions, 21 BYU J. Pub. L. 459, 463 (2007).*

Journal 2006 Discusses federal organ procurement policies. Proposes a plan under which the federal government guarantees equal distribution of organs, requires that all citizens act as default donors unless they opt out, and assumes all costs associated with transplantation. Quotes Opinion 2.155. Siegal & Bonnie, *Closing the Organ Gap: A Reciprocity-Based Social Contract Approach, 34 J. L. Med. & Ethics 415, 415 (2006).*

Journal 2006 Examines the organ donation system in the US. Concludes that a mandated choice system should be adopted along with an optimized allocation system. References Opinion 2.155. Spellman, *Encouragement Is Not Enough: The Benefits of Instituting a Mandated Choice Organ Procurement System, 56 Syracuse L. Rev. 353, 371 (2006).*

Journal 2003 Explores the ethical, legal, and clinical implications of non–heart-beating organ donation. Concludes that, if ambiguities are clarified, non–heart-beating organ donation can achieve an ethical good. References Opinions 2.155 and 2.162. Bell, *Non–Heart Beating Organ Donation: Old Procurement Strategy—New Ethical Problems, 29 J. Med. Ethics 176, 181 (2003).*

Journal 2003 Recommends a modified version of mandated choice for organ procurement. Concludes that the modified version recognizes arguments favoring mandated donation while still relying on the importance of individual consent. References Opinion 2.155. Chouhan & Draper, *Modified Mandated Choice for Organ Procurement, 29 J. Med. Ethics 157, 162 (2003).*

Journal 2003 Proposes a moral, communitarian approach to address organ shortages. Concludes the next step should involve a demonstration that the communitarian approach can succeed. Quotes Opinion 2.155. Cites Opinion 2.15. Etzioni, *Organ Donation: A Communitarian Approach, 13 Kennedy Inst. Ethics J. 1, 3, 4, 16 (March 2003).*

Journal 2002 Considers ethical incentives to increase organ donation. Concludes that market-based incentives are unethical. References Opinion 2.155. Delmonico, Arnold, Scheper-Hughes, Siminoff, Kahn, & Youngner, *Ethical Incentives—Not Payment—for Organ Donation, 346 New Eng. J. Med. 2002, 2005 (2002).*

Journal 2001 Explores ways to overcome barriers to organ donation. Clarifies ethical constraints affecting societal efforts to increase the supply of organs. Supports the rights of individuals to make organ donation decisions, but emphasizes the importance of doing so as members of communities—particularly small communities of families. Quotes Opinion 2.155. Childress, *The Failure to Give: Reducing Barriers to Organ Donation, 11 Kennedy Inst. Ethics J. 1, 13, 14 (2001).*

Journal 1997 Explores the current policies on cadaveric organ procurement in the US. Offers improvements to help save lives and end the waste of suitable organs. Discusses pertinent ethical and legal issues. References Opinion 2.155. MacDonald, *Organ Donation: The Time Has Come to Refocus the Ethical Spotlight,* 8 Stan. L. & Pol'y Rev. 177, 179, 185 (1997).

2.157 Organ Donation After Cardiac Death

Given the increasing need for donor organs, protocols for donation after cardiac death (DCD) have been developed. Controlled DCD allows patients who have agreed to be taken off of life support or their surrogate decision makers the opportunity to donate the patients' organs once death has been declared. In these cases, life support is discontinued in or near the operating room so that organs can be removed promptly after death is pronounced. DCD also may be considered from patients who suffer unexpected cardiac death (uncontrolled DCD). It requires that they be cannulated and perfused with cold preservation fluid (in situ preservation) within minutes after death to maintain the viability of organs. Both of these methods may be ethically permissible, with attention to certain safeguards.

(1) Hospital policies should specify important details of the DCD process, such as the required time delay before death can be pronounced after cardiac arrest.

(2) In all instances, it is critical to avoid perceived or actual conflicts of interest in the health care team with respect to caring for the patient versus facilitating organ donation. The health care professionals providing care at the end of life should be distinct from those participating on the transplant team. No member of the transplant team may have any role in the decision to withdraw life support or in the process leading to pronouncement of death.

(3) Clear clinical criteria should be in place to ensure that only appropriate candidates, whose organs are reasonably likely to be suitable for transplantation, are considered eligible to donate organs under these protocols.

(4) Palliative care for DCD candidates should continue after removal of life support until death is declared.

(5) In controlled DCD, the decision to withdraw life support should be made by the patient or the patient's surrogate decision maker before any mention of organ donation (unless the patient or surrogate spontaneously broaches the subject). This is meant to ensure that withdrawal of life support is not influenced by the prospect of organ donation.

The informed consent for controlled DCD should include specific discussion of premortem interventions aimed at organ preservation, to improve the opportunity for successful transplantation, rather than to benefit the patient. Interventions that are likely to hasten death must not be used.

(6) In cases of uncontrolled DCD, prior consent of the decedent or consent of the decedent's surrogate decision maker is ethically required. Perfusion without consent to organ donation violates requirements of informed consent for medical procedures and is not permissible. (I, III, V)

Issued June 1996 based on the reports "Ethical Issues in the Procurement of Organs Following Cardiac Death: The Pittsburgh Protocol" and "Ethical Issues in Organ Procurement Following Cardiac Death: In Situ Preservation of Cadaveric Organs," adopted December 1994.

Updated November 2005 based on the report "Organ Procurement Following Cardiac Death, *Amendment*," adopted June 2005.

Journal 2010 Argues that a precise definition of death is needed to counteract the focus on reducing medical costs and increasing organ supplies for transplantations. Concludes that allowing dying patients more autonomy to determine conditions for organ donation will foster an atmosphere of trust in which more people will be willing to donate earlier in the dying process. Quotes Opinion 2.157. Cites Opinion 10.01. Fry-Revere, Ray, & Reher, *Death: A New Legal Perspective, 27 J. Contemp. Health L. & Pol'y 1, 11, 50, 53 (2010).*

Journal 2008 Argues preservation of individuals who die of uncontrolled cardiac death is authorized by the Uniform Anatomical Gift Act and does not violate the rights of family members. Concludes that organ donor population should be expanded to include individuals who die uncontrolled cardiac deaths to increase the number of organs available for transplant. Cites Opinions 2.157 and 8.181. Bonnie, Wright, & Dineen, *Legal Authority to Preserve Organs in Cases of Uncontrolled Cardiac Death: Preserving Family Choice, 36 J. L. Med. & Ethics 741, 743 (2008).*

2.16   Organ Transplantation Guidelines

The following statement is offered for guidance of physicians as they seek to maintain the highest level of ethical conduct in the transplanting of human organs.

(1) In all professional relationships between a physician and a patient, the physician's primary concern must be the health of the patient. The physician owes the patient primary allegiance. This concern and allegiance must be preserved in all medical procedures, including those which involve the transplantation of an organ from one person to another where both donor and recipient are patients. Care must, therefore, be taken to protect the rights of both the donor and the recipient, and no physician may assume a responsibility in organ transplantation unless the rights of both donor and recipient are equally protected. A prospective organ transplant offers no justification for a relaxation of the usual standard of medical care for the potential donor.

(2) When a vital, single organ is to be transplanted, the death of the donor shall have been determined by at least one physician other than the recipient's physician. Death shall be determined by the clinical judgment of the physician, who should rely on currently accepted and available scientific tests.

(3) Full discussion of the proposed procedure with the donor and the recipient or their responsible relatives or representatives is mandatory. The physician should ensure that consent to the procedure is fully informed and voluntary, in accordance with the Council's guidelines on informed consent. The physician's interest in advancing scientific knowledge must always be secondary to his or her concern for the patient.

(4) Transplant procedures of body organs should be undertaken (a) only by physicians who possess special medical knowledge and technical competence developed through special training, study, and laboratory experience and practice, and (b) in medical institutions with facilities adequate to protect the health and well-being of the parties to the procedure.

(5) Recipients of organs for transplantation should be determined in accordance with the Council's guidelines on the allocation of limited medical resources.

(6) Organs should be considered a national, rather than a local or regional, resource. Geographical priorities in the allocation of organs should be prohibited except when transportation of organs would threaten their suitability for transplantation.

(7) Patients should not be placed on the waiting lists of multiple local transplant centers, but rather on a single waiting list for each type of organ.
(I, III, V)

Issued prior to April 1977. Updated June 1994 based on the report "Ethical Considerations in the Allocation of Organs and Other Scarce Medical Resources Among Patients," adopted June 1993.

Journal 2006 Examines the problem of organ donor shortage in New York. Concludes that the legislature should establish a financial incentive program of "modest value" to increase the rate of donations. References Opinions 2.151 and 2.16. Flamholz, *A Penny for Your Organs: Revising New York's Policy on Offering Financial Incentives for Organ Donation*, 14 J. L. & Pol'y 329, 330, 374 (2006).

Journal 2003 Considers the cause of persistent shortages of vaccines and other critical drugs. Concludes that government should take specific steps to encourage pharmaceutical manufacturers to supply these essential products. References Opinion 2.16. Noah, *Triage in the Nation's Medicine Cabinet: The Puzzling Scarcity of Vaccines and Other Drugs*, 54 S. C. L. Rev. 741, 755 (2003).

Journal 2003 Provides a moral and legal framework for considering the possibility of progress in managing technology applicable to organ transplantation. Concludes that progress in increasing the supply of organs will require an evolution in moral thinking. Quotes Opinion 2.16. Shapiro, *On the Possibility of "Progress" in Managing Biomedical Technologies: Markets, Lotteries, and Rational Moral Standards in Organ Transplantation*, 31 Cap. U. L. Rev. 13, 29 (2003).

Journal 2002 Provides ethical arguments in favor of transplantation in HIV-infected patients. Concludes that preventing such transplants is unethical and discriminatory. References Opinions 2.16 and 9.131. Halpern, Ubel, & Caplan, *Solid-Organ Transplantation in HIV-Infected Patients*, 347 New Eng. J. Med. 284, 287 (2002).

Journal 2000 Examines the criteria for organ transplantation. Explores the use of cognitive ability as an exclusion criterion for organ transplantation in children. Concludes that other useful neurologic criteria can be established to inform equitable allocation decisions. References Opinion 2.16. Orr, Johnston, Ashwal, & Bailey, *Should Children With Severe Cognitive Impairment Receive Solid Organ Transplants?* 11 J. Clinical Ethics 219, 222-23, 228 (2000).

Journal 1999 Examines the new federal rule mandating broader organ allocation. Raises various constitutional questions, particularly with respect to state laws regulating allocation of organs. Suggests that Congress needs to develop clearer guidelines in this area. Quotes Opinion 2.16. Chen, *Organ Allocation and the States: Can the States Restrict Broader Organ Sharing?* 49 Duke L. J. 261, 273 (1999).

Journal 1999 Attributes distrust and dissatisfaction with managed care organizations to individualism and cynicism in society. Argues that proposed reforms will not solve society's problems with managed care organizations. Recommends an alternative health care system that would strike a balance between considerations of patient autonomy and cost containment. References Opinion 2.16. Harris, *The Regulation of Managed Care: Conquering Individualism and Cynicism in America*, 6 Va. J. Soc. Pol'y. & L. 315, 329 (1999).

Journal 1999 Discusses the need for physicians to advocate on behalf of patients' rights in the context of health care delivery. Evaluates the nature and scope of the physician's role as advocate, noting that physicians cannot be expected to engage in attorney-like advocacy. Quotes Principles IV and VI, Fundamental Elements (2), (4), and (6) [now Opinion 10.01], Patient Responsibilities 5 [now Opinion 10.02], and Opinions 2.03, 2.07, 2.09, 2.16, 2.19, 3.06, 4.01, 4.04, 6.01, 7.02, 8.02, 8.03, 8.13, 8.132, 9.06, 9.07, and 9.131. Cites Opinions 5.05, 5.09, 7.01, 8.135, and 9.02. Sage, *Physicians as Advocates*, 35 Hous. L. Rev. 1529, 1537, 1541, 1542, 1552-53, 1554, 1556, 1557, 1559, 1561-62, 1564, 1571, 1574, 1576, 1580 (1999).

Journal 1987 Discusses the issue of the right of the individual to consent to organ removal and then examines the doctrine of informed consent as it is applied in the context of live organ donation. Evaluates the extent to which removal of nonregenerative organs disrupts the basis for application of the traditional informed consent model with special attention to children and incompetent patients. Quotes Opinion 2.15 (1986) [now Opinion 2.16]. Adams, *Live Organ Donors and Informed Consent: A Difficult Minuet, 8 J. Legal Med. 555, 560-61 (1987).*

2.161 Medical Applications of Fetal Tissue Transplantation

The principal ethical concern in the use of human fetal tissue for transplantation is the degree to which the decision to have an abortion might be influenced by the decision to donate the fetal tissue. In the application of fetal tissue transplantation the following safeguards should apply: (1) The Council on Ethical and Judicial Affairs' guidelines on clinical investigation and organ transplantation are followed, as they pertain to the recipient of the fetal tissue transplant (see Opinion 2.07, "Clinical Investigation," and Opinion 2.16, "Organ Transplantation Guidelines"); (2) a final decision regarding abortion is made before initiating a discussion of the transplantation use of fetal tissue; (3) decisions regarding the technique used to induce abortion, as well as the timing of the abortion in relation to the gestational age of the fetus, are based on concern for the safety of the pregnant woman; (4) fetal tissue is not provided in exchange for financial remuneration above that which is necessary to cover reasonable expenses; (5) the recipient of the tissue is not designated by the donor; (6) health care personnel involved in the termination of a particular pregnancy do not participate in or receive any benefit from the transplantation of tissue from the abortus of the same pregnancy; and (7) informed consent on behalf of both the donor and the recipient is obtained in accordance with applicable law. (I, IV, V)

Issued March 1992 based on the report "Medical Applications of Fetal Tissue Transplantation," adopted June 1989 (JAMA. 1990;263:565-570). Updated June 1996.

Journal 2002 Observes that changes in the health professions challenge certain assumptions about professional ethics. Concludes that these long-standing assumptions must be re-examined. Cites Opinion 2.161. References Opinion 8.13. Kelley, *The Meanings of Professional Life: Teaching Across the Health Professions, 27 J. Med. & Phil. 475, 485, 490, 491 (2002).*

Journal 1990 Presents an update on current medical research regarding Parkinson disease. Discusses the relevance of fetal tissue transplantation to this research. References Opinion 2.161. Joynt, *Neurology, 263 JAMA 2660 (1990).*

2.162 Anencephalic Neonates as Organ Donors

Anencephaly is a congenital absence of major portion of the brain, skull, and scalp. Anencephalic neonates are thought to be unique from other brain-damaged beings because of a lack of past consciousness with no potential for future consciousness.

Physicians may provide anencephalic neonates with ventilator assistance and other medical therapies that are necessary to sustain organ perfusion and viability until such time as a determination of death can be made in accordance with accepted medical standards, relevant law, and regional organ procurement organization policy. Retrieval and transplantation of the organs of anencephalic infants are ethically permissible only after such determination of death is made, and only in accordance with the Council's guidelines for transplantation. (I, III, V)

Issued March 1992 based on the report "Anencephalic Infants as Organ Donors," adopted December 1988. Updated June 1994; updated December 1994 based on the report "The Use of Anencephalic Neonates as Organ Donors," adopted December 1994 (*JAMA.* 1995;273:1614-1618); and updated June 1996 based on the report "Anencephalic Infants as Organ Donors— Reconsideration," adopted December 1995.

Journal 2009 Explores ethical concerns surrounding organ donation from anencephalic infants. Concludes that, by viewing anencephalic infants as having been born into a state of death, an infant's organs may be donated without violating the dead donor rule. Cites Opinion 2.147. References Opinion 2.162. Khan & Lea, *Paging King Solomon: Towards Allowing Organ Donation From Anencephalic Infants, 6 Ind. Health L. Rev. 17, 38 (2009).*

Journal 2007 Explores the idea of "legal personhood" in the context of scientific advancement. Concludes that this concept is still developing and suggests that a creative approach to this area of jurisprudence is required. Cites Opinion 2.162 and Opinion 2.162 (1994). Berg, *Of Elephants and Embryos: A Proposed Framework for Legal Personhood, 59 Hastings L. J. 369, 377-78 (2007).*

Journal 2007 Argues that death for potential organ donors should not be defined as brain death. Concludes that the current definition is likely to remain the same until new technology makes transplants from animals possible. References Opinion 2.162. Truog, *Brain Death—Too Flawed to Endure, Too Ingrained to Abandon, 35 J. L. Med. & Ethics 273, 280 (2007).*

Journal 2003 Explores the ethical, legal, and clinical implications of non–heart-beating organ donation. Concludes that, if ambiguities are clarified, non–heart-beating organ donation can achieve an ethical good. References Opinions 2.155 and 2.162. Bell, *Non–Heart Beating Organ Donation: Old Procurement Strategy—New Ethical Problems, 29 J. Med. Ethics 176, 181 (2003).*

Journal 2003 Discusses how legal norms can be challenged by advances in medical knowledge. Concludes that sources beyond the law should be considered to prevent untoward legal outcomes. References Opinion 2.162. Mayo, *Sex, Marriage, Medicine, and Law: "What Hope of Harmony?" 42 Washburn L. J. 269, 271 (2003).*

Journal 1999 Discusses legal, medical, social, and ethical issues regarding organ donation by anencephalic infants. Points out the dangers surrounding anencephalic organ donation versus parents' needs for good to come out of the lives of their anencephalic children. References Opinion 2.162. Bard, *The Diagnosis Is Anencephaly and the Parents Ask About Organ Donation: Now What? A Guide for Hospital Counsel and Ethics Committees, 21 W. New Eng. L. Rev. 49, 62 (1999).*

Journal 1999 Discusses the Uniform Declaration of Death Act and the dead-donor rule. Provides ethical justifications for sustaining current policies on non–heart-beating organ donation. Cites Opinions 2.06 and 2.162. DuBois, *Non–Heart-Beating Organ Donation: A Defense of the Required Determination of Death, 27 J. Law Med. & Ethics 126, 128 (1999).*

Journal 1999 Explains that shortages in available organs have prompted a movement that favors modifying the dead-donor rule. Discusses different proposals to amend the dead-donor rule. Suggests that even the slightest modification of the rule will prompt strong opposition. References Opinion 2.162. Robertson, *The Dead Donor Rule, 29 Hastings Center Rep. 6, 13 (Nov./ Dec. 1999).*

Journal 1999 Discusses national and international legislative proposals addressing human cloning. Considers human cloning for reproductive and nonreproductive reasons. Undertakes legal analysis and concludes that human cloning should not be banned completely. Cites Opinion 2.162. Smith, *Ignorance Is Not Bliss: Why a Ban on Human Cloning Is Unacceptable, 9 Health Matrix. 311, 330, 331 (1999).*

Journal 1998 Examines American and British views on the brain death test and advance directives. Points out that the brain death test has been criticized in cases where patients woke up after being in a coma for long periods of time. Argues that better utilization of advance directives may dissipate arguments for euthanasia. References Opinion 2.162. Trew, *Regulating Life and Death: The Modification and Commodification of Nature, 29 U. Tol. L. Rev. 271, 292 (1998).*

Journal 1996 Explores courses of treatment for infants born with hypoplastic left heart syndrome. Discusses the various treatment options available to infants and their frequency. Notes the controversy surrounding the AMA's opinion on anencephalic infants as organ donors. References Opinion 2.162 [subsequently amended]. Caplan, Cooper, Garcia-Prats, & Brody,

Diffusion of Innovative Approaches to Managing Hypoplastic Left Heart Syndrome, 150 Arch. Pediatr. Adolesc. Med. 487, 490 (1996).

Journal 1996 Describes the impact of federal laws on medical decisions for anencephalic infants. Discusses selective nontreatment of such infants and the debate regarding availability of their organs for transplantation. Quotes Opinions 2.162 (1994) [subsequently amended] and 2.17. Crossley, *Infants With Anencephaly, the ADA, and the Child Abuse Amendments, 11 Issues in Law & Med. 379, 385, 409 (1996).*

Journal 1996 Proposes an alternative method of capital punishment to allow for organ donation by executed prisoners. Provides justifications for this proposal. Concludes that physicians should be able to ethically participate in this process. Quotes Principle VII. Cites Opinion 2.06. References Opinion 2.162 (1994) [subsequently amended]. Patton, *A Call for Common Sense: Organ Donation and the Executed Prisoner, 3 Va. J. Soc. Pol'y & L. 387, 404, 405, 407-10 (1996).*

Journal 1996 Examines the recent trend in health care laws and ethics to focus on the alleviation of suffering. Expresses concern that such a focus may result in the valuation of one life over another. Emphasizes the need to evaluate multiple, diverse responses to suffering. Quotes Principle VI. References Opinion 2.162. Shepherd, *Sophie's Choices: Medical and Legal Responses to Suffering, 72 Notre Dame L. Rev. 103, 106, 133 (1996).*

Journal 1994 Criticizes both the White House's proposed National Bioethics Advisory Commission and certain purely private ethical advisory bodies. Proposes that an appropriately organized new federal advisory body could provide essential guidance in developing public bioethical policies, particularly if the meaningful input of ethics scholars at universities, ethics centers, and other private organizations and public commissions were sought. Cites Opinion 2.162. Capron, *Ethics: Public and Private, 24 Hastings Center Rep. 26, 27 (November/ December 1994).*

2.165   The previous Opinion 2.165, "Fetal Umbilical Cord Blood," issued June 1994, was replaced by the current Opinion 2.165, "Umbilical Cord Blood Banking."

2.165 Umbilical Cord Blood Banking

Umbilical cord blood stem cells are useful for some therapeutic purposes. Physicians providing obstetrical care should be prepared to inform pregnant women of the various options regarding cord blood donation or storage and the potential uses of donated samples. Collection procedures must not interfere with standard delivery practices and the safety of a newborn or the mother.

Informed consent for the collection of umbilical cord blood stem cells should be obtained, when feasible, before the onset of labor. Physicians' ties to public and private cord blood banks must be disclosed during the informed consent process. Physicians shall not accept financial or other inducements for providing samples to cord blood banks.

The utility of umbilical cord blood stem cells is greater when the donation is to a public rather than private bank. Therefore, physicians should encourage women who wish to donate cord blood to donate to a public bank if one is available. Doing so will result in greater availability of stem cells to patients from minority populations.

Private banking should be considered in the unusual circumstance when there exists a family predisposition to a condition in which umbilical cord stem cells are therapeutically indicated. However, because of its cost, limited likelihood of use, and inaccessibility to others, private banking should not be recommended to low-risk families.

Because safety and effectiveness of various methods of cord blood collection and use continue to evolve, physicians should monitor the results of ongoing research. (I, V)

Issued June 2008 based on the report "Umbilical Cord Blood Banking," adopted November 2007.

Journal 2011 Discusses the physician's role in educating and counseling patients on the donation and storage of umbilical cord blood. Concludes physicians should encourage patients to donate their newborn's umbilical cord blood to public banks or use the Related Donor Cord Blood Program to bank blood for the newborn's sibling, but cord blood should not be banked for an unidentified possible future use. Cites Opinion 2.165. Martin, Kurtzberg, & Hesse, *Umbilical Cord Blood: A Guide for Primary Care Physicians*, 84 Am. Fam. Physician 661, 661 (2011).

2.169 The Ethical Implications of Xenotransplantation

Xenotransplantation includes any procedure that involves the transplantation, implantation, or infusion into a human recipient of either (a) live cells, tissues, or organs from a nonhuman animal source or (b) human body fluids, cells, tissues or organs that have had ex vivo contact with live nonhuman animal cells, tissues, or organs. Although xenotransplantation offers a potential source of tissue and organs for medical procedures, research in this area may uncover physical and psychological conditions that require medical attention. As such, physicians need to be involved in developing and implementing guidelines for continued research. Therefore, the following guidelines are offered for the medical and scientific communities:

(1) Physicians should encourage education and public discussion of xenotransplantation because of the potential unique risks such procedures pose to individual patients and the public.

(2) The medical and scientific communities should support oversight for the development of clinical trial protocols and of ongoing xenotransplantation research.

(3) Given the uncertain risk xenotransplantation poses to society, participants in early clinical trials may have to agree to (a) postoperative measures such as lifelong surveillance, disclosure of sexual contacts, autopsy; and (b) a waiver of the traditional right to withdraw from a clinical trial until the risk of late xenozoonoses is reasonably known not to exist. These requirements may continue even if the transplanted tissue is rejected or removed. The informed consent process should include a discussion of the above issues as well as potential risks to third parties and psychological concerns associated with receiving an organ or tissue graft from an animal. Careful attention must be paid to both the content of the consent disclosure and the manner in which consent is obtained.

(4) It would be ethical to include children and incompetent adults in xenotransplantation research protocols only when the patients are terminally ill and alternative treatments are not available.

(5) Allocation protocols must be fair and in accordance with Opinion 2.03, "Allocation of Limited Medical Resources," which recommends that decisions regarding the allocation of medical resources among patients be based only on ethically appropriate criteria relating to medical need. These criteria include, but are not limited to, the likelihood of benefit, the urgency

of need, the change in quality of life, the duration of benefit, and, in some cases, the amount of resources required for treatment.

(6) Sponsors of xenotransplantation research should assure that adequate funding exists for lifelong surveillance and treatment of complications arising from xenotransplantation procedures on research subjects.

(7) At a minimum, all ongoing research should adhere to the Public Health Service Guideline on Infectious Disease Issues in Xenotransplantation, FDA guidelines relating to xenotransplantation, Opinion 2.07 "Clinical Investigation," and any additional precautionary measures believed to minimize potential risks to the public or to patients. It is inappropriate to participate in xenograft procedures outside federal guidelines.

(8) All xenotransplantation research should continue to promote high standards of care and humane treatment of all animals used in research (H-460.979, "Use of Animals in Research") and to apply these standards to the care and treatment of animals used as sources of transplantation material. (IV, VII)

Issued June 2001 based on the report "The Ethical Implications of Xenotransplantation," adopted December 2000.

2.17 Quality of Life

In the making of decisions for the treatment of seriously disabled newborns or of other persons who are severely disabled by injury or illness, the primary consideration should be what is best for the individual patient and not the avoidance of a burden to the family or to society. Quality of life, as defined by the patient's interests and values, is a factor to be considered in determining what is best for the individual. It is permissible to consider quality of life when deciding about life-sustaining treatment in accordance with Opinions 2.20, "Withholding or Withdrawing Life-Sustaining Medical Treatment," 2.215, "Treatment Decisions for Seriously Ill Newborns," and 2.22, "Do-Not-Resuscitate Orders." (I, III, IV)

Issued March 1981. Updated June 1994.

N.J. Super. 1983 Guardian of elderly nursing home patient suffering from severe organic brain syndrome sought to remove nasogastric tube from patient. Trial court granted guardian's petition, and patient's guardian ad litem appealed. Appellate court reversed, in part based upon Opinions 2.11 (1981) and 5.17 (1979) [now Opinions 2.17 and 2.20], and held that it is improper and would violate medical ethics to allow dehydration and starvation in a noncomatose, non–brain-dead patient not facing imminent death, not maintained by any life-support machine, and not able to speak for herself. *In re Conroy, 190 N.J. Super. 453, 464 A.2d 303, 313-15, rev'd, 98 N.J. 321, 486 A.2d 1209 (1985).*

Journal 2010 Discusses futility disputes where a patient's surrogate wishes to prolong treatment that the physician deems medically ineffective, and the current lack of legal remedies to resolve them. Concludes that states need to establish fair, impartial, and patient-centered methods of resolving futility disputes including independent medical boards that would operate under procedural and substantive regulations. Quotes Opinions 2.02 and 2.035. References Opinions 2.17 and 2.20. Bassel, *Order at the End of Life: Establishing a Clear and Fair Mechanism for the Resolution of Futility Disputes, 63 Vand. L. Rev. 491, 494, 523 (2010).*

Journal 2009 Examines therapeutic uses of cannabis and the legal and social controversies surrounding its legalization. Concludes changes in the regulation of medical cannabis are necessary to better care for patients and better utilize resources that are currently directed toward the war on drugs. Quotes Principle VIII and Opinion 2.17. DiFonzo, *The End of the Red Queen's Race: Medical Marijuana in the New Century*, 27 Quinnipiac L. Rev. 673, 736, 737 (2009).

Journal 2006 Examines the public reaction to the Terri Schiavo case. Concludes that public fears were misplaced and that all persons benefited from the decision. Quotes Opinions 2.03, 2.035, and 2.17. Cites Opinion 2.22. Cerminara, *Musings on the Need to Convince Some People With Disabilities That End-of-Life Decision-Making Advocates Are Not Out to Get Them*, 37 Loy. U. Chi. L. J. 343, 347 (2006).

Journal 2004 Analyzes use of medical marijuana within the framework of the physician-patient relationship. Concludes that permitting the use of medical marijuana in state-regulated programs may stop terminally ill patients from obtaining or growing it illegally. Quotes Opinion 2.17. McCarthy, *Conversations About Medical Marijuana Between Physicians and Their Patients*, 25 J. Legal Med. 333, 343 (2004).

Journal 2001 Observes that many aspects of managed care have increased the tensions between patients and their health care providers. Notes that patient dissatisfaction is on the rise for other reasons as well. Concludes that Congress should take a comprehensive legislative approach in addressing these issues. Quotes Opinion 2.17. Cites Opinion 2.035. References Opinions 2.037 and 2.22. Sanematsu, *Taking a Broader View of Treatment Disputes Beyond Managed Care: Are Recent Legislative Efforts the Cure?* 48 UCLA L. Rev. 1245, 1258, 1284 (2001).

Journal 1999 Advocates on behalf of allowing physicians to legally prescribe marijuana in certain medical situations. Discusses use of marijuana to slow the process of severe weight loss among AIDS patients. Argues in favor of reclassifying marijuana from a Schedule I drug to a Schedule II drug, thus allowing lawful prescription use. Cites Opinion 2.17. Wolfson, *A Quality of Mercy: The Struggle of the AIDS-Afflicted to Use Marijuana as Medicine*, 22 T. Jefferson L. Rev. 1, 24 (1999).

Journal 1999 Discusses the decision in *Conant v. McCaffrey*, which precluded the government from prosecuting physicians who recommended marijuana to patients for medical use. Examines the ramifications of removing physician judgment from medical decisions. Argues that the federal government should retract its restriction on the medical prescription and use of marijuana. Cites Opinion 2.17. Dixon, *Conant v. McCaffrey: Physicians, Marijuana, and the First Amendment*, 70 U. Colo. L. Rev. 975, 977 (1999).

Journal 1997 Considers percutaneous endoscopic gastrostomy tubes and the lack of standards for their placement. Discusses the medical and ethical problems involved, and creates a method for reconciling them. Recommends that patients in a persistent vegetative state not undergo the procedure. References Opinion 2.17. Rabeneck, McCullough, & Wray, *Ethically Justified, Clinically Comprehensive Guidelines for Percutaneous Endoscopic Gastrostomy Tube Placement*, 349 Lancet 496, 497, 498 (1997).

Journal 1996 Explores decision-making standards employed in the removal of medical treatment from incompetent patients. Suggests substituted judgment and best interests standards be replaced by a standard that focuses on patient dignity. Concludes that treatment should be removed when empirical evidence suggests a majority of individuals would want it removed. Cites Opinion 2.16 (1986) [now Opinion 2.17]. Cantor, *Discarding Substituted Judgment and Best Interests: Toward a Constructive Preference Standard for Dying, Previously Competent Patients Without Advance Instructions*, 48 Rutgers L. Rev. 1193, 1234, 1247 (1996).

Journal 1996 Examines the medical use of marijuana in a legal and ethical context. Posits that legal prohibitions against medical use of marijuana infringe upon patient autonomy and the physician-patient relationship. Concludes that societal laws should be modified to allow for regulated medical use of marijuana. Quotes Opinion 2.17. Comment, *Medical Use of Marijuana: Legal and Ethical Conflicts in the Patient-Physician Relationship*, 30 U. Rich. L. Rev. 249, 268-69 (1996).

Journal 1996 Describes the impact of federal laws on medical decisions for anencephalic infants. Discusses selective nontreatment of such infants and the debate regarding availability of their organs for transplantation. Quotes Opinions 2.162 (1994) [subsequently amended] and 2.17. Crossley, *Infants With Anencephaly, the ADA, and the Child Abuse Amendments*, 11 Issues in Law & Med. 379, 385, 409 (1996).

Journal 1994 Considers how greater patient autonomy has led to situations in which medical care may be viewed as futile. Suggests that the law has intruded too far into this area of medicine. Quotes Opinion 2.035. Cites Opinions 2.03, 2.095, 2.17, 2.19, 2.20, and 2.22. Cultice, *Medical Futility: When Is Enough, Enough? 27 J. Health & Hosp. Law 225, 230, 256 (1994).*

Journal 1993 Discusses the problem of physicians withholding needed medical treatment from HIV-infected infants. Concludes that current law should be expanded to eliminate this discrimination. Quotes Opinions 2.09, 2.17, 2.20, 2.22, 4.04, and 8.03. Crossley, *Of Diagnoses and Discrimination: Discriminatory Nontreatment of Infants With HIV Infection, 93 Columbia L. Rev. 1581, 1620, 1621 (1993).*

Journal 1993 Argues that society should not permit euthanasia because of lack of protection against potential abuses. Recommends that health care providers be taught to treat pain and more effectively care for dying patients, rather than to affirmatively end life. Quotes Opinions 2.17 and 2.20. Dickey, *Euthanasia: A Concept Whose Time Has Come? 8 Issues in Law & Med. 521, 523, 524 (1993).*

Journal 1992 Suggests that triage and cost-benefit analysis are the most effective means to evaluate issues associated with allocating scarce medical resources to disabled infants. Concludes both that selective treatment can never be considered murder and that governmental intrusion in this area should be minimal. Quotes Opinions 2.10 (1982) [now Opinion 2.17] and 2.18 (1986) [now Opinion 2.20]. Smith, *Murder, She Wrote or Was It Merely Selective Nontreatment? 8 J. Contemp. Health L. & Pol'y 49, 53 (1992).*

Journal 1990 Questions the value of medical treatment that is futile or may prolong suffering. Proposes that physicians be permitted to write do-not-resuscitate orders, in certain cases, without the consent of the family. Quotes Opinion 2.17. Hackler & Hiller, *Family Consent to Orders Not to Resuscitate: Reconsidering Hospital Policy, 264 JAMA 1281, 1282 (1990).*

Journal 1989 Examines the federal Baby Doe rule, and its implementing regulations, which require treatment of disabled infants in all but the most obviously hopeless cases. Concludes that the rule is insensitive to the complexities of the moral issue, and that state constitutions may prohibit local legislative adoption of the federal requirements. Quotes Opinion 2.14 (1984) [now Opinion 2.17]. Newman, *Baby Doe, Congress and the States: Challenging the Federal Treatment Standard for Impaired Infants, XV Am. J. Law and Med. 1, 42, 47 (1989).*

Journal 1986 Discusses the fact that the legal system has granted substantial professional autonomy to physicians. As a result, medical professionals have exerted dominance over individual health care decisions, particularly in the context of infanticide, or withholding of treatment from severely handicapped infants. Quotes Opinion 2.10 (1982) [now Opinion 2.17]. Malone, *Medical Authority and Infanticide, 1 J. Law & Health 77, 94, 96 (1985-86).*

Journal 1985 Discusses the constitutional rights of newborns with birth defects, noting that they are persons within the meaning of the Fourteenth Amendment. Observes that the fundamental right to life applies equally to healthy newborns as well as newborns with birth defects and concludes that the newborn's future quality of life with a disability should not be a factor in assessing whether medical treatment is in the child's best interest. Quotes from Opinion 2.10 (1982) [now Opinion 2.17]. Comment, *Withholding Life-saving Treatment From Defective Newborns: An Equal Protection Analysis, 29 St. Louis Univ. L. J. 853, 854 (1985).*

Journal 1982 From a legal viewpoint, focuses on the effect of abortion decisions on nontreatment of defective neonates issues as well as decisions that directly address the nontreatment issue. Also provides general discussion of the wide range of moral attitudes expressed by physicians on withholding treatment, the meaning of the terms ordinary and extraordinary care, and the question of who should bear the responsibility for deciding to treat or not to treat defective neonates. Quotes Opinion 2.10 (1981) [now Opinion 2.17]. Taub, *Withholding Treatment From Defective Newborns, 10 Law Med. & Health Care 4, 8 (Feb. 1982).*

Journal 1981 Discusses a Danville, Illinois, case in which the Illinois Department of Children and Family Services successfully opposed the decision of the physician and parents not to feed newborn Siamese twins. Focuses on both moral and legal aspects of nontreatment decisions, and discusses the common, yet controversial nature of decisions not to treat, categorization of birth defects for purposes of moral decision-making, the importance of medical and social information in nontreatment decisions, the legal duty to treat such children, and substantive and procedural criteria for nontreatment decisions. Quotes Opinion 2.10 (1981) [now Opinion 2.17]. Robertson, *Dilemma in Danville, 11 Hastings Center Rep. 5, 7 (Oct. 1981).*

2.18 Surrogate Mothers

"Surrogate" motherhood involves the artificial insemination of a woman who agrees, usually in return for payment, to give the resulting child to the child's father by surrendering her parental rights. Often, the father's infertile wife becomes the child's adoptive mother. The woman bearing the child is in most cases genetically related to the child, though gestational surrogacy (in which the ovum is provided by the father's infertile wife or other donor) is possible as well.

Ethical, social, and legal problems may arise in surrogacy arrangements. Surrogate motherhood may commodify children and women's reproductive capacities, exploit poor women whose decision to participate may not be wholly voluntary, and improperly discourage or interfere with the formation of a natural maternal-fetal or maternal-child bond. Psychological impairment may occur in a woman who deliberately conceives with the intention of bearing a child which she will give up. In addition, the woman who has contracted to bear the child may decide to have an abortion or to refuse to relinquish her parental rights. Alternatively, if there is a subsequent birth of a disabled child, prospective parents and the birth mother may not want to or will be unable to assume the responsibilities of parenthood.

On the other hand, surrogate motherhood arrangements are often the last hope of prospective parents to have a child that is genetically related to at least one of them. In addition, most surrogacy arrangements are believed by the parties involved to be mutually beneficial, and most are completed without mishap or dispute. In light of the concerns expressed above, however, some safeguards are necessary to protect the welfare of the child and the birth mother. The Council believes that surrogacy contracts, while permissible, should grant the birth mother the right to void the contract within a reasonable period of time after the birth of the child. If the contract is voided, custody of the child should be determined according to the child's best interests.

In gestational surrogacy, in which the surrogate mother has no genetic tie to the fetus, the justification for allowing the surrogate mother to void the contract becomes less clear. Gestational surrogacy contracts should be strictly enforceable (ie, not voidable by either party). (I, II, IV)

Issued December 1983. Updated June 1994.

Journal 2011 Discusses advancements in modern reproductive technologies and the need for legislation to regulate these technologies. Concludes that regulating these technologies may violate modern views of personal autonomy and therefore should focus on the safety of the technologies and not be used to "protect" women from their ability to freely contract. Quotes Opinions 2.18 and 10.05. Neal, *Protecting Women: Preserving Autonomy in the Commodification of Motherhood*, 17 Wm. & Mary J. Women & L. 611, 630, 635 (2011).

Journal 2000 Examines questions regarding the legality of such practices as voluntary stopping of eating and drinking (VSED), use of risky analgesics, and terminal sedation. Explores the distinctions between physician-assisted suicide and other palliative interventions. Concludes VSED, risky analgesics, and certain types of terminal sedation are lawful and should be made available to dying patients who make informed decisions to accept the risks involved. Quotes Opinions 2.21 and 2.211. Cites Opinions 2.18 and 2.20. Cantor & Thomas, *The Legal Bounds of Physician Conduct Hastening Death*, 48 Buff. L. Rev. 83, 110, 131, 158 (2000).

Journal 1990 Argues that gestational surrogacy, because of its inherent medical, ethical, and legal complications, is not an acceptable reproductive alternative. Discusses the California

Superior Court case of *Johnson v. Calvert* in which a gestational surrogacy contract was held valid and the genetic parents were found to have exclusive custody and parental rights. Quotes Opinion 2.18 (1988). Rothenberg, *Gestational Surrogacy and the Health Care Provider: Put Part of the IVF Genie Back Into the Bottle, 18 Law Med. & Health Care 345, 346 (1990).*

Journal 1987 Examines various ethical issues surrounding surrogate motherhood, artificial insemination, in vitro fertilization, and embryonic/fetal research. Reports on the positions of four ethics groups: the Warnock Committee of Inquiry Into Human Fertilization and Embryology; the AMA's Council on Ethical and Judicial Affairs; the Ethics Committee of the American Fertility Society; and the Ethics Committee of the American College of Obstetricians and Gynecologists. References Opinions 2.04, 2.05, and 2.13 (1986) [now Opinion 2.14]. Quotes Opinion 2.18. Rosner, Cassell, Friedland, Landolt, Loeb, Numann, Ora, Risemberg, & Sordillo, *Ethical Considerations of Reproductive Technologies, 87 N. Y. State J. Med. 398, 399-400 (1987).*

2.19 Unnecessary Medical Services

Physicians should not provide, prescribe, or seek compensation for medical services that they know are unnecessary. (II, VII)

Issued prior to April 1977. Updated June 1996 and December 2003.

Wis. Sup. 2010 State petitioned for involuntary administration of psychotropic medication for defendant who was in custody after acquittal due to mental illness. Defendant argued that Wisconsin statute allowing for such treatment unconstitutionally violated his due process rights. The majority quotes Opinions 2.065 and 2.19 in finding the Wisconsin statute in question facially valid on procedural due process grounds. *State v. Wood, 323 Wis. 2d 321, 780 N.W.2d 63, 82-83.*

Journal 1999 Discusses the need for physicians to advocate on behalf of patients' rights in the context of health care delivery. Evaluates the nature and scope of the physician's role as advocate, noting that physicians cannot be expected to engage in attorney-like advocacy. Quotes Principles IV and VI, Fundamental Elements (2), (4), and (6) [now Opinion 10.01], Patient Responsibilities 5 [now Opinion 10.02], and Opinions 2.03, 2.07, 2.09, 2.16, 2.19, 3.06, 4.01, 4.04, 6.01, 7.02, 8.02, 8.03, 8.13, 8.132, 9.06, 9.07, and 9.131. Cites Opinions 5.05, 5.09, 7.01, 8.135, and 9.02. Sage, *Physicians as Advocates, 35 Hous. L. Rev. 1529, 1537, 1541, 1542, 1552-53, 1554, 1556, 1557, 1559, 1561-62, 1564, 1571, 1574, 1576, 1580 (1999).*

Journal 1994 Considers how greater patient autonomy has led to situations in which medical care may be viewed as futile. Suggests that the law has intruded too far into this area of medicine. Quotes Opinion 2.035. Cites Opinions 2.03, 2.095, 2.17, 2.19, 2.20, and 2.22. Cultice, *Medical Futility: When Is Enough, Enough? 27 J. Health & Hosp. Law 225, 230, 256 (1994).*

Journal 1991 Looks at the physician as a fiduciary and the law governing fiduciary relationships. Concludes that fiduciary concepts are a valuable basis for establishing ethical and legal guidelines for physician behavior. Quotes Opinions 2.19, 8.03 (1989) [now Opinion 8.032], and 8.06. Healey & Dowling, *Controlling Conflicts of Interest in the Doctor-Patient Relationship: Lessons From Moore v. Regents of the University of California, 42 Mercer L. Rev. 989, 997, 998 (1991).*

Journal 1991 Examines the issues surrounding judicial use of professional ethics codes in private litigation. Concludes that judges should more extensively use professional ethics codes to define public policy, standards of care, and legal causes of action. Quotes Principle II and Opinion 2.19. Note, *Professional Ethics Codes in Court: Redefining the Social Contract Between the Public and the Professions, 25 Georgia L. Rev. 1327, 1335, 1351 (1991).*

Journal 1990 Discusses efforts of third-party payers to control health care expenditures for beneficiaries. Concludes that financial incentives to limit care and other cost-control techniques should be disclosed and that the rationale for such disclosure is compelling. Quotes Opinions 2.03, 2.09, and 8.03. Cites Opinions 2.19, 4.04, and 4.06. Hirshfeld, *Should Third Party Payors of Health Care Services Disclose Cost Control Mechanisms to Potential Beneficiaries? 14 Seton Hall Legis. J. 115, 130, 131, 144, 145, 146 (1990).*

Journal 1986 Discusses the Missouri living will statute and the Death-Prolonging Procedures Act. Examines the extent to which these laws ensure individuals the right to make choices regarding personal medical treatment in the event of terminal illness, even if they become incompetent. Quotes Opinion 2.12 (1981) [now Opinion 2.19]. Johnson, *The Death-Prolonging Procedures Act and Refusal of Treatment in Missouri*, 30 St. Louis Univ. L. J. 805, 816 (1986).

2.191   Advance Care Planning

The process of advance care planning is widely recognized as a way to support patient self-determination, facilitate decision making, and promote better care at the end of life. Although often thought of primarily for terminally ill patients or those with chronic medical conditions, advance care planning is valuable for everyone, regardless of age or current health status. Planning in advance for decisions about care in the event of a life-threatening illness or injury gives individuals the opportunity to reflect on and express the values they want to have govern their care, to articulate the factors that are important to them for quality of life, and to make clear any preferences they have with respect to specific interventions. Importantly, these discussions also give individuals the opportunity to identify who they would want to make decisions for them should they not have decision-making capacity.

Proactively discussing with patients what they would or would not want if recovery from illness or injury is improbable also gives physicians opportunity to address patients' concerns and expectations and clarify misunderstandings individuals may have about specific medical conditions or interventions. Encouraging patients to share their views with their families or other intimates and record them in advance directives, and to name a surrogate decision maker, helps to ensure that patients' own values, goals, and preferences will inform care decisions even when they cannot speak for themselves.

Physicians should routinely engage their patients in advance care planning in keeping with the following guidelines:

(a) Regularly encourage all patients, regardless of age or health status to:
   (i)   Think about their values and perspectives on quality of life and articulate what goals they would have for care if they faced a life-threatening illness or injury, including any preferences they may have about specific medical interventions (such as pain management, medically administered nutrition and hydration, mechanical ventilation, use of antibiotics, dialysis, or cardiopulmonary resuscitation);
   (ii) Identify someone they would want to have make decisions on their behalf if they did not have decision-making capacity;
   (iii) Make their views known to their designated surrogate and to (other) family members or intimates.

(b) Be prepared to answer questions about advance care planning, to help patients formulate their views, and to help them articulate their preferences for care (including their wishes regarding time-limited trials of interventions and surrogate decision maker). Physicians should also be prepared to refer patients to additional resources for further information and guidance if appropriate.

(c) Explain how advance directives, as written articulations of their preferences, are used as tools to help guide treatment decisions in collaboration with patients themselves when they have decision-making capacity, or with surrogates when they do not, and explain the surrogate's responsibilities in decision making. Involve the patient's surrogate in this conversation whenever possible.

(d) Incorporate notes from the advance care planning discussion in the medical record. Patient values, preferences for treatment, and designation of surrogate decision maker should be included in the notes to be used as guidance when the patient is unable to express his or her own decisions. If the patient has an advance directive document or written designation of proxy, include a copy (or note the existence of the directive) in the medical record and encourage the patient to give a copy to his or her surrogate and others to help ensure it will be available when needed.

(e) Periodically review with the patient his or her goals, preferences, and chosen decision maker, which often change over time or with changes in health status. Update the patient's medical records accordingly when preferences have changed to ensure that these continue to reflect the individual's current wishes. If applicable, assist the patient with updating his or her advance directive or designation of proxy forms. Involve the patient's surrogate in these reviews whenever possible. (I, IV)

Issued June 2011 based on the report "Advance Care Planning," adopted November 2010.

2.20 Withholding or Withdrawing Life-Sustaining Medical Treatment

The social commitment of the physician is to sustain life and relieve suffering. Where the performance of one duty conflicts with the other, the preferences of the patient should prevail. The principle of patient autonomy requires that physicians respect the decision to forgo life-sustaining treatment of a patient who possesses decision-making capacity. Life-sustaining treatment is any treatment that serves to prolong life without reversing the underlying medical condition. Life-sustaining treatment may include, but is not limited to, mechanical ventilation, renal dialysis, chemotherapy, antibiotics, and artificial nutrition and hydration.

There is no ethical distinction between withdrawing and withholding life-sustaining treatment.

A competent adult patient may, in advance, formulate and provide a valid consent to the withholding or withdrawal of life-support systems in the event that injury or illness renders that individual incompetent to make such a decision. A patient may also appoint a surrogate decision maker in accordance with state law.

If the patient receiving life-sustaining treatment is incompetent, a surrogate decision maker should be identified. Without an advance directive that designates a proxy, the patient's family should become the surrogate decision maker. Family includes persons with whom the patient is closely associated. In the case when there is no person closely associated with the patient, but there are persons who both care about the patient and have sufficient relevant knowledge of the patient, such persons may be appropriate surrogates. Physicians should provide all relevant medical information and explain to surrogate decision makers that decisions regarding withholding or withdrawing life-sustaining treatment should be based on substituted judgment (what the patient would have decided) when there is evidence of the patient's preferences and values. In making a substituted judgment, decision makers may consider the patient's advance directive (if any); the patient's values about life and the way it should be lived; and the patient's attitudes toward sickness, suffering, medical procedures, and death. If there is not adequate evidence of the incompetent patient's preferences and values, the decision should be based on the best interests of the patient (what outcome would most likely promote the patient's well-being).

Though the surrogate's decision for the incompetent patient should almost always be accepted by the physician, there are four situations that may require either institutional or judicial review and/or intervention in the decision-making process: (1) there is no available family member willing to be the patient's surrogate decision maker; (2) there is a dispute among family members and there is no decision maker designated in an advance directive; (3) a health care provider believes that the family's decision is clearly not what the patient would have decided if competent; and (4) a health care provider believes that the decision is not a decision that could reasonably be judged to be in the patient's best interests. When there are disputes among family members or between family and health care providers, the use of ethics committees specifically designed to facilitate sound decision making is recommended before resorting to the courts.

When a permanently unconscious patient was never competent or had not left any evidence of previous preferences or values, since there is no objective way to ascertain the best interests of the patient, the surrogate's decision should not be challenged as long as the decision is based on the decision maker's true concern for what would be best for the patient.

Physicians have an obligation to relieve pain and suffering and to promote the dignity and autonomy of dying patients in their care. This includes providing effective palliative treatment even though it may foreseeably hasten death.

Even if the patient is not terminally ill or permanently unconscious, it is not unethical to discontinue all means of life-sustaining medical treatment in accordance with a proper substituted judgment or best interests analysis. (I, III, IV, V)

Issued December 1984 as Opinion 2.18, Withholding or Withdrawing Life-Prolonging Medical Treatment, and Opinion 2.19, Withholding or Withdrawing Life-Prolonging Medical Treatment—Patients' Preferences. In 1989, these opinions were renumbered 2.20 and 2.21, respectively. Updated June 1994 based on the reports "Decisions Near the End of Life" and "Decisions to Forego Life-Sustaining Treatment for Incompetent Patients," both adopted June 1991 (Decisions Near the End of Life. JAMA. 1992;267:2229-2233). Updated June 1996. [In March, 1981, the Council on Ethical and Judicial Affairs issued Opinion 2.11, *Terminal Illness*. The opinion was renumbered 2.15 in 1984 and was deleted in 1986.]

U.S. 1997 Several physicians and terminally ill patients sued the state seeking a declaration that its prohibition against physician-assisted suicide violates the Fourteenth Amendment's Equal Protection Clause. The trial court disagreed, but the Second Circuit reversed, holding that the state accords different treatment to those terminally ill patients who wish to hasten their death by self-administering prescribed drugs and to those patients who wish to do so by directing the removal of life support systems. The Supreme Court reversed holding that the prohibition against assisting suicide does not violate the Equal Protection Clause. The Court concluded that there is a distinction between assisting suicide and withdrawing treatment quoting reports of the AMA Council on Ethical and Judicial Affairs [now Opinions 2.20 and 2.21]. *Vacco v. Quill*, 117 S. Ct. 2293, 2298, 138 L. Ed. 2d 834.

U.S. 1990 Parents of patient in persistent vegetative state appealed denial of request to discontinue gastrotomy feeding tube. The Supreme Court held that the federal constitution did not forbid the state's requirement of clear and convincing evidence of an incompetent patient's wishes regarding the withdrawal of life-prolonging treatment. The Court acknowledged that a competent person has a liberty interest under the due process clause in refusing unwanted medical care; however, the Court assumed the existence of a constitutionally protected right to refuse artificial hydration and nutrition only for purposes of the case. In a concurring opinion, Justice O'Connor cited Opinion 2.20 for the proposition that artificial feeding cannot be distinguished from other forms of medical treatment. In his dissent, Justice Brennan likewise cited Opinion 2.20 for this point. *Cruzan v. Director, Missouri Department of Health,* 497 U.S. 261.

9th Cir. 1996 Suit was brought by several physicians and not-for-profit corporation which provides information, assistance, and counseling to competent terminally ill adult patients contemplating suicide, asserting that a state statute making it a crime to aid anyone in attempting to commit suicide unconstitutionally prevents terminally ill patients from exercising their protected liberty interests. Appeals court, en banc, held that the choice of how and when to die is a liberty interest and that the statute violates the due process rights of competent, terminally ill adults who wish to hasten their deaths by obtaining medication prescribed by their physicians. Stating that physician-assisted suicide runs counter to medical ethics, the dissent cited Opinions 2.20, 2.21, and 2.211 and quoted Opinion 2.211. *Compassion in Dying v. Washington,* 79 F.3d 790, 840, 855, *replacing 49 F.3d 586 (9th Cir. 1995).*

E.D.N.Y. 2011 The court confronted the question of how to sentence young defendants whose drug addiction led to violations of criminal drug laws. In finding an ethical obligation of physicians to treat chronic pain, the court quotes Opinion 2.20. The court holds that where the defendant's drug addiction is causatively intertwined with a violation of criminal law, every effort should be made to minimize incarceration in favor of closely supervised, intensive medical treatment outside of prison. *United States v. Ilayayev,* 800 F. Supp. 2d 417, 435.

Ariz. 1987 Guardian of nursing home patient in persistent vegetative state sought removal of nasogastric tube and retention of do-not-resuscitate and do-not-hospitalize orders. Patient had not communicated desires regarding life-sustaining procedures while competent. In assessing whether safeguarding the integrity of the medical profession might be a state interest that outweighed the patient's right to refuse medical treatment, the court noted Opinion 2.18 (1986) [now Opinion 2.20] to support the view that the medical profession itself now recognizes that it is no longer obligated to provide medical treatment in all situations. Since the Opinion would allow the disputed orders for a patient suffering from an irreversible coma, the court concluded that the same action would be allowed in a case of irreversible chronic vegetative state and thus concluded that the case did not bring into disrepute the ethical integrity of the medical profession. *Rasmussen v. Fleming,* 154 Ariz. 207, 741 P.2d 674, 684, 685.

Ariz. App. 1986 Guardian of nursing home patient in persistent vegetative state sought removal of nasogastric tube and retention of do-not-resuscitate and do-not-hospitalize orders. Patient had not communicated her desires regarding life-sustaining procedures while competent. The court quoted Opinion 2.18 (1986) [now Opinion 2.20] in holding that competing state interests, including the ethical integrity of the medical profession, did not outweigh patient's constitutional right to privacy and held that rights of incompetent patient could be asserted vicariously. *Rasmussen v. Fleming,* 154 Ariz. 200, 741 P.2d 667, 671, 672, 673 n.4, *aff'd in part and rev'd in part,* 154 Ariz. 207, 741 P.2d 674 (1987).

Cal. App. 1988 Conservator sought an injunction requiring physician to remove nasogastric feeding tube from a patient who was in a persistent vegetative state. The court held that while a conservator may authorize withdrawal or withholding of medical treatment, he may not force a physician to do so against the physician's personal moral objections if the patient can be transferred to the care of a physician who will follow the directive. Citing Opinion 2.18 (1986) [now Opinion 2.20], the court noted that the physician's compliance with the conservator's decision would not have violated the ethical code of the medical profession. *Morrison v. Abramovice,* 206 Cal. App. 3d 304, 309, 253 Cal. Rptr. 530, 533.

Cal. App. 1988 Conservator of patient in persistent vegetative state sought permission for removal of nasogastric feeding tube claiming such relief would serve the patient's best interests. Patient had expressed a desire never to be kept alive through artificial means. The court held that a conservator is authorized to order that artificial life support be withdrawn after considering medical advice and the patient's best interests. In so holding, the court quoted Opinion 2.18

(1986) [now Opinion 2.20] showing support within the medical community for its analysis. *In re Drabick, 200 Cal. App. 3d 185, 245 Cal. Rptr. 840, 845 n.8.*

Cal. App. 1986 Mentally competent, physically debilitated patient sought authorization to discontinue forced feedings through nasogastric tube. Patient had dictated instructions to her lawyers and signed them with an x by means of a pen held in her mouth. In holding that a competent adult patient has the legal right to refuse medical treatment even though such refusal will hasten her death, the court quoted Opinion 2.18 (1986) [now Opinion 2.20]. *Bouvia v. Superior Court, 179 Cal. App. 3d 1127, 225 Cal. Rptr. 297, 303-04.*

Conn. 1989 Family of comatose, terminal patient in nursing home sought injunction to discontinue life support services. In holding that removal of a gastrostomy tube was authorized by statute and no compelling state interests outweighed the patient's rights, the court cited Opinion 2.18 (1986) [now Opinion 2.20] for its view that the provision of nutrition and hydration is a form of life-prolonging medical treatment. *McConnell v. Beverly Enterprises-Connecticut, Inc., 209 Conn. 692, 553 A.2d 596, 603 n.13.*

Fla. App. 1986 Husband of terminally ill patient in persistent vegetative state sought declaratory judgment to permit removal of nasogastric feeding tube. In recognizing a right to allow the natural consequence of removal of artificial life-sustaining measures, the court quoted Opinion 2.18 (1986) [now Opinion 2.20]. *Corbett v. D'Alessandro, 487 So. 2d 368, 371 n.1.*

Ill. 1989 Daughter of permanently unconscious patient petitioned to withdraw life-prolonging gastrotomy feeding tube. The court cited with approval Opinion 2.18 (1986) [now Opinion 2.20] that the AMA considers artificial hydration and nutrition to be medical treatments which may be withdrawn under certain circumstances. The court based the right to refuse life-prolonging procedures upon the state's common law of informed consent, probate law, and power of attorney for health care statute. The court established guidelines for a guardian's exercise of this right. The patient must be terminally ill, in a persistent vegetative state, and the guardian must exercise the substituted judgment of the patient as shown through clear and convincing evidence in a judicial proceeding. *In re Longeway, 133 Ill. 2d 33, 549 N.E.2d 292, 295-96.*

Ill. App. 1988 Guardian of patient in persistent vegetative state petitioned to withdraw artificial feeding tube. Prior to her incompetence, the patient had stated in writing and in conversations with friends that she desired no artificial means of treatment if there was no hope for her recovery, and had completed a living will form, but had failed to obtain the requisite number of witness signatures. The trial court dismissed the case upon the patient's death. On appeal, the court held that the guardian, using the doctrine of substituted judgment, could consent to the removal of a feeding tube from a patient in a persistent vegetative state. In so holding, the court quoted Opinion 2.18 [now Opinion 2.20], noting that it was within a physician's ethical parameters to discontinue such treatment. *In re Prange, 166 Ill. App. 3d 1091, 520 N.E.2d 946, vacated, 121 Ill. 2d 570, 527 N.E.2d 303 (1988).*

Ind. 1991 State statute provided procedures by which parents of an incompetent patient, in consultation with the patient's physician, could withhold or withdraw life-prolonging medical treatment. The court held that barring any challenge from the treating physician or interested parties, the family could make these decisions without a court proceeding. Quoting Opinion 2.20 (1989), the court concluded that medical treatment includes artificial nutrition and hydration. *In re Lawrance, 579 N.E.2d 32, 40.*

Kan. App. 1998 Physician was convicted of attempted murder of a terminally ill patient, and intentional and malicious second-degree murder of another terminally ill patient. The court quoted Opinion 2.22, to exemplify a physician's duty to provide cardiopulmonary resuscitation unless the physician believes that such action would be futile. Additionally, the court referenced Opinion 2.20, in support of a physician's duty to provide a terminally ill patient adequate pain relief. The court reversed the physician's convictions, stating that the jury could not disregard the testimony of several physicians who concurred with the defendant-physician's treatment of the deceased patients. *State v. Naramore, 25 Kan. App. 2d 302, 965 P.2d 211, 214, 216.*

Ky. 2004 Plaintiff challenged the constitutionality of a provision of the Kentucky Living Will Directive Act which allows a judicially appointed guardian or surrogate to decide to withhold or withdraw life-sustaining medical treatment from a patient in a persistent vegetative state or who is permanently unconscious. The Kentucky Supreme Court quoted Opinion 2.20 in determining that the challenged provision does not violate any modern legal, moral, or ethical standards. The court found the statute constitutional, but stated that if the family and the guardian disagree as to whether to withhold or withdraw life-sustaining treatment, those attempting to withhold or withdraw treatment must show by clear and convincing evidence that the patient is in a permanently unconscious or persistent vegetative state or that death is imminent and that withholding or withdrawing life-sustaining treatment is in the patient's best interest. *Woods v. Commonwealth, 142 S.W.3d 24, 46, 47.*

Ky. 1993 In a declaratory judgment action, the court was asked to allow a surrogate to exercise the right to withdraw life-prolonging treatment for a patient who had orally expressed her wishes not to be sustained artificially. Since common law recognizes a patient's right to withdraw or withhold medical treatment, the court held that a surrogate could rely on the patient's statement of choice made before patient became incompetent to exercise "substituted judgment." The court quoted from guidelines for state courts deciding life-sustaining medical treatment cases issued by the National Center for State Courts. Citing Opinion 2.20 and other sources, the Guidelines stated that a consensus had already been reached on the primary ethical issues relating to life-prolonging treatment. *DeGrella v. Elston, 858 S.W.2d 698, 707 n.5.*

Me. 1987 Guardian sought to have nasogastric feeding tube withdrawn from patient in persistent vegetative state. Investigation by a state agency corroborated evidence of patient's prior statements that he desired no life-sustaining procedures if in a persistent vegetative state. The court noted that under state's common law an individual has a personal right to refuse medical treatment, including life-sustaining procedures. The court held that where the patient had clearly and convincingly expressed his desire not to be maintained by life-sustaining procedures if in a persistent vegetative state, health professionals had a duty to respect that decision. The court cited Opinion 2.18 (1986) [now Opinion 2.20] for the concept that artificial hydration and nutrition should be equated with other life-sustaining treatments in delineating the patient's right to reject such treatment. *In re Gardner, 534 A.2d 947, 954.*

Md. Att'y Gen. 1988 Attorney general was asked whether persons with capacity to decide about medical care have a right to instruct that artificially administered sustenance not be provided if they become terminally ill or permanently comatose. An opinion was also requested regarding decision-making for incompetent persons who have given no prior instructions about artificial feeding. In response, Opinion 2.18 (1986) [now Opinion 2.20] is cited to support the view that no distinction should be drawn between artificial feeding and other forms of life-prolonging treatment. Further, in delineating procedures for deciding to forgo treatment for an incompetent, terminally ill patient who has given no prior instructions, Opinion 2.18 (1986) [now Opinion 2.20] is also cited in terms of the physician's role in advising whether withdrawal is medically proper. Finally, while disallowing family members, without court approval, to terminate tube feeding for a nonterminal, permanently comatose patient, it is recognized that under this Opinion it is not unethical to discontinue life-sustaining treatment for such a patient. *Maryland Att'y Gen. Op. No. 88-046, 73 Op. Att'y Gen. 162.*

Mass. 1992 Request of parents of a patient in a persistent vegetative state to employ "substituted judgment" in order to withdraw medical treatment was granted. Citing Opinion 2.18 (1986) [now Opinion 2.20], the court noted that medical treatment includes artificial hydration and nutrition. *In re Doe, 411 Mass. 512, 517 n.11, 583 N.E.2d 1263, 1267 n.11.*

Mass. 1986 Guardian of patient in persistent vegetative state who, according to trial court, would have declined food and water, sued for declaratory judgment requesting authority to have artificial hydration and nutrition discontinued. The court held that while the hospital had a right to refuse to participate in the removal of the gastrostomy tube, the guardian was authorized to transfer the patient to other physicians who would honor the guardian's request. The court cited Opinion 2.18 (1986) [now Opinion 2.20] in finding that the patient's right to refuse medical treatment did not violate the state's interest in the maintenance of the ethical integrity of the medical profession as long as the hospital was not forced to participate in the removal or clamping of the gastronomy tube. *Brophy v. New England Sinai Hosp., Inc., 398 Mass. 417, 497 N.E.2d 626, 638-39 n.38.*

Mich. App. 2001 State brought criminal action against physician for the murder of a patient by lethal injection. The trial court convicted the physician of second-degree murder and delivering a controlled substance. On appeal, the trial court decision was affirmed. The physician asked the appellate court to conclude that euthanasia is legal and to reverse his conviction on constitutional grounds. The appellate court relied on *Washington v. Glucksberg, 521 U.S. 702 (1997)* in determining there is no constitutional right to commit euthanasia, so that an individual can be free from intolerable and irremediable suffering. In discussing Glucksberg, the court observed that a state has a legitimate interest in protecting the integrity and ethics of the medical profession. The court noted Glucksberg's reference to Opinions 2.20, 2.21, and 2.211 in this regard. *People v. Kevorkian, 248 Mich. App. 373, 639 N.W.2d 291, 305 n. 42.*

Mo. 1988 Parents-guardians of a nonterminal patient in a persistent vegetative state sought a declaratory judgment after a state hospital refused to terminate artificial hydration and nutrition. The court found that the patient's burden in being fed through gastronomy tube did not outweigh the state's interest in preserving life and that guardians could not order withdrawal of hydration and nutrition. The court, in refusing to classify artificial hydration and nutrition as medical treatment, rejected Opinion 2.18 (1986) [now Opinion 2.20] which expresses a contrary view. *Cruzan v. Harmon, 760 S.W.2d 408, 423 n.18, aff'd, 497 U.S. 261.*

N.J. 1987 Husband applied to court for authorization to discontinue wife's hydration and nutrition after nursing home refused his request to do so. The court held that the right of a patient in an irreversible vegetative state to refuse life-sustaining procedures may be exercised by the patient's family or close friend after two independent neurologists have confirmed the diagnosis and prognosis. The court further stated that the processes of surrogate decision-making should be substantially the same regardless of type of medical facility. In so holding, the court cited Opinion 2.18 (1986) [now Opinion 2.20] with approval. *In re Jobes, 108 N.J. 394, 529 A.2d 434, 446.*

N.J. 1987 Elderly nursing home patient was comatose in a persistent vegetative state. Patient's designee, under power of attorney for health care decisions, sought appointment as guardian and authorization for removal of patient's artificial nutrition and hydration. The court held that where there is clear and convincing proof that patient would refuse such treatment if competent, a surrogate may effect that decision regardless of the patient's life expectancy. The court quoted with approval Opinion 2.18 (1986) [now Opinion 2.20] stating that artificial hydration and nutrition is a form of medical treatment. *In re Peter, 108 N.J. 365, 529 A.2d 419, 427-28.*

N.J. 1987 Husband of competent, terminally ill patient applied to be special medical guardian to effectuate patient's desire to remove respirator. In holding that the right of a competent, terminally ill patient to decline medical treatment outweighed the state's interests in preserving life, preventing suicide, protecting innocent third parties, and safeguarding the integrity of the medical profession, the court cited as reflective of the views of the medical profession the Judicial Council's report at 253 JAMA 2424 (1985) [now Opinion 2.20]. *In re Farrell, 108 N.J. 335, 529 A.2d 404, 412.*

N.J. Super. 1983 Guardian of elderly nursing home patient suffering from severe organic brain syndrome sought to remove nasogastric tube from patient. Trial court granted guardian's petition, and patient's guardian ad litem appealed. Appellate court reversed, in part based upon Opinions 2.11 (1981) and 5.17 (1979) [now Opinions 2.17 and 2.20], and held that it is improper and would violate medical ethics to allow dehydration and starvation in a noncomatose, non–brain-dead patient not facing imminent death, not maintained by any life-support machine, and not able to speak for herself. *In re Conroy, 190 N.J. Super. 453, 464 A.2d 303, 313-15, rev'd, 98 N.J. 321, 486 A.2d 1209 (1985).*

N.Y. 1990 Jehovah's Witness was given blood transfusion against her express wishes. The court held that the lower court erred in ordering the transfusions without giving the patient or her family notice and a hearing. Barring any superior interest of the state, the patient had a right to determine the course of her own treatment. Concurring opinion argued that the majority rule created an absolute right to refuse treatment. Quoting from Opinion 2.21 (1989) [now Opinion 2.20], the concurring opinion held that a physician had a corresponding ethical duty to render treatment which, in his judgment, benefits the patient. Note that Opinion 2.20 does not retain the specific language of former Opinion 2.21 relied on by concurring judge. *Fosmire v. Nicoleau, 75 N.Y.2d 218, 236 n.2, 551 N.E.2d 77, 87 n.2, 551 N.Y.S.2d 876, 886 n.2.*

N.Y. Sup. 2003 Mother petitioned court to remove her daughter from a respirator. Hospital policy denied mother the authorization to withdraw care. Court granted petition and held parents have a right to refuse medical treatment for their children. Applying the best interest test, the court held that the burdens of prolonging life exceeded the benefits and that, absent extraordinary circumstances or disagreement between parents, judicial intervention is not required to withhold medical treatment from a minor in a vegetative state. Quotes Opinion 2.215. References Opinion 2.20. *In re AB, 196 Misc. 2d 940, 768 N.Y.S. 2d 256, 268-69.*

N.Y. Sup. 1986 Plaintiff petitioned for judicial authorization to remove feeding tube from her 33-year-old husband, a patient in a permanent chronic vegetative state. In denying the petition, the court noted the AMA's position set out in 245 JAMA 819 (1981), later included as Opinion

2.11 (1981) [now Opinion 2.20] that, in such cases, members of the family and physicians should decide whether to continue treatment. However, the court concluded that the legislature must resolve the issue and denied the petition. *Delio v. Westchester County Medical Center, 134 Misc. 2d 206, 510 N.Y.S.2d 415, 419, rev'd, 129 A.D. 2d 1, 516 N.Y.S. 2d 677 (1987).*

Ohio App. 1989 The divorced parents of a patient in a persistent vegetative state each petitioned to be appointed guardian of their son. The mother was initially appointed guardian and testified that it would be in the best interests of her son, and consistent with his wishes, to terminate nutrition and hydration. Over the father's objections, the probate court granted the mother, as guardian, the right to make decisions regarding her son's treatment and care. On appeal, the appellate court modified the lower court's order, pursuant to a state statute enacted after that order was entered. Although recognizing that the lower court's decision was consistent with the position of the AMA as articulated in Opinion 2.20, the appellate court held that to allow termination of nutrition and hydration in this case would violate the public policy as expressed in recent legislation. *Couture v. Couture, 48 Ohio App. 3d 208, 549 N.E.2d 571, 574.*

Pa. Super. 1995 Parent of nursing home patient in persistent vegetative state sought removal of gastrostomy tube. Nursing home refused to comply with request without court order. Trial court, applying best interests test, authorized removal of tube. On appeal, court held that consent of close family member, with approval of two qualified physicians, is sufficient without court order to terminate life-sustaining treatment for patient in a long-term persistent vegetative state. Court referred to *In re Grant*, 109 Wash. 2d 545, 747 P.2d 445 (1987) citing Opinion 2.18 [now Opinion 2.20] for proposition that medical ethical principles permit withdrawal of nutrition and hydration for patient in persistent vegetative state. *In re Fiori, 438 Pa. Super. 610, 652 A.2d 1350, 1354, app. granted, 655 A.2d 989 (Pa. 1995).*

Phila. Co. 1987 In a declaratory judgment action, the court held that a patient has a right to withhold or withdraw medical treatment. This right is subject to the state's interest in (1) the preservation of life, (2) protection of innocent third parties, (3) prevention of suicide, and (4) protecting the ethical integrity of the medical profession. The court held that the withholding or withdrawal of life support by a physician or hospital or their agents did not constitute a criminal act or give rise to any civil liability. Citing Opinion 2.18 (1986) [now Opinion 2.20]), the court noted that respect for a patient's autonomy and decision to withdraw life support was consistent with medical ethics. *In re Doe, 16 Phila. 229, 1987 Phila. Cty. Rptr. LEXIS 30 (1987).*

Tenn. App. 2002 Patient was in a vegetative state and had metastasized breast cancer. Her family sought to terminate nutrition and hydration. Trial court found clear and convincing evidence showed patient did not want to live by artificial nutrition. However, court also ruled that state statute required a valid written document in order for an incompetent person to refuse nutrition and hydration. Appellate court reversed, holding that lower court misinterpreted the statute. The court held that patient had an inherent fundamental right to refuse medical treatment. Quotes Opinion 2.18 [now Opinion 2.20]. *San Juan-Torregosa v. Garcia, 80 S.W.3d 539, 543.*

Va. Att'y Gen. 1990 Attorney general answered in the affirmative when asked whether a competent adult could create a document authorizing a surrogate to consent to the withholding or withdrawal of medical treatment if the person later enters a persistent vegetative state but is not terminally ill. Quoting Opinion 2.18 (1986) [now Opinion 2.20], the attorney general concluded that medical treatment includes artificial hydration and nutrition. *Va. Att'y Gen. Op., 1990 Va. AG LEXIS 63.*

Wash. 1987 Court authorization sought by guardian to withhold mechanical or artificial life-sustaining procedures from incompetent patient with terminal disorder. Trial court denied request as premature because patient was not yet comatose or vegetative, and did not yet need intrusive medical procedures. Supreme Court held that an incompetent patient in an advanced stage of a terminal illness has right to have life-sustaining treatment withheld, a right which stems from the constitutional right of privacy and the common law right to be free of bodily invasion. Court quoted Opinion 2.18 (1986) [now Opinion 2.20] in support of the right of a terminally ill, noncomatose patient to have life-sustaining procedures withheld including the right to withhold artificial means of nutrition and hydration. *In re Grant, 109 Wash. 2d 545, 747 P.2d 445, 450, 454.*

Wis. 1992 Guardian may consent to the withholding or withdrawal of life-prolonging medical treatment on behalf of an incompetent patient and/or a patient for whom the guardian cannot reasonably make a "substituted judgment" where (1) the patient is in a persistent vegetative state with no reasonable chance of recovery, and (2) the guardian in good faith determines that it is in the patient's "best interest." The court referred to the concurring opinion in *Cruzan v. Director, Missouri Dept. of Health*, 497 U.S. 261 (1990) which quoted Opinion 2.20 (1989) in holding that medical treatment includes nutrition and hydration. Further, citing Opinion 2.18 (1986) [now Opinion 2.20], the court found the actions here consistent with current medical ethics. Thus, the state's interest in protecting the integrity of the medical profession was not implicated. *L.W. v. L.E. Phillips Career Dev. Ctr.*, 167 Wis. 2d 53, 71, 72, 91, 482 N.W.2d 60, 66, 74.

Journal 2011 Analyzes the development of Italian end-of-life decision-making law. Concludes that, while Italian law more closely resembles that of the U.S. than one might predict given the countries' differing cultural backgrounds and political-legal systems, substantial differences remain. References Opinions 2.20. Cerminara, Pizzetti, & Photangtham, *Schiavo Revisited? The Struggle for Autonomy at the End of Life in Italy*, 12 Marq. Elder's Advisor 295, 308 (2011).

Journal 2010 Discusses futility disputes where a patient's surrogate wishes to prolong treatment that the physician deems medically ineffective, and the current lack of legal remedies to resolve them. Concludes that states need to establish fair, impartial, and patient-centered methods of resolving futility disputes including independent medical boards that would operate under procedural and substantive regulations. Quotes Opinions 2.02 and 2.035. References Opinions 2.17 and 2.20. Bassel, *Order at the End of Life: Establishing a Clear and Fair Mechanism for the Resolution of Futility Disputes*, 63 Vand. L. Rev. 491, 494, 523 (2010).

Journal 2010 Discusses conflicts between surrogates and health care professionals in the context of "futile" care for patients. Further, discusses how "surrogate selection" laws may be used to replace a surrogate demanding inappropriately aggressive end-of-life treatment. Concludes that while surrogate selection has resolved some futility issues, an increase in independent ethics committees would be beneficial in dispelling other major issues. Quotes and cites Opinions 2.20 and 8.081. Pope, *Surrogate Selection: An Increasingly Viable, but Limited, Solution to Intractable Futility Disputes*, 3 St. Louis U. J. Health L. & Pol'y 183, 207, 208, 211-214, 224, 228 (2010).

Journal 2010 Examines whether standards and practices regarding euthanasia, other than those which have been legally and ethically established, should be applied in extreme emergency situations. Concludes that creating an exception to the prohibition against euthanasia in such situations has no legal or ethical foundation and is not necessary as a means to cope with disasters. Argues for the development of disaster planning consistent with established legal and ethical principles. Quotes Opinion 8.08. Cites Opinions 2.20 and 2.21. Shea, *Hurricane Katrina and the Legal and Bioethical Implications of Involuntary Euthanasia as a Component of Disaster Management in Extreme Emergency Situations*, 19 Annals Health L. 133, 137-138 (2010).

Journal 2009 Argues that adults have the right to procreate using assisted reproductive technologies that create embryos, and that such embryos are morally equivalent to individuals on life support. Further argues that, just as families of an individual being removed from life support can consent to the donation of that individual's organs, parents of an embryo can consent to the donation of that embryo's cells for research. Concludes the philosophical notion that life begins at conception can be reconciled with support for embryonic stem cell research if the full humanity of the embryo is recognized throughout the process. Quotes Opinion 2.20. References Opinion 2.20. Dolin, *A Defense of Embryonic Stem Cell Research*, 84 Ind. L. J. 1203, 1223, 1227 (2009).

Journal 2009 Discusses the avoidable consequences rule in the context of awards for pain and suffering. Suggests courts should reevaluate the noneconomic nature of emotional harm to recharacterize some pain and suffering damages as medical expenses. Quotes Opinion 2.20. Noah, *Comfortably Numb: Medicalizing (and Mitigating) Pain-and-Suffering Damages*, 42 U. Mich. J. L. Reform 431, 435 (2009).

Journal 2008 Discusses medical options when the physician can do nothing further to cure the patient and examines the Texas Advance Directives Act, a medical futility statute. Concludes conflicts may be reduced if physician-patient communication is initiated when treatment begins rather than when further treatment becomes futile. Cites the Texas medical futility process as an example for providing physicians a mechanism for resolving conflicts with patients. Quotes Opinions 2.035, 2.037, and 2.20. Dahm, *Medical Futility and the Texas Medical Futility Statute: A Model to Follow or One to Avoid?* 20 Health Law 25, 26 (Aug. 2008).

Journal 2008 Discusses patient autonomy, pain, and the current law governing the right to die. Argues pain management is essential to ensure patients possess the requisite autonomy to make end-of-life care decisions. Quotes Opinion 2.20. Lasken, *The Incoherent Right to Die*, 4 NAELA J. 167, 176 (2008).

Journal 2007 Compares US and international policy on end-of-life decision making. Concludes that interests of patient autonomy should be balanced with family interests and advocates a comprehensive "best interest" model. Quotes Opinion 2.037. Cites Opinions 2.035 and 2.20. Rode, *End-of-Life Decision Making for Patients in Persistent Vegetative States: A Comparative Analysis*, 30 Hastings Int'l & Comp. L. Rev. 477, 499, 500 (2007).

Journal 2007 Discusses patients' right to refuse medical treatment and the corresponding duties of health care professionals. Concludes that detailed, carefully prepared advance directives are necessary to fulfill patients' wishes. Quotes Ch. II (1940) [now Opinions 8.08 and 8.082] and Opinions 2.035, 2.037, 2.20, 2.225, 8.081, and 10.015. Cites Opinions 9.11 and 9.115. Stamatakis, *Beyond Advance Directives: Personal Autonomy and the Right to Refuse Life-Sustaining Medical Treatment*, 47 N. H. B. J. 20, 29-30 (2007).

Journal 2007 Argues that Drug Enforcement Agency (DEA) regulation of physicians has resulted in a denial of palliative care to patients. Concludes that in regulating controlled substances, federal and state government must not lose sight of patient need for palliative care. Quotes Opinion 2.20. Trehan, *Fear of Prescribing: How the DEA Is Infringing on Patients' Right to Palliative Care*, 61 U. Miami L. Rev. 961, 975 (2007).

Journal 2006 Discusses an attorney's responsibility to a client on death row who wishes to volunteer for execution. Concludes that an attorney should never assist a client in waiving an appeal. Quotes Opinions 2.20 and 2.211. Oleson, *Swilling Hemlock: The Legal Ethics of Defending a Client Who Wishes to Volunteer for Execution*, 63 Wash. & Lee L. Rev. 147, 277, 325 (2006).

Journal 2006 Examines current policy governing removal of a feeding tube from a patient in a permanent vegetative state. Proposes a policy of a rebuttable presumption that the feeding tube may be removed. References Opinion 2.20. Shepherd, *In Respect of People Living in a Permanent Vegetative State—And Allowing Them to Die*, 16 Health Matrix 631, 671 (2006).

Journal 2006 Reviews legislation and case law governing conscience clauses for medical professionals. Concludes that conscientious objections to providing care should be permitted only when based on accepted principles of medical ethics. Quotes Opinion 2.18 (1986) [now Opinion 2.20]. References Opinion 8.032. Swartz, *"Conscience Clauses" or "Unconscionable Clauses": Personal Beliefs Versus Professional Responsibilities*, 6 Yale J. Health Pol'y, L. & Ethics 269, 317, 347 (2006).

Journal 2005 Discusses the "best interest" standard used in making end-of-life decisions. Concludes that this standard allows for humane end-of-life decisions to be made on behalf of never-competent patients. Cites Opinion 2.20. Cantor, *The Bane of Surrogate Decision-Making: Defining the Best Interests of Never-Competent Persons*, 26 J. Legal Med. 155, 160 (2005).

Journal 2005 Discusses the facts and history of the *Schiavo* case. Concludes that patient autonomy, family privacy, and patient dignity should prevail in making decisions to withhold life-sustaining treatment. References Opinion 2.20. Gostin, *Ethics, the Constitution, and the Dying Process: The Case of Theresa Marie Schiavo*, 293 JAMA 2403, 2405 (2005).

Journal 2005 Discusses the moral and ethical justifications for the Supreme Court's use of the doctrine of double effect in *Vacco v. Quill*. Concludes that the Court's use of the principle of double effect conforms with widely accepted clinical and ethical norms and is supported by American case law. Quotes Opinion 2.20. Lyons, *In Incognito—The Principle of Double Effect in American Constitutional Law*, 57 Fla. L. Rev. 469, 474 (2005).

Journal 2005 Discusses the evidentiary standards utilized to permit withdrawal of life-sustaining treatment by substitute decision-makers when patients are in a persistent vegetative state. Concludes that a futility rationale for making end-of-life decisions may represent the best approach in these situations. Quotes Opinion 2.035. Cites Opinion 2.20. Mareiniss, *A Comparison of Cruzan and Schiavo: The Burden of Proof, Due Process, and Autonomy in the Persistently Vegetative Patient*, 26 J. Legal Med. 233, 248, 250 (2005).

Journal 2004 Considers whether profoundly mentally disabled persons have the same constitutional rights as competent individuals to refuse life-sustaining medical treatment. Concludes that through the use of a surrogate, these individuals have similar but not identical rights in this context. Cites Opinion 2.20. Cantor, *The Relation Between Autonomy-Based Rights and Profoundly Mentally Disabled Persons*, 13 Annals Health L. 37, 70 (2004).

Journal 2004 Analyzes various issues relating to the role of mental health professionals in capital punishment in light of Albert Bandura's model of "mechanisms of moral disengagement."

Concludes that facilitating participation of mental health professionals in executions creates conflicts with the humanistic norms of the profession. Quotes Preamble and Opinions 1.01, 1.02, 2.06, 2.067, 2.20, 2.21, 2.211, and 8.14. Judges, *The Role of Mental Health Professionals in Capital Punishment: An Exercise in Moral Disengagement*, 41 Hous. L. Rev. 515, 562, 568, 569, 570, 571-72, 581, 586, 588, 598 (2004).

Journal 2003 Discusses whether patients may assert a claim of medical malpractice for inadequate treatment of pain. Concludes courts should find that failure to adequately treat pain constitutes negligence. Quotes Opinion 2.20. Mayer, *Bergman v. Chin: Why an Elder Abuse Case Is a Stride in the Direction of Civil Culpability for Physicians Who Undertreat Patients Suffering From Terminal Pain*, 37 New Eng. L. Rev. 313, 340 (2003).

Journal 2003 Identifies legal obstacles to adequate pain care in long-term care facilities. Concludes that the government must take action to ensure effective pain management for patients in these facilities. Quotes Opinion 2.20. Seng, *Legal and Regulatory Barriers to Adequate Pain Control for Elders in Long-Term Care Facilities*, 6 N. Y. City L. Rev. 95, 97 (2003).

Journal 2002 Suggests a reconceptualization for bioethics that integrates an analysis of the history of moral change. Concludes that bioethical textbooks should include discussion about the history of bioethics and medical ethics. Quotes Opinion 2.20. References Opinions 6.02, 6.03, 6.04 [now Opinion 8.06], and 8.032. Baker, *Bioethics and History*, 27 J. Med. & Phil. 447, 455, 469 (2002).

Journal 2002 Explores the implications of withholding medical treatment when abortion results in a live birth. Concludes that, in these situations, abortive parents and physicians should not solely decide the child's best interest. Quotes Preamble, Principles I and III, and Opinions 2.035, 2.20, and 2.215. Casagrande, *Children Not Meant to Be: Protecting the Interests of the Child When Abortion Results in Live Birth*, 6 Quinnipiac Health L. J. 19, 44, 45, 47-48 (2002).

Journal 2002 Considers a judicial model to evaluate the relationship between law and bioethics. Concludes that, in this regard, ethics may justify court decisions but likely will not break new ground. Quotes Opinion 2.20. Gross, *Wagging the Watchdog: Law and the Emergence of Bioethical Norms*, 21 Med. & L. 687, 702 (2002).

Journal 2002 Considers the use of nonlegal materials in US Supreme Court decisions. Concludes that law alone cannot answer complex legal questions. Cites Opinions 2.20 and 2.211. Hasko, *Persuasion in the Court: Nonlegal Materials in U.S. Supreme Court Opinions*, 94 Law Libr. J. 427, 444, 453 (2002).

Journal 2002 Examines competing interests regarding genetic testing. Argues that testing of employees should be banned. Concludes that Congress should pass legislation prohibiting genetic testing in the workplace. Quotes Opinion 2.20. Krumm, *Genetic Discrimination: Why Congress Must Ban Genetic Testing in the Workplace*, 23 J. Legal Med. 491, 506 (2002).

Journal 2002 Evaluates pain management treatment for prisoners. Concludes that withholding treatment for, or failing to adequately treat, pain violates the Eighth Amendment. Quotes Principle V and Opinion 2.20. McGrath, *Raising the "Civilized Minimum" of Pain Amelioration for Prisoners to Avoid Cruel and Unusual Punishment*, 54 Rutgers L. Rev. 649, 657, 660 (2002).

Journal 2002 Examines key factors that led to the current palliative care crisis. Analyzes state legislative and judicial efforts to improve palliative care. Concludes with model legislation that holds physicians accountable for inadequate palliative care. Quotes Opinions 2.21 and 2.211. References Opinion 2.20. Oken, *Curing Healthcare Providers' Failure to Administer Opioids in the Treatment of Severe Pain*, 23 Cardozo L. Rev. 1917, 1925-26, 1952, 1954 (2002).

Journal 2001 Explores the similarities and differences among active voluntary euthanasia, terminal sedation, and assisted suicide. Examines the problems with making moral distinctions based on physicians' intentions. Concludes that, with proper safeguards, active voluntary euthanasia and assisted suicide are more protective of patient self-determination. Quotes Opinions 2.20 and 2.21. Gauthier, *Active Voluntary Euthanasia, Terminal Sedation, and Assisted Suicide*, 12 J. Clinical Ethics 43, 43-44, 49 (2001).

Journal 2001 Examines the role of telemedicine in end-of-life decision-making. Concludes that telemedicine should not be used as a substitute for face-to-face discussions, but as a method to supplement such discussions with input from other experienced clinicians. Cites Opinion 2.20. Pronovost & Williams, *Telemedicine and End-of-Life Care: What's Wrong With This Picture?* 12 J. Clinical Ethics 64, 68 (2001).

Journal 2001 Discusses the North Carolina case of *In Re Cartrette*, which focuses on a mother's decision to terminate life support for her incompetent daughter, who is neither terminally ill nor in a persistent vegetative state (PVS). Argues against sole reliance on a quality-of-life assessment as a predicate for surrogate decision-making for a patient who has never been competent. Urges adoption of best interests standard. Quotes Opinion 2.20. Sabo, *Limiting a Surrogate's Authority to Terminate Life-Support for an Incompetent Adult*, 79 N. C. L. Rev. 1815, 1815 (2001).

Journal 2000 Examines questions regarding the legality of such practices as voluntary stopping of eating and drinking (VSED), use of risky analgesics, and terminal sedation. Explores the distinctions between physician-assisted suicide and other palliative interventions. Concludes VSED, risky analgesics, and certain types of terminal sedation are lawful and should be made available to dying patients who make informed decisions to accept the risks involved. Quotes Opinions 2.21 and 2.211. Cites Opinions 2.18 and 2.20. Cantor & Thomas, *The Legal Bounds of Physician Conduct Hastening Death*, 48 Buff. L. Rev. 83, 110, 131, 158 (2000).

Journal 2000 Examines various laws associated with physician-assisted suicide, including the Oregon Death with Dignity Act, the Legal Drug Abuse and Prevention Act of 1998, and the Pain Relief Promotion Act of 1999 (PRPA). Argues that the Supreme Court should declare the PRPA unconstitutional. References Opinion 2.20. Fallek, *The Pain Relief Promotion Act: Will It Spell Death to "Death With Dignity" or Is It Unconstitutional?* 27 Fordham Urb. L. J. 1739, 1755 (2000).

Journal 2000 Considers the question of whether physician-assisted suicide and euthanasia should be legalized. Concludes that, under basic moral and common law principles, the intentional taking of human life by a private person is wrong. References Opinions 2.20, 2.21, and 2.211. Gorsuch, *The Right to Assisted Suicide and Euthanasia*, 23 Harv. J. L. & Pub. Pol'y 599, 653, 707 (2000).

Journal 2000 Examines advance directive pregnancy provisions. Discusses the right to refuse medical treatment and the right to terminate pregnancy. Concludes the Minnesota advance directive pregnancy presumption balances the woman's right to terminate a pregnancy and the right to refuse medical treatment with the state interest in potential life. References Opinion 2.20. Jerdee, *Breaking Through the Silence: Minnesota's Pregnancy Presumption and the Right to Refuse Medical Treatment*, 84 Minn. L. Rev. 971, 980 (2000).

Journal 2000 Examines legal and ethical issues bearing upon pain management. Asserts that health care professionals have a legal and ethical duty to relieve pain and suffering of patients whenever possible. Suggests that this duty is legally enforceable. Quotes Principle V and Opinions 2.20 and 9.011. Rich, *A Prescription for the Pain: The Emerging Standard of Care for Pain Management*, 26 Wm. Mitchell L. Rev. 1, 35-36, 85 (2000).

Journal 2000 Examines existing law governing a parent's authority to make health care decisions for a child. Concludes that, consistent with principles of beneficence and autonomy, parents generally should retain their status as primary decision-makers for their children. Cites Opinion 2.20. Rosato, *Using Bioethics Discourse to Determine When Parents Should Make Health Care Decisions for Their Children: Is Deference Justified?* 73 Temp. L. Rev. 1, 40, 44 (2000).

Journal 1999 States that a distrust of the medical profession arose from changes in the health care system and federal law. Explains how legislation may help alleviate some of the distrust. Suggests that people need more access to information about their health plans. References Opinions 2.20 and 2.225. Cerminara, *Protecting Participants in and Beneficiaries of ERISA-Governed Managed Health Care Plans*, 29 U. Mem. L. Rev. 317, 324 (1999).

Journal 1999 Discusses use of the hierarchical decision-making model for end-of-life decisions. Proposes that a consensus-based decision-making model, which synthesizes therapeutic jurisprudence and preventive law, should replace the hierarchical decision-making model. Argues that the consensus-based model would decrease court involvement and advance the interests of those affected by the decision. Quotes Opinion 2.20. Hafemeister, *End-of-Life Decision Making, Therapeutic Jurisprudence, and Preventive Law: Hierarchical v. Consensus-Based Decision-Making Model*, 41 Ariz. L. Rev. 329 (1999).

Journal 1999 States that the Patient Self-Determination Act is the medical field's version of the Miranda warning. Suggests that, although the act is followed, many patients do not understand how to exercise their right to medical self-determination. Argues that informed consent should be required in relation to advance directives. Cites Opinion 2.20. Pope, *The Maladaptation of Miranda to Advance Directives: A Critique of the Implementation of the Patient Self-Determination Act*, 9 Health Matrix 139, 178 (1999).

Journal 1999 Examines legal and policy issues regarding physician-assisted suicide. Distinguishes between refusing treatment and assisted suicide. Concludes that there are too many dangers posed by physician-assisted suicide to warrant legalization. Quotes Opinion 2.211. Cites Opinions 2.20 and 2.21. Pratt, *Too Many Physicians: Physician-Assisted Suicide After Glucksberg/Quill, 9 Alb. L. J. Sci. & Tech. 161, 208 (1999).*

Journal 1999 Evaluates liability theories used in cases alleging failure to follow do-not-resuscitate orders and advance directives. Analyzes the impact of legal liability as a means to ensure compliance with such orders and directives. Concludes that there is an increased need for open communication among physicians, patients, and patients' family members. Quotes Opinion 2.20. Rodriguez, *Suing Health Care Providers for Saving Lives: Liability for Providing Unwanted Life-Sustaining Treatment, 20 J. Legal Med. 1, 62 (1999).*

Journal 1999 Explains the rule of double effect. Distinguishes between assisted suicide and pain control for terminally ill patients. Suggests that the rule of double effect needs to be adequately defined so physicians will understand that they can ethically give terminally ill patients drugs that will alleviate their pain, but that also may hasten their death. Cites Opinion 2.20. Sulmasy & Pellegrino, *The Rule of Double Effect: Clearing Up the Double Talk, 159 Arch. Intern. Med. 545, 550 (1999).*

Journal 1998 Explains that the US Supreme Court's decisions in *Washington* and *Vacco* left the door open for future constitutional challenges regarding the right to physician-assisted suicide. States that the Court did not explicitly deny the existence of a right to physician-assisted suicide. Quotes Opinion 2.20. Cites Opinion 2.211. Cohen, *The Open Door: Will the Right to Die Survive Washington v. Glucksberg and Vacco v. Quill? 16 In Pub. Interest 79, 94 (1998).*

Journal 1998 Describes a survey regarding physician-assisted suicide given to members of the Group for the Advancement of Psychiatry. Discusses the results of the survey, noting that most surveyed psychiatrists oppose assisting patients to die. Cites Opinions 2.06 and 2.20. Kramer, Gruenberg, & Fidler, *Psychiatrists' Attitudes Toward Physician-Assisted Suicide: A Survey, 19 Am. J. Forensic Psychiatry 81, 87, 90 (1998).*

Journal 1998 Discusses legal aspects of physician-assisted suicide. Identifies acceptable end-of-life choices and compares them to physician-assisted suicide. Points out that physician-assisted suicide has the potential for abuse and that safeguards have not been implemented to protect people from that risk. Quotes Opinion 2.211. Cites Opinions 2.20 and 8.08. Mitchell, *Physician-Assisted Suicide: A Survey of the Issues Surrounding Legalization, 74 N. D. L. Rev. 341, 349 (1998).*

Journal 1998 Points out that the court in *Vacco v. Quill* did not reject the practice of physician-assisted suicide and left the subject open for state experimentation. Discusses routes some states have taken regarding assisted suicide. Concludes that access to assisted suicide is outweighed by the risk it will be utilized by depressed and mentally ill people. Quotes Opinions 2.20 and 2.211. Moore, *Physician-Assisted Suicide: Does "The End" Justify the Means? 40 Ariz. L. Rev. 1471, 1472, 1481-82, 1491 (1998).*

Journal 1998 Discusses consequences physician-assisted suicide may have on disabled individuals. Weighs potential benefits and disadvantages stemming from physician-assisted suicide. Concludes that only a small number of people with disabilities would benefit from physician-assisted suicide and that the benefits are outweighed by the risk of abuse. Cites Opinion 2.20. National Council on Disability, *Assisted Suicide: A Disability Perspective, 14 Issues L. & Med. 273, 292 (1998).*

Journal 1998 Observes that the Patient Self-Determination Act does not obligate physicians to discuss advance directives with patients. Explains that physicians may elect not to discuss advance directives with patients because of lack of time and reimbursement for such discussions. Emphasizes that patients, physicians, and health care providers may benefit from advance directives. Quotes Opinion 2.20. Rich, *Advance Directives: The Next Generation, 19 J. Legal Med. 63, 79 (1998).*

Journal 1998 Provides a historical view on parents' rights to make medical decisions for their children. Argues that parents have the right to make medical decisions for their children when the decisions are supported by medical evidence. This right extends to decisions regarding life-sustaining medical treatment. Quotes Opinion 2.20. Walters, *Life-Sustaining Medical Decisions Involving Children: Father Knows Best, 15 T. M. Cooley L. Rev. 115, 128, 138, 151 (1998).*

Journal 1997 Reviews the criminalization of physician-assisted suicide. Discusses informed consent, the double effect, and the right to die. Explains the current state of the law and the position

Illinois has taken. Advocates the adoption of a law authorizing physician-assisted suicide in Illinois. References Opinion 2.20. Comment, *An Illinois Physician-Assisted Suicide Act: A Merciful End to a Terminally Ill Criminal Tradition*, 28 Loy. U. Chi. L. J. 763, 775 (1997).

Journal 1997 Discusses Pennsylvania Supreme Court case of *In Re Fiori*. Explains that the court extended the right to refuse medical treatment to patients in permanent vegetative states. Notes that the court now allows family members to exercise this right on behalf of such patients. Quotes Opinion 2.20. Comment, *Surrogate Health Care Decision Making: The Pennsylvania Supreme Court Recognizes the Right of an Individual in a Permanent Vegetative State to Refuse Life-Sustaining Measures Through a Surrogate Decision Maker*, 35 Duq. L. Rev. 849, 859-60 (1997).

Journal 1997 Discusses goals of care included in advance directives and whether they can be used to predict specific interventions and results. Offers insights provided by survey of physicians at Massachusetts General Hospital. Cites Opinions 2.20 and 2.21. Fischer, Alpert, Stoeckle, & Emanuel, *Can Goals of Care Be Used to Predict Intervention Preferences in an Advance Directive?* 157 Arch. Intern. Med. 801, 807 (1997).

Journal 1997 Examines the evolution of the Indiana health care system. Discusses developments in Indiana jurisprudence regarding the physician-patient relationship. Explores various challenges facing the relationship and recognizes the need for legal rules to help address these challenges. Quotes Opinion 8.08. Cites Opinions 2.20, 9.06, and 9.12. Kinney & Selby, *History and Jurisprudence of the Physician-Patient Relationship in Indiana*, 30 Ind. L. Rev. 263, 269, 272, 276 (1997).

Journal 1996 Proposes a model state statute allowing and controlling physician-assisted suicide. Analyzes the constitutionality of the act and offers public policy justifications for the act's provisions. Concludes that proponents of physician-assisted suicide should provide precise, carefully tailored examples of regulations. Quotes Opinion 2.211. Cites Opinion 2.20. Baron, Bergstresser, Brock, Cole, Dorfman, Johnson, Schnipper, Vorenberg, & Wanzer, *A Model State Act to Authorize and Regulate Physician-Assisted Suicide*, 33 Harv. J. Legis. 1, 2, 7 (1996).

Journal 1996 Explores the issue of legalizing physician-assisted suicide. Opines that the current state of technology increases life expectancy but with a concomitant decrease in dignity and autonomy surrounding one's death. Notes that the elderly are committing suicide at an increasing rate. Cites Opinions 2.20, 2.21, and 2.211. Morgan & Sutherland, *Last Rights? Confronting Physician-Assisted Suicide in Law and Society: Legal Liturgies on Physician-Assisted Suicide*, 26 Stetson L. Rev. 481, 484 (1996).

Journal 1996 Considers the right to death with dignity. Suggests that the AMA's position undermines mitigation of suffering and the individuals' right to self-determination. Concludes that restrictions on the right to death with dignity may be constitutionally impermissible. Quotes Opinion 2.211. Cites Opinion 2.20. Note, *Who Decides if There Is Triumph in the Ultimate Agony? Constitutional Theory and the Emerging Right to Die With Dignity*, 37 Wm. & Mary L. Rev. 827, 829 (1996).

Journal 1996 Discusses the physician's duty to relieve pain. Considers current attitudes toward pain management. Concludes that, consistent with principles of beneficence, physicians are obligated to provide pain relief and palliation. Quotes Opinion 2.20. Post, Blustein, Gordon, & Dubler, *Pain: Ethics, Culture, and Informed Consent to Relief*, 24 J. Law Med. & Ethics 348, 349, 356 (1996).

Journal 1996 Discusses children's rights to consent to or refuse life-sustaining medical treatment. Compares the rights of children to those of adults in a medical decision-making context. Proposes reforms to allow minors legal rights to make decisions regarding withdrawal of life-sustaining treatment. Quotes Opinion 2.20. Rosato, *The Ultimate Test of Autonomy: Should Minors Have a Right to Make Decisions Regarding Life-Sustaining Treatment?* 49 Rutgers L. Rev. 1, 80-81, 82 (1996).

Journal 1995 Explores reluctance of long-term care facilities to allow patients to forgo life-sustaining tube feeding. Concludes that policies must be adopted to ensure that patients' rights to refuse artificial nutrition and hydration are protected. Cites Opinion 2.20. Meisel, *Barriers to Forgoing Nutrition and Hydration in Nursing Homes*, XXI Am. J. Law & Med. 335, 353-54 (1995).

Journal 1995 Examines the problem of determining when a patient has lost decision-making capacity. Compares the authority of the treating physician with that of the patient's designated agent in making such a determination. Cites Opinion 2.20. Schneiderman, Teetzel, & Kalmanson, *Who Decides Who Decides? When Disagreement Occurs Between the Physician and the*

Patient's Appointed Proxy About the Patient's Decision-Making Capacity, 155 Arch. Intern. Med. 793, 796 (1995).

Journal 1995 Offers relevant historical perspectives and provides comprehensive ethical and legal discussion of physician-assisted suicide and euthanasia. Highlights important legislative developments, including the Oregon Death with Dignity Act, and analyzes significant judicial opinions. Quotes Principles III, IV, and VI and Opinions 2.21 and 9.12. Cites Opinions 2.20 and 8.11. Stone & Winslade, *Physician-Assisted Suicide and Euthanasia in the United States: Legal and Ethical Observations*, 16 J. Legal Med. 481, 483, 490, 497, 498, 499 (1995).

Journal 1994 Considers how greater patient autonomy has led to situations in which medical care may be viewed as futile. Suggests that the law has intruded too far into this area of medicine. Quotes Opinion 2.035. Cites Opinions 2.03, 2.095, 2.17, 2.19, 2.20, and 2.22. Cultice, *Medical Futility: When Is Enough, Enough?* 27 J. Health & Hosp. Law 225, 230, 256 (1994).

Journal 1994 Discusses whether a patient's prior expression of treatment choices in an advance directive accurately represents future choices. Concludes that patients are capable of making stable scenario- and treatment-specific advance directives, that their choices become more stable with repeated consideration, and that illness has little effect on stability of choices. Cites Opinion 2.20. Emanuel, Emanuel, Stoeckle, Hummel, & Barry, *Advance Directives: Stability of Patients' Treatment Choices*, 154 Arch. Intern. Med. 209, 217 (1994).

Journal 1994 Analyzes physicians' attitudes about whether to initiate or withhold tube feeding when patients' preferences are unknown. Concludes that patient prognosis and quality of life are the most important influences on physician decisions about tube feeding. Cites Opinion 2.20. Hodges, Tolle, Stocking, & Cassel, *Tube Feeding: Internists' Attitudes Regarding Ethical Obligations*, 154 Arch. Intern. Med. 1013, 1020 (1994).

Journal 1994 Examines the various types of advance health care directives and reviews pertinent Arkansas law. Concludes that directives should conform to each person's values, health status, and medical prognosis. Cites Opinion 2.20. Leflar, *Advance Health Care Directives Under Arkansas Law*, 1994 Ark. L. Notes 37, 42.

Journal 1994 Examines how state laws have accommodated medical developments in the area of treatment decisions and how they serve to resolve and encourage conflict in health care decision-making. Considers the roles of physicians, hospitals, and families and how their wishes may conflict with those of the patient. Cites Opinion 2.20. Tarantino, *Withdrawal of Life Support: Conflict Among Patient Wishes, Family, Physicians, Courts and Statutes, and the Law*, 42 Buff. L. Rev. 623, 638, 639, 646 (1994).

Journal 1994 Determines that physicians are not taking the responsibility for initiating discussions about end-of-life medical treatment and that many patients falsely assume that their physicians would know what kind of treatments they would want. Concludes that physician-patient communication is improved slightly when there is an advance directive, but that there is still a lack of detailed discussion about end-of-life treatments. Cites Opinion 2.20. Virmani, Schneiderman, & Kaplan, *Relationship of Advance Directives to Physician-Patient Communication*, 154 Arch. Intern. Med. 909, 913 (1994).

Journal 1993 Analyzes the implications of giving patients and their families an absolute right to control medical treatment. Argues that courts should refrain from ordering physicians to treat patients when physicians believe that treatment would be ineffective. Quotes Fundamental Elements (5) and Opinions 2.11 (1982) [now Opinion 2.20] and 2.18 (1986) [now Opinion 2.20]. Comment, *Beyond Autonomy: Judicial Restraint and the Legal Limits Necessary to Uphold the Hippocratic Tradition and Preserve the Ethical Integrity of the Medical Profession*, 9 J. Contemp. Health L. & Pol'y 451, 467, 468 (1993).

Journal 1993 Discusses Ohio's living will statute in light of the Cruzan decision. Presents the medical implications of the persistent vegetative state patient. Quotes Opinion 2.18 (1986) [now Opinion 2.20]. Comment, *One Step Forward, Two Steps Back: A Constitutional and Critical Look at Ohio's New Living Will Statute*, 54 Ohio St. L. J. 445, 447, 460, 470 (1993).

Journal 1993 Discusses the problem of physicians withholding needed medical treatment from HIV-infected infants. Concludes that current law should be expanded to eliminate this discrimination. Quotes Opinions 2.09, 2.17, 2.20, 2.22, 4.04, and 8.03. Crossley, *Of Diagnoses and Discrimination: Discriminatory Nontreatment of Infants With HIV Infection*, 93 Columbia L. Rev. 1581, 1620, 1621 (1993).

Journal 1993 Discusses the relationship between a physician's professional conscience and end of life decision-making. Considers the issue of futile medical treatment. Examines case law concerning a patient's right to demand treatment and a physician's obligation to provide it. References Opinions 2.20 and 2.22. Daar, *A Clash at the Bedside: Patient Autonomy v. a Physician's Professional Conscience, 44 Hastings L. J. 1241, 1257, 1268, 1286 (1993).*

Journal 1993 Argues that society should not permit euthanasia because of lack of protection against potential abuses. Recommends that health care providers be taught to treat pain and more effectively care for dying patients, rather than to affirmatively end life. Quotes Opinions 2.17 and 2.20. Dickey, *Euthanasia: A Concept Whose Time Has Come? 8 Issues in Law & Med. 521, 523, 524 (1993).*

Journal 1993 Discusses the legal distinction between "the right to die" and physician-assisted suicide. Examines how the law is applied and whether it should be reformed in light of public opinion and changing ethical standards. References Opinion 2.20. Gostin, *Drawing a Line Between Killing and Letting Die: The Law, and Law Reform, on Medically Assisted Dying, 21 J. Law Med. & Ethics 94, 98 (1993).*

Journal 1993 Considers how life-sustaining treatments have led to prolonged life under unacceptable circumstances. Recommends quality assurance programs that promote discussion between physicians and patients regarding life-sustaining treatment problems. Cites Opinions 2.20 and 2.21. Pearlman, Cain, Patrick, Appelbaum-Maizel, Starks, Jecker, & Uhlmann, *Insights Pertaining to Patient Assessments of States Worse Than Death, 4 J. Clinical Ethics 33, 40 (1993).*

Journal 1993 Considers whether criminal penalties should be imposed on a physician who assists in the suicide of a competent, nonterminal patient who requested such assistance. Presents the arguments for and against active euthanasia, with emphasis on the "slippery slope" argument. References Opinions 2.06 and 2.20. Persels, *Forcing the Issue of Physician-Assisted Suicide: Impact of the Kevorkian Case on the Euthanasia Debate, 14 J. Legal Med. 93, 115 (1993).*

Journal 1993 Discusses legal and ethical issues raised by physician aid-in-dying. Concludes that passive euthanasia for competent, terminal adults is the accepted norm and physician aid-in-dying is the new frontier. Quotes Opinion 2.18 (1986) [now Opinion 2.20]. Risley, *Ethical and Legal Issues in the Individual's Right to Die, 20 Ohio N. U. L. Rev. 597, 605 (1993).*

Journal 1992 Considers when it is appropriate to withdraw artificial food and nutrition from an incompetent patient under the Indiana "Living Wills" statute. Concludes that, in Indiana, it is appropriate to remove artificial nutrition and hydration that only "prolongs the dying process." Quotes Opinion 2.20. Anderson, *A Medical-Legal Dilemma: When Can "Inappropriate" Nutrition and Hydration Be Removed in Indiana? 67 Ind. L. J. 479, 480 (1992).*

Journal 1992 Analyzes the arguments for and against active euthanasia, including ethical concerns, the slippery slope argument, and the proper role of the physician. Suggests that active euthanasia may be acceptable when its administration is restricted to physicians. References Opinions 2.20 and 2.21. Brock, *Voluntary Active Euthanasia, 22 Hastings Center Rep. 10 (March/April 1992).*

Journal 1992 Examines several issues regarding persistent vegetative state (PVS) patients, including whether PVS patients are really dead, whether nutrition and hydration should be withheld, whether life-sustaining treatments are futile or medically inappropriate, and whether ordinary standards for decision-making should be applied to PVS patients. Concludes that life-sustaining therapy may be withheld or continued, but that withdrawal of nutrition and hydration, as well as active euthanasia, present more difficult questions. References Opinions 2.20 and 2.22. Brody, *Special Ethical Issues in the Management of PVS Patients, 20 Law Med. & Health Care 104, 109 (1992).*

Journal 1992 Examines ethical and legal issues surrounding cardiopulmonary resuscitation and emergency cardiac care. Discusses advance directives and proxy decision-making, medical futility, resource allocation, and do-not-resuscitate orders. References Opinions 2.20 and 2.22. Comment, *Ethical Considerations in Resuscitation, 268 JAMA 2282, 2283, 2287 (1992).*

Journal 1992 Defines the right of terminally ill, competent patients to die with the assistance of a physician and argues that it is essentially the same as the right to die by refusing life-sustaining medical treatment. Concludes that courts should balance patients' rights with compelling state interests in assessing the scope of this right. Cites Opinion 2.20. Comment, *Physician Assisted Suicide and the Right to Die With Assistance, 105 Harvard L. Rev. 2021, 2027, 2035 (1992).*

Journal 1992 Discusses the Iowa living will statute, comparing it to similar laws in other states. Proposes a revised statute to address problems arising in light of recent court decisions. References Opinion 2.20. Goldman, *Revising Iowa's Life-Sustaining Procedures Act: Creating a Practical Guide to Living Wills in Iowa*, 76 Iowa L. Rev. 1137, 1149 (1992).

Journal 1992 Explores various health policy issues addressed by the Indiana state legislature. Considers Indiana lawmakers' responses to the following concerns: health care access, tort reform, the right to die, Medicaid reimbursements, and discrimination against AIDS patients. Cites Opinion 2.18 (1986) [now Opinion 2.20]. Kumar & Kinney, *Indiana Lawmakers Face National Health Policy Issues*, 25 Indiana L. Rev. 1271, 1275, 1276 (1992).

Journal 1992 Discusses the need for a policy governing life-sustaining treatment decisions for incompetent adult wards of the state. Provides a basic outline for such a policy and proposes a model policy statement. Quotes Opinion 2.20. McKnight & Bollis, *Foregoing Life-Sustaining Treatment for Adult Developmentally Disabled, Public Wards: A Proposed Statute*, XVIII Am. J. Law & Med. 203, 206, 220, 227 (1992).

Journal 1992 Observes that the fundamental question in *Cruzan* was whether there should be judicial oversight regarding decisions to forgo life-sustaining treatment. Concludes that *Cruzan* did not resolve this issue. Cites Opinion 2.18 (1986) [now Opinion 2.20]. Meisel, *A Retrospective on Cruzan*, 20 Law Med. & Health Care 340, 345 (1992).

Journal 1992 Explores evolution of the legal consensus that terminating life support is legitimate under some circumstances. Suggests that the consensus will continue to spread in the absence of opposition and may extend to mercy killing and futility cases. Quotes Opinion 2.18 (1986) [now Opinion 2.20]. Meisel, *The Legal Consensus About Forgoing Life-Sustaining Treatment: Its Status and Its Prospects*, 2 Kennedy Inst. Ethics J. 309, 325 (1992).

Journal 1992 Considers the debate surrounding medical futility. Observes that this debate is encouraging reexamination of the nature of patient entitlement to medical care as well as the "ends of medicine." References Opinions 2.20, 2.21, and 2.22. Miles, *Medical Futility*, 20 Law Med. & Health Care 310, 311, 313 (1992).

Journal 1992 Analyzes North Carolina's living will and health care power of attorney statutes in light of the *Cruzan* case. Notes recent changes to both statutes and problems that continue to exist. Quotes Opinion 2.21 (1992) [now Opinion 2.20]. Note, *Exercising the Right to Die: North Carolina's Amended Natural Death Act and the 1991 Health Care Power of Attorney Act*, 70 No. Carolina L. Rev. 2108, 2116 (1992).

Journal 1992 Explains how the "terminal condition" requirement in natural death acts may reduce the number of people who fall within the scope of coverage. Also indicates that omission of nutrition and hydration from the list of treatments that may be withdrawn limits patient choices. Quotes Opinion 2.20. References Opinion 2.22. Note, *State Natural Death Acts: Illusory Protection of Individuals' Life-Sustaining Treatment Decisions*, 29 Harvard J. Legis. 175, 186, 194, 195, 201 (1992).

Journal 1992 Discusses the impact of physicians' values on end-of-life decision making for patients. Examines how and why physician values may become dominant. References Opinions 2.20, 2.22, and 9.121. Orentlicher, *The Illusion of Patient Choice in End-Of-Life Decisions*, 267 JAMA 2101, 2102 (1992).

Journal 1992 Contrasts physician-assisted suicide and voluntary euthanasia. Recommends legalization of physician-assisted suicide and proposes guidelines for implementation. References Opinion 2.20. Quill, Cassel, & Meier, *Care of the Hopelessly Ill: Proposed Clinical Criteria for Physician-Assisted Suicide*, 327 New Eng. J. Med. 1380, 1381 (1992).

Journal 1992 Suggests that triage and cost-benefit analysis are the most effective means to evaluate issues associated with allocating scarce medical resources to disabled infants. Concludes both that selective treatment can never be considered murder and that governmental intrusion in this area should be minimal. Quotes Opinions 2.10 (1982) [now Opinion 2.17] and 2.18 (1986) [now Opinion 2.20]. Smith, *Murder, She Wrote or Was It Merely Selective Nontreatment?* 8 J. Contemp. Health L. & Pol'y 49, 53 (1992).

Journal 1991 Discusses the manner in which competent and incompetent patients could exercise the right to refuse life-sustaining medical treatment prior to *Cruzan*. Analyzes the effect *Cruzan* had on these rights. Concludes that *Cruzan* had limited far-reaching impact and failed to answer several important questions. Cites Opinion 2.20. Albert, *Cruzan v. Director, Missouri Department of Health: Too Much Ado, 12 J. Legal Med. 331, 338, 343 (1991).*

Journal 1991 Discusses why families of persistent vegetative state patients should not make decisions regarding whether to withdraw life support. Observes that leaving decisions to families creates the possibility they will decide in opposition of the patient. References Opinion 2.20. Baron, *Why Withdrawal of Life-Support for PVS Patients Is Not a Family Decision, 19 Law Med. & Health Care 73 (1991).*

Journal 1991 Considers the issue of how courts should decide right-to-die cases in Massachusetts. Concludes that there are no clear standards for physicians to follow and recommends that physicians obtain court approval before withdrawing artificial nutrition and hydration from a patient in a persistent vegetative state. Quotes Opinion 2.20. Comment, *A Right to Die: Can a Massachusetts Physician Withdraw Artificial Nutrition and Hydration From a Persistently Vegetative Patient Following Cruzan v. Director, Missouri Department of Health? 26 New Eng. L. Rev. 199, 216, 220 (1991).*

Journal 1991 Discusses major neurologic syndromes in life-sustaining medical treatment decisions. Concludes with a survey of the major legal developments in the area since *Cruzan*. References Opinion 2.20. Cranford, *Neurologic Syndromes and Prolonged Survival: When Can Artificial Nutrition and Hydration Be Foregone? 19 Law Med. & Health Care 13, 14, 16, 17 (1991).*

Journal 1991 Reports that most individuals surveyed favor use of advance directives and would not desire life-sustaining treatment if faced with a poor prognosis. Recommends that physicians routinely discuss advance directives with patients. Cites Opinion 2.20. Emanuel, Barry, Stoeckle, Ettelson, & Emanuel, *Advance Directives for Medical Care—A Case for Greater Use, 324 New Eng. J. Med. 889 (1991).*

Journal 1991 Discusses the "slippery slope" argument against expanding the right to die. Concludes that society seems to be sliding down the slippery slope toward euthanasia. Cites Opinion 2.18 (1986) [now Opinion 2.20]. Kamisar, *When Is There A Constitutional "Right to Die?" When Is There No Constitutional "Right to Live?" 25 Georgia L. Rev. 1203, 1207, 1208, 1222 (1991).*

Journal 1991 Discusses common misperceptions about legal implications of terminating life support. Emphasizes importance of educating physicians about these medical-legal considerations. References Opinion 2.20. Meisel, *Legal Myths About Terminating Life Support, 151 Arch. Intern. Med. 1497, 1499 (1991).*

Journal 1991 Discusses health care decision-making for terminally ill incompetent patients in Ohio. Argues that Ohio is one of the few remaining states that does not adequately protect the rights of incompetent terminally ill patients. Cites Opinion 2.18 (1986) [now Opinion 2.20]. Mullins, *The Need for Guidance in Decisionmaking for Terminally Ill Incompetents: Is the Ohio Legislature in a "Persistent Vegetative State?" 17 Ohio No. Univ. L. Rev. 827, 844 (1991).*

Journal 1991 Discusses the major issues contained in the *Cruzan* decision. Analyzes the legal predicates for an incompetent patient's right to refuse life-sustaining treatment. References Opinion 2.20. Note, *Cruzan v. Director, Missouri Department of Health: To Die or Not to Die: That Is the Question—But Who Decides? 51 Louisiana L. Rev. 1307, 1327, 1333 (1991).*

Journal 1991 Explores the growth of "right to die" jurisprudence with particular emphasis on post-*Cruzan* developments. Notes that the New York "Health Care Proxy Law" does not apply to situations in which a patient is incompetent, but did not appoint an agent. References Opinion 2.20. Note, *Health Care Proxies: New York's Attempt to Resolve the Right to Die Dilemma, 57 Brooklyn L. Rev. 145, 168 (1991).*

Journal 1991 Analyzes the Illinois Supreme Court case of *In re Estate of Longeway*, where the court decided that, absent an advance directive, the guardian of an incompetent patient could authorize the withdrawal of artificial nutrition and hydration. Concludes that written directives other than living wills may best secure patients' rights. Cites Opinion 2.18 (1986) [now Opinion 2.20]. Note, *Redefining the Right to Die in Illinois, 15 So. Ill. Univ. L. J. 1261, 1273 (1991).*

Journal 1991 Discusses applicable law regarding patients in a persistent vegetative state. Compares *Cruzan* with other right-to-die cases, arguing that the *Cruzan* decision makes it more difficult for individuals to secure this right. Quotes Opinion 2.20. Note, *Something Worth Writing Home About: Clear and Convincing Evidence, Living Wills, and Cruzan v. Director, Missouri Department of Health, 22 Univ. Toledo L. Rev. 871, 879 (1991).*

Journal 1991 Examines the living will and durable power of attorney as health care planning devices in South Carolina. Considers both statutory and nonstatutory forms of the living will. References Opinion 2.20. Patterson, *Planning for Health Care Using Living Wills and Durable Powers of Attorney: A Guide for the South Carolina Attorney, 42 So. Carolina L. Rev. 525, 535, 541, 547, 548 (1991).*

Journal 1991 Explains the contractual nature of the physician-patient relationship and how it has been ignored by many courts in right-to-die cases. Concludes there is a constitutional right to privacy in health care decision-making. Cites Opinion 2.18 (1986) [now Opinion 2.20]. Rich, *The Assault on Privacy on Healthcare Decisionmaking, 68 Denver L. Rev. 1, 10 (1991).*

Journal 1991 Considers the limits of patient autonomy in demanding treatment that the physician feels provides no medical benefit. Discusses these issues in light of the Helga Wanglie case. References Opinion 2.20. Rie, *The Limits of a Wish, 21 Hastings Center Rep. 24 (July/August 1991).*

Journal 1991 Analyzes three important right-to-die cases: *Cruzan, Wanglie,* and *Busalacchi.* Concludes that there should be a nationwide system to address right-to-die cases. References Opinion 2.20. Roach, *Paradox and Pandora's Box: The Tragedy of Current Right-to-Die Jurisprudence, 25 Univ. Mich. J. Law Reform 133, 137, 158 (1991).*

Journal 1990 Argues that *Roe v. Wade* not only protects a woman's right to choose, but also preserves a physician's right to treat. Observes that this protected relationship extends into the arena of right-to-die cases. Cites Opinion 2.20. Annas, Glantz, & Mariner, *The Right of Privacy Protects the Doctor-Patient Relationship, 263 JAMA 858, 861 (1990).*

Journal 1990 Discusses the connection between law and medicine in the context of health care decision-making. Presents several illustrations, noting the involvement of courts and judges. Quotes Opinion 2.18 [now Opinion 2.20]. Bellacosa, *The Fusion of Medicine and Law for In Extremis Health and Medical Decisions: Does It Produce Energy and Light or Just Cosmic Debris? 18 Bull. Am. Acad. Psychiatry Law 5, 9 (1990).*

Journal 1990 Finds that a vast majority of North Carolina nursing homes have written cardio-pulmonary resuscitation policies, but that there is substantial variation among them. Concludes that such variations risk limiting or ignoring the personal rights of residents. References Opinions 2.20 and 2.22. Brunetti, Weiss, Studenski, & Clipp, *Cardiopulmonary Resuscitation Policies and Practices: A Statewide Nursing Home Study, 150 Arch. Intern. Med. 121, 122 (1990).*

Journal 1990 Discusses the importance of living wills and society's acceptance of terminating medical care in appropriate situations. Proposes a living will that addresses the shortcomings of current living will statutes. Cites Opinion 2.18 (1986) [now Opinion 2.20]. Cantor, *My Annotated Living Will, 18 Law Med. & Health Care 114 (1990).*

Journal 1990 Discusses the "living will" and its role in American society. Concludes that legislators need to be more aware of the goals of living wills when drafting statutes. Quotes Opinion 2.20. Comment, *The Living Will: Preservation of the Right-To-Die Demands Clarity and Consistency, 95 Dickinson L. Rev. 209, 217 (1990).*

Journal 1990 Explores current law governing the right of a person to withdraw artificial hydration and nutrition, with emphasis on Oklahoma law, which omits artificial nutrition and hydration from the list of treatments that may be withdrawn. Concludes that individuals have a right to withdraw such treatment and that Oklahoma law may be unconstitutional. Quotes Opinion 2.18 (1986) [now Opinion 2.20]. Comment, *Right to Die: Oklahoma's Position on Nutrition and Hydration: Confusing or Unconstitutional? 43 Okla. L. Rev. 143, 151 (1990).*

Journal 1990 Examines the right of competent patients to refuse treatment on the basis of a common law right of bodily integrity, the right to privacy, and statutory provisions such as natural death acts. Concludes that the law is unsettled with respect to the right of incompetent, nonterminal patients to refuse medical care. Quotes Opinion 2.18 (1986) [now Opinion 2.20]. Comment, *The Right to Refuse Life Sustaining Medical Treatment and the Nonterminally Ill Patient: An Analysis of Abridgment and Anarchy, 17 Pepperdine L. Rev. 461, 462 (1990).*

Journal 1990 Discusses how the imprecise language of euthanasia muddles public discussion of the issue. Concludes that medical ethics must distinguish between acts and omissions undertaken to cause death and those considered reasonable treatment under the circumstances. Quotes Opinion 2.20 (1989). Devettere, *The Imprecise Language of Euthanasia and Causing Death, 1 J. Clinical Ethics 268, 268 (1990).*

Journal 1990 Discusses the proposition that an objective standard should govern end-of-life decision-making instead of living wills or similar instruments. Concludes that an objective standard is preferable and recommends that courts adopt such a standard. References Opinion 2.20. Dresser, *Relitigating Life and Death, 51 Ohio St. L. J. 425, 436 (1990).*

Journal 1990 Discusses the development of the law regarding the withdrawal of life-sustaining medical treatment from incompetent patients since the *Quinlan* case. Concludes that *Cruzan* did not resolve a number of important questions concerning the right to die. Quotes Opinion 2.18 (1986) [now Opinion 2.20]. McNoble, *The Cruzan Decision—A Surgeon's Perspective, 20 Memphis State Univ. L. Rev. 569, 581, 600, 601 (1990).*

Journal 1990 Considers how the case may be misperceived. Proposes that health care professionals should routinely advise patients of the necessity of making their wishes about life-sustaining treatment known. Quotes Opinion 2.18 (1986) [now Opinion 2.20]. Meisel, *Lessons From Cruzan, 1 J. Clinical Ethics 245, 248 (1990).*

Journal 1990 Discusses the right of physicians to refrain from participating in the withdrawal or removal of life-sustaining treatment. Concludes that federal and state legislation is needed to protect the right of conscience of medical personnel in this context. Quotes Opinion 2.20. Note, *I Have A Conscience, Too: The Plight of Medical Personnel Confronting the Right to Die, 65 Notre Dame L. Rev. 699, 706 (1990).*

Journal 1990 Discusses advance medical directives including living wills and durable powers of attorney. Concludes by examining the physician's role in implementing patient preferences. Cites Opinion 2.20. Orentlicher, *Advance Medical Directives, 263 JAMA 2365 (1990).*

Journal 1990 Discusses the moral dilemma in deciding whether to withdraw artificial nutrition and hydration from a patient and the appropriate role of the judiciary. Concludes that judicial decisions do not represent the moral viewpoint of society and that moral pronouncements should not be made in the courtroom. Quotes Preamble, Principles I, II, III, IV, V, VI, and VII, and Opinion 2.20. Peccarelli, *A Moral Dilemma: The Role of Judicial Intervention in Withholding or Withdrawing Nutrition and Hydration, 23 John Marshall L. Rev. 537, 539, 540, 541 (1990).*

Journal 1990 Explores how recent advances in medical science and technology have resulted in changing views concerning withdrawing and withholding of life support. Concludes that morality plays a key role in dealing with this issue and that physicians should rely upon fundamental principles of medicine for guidance. Quotes Opinion 2.20. Sprung, *Changing Attitudes and Practices in Forgoing Life-Sustaining Treatments, 263 JAMA 2211, 2213 (1990).*

Journal 1990 Looks into the appropriateness of terminating life-prolonging treatment for patients lacking decision-making abilities. Concludes that physicians do not risk serious liability for withdrawing life support. References Opinion 2.20. Weir & Gostin, *Decisions to Abate Life-Sustaining Treatment for Nonautonomous Patients: Ethical Standards and Legal Liability for Physicians After Cruzan, 264 JAMA 1846, 1849, 1850 (1990).*

Journal 1989 Challenges the notion that removal of artificial nutrition from permanently unconscious patients constitutes active euthanasia. Concludes by observing that the traditional judicial approach, which permits withdrawal of artificial nutrition, is entirely consistent with accepted medical, legal, and ethical doctrines. Cites Opinion 2.18 (1986) [now Opinion 2.20]. Cantor, *The Permanently Unconscious Patient, Non-Feeding and Euthanasia, XV Am. J. Law & Med. 381, 385 (1989).*

Journal 1989 Examines and criticizes the legal advice that was rendered by hospital counsel in the context of the Samuel Linares case which occurred at Rush-Presbyterian-St. Luke's Medical Center in Chicago, Illinois. Focusing on such issues as whether forgoing ventilator assistance constitutes murder or child abuse and neglect, concludes that ultraconservative legal advice led to moral paralysis, thereby precipitating the tragic and unnecessary action of the child's father. References Opinion 2.20. Nelson & Cranford, *Legal Advice, Moral Paralysis and the Death of Samuel Linares, 17 Law Med. & Health Care 316, 319 (1989).*

Journal 1989 Observes that, while new policies regarding physician care of hopelessly ill patients have developed, there is a significant gap between development and implementation of those policies. Urges that this gap be closed and that an overall doctrine of flexible care be developed. References Opinion 2.20. Wanzer, Federman, Adelstein, Cassel, Cassem, Cranford, Hook, Lo, Moertel, Safar, Stone, & Van Eys, *The Physician's Responsibility Toward Hopelessly Ill Patients: A Second Look, 320 New Eng. J. Med. 844, 844 (1989).*

Journal 1988 Considers and challenges certain presumed implications of the definition of *death* as brain death. Points to the importance of the distinction between death of the person as contrasted with death of the body. References Opinion 2.18 (1986) [now Opinion 2.20]. Brody, *Ethical Questions Raised by the Persistent Vegetative Patient*, 18 Hastings Center Rep. 33, 34 (Feb./ March 1988).

Journal 1988 Explores the revitalization of the hospice concept and the various structural models available for providing care to the terminally ill. Examines the cost-effectiveness of hospice care, including withholding or withdrawing life-prolonging medical treatment. References Opinion 2.18 (1986) [now Opinion 2.20]. Comment, *The Hospice Movement: A Renewed View of the Death Process*, 4 J. Contemp. Health L. & Pol'y 295, 312 (1988).

Journal 1988 Focuses on the issue of removal of life-sustaining medical treatment from incompetent patients whose wishes are unknown. The importance of quality-of-life considerations as an aspect of surrogate decision-making in this context is emphasized. References Opinion 2.18 (1986) [now Opinion 2.20]. Quinn, *The Best Interests of Incompetent Patients: The Capacity for Interpersonal Relationships as a Standard for Decisionmaking*, 76 Cal. L. Rev. 897, 906 (1988).

Journal 1988 Examines the meaning and scope of the phrase *artificial feeding*, the distinction between ordinary and extraordinary care, and the impact of medical condition and competency on the patient's right to refuse treatment. Concludes that the value of patient autonomy is not the controlling factor in such cases, but only one factor that must be balanced against the nature and probable results of the proposed treatment. Quotes Opinion 2.18 (1986) [now Opinion 2.20]. Snyder, *Artificial Feeding and the Right to Die: The Legal Issues*, 9 J. Legal Med. 349, 351, 352, 357 (1988).

Journal 1988 Discusses numerous judicial decisions in which the courts have focused, among other things, on the withdrawal of artificial feeding from incompetent adult patients. Practical suggestions are offered to caregivers and relevant policy implications and other unresolved issues are addressed. Quotes from Opinion 2.18 (1986) [now Opinion 2.20]. Steinbrook & Lo, *Artificial Feeding Solid Ground, Not a Slippery Slope*, 318 New Eng. J. Med. 286, 288 (1988).

Journal 1988 Discusses moral justification for limited respirator use in prolonging anencephalic infants as organ donors for neonates, problems in determining brain death, and the need for additional research relative to anencephalic newborns. Ethical justifications for withdrawal of artificial life support from adult patients who are permanently comatose are offered, by way of analogy, for the purpose of demonstrating the ethical and medical propriety of attaching volunteered, select anencephalic infants to respirators in an effort to obtain scarce organs. Cites Opinion 2.18 (1986) [now Opinion 2.20]. Walters & Ashwal, *Organ Prolongation in Anencephalic Infants: Ethical and Medical Issues*, 18 Hastings Center Rep. 19, 21 (Oct./Nov. 1988).

Journal 1987 Focuses on the issue of withholding nutrition and hydration from comatose patients with emphasis on the questions of what constitutes medical treeatment and when it may properly be withheld. Briefly discusses the often cited cases that have addressed these issues, noting the importance of the position of the AMA regarding withholding or withdrawing life-prolonging medical treatment. References Opinion 2.18 (1986) [now Opinion 2.20]. Comment, *Hold on Courts: May a Comatose Patient Be Denied Food and Water*, 31 St. Louis Univ. L. J. 749, 750 (1987).

Journal 1987 Following comprehensive analysis of existing common law, notes a trend toward granting families greater autonomy in making decisions for incompetent adult patients. Supports this trend and advocates recognition of a more prominent role for the family in these situations. References Opinion 2.18 (1986) [now Opinion 2.20]. Comment, *The Role of the Family in Medical Decisionmaking for Incompetent Adult Patients: A Historical Perspective and Case Analysis*, 48 U. Pittsburgh L. Rev. 539, 571, 607, 610-11 (1987).

Journal 1986 Discusses the distinction between the persistent vegetative state and coma, pointing out the confusion of these concepts in various leading right-to-die cases. Addresses philosophical and ethical predicates for withholding treatment noting that, in the final analysis, a balancing of the benefits and burdens of treatment should involve the patient, the family, and the physician. Cites Opinion 2.11 (1981) [now Opinion 2.20]. Berrol, *Considerations for Management of the Persistent Vegetative State*, 67 Arch. Phys. Med. Rehabil. 283, 285 (1986).

Journal 1986 Observes that life-sustaining medical treatment includes artificial nutrition and hydration and that patients have a right to forgo such treatment under the Washington State

Constitution, applicable common law, and the Washington Natural Death Act. Notes that available judicial standards for surrogate decision-making in this context are inadequate, and proposes substantive guidelines for the making of such decisions. References Opinion 2.18 (1986) [now Opinion 2.20]. Comment, *Artificial Nutrition and the Terminally Ill: How Should Washington Decide? 61 Wash. L. Rev. 419, 421, 447 (1986).*

Journal 1986 Analyzes the law's approach to death by evaluating various legal issues that arise in the context of efforts to define death. Asserts that neocortical death should be viewed as death of the person for all legal purposes. References Opinion 2.18 (1986) [now Opinion 2.20]. Smith, *Legal Recognition of Neocortical Death, 71 Cornell L. Rev. 850, 860, 876-77 (1986).*

Journal 1985 Focuses on the issue of withholding medical care and treatment from infants for whom there is little reasonable expectation of normal development. Urges that parents should assume principal decision-making responsibility and offers framework for limited state intervention. References Opinion 2.18 (1986) [now Opinion 2.20]. Haddon, *Baby Doe Cases: Compromise and Moral Dilemma, 34 Emory L. J. 545, 556 (1985).*

Journal 1984 Evaluates two divergent approaches to the legal treatment of withdrawing nourishment. Favors the patient's rights to privacy and to treatment as the primary factors in resolving the issue of withdrawing nourishment. Quotes Opinion 2.11 (1982) [now Opinion 2.20]. Horan & Grant, *The Legal Aspects of Withdrawing Nourishment, 5 J. Legal Med. 595, 626 (1984).*

2.201 Sedation to Unconsciousness in End-of-Life Care

The duty to relieve pain and suffering is central to the physician's role as healer and is an obligation physicians have to their patients. Palliative sedation to unconsciousness is the administration of sedative medication to the point of unconsciousness in a terminally ill patient. It is an intervention of last resort to reduce severe, refractory pain or other distressing clinical symptoms that do not respond to aggressive symptom-specific palliation. It is an accepted and appropriate component of end-of-life care under specific, relatively rare circumstances. When symptoms cannot be diminished through all other means of palliation, including symptom-specific treatments, it is the ethical obligation of a physician to offer palliative sedation to unconsciousness as an option for the relief of intractable symptoms. When considering the use of palliative sedation, the following ethical guidelines are recommended:

(1) Patients may be offered palliative sedation to unconsciousness when they are in the final stages of terminal illness. The rationale for all palliative care measures should be documented in the medical record.

(2) Palliative sedation to unconsciousness may be considered for those terminally ill patients whose clinical symptoms have been unresponsive to aggressive, symptom-specific treatments.

(3) Physicians should ensure that the patient and/or the patient's surrogate have given informed consent for palliative sedation to unconsciousness.

(4) Physicians should consult with a multidisciplinary team, if available, including an expert in the field of palliative care, to ensure that symptom-specific treatments have been sufficiently employed and that palliative sedation to unconsciousness is now the most appropriate course of treatment.

(5) Physicians should discuss with their patients considering palliative sedation the care plan relative to degree and length (intermittent or constant) of sedation, and the specific expectations for continuing, withdrawing, or withholding future life-sustaining treatments.

(6) Once palliative sedation is begun, a process must be implemented to monitor for appropriate care.

(7) Palliative sedation is not an appropriate response to suffering that is primarily existential, defined as the experience of agony and distress that may arise from such issues as death anxiety, isolation, and loss of control. Existential suffering is better addressed by other interventions. For example, palliative sedation is not the way to address suffering created by social isolation and loneliness; such suffering should be addressed by providing the patient with needed social support.

(8) Palliative sedation must never be used to intentionally cause a patient's death. (I, VII)

Issued November 2008 based on the report "Sedation to Unconsciousness in End-of-Life Care," adopted June 2008.

2.21   The previous Opinion 2.21, "Withholding or Withdrawing Life-Prolonging Medical Treatment—Patients' Preferences," was deleted in 1994 and combined with the current Opinion 2.20, "Withholding or Withdrawing Life-Sustaining Medical Treatment."

2.21   Euthanasia

Euthanasia is the administration of a lethal agent by another person to a patient for the purpose of relieving the patient's intolerable and incurable suffering.

It is understandable, though tragic, that some patients in extreme duress—such as those suffering from a terminal, painful, debilitating illness—may come to decide that death is preferable to life. However, permitting physicians to engage in euthanasia would ultimately cause more harm than good. Euthanasia is fundamentally incompatible with the physician's role as healer, would be difficult or impossible to control, and would pose serious societal risks.

The involvement of physicians in euthanasia heightens the significance of its ethical prohibition. The physician who performs euthanasia assumes unique responsibility for the act of ending the patient's life. Euthanasia could also readily be extended to incompetent patients and other vulnerable populations.

Instead of engaging in euthanasia, physicians must aggressively respond to the needs of patients at the end of life. Patients should not be abandoned once it is determined that cure is impossible. Patients near the end of life must continue to receive emotional support, comfort care, adequate pain control, respect for patient autonomy, and good communication. (I, IV)

Issued June 1994 based on the report "Decisions Near the End of Life," adopted June 1991 (JAMA. 1992;267:2229-2233). Updated June 1996.

9th Cir. 1996 Suit was brought by several physicians and not-for-profit corporation which provides information, assistance, and counseling to competent terminally ill adult patients contemplating suicide, asserting that a state statute making it a crime to aid anyone in attempting to commit suicide unconstitutionally prevents terminally ill patients from exercising their protected liberty interests. Appeals court, en banc, held that the choice of how and when to die is a liberty interest and that the statute violates the due process rights of competent, terminally ill adults who wish to hasten their deaths by obtaining medication prescribed by their physicians. Stating that physician-assisted suicide runs counter to medical ethics, the dissent cited Opinions 2.20,

2.21, and 2.211 and quoted Opinion 2.211. *Compassion in Dying v. Washington, 79 F.3d 790, 840, 855 replacing, 49 F.3d 586 (9th Cir. 1995).*

Mich. App. 2001 State brought criminal action against physician for the murder of a patient by lethal injection. The trial court convicted the physician of second-degree murder and delivering a controlled substance. On appeal, the trial court decision was affirmed. The physician asked the appellate court to conclude that euthanasia is legal and to reverse his conviction on constitutional grounds. The appellate court relied on *Washington v. Glucksberg,* 521 U.S. 702 (1997) in determining there is no constitutional right to commit euthanasia, so that an individual can be free from intolerable and irremediable suffering. In discussing *Glucksberg,* the court observed that a state has a legitimate interest in protecting the integrity and ethics of the medical profession. The court noted *Glucksberg's* reference to Opinions 2.20, 2.21, and 2.211 in this regard. *People v. Kevorkian, 248 Mich. App. 373, 639 N.W.2d 291, 305 n. 42.*

Journal 2010 Examines whether standards and practices regarding euthanasia, other than those which have been legally and ethically established, should be applied in extreme emergency situations. Concludes that creating an exception to the prohibition against euthanasia in such situations has no legal or ethical foundation and is not necessary as a means to cope with disasters. Argues for the development of disaster planning consistent with established legal and ethical principles. Quotes Opinion 8.08. Cites Opinions 2.20 and 2.21. Shea, *Hurricane Katrina and the Legal and Bioethical Implications of Involuntary Euthanasia as a Component of Disaster Management in Extreme Emergency Situations, 19 Annals Health L. 133, 137-138 (2010).*

Journal 2008 Explores the question of whether physician-assisted dying is ethically and legally appropriate by using empirical research to address concerns and objections. Concludes more research is needed to better understand the pressures experienced by patients facing end-of-life decisions. Quotes Opinions 2.21 and 2.211. Battin, *Physician-Assisted Dying and the Slippery Slope: The Challenge of Empirical Evidence, 45 Willamette L. Rev. 91, 98-99 (2008).*

Journal 2006 Argues that current law and ethics governing physician-assisted suicide are too simplistic. Concludes there are a number of legal ways for terminally ill patients to hasten death. Quotes Opinion 2.21. Cantor, *On Hastening Death Without Violating Legal and Moral Prohibitions, 37 Loy. U. Chi. L. J. 407, 427 (2006).*

Journal 2005 Examines the legal and ethical aspects of physician participation in capital punishment. Concludes that federal and state laws addressing this practice must be amended to harmonize the law with applicable principles of medical ethics. Quotes Opinion 2.06. Cites Opinion 2.21. References Opinion 2.01. Levy, *Conflict of Duty: Capital Punishment Regulations and AMA Medical Ethics, 26 J. Legal Med. 261, 268, 269, 270, 273 (2005).*

Journal 2004 Reviews empirical data and the arguments on both sides of the physician-assisted suicide debate. Concludes that weighing the costs and benefits associated with legalizing assisted suicide likely will not resolve the debate. References Opinion 2.211. Gorsuch, *The Legalization of Assisted Suicide and the Law of Unintended Consequences: A Review of the Dutch and Oregon Experiments and Leading Utilitarian Arguments for Legal Change, 2004 Wis. L. Rev. 1347, 1379 (2004).*

Journal 2004 Analyzes various issues relating to the role of mental health professionals in capital punishment in light of Albert Bandura's model of "mechanisms of moral disengagement." Concludes that facilitating participation of mental health professionals in executions creates conflicts with the humanistic norms of the profession. Quotes Preamble and Opinions 1.01, 1.02, 2.06, 2.067, 2.20, 2.21, 2.211, and 8.14. Judges, *The Role of Mental Health Professionals in Capital Punishment: An Exercise in Moral Disengagement, 41 Hous. L. Rev. 515, 562, 568, 569, 570, 571-72, 581, 586, 588, 598 (2004).*

Journal 2003 Analyzes the objective and subjective tests used to determine which individuals qualify for physician-assisted suicide (PAS) and euthanasia in the US and the Netherlands. Concludes that both tests provide sufficient safeguards to protect vulnerable groups. Quotes Opinions 2.21 and 2.211. Green, *Physician-Assisted Suicide and Euthanasia: Safeguarding Against the "Slippery Slope"—The Netherlands Versus the United States, 13 Ind. Int'l & Comp. L. Rev. 639, 662 (2003).*

Journal 2002 Examines key factors that led to the current palliative care crisis. Analyzes state legislative and judicial efforts to improve palliative care. Concludes with model legislation that holds physicians accountable for inadequate palliative care. Quotes Opinions 2.21 and 2.211. References Opinion 2.20. Oken, *Curing Healthcare Providers' Failure to Administer Opioids in the Treatment of Severe Pain, 23 Cardozo L. Rev. 1917, 1925-26, 1952, 1954 (2002).*

Journal 2002 Reviews the ethical and legal issues arising in connection with the development of standards for pain management. Concludes that appropriate guidelines for pain management should be established by the medical profession. Cites Opinions 2.21 and 2.211. Stark, *Bio-Ethics and Physician Liability: The Liability Effects of Developing Pain Management Standards, 14 St. Thomas L. Rev. 601, 631 (2002).*

Journal 2001 Explores the similarities and differences among active voluntary euthanasia, terminal sedation, and assisted suicide. Examines the problems with making moral distinctions based on physicians' intentions. Concludes that, with proper safeguards, active voluntary euthanasia and assisted suicide are more protective of patient self-determination. Quotes Opinions 2.20 and 2.21. Gauthier, *Active Voluntary Euthanasia, Terminal Sedation, and Assisted Suicide, 12 J. Clinical Ethics 43, 43-44, 49 (2001).*

Journal 2000 Examines questions regarding the legality of such practices as voluntary stopping of eating and drinking (VSED), use of risky analgesics, and terminal sedation. Explores the distinctions between physician-assisted suicide and other palliative interventions. Concludes VSED, risky analgesics, and certain types of terminal sedation are lawful and should be made available to dying patients who make informed decisions to accept the risks involved. Quotes Opinions 2.21 and 2.211. Cites Opinions 2.18 and 2.20. Cantor & Thomas, *The Legal Bounds of Physician Conduct Hastening Death, 48 Buff. L. Rev. 83, 110, 131, 158 (2000).*

Journal 2000 Considers the question of whether physician-assisted suicide and euthanasia should be legalized. Concludes that, under basic moral and common law principles, the intentional taking of human life by a private person is wrong. References Opinions 2.20, 2.21, and 2.211. Gorsuch, *The Right to Assisted Suicide and Euthanasia, 23 Harv. J. L. & Pub. Pol'y 599, 653, 707 (2000).*

Journal 2000 Explores the ongoing debate surrounding the legalization of assisted suicide. Defines and distinguishes assisted suicide and euthanasia from other ethical acts. Concludes most of the critical research questions that bear on current policy debates regarding legalization of assisted suicide remain unanswered. References Opinions 2.21 and 2.211. Rosenfeld, *Assisted Suicide, Depression, and the Right to Die, 6 Psychol. Pub. Pol'y & L. 467, 469 (2000).*

Journal 1999 Examines legal and policy issues regarding physician-assisted suicide. Distinguishes between refusing treatment and assisted suicide. Concludes that there are too many dangers posed by physician-assisted suicide to warrant legalization. Quotes Opinion 2.211. Cites Opinions 2.20 and 2.21. Pratt, *Too Many Physicians: Physician-Assisted Suicide After Glucksberg/Quill, 9 Alb. L. J. Sci. & Tech. 161, 208 (1999).*

Journal 1997 Considers the legal and ethical issues involved with physician-assisted suicide and euthanasia. Explores recent legal developments in the courts. Opines that Texas should allow physician-assisted suicide, at least for the terminally ill. Asserts that banning such a practice is unconstitutional. Quotes Opinion 2.211. References Opinion 2.21. Comment, *Physician-Assisted Suicide: Should Texas Be Different? 33 Hous. L. Rev. 1475, 1480, 1488 (1997).*

Journal 1997 Discusses goals of care included in advance directives and whether they can be used to predict specific interventions and results. Offers insights provided by survey of physicians at Massachusetts General Hospital. Cites Opinions 2.20 and 2.21. Fischer, Alpert, Stoeckle, & Emanuel, *Can Goals of Care Be Used to Predict Intervention Preferences in an Advance Directive? 157 Arch. Intern. Med. 801, 807 (1997).*

Journal 1996 Examines the issue of physician-assisted suicide. Observes that it is important to consider not only whether some form of physician-assisted suicide should enjoy legal and ethical support in our society, but also whether physicians should be involved. Concludes that physicians, as a profession, probably are not the proper individuals to perform this function. Cites Opinions 2.21 and 2.211. Clark, *Autonomy and Death, 71 Tul. L. Rev. 45, 89 (1996).*

Journal 1996 Explores the issue of legalizing physician-assisted suicide. Opines that the current state of technology increases life expectancy but with a concomitant decrease in dignity and autonomy surrounding one's death. Notes that the elderly are committing suicide at an increasing rate. Cites Opinions 2.20, 2.21, and 2.211. Morgan & Sutherland, *Last Rights? Confronting Physician-Assisted Suicide in Law and Society: Legal Liturgies on Physician-Assisted Suicide, 26 Stetson L. Rev. 481, 484 (1996).*

Journal 1995 Analyzes the case of *Compassion in Dying v. Washington* in which a federal district court judge held that certain people have a constitutional right to physician-assisted suicide. Criticizes the decision for being too broad in that it would protect active euthanasia by physicians on patients who are physically unable to perform the act themselves. Quotes Opinion 2.21. References Opinion 2.211. Larson, *Prescription for Death: A Second Opinion*, 44 *DePaul L. Rev.* 461, 472 (1995).

Journal 1995 Offers relevant historical perspectives and provides comprehensive ethical and legal discussion of physician-assisted suicide and euthanasia. Highlights important legislative developments, including the Oregon Death with Dignity Act, and analyzes significant judicial opinions. Quotes Principles III, IV, and VI and Opinions 2.21 and 9.12. Cites Opinions 2.20 and 8.11. Stone & Winslade, *Physician-Assisted Suicide and Euthanasia in the United States: Legal and Ethical Observations*, 16 *J. Legal Med.* 481, 483, 490, 497, 498, 499 (1995).

Journal 1993 Considers how life-sustaining treatments have led to prolonged life under unacceptable circumstances. Recommends quality assurance programs that promote discussion between physicians and patients regarding life-sustaining treatment problems. Cites Opinions 2.20 and 2.21. Pearlman, Cain, Patrick, Appelbaum-Maizel, Starks, Jecker, & Uhlmann, *Insights Pertaining to Patient Assessments of States Worse Than Death*, 4 *J. Clinical Ethics* 33, 40 (1993).

Journal 1992 Analyzes the arguments for and against active euthanasia, including ethical concerns, the slippery slope argument, and the proper role of the physician. Suggests that active euthanasia may be acceptable when its administration is restricted to physicians. References Opinions 2.20 and 2.21. Brock, *Voluntary Active Euthanasia*, 22 *Hastings Center Rep.* 10 (March/April 1992).

Journal 1992 Considers the debate surrounding medical futility. Observes that this debate is encouraging reexamination of the nature of patient entitlement to medical care as well as the "ends of medicine." References Opinions 2.20, 2.21, and 2.22. Miles, *Medical Futility*, 20 *Law Med. & Health Care* 310, 311, 313 (1992).

Journal 1992 Examines the history of the right an individual has over his or her own body, and how the right to commit suicide has evolved from that concept. Concludes that the right of an incurably ill person to commit suicide is a personal issue to be decided outside of the judicial system. References Opinions 2.21 and 2.211. Morgan, Marks, & Harty-Golder, *The Issue of Personal Choice: The Competent Incurable Patient and the Right to Commit Suicide?* 57 *Mo. L. Rev.* 1, 44, 45 (1992).

2.211 Physician-Assisted Suicide

Physician-assisted suicide occurs when a physician facilitates a patient's death by providing the necessary means and/or information to enable the patient to perform the life-ending act (eg, the physician provides sleeping pills and information about the lethal dose, while aware that the patient may commit suicide).

It is understandable, though tragic, that some patients in extreme duress—such as those suffering from a terminal, painful, debilitating illness—may come to decide that death is preferable to life. However, allowing physicians to participate in assisted suicide would cause more harm than good. Physician-assisted suicide is fundamentally incompatible with the physician's role as healer, would be difficult or impossible to control, and would pose serious societal risks.

Instead of participating in assisted suicide, physicians must aggressively respond to the needs of patients at the end of life. Patients should not be abandoned once it is determined that cure is impossible. Multidisciplinary interventions should be sought including specialty consultation, hospice care, pastoral support, family counseling, and other modalities. Patients near the end of life must continue to receive emotional support, comfort care, adequate pain control, respect for patient autonomy, and good communication. (I, IV)

Issued 1994 based on the reports "Decisions Near the End of Life," adopted June 1991 (JAMA. 1992;267:2229-2233) and "Physician-Assisted Suicide," adopted December 1993. Updated June 1996.

U.S. 2006 State of Oregon brought suit seeking declaratory and injunctive relief from enforcement of an interpretive rule of a US Attorney General's opinion, which stated that physicians who assist patients in suicide under the authority of the Oregon Death with Dignity Act (ODWDA) violate the federal Controlled Substances Act (CSA). The Ninth Circuit Court of Appeals found the rule invalid. Appeal to the Supreme Court followed. In affirming, the majority held that the interpretive rule is not entitled to deference and that the CSA does not allow the attorney general to prohibit physicians from prescribing drugs for use in assisted suicide pursuant to state law. Quoting Opinion 2.211, the dissent stated that assisted suicide is incompatible with a physician's role as a healer and does not serve a legitimate medical purpose. *Gonzales v. Oregon, 126 S. Ct. 904, 932.*

U.S. 1997 Several physicians and terminally ill patients sued the state seeking a declaration that its prohibition against physician-assisted suicide violates the Fourteenth Amendment's Equal Protection Clause. The trial court disagreed, but the Second Circuit reversed, holding that the state accords different treatment to those terminally ill patients who wish to hasten their death by self-administering prescribed drugs and to those patients who wish to do so by directing the removal of life support systems. The Supreme Court reversed holding that the prohibition against assisting suicide does not violate the Equal Protection Clause. The Court concluded that there is a distinction between assisting suicide and withdrawing treatment quoting reports of the AMA Council on Ethical and Judicial Affairs [now Opinions 2.20 and 2.211]. *Vacco v. Quill, 117 S. Ct. 2293, 2298, 138 L. Ed. 2d 834.*

U.S. 1997 Several Washington physicians, terminally ill patients, and a not-for-profit organization that counsels people considering physician-assisted suicide sued the state seeking to have statutory ban on physician-assisted suicide declared unconstitutional. The trial court agreed and the Ninth Circuit affirmed. The Supreme Court, in reversing the decision, held that prohibition against causing or aiding a suicide does not violate the Due Process Clause. The Court also noted that the prohibition was rationally related to legitimate state interests in protecting the integrity and ethics of the medical profession quoting from Opinion 2.211. *Washington v. Glucksberg, 117 S. Ct. 2258, 2273, 138 L. Ed. 2d 772.*

9th Cir. 1996 Suit was brought by several physicians and not-for-profit corporation which provides information, assistance, and counseling to competent terminally ill adult patients contemplating suicide, asserting that a state statute making it a crime to aid anyone in attempting to commit suicide unconstitutionally prevents terminally ill patients from exercising their protected liberty interests. Appeals court, en banc, held that the choice of how and when to die is a liberty interest and that the statute violates the due process rights of competent, terminally ill adults who wish to hasten their deaths by obtaining medication prescribed by their physicians. Stating that physician-assisted suicide runs counter to medical ethics, the dissent cited Opinions 2.20, 2.21, and 2.211 and quoted Opinion 2.211. *Compassion in Dying v. Washington, 79 F.3d 790, 840, 855 replacing, 49 F.3d 586 (9th Cir. 1995).*

9th Cir. 1995 A not-for-profit corporation organized to assist terminally ill persons in committing suicide and several physicians alleged that a state statute making aiding a suicide attempt a crime violated 42 USC § 1983 and the Constitution. In upholding the statute, the court quoted Opinion 2.211 as articulating the ethical position of the medical profession against assisted suicide. In turn, the court found upholding the ethical integrity of the medical profession to be one of the many state interests outweighing the alleged liberty interest in medically assisted suicide. *Compassion in Dying v. Washington, 49 F.3d 586, 592, replaced, 79 F.3d 790 (9th Cir. 1996).*

Alaska 2001 Two mentally competent, terminally ill adults filed suit, asking the superior court to declare Alaska's manslaughter statute invalid so that their physicians could assist them in committing suicide. The superior court entered summary judgment against the patients and the Alaska Supreme Court affirmed. In concluding that Alaska's constitutional rights of privacy and liberty do not afford terminally ill patients the right to a physician's assistance in committing suicide, the court quoted Opinion 2.211 in support of the state's interest in protecting the integrity of the medical profession. *Sampson v. State, 31 P.3d 88, 96, 97.*

Fla. 1997 A patient, suffering from acquired immune deficiency syndrome (AIDS), and his physician filed suit for a declaratory judgment that state law prohibiting assisted suicide violated the privacy clause of the state constitution, as well as the due process and equal protection clauses of the Fourteenth Amendment to the US Constitution. The trial court concluded that the law was unconstitutional. On appeal the state Supreme Court, relying on the US Supreme Court's rulings in *Washington v. Glucksberg,* 117 S.Ct. 2258 (1997) and *Vacco v. Quill,* 117 S.Ct. 2293 (1997), held that the state's ban was not unconstitutional. In determining that the right to assisted suicide is not included in the state's guarantee of privacy, the court quoted from Opinion 2.211. *Krischer v. McIver, 697 So. 2d 97, 103.*

Mich. App. 2001 State brought criminal action against physician for the murder of a patient by lethal injection. The trial court convicted the physician of second-degree murder and delivering a controlled substance. On appeal, the trial court decision was affirmed. The physician asked the appellate court to conclude that euthanasia is legal and to reverse his conviction on constitutional grounds. The appellate court relied on *Washington v. Glucksberg,* 521 U.S. 702 (1997) in determining there is no constitutional right to commit euthanasia, so that an individual can be free from intolerable and irremediable suffering. In discussing *Glucksberg,* the court observed that a state has a legitimate interest in protecting the integrity and ethics of the medical profession. The court noted *Glucksberg's* reference to Opinions 2.20, 2.21, and 2.211 in this regard. *People v. Kevorkian, 248 Mich. App. 373, 639 N.W.2d 291, 305 n. 42.*

Journal 2011 Discusses physician-assisted suicide as permitted in Oregon and Washington and examines 2009 legislative proposal allowing physician-assisted suicide in Vermont. Concludes that legalizing physician-assisted suicides would promote elder abuse and would also devalue the lives of the disabled. Quotes Opinion 2.211. Dore, *Physician-Assisted Suicide: A Recipe for Elder Abuse and the Illusion of Personal Choice, 36 Vt. B. J. 53, 53 (Winter 2011).*

Journal 2011 Argues physicians should have the choice to participate in lethal injection executions. Concludes that although executions may proceed without physician involvement and the integrity and ethics of the medical profession must be protected, because executions performed without a physician have been mishandled, physician involvement is needed. Quotes Opinion 2.211. References Opinion 2.06. Nelson & Ashby, *Rethinking the Ethics of Physician Participation in Lethal Injection Execution, 41 Hastings Center Rep., 28, 29, 35 (May-June 2011).*

Journal 2011 Analyzes and criticizes changes in Britain's assisted suicide law and policy. Argues that recent changes mistakenly view the value of human life from a human-centered, morally relative legal positivist perspective. Cites Opinion 2.211. Wagner, Kane, & Kallman, *Suicide Killing of Human Life as a Human Right, 6 Liberty U. L. Rev. 27, 38 (2011).*

Journal 2010 Examines aid in dying or physician-assisted suicide in Idaho. Concludes physician-assisted suicide is not legal in Idaho and any physician engaging in this practice may face criminal and civil liability. Quotes Opinion 2.211. Dore, *Aid in Dying: Not Legal in Idaho; Not About Choice, 53 The Advocate 18 (Sept. 2010).*

Journal 2010 Discusses the need for statutory regulation in the context of physician-assisted death. Concludes that states should proactively regulate this practice to prevent abuse and misuse and proposes a statutory framework. Quotes Opinion 2.211. Mason, *Ignoring It Will Not Make It Go Away: Guidelines for Statutory Regulation of Physician-Assisted Death, 45 New Eng. L. Rev. 139, 142 (2010).*

Journal 2009 Argues there is no basis for distinguishing the right to refuse life-sustaining treatment and the right to physician-assisted suicide. Concludes physician-assisted suicide should be permitted as a constitutionally protected right for mentally competent, terminally ill patients, in accordance with the American values of individualism and self-determination. Quotes Opinion 2.211. Chamberlain, *Looking for a "Good Death": The Elderly Terminally Ill's Right to Die by Physician-Assisted Suicide, 17 Elder L. J. 61, 81 (2009).*

Journal 2008 Explores the question of whether physician-assisted dying is ethically and legally appropriate by using empirical research to address concerns and objections. Concludes more research is needed to better understand the pressures experienced by patients facing end-of-life decisions. Quotes Opinions 2.21 and 2.211. Battin, *Physician-Assisted Dying and the Slippery Slope: The Challenge of Empirical Evidence, 45 Willamette L. Rev. 91, 98-99 (2008).*

Journal 2008 Examines patient-familial concerns in physician-assisted suicide (PAS) and existing case law. Concludes legislators must focus on families of terminally ill patients when proposing PAS legislation. Quotes Opinion 2.211. Economou, *What About Families? A Different Perspective on Physician Assisted Suicide in California, 7 Whittier J. Child & Fam. Advoc. 253, 259 (2008).*

Journal 2007 Examines the role of the medical profession in participating in state-sanctioned lethal injection. Concludes that any participation is unethical because it causes harm and undermines trust. Cites Opinion 2.06. References Opinions 2.211 and 9.02. Black & Sade, *Lethal Injection and Physicians: State Law vs Medical Ethics, 298 JAMA 2779, 2780, 2781 (2007).*

Journal 2007 Discusses the impact of *Gonzales v. Oregon* on palliative care policies. Concludes Gonzales paves the way for ethical provision of palliative care. Quotes Opinion 2.211. Hilliard, *The Politics of Palliative Care and the Ethical Boundaries of Medicine: Gonzales v. Oregon as a Cautionary Tale, 35 J. L. Med. & Ethics 158, 170 (2007).*

Journal 2007 Reviews recent US Supreme Court decisions on physician-assisted suicide. Concludes that the most important public policy question to be considered is the motivation of patients in electing to end their lives. Quotes Opinion 2.211. Levy, *Gonzales v. Oregon and Physician-Assisted Suicide: Ethical and Policy Issues, 42 Tulsa L. Rev. 699, 699 (2007).*

Journal 2007 Examines the existence of a right to physician-assisted suicide. Concludes that terminally ill patients deserve the availability of a means to alleviate their suffering and preserve their dignity. Quotes Opinion 2.211. Urofsky, *Do Go Gentle Into That Good Night: Thoughts on Death, Suicide, Morality and the Law, 59 Ark. L. Rev. 819, 832 (2007).*

Journal 2006 Discusses legal and political issues surrounding physician-assisted suicide. Concludes that palliative care is sufficient to allow for a death with dignity. Quotes Opinion 2.211. Aden, *End of Life Decision Making: The Right to Die? You Can Go Your Own Way: Exploring the Relationship Between Personal and Political Autonomy in Gonzales v. Oregon, 15 Temp. Pol. & Civ. Rts. L. Rev. 323, 329 (2006).*

Journal 2006 Analyzes the proceedings and decision in *Gonzales v. Oregon.* Concludes the Court's holding is correct and that other states should adopt statutes similar to the Oregon Death with Dignity Act. Quotes Opinion 2.211. Chand, *Deconstructing Gonzales v. Oregon: When Political Agendas Yield to Rudimentary Notions of Federalism and Statutory Interpretation, 50 How. L. J. 229, 239-40 (2006).*

Journal 2006 Reviews government responses to euthanasia after passage of Oregon's Death with Dignity Act. Concludes that palliative care should be embraced by lawmakers as an alternative to euthanasia. References Opinion 2.211. Clark, *Oregon's Death with Dignity Act and Alleged Patient Euthanasia After Hurricane Katrina—The Government's Role, 18 Health Lawyer 1, 8 (2006).*

Journal 2006 Reviews physician-assisted suicide jurisprudence. Predicted that the Supreme Court would likely strike down Oregon's Death with Dignity Act in 2006. Quotes Opinion 2.211. Danino, *Dodging the Issue of Physician Assisted Suicide: The Supreme Court's Likely Response in Gonzales v. Oregon, 10 Mich. St. U. J. Med. & L. 299, 305 (2006).*

Journal 2006 Reviews *Gonzales v. Oregon* and discusses its impact on the field of medicine. Concludes that palliative care is an important consideration in end-of-life care. Quotes Opinion 2.211 (1993). Gostin, *Physician-Assisted Suicide: A Legitimate Medical Practice? 295 JAMA 1941, 1942 (2006).*

Journal 2006 Reviews the role of the judiciary and the medical profession in deciding what purposes medicine should serve. Concludes the medical profession's ability to address patient need rests on its authority to act as a self-governing profession. References Opinion 2.211. Gregg, *The Supreme Court and the Purposes of Medicine, 354 New Eng. J. Med. 993, 994 (2006).*

Journal 2006 Discusses whether, under the Oregon Death with Dignity Act, physician-assisted suicide serves a "legitimate medical purpose" within the meaning of the Controlled Substances Act. Concludes that it does. Quotes Opinion 2.211. Hughes, *The Oregon Death with Dignity Act: Relief of Suffering at the End of Medicine's Ability to Heal, 95 Geo. L. J. 207, 219 (2006).*

Journal 2006 Discusses surrogate decision making and an individual's right to refuse medical treatment. Concludes that the *Cruzan* clear and convincing evidence standard should serve as the constitutional minimum test for withdrawing life support. References Opinion 2.211. Lapertosa, *End of Life Decision Making: The Right to Die? Preventing the "Right to Refuse" From Becoming a License to Kill: Adopting a Constitutional Minimum Standard for Approving Withdrawal of Life Support for Legally Incompetent Patients, 15 Temp. Pol. & Civ. Rts. L. Rev. 483, 488 (2006).*

Journal 2006 Considers current laws governing physician-assisted suicide. Concludes that Hawaii should adopt a law analogous to Oregon's Death with Dignity Act. Quotes Opinion 2.211. McAneeley, *Physician-Assisted Suicide: Expanding the Laboratory to the State of Hawai'i, 29 Hawaii L. Rev. 269, 294 (2006).*

Journal 2006 Discusses political philosophies which support an individual's constitutional right to die. Concludes that individuals past the age of retirement should be able to choose physician-assisted suicide. References Opinion 2.211. Mitchell, *My Father, John Locke, and Assisted Suicide: The Real Constitutional Right, 3 Ind. Health L. Rev. 45, 60 (2006).*

Journal 2006 Discusses an attorney's responsibility to a client on death row who wishes to volunteer for execution. Concludes that an attorney should never assist a client in waiving an appeal. Quotes Opinions 2.20 and 2.211. Oleson, *Swilling Hemlock: The Legal Ethics of Defending a Client Who Wishes to Volunteer for Execution*, 63 Wash. & Lee L. Rev. 147, 277, 325 (2006).

Journal 2006 Discusses the ethical controversy surrounding physician-assisted suicide. Concludes that natural law and individual autonomy are important considerations in the ethical debate. Quotes Opinion 2.211. Cites Opinion 2.035. Wong, *Whose Life Is It Anyway?* 5 Cardozo Pub. L. Pol'y & Ethics J. 233, 271-72 (2006).

Journal 2005 Provides the morals rationale for the Partial-Birth Abortion Ban Act of 2003. Concludes that the Supreme Court's decision in *Lawrence v. Texas* does not prohibit morals legislation where the proscribed conduct may broadly affect societal morals. Quotes 2.211. Johnson, *Habit and Discernment in Abortion Practice: The Partial-Birth Abortion Ban Act of 2003 as Morals Legislation*, 36 Rutgers L. J. 549, 582 (2005).

Journal 2004 Analyzes various issues relating to the role of mental health professionals in capital punishment in light of Albert Bandura's model of "mechanisms of moral disengagement." Concludes that facilitating participation of mental health professionals in executions creates conflicts with the humanistic norms of the profession. Quotes Preamble and Opinions 1.01, 1.02, 2.06, 2.067, 2.20, 2.21, 2.211, and 8.14. Judges, *The Role of Mental Health Professionals in Capital Punishment: An Exercise in Moral Disengagement*, 41 Hous. L. Rev. 515, 562, 568, 569, 570, 571-72, 581, 586, 588, 598 (2004).

Journal 2003 Analyzes the objective and subjective tests used to determine which individuals qualify for PAS and euthanasia in the US and the Netherlands. Concludes that both tests provide sufficient safeguards to protect vulnerable groups. Quotes Opinions 2.21 and 2.211. Green, *Physician-Assisted Suicide and Euthanasia: Safeguarding Against the "Slippery Slope"—The Netherlands Versus the United States*, 13 Ind. Int'l & Comp. L. Rev. 639, 662 (2003).

Journal 2003 Discusses the inconsistent governmental regulation of drugs used in physician-assisted suicide (PAS) and lethal injections. Concludes that the FDA should regulate drugs used in lethal injections in the same manner it has attempted to regulate drugs used in PAS. Quotes Opinions 2.06 and 2.211. Miller, *A Death by Any Other Name: The Federal Government's Inconsistent Treatment of Drugs Used in Lethal Injections and Physician-Assisted Suicide*, 17 J. L. & Health 217, 234-35 (2003).

Journal 2003 Considers societal harm as a justification for statutes prohibiting otherwise harmless conduct. Concludes that moral reaction patterns, which typically prevent humans from injuring one another, are important fibers in the fabric of society. Quotes Opinion 2.211. Johnson, *Harm to the "Fabric of Society" as a Basis for Regulating Otherwise Harmless Conduct: Notes on a Theme From Ravin v. State*, 27 Seattle U. L. Rev. 41, 55 (2003).

Journal 2003 Examines the individual rights arguments in the physician-assisted suicide and euthanasia debate. Concludes that collective rather than individual rationality should determine the path that society takes on these issues. Quotes Opinion 2.211. Wong, *A Matter of Life and Death: A Very Personal Discourse*, 1 Geo. J. L. & Pub. Pol'y 339, 350 (2003).

Journal 2002 Considers the use of nonlegal materials in US Supreme Court decisions. Concludes that law alone cannot answer complex legal questions. Cites Opinions 2.20 and 2.211. Hasko, *Persuasion in the Court: Nonlegal Materials in U.S. Supreme Court Opinions*, 94 Law Libr. J. 427, 444, 453 (2002).

Journal 2002 Examines key factors that led to the current palliative care crisis. Analyzes state legislative and judicial efforts to improve palliative care. Concludes with model legislation that holds physicians accountable for inadequate palliative care. Quotes Opinions 2.21 and 2.211. References Opinion 2.20. Oken, *Curing Healthcare Providers' Failure to Administer Opioids in the Treatment of Severe Pain*, 23 Cardozo L. Rev. 1917, 1925-26, 1952, 1954 (2002).

Journal 2002 Proposes an ethical argument for suppressing agonal respiration in dying patients under rare circumstances. Concludes that using neuromuscular block agents in terminally ill, well-sedated, gasping patients can allow for a good death. References Opinion 2.211. Perkin & Resnik, *The Agony of Agonal Respiration: Is the Last Gasp Necessary?* 28 J. Med. Ethics 164, 169 (2002).

Journal 2002 Reviews the ethical and legal issues arising in connection with the development of standards for pain management. Concludes that appropriate guidelines for pain management should be established by the medical profession. Cites Opinions 2.21 and 2.211. Stark, *Bio-Ethics and Physician Liability: The Liability Effects of Developing Pain Management Standards*, 14 St. Thomas L. Rev. 601, 631 (2002).

Journal 2000 Examines questions regarding the legality of such practices as voluntary stopping of eating and drinking (VSED), use of risky analgesics, and terminal sedation. Explores the distinctions between physician-assisted suicide and other palliative interventions. Concludes VSED, risky analgesics, and certain types of terminal sedation are lawful and should be made available to dying patients who make informed decisions to accept the risks involved. Quotes Opinions 2.21 and 2.211. Cites Opinions 2.18 and 2.20. Cantor & Thomas, *The Legal Bounds of Physician Conduct Hastening Death*, 48 Buff. L. Rev. 83, 110, 131, 158 (2000).

Journal 2000 Considers the question of whether physician-assisted suicide and euthanasia should be legalized. Concludes that, under basic moral and common law principles, the intentional taking of human life by a private person is wrong. References Opinions 2.20, 2.21, and 2.211. Gorsuch, *The Right to Assisted Suicide and Euthanasia*, 23 Harv. J. L. & Pub. Pol'y 599, 653, 707 (2000).

Journal 2000 Examines British pharmacists' views on physician-assisted suicide (PAS), including such topics as professional responsibility, personal beliefs, and relevant legal and ethical guidelines. Concludes that most pharmacists view their professional responsibilities regarding PAS differently from physicians. Cites Opinion 2.211. Hanlon, Weiss, & Rees, *British Community Pharmacists' Views of Physician-Assisted Suicide (PAS)*, 26 J. Med. Ethics 363, 367, 369 (2000).

Journal 2000 Discusses ways in which courts and society can take steps to ensure ethical integrity in the medical profession (EIMP). Reviews the case of *Washington v. Glucksberg*, discussing its role in advocating EIMP as a state interest in assisted suicide law. Quotes Opinion 2.211. Kalt, *Death, Ethics, and the State*, 23 Harv. J. L. & Pub. Pol'y 487, 537, 539 (2000).

Journal 2000 Discusses the debate regarding whether physicians should legally participate in hastening or causing death. Explores laws against assisted suicide. Evaluates ethical and social concerns associated with assisted suicide. Quotes Opinion 2.211. Larson, *Tales of Death: Storytelling in the Physician-Assisted Suicide Litigation*, 39 Washburn L. J. 159, 177 (2000).

Journal 2000 Explores the ongoing debate surrounding the legalization of assisted suicide. Defines and distinguishes assisted suicide and euthanasia from other ethical acts. Concludes most of the critical research questions that bear on current policy debates regarding legalization of assisted suicide remain unanswered. References Opinions 2.21 and 2.211. Rosenfeld, *Assisted Suicide, Depression, and the Right to Die*, 6 Psychol. Pub. Pol'y & L. 467, 469 (2000).

Journal 2000 Examines the background of assisted suicide and Michigan's attempt to ban it. Discusses *Cooley v. Granholm*, which is Michigan's most recent constitutional challenge. Concludes that the issue of physician-assisted suicide likely would not arise if society did a better job of providing end-of-life care. Quotes Opinion 2.211. Santayana, *The Michigan Legislature Persists in Prohibiting Assisted Suicide*, 77 U. Det. Mercy L. Rev. 875, 886 (2000).

Journal 2000 Explores the debate regarding physician-assisted suicide. Concludes that autonomy should be respected and that an individual's wishes for assisted suicide should be honored, unless the individual is misinformed or legally incompetent. Quotes Opinion 2.211. References Opinion 2.06. Urofsky, *Justifying Assisted Suicide: Comments on the Ongoing Debate*, 14 Notre Dame J. L. Ethics & Pub. Pol'y 893, 918, 923 (2000).

Journal 1999 Points out that a majority of people favor legalizing physician-assisted suicide. Discusses the right to die under the Ninth Amendment. Explains that a Ninth Amendment claim to the right to die has not been addressed by the US Supreme Court. Quotes Opinion 2.211. Hardaway, Peterson, & Mann, *The Right to Die and the Ninth Amendment: Compassion and Dying After Glucksberg and Vacco*, 7 Geo. Mason L. Rev. 313, 342 (1999).

Journal 1999 Examines legal and policy issues regarding physician-assisted suicide. Distinguishes between refusing treatment and assisted suicide. Concludes that there are too many dangers posed by physician-assisted suicide to warrant legalization. Quotes Opinion 2.211. Cites Opinions 2.20 and 2.21. Pratt, *Too Many Physicians: Physician-Assisted Suicide After Glucksberg/Quill*, 9 Alb. L. J. Sci. & Tech. 161, 208 (1999).

Journal 1998 Evaluates recent Supreme Court decisions denying a constitutional right to physician-assisted suicide. Explains that, if society adopts Oregon's view on physician-assisted suicide, then the focus will shift to when it is acceptable to end someone's life. Suggests that the debate over physician-assisted suicide does not concern death, but rather how society will care for people at the end of their lives. Quotes Opinion 2.211. Chopko, *Responsible Public Policy at the End of Life*, 75 U. Det. Mercy L. Rev. 557, 573 (1998).

Journal 1998 Explains that the US Supreme Court's decisions in *Washington* and *Vacco* left the door open for future constitutional challenges regarding the right to physician-assisted suicide. States that the Court did not explicitly deny the existence of a right to physician-assisted suicide. Quotes Opinion 2.20. Cites Opinion 2.211. Cohen, *The Open Door: Will the Right to Die Survive Washington v. Glucksberg and Vacco v. Quill?* 16 In Pub. Interest 79, 94 (1998).

Journal 1998 Examines ethical issues surrounding physician-assisted suicide. Explores physician-assisted suicide in the context of the influence of psychodynamic psychiatry on the physician-patient relationship. Concludes that if physicians approved of physician-assisted suicide, then it would undermine the physician-patient relationship. Quotes Opinion 2.211. Hamilton, Edwards, Boehnlein, & Hamilton, *The Doctor-Patient Relationship and Assisted Suicide: A Contribution From Dynamic Psychiatry*, 19 Am. J. Forensic Psychiatry 59, 60 (1998).

Journal 1998 Analyzes recent US Supreme Court decisions on physician-assisted suicide. Discusses amicus briefs that may have affected the Supreme Court's decisions. Theorizes that the Supreme Court will confront the subject of physician-assisted suicide in the future. References Opinion 2.211. Kamisar, *On the Meaning and Impact of the Physician-Assisted Suicide Cases*, 82 Minn. L. Rev. 895, 909, 918 (1998).

Journal 1998 Explains that a determination of mental capacity to consent must be made when a person requests physician-assisted suicide in a jurisdiction where such practice is legal. Explores the potential for liability in the context of making such a determination. Argues that standards regarding determination of mental capacity must be established by case law or legislation. Cites Opinion 2.211. References Opinion 2.06. Lipschitz, *Psychiatry and Consent for Physician-Assisted Suicide*, 19 Am. J. Forensic Psychiatry 91, 103, 104 (1998).

Journal 1998 Discusses legal aspects of physician-assisted suicide. Identifies acceptable end-of-life choices and compares them to physician-assisted suicide. Points out that physician-assisted suicide has the potential for abuse and that safeguards have not been implemented to protect people from that risk. Quotes Opinion 2.211. Cites Opinions 2.20 and 8.08. Mitchell, *Physician-Assisted Suicide: A Survey of the Issues Surrounding Legalization*, 74 N. D. L. Rev. 341, 349 (1998).

Journal 1998 Points out that the court in *Vacco v. Quill* did not reject the practice of physician-assisted suicide and left the subject open for state experimentation. Discusses routes some states have taken regarding assisted suicide. Concludes that access to assisted suicide is outweighed by the risk it will be utilized by depressed and mentally ill people. Quotes Opinions 2.20 and 2.211. Moore, *Physician-Assisted Suicide: Does "The End" Justify the Means?* 40 Ariz. L. Rev. 1471, 1472, 1481-82, 1491 (1998).

Journal 1998 Points out that psychiatrists have a limited ability to make assessments regarding the requests of terminally ill patients for physician-assisted suicide. Argues that psychiatrists must oppose physician-assisted suicide because its practice would be detrimental to the profession of medicine and would adversely affect the practice of psychiatry. Quotes Opinion 2.211. Orr & Bishop, *Why Psychiatrists Should Not Participate in Euthanasia and Physician-Assisted Suicide*, 19 Am. J. Forensic Psychiatry 35, 36 (1998).

Journal 1998 Analyzes arguments for and against physician-assisted suicide. Distinguishes between killing and allowing a person to die. Concludes that the issue of assisted suicide should be addressed in the political arena rather than in the federal court system. Cites Opinion 2.211. Park, *Physician-Assisted Suicide: State Legislation Teetering at the Pinnacle of a Slippery Slope*, 7 Wm. & Mary Bill Rts. J. 277, 292, 293 (1998).

Journal 1998 Argues that physician-assisted suicide should be available for terminally ill patients whose pain is not alleviated through medications. Analyzes the effects of state regulation of physician-assisted suicide. Explores the possibility of using Thirteenth Amendment claims to abolish possible racially discriminatory use of physician-assisted suicide. Quotes Opinion 2.211. Pittman, *Physician-Assisted Suicide in the Dark Ward: The Intersection of the Thirteenth Amendment and Health Care Treatments Having Disproportionate Impacts on Disfavored Groups*, 28 Seton Hall L. Rev. 774, 784 (1998).

Journal 1998 Explains that physician-assisted suicide diametrically opposes the ideals of the medical profession. States that referendums are not good ways to make public policy. Suggests that patients should discuss their wishes regarding withholding or withdrawing life-sustaining medical treatment with their physicians and families. References Opinion 2.211. Reardon, *American Medical Association Perspective on Physician Assisted Suicide, 75 U. Det. Mercy L. Rev. 515 (1998).*

Journal 1998 Analyzes the Supreme Court's decision in *Washington v. Glucksberg.* Explains how the state's interest in preserving life can be viewed as an interest in preserving the sanctity of personal autonomy. Argues that physician-assisted suicide would preserve individual freedom and the sanctity of life. Quotes Opinion 2.211. Staihar, *The State's Unqualified Interest in Preserving Life: A Critique of the Formulations of Life's Sanctity in Washington v. Glucksberg, 34 Idaho L. Rev. 401, 415 (1998).*

Journal 1998 Discusses the US Supreme Court's decision in *Washington v. Glucksberg.* Points out that the Supreme Court left many unresolved issues concerning physician-assisted suicide. Provides criteria that could be used by state legislatures in drafting pertinent statutes. Cites Opinion 2.211. Testa, *Sentenced to Life? An Analysis of the United States Supreme Court's Decision in Washington v. Glucksberg, 22 Nova L. Rev. 821, 839 (1998).*

Journal 1998 Examines society's increasing acceptance of the belief in an individual's right to die. Discusses issues surrounding physician-assisted suicide. Evaluates the impact of US Supreme Court decisions on physician-assisted suicide. Quotes Opinion 2.211. Urofsky, *Leaving the Door Ajar: The Supreme Court and Assisted Suicide, 32 U. Rich. L. Rev. 313, 336 (1998).*

Journal 1997 Reviews the arguments made in *amicus curiae* briefs submitted to the Supreme Court on the topic of assisted suicide. Focuses on key insights into the debate offered by the various *amici curiae.* Quotes Opinion 2.211. Coleson, *The Glucksberg & Quill Amicus Curiae Briefs: Verbatim Arguments Opposing Assisted Suicide, 13 Issues in Law & Med. 3, 67 (1997).*

Journal 1997 Considers the legal and ethical issues involved with physician-assisted suicide and euthanasia. Explores recent legal developments in the courts. Opines that Texas should allow physician-assisted suicide, at least for the terminally ill. Asserts that banning such a practice is unconstitutional. Quotes Opinion 2.211. References Opinion 2.21. Comment, *Physician-Assisted Suicide: Should Texas Be Different? 33 Hous. L. Rev. 1475, 1480, 1488 (1997).*

Journal 1997 Discusses the consequences of physician-assisted suicide. Argues that assisted suicide would divide the medical community. Concludes that physician-assisted suicide does not enhance freedom. Quotes Opinion 2.211. FitzGibbon, *The Failure of the Freedom-Based and Utilitarian Arguments for Assisted Suicide, 42 Am. J. Juris. 211, 252 (1997).*

Journal 1997 Explores a model physician-assisted suicide statute. Explains its history, provisions, and effects. Posits that the Act reaches further than one may suspect. Notes the AMA's position on assisted death and concludes that the Act fails to account for moral tradition. Quotes Opinion 2.211. FitzGibbon & Lai, *The Model Physician-Assisted Suicide Act and the Jurisprudence of Death, 13 Issues in Law & Med. 173, 203-04 (1997).*

Journal 1997 Considers US Supreme Court decisions regarding physician-assisted suicide. Argues that state legislatures should enact statutes to legalize physician-assisted suicide. Proposes a model act on physician-assisted suicide. Cites Opinion 2.211. Glynn, *Turning to State Legislatures to Legalize Physician-Assisted Suicide for Seriously Ill, Non-Terminal Patients After Vacco v. Quill and Washington v. Glucksberg, 6 J. L. & Pol'y. 329, 345 (1997).*

Journal 1997 Considers the right to die. Discusses the extension of the right to refuse treatment to decisions affecting life and death. Explains that courts distinguish between withdrawing life-sustaining treatment and euthanasia or assisted suicide. Emphasizes the importance of quality end-of-life care. Cites Opinion 2.211. Gostin, *Deciding Life and Death in the Courtroom: From Quinlan to Cruzan, Glucksberg, and Vacco—A Brief History and Analysis of Constitutional Protection of the Right to Die, 278 JAMA 1523, 1525, 1528 (1997).*

Journal 1997 States that the US Supreme Court has ended the *Roe v. Wade* era in which the Court made decisions on social policy based on normative judgments. Discusses the dangers posed by physician-assisted suicide. Argues that the decision in *Washington v. Glucksberg* averted the danger of abuse posed by physician-assisted suicide. Quotes Opinion 2.211. McConnell, *The Right to Die and the Jurisprudence of Tradition, 1997 Utah L. Rev. 665, 703-04 (1997).*

Journal 1997 Examines possible legalization of euthanasia, observing that any form of euthanasia will be a step toward horrible death. Posits that legalizing euthanasia will create unsolvable mortal dangers that conflict with universal values of life. Concludes that physician-assisted suicide would create many victims. Cites Opinion 2.211. McGonnigal, *This Is Who Will Die When Doctors Are Allowed to Kill Their Patients, 31 J. Marshall L. Rev. 95, 103 (1997).*

Journal 1997 Explores the ethical and legal debate over assisted suicide. Examines cases dealing with prohibitions against physician-assisted suicide. Considers the Oregon Death with Dignity Act in light of the ruling in *Lee v. Oregon*. Quotes Opinion 2.211. Note, *Constitutional Aspects of Physician-Assisted Suicide After Lee v. Oregon, XXIII Am. J. Law & Med. 69 (1997)*.

Journal 1997 Discusses the difference between physician-assisted suicide and the withdrawal of life-sustaining medical treatment. Posits that traditional moral arguments cannot justify the distinction. Examines how a right to assisted suicide for terminal patients brings right-to-die laws into alignment with underlying ethical precepts. References Opinion 2.211. Orentlicher, *The Legalization of Physician Assisted Suicide: A Very Modest Revolution, 38 B. C. L. Rev. 443, 459-60 (1997)*.

Journal 1997 Considers the perspectives of medical residents about end-of-life issues. Investigates the differences of opinion held by residents in psychiatry, internal medicine, and emergency medicine. References Opinion 2.211. Roberts, Roberts, Warner, Solomon, Hardee, & McCarty, *Internal Medicine, Psychiatry, and Emergency Medicine Residents' Views of Assisted Death Practices, 157 Arch. Intern. Med. 1603, 1609 (1997)*.

Journal 1996 Proposes a model state statute allowing and controlling physician-assisted suicide. Analyzes the constitutionality of the act and offers public policy justifications for the act's provisions. Concludes that proponents of physician-assisted suicide should provide precise, carefully tailored examples of regulations. Quotes Opinion 2.211. Cites Opinion 2.20. Baron, Bergstresser, Brock, Cole, Dorfman, Johnson, Schnipper, Vorenberg, & Wanzer, *A Model State Act to Authorize and Regulate Physician-Assisted Suicide, 33 Harv. J. Legis. 1, 2, 7 (1996)*.

Journal 1996 Examines the issue of physician-assisted suicide. Observes that it is important to consider not only whether some form of physician-assisted suicide should enjoy legal and ethical support in our society, but also whether physicians should be involved. Concludes that physicians, as a profession, probably are not the proper individuals to perform this function. Cites Opinions 2.21 and 2.211. Clark, *Autonomy and Death, 71 Tul. L. Rev. 45, 89 (1996)*.

Journal 1996 Criticizes the circuit court's opinion in *Compassion in Dying*. Suggests that the opinion fails to fully consider the ethical prohibitions against physician-assisted suicide. Concludes that the court's opinion is not based on a complete and accurate presentation of historical views and attitudes about suicide. Quotes Opinion 2.211. Duncan & Lubin, *The Use and Abuse of History in Compassion in Dying, 20 Harv. J. L. & Pub. Pol'y 175, 183 (1996)*.

Journal 1996 Examines ethical and legal issues involved in physician-assisted suicide. Asserts that the judiciary is not the proper forum for establishing guidelines regarding these issues. Concludes that individual state legislative enactments are the proper vehicles for delineating appropriate guidelines. Quotes Opinion 2.211. Kass & Lund, *Physician-Assisted Suicide, Medical Ethics and the Future of the Medical Profession, 35 Duq. L. Rev. 395, 404 (1996)*.

Journal 1996 Discusses the historical development of the right to die. Considers patient autonomy and paternalism and the role physicians play in end-of-life decisions. Explains the issue in the context of federal cases. Examines the true extent of a protected right to die. Cites Opinion 2.211. Kelly, *The "Right to Die" in America: The Ninth Circuit's Decision in Compassion in Dying v. the State of Washington, 29 J. Health & Hosp. L. 246, 255 (1996)*.

Journal 1996 Explores the issue of legalizing physician-assisted suicide. Opines that the current state of technology increases life expectancy but with a concomitant decrease in dignity and autonomy surrounding one's death. Notes that the elderly are committing suicide at an increasing rate. Cites Opinions 2.20, 2.21, and 2.211. Morgan & Sutherland, *Last Rights? Confronting Physician-Assisted Suicide in Law and Society: Legal Liturgies on Physician-Assisted Suicide, 26 Stetson L. Rev. 481, 484 (1996)*.

Journal 1996 Considers the right to death with dignity. Suggests that the AMA's position undermines mitigation of suffering and the individuals' right to self-determination. Concludes that restrictions on the right to death with dignity may be constitutionally impermissible. Quotes Opinion 2.211. Cites Opinion 2.20. Note, *Who Decides if There Is Triumph in the Ultimate Agony? Constitutional Theory and the Emerging Right to Die With Dignity, 37 Wm. & Mary L. Rev. 827, 829 (1996)*.

Journal 1996 Explores ethical problems accompanying the power to prolong and preserve life past points previously achievable. Questions whether physician-assisted suicide is a proper and ethically desirable course of treatment. Discusses recent developments and arguments surrounding physician-assisted suicide. References Opinion 2.211. Thomasma, *When Physicians Choose to*

Participate in the Death of Their Patients: Ethics and Physician-Assisted Suicide, 24 J. Law Med. & Ethics 183, 184, 195 (1996).

Journal 1995 Suggests that people seeking suicide need life-affirming treatment, not aid in dying. Concludes that the US Constitution does not require society to stand by while a person seeks suicide. Cites Opinion 2.211. Bopp & Coleson, *The Constitutional Case Against Permitting Physician-Assisted Suicide for Competent Adults With Terminal Conditions, 11 Issues in Law & Med. 239, 250 (1995).*

Journal 1995 Examines four essential principles of bioethics—patient autonomy, nonmalefi-cence, beneficence. and justice—and describes the application of these in clinical settings according to bioethical norms and AMA opinions. Concludes that such an approach promotes compassionate medical caregiving and that laws should reflect these values. Quotes Opinions 2.01 and 8.18. References Opinion 2.211. Cohen, *Toward a Bioethics of Compassion, 28 Ind. L. Rev. 667, 673, 681-82, 683 (1995).*

Journal 1995 Analyzes the case of *Compassion in Dying v. Washington* in which a federal district court judge held that certain people have a constitutional right to physician-assisted suicide. Criticizes the decision for being too broad in that it would protect active euthanasia by physi-cians on patients who are physically unable to perform the act themselves. Quotes Opinion 2.21. References Opinion 2.211. Larson, *Prescription for Death: A Second Opinion, 44 DePaul L. Rev. 461, 472 (1995).*

Journal 1994 Argues that assisted suicide is not an implicit right under the Fourteenth Amendment's liberty guarantee. Suggests that giving physicians the authority to determine the appropriateness of assisted suicide furthers no legitimate state interest. Cites Opinion 2.06. References Opinion 2.211. Marzen, *Out, Out Brief Candle: Constitutionally Prescribed Suicide for the Terminally Ill, 21 Hastings Const. L. Q. 799, 821 (1994).*

Journal 1992 Examines the history of the right an individual has over his or her own body, and how the right to commit suicide has evolved from that concept. Concludes that the right of an incurably ill person to commit suicide is a personal issue to be decided outside of the judicial sys-tem. References Opinions 2.21 and 2.211. Morgan, Marks, & Harty-Golder, *The Issue of Personal Choice: The Competent Incurable Patient and the Right to Commit Suicide? 57 Mo. L. Rev. 1, 44, 45 (1992).*

Journal 1992 Discusses the historical, legal, and social arguments both for and against assisted suicide and voluntary active euthanasia. Concludes that only physician-assisted suicide should be legalized. References Opinion 2.211. Note, *Aid-in-Dying: Should We Decriminalize Physician-Assisted Suicide and Physician-Committed Euthanasia? XVIII Am. J. Law & Med. 369, 370 (1992).*

2.215 Treatment Decisions for Seriously Ill Newborns

The primary consideration for decisions regarding life-sustaining treatment for seriously ill newborns should be what is best for the newborn. Factors that should be weighed are (1) the chance that therapy will succeed, (2) the risks involved with treatment and nontreatment, (3) the degree to which the ther-apy, if successful, will extend life, (4) the pain and discomfort associated with the therapy, and (5) the anticipated quality of life for the newborn with and without treatment.

Care must be taken to evaluate the newborn's expected quality of life from the child's perspective. Life-sustaining treatment may be withheld or with-drawn from a newborn when the pain and suffering expected to be endured by the child will overwhelm any potential for joy during his or her life. When an infant suffers extreme neurological damage, and is consequently not capable of experiencing either suffering or joy, a decision may be made to withhold or withdraw life-sustaining treatment. When life-sustaining treatment is withheld or withdrawn, comfort care must not be discontinued.

When an infant's prognosis is largely uncertain, as is often the case with extremely premature newborns, all life-sustaining and life-enhancing treatment should be initiated. Decisions about life-sustaining treatment should be made once the prognosis becomes more certain. It is not necessary to attain absolute or near absolute prognostic certainty before life-sustaining treatment is withdrawn, since this goal is often unattainable and risks unnecessarily prolonging the infant's suffering.

Physicians must provide full information to parents of seriously ill newborns regarding the nature of treatments, therapeutic options, and expected prognosis with and without therapy, so that parents can make informed decisions for their children about life-sustaining treatment. Counseling services and an opportunity to talk with persons who have had to make similar decisions should be available to parents. Ethics committees or infant review committees should also be utilized to facilitate parental decision making. These committees should help mediate resolutions of conflicts that may arise among parents, physicians, and others involved in the care of the infant. These committees should also be responsible for referring cases to the appropriate public agencies when it is concluded that the parents' decision is not a decision that could reasonably be judged to be in the best interests of the infant. (I, III, IV, V)

Issued June 1994 based on the report "Treatment Decisions for Seriously Ill Newborns," adopted June 1992.

N.Y. Sup. 2003 Mother petitioned court to remove her daughter from a respirator. Hospital policy denied mother the authorization to withdraw care. Court granted petition and held parents have a right to refuse medical treatment for their children. Applying the best interest test, the court held that the burdens of prolonging life exceeded the benefits and that, absent extraordinary circumstances or disagreement between parents, judicial intervention is not required to withhold medical treatment from a minor in a vegetative state. Quotes Opinion 2.215. References Opinion 2.20. *In re AB, 196 Misc. 2d 940, 768 N.Y.S. 2d 256, 268-69.*

Journal 2004 Discusses the lack of a rational basis for a distinction between physician-assisted suicide and a physician's cooperation with a patient's refusal of life-sustaining treatment. Concludes that once legally permissible means of hastening death are widely known by physicians, restrictions on physician-assisted death may become anomalous. Cites Opinion 2.215. Cantor, *On Kamisar, Killing, and the Future of Physician-Assisted Death, 102 Mich. L. Rev. 1793, 1825 (2004).*

Journal 2002 Explores the implications of withholding medical treatment when abortion results in a live birth. Concludes that, in these situations, abortive parents and physicians should not solely decide the child's best interest. Quotes Preamble, Principles I and III, and Opinions 2.035, 2.20, and 2.215. Casagrande, *Children Not Meant to Be: Protecting the Interests of the Child When Abortion Results in Live Birth, 6 Quinnipiac Health L. J. 19, 44, 45, 47-48 (2002).*

Journal 2001 Examines end-of-life care given to infants under the age of one. Concludes that palliative care consultations may improve the end-of-life care that terminally ill infants and their families currently receive. References Opinion 2.215. Pierucci, Kirby, & Leuthner, *End-of-Life Care for Neonates and Infants: The Experience and Effects of a Palliative Care Consultation Service, 108 Pediatrics 653, 659 (2001).*

Journal 2001 Discusses neonatal euthanasia and the related moral dilemmas. Explores the background and current legal status of neonatal euthanasia in the US. Concludes that the moral and legal status of passive neonatal euthanasia is unclear and should be reviewed and clarified. Quotes Opinion 2.215. Sklansky, *Neonatal Euthanasia: Moral Considerations and Criminal Liability, 27 J. Med. Ethics 5, 8, 9 (2001).*

2.22 Do-Not-Resuscitate Orders

When a patient suffers cardiac or respiratory arrest, attempts should be made to resuscitate the patient, except when cardiopulmonary resuscitation (CPR) is not in accord with the patient's expressed desires or is clinically inappropriate.

All patients should be encouraged to express in advance their preferences regarding the extent of treatment after cardiopulmonary arrest, especially patients at substantial risk of such an event. During discussions regarding patients' preferences, physicians should include a description of the procedures encompassed by CPR. Patients' preferences should be documented as early as possible and should be revisited and revised as appropriate.

Advance directives stating patients' refusals of CPR should be honored whether patients are in or out of hospital. When patients refuse CPR, physicians should not permit their personal value judgments to obstruct implementation of the refusals.

If a patient lacks the ability to make or cannot communicate a decision regarding the use of CPR, a surrogate decision maker may make a decision based upon the previously expressed preferences of the patient. If such preferences are unknown, decisions should be made in accordance with the patient's best interests. If no surrogate decision maker is available, an attending physician contemplating a "do-not-resuscitate" (DNR) order should consult another physician or a hospital ethics committee, if one is available. (See Opinion 8.081, "Surrogate Decision Making.")

If a patient (either directly or through an advance directive) or the patient's surrogate requests resuscitation that the physician determines would not be medically effective, the physician should seek to resolve the conflict through a fair decision-making process, when time permits. (See Opinion 2.037, "Medical Futility in End-of-Life Care.") In hospitals and other health care organizations, medical staffs or, in their absence, medical directors should adopt and disseminate policies regarding the form and function of DNR orders and a process for resolving conflicts.

DNR orders, as well as the basis for their implementation, should be entered by the attending physician in the patient's medical record.

DNR orders and a patient's advance refusal of CPR preclude only resuscitative efforts after cardiopulmonary arrest and should not influence other medically appropriate interventions, such as pharmacologic circulatory support and antibiotics, unless they also are specifically refused. (See Opinion 2.225, "Optimal Use of Orders Not-to-Intervene and Advance Directives.") (I, IV, VIII)

Issued March 1992 based on the report "Guidelines for the Appropriate Use of Do-Not-Resuscitate Orders," adopted December 1990 (JAMA. 1991;265:1868-1871). Updated June 1994 and November 2005 based on the report "Universal Out-of-Hospital DNR Systems," adopted June 2005.

Kan. App. 1998 Physician was convicted of attempted murder of a terminally ill patient, and intentional and malicious second-degree murder of another terminally ill patient. The court quoted Opinion 2.22, to exemplify a physician's duty to provide cardiopulmonary resuscitation unless the physician believes that such action would be futile. Additionally, the court referenced Opinion 2.20, in support of a physician's duty to provide a terminally ill patient adequate pain relief. The court reversed the physician's convictions, stating that the jury could not disregard the testimony of several physicians who concurred with the defendant-physician's treatment of the deceased patients. *State v. Naramore, 25 Kan. App. 2d 302, 965 P.2d 211, 214, 216.*

Journal 2006 Examines the public reaction to the Terri Schiavo case. Concludes that public fears were misplaced and that all persons benefited from the decision. Quotes Opinions 2.03, 2.035, and 2.17. Cites Opinion 2.22. Cerminara, *Musings on the Need to Convince Some People With Disabilities That End-of-Life Decision-Making Advocates Are Not Out to Get Them, 37 Loy. U. Chi. L. J. 343, 347 (2006).*

Journal 2006 Argues for an alternative framework by which health ethics, policy, and law can address equitable distribution of health care. Concludes that a new paradigm would lead to a more efficient and compassionate system. References Opinions 2.22 and 8.13. Ruger, *Health, Capability, and Justice: Toward a New Paradigm of Health Ethics, Policy and Law, 15 Cornell J. L. & Pub. Pol'y 403, 425, 465 (2006).*

Journal 2004 Examines conflicts that arise when a hospice may be obligated to resuscitate a patient who has not executed an advance directive regarding CPR. Concludes that the Patient Self-Determination Act must be amended to allow hospice providers to administer CPR in only a limited number of circumstances. References Opinions 2.035 and 2.22. Rutkow, *Dying to Live: The Effect of the Patient Self-determination Act on Hospice Care, 7 N. Y. U. J. Legis. & Pub. Pol'y 393, 413, 430 (2004).*

Journal 2001 Observes that many aspects of managed care have increased the tensions between patients and their health care providers. Notes that patient dissatisfaction is on the rise for other reasons as well. Concludes that Congress should take a comprehensive legislative approach in addressing these issues. Quotes Opinion 2.17. Cites Opinion 2.035. References Opinions 2.037 and 2.22. Sanematsu, *Taking a Broader View of Treatment Disputes Beyond Managed Care: Are Recent Legislative Efforts the Cure? 48 UCLA L. Rev. 1245, 1258, 1284 (2001).*

Journal 2000 Discusses a medical-ethical strategy for managing iatrogenic cardiac arrests in DNR patients. Suggests that many factors must be taken into account before withholding resuscitation in certain unanticipated situations, such as an iatrogenic catastrophe. References Opinion 2.22. Christensen & Orlowski, *Iatrogenic Cardiopulmonary Arrests in DNR Patients, 11 J. Clinical Ethics 14, 15, 20 (2000).*

Journal 2000 Discusses euphemisms used through medical codes in hospitals regarding end-of-life patient care. Examines how the fear of medical failure and the fear of litigation mold decision-making in critical care units. Concludes that health care providers often lack the courage to let a patient die. References Opinion 2.22. Smith, *Euphemistic Codes and Tell-Tale Hearts: Humane Assistance in End-of-Life Cases, 10 Health Matrix 175, 177 (2000).*

Journal 2000 Discusses current law governing consent to sperm retrieval and insemination after death or persistent vegetative state. Identifies gaps in the law. Concludes that sperm retrieval and insemination in these situations should be permitted, provided there is express prior consent or sufficient evidence from which consent may be implied. Cites Opinion 2.22. Strong, *Consent to Sperm Retrieval and Insemination After Death or Persistent Vegetative State, 14 J. L. & Health 243, 248 (2000).*

Journal 1998 Explains when a surrogate is required to make health care decisions. Discusses limitations of a surrogate's authority. Emphasizes that the health care provider must recognize that ultimate decision-making regarding care first belongs to the patient, and then to the surrogate. Quotes Opinion 2.035. Cites Opinion 8.11. References Opinion 2.22. O'Neill, *Surrogate Health Care Decisions for Adults in Illinois—Answers to the Legal Questions That Health Care Providers Face on a Daily Basis, 29 Loy. Univ. Chi. L. J. 411, 445, 448 (1998).*

Journal 1998 Discusses various ways theorists define medical futility. Evaluates the impact of *In re Baby K* on the correct notion of medical futility. Examines how futility affects patient autonomy. Quotes Opinion 2.22. Strasser, *The Futility of Futility? On Life, Death, and Reasoned Public Policy, 57 Md. L. Rev. 505, 523, 552, 553 (1998).*

Journal 1997 Examines case law pertaining to medical futility disputes. Reviews hospital policies regarding futility and notes a variety of definitions and guidelines. Concludes that, absent a clear consensus, physicians should not act solely to decide questions of futility. References Opinions 2.035 and 2.22. Johnson, Gibbons, Goldner, Wiener, & Eton, *Legal and Institutional Policy Responses to Medical Futility, 30 J. Health & Hosp. L. 21, 26, 31, 35, 36 (1997).*

Journal 1997 Explores the meaning of cardiopulmonary resuscitation and legal issues involving DNR orders. Considers problems created by DNR orders in operating rooms in light of patients' rights. Concludes that hospitals must adopt clear policies for their surgical teams to follow. Quotes Opinion 8.08. References Opinion 2.22. Lonchyna, *To Resuscitate or Not . . . In the Operating Room: The Need for Hospital Policies for Surgeons Regarding DNR Orders, 6 Annals Health L. 209, 215, 217 (1997).*

Journal 1997 Considers individuals' right to die and the value of a wrongful living tort. Proposes that courts should reject any cause of action for wrongful living in situations where patient advance directives are not honored by physicians. References Opinion 2.22. Milani, *Better Off Dead Than Disabled? Should Courts Recognize a Wrongful Living Cause of Action When Doctors Fail to Honor Patients' Advance Directives? 54 Wash. & Lee L. Rev. 149, 151-52 (1997).*

Journal 1994 Considers how greater patient autonomy has led to situations in which medical care may be viewed as futile. Suggests that the law has intruded too far into this area of medicine. Quotes Opinion 2.035. Cites Opinions 2.03, 2.095, 2.17, 2.19, 2.20, and 2.22. Cultice, *Medical Futility: When Is Enough, Enough? 27 J. Health & Hosp. Law 225, 230, 256 (1994).*

Journal 1993 Discusses physician, patient, and societal concerns about futility. Concludes that futility decisions should be left to physicians. Cites Opinion 2.22. Bennett, *When Is Medical Treatment Futile? 9 Issues in Law & Med. 35, 39 (1993).*

Journal 1993 Considers how patient self-determination may be affected by cardiopulmonary resuscitation and do-not-resuscitate policies. Opposes a "futility" exception to informed consent as being violative of a physician's fiduciary duties to patients. Cites Opinion 8.07 (1986) [now Opinion 8.08]. References Opinion 2.22. Boozang, *Death Wish: Resuscitating Self-Determination for the Critically Ill, 35 Ariz. L. Rev. 23, 24, 28, 52 (1993).*

Journal 1993 Discusses the problem of physicians withholding needed medical treatment from HIV-infected infants. Concludes that current law should be expanded to eliminate this discrimination. Quotes Opinions 2.09, 2.17, 2.20, 2.22, 4.04, and 8.03. Crossley, *Of Diagnoses and Discrimination: Discriminatory Nontreatment of Infants With HIV Infection, 93 Columbia L. Rev. 1581, 1620, 1621 (1993).*

Journal 1993 Discusses the relationship between a physician's professional conscience and end-of-life decision-making. Considers the issue of futile medical treatment. Examines case law concerning a patient's right to demand treatment and a physician's obligation to provide it. References Opinions 2.20 and 2.22. Daar, *A Clash at the Bedside: Patient Autonomy v. a Physician's Professional Conscience, 44 Hastings L. J. 1241, 1257, 1268, 1286 (1993).*

Journal 1993 Discusses the American Heart Association's acknowledgment of medical futility, but questions whether its views adequately reflect current ethical perceptions. Proposes ways in which the guidelines should be reformed. References Opinion 2.22. Jecker & Schneiderman, *An Ethical Analysis of the Use of "Futility" in the 1992 American Heart Association Guidelines for Cardiopulmonary Resuscitation and Emergency Cardiac Care, 153 Arch. Intern. Med. 2195, 2197 (1993).*

Journal 1993 Examines the American Heart Association's guidelines for withholding cardiopulmonary resuscitation in emergency medical service systems and criticizes them for being too strict. Argues that a mechanism should be created to facilitate prehospital DNR orders and ensure that they are followed. References Opinion 2.22. McIntyre, *Loosening Criteria for Withholding Prehospital Cardiopulmonary Resuscitation, 153 Arch. Intern. Med. 2189, 2190 (1993).*

Journal 1992 Examines several issues regarding persistent vegetative state (PVS) patients, including whether PVS patients are really dead, whether nutrition and hydration should be withheld, whether life-sustaining treatments are futile or medically inappropriate, and whether ordinary standards for decision-making should be applied to PVS patients. Concludes that life-sustaining therapy may be withheld or continued, but that withdrawal of nutrition and hydration, as well as active euthanasia, present more difficult questions. References Opinions 2.20 and 2.22. Brody, *Special Ethical Issues in the Management of PVS Patients, 20 Law Med. & Health Care 104, 109 (1992).*

Journal 1992 Discusses "do-not-resuscitate" (DNR) orders in light of the Patient Self-Determination Act. Proposes a policy of required reconsideration of DNR orders in hospitals when a patient enters a treatment setting in which discreet, time-limited therapies are offered that may precipitate cardiac arrest. References Opinion 2.22. Cohen & Cohen, *Required Reconsideration of "Do-Not-Resuscitate" Orders in the Operating Room and Certain Other Treatment Settings, 20 Law Med. & Health Care 354, 356 (1992).*

Journal 1992 Examines ethical and legal issues surrounding cardiopulmonary resuscitation and emergency cardiac care. Discusses advance directives and proxy decision-making, medical futility, resource allocation, and do-not-resuscitate orders. References Opinions 2.20 and 2.22. Comment, *Ethical Considerations in Resuscitation*, 268 JAMA 2282, 2283, 2287 (1992).

Journal 1992 Considers the debate surrounding medical futility. Observes that this debate is encouraging reexamination of the nature of patient entitlement to medical care as well as the "ends of medicine." References Opinions 2.20, 2.21, and 2.22. Miles, *Medical Futility*, 20 Law Med. & Health Care 310, 311, 313 (1992).

Journal 1992 Explains how the "terminal condition" requirement in natural death acts may reduce the number of people who fall within the scope of coverage. Also indicates that omission of nutrition and hydration from the list of treatments that may be withdrawn limits patient choices. Quotes Opinion 2.20. References Opinion 2.22. Note, *State Natural Death Acts: Illusory Protection of Individuals' Life-Sustaining Treatment Decisions*, 29 Harvard J. Legis. 175, 186, 194, 195, 201 (1992).

Journal 1992 Discusses the impact of physicians' values on end-of-life decision making for patients. Examines how and why physician values may become dominant. References Opinions 2.20, 2.22, and 9.121. Orentlicher, *The Illusion of Patient Choice in End-of-Life Decisions*, 267 JAMA 2101, 2102 (1992).

Journal 1992 Discusses results of a study that evaluated the impact of ethics education on do-not-resuscitate (DNR) practices by house officers. Concludes that educational programs improve care for DNR patients. References Opinion 2.22. Sulmasy, Geller, Faden, & Levine, *The Quality of Mercy: Caring for Patients With "Do-Not-Resuscitate" Orders*, 267 JAMA 682 (1992).

Journal 1991 Examines the involvement of the legal system in end-of-life medical decision-making. Questions whether the law should intrude into the domain. Concludes that judges should become involved primarily to address the "terms of reconciliation" between physicians and patients. References Opinion 2.22. Flick, *The Due Process of Dying*, 79 Cal. L. Rev. 1121, 1152 (1991).

Journal 1990 Finds that a vast majority of North Carolina nursing homes have written cardiopulmonary resuscitation policies, but that there is substantial variation among them. Concludes that such variations risk limiting or ignoring the personal rights of residents. References Opinions 2.20 and 2.22. Brunetti, Weiss, Studenski, & Clipp, *Cardiopulmonary Resuscitation Policies and Practices: A Statewide Nursing Home Study*, 150 Arch. Intern. Med. 121, 122 (1990).

2.225 Optimal Use of Orders Not-to-Intervene and Advance Directives

More rigorous efforts in advance care planning are required in order to tailor end-of-life care to the preferences of patients so that they can experience a satisfactory last chapter in their lives. There is need for better availability and tracking of advance directives, and more uniform adoption of form documents that can be honored in all states of the United States. The discouraging evidence of inadequate end-of-life decision-making indicates the necessity of several improvement strategies:

(1) Patients and physicians should make use of advisory as well as statutory documents. Advisory documents aim to accurately represent a patient's wishes and are legally binding under law. Statutory documents give physicians immunity from malpractice for following a patient's wishes. If a form is not available that combines the two, an advisory document should be appended to the state statutory form.

(2) Advisory documents should be based on validated worksheets, thus ensuring reasonable confidence that preferences for end-of-life treatment can be fairly and effectively elicited and recorded, and that they are applicable to medical decisions.

(3) Physicians should directly discuss the patient's preferences with the patient and the patient's proxy. These discussions should be held ahead of time wherever possible. The key steps of structuring a core discussion and of signing and recording the document in the medical record should not be delegated to a junior member of the health care team.

(4) Central repositories should be established so that completed advisory documents, state statutory documents, identification of a proxy, and identification of the primary physician can be obtained efficiently in emergency and urgent circumstances as well as routinely.

(5) Health care facilities should honor, and physicians use, a range of orders on the doctor's order sheet to indicate patient wishes regarding avoidable treatments that might otherwise be given on an emergency basis or by a covering physician with less knowledge of the patient's wishes. Treatment avoidance orders might include, along with a do-not-resuscitate (DNR) order, some of the following: full comfort care only (FCCO); do not intubate (DNI); do not defibrillate (DND); do not leave home (DNLH); do not transfer (DNTransfer); no intravenous lines (NIL); no blood draws (NBD); no feeding tube (NFT); no vital signs (NVS); and so forth. One common new order, do not treat (DNT), is specifically not included in this list, since it may unintentionally convey the message that no care should be given and the patient may lose the intense attention due to a dying person; FCCO serves the same purpose without the likely misinterpretation. As with DNR orders, these treatment avoidance orders should be revisited periodically to ensure their continued applicability. Active comfort care orders might include allow visitors extended hours (AVEH) and inquire about comfort (IAC) bid (twice daily). (I, IV)

Issued June 1998 based on the report "Optimal Use of Orders-Not-to-Intervene and Advance Directives," adopted June 1997 (*Psych, Pub Pol'y, and Law*. 1998;4:668-675).

Journal 2009 Argues new physician orders for life-sustaining treatment (POLST) legislation should be enacted in Florida because the POLST form can more effectively achieve the purposes of advance directives. Concludes the POLST form will reduce problems with advance directives by creating a system to translate a patient's wishes into standardized physician's orders. Quotes Opinion 2.225. Sonderling, *POLST: A Cure for the Common Advance Directive—It's Just What the Doctor Ordered*, 33 Nova L. Rev. 451, 470, 478 (2009).

Journal 2007 Discusses patients' right to refuse medical treatment and the corresponding duties of health care professionals. Concludes that detailed, carefully prepared advance directives are necessary to fulfill patients' wishes. Quotes Ch. II (1940) [now Opinions 8.08 and 8.082] and Opinions 2.035, 2.037, 2.20, 2.225, 8.081, and 10.015. Cites Opinions 9.11 and 9.115. Stamatakis, *Beyond Advance Directives: Personal Autonomy and the Right to Refuse Life-Sustaining Medical Treatment*, 47 N. H. B. J. 20, 29-30 (2007).

Journal 2000 Discusses the process of advance care planning. Identifies five steps for success: appropriate introduction of the topic; structured discussions covering specific situations; documentation of patient preferences; updating of directives; and application of directives when indicated. References Opinion 2.225. Emanuel, von Gunten, & Ferris, *Advance Care Planning*, 9 Arch. Fam. Med. 1181, 1181 (2000).

Journal 1999 States that a distrust of the medical profession arose from changes in the health care system and federal law. Explains how legislation may help alleviate some of the distrust. Suggests that people need more access to information about their health plans. References Opinions 2.20 and 2.225. Cerminara, *Protecting Participants in and Beneficiaries of ERISA-Governed Managed Health Care Plans*, 29 U. Mem. L. Rev. 317, 324 (1999).

2.23   Opinion 2.23, "HIV Testing," originally issued March 1992, was replaced by
        Opinion 2.23, "HIV Testing," June 2008, which was replaced by the current
        Opinion 2.23, "HIV Testing," November 2010.

2.23   HIV Testing

Physicians' duties to promote patients' welfare and to improve the public's
health are fostered by routinely testing their adult patients for HIV. Physicians
must balance these obligations with their concurrent duties to their individual
patients' best interest by following the guidelines below:

(1) In order to protect patients, avoid injury to third parties, and promote pub-
     lic health, physicians should support routine universal screening for HIV
     with opt-out provisions.

(2) Although medical and social advances have minimized the need for spe-
     cific written consent prior to HIV testing, the ethical tenets of respect for
     autonomy and informed consent require that physicians continue to seek
     patients' informed consent to undergo any form of medical treatment,
     including refusal of HIV testing. Given the potential benefits to a patient
     (and the patient's intimate others) of knowing his/her HIV status, it is
     appropriate for physicians to make efforts to persuade reluctant patients to
     be screened. Physicians should, however, respect the decision of a patient
     who "opts out." Unless required by law, patients' consent to HIV testing
     does not need to be documented in writing. However, the conversation
     concerning testing should be documented in the patient's chart. It is justifi-
     able to test patients without prior consent only in limited cases where the
     harms to individual autonomy are offset by significant benefits to known
     third parties. Such exceptions include testing for the protection of occupa-
     tionally exposed health care professionals or patients.

(3) Physicians must work to ensure that patients identified as being HIV posi-
     tive receive appropriate follow-up care and counseling.

(4) Physicians must comply with all applicable disease reporting laws while
     taking appropriate measures to safeguard the confidentiality of patients'
     medical information to the extent possible.

(5) Physicians must honor their obligation to promote the public's health by
     working to prevent HIV-positive individuals from infecting third parties
     within the constraints of the law. If an HIV-positive individual poses a sig-
     nificant threat of infecting an identifiable third party, the physician should:
     (a) notify the public health authorities, if required by law;
     (b) attempt to persuade the infected patient to cease endangering the
          third party; and
     (c) if permitted by state law, notify the endangered third party without
          revealing the identity of the source person. (I, IV, VII)

Issued November 2010 based on the report "Amendment to E-2.23, 'HIV Testing,'" adopted
June 2010.

Journal 2010 Examines published resources within the medical and legal fields that focus on
confidentiality and evaluates those resources to determine if they help clarify confidentiality issues. Further, discusses differences between these professions that may be hindrances
when serving the same patient or client. Concludes that, while both professions guard against

disclosure of patient/client communications, they also allow for disclosure in certain instances such as imminent death, harm, or injury. References Principle IV and cites Opinions 2.02, 2.23, 2.24, and 5.05. Johns, *Multidisciplinary Practice and Ethics Part II—Lawyers, Doctors, and Confidentiality*, 6 NAELA J. 55, 57-65, 68 (2010).

Journal 2009 Examines the role of physicians during natural and man-made disasters. Concludes hospitals must make plans to define disaster response procedures that shift responsibility for survival from the physician to the community. Quotes Code of Ethics, Ch. III, Art. I §1 (1847) [now Opinion 9.067], Principle 5 (1957) [now Principle VI], Principle VI, and Opinions 2.23, 9.067, and 9.131. Cites Opinions 9.06, 9.067, and 9.12. Ahronheim, *Service by Health Care Providers in a Public Health Emergency: The Physician's Duty and the Law*, 12 J. Health Care L. & Pol'y 195, 209-11, 215, 225 (2009).

Journal 2007 Considers whether health care providers should initiate discussions of HIV testing for their patients. Concludes that adopting such a policy, with specialized informed consent, would help limit the spread of HIV. Quotes Opinion 2.23. Rajkumar, *A Human Rights Approach to Routine Provider-Initiated HIV Testing*, 7 Yale J. Health Pol'y L. & Ethics 319, 371 (2007).

Journal 2001 Compares the American system of patient confidentiality to the Austrian system. Discusses the debate between patients' rights and public safety. Concludes that the duty to warn third parties of dangerous patients should be discretionary instead of mandatory, except in cases of HIV seropositivity, which should involve mandatory disclosure to public health officials. Quotes Opinions 2.23, 5.05, and 5.06. Kenworthy, *The Austrian Psychotherapy Act: No Legal Duty to Warn*, 11 Ind. Int'l & Comp. L. Rev. 469, 480-81, 485, 490, 496 (2001).

Journal 2000 Examines the effect of HIV/AIDS on the relationship between the general public and health care professionals (HCPs). Discusses the importance of creating an environment in which HIV-positive patients do not fear disclosing their HIV status. Discusses policies and guidelines that address methods to prevent transmission of HIV from HCPs to patients. Quotes Opinion 2.23. References Opinions 9.13 and 9.131. Rediger, *Living in a World With HIV: Balancing Privacy, Privilege and the Right to Know Between Patients and Health Care Professionals*, 21 Hamline J. Pub. L. & Pol'y 443, 456-57, 461, 472 (2000).

Journal 1999 Explores the possibility of genetic testing in the managed care setting. Points out that genetic testing is not likely to reduce health care costs, but may improve health. Recommends ways in which genetic medicine can be practiced in the managed care context. Quotes Opinion 2.23. Rothstein & Hoffman, *Genetic Testing, Genetic Medicine, and Managed Care*, 34 Wake Forest L. Rev. 849, 883 (1999).

Journal 1999 Discusses whether health care professionals have the right to refuse to treat patients under common law and federal statutes and regulations. Explores the impact of the Americans with Disabilities Act and the US Supreme Court decision in *Bragdon v. Abbott* on the duties of health care professionals in the context of providing treatment to HIV-positive patients. Quotes Principle VI and Opinions 2.23 and 9.131. White, *Health Care Professionals and Treatment of HIV-Positive Patients*, 20 J. Legal Med. 67, 86 (1999).

Journal 1998 Compares the New York AIDS confidentiality statute with statutes that mandate testing for other communicable diseases. Discusses whether the legal response to AIDS will serve as a model for responses to undiscovered diseases. Suggests that the prohibition on involuntary HIV testing should be reconsidered. Cites Opinion 2.23. Fernandez, *Is AIDS Different?* 61 Alb. L. Rev. 1053 (1998).

Journal 1996 Discusses conflict between physicians' duty of confidentiality to patients and physicians' obligation to warn third parties of foreseeable injuries. Examines physicians' current legal responsibility to breach confidentiality to prevent the spread of infectious diseases, including AIDS. Identifies guidelines for physicians. Cites Opinions 2.23 and 5.057. Comment, *Taking Tarasoff Where No One Has Gone Before: Looking at Duty to Warn Under the AIDS Crisis*, 15 St. Louis U. Pub. L. Rev. 471, 499 (1996).

Journal 1995 Observes that statutes criminalizing HIV transmission would pose a disincentive for testing and also infringe upon the patient's right to confidentiality because criminal prosecutions are a matter of public record. Concludes that legislatures must carefully consider such issues when drafting legislation to prevent the spread of HIV. Quotes Opinion 2.23. O'Toole, *HIV-Specific Crime Legislation: Targeting an Epidemic for Criminal Prosecution*, 10 J. L. & Health 183, 195, 199 (1995).

Journal 1990 Explores potential physician tort liability for failure to warn at-risk individuals of the danger of being infected by the physician's HIV-positive patient. Concludes that there is a legal duty requiring health care professionals to warn those persons foreseeably at risk of being infected by an HIV-positive patient. References Opinion 2.23. Labowitz, *Beyond Tarasoff: AIDS and the Obligation to Breach Confidentiality*, 9 St. Louis Univ. Pub. L. Rev. 495, 514 (1990).

Journal 1990 Considers the tension between confidentiality and the duty to warn in the context of AIDS and HIV. Considers the appropriateness of mandatory reporting and partner notification and proposes legal reforms in this area. References Opinion 2.23. Price, *Between Scylla and Charybdis: Charting a Course to Reconcile the Duty of Confidentiality and the Duty to Warn in the AIDS Context*, 94 Dickinson L. Rev. 435, 477 (1990).

2.24 Impaired Drivers and Their Physicians

The purpose of this report is to articulate physicians' responsibility to recognize impairments in patients' driving ability that pose a strong threat to public safety and which ultimately may need to be reported to the department of motor vehicles. It does not address the reporting of medical information for the purpose of punishment or criminal prosecution.

(1) Physicians should assess patients' physical or mental impairments that might adversely affect driving abilities. Each case must be evaluated individually since not all impairments may give rise to an obligation on the part of the physician. Nor may all physicians be in a position to evaluate the extent or the effect of an impairment (eg, physicians who treat patients on a short-term basis). In making evaluations, physicians should consider the following factors:

(a) The physician must be able to identify and document physical or mental impairments that clearly relate to the ability to drive.

(b) The driver must pose a clear risk to public safety.

(2) Before reporting, there are a number of initial steps physicians should take. A tactful but candid discussion with the patient and family about the risks of driving is of primary importance. Depending on the patient's medical condition, the physician may suggest to the patient that he or she seek further treatment, such as substance abuse treatment or occupational therapy. Physicians also may encourage the patient and the family to decide on a restricted driving schedule. Efforts made by physicians to inform patients and their families, advise them of their options, and negotiate a workable plan may render reporting unnecessary.

(3) Physicians should use their best judgment when determining when to report impairments that could limit a patient's ability to drive safely. In situations where clear evidence of substantial driving impairment implies a strong threat to patient and public safety, and where the physician's advice to discontinue driving privileges is ignored, it is desirable and ethical to notify the department of motor vehicles.

(4) The physician's role is to report medical conditions that would impair safe driving as dictated by his or her state's mandatory reporting laws and standards of medical practice. The determination of the inability to drive safely should be made by the state's department of motor vehicles.

(5) Physicians should disclose and explain to their patients this responsibility to report.

(6) Physicians should protect patient confidentiality by ensuring that only the minimal amount of information is reported and that reasonable security measures are used in handling that information.

(7) Physicians should work with their state medical societies to create statutes that uphold the best interests of patients and community and that safeguard physicians from liability when reporting in good faith. (I, III, IV, VII)

Issued June 2000 based on the report "Impaired Drivers and Their Physicians," adopted December 1999.

Journal 2010 Examines published resources within the medical and legal fields that focus on confidentiality and evaluates those resources to determine if they help clarify confidentiality issues. Further, discusses differences between these professions that may be hindrances when serving the same patient or client. Concludes that, while both professions guard against disclosure of patient/client communications, they also allow for disclosure in certain instances such as imminent death, harm, or injury. References Principle IV and cites Opinions 2.02, 2.23, 2.24, and 5.05. Johns, *Multidisciplinary Practice and Ethics Part II—Lawyers, Doctors, and Confidentiality*, 6 *NAELA J.* 55, 57-65, 68 (2010).

Journal 2004 Considers third-party liability in situations where an elderly impaired driver negligently injures another. Discusses the impact on family members who occupy a special relationship with the driver. Concludes that a proper balance must be struck to encourage active family support. Quotes Opinion 2.24. Martin, *Who Will Take the Keys From Grandpa?* 21 T. M. *Cooley L. Rev.* 257, 263, 264 (2004).

Journal 2002 Discusses issues regarding regulation of elderly drivers. Concludes that mandating physicians to report unfit elderly patients will protect the public and help resolve ethical and legal dilemmas. Quotes Opinions 1.02, 2.24, 5.05, and 10.01. Kane, *Driving Into the Sunset: A Proposal for Mandatory Reporting to the DMV by Physicians Treating Unsafe Elderly Drivers*, 25 U. *Haw. L. Rev.* 59, 59, 61, 62, 67, 69, 82, 83 (2002).

Journal 2002 Discusses malpractice liability in connection with treatment and diagnosis of dementia. Concludes that physicians must stay aware of new diagnostic and treatment developments in order to reduce risk. Cites Opinion 2.24. Kapp, *Legal Standards for the Medical Diagnosis and Treatment of Dementia*, 23 J. *Legal Med.* 359, 382 (2002).

Journal 2000 Explores physician involvement in the care of cognitively impaired elderly people who operate motor vehicles. Discusses conflicts that arise in fulfilling obligations to the patient, while upholding obligations to the welfare of the community. Cites Opinion 2.24. Berger & Rosner, *Ethical Challenges Posed by Dementia and Driving*, 11 J. *Clinical Ethics* 304, 307, 308 (2000).

2.25 The Use of Quarantine and Isolation as Public Health Interventions

Quarantine and isolation to protect the population's health potentially conflict with the individual rights of liberty and self-determination. The medical profession, in collaboration with public health colleagues, must take an active role in ensuring that those interventions are based on science and are applied according to certain ethical considerations.

(1) To this end, the medical profession should:

(a) seek an appropriate balance of public needs and individual restraints so that quarantine and isolation use the least restrictive measures available that will minimize negative effects on the community through disease control while providing protections for individual rights;

(b) help ensure that quarantine and isolation are based upon valid science and do not arbitrarily target socioeconomic, racial, or ethnic groups;

(c) advocate for the highest possible level of confidentiality of personal health information whenever clinical information is transmitted in the context of public health reporting;

(d) advocate for access to public health services to ensure timely detection of risks and prevent undue delays in the implementation of quarantine and isolation;

(e) help to educate patients and the public about quarantine and isolation through the development of educational materials and participation in educational programs;

(f) advocate for the availability of protective and preventive measures for physicians and others caring for patients with communicable diseases.

(2) Individual physicians should participate in the implementation of appropriate quarantine and isolation measures as part of their obligation to provide medical care during epidemics (see Opinion E-9.067, "Physician Obligation in Disaster Preparedness and Response"). In doing so, advocacy for their individual patients' best interests remains paramount (see Opinion E-10.015, "The Patient-Physician Relationship"). Accordingly, physicians should:

(a) encourage patients to adhere voluntarily to scientifically grounded quarantine and isolation measures by educating them about the nature of the threat to public health, the potential harm that it poses to the patient and others, and the personal and public benefits to be derived from quarantine or isolation. If the patient fails to comply voluntarily with such measures, the physician should support mandatory quarantine and isolation for the noncompliant patient;

(b) comply with mandatory reporting requirements when appropriate and inform patients of such reports when feasible;

(c) minimize the risk of transmitting infectious diseases from physician to patient and ensure that they remain available to provide necessary medical services by using appropriate protective and preventive measures, seeking medical evaluation and treatment if they suspect themselves to be infected, and adhering to mandated public health measures.

(3) Frontline physicians have an increased ethical obligation to avail themselves of safe and effective protective and preventive measures (for example, influenza vaccine). (I, III, VI, VII, VIII,)

Issued June 2006 based on the report "The Use of Quarantine and Isolation as Public Health Interventions," adopted November 2005.

Journal 2008 Examines the ethical reasons why physicians choose to provide treatment in disaster situations, even at great risk to themselves. Concludes that individual values play a substantial role in such decision making. Quotes Preamble, Opinion 9.131, and Ch. III, Art. 1, Sec. 1 (May 1847) [now Opinions 2.25 and 9.067]. Iserson, Heine, Larkin, Moskop, Baruch, & Aswegan, *Fight or Flight: The Ethics of Emergency Physician Disaster Response*, 51 Annals of Emergency Med. 345-353 (2008).

Journal 2008 Discusses the duty of physicians to participate in pandemic care. Concludes that the extent of personal risk a physician is obligated to take has a limit, although the limit has yet to be clearly defined. Quotes Ch. III, Art. I, Sec. 1 (1847) [now Opinions 2.25 and 9.067]. Meerschaert, *Physicians' Duty to Participate in Pandemic Care*, 300 JAMA 284, 284 (2008).

Journal 2007 Discusses the role of job security and income reimbursement in ensuring voluntary compliance with quarantine orders in the US, and analyzes the adequacy of current laws to address such concerns. Concludes that existing statutes would be inadequate and proposes new model legislation. Cites Ch. III, Art. I, Sec. I (May 1847) [now Opinion 2.25]. Rothstein & Talbott, *Job Security and Income Replacement for Individuals in Quarantine: The Need for Legislation*, 10 J. Health Care L. & Pol'y 239, 239-40 (2007).

Journal 2007 Examines physicians' duty to treat victims of highly infectious diseases during an epidemic. Concludes that no clear duty exists, and that if physicians are compelled to provide care by law they must be afforded sufficient due process to protect their property interests in their medical licenses. Quotes Ch. III, Art. I, Sec. I (May 1847) [now Opinions 2.25 and 9.067] and Opinion 9.131. References Principle 10 (1957) [now Principle VII]. Schwartz, *Doubtful Duty: Physicians' Legal Obligation to Treat During an Epidemic*, 60 Stan. L. Rev. 657, 662, 663 (2007).

Journal 2007 Speculates on the availability of funding for hospitals confronted with an infectious disease pandemic. Concludes that new legislation is required to ensure adequate funding for hospitals in such a situation. Quotes Ch. III, Art. I, Sec. 1 (May 1847) [now Opinions 2.25 and 9.067]. Williams, *Fluconomics: Preserving Our Hospital Infrastructure During and After a Pandemic*, 7 Yale J. Health Pol'y L. & Ethics 99, 115 (2007).

2.30   Information From Unethical Experiments

All proposed experiments using human subjects should undergo proper ethical evaluation by a human studies review board before being undertaken.

Responsibility for revealing that the data are from unethical experiments lies in the hands of authors, peer reviewers, and editors of medical texts that publish results of experimental studies. Each publication should adopt a standard regarding publication of data from unethical experiments.

If data from unethical experiments can be replaced by existing ethically sound data and achieve the same ends, then such must be done. If ethically tainted data that have been validated by rigorous scientific analysis are the only data of that nature available, and such data are necessary in order to save lives, then the utilization of such data by physicians and editors may be appropriate.

Should editors and/or authors decide to publish an experiment or data from an experiment that does not reach standards of contemporary ethical conduct, a disclaimer should be included. Such disclosure would by no means rectify unethical conduct or legitimize the methods of collection of data gathered from unethical experimentation. This disclaimer should: (1) clearly describe the unethical nature of the origin of any material being published; (2) clearly state that publication of the data is needed in order to save human lives; (3) pay respect to the victims; (4) avoid trivializing trauma suffered by the participants; (5) acknowledge the unacceptable nature of the experiments; and (6) endorse higher ethical standards.

Based on both scientific and moral grounds, data obtained from cruel and inhumane experiments, such as data collected from the Nazi experiments and data collected from the Tuskegee Study, should virtually never be published or cited. In the extremely rare case when no other data exist and human lives would certainly be lost without the knowledge obtained from use of such data, publication or citation is permissible. In such a case, the disclosure should cite the specific reasons and clearly justify the necessity for citation.

Certain generally accepted historical data may be cited without a disclaimer, though a disclosure of the ethical issues would be valuable and desirable. (II, V, VII)

Issued December 1998 based on the report "Information From Unethical Experiments," adopted June 1998.

Journal 2001 Focuses on the moral dilemmas raised by stem cell research. Concludes that problems arising as a result of use of embryonic stem cells may be avoided if adult stem cells are used instead. Quotes Opinion 2.30. Orr & Hook, *Stem Cell Research: Magical Promise v. Moral Peril, 2 Yale J. Health Pol'y, Law & Ethics 189, 197 (2001).*

2.40 Radio-Frequency ID Devices in Humans

Radio-frequency identification (RFID) devices may help to identify patients, thereby improving the safety and efficiency of patient care, and may be used to enable secure access to patient clinical information. However, their efficacy and security have not been established. Therefore, physicians implanting such devices should take certain precautions:

(1) The informed consent process must include disclosure of medical uncertainties associated with these devices.

(2) Physicians should strive to protect patients' privacy by storing confidential information only on RFID devices with informational security similar to that required of medical records.

(3) Physicians should support research into the safety, efficacy, and potential nonmedical uses of RFID devices in human beings. (I, III, V)

Issued November 2007 based on the report "Radio Frequency ID Devices in Humans," adopted June 2007.

3.00 # Opinions on Interprofessional Relations

3.01 ## Nonscientific Practitioners

It is unethical to engage in or to aid and abet in treatment which has no scientific basis and is dangerous, is calculated to deceive the patient by giving false hope, or which may cause the patient to delay in seeking proper care.

Physicians should also be mindful of state laws which prohibit a physician from aiding and abetting an unlicensed person in the practice of medicine, aiding or abetting a person with a limited license in providing services beyond the scope of his or her license, or undertaking the joint medical treatment of patients under the foregoing circumstances.

Physicians are otherwise free to accept or decline to serve anyone who seeks their services, regardless of who has recommended that the individual see the physician. (III, VI)

Issued prior to April 1977. Updated June 1994 and June 1996.

3d Cir. 1984 Osteopathic physician brought class action against hospital and medical staff alleging violation of antitrust statute after hospital refused to grant staff privileges. In determining that the per se rule should be used to determine whether the medical staff had violated restraint of trade section of antitrust statute, the court distinguished in a footnote an earlier case which had employed the rule of reason analysis in a boycott case involving physicians and chiropractors. The earlier case had concluded that since there was no per se illegal purpose for Principle 3 (1957) [now Opinion 3.01], rule of reason analysis was appropriate because defendants were asserting a public service/ethical norm justification for their actions; no such rationale for their discriminatory treatment was raised by defendants in the instant case. *Weiss v. York Hosp., 745 F.2d 786, 821 n.61, cert. denied, 470 US 1060 (1985).*

6th Cir. 1989 Plaintiff, a chiropractic association, alleged that the AMA and several other professional associations violated antitrust law by conspiring to contain and ultimately eliminate the practice of chiropractic. The court provided an historical overview of the AMA's gradual, but incomplete, recognition of chiropractors and limited licensed practitioners referring specifically to Principle 3 (1957) as well as to the Opinions and Reports of the Judicial Council Sec. 3, Para. 8 (1969) and to the Opinions and Reports 3.60 and 3.70 (1977) [now Principles VI and Opinions 3.01 and 3.04]. Based on its reading of these Principles and Opinions, the court reversed the trial court's grant of summary judgment to the AMA because there remained a material issue of fact of whether it had continued to illegally boycott chiropractic. *Chiropractic Coop. Ass'n v. AMA, 867 F.2d 270, 272-75.*

7th Cir. 1990 Appellate court affirmed district court ruling that AMA and other national professional associations violated federal antitrust laws by illegal conspiracy against chiropractors. Plaintiff alleged in lower court that Association sought by means of boycott to eliminate chiropractic through application of Principle 3 (1957) [now Opinion 3.01] labeling chiropractors as unscientific practitioners. The appellate court traced the history of the AMA's position regarding chiropractic including references to Principle 3 and Opinion 3.50 (1977) as revised by Opinion

3.01 (1981). The court found the evidence supported finding of an illegal boycott and that injunctive relief was appropriate. *Wilk v. American Medical Ass'n, 895 F.2d 352, 355 n.1, 356-58, 361-63, 364 n.2, 365-66, 368-69, 369 n.4.*

7th Cir. 1983 Defendants in antitrust suit appealed the denial of their directed verdict, claiming that the evidence presented by plaintiff failed to show the existence of a conspiracy to eliminate the practice of chiropractic. The Seventh Circuit affirmed the lower court's decision, noting that the adoption of Principle 3 (1957) [now Opinion 3.01], which condemned professional association with any one practicing a method of healing that was not scientifically based, in concert with other actions, might have allowed a jury to reasonably conclude that the defendant orthopaedic association conspired to discourage medical doctors from associating with chiropractors. *Wilk v. American Medical Ass'n, 735 F.2d 217, 219, cert. denied, 467 US 1210 (1984).*

7th Cir. 1983 Plaintiff-chiropractors alleged that AMA and others conspired to induce physicians to forgo any professional association with chiropractors, to induce hospitals to deny access to chiropractors, and to induce patients to avoid chiropractors, all in violation of the Sherman Act. Plaintiffs argued that Principle 3 (1957) and a 1966 House of Delegates resolution later included in Opinions and Reports of the Judicial Council Sec. 3, Para. 8 (1969) [now Opinion 3.01] reflected defendants' behavior. In response, defendants asserted that their actions were noncommercial and had been taken in the interest of public health, safety, and welfare in the good faith belief that chiropractic was dangerous to patients. The appellate court found the case inappropriate for application of the per se rule applying instead the rule of reason focusing on whether the challenged activities were anticompetitive. Further, as to the rule of reason, the court found the defendants could possibly avoid antitrust liability by showing that the dominant motive in their actions was a genuine concern for patient care. However, the court held that only such patient care concerns, and not a generalized public interest motive, could be used as an antitrust defense. *Wilk v. American Medical Ass'n, 719 F.2d 207, 213-15, 225-27, 233, cert. denied, 467 US 1210 (1984).*

N.D. Ill. 1987 Plaintiffs, licensed chiropractors, sued defendant medical associations for violation of antitrust laws. With regard to defendant AMA, plaintiffs alleged that through Principle 3 (1957) [now Opinion 3.01], the AMA had successfully precluded physicians from associating professionally with chiropractors. The AMA asserted that with the 1980 revision of its Principles, which eliminated the offending portions of Principle 3, any alleged boycott activity directed toward chiropractors had ceased. The court found, however, that plaintiffs did in fact suffer professional rejections and lost opportunities due to lingering effects of the boycott, traceable to the AMA's actions. The court also noted that the revised stance of the AMA on the legitimacy of chiropractic as reflected in Opinion 3.01 fell short of being an affirmative statement that physicians could professionally associate with chiropractors without fear of reprisal. *Wilk v. American Medical Ass'n., 671 F. Supp 1465, 1470, 1473, 1474, 1475, aff'd, 895 F.2d 352 (7th Cir. 1990).*

N.D. Ill. 1986 In case involving antitrust challenge to rule promulgated by American College of Surgeons, the court concluded that the rule was a facially legitimate ethical canon and therefore it would apply the rule of reason in deciding the case. The court also rejected defendant's argument that the modified rule of reason test in *Wilk v. AMA, 719 F.2d 207 (7th Cir. 1983),* cert. denied, 467 US 1210 (1984), allowing a defense based upon a patient care motive exception to otherwise illegal restraint, should be applicable in this case. The court found that the *Wilk* exception was limited to Principle 3 (1957) [now Opinion 3.01] pertaining to the importance of scientific method in patient care. *Koefoot v. American College of Surgeons, 652 F. Supp. 882, 889, 890, 891.*

E.D. Mich. 1986 Plaintiff-chiropractors claimed violation of the Sherman Antitrust Act alleging that the AMA conspired with others to injure them professionally and financially. In support of their claim, plaintiffs cited Principle 3 (1957) and the Opinions and Reports of the Judicial Council Sec. 3, Para. 8 (1969) [now Principle VI and Opinions 3.01 and 3.04]. The court, noting the 1977 change in the AMA's position regarding chiropractic, reflected in the Opinions and Reports of the Judicial Council 3.60 and 3.70 (1977) [now Opinion 3.04] held that plaintiffs failed to demonstrate evidence of an overt act by the AMA within the statutory limitations period. Summary judgment entered for AMA. *Chiropractic Coop. Ass'n v. AMA, 1986-2 Trade Cas. (CCH) & 67,294, aff'd in part and rev'd in part, 867 F.2d 270 (6th Cir. 1989).*

E.D. Mich. 1985 In an antitrust case brought by plaintiff-chiropractic association against the AMA, plaintiffs presented the court with a motion in limine asking that the court strike defendant's affirmative defense of a good faith concern with public health and patient care. Plaintiffs argued that the defense was unprecedented, in conflict with existing law, and dramatically wrong. Plaintiffs referred to Principle 3 (1957) [now Principle VI and Opinions 3.01 and 3.04] as the source of the AMA's antitrust violations. The court denied plaintiffs' motion to strike, stating that under the rule of reason test, the AMA had the right to present evidence that its actions furthered the public interest and patient care. *Chiropractic Coop. Ass'n v. AMA, 617 F. Supp. 264, 266, aff'd in part and rev'd in part, 867 F.2d 270 (6th Cir. 1989).*

D.N.M. 1987 In an antitrust action against major health insurance provider and state medical society, group of chiropractors alleged that a conspiracy existed in which the insurer refused to provide health cost reimbursement coverage for chiropractic services. Plaintiffs urged court to apply a per se analysis, rather than the rule of reason analysis, to determine the legality of defendants' restrictive practices. The court declined to apply the per se test. In part, court's conclusion was based on view that concerns of defendant-physicians about relationship with chiropractors because of ethical restrictions imposed by Principle 3 (1957) [now Principle VI and Opinions 3.01 and 3.04] deserved more consideration than the per se test would afford. *Johnson v. Blue Cross/ Blue Shield, 677 F. Supp. 1112, 1118.*

Ariz. 1965 Physician appealed denial of medical license which was based on alleged violations of local medical society rules and Principles 3, 5, and 10 (1957) [now Principles III and VII and Opinions 3.01, 8.11, and 9.06]. Alleged violations included treating a patient without first obtaining a prior treating physician's permission, inadequate patient care, performing operations without hospital privileges, and signing the medical record of a deceased patient who had been treated by interns. The court held that the evidence failed to show any clear violation of the Principles and that a local medical society had no right to prescribe a code of ethics for state licensing purposes. *Arizona State Bd. of Medical Examiners v. Clark, 97 Ariz. 205, 398 P.2d 908, 914-915, 915 n.3.*

N.J. 1963 Plaintiff, an osteopath fully licensed to practice medicine and surgery by the state, sought to apply for staff privileges at defendant-hospital, a private, not-for-profit, general hospital. Defendant refused application based on a by-law requiring staff members to be graduates of medical schools approved by the AMA and members of the county medical society. In plaintiff's action challenging refusal of the application, the court held that the hospital's power to pass upon staff applications was a fiduciary power, and that plaintiff's application was to be considered on its own merit without regard to the by-law provision. In its opinion, the court noted the historic opposition of the AMA to osteopathy. The court also referred to a position adopted by the AMA in 1961, later reflected in Opinions and Reports of the Judicial Council Sec. 3, Para. 7 (1965) [now Opinion 3.01], allowing for association with osteopaths who follow scientific principles. *Greisman v. Newcomb Hosp., 40 N.J. 389, 192 A.2d 817, 819.*

N.J. Super. 1960 Plaintiff, a graduate of a school of osteopathy and licensed to practice medicine and surgery in New Jersey, sought to compel the defendant medical society to admit him to full membership. Defendant claimed as an affirmative defense that to admit plaintiff would violate Principle 3 (1957) [now Principle VI and Opinion 3.01] because plaintiff possessed a degree in osteopathy rather than an MD. The court noted that the defendant society had virtually monopolistic control of medical practice in the state and that exclusion from membership caused substantial injury. In view of this, the court ordered the defendant society to admit plaintiff to its membership. To bar membership of a licensed graduate of an approved school of osteopathy would, the court held, violate public policy. *Falcone v. Middlesex County Medical Soc'y, 62 N.J. Super. 184, 162 A.2d 324, 328-329, aff'd, 34 N.J. 582, 170 A.2d 791 (1961).*

Journal 2009 Discusses need for accreditation of programs in the field of bioethics and the creation of a code of ethics for the field. Concludes that professionalization of the field is occurring at a reasonable pace. Quotes Ch. II, Art. IV, Sec. 1 (1847) [now Opinion 3.01]. Baker, *In Defense of Bioethics, 37 J. of Law Med. and Ethics 83, 87 (2009).*

Journal 2008 Questions what entity should be responsible for critically evaluating chiropractors. Concludes that chiropractic should be a self-regulated profession. Quotes Introduction (1847) [now Opinions 1.01 and 1.02]. References Ch. II, Art. I, Sec. 3 (1847) [now Opinion 5.02] and Ch. II, Art. IV, Sec. 1 (May 1847) [now Opinion 3.01]. Johnson, *Keeping a Critical Eye on Chiropractic, 31 J. of Manipulative and Physiological Therapeutics 559, 559 (2008).*

Journal 1999 Explores the use of alternative therapies in the Caribbean due to the high cost of medical care. Compares the AMA and the Commonwealth Medical Association views on nonscientific practitioners. Observes that Caribbean societies should implement standards for conducting research on alternative forms of treatment and should establish practice guidelines for utilization of these types of therapy. Quotes Opinion 3.01. Aarons, *Medicine* *and Its Alternatives: Health Care Priorities in the Caribbean,* 29 Hastings Center Rep. 23, 25 (July-Aug. 1999).

Journal 1996 Explores the incorporation of holistic health care into modern medical practice. Observes that the AMA previously condemned association with chiropractors as unethical. Concludes that alternative health care methods need to be further integrated into patient treatment plans where warranted. Quotes Principle 3 (1956) [amended and now Opinion 3.01]. Cohen, *Holistic Health Care: Including Alternative and Complementary Medicine in Insurance and Regulatory Schemes,* 38 Ariz. L. Rev. 83, 92 (1996).

3.02 Nurses

The primary bond between the practices of medicine and nursing is mutual ethical concern for patients. One of the duties in providing reasonable care is fulfilled by a nurse who carries out the orders of the attending physician. Where orders appear to the nurse to be in error or contrary to customary medical and nursing practice, the physician has an ethical obligation to hear the nurse's concern and explain those orders to the nurse involved. The ethical physician should neither expect nor insist that nurses follow orders contrary to standards of good medical and nursing practice. In emergencies, when prompt action is necessary and the physician is not immediately available, a nurse may be justified in acting contrary to the physician's standing orders for the safety of the patient. Such occurrences should not be considered to be a breakdown in professional relations. (IV, V)

Issued June 1983. Updated June 1994.

Journal 2010 Observes that miscommunicated, misunderstood, and forgotten information among physicians, nurses, and other hospital staff leads to serious patient injury. Concludes that to assess if a client's injury resulted from a miscommunication among hospital staff, attorneys must examine hospital policies and procedures, medical ethics, and communications technology in relation to information sharing. Quotes Opinions 3.02 and 9.045. Cohen, Dicecco, & Levin, *Failure to Communicate: When It Comes to Hospital Patient Care, Communication Between Doctor and Nurse Should Be Seamless. If It's Not, Patients Suffer. Here's How to Find Out if a Miscommunication Is at the Core of Your Client's Case,* 46 Trial 38, 40-41 (May 2010).

3.03 The previous Opinion 3.03, "Optometry," was deleted in June 1994.

3.03 Allied Health Professionals

Physicians often practice in concert with allied health professionals such as, but not limited to, optometrists, nurse anesthetists, nurse midwives, and physician assistants in the course of delivering appropriate medical care to their patients. In doing so, physicians should be guided by the following principles:

(1) It is ethical for a physician to work in consultation with or employ allied health professionals, as long as they are appropriately trained and duly licensed to perform the activities being requested.

(2) Physicians have an ethical obligation to the patients for whom they are responsible to ensure that medical and surgical conditions are appropriately evaluated and treated.

(3) Physicians may teach in recognized schools for the allied health professionals for the purpose of improving the quality of their education. The scope of teaching may embrace subjects which are within the legitimate scope of

the allied health profession and which are designed to prepare students to engage in the practice of the profession within the limits prescribed by law.

(4) It is inappropriate to substitute the services of an allied health professional for those of a physician when the allied health professional is not appropriately trained and duly licensed to provide the medical services being requested. (I, V, VII)

Issued December 1997.

Journal 2008 Questions whether it is ethical for ophthalmologists to teach surgery to optometrists. Concludes that the welfare of the patient must be the primary consideration in making this determination. Quotes Opinion 3.03. Packer, Parke II, & Pellegrino, *Should Ophthalmologists Teach Surgery to Optometrists? 126 Arch. Ophthalmol. 1458, 1458 (2008).*

Journal 2006 Discusses the evolution of health law in Virginia. Concludes that the area of health law continues to expand, develop, and be refined. Cites Opinions 3.03, 3.08, 5.01, 5.015, 5.02, 5.04, 5.055, 6.02, 6.021, 6.03, 6.04, 7.03, 7.04, 7.05, 8.054, 8.08, 8.081, 8.085, 8.115, 8.12, 8.14, 8.145, 8.19, and 9.045. Guanzon, *Health Care Law, 41 U. Rich. L. Rev. 179, 199 (2006).*

3.04 Referral of Patients

A physician may refer a patient for diagnostic or therapeutic services to another physician, limited practitioner, or any other provider of health care services permitted by law to furnish such services, whenever he or she believes that this may benefit the patient. As in the case of referrals to physician-specialists, referrals to limited practitioners should be based on their individual competence and ability to perform the services needed by the patient. A physician should not so refer a patient unless the physician is confident that the services provided on referral will be performed competently and in accordance with accepted scientific standards and legal requirements. (V, VI)

Issued prior to April 1977.

6th Cir. 1989 Plaintiff, a chiropractic association, alleged that the AMA and several other professional associations violated antitrust law by conspiring to contain and ultimately eliminate the practice of chiropractic. The court provided an historical overview of the AMA's gradual, but incomplete, recognition of chiropractors and limited licensed practitioners referring specifically to Principle 3 (1957) as well as to the Opinions and Reports of the Judicial Council Sec. 3, Para. 8 (1969) and to the Opinions and Reports 3.60 and 3.70 (1977) [now Principle VI and Opinions 3.01 and 3.04]. Based on its reading of these Principles and Opinions, the court reversed the trial court's grant of summary judgment to the AMA because there remained a material issue of fact of whether it had continued to illegally boycott chiropractic. *Chiropractic Coop. Ass'n v. AMA, 867 F.2d 270, 272-75.*

E.D. Mich. 1986 Plaintiff-chiropractors claimed violation of the Sherman Antitrust Act alleging that the AMA conspired with others to injure them professionally and financially. In support of their claim, plaintiffs cited Principle 3 (1957) and the Opinions and Reports of the Judicial Council Sec. 3, Para. 8 (1969) [now Principles VI and Opinions 3.01 and 3.04]. The court, noting the 1977 change in the AMA's position regarding chiropractic reflected in the Opinions and Reports of the Judicial Council 3.60 and 3.70 (1977) [now Opinion 3.04] held that plaintiffs failed to demonstrate evidence of an overt act by the AMA within the statutory limitations period. Summary judgment entered for AMA. *Chiropractic Coop. Ass'n v. AMA, 1986-2 Trade Cas. (CCH) & 67,294, aff'd in part and rev'd in part, 867 F.2d 270 (6th Cir. 1989).*

E.D. Mich. 1985 In an antitrust case brought by plaintiff-chiropractic association against the AMA, plaintiffs presented the court with a motion in limine asking that the court strike defendant's affirmative defense of a good faith concern with public health and patient care. Plaintiffs argued that the defense was unprecedented, in conflict with existing law, and dramatically wrong. Plaintiffs referred to Principle 3 (1957) [now Principle VI and Opinions 3.01 and 3.04] as the source of the AMA's antitrust violations. The court denied plaintiffs' motion to strike, stating that under the rule of reason test, the AMA had the right to present evidence that its actions furthered the public interest and patient care. *Chiropractic Coop. Ass'n v. AMA, 617 F. Supp. 264, 266, aff'd in part and rev'd in part, 867 F.2d 270 (6th Cir. 1989).*

D.N.M. 1987 In an antitrust action against major health insurance provider and state medical society, group of chiropractors alleged that a conspiracy existed in which the insurer refused to provide health cost reimbursement coverage for chiropractic services. Plaintiffs urged court to apply a per se analysis, rather than the rule of reason analysis to determine the legality of defendants' restrictive practices. The court declined to apply the per se test. In part, court's conclusion was based on view that concerns of defendant-physicians about relationship with chiropractors because of ethical restrictions imposed by Principle 3 (1957) [now Principle VI and Opinions 3.01 and 3.04] deserved more consideration than the per se test would afford. *Johnson v. Blue Cross/ Blue Shield, 677 F. Supp. 1112, 1118.*

S.D. Ohio 1995 Physician accused of soliciting bribes in return for referring patients to Medicaid provider moved to dismiss the indictment which alleged mail fraud and violations of Medicaid antikickback statute. In denying physician's motion to dismiss indictment, the court noted that physician's fiduciary duty under Opinion 3.04 supported an intangible rights mail fraud charge. *United States v. Neufeld, 908 F. Supp. 491, 500.*

Journal 1994 Focuses on physicians' legal and ethical duties to pregnant women to provide medical information relevant to patient choice regarding abortion and to make referrals for services that physicians are unable or unwilling to perform. Concludes that medical educators, professional associations, women's groups, and state legislatures should address these issues. Cites Opinions 3.04 and 8.04. Law, *Silent No More: Physicians' Legal and Ethical Obligations to Patients Seeking Abortions, 21 N. Y. U. Rev. L. & Soc. Change 279, 289, 290, 300 (1994).*

Journal 1993 Focuses on how antitrust laws might be used to prevent exclusion of chiropractors by health maintenance organizations (HMOs) by discussing two theories under which it might be illegal. Concludes that chiropractors challenging their exclusion from HMOs may establish an antitrust claim under the theories of "structural conspiracy" and "tacit collusion" if certain criteria are met. Quotes Opinion 3.04. Note, *HMO Exclusion of Chiropractors, 66 So. Cal. L. Rev. 807, 823 (1993).*

3.041 Chiropractic

It is ethical for a physician to associate professionally with chiropractors provided that the physician believes that such association is in the best interests of his or her patient. A physician may refer a patient for diagnostic or therapeutic services to a chiropractor permitted by law to furnish such services whenever the physician believes that this may benefit his or her patient. Physicians may also ethically teach in recognized schools of chiropractic. (V, VI)

Issued March 1992.

W.D. Pa. 2008 Plaintiff filed a Social Security appeal, challenging an administrative decision that her severe impairments did not preclude her from performing sedentary work with a sit-stand option. The court quoted Opinion 3.041 in deciding that the plaintiff should not be faulted for seeking chiropractic care for her back injury. The court adopted the magistrate judge's recommendation that plaintiff's motion for summary judgment be granted and the case remanded for further administrative proceedings. *Thompson v. Astrue, 2008 WL 2444532, 3, n. 3.*

E.D.N.Y. 2004 Plaintiffs sued the US for injuries sustained in a collision with a postal inspector's vehicle. The court held that the inspector's vehicle was a police vehicle within the meaning of a state statute and as that such, it was exempt from following traffic laws in certain situations. The court said it was reasonable for the postal inspector to follow a suspect through a red light. During the proceedings, the US questioned whether the testimony of a chiropractor regarding plaintiff's injuries was admissible. The court, citing Opinion 3.041, found that techniques used by chiropractors have gained acceptance in the medical community and that the testimony was admissible. However, the court denied recover. *Hodder v. U.S., 328 F. Supp. 2d 335, 347.*

3.05   The previous Opinion 3.05, "Specialists," issued in 1994 was deleted and replaced by the current Opinion 3.05, "Physician Employment by a Nonphysician Supervisee."

3.05   Physician Employment by a Nonphysician Supervisee

Physicians' relationships with midlevel practitioners must be based on mutual respect and trust as well as their shared commitment to patient well-being. Health care professionals recognize that clinical tasks should be shared and delegated in keeping with each practitioner's training and scope of practice. Given their comprehensive training and broad scope of practice, physicians have a professional responsibility for the quality of overall care that patients receive, even when aspects of that care are delivered by nonphysician clinicians.

When nonphysicians employ physicians to supervise the employer's clinical practice, conditions are created that can lead to ethical dilemmas for the physician. If maintaining an employment relationship with a midlevel practitioner contributes significantly to the physician's livelihood, a physician's personal and financial interests can be put at odds with patient care interests. Similarly, the administrative and financial influence that employer status confers creates an inherent conflict for a physician who is simultaneously an employee and a clinical supervisor of his or her employer.

Physicians in such arrangements must give precedence to their ethical obligation to act in the patient's best interest by always exercising independent professional judgment, even if that puts the physician at odds with the employer/supervisee. (II, VI, VIII)

Issued November 2009 based on the report "Physician Employment by a Nonphysician Supervisee," adopted June 2009.

3.06   Sports Medicine

Physicians should assist athletes to make informed decisions about their participation in amateur and professional contact sports which entail risks of bodily injury.

The professional responsibility of the physician who serves in a medical capacity at an athletic contest or sporting event is to protect the health and safety of the contestants. The desire of spectators, promoters of the event, or even the injured athlete that he or she not be removed from the contest should not be controlling. The physician's judgment should be governed only by medical considerations. (I, VII)

Issued June 1983. Updated June 1994.

Journal 2008 Discusses medical and legal issues facing the National Football League stemming from concussions sustained by players. Argues steps must be taken to minimize the impact of concussions on active players and increase assistance for former injured players. Quotes Opinion 3.06. Lipsky, *Dealing With the NFL's Concussion Problems of Yesterday, Today, and Tomorrow*, 18 *Fordham Intell. Prop. Media & Ent. L. J.* 959, 988 (2008).

Journal 2007 Examines ethical issues that arise when physicians are employed by sports teams. Concludes that for team physicians, special guidelines apply to informed consent, advertising, confidentiality, and third-party influences. Quotes Opinion 3.06. Dunn, George, Churchill, & Spindler, *Ethics in Sports Medicine*, 35 *The Am. J. of Sports Med.* 840, 841, 842 (2007).

Journal 1999 Describes conflicts of interest faced by professional sports team physicians. Examines cases where athletes have sued team physicians for failing to follow the proper standard of care. Provides a clear standard of care and suggests ways team physicians can reduce conflicts of interest. Quotes Opinion 3.06. Keim, *Physicians for Professional Sports Teams: Health Care Under the Pressure of Economic and Commercial Interests*, 9 Seton Hall. J. Sport L. 196, 218-19 (1999).

Journal 1999 Discusses the need for physicians to advocate on behalf of patients' rights in the context of health care delivery. Evaluates the nature and scope of the physician's role as advocate, noting that physicians cannot be expected to engage in attorney-like advocacy. Quotes Principles IV and VI, Fundamental Elements (2), (4), and (6) [now Opinion 10.01], Patient Responsibilities 5 [now Opinion 10.02], and Opinions 2.03, 2.07, 2.09, 2.16, 2.19, 3.06, 4.01, 4.04, 6.01, 7.02, 8.02, 8.03, 8.13, 8.132, 9.06, 9.07, and 9.131. Cites Opinions 5.05, 5.09, 7.01, 8.135, and 9.02. Sage, *Physicians as Advocates*, 35 Hous. L. Rev. 1529, 1537, 1541, 1542, 1552-53, 1554, 1556, 1557, 1559, 1561-62, 1564, 1571, 1574, 1576, 1580 (1999).

Journal 1993 Discusses an athlete's rights to assume serious health risks by playing a sport, despite a physical abnormality or medical condition. Considers the team physician's conflicting duties toward the patient/player and the team. Concludes that physicians or athletes should bear legal responsibility if either violates their obligations in this context. Cites Opinion 3.06. Mitten, *Team Physicians and Competitive Athletes: Allocating Legal Responsibility for Athletic Injuries*, 55 U. Pitt. L. Rev. 129, 140 (1993).

3.07   The previous Opinion 3.07, "Teaching," was deleted in June 1994.

3.08   Sexual Harassment and Exploitation Between Medical Supervisors and Trainees

Sexual harassment may be defined as sexual advances, requests for sexual favors, and other verbal or physical conduct of a sexual nature when (1) such conduct interferes with an individual's work or academic performance or creates an intimidating, hostile, or offensive work or academic environment or (2) accepting or rejecting such conduct affects or may be perceived to affect employment decisions or academic evaluations concerning the individual. Sexual harassment is unethical.

Sexual relationships between medical supervisors and their medical trainees raise concerns because of inherent inequalities in the status and power that medical supervisors wield in relation to medical trainees and may adversely affect patient care. Sexual relationships between a medical trainee and a supervisor even when consensual are not acceptable regardless of the degree of supervision in any given situation. The supervisory role should be eliminated if the parties involved wish to pursue their relationship. (II, IV, VII)

Issued March 1992 based on the report "Sexual Harassment and Exploitation Between Medical Supervisors and Trainees," adopted June 1989. Updated June 1994.

Va. App. 2003 Physician appealed board of medicine's license probation order for unprofessional conduct. Board found the physician's pattern of inappropriate advances toward medical students violated medical ethical standards. Appellate court reversed, holding that the evidence was insufficient to support board's finding, since the ethical standards by which the physician should be adjudicated were not established by competent evidence. Quotes Opinions 3.08 and 9.05. *Goad v. Virginia Board of Medicine*, 40 Va. App. 621, 580 S.E.2d 494, 498, n.7, 499, n.9.

Journal 2006 Discusses the evolution of health law in Virginia. Concludes that the area of health law continues to expand, develop, and be refined. Cites Opinions 3.03, 3.08, 5.01, 5.015,

5.02, 5.04, 5.055, 6.02, 6.021, 6.03, 6.04, 7.03, 7.04, 7.05, 8.054, 8.08, 8.081, 8.085, 8.115, 8.12, 8.14, 8.145, 8.19, and 9.045. Guanzon, *Health Care Law, 41 U. Rich. L. Rev. 179, 199 (2006).*

Journal 2006 Considers prisoners' rights to expression of sexuality and the state's legitimate interest in regulating that expression. Concludes that states should encourage healthy expressions of sexuality while protecting the goals of the Prison Rape Elimination Act. Cites Opinions 3.08, 8.14, 8.145, and 10.015. Smith, *Rethinking Prison Sex: Self-expression and Safety,* 15 Colum. J. Gender & L. 185, 202 (2006).

3.09 Medical Students Performing Procedures on Fellow Students

(1) In the context of learning basic clinical skills, medical students must be asked specifically to consent to procedures being performed by fellow students. The stringency of standards for ensuring the explicit and non-coerced informed consent increases as the invasiveness and intimacy of the procedure increase.

(2) Instructors should explain to students how the procedures will be performed, making certain that students are not placed in situations that violate their privacy or sense of propriety. The confidentiality, consequences, and appropriate management of a diagnostic finding should also be discussed.

(3) Students should be given the choice of whether to participate prior to entering the classroom and there should be no requirement that the students provide a reason for their unwillingness to participate.

(4) Students should not be penalized for refusal to participate. Thus instructors must refrain from evaluating students' overall performance in terms of their willingness to volunteer as "patients." (IV, V)

Issued June 2000 based on the report "Medical Students Performing Procedures on Fellow Students," adopted December 1999.

4.00 **Opinions on Hospital Relations**

4.01   Admission Fee

Charging a separate and distinct fee for the incidental, administrative, non-medical service the physician performs in securing the admission of a patient to a hospital is unethical. Physicians should derive their income from medical services rendered, in keeping with the traditions of the American Medical Association. (IV)

Issued prior to April 1977. Updated June 1994.

Journal 2007 Highlights inconsistencies in applying judicial deference to medical ethics. Concludes that courts should afford greater deference to established medical ethics standards. Quotes Principle I and Opinions 2.06 and Ch. II, Art. I, Sec. 3 (May 1847) [now Opinion 5.02]. Cites Opinions 4.01 and 7.05. Lerman, *Second Opinion: Inconsistent Deference to Medical Ethics in Death Penalty Jurisprudence*, 95 Geo. L. J. 1941, 1945, 1974-75, 1976, 1977 (2007).

Journal 2006 Discusses health care service fees and the Maryland "Hold Harmless" statute. Concludes that physicians may charge administrative fees for services not covered by insurance as long as they do not violate a statute or impede proper care. Quotes Opinions 4.01 and 8.055. Doherty & Freed, *User Fees in Health Care*, 39 Md. B.J. 5, 9 (April 2006).

Journal 1999 Discusses the need for physicians to advocate on behalf of patients' rights in the context of health care delivery. Evaluates the nature and scope of the physician's role as advocate, noting that physicians cannot be expected to engage in attorney-like advocacy. Quotes Principles IV and VI, Fundamental Elements (2), (4), and (6) [now Opinion 10.01], Patient Responsibilities 5 [now Opinion 10.02], and Opinions 2.03, 2.07, 2.09, 2.16, 2.19, 3.06, 4.01, 4.04, 6.01, 7.02, 8.02, 8.03, 8.13, 8.132, 9.06, 9.07, and 9.131. Cites Opinions 5.05, 5.09, 7.01, 8.135, and 9.02. Sage, *Physicians as Advocates*, 35 Hous. L. Rev. 1529, 1537, 1541, 1542, 1552-53, 1554, 1556, 1557, 1559, 1561-62, 1564, 1571, 1574, 1576, 1580 (1999).

4.02   Assessments, Compulsory

It is improper to condition medical staff membership or privileges on compulsory assessments for any purpose. However, self-imposed assessments by vote of the medical staff are acceptable. (IV)

Issued prior to April 1977. Updated June 1994.

4.03   Billing for Housestaff and Student Services

When a physician assumes responsibility for the services rendered to a patient by a resident or student, the physician may ethically bill the patient for services which were performed under the physician's direct personal observation, direction, and supervision. (II)

Issued prior to April 1977. Updated June 1994.

4.04   Economic Incentives and Levels of Care

The primary obligation of the hospital medical staff is to safeguard the quality of care provided within the institution. The medical staff has the responsibility to perform essential functions on behalf of the hospital in accordance with licensing laws and accreditation requirements. Treatment or hospitalization that is willfully excessive or inadequate constitutes unethical practice. The organized medical staff has an obligation to avoid wasteful practices and unnecessary treatment that may cause the hospital needless expense. In a situation where the economic interests of the hospital are in conflict with patient welfare, patient welfare takes priority. (I, II, IV, V, VI)

Issued June 1986.

Journal 2003 Discusses the practice of gainsharing and argues that providing physicians and hospitals with certain financial incentives to reduce health costs may be of value in health care reform. Concludes with suggestions for how best to proceed in this difficult context. Quotes Opinions 2.03, 2.09, 4.04, and 8.03. References Opinion 8.13. Saver, *Squandering the Gain: Gainsharing and the Continuing Dilemma of Physician Financial Incentives*, 98 Nw. U. L. Rev. 145, 219, 221, 222 (2003).

Journal 1999 Discusses the need for physicians to advocate on behalf of patients' rights in the context of health care delivery. Evaluates the nature and scope of the physician's role as advocate, noting that physicians cannot be expected to engage in attorney-like advocacy. Quotes Principles IV and VI, Fundamental Elements (2), (4), and (6) [now Opinion 10.01], Patient Responsibilities 5 [now Opinion 10.02], and Opinions 2.03, 2.07, 2.09, 2.16, 2.19, 3.06, 4.01, 4.04, 6.01, 7.02, 8.02, 8.03, 8.13, 8.132, 9.06, 9.07, and 9.131. Cites Opinions 5.05, 5.09, 7.01, 8.135, and 9.02. Sage, *Physicians as Advocates*, 35 Hous. L. Rev. 1529, 1537, 1541, 1542, 1552-53, 1554, 1556, 1557, 1559, 1561-62, 1564, 1571, 1574, 1576, 1580 (1999).

Journal 1998 Discusses conflicts of interest in the physician-patient relationship arising out of use of financial incentives by managed care organizations. Considers how such conflicts are dealt with in the attorney-client relationship. Suggests that a financial incentive should be legally denounced if it unreasonably interferes with a physician's duty to properly care for and treat patients. Quotes Preamble, Fundamental Elements (1) [now Opinion 10.01] and Opinions 4.04, 5.01, 8.03, 8.13, and 9.06. Cites Fundamental Elements (4) [now Opinion 10.01], and Opinions 2.07, 2.08, and 2.132. Hall, *Third-Party Payor Conflicts of Interest in Managed Care: A Proposal for Regulation Based on the Model Rules of Professional Conduct*, 29 Seton Hall L. Rev. 95, 96, 107, 108, 109, 110, 111, 112, 134, 135, 136 (1998).

Journal 1996 Considers the change from traditional medical care systems to managed care, noting the conflicts of interest this creates between physicians' ethical obligations and financial concerns. Discusses these issues in the context of managed behavioral health care. Suggests community-based care and social supports as a solution. Quotes Opinions 2.03 and 4.04. Petrila, *Ethics, Money, and the Problem of Coercion in Managed Behavioral Health Care*, 40 St. Louis U. L. J. 359, 377 (1996).

Journal 1994 Observes that health care reform proposals present significant challenges to the role and ethics of attending physicians. Emphasizes that reform proposals must set forth the role envisioned for physicians and must articulate an acceptable ethical framework within which physicians may fulfill that role. Quotes Opinions 4.04, 9.121, and 9.122. Cites Opinions 2.03, 2.09, 5.01, and 8.03. Wolf, *Health Care Reform and the Future of Physician Ethics*, 24 Hastings Center Rep. 28, 32, 40 (March/April 1994).

Journal 1993 Discusses the problem of physicians withholding needed medical treatment from HIV-infected infants. Concludes that current law should be expanded to eliminate this discrimination. Quotes Opinions 2.09, 2.17, 2.20, 2.22, 4.04, and 8.03. Crossley, *Of Diagnoses and Discrimination: Discriminatory Nontreatment of Infants With HIV Infection*, 93 Columbia L. Rev. 1581, 1620, 1621 (1993).

Journal 1992 Examines the major health care rationing issues facing the US including increasing costs and decreasing access. Concludes that the standard of care should not be changed and that rationing should be a separate enterprise undertaken pursuant to explicit criteria. Quotes

Opinions 2.03, 2.09, and 4.04. Hirshfeld, *Should Ethical and Legal Standards for Physicians Be Changed to Accommodate New Models for Rationing Health Care?* 140 Univ. Pa. L. Rev. 1809, 1816 (1992).

Journal 1990 Discusses efforts of third-party payers to control health care expenditures for beneficiaries. Concludes that financial incentives to limit care and other cost-control techniques should be disclosed and that the rationale for such disclosure is compelling. Quotes Opinions 2.03, 2.09, and 8.03. Cites Opinions 2.19, 4.04, and 4.06. Hirshfeld, *Should Third Party Payors of Health Care Services Disclose Cost Control Mechanisms to Potential Beneficiaries?* 14 Seton Hall Legis. J. 115, 130, 131, 144, 145, 146 (1990).

4.05 Organized Medical Staff

The organized medical staff performs essential hospital functions even though it may often consist primarily of independent practicing physicians who are not hospital employees. The core responsibilities of the organized medical staff are the promotion of patient safety and the quality of care. Members of the organized medical staff may choose to act as a group for the purpose of communicating and dealing with the governing board and others with respect to matters that concern the interests of the organized medical staff and its members. This is ethical so long as there is no adverse effect on patient safety and the quality of care. (IV, VI)

Issued July 1983; updated June 1994 and June 2004.

4.06 Physician-Hospital Contractual Relations

There are various financial or contractual arrangements that physicians and hospitals may enter into and find mutually satisfactory. A physician may, for example, be a hospital employee, a hospital-associated medical specialist, or an independent practitioner with staff privileges. The form of the contractual or financial arrangement between physicians and hospitals depends on the facts and circumstances of each situation. A physician may be employed by a hospital for a fixed annual amount, for a certain amount per hour, or pursuant to other similar arrangements that are related to the professional services, skill, education, expertise, or time involved. (VI)

Issued March 1981. Updated June 1994.

Journal 1990 Discusses efforts of third-party payers to control health care expenditures for beneficiaries. Concludes that financial incentives to limit care and other cost-control techniques should be disclosed and that the rationale for such disclosure is compelling. Quotes Opinions 2.03, 2.09, and 8.03. Cites Opinions 2.19, 4.04, and 4.06. Hirshfeld, *Should Third Party Payors of Health Care Services Disclose Cost Control Mechanisms to Potential Beneficiaries?* 14 Seton Hall Legis. J. 115, 130, 131, 144, 145, 146 (1990).

4.07 Staff Privileges

The mutual objective of both the governing board and the medical staff is to improve the quality and efficiency of patient care in the hospital. Decisions regarding hospital privileges should be based upon the training, experience, and demonstrated competence of candidates, taking into consideration the availability of facilities and the overall medical needs of the community, the hospital, and especially patients. Privileges should not be based on numbers of patients admitted to the facility or the economic or insurance status of the patient. Personal friendships, antagonisms, jurisdictional disputes, or fear of competition should not play a role in making these decisions. Physicians who are involved in the granting, denying, or termination of hospital privileges have an ethical responsibility to be guided primarily by concern for the welfare and best interests of patients in discharging this responsibility. (IV, VI, VII)

Issued July 1983. Updated June 1994.

Journal 2006 Discusses the efficacy of peer-review programs in preventing medical malpractice. Concludes that peer review is effective and that confidentiality of peer review must remain protected by law. Quotes Opinion 4.07. Cites Opinions 4.07 and 9.10. Moore, Pichert, Hickson, Federspiel, & Blackford, *Rethinking Peer Review: Detecting and Addressing Medical Malpractice Claims Risk, 59 Vand. L. Rev. 1175, 1144 (2006).*

Journal 1990 Presents current issues, policies, legislation, and judicial decisions regarding impaired physicians. Concludes by proposing enhanced confidentiality requirements in disciplinary proceedings and nationwide adoption of a uniform law in this area. Quotes Opinion 4.07. References Principle IV. Walzer, *Impaired Physicians: An Overview and Update of the Legal Issues, 11 J. Legal Med. 131, 174, 192 (1990).*

5.00 **Opinions on Confidentiality, Advertising, and Communications Media Relations**

5.01 **Advertising and Managed Care Organizations**

A physician may provide medical services to members of a prepaid medical care plan or to members of a health maintenance organization which seeks members or subscribers through advertising. Physicians practicing in prepaid plans or managed care organizations are subject to the same ethical principles as other physicians. Advertising which would lead prospective members or subscribers to believe that the services of a named physician who has a reputation for outstanding skill would be routinely available to all members or subscribers, if in fact this is not so, is deceptive. However, the publication by name of the roster of physicians who provide services to members, the type of practice in which each is engaged, and biographical and other relevant information is not a deceptive practice. (II, VI)

Issued prior to April 1977. Updated June 1996.

Journal 2006 Discusses the evolution of health law in Virginia. Concludes that the area of health law continues to expand, develop, and be refined. Cites Opinions 3.03, 3.08, 5.01, 5.015, 5.02, 5.04, 5.055, 6.02, 6.021, 6.03, 6.04, 7.03, 7.04, 7.05, 8.054, 8.08, 8.081, 8.085, 8.115, 8.12, 8.14, 8.145, 8.19, and 9.045. Guanzon, *Health Care Law, 41 U. Rich. L. Rev. 179, 199 (2006).*

Journal 1998 Discusses conflicts of interest in the physician-patient relationship arising out of use of financial incentives by managed care organizations. Considers how such conflicts are dealt with in the attorney-client relationship. Suggests that a financial incentive should be legally denounced if it unreasonably interferes with a physician's duty to properly care for and treat patients. Quotes Preamble, Fundamental Elements (1) [now Opinion 10.01], and Opinions 4.04, 5.01, 8.03, 8.13, and 9.06. Cites Fundamental Elements (4) [now Opinion 10.01] and Opinions 2.07, 2.08, and 2.132. Hall, *Third-Party Payor Conflicts of Interest in Managed Care: A Proposal for Regulation Based on the Model Rules of Professional Conduct, 29 Seton Hall L. Rev. 95, 96, 107, 108, 109, 110, 111, 112, 134, 135, 136 (1998).*

Journal 1994 Observes that health care reform proposals present significant challenges to the role and ethics of attending physicians. Emphasizes that reform proposals must set forth the role envisioned for physicians and must articulate an acceptable ethical framework within which physicians may fulfill that role. Quotes Opinions 4.04, 9.121, and 9.122. Cites Opinions 2.03, 2.09, 5.01, and 8.03. Wolf, *Health Care Reform and the Future of Physician Ethics, 24 Hastings Center Rep. 28, 32, 40 (March/April 1994).*

5.015 Direct-to-Consumer Advertisements of Prescription Drugs

The medical profession needs to take an active role in ensuring that proper advertising guidelines are enforced and that the care patients receive is not compromised as a result of direct-to-consumer advertising. Since the Food and Drug Administration (FDA) has a critical role in determining future directions of direct-to-consumer advertising of prescription drugs, physicians should work to ensure that the FDA remains committed to advertising standards that protect patients' health and safety. Moreover, physicians should encourage and engage in studies regarding the effect of direct-to-consumer advertising on patient health and medical care. Such studies should examine whether direct-to-consumer advertising improves the communication of health information; enhances the patient-physician relationship; and contains accurate and reasonable information on risks, precautions, adverse reactions, and costs.

Physicians must maintain professional standards of informed consent when prescribing. When a patient comes to a physician with a request for a drug he or she has seen advertised, the physician and the patient should engage in a dialogue that would assess and enhance the patient's understanding of the treatment. Although physicians should not be biased against drugs that are advertised, physicians should resist commercially induced pressure to prescribe drugs that may not be indicated. Physicians should deny requests for inappropriate prescriptions and educate patients as to why certain advertised drugs may not be suitable treatment options, providing, when available, information on the cost-effectiveness of different options.

Physicians must remain vigilant to assure that direct-to-consumer advertising does not promote false expectations. Physicians should be concerned about advertisements that do not enhance consumer education; do not convey a clear, accurate, and responsible health education message; do not refer patients to their physicians for more information; do not identify the target population at risk; and fail to discourage consumer self-diagnosis and self-treatment. Physicians may choose to report these concerns directly to the pharmaceutical company that sponsored the advertisement.

To assist the FDA in enforcing existing law and tracking the effects of direct-to-consumer advertising, physicians should, whenever reasonably possible, report to them advertisements that (1) do not provide a fair and balanced discussion of the use of the drug product for the disease, disorder, or condition; (2) do not clearly explain warnings, precautions, and potential adverse reactions associated with the drug product; (3) do not present summary information in language that can be understood by the consumer; (4) do not comply with applicable FDA rules, regulations, policies, and guidelines as provided by the FDA; or (5) do not provide collateral materials to educate both physicians and consumers. (II, III)

Issued June 1999 based on the report "Direct-to-Consumer Advertisements of Prescription Drugs," adopted December 1998 (*Food & Drug L. J.* 2000;55:119-124).

Journal 2009 Reviews the history of pharmaceutical marketing, the creation of the FDA, and advertising regulation and laws. Concludes direct-to-consumer advertising has not fundamentally changed the relationship between pharmaceutical manufacturers and physicians, with physicians maintaining their essential role as the learned intermediary. Quotes Opinion 5.015. Schwartz,

Silverman, Hulka, & Appel, *Marketing Pharmaceutical Products in the Twenty-First Century: An Analysis of the Continued Viability of Traditional Principles of Law in the Age of Direct-to-Consumer Advertising*, 32 Harv. J. L. & Pub. Pol'y 333, 365 (2009).

Journal 2007 Questions FDA restrictions prohibiting drug manufacturers from discussing off-label uses of their products. Concludes that such restrictions on speech violate the First Amendment under the *Central Hudson* test. References Opinion 5.015. Hall & Sobotka, *Inconsistent Government Policies: Why FDA Off-Label Regulation Cannot Survive First Amendment Review Under Greater New Orleans*, 62 Food Drug L. J. 1, 31 (2007).

Journal 2006 Discusses the evolution of health law in Virginia. Concludes that the area of health law continues to expand, develop, and be refined. Cites Opinions 3.03, 3.08, 5.01, 5.015, 5.02, 5.04, 5.055, 6.02, 6.021, 6.03, 6.04, 7.03, 7.04, 7.05, 8.054, 8.08, 8.081, 8.085, 8.115, 8.12, 8.14, 8.145, 8.19, and 9.045. Guanzon, *Health Care Law*, 41 U. Rich. L. Rev. 179, 199 (2006).

Journal 2004 Discusses whether the government may legally restrain direct-to-consumer advertising of genetic tests. Concludes that any such restraint on truthful and nonmisleading advertising in this context would be unconstitutional. References Opinion 5.015. Javitt, Stanley, & Hudson, *Direct-to-Consumer Genetic Tests, Government Oversight, and the First Amendment: What the Government Can (and Can't) Do to Protect the Public's Health*, 57 Okla. L. Rev. 251, 280 (2004).

Journal 2003 Discusses the pharmaceutical industry's direct-to-consumer (DTC) Internet advertising program. Concludes that reforms to Internet-based DTC advertising practices are necessary, with emphasis on the physician-patient relationship. References Opinion 5.015. Hall, *The Promise and Peril of Direct-to-Consumer Prescription Drug Promotion on the Internet*, 7 DePaul J. Health Care L. 1, 35 (2003).

Journal 2002 Examines the legal, ethical, and social implications of Internet direct-to-consumer advertising of health products. Concludes that such advertising may be worthwhile, but privacy, product liability, and corporate responsibility issues must be addressed. References Opinion 5.015. Kao & Linden, *Direct-to-Consumer Advertising and the Internet: Informational Privacy, Product Liability and Organizational Responsibility*, 46 St. Louis U. L. J. 157, 170 (2002).

5.02 Advertising and Publicity

There are no restrictions on advertising by physicians except those that can be specifically justified to protect the public from deceptive practices. A physician may publicize himself or herself as a physician through any commercial publicity or other form of public communication (including any newspaper, magazine, telephone directory, radio, television, direct mail, or other advertising) provided that the communication shall not be misleading because of the omission of necessary material information, shall not contain any false or misleading statement, or shall not otherwise operate to deceive.

Because the public can sometimes be deceived by the use of medical terms or illustrations that are difficult to understand, physicians should design the form of communication to communicate the information contained therein to the public in a readily comprehensible manner. Aggressive, high-pressure advertising and publicity should be avoided if they create unjustified medical expectations or are accompanied by deceptive claims. The key issue, however, is whether advertising or publicity, regardless of format or content, is true and not materially misleading.

The communication may include (1) the educational background of the physician, (2) the basis on which fees are determined (including charges for specific services), (3) available credit or other methods of payment, and (4) any other nondeceptive information.

Nothing in this opinion is intended to discourage or to limit advertising and representations which are not false or deceptive within the meaning of Section 5 of the Federal Trade Commission Act. At the same time, however, physicians are advised that certain types of communications have a significant potential for deception and should therefore receive special attention. For example, testimonials of patients as to the physician's skill or the quality of the physician's professional services tend to be deceptive when they do not reflect the results that patients with conditions comparable to the testimoniant's condition generally receive.

Objective claims regarding experience, competence, and the quality of physicians and the services they provide may be made only if they are factually supportable. Similarly, generalized statements of satisfaction with a physician's services may be made if they are representative of the experiences of that physician's patients.

Because physicians have an ethical obligation to share medical advances, it is unlikely that a physician will have a truly exclusive or unique skill or remedy. Claims that imply such a skill or remedy therefore can be deceptive. Statements that a physician has an exclusive or unique skill or remedy in a particular geographic area, if true, however, are permissible. Similarly, a statement that a physician has cured or successfully treated a large number of cases involving a particular serious ailment is deceptive if it implies a certainty of result and creates unjustified and misleading expectations in prospective patients.

Consistent with federal regulatory standards which apply to commercial advertising, a physician who is considering the placement of an advertisement or publicity release, whether in print, radio, or television, should determine in advance that the communication or message is explicitly and implicitly truthful and not misleading. These standards require the advertiser to have a reasonable basis for claims before they are used in advertising. The reasonable basis must be established by those facts known to the advertiser, and those which a reasonable, prudent advertiser should have discovered. Inclusion of the physician's name in advertising may help to assure that these guidelines are being met. (II)

Issued prior to April 1977. Updated June 1996.

US 1977 Disciplinary sanctions were imposed by state bar against attorneys who violated state rule prohibiting advertising. After state court upheld sanctions, attorneys appealed to Supreme Court arguing that state rule violated federal antitrust laws and was unconstitutional. State bar argued that rule prohibiting advertising was justified to prevent adverse impact on the legal profession. In questioning this assertion, the Court referred to the position of the AMA announced in 235 JAMA 2328 (1976) and included in Opinions and Reports of the Judicial Council 6.00 (1977) [now Opinion 5.02], that the medical profession permits advertising by physicians. The Court held that the state may regulate some aspects of advertising, but that a blanket prohibition against advertising by attorneys was unconstitutional as a violation of the First Amendment. *Bates v. State Bar of Ariz., 433 US 350, 369-70 n.20.*

1st Cir. 1966 Physician sued electric shaver manufacturer for libel on basis of its use of reprints of an article quoting a study favorably mentioning manufacturer which allegedly falsely indicated that physician was one of the coauthors of the research study. Plaintiff asserted that he had agreed to participate in the research only if his name was not used in advertising claims since this would be a violation of established rules of ethics of the AMA, Opinions and Reports of the Judicial Council Sec. 5, Para. 29 (1965) [now Opinion 5.02]. These facts were considered sufficient to submit to the jury. *Sperry Rand Corp. v. Hill, 356 F.2d 181, 184, cert. denied, 384 US 973 (1966).*

2d Cir. 1980 Federal Trade Commission ordered AMA and others to cease, with some exceptions, imposing restraints on advertising and contract practice by physicians, as well as on business relations between physicians and laypersons. Commission found restraints violated 15 USC Sec. 45 (a) (1). See 94 FTC 701 (1979). AMA petitioned for judicial review of Commission's order. Court reviewed order, noting specific ethical pronouncements of AMA which Commission found improper, including the following: restrictions upon advertising and solicitation, Principle 5 (1957) and Opinions and Reports of the Judicial Council Sec. 5, Para. 11 (1971) [now Opinion 5.02]; restrictions on contract practice, Principle 6 (1957) and Opinions and Reports of the Judicial Council Sec. 6, Paras. 3, 4, and 5 (1971) [now Opinion 8.05]; and restrictions on business organizations and relations with laypersons, Opinions and Reports of the Judicial Council, Sec.6, Paras. 14 and 15 (1971). The court rejected the AMA's argument that its ethical rules did not provide impetus for local and state medical societies to act against physicians violating its rules. Further, the court rejected the AMA's position that liability should be precluded because of revisions in the Opinions in 1977 and the Principles in 1980. Specifically, the court found that removal of the ban on patient solicitation and changes reflected in Principles II and IV (1980) did not render Commission's order moot. The order was therefore enforced with modifications. Dissenting judge, referring to 1980 revisions in Principles and to Opinions and Reports of the Judicial Council 4.05 and 6.00 (1977) [now Opinions 5.02 and 8.05], concluded order should not be enforced on grounds of mootness. *American Medical Ass'n v. FTC, 638 F.2d 443, 446, 446 n.1, 448, 449, 449 n.5, 450, 451, 455-57, aff'd, 455 US 676 (1982).*

D.C. Cir. 1980 Professional associations, including AMA, filed for judicial review of a Federal Trade Commission rule limiting the ability of states and professional associations to restrict advertising of eye exams as well as ophthalmic goods and services. Since the US Supreme Court had found certain restrictions on lawyer advertising unconstitutional while the case was pending, the court remanded the case for further consideration by the Commission. In its analysis of advertising in the eye care profession, the court quoted Principle 5 (1957) and the Opinions and Reports of the Judicial Council Sec. 10, Para. 4 (1971) which prohibited solicitation and advertising. However, the court also noted the intervening changes in the AMA's position regarding advertising, quoting the Opinions and Reports of the Judicial Council 6.00 (1977) [now Opinion 5.02] which permitted nondeceptive advertising. *American Optometric Ass'n v. F.T.C., 626 F.2d 896, 900-01, 913, 914, 914 n.11.*

E.D. Va. 1976 Health planning agency, which sought to compile directory of services and fees of community physicians, and consumer group interested in obtaining such information, challenged state statute which prohibited direct or indirect advertisement by physicians. In holding that the statute violated First Amendment rights, court noted that to protect the public from being misled as to medical quality, directory was designed in conformity with AMA advertising guidelines. Court quoted Judicial Council position published in 235 JAMA 2328 (1976), later included in Opinions and Reports of the Judicial Council 6.00 (1977) [now Opinion 5.02] to support analysis. *Health Sys. Agency v. Virginia State Bd. of Medicine, 424 F. Supp. 267, 274, 275 n.11, 276 Appendix B.*

Cal. App. 1968 Plaintiff-physician sought dissolution of a medical partnership with defendant's decedent, and also sought a larger percentage of the partnership receipts based upon an alleged oral agreement. Defendant cross-claimed to enjoin plaintiff from taking physical control of the partnership offices and patient records. The trial court enjoined plaintiff from treating previous patients, requiring that he return all medical records and pay defendant all fees received from patients he had treated during the time of dispute. The appellate court reversed insofar as the injunction prohibited plaintiff from treating the patient who desired to continue to receive his services or prevented access to medical records essential for this purpose, citing Opinions and Reports of the Judicial Council Sec. 7, Para. 16, Sec. 5, Para. 21, and Sec. 9 (1966) [now Opinions 6.08, 5.02, and 5.05] to support view that patients may not be regarded as the subject of ownership. *Jones v. Fakehany, 261 Cal. App. 2d 298, 67 Cal. Rptr. 810, 815, 816 n.1.*

Fla. App. 1968 Physician sued to enjoin county medical association and telephone company from eliminating medical specialty headings in classified section of directory pursuant to guidelines issued by AMA's Judicial Council in June, 1966 [now Opinion 5.02]. The court held that where medical association had no statutory authority to dictate directory listings, association's restrictions interfered with individual physicians' right to contract and deprived them of due process. *Dade County Medical Ass'n v. Samartino, 213 So. 2d 627, 629, n.2, 631.*

Mich. Att'y Gen. 1978 Opinion was requested from state attorney general as to constitutionality of blanket statutory prohibition of advertising by physicians and as to legality of expulsion of a member of a professional society for advertising that is otherwise proper. In finding the statutory restrictions unconstitutional, the opinion refers to the Judicial Council's advertising statement at 235 JAMA 2328 (1976) included as Opinion 6.00 (1977) [now Opinion 5.02]. *Michigan Att'y. Gen. Opinion N. 5024, 1977-78 Att'y Gen. Op. 299, 303.*

N.Y. Sup. 1965 Physician sued publishing company to bar insertion of advertisement for baby and child care products in physician's book, seeking declaration that book contract was void to the extent that it allowed inclusion of such an advertisement. Physician asserted that the advertisement was contrary to public policy, citing Opinions and Reports of the Judicial Council Sec. 5, Para. 29 (1965) [now Opinion 5.02] which stated that a doctor should not lend his name to any product. In rejecting the physician's claim, the court was willing to give careful consideration to the AMA's view but concluded that it did not, in itself, constitute an expression of public policy. *Spock v. Pocket Books, Inc., 48 Misc. 2d 812, 266 N.Y.S.2d 77, 79.*

Journal 2009 Discusses the judicial standard for reviewing physician noncompete covenants. Concludes courts should apply a strict standard to such covenants, rather than declare the covenants per se invalid. Quotes Principles IV and VII, Principles of Medical Ethics §5 (1957) [now Principle VI], Code of Medical Ethics Ch. II, Art. I §3 (1847) [now Opinion 5.02], Opinion 9.02, and Code of Medical Ethics Ch. II, Art. I §4 (1847) [now Opinion 9.09]. Cites Opinions 8.041, 8.115, 9.02, 9.06, 9.065, 9.067, 10.01, and 10.015. Koons, *Physician Employee Non-Compete Agreements on the Examining Table: The Need to Better Protect Patients' and the Public's Interests in Indiana,* 6 Ind. Health L. Rev. 253, 272-77, 280-81 (2009).

Journal 2008 Questions what entity should be responsible for critically evaluating chiropractors. Concludes that chiropractic should be a self-regulated profession. Quotes Introduction (1847) [now Opinions 1.01 and 1.02]. References Ch. II, Art. I, Sec. 3 (1847) [now Opinion 5.02] and Ch. II, Art. IV, Sec. 1 (May 1847) [now Opinion 3.01]. Johnson, *Keeping a Critical Eye on Chiropractic,* 31 J. of Manipulative and Physiological Therapeutics 559, 559 (2008).

Journal 2007 Highlights inconsistencies in applying judicial deference to medical ethics. Concludes that courts should afford greater deference to established medical ethics standards. Quotes Principle I and Opinions 2.06 and Ch. II, Art. I, Sec. 3 (May 1847) [now Opinion 5.02]. Cites Opinions 4.01 and 7.05. Lerman, *Second Opinion: Inconsistent Deference to Medical Ethics in Death Penalty Jurisprudence,* 95 Geo. L. J. 1941, 1945, 1974-75, 1976, 1977 (2007).

Journal 2006 Discusses the evolution of health law in Virginia. Concludes that the area of health law continues to expand, develop, and be refined. Cites Opinions 3.03, 3.08, 5.01, 5.015, 5.02, 5.04, 5.055, 6.02, 6.021, 6.03, 6.04, 7.03, 7.04, 7.05, 8.054, 8.08, 8.081, 8.085, 8.115, 8.12, 8.14, 8.145, 8.19, and 9.045. Guanzon, *Health Care Law,* 41 U. Rich. L. Rev. 179, 199 (2006).

Journal 2001 Compares and contrasts certain ethical positions articulated by the legal and medical professions. Concludes that both professions generally agree on ethical principles, but sometimes differ in the manner of implementation. Quotes Principle II. Cites Opinion 5.02. Needell, *Legal Ethics in Medicine: Are Medical Ethics Different From Legal Ethics?* 14 St. Thomas L. Rev. 31, 35, 50 (2001).

Journal 1999 Explains modern jurisdictional analysis and how it applies in medical malpractice cases. Examines the impact of physician advertising, referrals, consultations, prescribing practices, and involvement in state programs on personal jurisdiction in medical malpractice cases. Cites Opinion 5.02. Booker, *Physicians, Malpractice, and State Lines: A Guide to Personal Jurisdiction in Medical Malpractice Lawsuits,* 20 J. Legal Med. 385, 394 (1999).

Journal 1990 Provides an overview of the recent developments in the area of physician advertising. Proposes alternative solutions to the practical and ethical problems raised. Quotes Opinion 5.02. Olson, *Physician Specialty Advertising: The Tendency to Deceive?* 11 J. Legal Med. 351, 354 (1990).

Journal 1984 Discusses the AMA policy on physician advertising and identifies several factors that may affect the decision to advertise. Among the important factors are variations in prominence of physician advertising from region to region and state to state, local attitudes of patients and physicians toward physician advertising, and acceptable forms of physician advertising. Quotes Opinion 5.01 (1984) [now Opinion 5.02]. Porter, *Physician Advertising—What Is Legal? What Is Ethical? What Is Acceptable?* 80 Ohio State Med. J. 437, 437, 439 (1984).

5.025 Physician Advisory or Referral Services by Telecommunication

Telecommunication advisory services, by way of phone, fax, or computer, distinct from an existing patient-physician relationship can be a helpful source of medical information for the public. Often, people are not sure where to turn for information of a general medical nature or do not have easy access to other sources of information. Individuals also may be embarrassed about directly bringing up certain questions with their physicians. Although telecommunication advisory services can provide only limited medical services, they can be a useful complement to more comprehensive services, if used properly.

Any telecommunication advisory service should employ certain safeguards to prevent misuse. For example, the physician responding to the call should not make a clinical diagnosis. Diagnosis by telecommunication is done without the benefit of a physician examination or even a face-to-face meeting with the caller. Critical medical data may be unavailable to the physician. Physicians who respond to callers should therefore act within the limitations of telecommunication services and ensure that callers understand the limitations of the services. Under no circumstances should medications be prescribed.

Physicians who respond to the calls should elicit all necessary information from the callers. When callers are charged by the minute, they may try to hurry their calls to limit their costs. As a result, important information may not be disclosed to the physician. Physicians should also ensure that callers do not incur large bills inadvertently or without understanding the billing system.

Physician referral services can also offer important information to the public. Referral services are often provided by medical societies, hospitals, and for-profit entities. To ensure that the service bases its recommendation on medically legitimate considerations rather than the likelihood of being paid by the physician, when the service charges physicians a fee to participate, physicians should not pay the service per referral. Also, callers should be told how the list is created. For example, callers should be informed whether the list includes physicians who pay a flat fee to be listed, members of a particular hospital staff or medical society, or physicians who meet some general quality-based criteria.

While these safeguards are described as applying primarily to telephone services, they should be considered equally applicable to any other communication media, such as radio or television, in which the physician and patient do not meet face-to-face. (I, IV, VI)

Issued June 1994. Updated June 1996.

5.026 The Use of Electronic Mail

Electronic mail (e-mail) can be a useful tool in the practice of medicine and can facilitate communication within a patient-physician relationship. When communicating with patients via e-mail, physicians should take the same precautions used when sending faxes to patients. These precautions are presented in the following considerations:

(1) E-mail correspondence should not be used to establish a patient-physician relationship. Rather, e-mail should supplement other, more personal, encounters.

(2) When using e-mail communication, physicians hold the same ethical responsibilities to their patients as they do during other encounters. Whenever communicating medical information, physicians must present the information in a manner that meets professional standards. To this end, specialty societies can provide specific guidance as to the appropriateness of offering specialty care or advice through e-mail communication.

(3) Physicians should engage in e-mail communication with proper notification of e-mail's inherent limitations. Such notice should include information regarding potential breaches of privacy and confidentiality, difficulties in validating the identity of the parties, and delays in responses. Patients should have the opportunity to accept these limitations prior to the communication of privileged information. Disclaimers alone cannot absolve physicians of the ethical responsibility to protect patients' interests.

(4) Proper notification of e-mail's inherent limitations can be communicated during a prior patient encounter or in the initial e-mail communication with a patient. This is similar to checking with a patient about the privacy or security of a particular fax machine prior to faxing sensitive medical information. If a patient initiates e-mail communication, the physician's initial response should include information regarding the limitations of e-mail and ask for the patient's consent to continue the e-mail conversation. Medical advice or information specific to the patient's condition should not be transmitted prior to obtaining the patient's authorization. (I, IV, VI, VIII)

Issued June 2003 based on the report "Ethical Guidelines for the Use of Electronic Mail Between Patients and Physicians," adopted December 2002 (*AJOB* 2003;3(3)).

Wash. App. 2007 The defendant-physician resided in New Jersey and was licensed to practice medicine in Washington. Complaints were filed alleging he had prescribed pharmaceuticals over the Internet without any direct contact with patients. His license was revoked by the State Department of Health for unprofessional conduct. Defendant appealed, challenging the sufficiency of the evidence proving he created an unreasonable risk of harm to patients. With apparent reference to Opinions 5.026 and 5.027, the court found that defendant violated the AMA's ethical guidelines. The court reasoned that the Opinions are incorporated into state guidelines and are highly persuasive. The court found ample evidence to show defendant created an unreasonable risk to patients. *Ancier v. State Dept. of Health, 140 Wash. App 564, 166 P.3d 829, 833, 836, 837.*

Journal 2010 Explores how participation in online social networks may blur boundaries between personal and professional relationships for health care professionals and how such risks may be mitigated by use of network privacy and security settings. Suggests that health care institutions are likely to institute online social-networking policies for employees. Quotes Opinions 5.026, 5.027, 5.045, 5.046, 5.05, 5.059, 5.0591, 8.14, 9.08, and 9.123. Cites Opinions 5.026, 9.031, and 9.12. Terry, *Physicians and Patients Who "Friend" or "Tweet": Constructing a Legal Framework for Social Networking in a Highly Regulated Domain, 43 Ind. L. Rev. 285, 314-16, 319, 334-36, 338 (2010).*

Journal 2006 Argues that state and federal law enforcement agencies are unable to regulate online sale of pharmaceuticals. Concludes that alternative tactics must be used, such as controlling the price of pharmaceuticals. Quotes Opinion 5.026 (incorrectly cited as 5.06). Castronova, *Operation Cyber Chase and Other Agency Efforts to Control Internet Drug Trafficking, 27 J. Legal Med. 207, 219 (2006).*

Journal 2006 Argues that states have authority to regulate Internet pharmacies within the constraints of the Dormant Commerce Clause. Concludes that the federal government does not have sole authority to regulate Internet pharmacies. References Opinion 5.026. Vanderstappen, *Internet Pharmacies and the Specter of the Dormant Commerce Clause, 22 Wash. U. J. L. & Pol'y 619, 628 (2006).*

Journal 2004 Discusses legal and policy issues surrounding Internet drug prescribing and dispensing. Concludes that the current regulatory scheme may impede development of innovative and efficient online prescription models. Quotes Opinion 5.026. References 5.027. Terry, *Prescriptions sans Frontières (or How I Stopped Worrying About Viagra on the Web but Grew Concerned About the Future of Healthcare Delivery)*, 4 Yale J. Health Pol'y L. & Ethics 183, 240, 244, 251 (2004).

5.027 Use of Health-Related Online Sites

As Internet prevalence and access rapidly increase, individuals turn to the Internet to find health-related information quickly and efficiently. Online users can access innumerable informational or interactive online sites, many of which are maintained by physicians or rely on their services. Physician involvement should be guided by the following considerations:

(1) Physicians responsible for the health-related content of an online site should ensure that the information is accurate, timely, reliable, and scientifically sound, and includes appropriate scientific references.

(2) The provision of diagnostic or therapeutic services through interactive online sites, including advice to online users with whom the physician does not have a pre-existing relationship or the use of decision-support programs that generate personalized information directly transmitted to users, should be consistent with general and specialty-specific standards. General standards include truthfulness, protection of privacy, principles of informed consent, and disclosures such as limitations inherent in the technology.

(3) When participating in interactive online sites that offer e-mail communication, physicians should follow guidelines established in Opinion 5.026, "The Use of Electronic Mail."

(4) Physicians who establish or are involved in health-related online sites must minimize conflicts of interest and commercial biases. This can be achieved through safeguards for disclosure and honesty in funding and advertising. It also requires that physicians not place commercial interests ahead of patient health; therefore, physicians must not use health-related online sites to promote unnecessary services, refer patients to entities in which they have ownership interests, or sell products outside of established ethical guidelines. (See Opinions 2.19, "Unnecessary Medical Services"; 8.032, "Conflicts of Interest: Health Facility Ownership by a Physician;" 8.062, "Sale of Non–Health-Related Goods from Physicians' Offices;" and 8.063, "Sale of Health-Related Products from Physicians' Offices.") Promotional claims on online sites must conform to Opinion 5.02, "Advertising and Publicity."

(5) Physicians who establish or are involved in health-related online sites that use patient-specific information must provide high-level security protections, as well as privacy and confidentiality safeguards. (I, II, IV, V, VI)

Issued December 2003 based on the report "Use of Health-Related Online Sites," adopted June 2003 (*AJOB* 2003;3(3)).

Wash. App. 2007 The defendant-physician resided in New Jersey and was licensed to practice medicine in Washington. Complaints were filed alleging he had prescribed pharmaceuticals over the Internet without any direct contact with patients. His license was revoked by the State Department of Health for unprofessional conduct. Defendant appealed, challenging the sufficiency of the evidence proving he created an unreasonable risk of harm to patients. With apparent reference to Opinions 5.026 and 5.027, the court found that defendant violated the AMA's ethical guidelines. The court reasoned that the Opinions are incorporated into state guidelines and are highly persuasive. The court found ample evidence to show defendant created an unreasonable risk to patients. *Ancier v. State Dept. of Health*, 140 Wash. App 564, 166 P.3d 829, 833, 836, 837.

Journal 2010 Explores how participation in online social networks may blur boundaries between personal and professional relationships for health care professionals and how such risks may be mitigated by use of network privacy and security settings. Suggests that health care institutions are likely to institute online social-networking policies for employees. Quotes Opinions 5.026, 5.027, 5.045, 5.046, 5.05, 5.059, 5.0591, 8.14, 9.08, and 9.123. Cites Opinions 5.026, 9.031, and 9.12. Terry, *Physicians and Patients Who "Friend" or "Tweet": Constructing a Legal Framework for Social Networking in a Highly Regulated Domain*, 43 Ind. L. Rev. 285, 314-16, 319, 334-36, 338 (2010).

Journal 2004 Explores whether treatment of patients over the Internet without a prior physician-patient relationship is a violation of conventional standards of care. Concludes that the Federation of State Medical Boards must address this concern and that uniform online medicine guidelines must be adopted by the states. References Opinion 5.027. Reed, *Cybermedicine: Defying and Redefining Patient Standards of Care*, 37 Ind. L. Rev. 845, 850, 859, 862 (2004).

Journal 2004 Discusses legal and policy issues surrounding Internet drug prescribing and dispensing. Concludes that the current regulatory scheme may impede development of innovative and efficient online prescription models. Quotes Opinion 5.026. References 5.027. Terry, *Prescriptions sans Frontières (or How I Stopped Worrying About Viagra on the Web but Grew Concerned About the Future of Healthcare Delivery)*, 4 Yale J. Health Pol'y L. & Ethics 183, 240, 244, 251 (2004).

5.03   The previous Opinion 5.03, "Communications Media: Press Relations," issued prior to April 1977, was deleted in June 1996 and combined with Opinion 5.04, "Communications Media: Standards of Professional Responsibility."

5.04   Communications Media: Standards of Professional Responsibility

Physicians are ethically and legally required to protect the personal privacy and other legal rights of patients. When information concerning a specific patient is requested by the media, the physician must obtain the consent of the patient or an authorized representative before releasing such information. The physician may release only the authorized information or that which is public knowledge. The patient-physician relationship and its confidential nature must be maintained.

With these considerations in mind, the physician may assist the representatives of the media in every way possible. When the patient or authorized representative consents to the release of information, physicians should cooperate with the press to ensure that medical news is available more promptly and more accurately than would be possible without their assistance. Inasmuch as a diagnosis may be made only by a physician and may depend upon X-ray and laboratory studies, no statement regarding diagnosis should be made except by or on behalf of the attending physician. For the same reason, prognosis will be given only by the attending physician or at the attending physician's direction.

Statements regarding the circumstances surrounding shootings, knifings, and poisonings are properly police matters, and questions whether they were accidental should be referred to the appropriate authorities.

Certain news that is part of the public record, such as deaths, may be made available without the consent of the patient or authorized representative. (IV)

Issued prior to 1977. Updated June 1994 and June 1996.

Journal 2006 Discusses the evolution of health law in Virginia. Concludes that the area of health law continues to expand, develop, and be refined. Cites Opinions 3.03, 3.08, 5.01, 5.015, 5.02, 5.04, 5.055, 6.02, 6.021, 6.03, 6.04, 7.03, 7.04, 7.05, 8.054, 8.08, 8.081, 8.085, 8.115, 8.12, 8.14, 8.145, 8.19, and 9.045. Guanzon, *Health Care Law, 41 U. Rich. L. Rev. 179, 199 (2006).*

Journal 1999 Explores the increased use of physician-patient communication through e-mail. Analyzes current laws regarding medical privacy. Suggests that patients' communications to their physicians are part of their medical record and should be given the same protections. Quotes Opinions 5.05 and 5.07. Cites Opinions 5.04 and 5.06. Spielberg, *Online Without a Net: Physician-Patient Communication by Electronic Mail, 25 Am. J. Law & Med. 267, 284-85 (1999).*

Journal 1998 Examines the use of e-mail in the physician-patient relationship. Focuses on privacy concerns stemming from the use of e-mail in the medical context. Suggests that physicians should discuss the implications of communicating through e-mail with their patients and should obtain informed consent prior to communicating in this manner. Cites Opinions 5.04, 5.05, 5.057, 5.07, 5.075, and 5.08. Spielberg, *On Call and Online: Sociohistorical, Legal, and Ethical Implications of E-mail for the Patient-Physician Relationship, 280 JAMA 1353, 1356 (1998).*

Journal 1995 Addresses presidential disability, its past impact on American government, and possible solutions to potential problems. Proposes enhancement of the role of the President's physician. Quotes Opinion 8.03. Cites Opinions 5.04 and 5.05. Abrams, *The Vulnerable President and the Twenty-Fifth Amendment, With Observations on Guidelines, a Health Commission, and the Role of the President's Physician, 30 Wake Forest L. Rev. 453, 466, 471 (1995).*

Journal 1984 Observes that available ethical and legal guidelines are insufficient to aid physicians in addressing issues of patient privacy and confidentiality. Concludes that there is need for legislation in order to provide suitable guidance to physicians who fulfill an important role in protecting patient privacy. Cites 1982 Opinions 5.03 [now Opinion 5.04], 5.04, 5.05 [now Opinion 5.06], 5.06 [now Opinion 5.07], 5.07 [now Opinion 5.08], and 5.08 [now Opinion 5.09]. Gellman, *Prescribing Privacy: The Uncertain Role of the Physician in the Protection of Patient Privacy, 62 No. Carolina L. Rev. 255, 271 (1984).*

5.045 Filming Patients in Health Care Settings

The use of any medium to film, videotape, or otherwise record (hereafter film) patient interactions with health care providers requires the utmost respect for the privacy and confidentiality of the patient. The following guidelines are offered to help ensure that the rights of patients are protected when filming occurs. These guidelines specifically address filming with the intent of broadcast for public viewing. As such, they consider physicians' role in striving to deliver information to the public that is both complete and accurate. They do not address other uses such as filming for medical education (see Opinion 5.046), forensic or diagnostic filming, or the use of security cameras.

(1) Educating the public about the health care system should be encouraged, and filming of patients may be one way to accomplish this. This educational objective can be achieved ethically by filming only patients who can consent.

(2) Filming patients without consent is a violation of the patient's privacy. Consent is therefore an ethical requirement for both initial filming and subsequent broadcast for public viewing. Because filming cannot benefit a patient medically and may cause harm, filming should be done only if the patient being filmed can explicitly consent. When patients cannot consent, dramatic reenactments utilizing actors should be considered instead of violating patient privacy.

Consent by a surrogate medical decision-maker is not an ethically appropriate substitute for consent by the patient because the role of such surrogates is to make medically necessary decisions, and whether to film for public broadcast is not a medical decision. A possible exception exists when the person in question is permanently or indefinitely incapacitated (eg, a patient in a persistent vegetative state) or is a minor child, in which case the consent should be obtained from a parent or legal guardian who has the authority to make nonmedical decisions.

(a) Patients should have the right to have filming stopped upon request at any time and the film crew removed from the area. Also, persons involved in the direct medical care of the patient who feel that the filming may jeopardize patient care should request that the film crew be removed from the patient care area.

(b) The initial granting of consent does not preclude the patient from withdrawing consent at a later time. After filming has occurred, patients who have been filmed should have the opportunity to rescind their consent up until a reasonable time period before broadcast for public viewing. The consent process should include a full disclosure of whether the tape will be destroyed if consent is rescinded, and the degree to which the patient is allowed to view and edit the final footage before broadcast for public viewing.

(c) Due to the potential conflict of interest, informed consent should be obtained by a disinterested third party, and not a member of the film crew or production team.

(3) Information obtained in the course of filming medical encounters between patients and physicians is confidential. Persons who are not members of the health care team, but who may be present for filming purposes, must demonstrate that they understand the confidential nature of the information and are committed to respecting it. If possible, it is desirable for stationary cameras or health care professionals to perform the filming.

(4) Physicians retain their responsibility to maintain professional standards whenever medical or surgical encounters are filmed for public broadcast. They should be mindful that the educational content of the finished product may become marginalized, potentially distorting the portrayal of the patient-physician encounter and of the medical procedures. Physicians should accurately convey the risks, benefits, and alternatives of treatments to an audience of prospective patients, and should refuse to participate in programs that foster misperceptions or are otherwise misleading.

(5) Independent peer groups, such as medical specialty societies, also may help prevent misleading information from reaching the public by making themselves available to producers to assess the accuracy of program content. They may help dispel misperception by providing educational resources and, if necessary, taking corrective or disciplinary action.

(6) As advocates for their patients, physicians should not allow the care they provide or their advice to patients regarding participation in filming to be influenced by financial gain or promotional benefit to themselves, their patients, or their health care institutions.

(7) If a physician is compensated beyond services to the patient, the amount and conditions of compensation must be disclosed to the patient.

(8) To protect the best interests of patients, physicians should participate in institutional review of requests to film.

(9) Programs regarding various aspects of health care are commonly televised; therefore, physicians should recognize that their patients may have pre-formed expectations from public broadcasts that may need to be addressed. (I, IV, VII, VIII)

Issued December 2001 based on the report "Filming Patients in Health Care Settings," adopted June 2001. Updated June 2006 based on the report "Ethics of Physician Participation in Reality Television for Entertainment," adopted November 2005.

Journal 2010 Explores how participation in online social networks may blur boundaries between personal and professional relationships for health care professionals and how such risks may be mitigated by use of network privacy and security settings. Suggests that health care institutions are likely to institute online social-networking policies for employees. Quotes Opinions 5.026, 5.027, 5.045, 5.046, 5.05, 5.059, 5.0591, 8.14, 9.08, and 9.123. Cites Opinions 5.026, 9.031, and 9.12. Terry, *Physicians and Patients Who "Friend" or "Tweet": Constructing a Legal Framework for Social Networking in a Highly Regulated Domain*, 43 Ind. L. Rev. 285, 314-16, 319, 334-36, 338 (2010).

5.046 Filming Patients for the Education of Health Professionals

It is important to recognize that filming patients for educational purposes has direct implications in relation to privacy, which itself has become the object of recent detailed federal regulations. Therefore, filming for educational purposes in the health care setting should comply with relevant laws and regulations. In addition, filming for educational purposes should be analyzed from the perspective of the ethics of the patient-physician relationship. In this regard, an important distinction can be drawn between filming for commercial purposes (see Opinion 5.045, "Filming Patients in Health Care Settings") and filming for educational purposes, since the latter is performed and viewed by members of the health care team, who are bound by ethical responsibilities regarding patient autonomy, privacy, and confidentiality. Specifically:

(1) Informed consent should be obtained before filming whenever possible. If it is not possible to obtain consent from the patient before filming, then consent must be obtained before the film is used for educational purposes. A surrogate decision-maker may give consent for filming only if the patient temporarily lacks capacity to give consent before the filming. When the patient regains decision-making capacity, his or her consent should be obtained before the film is used. In the case of minor children or permanently incompetent adults, consent may be obtained from the patient's parent or guardian. (See Opinion 5.045, "Filming Patients in Health Care Settings.")

(2) When obtaining consent, physicians should disclose information similar to that provided for other medical interventions, including an explanation of the educational purpose of film, potential benefits and harms (such as breaches of privacy and confidentiality), as well as a clear statement that participation in filming is voluntary and that the decision will not affect the medical care the patient receives. Moreover, physicians should be aware that filming may affect patient behavior during a clinical encounter. The

patient should be given ample opportunity to discuss concerns about the film, before and after filming, and a decision to withdraw consent must be respected.

(3) Information contained in educational films must be held to the same standards of confidentiality as other patient information. If filming requires the presence of nonclinical persons, these persons must agree to protect the patient's privacy and confidentiality. Viewing must be limited to health professionals, professionals-in-training, and students in the health professions, unless it has been disclosed to the patient that non–health professionals would view the film and the patient has consented to such viewing. If the film is to be distributed outside the institution in which it was produced, disclosure of the distribution must be made and explicit consent obtained.

(4) Films contain a record of personal patient information. Depending on its content, a film may or may not be considered part of the patient's medical record, and may be protected under privacy law. Irrespective of these legal standards, films should be securely stored and final disposal should ensure that they are properly destroyed. (I, IV, V, VIII)

Issued December 2003 based on the report "Filming Patients for Educational Purposes," adopted June 2003.

Journal 2010 Explores how participation in online social networks may blur boundaries between personal and professional relationships for health care professionals and how such risks may be mitigated by use of network privacy and security settings. Suggests that health care institutions are likely to institute online social-networking policies for employees. Quotes Opinions 5.026, 5.027, 5.045, 5.046, 5.05, 5.059, 5.0591, 8.14, 9.08, and 9.123. Cites Opinions 5.026, 9.031, and 9.12. Terry, *Physicians and Patients Who "Friend" or "Tweet": Constructing a Legal Framework for Social Networking in a Highly Regulated Domain*, 43 Ind. L. Rev. 285, 314-16, 319, 334-36, 338 (2010).

5.05 Confidentiality

The information disclosed to a physician by a patient should be held in confidence. The patient should feel free to make a full disclosure of information to the physician in order that the physician may most effectively provide needed services. The patient should be able to make this disclosure with the knowledge that the physician will respect the confidential nature of the communication. The physician should not reveal confidential information without the express consent of the patient, subject to certain exceptions which are ethically justified because of overriding considerations.

When a patient threatens to inflict serious physical harm to another person or to himself or herself and there is a reasonable probability that the patient may carry out the threat, the physician should take reasonable precautions for the protection of the intended victim, which may include notification of law enforcement authorities.

When the disclosure of confidential information is required by law or court order, physicians generally should notify the patient. Physicians should disclose the minimal information required by law, advocate for the protection of confidential information, and, if appropriate, seek a change in the law. (III, IV, VII, VIII)

Issued December 1983. Updated June 1994. Updated June 2007 based on the report "Opinion E-5.05, 'Confidentiality,' Amendment," adopted November 2006.

US 2001 Obstetrical patients at a state university hospital who were arrested after testing positive for cocaine, filed suit challenging the nonconsensual drug tests given to them by the hospital and later used for law enforcement purposes. The lower courts found for the respondents. The Supreme Court reversed, finding the searches unconstitutional and not within the "special needs" category of constitutional, nonconsensual searches. The Court quoted Opinion 5.05, noting that this was not a case where the physicians were required to report to law enforcement the threat of harm by a patient. *Ferguson v. City of Charleston, 532 US 67, 121 S. Ct. 1281, 1290.*

E.D. Ark. 1992 Plaintiff sought an injunction to prevent defendant's attorneys from contacting patient's nonparty treating physicians and interviewing them privately without the patient's consent. Quoting Opinion 5.05, the court stated that patients have a right not to have privileged information disclosed by their physician without express authorization. While the privilege may be partially waived where the patient's medical condition is put in issue by the filing of a lawsuit, patients still retain the right to insist that disclosure be made pursuant to formal discovery methods, absent express consent to ex parte contact. *Harlan v. Lewis, 141 F.R.D. 107, 109 n.5.*

D. Kan. 1991 With apparent reliance on Principle IV and Opinion 5.05, plaintiff claimed that other than in discovery or judicial proceedings, the physician-patient privilege is absolute and precludes ex parte communications with defense counsel. While recognizing the confidential nature of the physician-patient relationship, the court held that the ethical standards promulgated by the AMA are not binding law and that, where a litigant-patient has placed his or her medical status in issue, the physician is released from the constraints imposed by the physician-patient relationship for the purposes of the litigation. *Bryant v. Hilst, 136 F.R.D. 487, 490.*

E.D. La. 2005 Plaintiff filed a motion to modify the district court's order requiring five days' notice to opposing counsel before interviewing plaintiff's prescribing physician. The court quoted Opinion 5.05 and cited Principle IV when discussing the physician-patient relationship and the physician's duty to protect confidences revealed by a patient. The court granted the plaintiff's motion and modified the order to ensure that defendants were faced with the same restrictions as the plaintiff and that plaintiff could conduct ex parte interviews with physicians not named as defendants. *In re Vioxx Products Liability Litigation, 230 F.R.D. 473, 476 n. 17.*

E.D. Pa. 1992 Patient sued state mental institution and psychiatrist for violation of her right to privacy under the Fourteenth Amendment. Defendants had disclosed to law enforcement personnel and to plaintiff's supervisor threats made by plaintiff during the course of her treatment. While recognizing a strong public policy against breaches of confidentiality, the court held that the state's interest in protecting its citizens from serious bodily harm was overriding. The court noted that the limits placed on patient-therapist confidentiality by Opinion 5.05 (1989) are in accordance with the judicially recognized duty that a mental health professional take reasonable steps to prevent harm to others threatened by his or her patient. *Ms. B. v. Montgomery County Emergency Service, Inc., 799 F. Supp. 534, 539 cert denied, 114 S.Ct. 174 (1993).*

M.D. Pa. 1987 Plaintiff in a medical malpractice action sought to preclude his treating physicians from serving as defendant's expert witnesses at trial. The court held that defense counsel's failure to provide prior notice of ex parte communication with plaintiff's treating physicians barred their use as defense experts. Referring to *Petrillo v. Syntex Laboratories, Inc.,* 148 Ill. App. 3d 581, 499 N.E.2d 952 (1986), the court noted that the court there favorably cited Principle IV and Opinions 5.05, 5.06, and 5.07 (1984) in support of a public policy protecting confidentiality between physician and patient and against ex parte discussion. *Manion v. N.P.W. Medical Center of N.E. Pa., Inc., 676 F. Supp. 585, 591.*

Ala. 1973 Physician revealed patient information to the patient's employer, contrary to instructions of patient. Patient sued for breach of fiduciary duty. Citing Principle 9 (1957) [now Principle IV and Opinion 5.05] as well as cases from other states, the court held that even in the absence of a testimonial privilege statute, as a matter of public policy, a physician has a fiduciary duty not to make extrajudicial disclosures of patient information acquired in the course of treatment unless the public interest or the private interest of the patient demands otherwise. In holding that the physician had breached his contract with patient, the court found the Principles together with state licensing requirements sufficient to establish the public policy of confidentiality. *Horne v. Patton, 291 Ala. 701, 287 So. 2d 824, 829, 832.*

Alaska 1977 Physician–school board member failed to fully comply with state's conflict of interest law by refusing to reveal the names of patients from whom he had received over $100 in income. The physician claimed a legal privilege or ethical duty not to disclose the information under Principle 9 (1957) [now Principle IV and Opinion 5.05] and, alternatively, that the conflict of interest law unconstitutionally invaded a patient's right to privacy. The court held that disclosure was not barred by a legal privilege or ethical mandate, but that the conflict of interest law unconstitutionally invaded patient privacy due to the absence of protective regulations. In ruling on the ethical duty issue, the court noted that under Alaska law, a physician's license may be revoked for violating the Principles. However, the court found this licensing provision irrelevant to the privileged relationship exception in the conflict of interest law. The court found that otherwise the privilege exception in the statute could be changed by the AMA, a private organization, simply by amending the Principles. *Falcon v. Alaska Pub. Offices Comm'n, 570 P.2d 469, 474 n.13.*

Ariz. App. 1989 In a medical malpractice action, defense counsel interviewed several of plaintiff's treating physicians ex parte and notified plaintiff of this in preparation for a medical liability review panel hearing. Plaintiff moved to bar all testimony by those physicians and to disqualify defense counsel from representing defendants. The appellate court noted a physician's obligation of confidentiality pursuant to Principle IV and Opinion 5.05 and held that defense counsel in a medical malpractice action may not engage in nonconsensual ex parte communications with plaintiff's treating physicians. *Duquette v. Superior Court, 161 Ariz. 269, 778 P.2d 634, 641.*

Cal. 1994 Plaintiff alleged that treating physician and medical group violated her statutory and constitutional right to privacy by engaging in ex parte communications with original physician's insurance company during discovery in a medical malpractice action against her original physician. The court concluded that state law clearly exempts the defendants from liability and that plaintiff failed to allege a sufficiently serious invasion of privacy to warrant relief. The dissent quoted Opinion 5.05 to emphasize the fiduciary nature of the physician-patient relationship. *Heller v. Norcal Mutual Ins. Co., 8 Cal. 4th 30, 876 P.2d 999, 32 Cal. Rptr. 2d 200, 220, cert. denied, 115 S. Ct. 669, 130 L. Ed. 2d 602 (1994).*

Cal. 1976 Parents sued psychotherapists to recover for murder of daughter by psychiatric patient, alleging that failure to warn victim of patient's violent threat was a proximate cause of her death. In considering whether such a revelation would have been a violation of professional ethics, the court noted that Principle 9 (1957) [now Principle IV and Opinion 5.05] recognized that the confidential nature of a physician-patient communication must yield when disclosure is necessary to protect an individual or community as a whole. The court concluded that, in the circumstances of this case, disclosure would not have violated medical ethics and held that psychotherapists are under a duty to warn when they determine or should determine that a patient poses a serious danger of violence to someone else. *Tarasoff v. Regents of Univ. of Cal., 17 Cal. 3d 425, 551 P.2d 334, 347, 131 Cal. Rptr. 14, 27.*

Cal. 1970 Psychiatrist-witness in civil assault case applied for writ of habeas corpus after being held in contempt of court for refusing to produce patient's psychiatric records. Patient, plaintiff in the assault action, neither expressly claimed nor waived the statutory psychotherapist-patient privilege. The court held that the litigant-patient exception to the statutory psychotherapist-patient privilege does not unconstitutionally infringe rights of privacy of either psychotherapists or their patients. The court noted that in such a context a psychiatrist does not violate Principle 9 (1957) [now Principle IV and Opinion 5.05] since the Principle allows for legally compelled disclosure. *In re Lifschutz, 2 Cal. 3d 415, 467 P.2d 557, 565-66 n.9, 85 Cal. Rptr. 829, 837-38 n.9.*

Cal. App. 1982 Defendant was convicted of lewd act with a child and child molestation or annoyance, after licensed clinical psychologist reported defendant's admission of sexual conduct to authorities. The court held that the psychologist's testimony was properly admitted since a statute requiring the reporting of actual or suspected child abuse expressly made the psychotherapist-patient privilege inapplicable. The court quoted Principle 9 (1957) [now Principle IV and Opinions 2.02 and 5.05] in concluding the disclosure was not a breach of professional ethics. *People v. Stritzinger, 126 Cal. App. 3d 135, 186 Cal. Rptr. 750, 752 rev'd, 34 Cal. 3d 505, 668 P.2d 738, 194 Cal. Rptr. 431 (1983).*

Cal. App. 1968 Plaintiff-physician sought dissolution of a medical partnership with defendant's decedent, and also sought a larger percentage of the partnership receipts based upon an alleged oral agreement. Defendant cross-claimed to enjoin plaintiff from taking physical control of the partnership offices and patient records. The trial court enjoined plaintiff from treating previous patients, requiring that he return all medical records and pay defendant all fees received from patients he had treated during the time of dispute. The appellate court reversed insofar as the injunction prohibited the plaintiff from treating patient who desired to continue to receive his services or prevented access to medical records essential for this purpose, citing Opinions and Reports of the Judicial Council Sec. 7, Para. 16, Sec. 5, Para. 21, and Sec. 9 (1966) [now Opinions 6.08, 5.02, and 5.05] to support view that patients may not be regarded as the subject of ownership. *Jones v. Fakehany, 261 Cal. App. 2d 298, 67 Cal. Rptr. 810, 815, 816 n.1.*

Colo. 1989 Spouse of police officer killed by released psychiatric patient sued state mental hospital and psychiatrist for negligence. Patient had blamed police for his misfortunes during repeated involuntary commitments for paranoid schizophrenia, and psychiatrist knew that patient would have access to a gun after release. The court held that a psychiatrist owed a duty of care in determining whether patient had propensity for violence and posed unreasonable risk of serious bodily harm to others. In so holding, the court cited Principle 9 (1957) [now Principle IV and Opinion 5.05], in support of the view that there are situations in which the need to protect an individual or the community from the threat of harm from a patient may outweigh the strong policy in favor of nondisclosure of patient confidences. *Perreira v. State, 768 P.2d 1198, 1210 n.7.*

D.C. App. 1985 Patient sued plastic surgeon for breach of confidential physician-patient relationship following surgeon's use of before and after photographs of her plastic surgery in a department store presentation. In considering whether such a breach was an actionable tort, the court made reference to an earlier case quoting Principles Ch. II, Sec. 2 (1947) [erroneously cited in the earlier case as Ch. II, Sec. 1 (1943)] [now Principle IV and Opinion 5.05], as evidence of the strong public policy which exists in favor of maintaining a patient's confidences. *Vassiliades v. Garfinckel's, Brooks Bros., 492 A.2d 580, 590, 591.*

Fla. App. 1995 The court considered the issue of the effect of § 455.241(2) of the Florida Statutes on right of defense in a medical malpractice action to engage in ex parte communications with plaintiff's nonparty treating physician. The court held that a 1988 amendment to § 455.241(2) negated the applicability of the statute to medical malpractice cases. The dissent, citing *Petrillo v. Syntex Laboratories, Inc.,* 148 Ill. App. 3d 581, 499 N.E.2d 952 (1986), quoted Principles II and IV and Opinions 5.05, 5.06, and 5.08 as strong public policy support for its position that ex parte communications should be barred altogether. *Castillo-Plaza v. Green, 655 So. 2d 197, 206 n.4.*

Ill. 1997 Trial court held various statutory sections, including those permitting unlimited disclosure of a patient's medical records, unconstitutional. On appeal, state Supreme Court affirmed. Regarding provisions mandating consent to the disclosure of medical records, the court noted, with reference to Principle IV and Opinion 5.05, the crucial importance of confidentiality in the physician-patient relationship. *Best v. Taylor Machine Works, 179 Ill. 2d 367, 689 N.E. 2d 1057, 1099.*

Ill. App. 1987 In appeal of malpractice action, an issue was whether expert testimony of plaintiff's treating physician, based upon discussions with the defense counsel without patient's consent, was admissible. The court held that ex parte communications between a plaintiff's treating physician and legal adversary violated public policy. In determining the existence of such a policy favoring the sanctity of the doctor-patient relationship, the court noted *Petrillo v. Syntex Laboratories, Inc.,* 148 Ill. App. 3d 581, 499 N.E.2d 952 (1st Dist. 1986) and its reference to the Principles and Opinions, namely Principle IV and Opinion 5.05 (1984), which establish an ethical obligation to keep physician-patient communications confidential, generally requiring a patient's consent before information is released. *Yates v. El-Deiry, 160 Ill. App. 3d 198, 513 N.E.2d 519, 522.*

Ill. App. 1986 Defense attorney in product liability suit was held in contempt of court for conducting ex parte discussions with plaintiff-patient's treating physician without patient's consent and contrary to authorized methods of discovery. The court held that the strong public policy favoring physician-patient confidentiality articulated in Principles II and IV and Opinions 5.05, 5.06, 5.07, and 5.08 (1984) justified a rule against such ex parte discussions. Further, the court held that the public has the right to rely on physicians to faithfully execute their ethical obligations. *Petrillo v. Syntex Laboratories, Inc., 148 Ill. App. 3d 581, 499 N.E.2d 952, 957, 958, 959, cert. denied, 483 US 1007 (1987).*

Ill. App. 1979 Patient filed suit against physician for breach of contract and breach of confidential relationship after physician's employee disclosed patient's name to police. Patient alleged that implied contract arose out of a statutory physician-patient privilege, and provisions of the Canons of Medical Ethics, with apparent reference to Principle 9 (1957) [now Principle IV and

Opinion 5.05]. The court held that disclosure of patient's name alone by a physician or the physician's agents is insufficient to state a cause of action in contract and does not violate the physician-patient privilege. *Geisberger v. Willuhn, 72 Ill. App. 3d 435, 390 N.E.2d 945, 946, 948.*

Ind. App. 1996 A patient filed suit against a mental health counseling center for disclosing to a third party death threats made by the patient during therapy. The patient claimed this was a breach of the standard of care owed to her. The trial court found that the counseling center was not statutorily prohibited from disclosing death threats the patient made. On appeal, the court affirmed the decision. It noted, with apparent reference to Principle IV and Opinion 5.05, that physicians may disclose confidential information to ensure the safety of the public or of individuals. In clarifying its holding, the court observed that while free and frank communication should be promoted to aid proper diagnosis and treatment, public policy supports disclosure of confidential information when appropriate. *Rocca v. Southern Hills Counseling Center, Inc., 671 N.E. 2d 913, 916.*

La. App. 2009 Accused criminal sued emergency room physician for defamation and false arrest and imprisonment after he was charged with second-degree murder based on physician's report to police that accused's deceased girlfriend had been shot. The court, quoting Opinion 5.05, noted that while a physician has a duty of confidentiality to a patient, because state law required report of gunshot wounds to local law enforcement, and because the physician did not fabricate the report, the physician was immune from liability. *Mitchell v. Villien, 19 So. 3d 557, 567, n. 14.*

Md. App. 2007 In an espionage case, a psychiatrist was engaged to evaluate defendant's competency. Defendant disclosed confidential information which the psychiatrist later disclosed to defendant's wife and the media. Defendant and his wife filed a complaint for breach of confidentiality with the State Board of Physicians which revoked the psychiatrist's medical license. On appeal, the psychiatrist denied any unprofessional conduct. The court, quoting Principle IV, found the psychiatrist's behavior was unethical and unprofessional. With apparent reference to Opinion 5.05, the psychiatrist argued there was an exception to the duty of confidentiality when disclosure would protect the "community interest." The court found no such "community interest" exception. *Salerian v. Maryland State Board of Physicians, 176 Md. App. 231, 932 A.2d 1225, 1235-36, 1241-42.*

Ky. 2002 Patient appealed denial of writ to prevent release to grand jury of psychiatric treatment records. Records were requested to demonstrate that patient had visited multiple physicians to obtain the same prescription drugs. Trial judge reviewed the records in camera and denied writ. The Supreme Court of Kentucky reversed, holding that the evidence reviewed in camera was inadmissible. The court found that a sufficient evidentiary basis must be shown to permit in camera review of privileged records. Concurring judge quotes Opinion 5.05. *Stidham v. Clark, 74 S.W.3d 719, 729, 730.*

Md. Att'y Gen. 1977 Opinion addresses the obligation of a psychiatrist to report child abuse information obtained from a parent-patient. Referring to state statutes and to Principle 9 (1957) [now Principle IV and Opinions 2.02 and 5.05] the opinion concludes that the question of whether to disclose suspected child abuse is a matter left to the individual psychiatrist's professional and moral judgment. *Maryland Att'y. Gen. Opinion, 62 Op. Att'y Gen. Md. 157, 160.*

Mass. 1984 Employee sued employer for libel and invasion of privacy following disclosure of medical facts about employee to other employees. In part, claim involved disclosure of opinion about employee's mental state to his supervisor by physician retained by employer. Citing Principle 9 (1957) [now Principle IV and Opinions 5.05 and 5.09], the court held that a physician retained by an employer may disclose to the employer information concerning an employee if receipt of the information is reasonably necessary to serve a substantial and valid business interest of the employer. *Bratt v. Int'l Business Mach. Corp., 392 Mass. 508, 467 N.E.2d 126, 137 n.23.*

Minn. 1976 Plaintiff-patient in malpractice action appealed trial court's order to provide authorization for private, informal interview between defense counsel and patient's treating physician. In holding that formal pretrial discovery provided the exclusive procedure by which defendant could obtain medical testimony, the court noted, without deciding the issue, that a physician who discloses confidential patient information in a private interview may be subject to tort liability for breach of patient's right to privacy or professional discipline for unprofessional conduct, citing Principle 9 (1957) [now Principle IV and Opinion 5.05]. *Wenninger v. Muesing, 240 N.W.2d 333, 337 n.3.*

Mo. 1993 Patient sued physicians alleging a breach of fiduciary duty of confidentiality for participating in an unauthorized ex parte discussion with defendant's attorney. While recognizing this duty, the court held that, where the plaintiff's medical condition is in issue, this constitutes a waiver of both the testimonial privilege and the physician's fiduciary duty in so far as the information is related to the medical issues. Quoting Opinion 5.05 and citing Principle IV, the court stated that courts may apply ethical principles to frame the specific limits of the legal duty of confidentiality. *Brandt v. Medical Defense Assoc., 856 S.W.2d 667, 671 n.1.*

Mo. 1989 In a personal injury suit, plaintiff challenged trial court's authority to compel plaintiff to authorize ex parte meetings between defendant insurance company and plaintiff's treating physician. Applying a balancing test between preserving the physician-patient confidential and fiduciary relationship, the physician-patient testimonal privilege, and the quest for truth in civil litigation, the court held that such information could be obtained through the methods of formal discovery. The court quoted Principle IV and Opinion 5.05 (1984) as statements of the policy underlying medical confidentiality and a basis for a patient's affirmative right to rely on the confidential nature of disclosures to a treating physician. *State ex. rel. Woytus v. Ryan, 776 S.W.2d 389, 392-93.*

Mo. App. 1985 In a prohibition proceeding arising from a medical malpractice action, defense attorneys sought order compelling plaintiff to authorize a private interview between defense attorneys and physician who treated plaintiff for injuries allegedly caused by defendant-physician. The appellate court, after discussing Principle IV and Opinion 5.05 (1984), held that the defense attorneys had the right to seek an ex parte interview with the treating physician, subject to the willingness of the physician to grant the interview. Furthermore, the court noted that Opinion 5.05 prevents a physician from revealing a patient's confidences only where there is a lack of consent from the patient and found that consent did exist here in the form of a medical authorization executed by plaintiff during pendency of the malpractice action. *State ex rel. Stufflebam v. Appelquist, 694 S.W.2d 882, 886, 888 n.7, overruled by State ex. rel. Woytus v. Ryan, 776 S.W.2d 389 (Mo. 1989).*

N.J. 1985 Plaintiff provided authorization for release of decedent's medical records from former treating physicians but refused to consent to depositions or interviews between defense counsel and physicians. The court noted physicians' ethical duty to avoid unauthorized disclosure, as stated in Principle 9 (1957) [now Principle IV and Opinion 5.05], but recognized that a patient's right to confidentiality was not absolute. After balancing the competing interests involved, the court held that defense counsel had a right to seek ex parte interviews of decedent's other treating physicians regarding litigation matters, provided procedural safeguards were met including clear statements that participation in such an interview is voluntary on the part of a physician. *Stempler v. Speidell, 100 N.J. 368, 495 A.2d 857, 860, cert. denied, 483 US 1007 (1987).*

N.J. 1979 In wrongful death action against a psychiatrist whose patient murdered plaintiff's decedent, the court concluded, in accord with Principle 9 (1957) [now Principle IV], that a psychiatrist may owe a duty to warn potential victims of possible danger from psychiatrist's patient despite the general emphasis on confidentiality. The court also noted the Preamble and Principles 1 and 3 (1957) [now revised Preamble, Principle I, and Opinion 5.05] in discussing the psychiatrist-patient relationship. *McIntosh v. Milano, 168 N.J. Super. 466, 403 A.2d 500, 510, 512-13.*

N.J. 1962 Parents sued pediatrician for unauthorized disclosure to life insurer of deceased infant's congenital heart defect. The court quoted Principle 9 (1957) [now Principle IV and Opinion 5.05] as an articulation of a physician's legal duty to his or her patient subject to exceptions of compelling social or patient interests. The court held that the parents had lost their limited right to nondisclosure by filing an insurance claim. *Hague v. Williams, 37 N.J. 328, 181 A.2d 345, 347.*

N.J. Super. 1991 Physician's estate sued hospital alleging that it violated state law against discrimination by restricting the physician's surgery privileges and requiring him to inform patients of his HIV-infected status before performing invasive procedures. The defendant hospital was also alleged to have breached its duty to maintain confidentiality of his seropositive diagnosis. The court held that the hospital had not discriminated against the physician since the hospital had relied on ethical and professional standards, including a report of the Council on Ethical and Judicial Affairs of the AMA dealing with the issue of AIDS [now Opinions 9.13 and 9.131]. However, the hospital was held to have breached its fiduciary duty to maintain the confidentiality of the physician's medical records. Referring to *McIntosh v. Milano, 168 N.J. Super. 466, 403 A.2d 500 (1979)* which had quoted AMA Principles of Medical Ethics sec. 9 (1957) [now Principle IV and Opinion 5.05] in applying the "duty to warn" exception, the court noted that the disclosure in this case went far beyond the medical personnel directly involved in the treatment of the physician and those patients entitled to informed consent. *Estate of Behringer v. Medical Ctr.*, 249 N.J. Super. 597, 614, 633, 592 A.2d 1251, 1259, 1268.

N.J. Super. 1988 Several portions of state department of corrections regulations concerning exceptions to privileged communications between psychologist and inmates were invalidated by appellate court because they permitted disclosure of confidences that did not present clear and imminent danger to the inmate or others, or failed to identify any intended victim. Court made general reference (with erroneous quotation) to Principle 9 (1957) [now Principle IV and Opinion 5.05]. *In re Rules Adoption*, 224 N.J. Super. 252, 540 A.2d 212, 215.

N.J. Super. 1987 Defendant in a personal injury suit sought to offer testimony from plaintiff's treating physician regarding plaintiff's prognosis. The court denied plaintiff's motion to exclude that evidence, despite the ethical obligation of physicians to uphold patients' communications as confidential under Principle 9 (1957) [now Principle IV and Opinion 5.05]. The court's decision was based on New Jersey case law permitting disclosure of a patient's medical condition to someone having a legitimate interest where the physical condition of the patient is made an element of a claim. *Kurdek v. West Orange Bd. of Educ.*, 222 N.J. Super. 218, 536 A.2d 332, 335.

N.J. Super. 1967 In a suit for separate maintenance, communications between plaintiff-wife and her psychiatrist were not protected from disclosure during depositions, despite Principle 9 (1957) [now Principle IV and Opinion 5.05] which prohibited physicians from disclosing patient confidences except where necessary to protect the welfare of the individual or of the community. The court concluded that the patient had only a limited right of nondisclosure, subject to exceptions created by supervening interest of society and that the institution of litigation by the patient constituted a vitiation of that right. *Ritt v. Ritt*, 98 N.J. Super. 590, 238 A.2d 196, 199, rev'd, 52 N.J. 177, 244 A.2d 497 (1968).

N.Y. Sup. 2000 Physician brought wrongful discharge claim against corporate employer. The physician alleged she was discharged because she refused to reveal confidential medical information regarding employees. With apparent reference to Principle IV and Opinions 5.05 and 5.09, the affidavit filed by the physician claimed she had an ethical and legal duty to protect patient confidentiality. The court found termination of an employee at will based upon such grounds is sufficient to state a cause of action for breach of contract. The court ruled that obligations of good faith and fair dealing may be implied in a contract for the employment of a physician and that no physician should be placed in the position of choosing between retaining employment and violating ethical standards. *Horn v. New York Times*, 186 Misc. 2d 469, 719 N.Y.S. 2d 471, 474.

N.Y. Sup. 1977 Plaintiff, a psychiatric patient, sued her psychiatrist and the psychiatrist's spouse for violating several state statutes and her privacy rights by publishing a book about the intimate details of plaintiff's psychotherapy. The court found for plaintiff, basing its decision in part upon Principle 9 (1957) [now Principle IV and Opinion 5.05] which requires a physician to uphold the confidences of a patient. *Doe v. Roe*, 93 Misc. 2d 201, 400 N.Y.S.2d 668, 674.

N.Y. Surr. 1977 In a discovery proceeding, respondent-psychiatrist, who had treated some patients of deceased psychiatrist subsequent to his death, allegedly misappropriated decedent's patient records. Estate petitioned court for return of records and damages for injury to value of decedent's practice. Respondent sought dismissal of claim arguing that estate could not sell patient records. The court rejected respondent's request. In so ruling, the court noted that under Principle 9 (1957) [now Principle IV and Opinion 5.05] prohibiting physicians from revealing patient confidences, various guidelines had been issued regarding sale of a medical practice [now Opinion 7.04]. Whether respondent's actions had interfered with the estate's efforts to dispose of decedent's practice in keeping with these guidelines presented the court with factual issues for later resolution. *Estate of Finkle*, 90 Misc. 2d 550, 395 N.Y.S.2d 343, 346.

N.C. 1990 Plaintiff in a malpractice case was granted an order prohibiting ex parte conferences between defendant's attorney and nonparty treating physicians. The court noted that both the Principles of Medical Ethics and Current Opinions affirm the physician's duty to protect patient confidentiality, in apparent reference to Principle IV and Opinion 5.05. In consideration of (1) the patient's right to privacy, (2) physician-patient confidentiality, (3) the adequacy of formal discovery procedures, and (4) the dilemma in which nonparty treating physicians are placed by ex parte conferences, the court held that an attorney may not interview a patient's nonparty treating physicians privately without express authorization. *Crist v. Moffatt*, 326 N.C. 326, 333, 389 S.E.2d 41, 46.

N.C. App. 1999 Plaintiff appealed industrial commission's finding for the plaintiff's employer on the grounds that there was insufficient medical evidence to find that the plaintiff's absence from work was attributed to injury. The plaintiff in part alleged that his employer engaged in ex parte communications with the plaintiff's treating physician. The court held that the commission erroneously placed on the plaintiff the burden of proving that the medical treatment he sought related to his injury. The court quoted Opinion 5.05, noting that it is improper for a physician to engage in ex parte communications with a defendant. The court stated, however, that the plaintiff failed to present evidence of such ex parte communications. *Reinninger v. Prestige Fabricators, Inc., 523 S.E.2d 720, 724.*

Ohio 1999 Patients brought a class action suit against hospital on grounds that the hospital disclosed patients' confidential medical information to the hospital's law firm, in order to determine whether the patients were eligible for government benefits to pay for unpaid hospital bills. The trial court granted defendants' motion for summary judgment. On appeal, the court held that a physician or a hospital can be held liable for unauthorized out-of-court disclosure of patients' confidential information. Additionally, the court found that an independent tort exists for unauthorized, unprivileged disclosure of patients' private medical information to a third party. The court cited Principle 9 (1957) [now Principle IV and Opinion 5.05], noting that courts have looked to such sources in providing a cause of action for breach of patient confidentiality. *Biddle v. Warren General Hospital, 86 Ohio St. 3d 395, 715 N.E.2d 518, 523.*

Ohio 1997 Estates of victims who were killed by their mentally ill son brought suit against son's psychotherapist for failing to disclose potential for violence. Son had been institutionalized and treated for schizophrenia. After release, he continued to take medication and see a psychotherapist. Despite parents' objections and attempts to have him involuntarily recommitted, psychotherapist reduced his medication and continued to recommend outpatient treatment. The court held that the psychotherapist had a duty to exercise reasonable care to control the son so as to prevent him from causing harm to his family. The court expressed concern for safeguarding the confidentiality of psychotherapeutic communications but noted that Principle 9 (1957) [now Principle IV and Opinion 5.05] has long allowed breaches of confidence when it becomes necessary to protect the welfare of the individual or the community. *Estates of Morgan v. Fairfield Family Counseling Center, 77 Ohio St. 3d 284, 303, 673 N.E.2d 1311, 1326.*

Ohio 1988 Administrator sued psychiatrist for wrongful death after recently discharged patient killed her infant daughter. In determining whether a professional judgment rule should be adopted in the malpractice standard of care where the prediction of violent behavior is involved, the court referred favorably to Principle 9 (1957) [now Principle IV and Opinion 5.05] which allows breaches of patient confidences when necessary to protect potential victims. *Littleton v. Good Samaritan Hospital, 39 Ohio St. 3d 86, 529 N.E.2d 449, 459 n.19.*

Okla. 1988 In response to a police request, physician reported patient treated for a penile bite. Patient sued physician for negligence after information furnished by physician led to patient's arrest and conviction for rape. Patient alleged a tortious breach of the physician-patient confidential relationship, breach of contract, violation of licensing statute, and breach of Principle 9 (1957) [now Principle IV and Opinion 5.05]. The court reasoned that the benefit of the divulgence inured to the public at large and thus fell within the public policy exception to the testimonial privilege, created no liability in tort or contract, and was not a breach of medical ethics under the licensing statute or the Principles. *Bryson v. Tillinghast, 749 P.2d 110, 113, 114.*

Pa. 1999 Administratrix of estate of victim murdered by a mental patient filed suit against the mental health center and member of professional staff. The trial court found in favor of the defendants. The Pennsylvania Supreme Court held that mental health professionals have a duty to warn a third party who is the subject of patient's threats when there is a immediate risk of serious bodily harm. The court quoted Opinion 5.05, noting that the AMA allows an exception to the duty of confidentiality when safety is a reasonable concern. The court found that the defendants had the duty to warn the victim and had fulfilled that duty when the victim was warned not to go to the patient's apartment. *Emerich v. Philadelphia Center for Human Development, Inc., 554 Pa. 209, 720 A.2d 1032, 1043.*

Pa. 1973 Plaintiff in personal injury suit resulting from auto accident claimed that trial court should have allowed showing on cross-examination that defendant's expert medical witness, who had treated plaintiff, violated Principle 9 (1957) [now Principle IV and Opinion 5.05] by ex parte communications with defense counsel, in order to impeach his medical testimony. The court held that any connection between an alleged breach of medical ethics and the credibility of a physician on the witness stand was tenuous. Therefore, the trial court's decision barring further inquiry in this regard was proper. *Downey v. Weston, 451 Pa. 259, 301 A.2d 635, 638.*

Pa. Super. 1998 The court denied a social worker's motion to quash a subpoena compelling her to testify before a grand jury regarding a client's murder. The court explained that the duty of confidentiality should be waived because the deceased client was not a crime suspect and because the information was necessary to solve a crime. The court further reasoned that disclosure of the confidential information was in the client's best interest because it would aid in solving the client's murder. The court, citing an earlier case, referenced Opinion 5.05, in support of the notion that confidentiality may be waived under special circumstances such as overriding public safety concerns. *In re Subpoena No. 22., Appeal of A.B., 709 A.2d 385, 391.*

Pa. Super. 1988 Plaintiff-patient sued her physician for breach of confidentiality when physician conferred with defense counsel in plaintiff's malpractice suit against the hospital (physician's employer). In its majority opinion, the court cited Principle IV, commenting that it gave very little guidance to physicians but nonetheless was not violated by the physician. The court also noted Opinion 5.07 (1986) finding that the plaintiff's suit minimized her expectations of confidentiality. The dissent, however, interpreted these same provisions, along with Opinion 5.05 (1986), as protecting plaintiff's expectations of confidentiality. *Moses v. McWilliams, 379 Pa. Super. 150, 549 A.2d 950, 956, 962 (dissent), appeal denied, 521 Pa. 630, 558 A.2d 532 (1989).*

Tenn. App. 1994 Plaintiff sought damages for wrongful death from defendant-surgeon. Defendant requested that the court require plaintiff to sign a form authorizing release of medical records and information to defense counsel. Trial court denied defendant's motion noting, with apparent reference to Principle IV and Opinion 5.05, that confidential relationship exists between physician and patient. Appellate court affirmed although it did not reach the ethical issue of the propriety of disclosures by a physician. *Wright v. Wasudev, 1994 Tenn. App. LEXIS 657.*

Utah App. 2006 Following an automobile accident, plaintiff filed a personal injury suit against the driver. Plaintiff discovered that his treating physician had been subpoenaed by the driver's lawyer, had agreed to testify against plaintiff, and had engaged in ex parte communications with defense counsel. Plaintiff sued the physician. With apparent reference to Opinions 5.05 and 5.059 plaintiff relied in part on the AMA ethical principles to establish the standard of care. The court of appeals held that the physician could be liable for breach of the fiduciary duty of confidentiality as well as for intentional infliction of emotional distress. *Sorensen v. Barbuto, 143 P.3d 295, 299.*

Utah Att'y Gen. 1978 A physician who, acting in good faith, discloses confidential information to proper authorities concerning a patient's unfitness to drive is not liable for doing so. Reference is made to Principle 9 (1957) [now Principle IV and Opinion 5.05] to support propriety of such disclosure where the public interest is involved. *Utah Att'y Gen. Op. No. 77-294.*

Wash. 1988 Personal representative brought wrongful death action against decedent's physicians. At issue was whether defense counsel in a personal injury action may communicate ex parte with plaintiff's treating physician where plaintiff has waived the physician-patient relationship. In holding that defense counsel may not engage in ex parte communication, and is limited to formal discovery methods, the court cited Principle IV and Opinion 5.05 (1986) with approval, reasoning that the mere threat of disclosure of private conversations between a physician and defense counsel would chill the physician-patient relationship and hinder further treatment. *Loudon v. Mhyre, 110 Wash. 2d 675, 756 P.2d 138, 141, 141 n.3.*

W. Va. 1993 Plaintiff, in a malpractice action, sought a writ of prohibition to prevent the enforcement of a trial court order allowing ex parte interviews. The court, in granting the writ, held that any benefit from ex parte interviews that occurs is minimal compared to the danger that they will undermine the confidential nature of the physician-patient relationship. Quoting Principles of Medical Ethics Ch. II, sec. 1 (1943) [now Principle IV and Opinion 5.05], the court noted that the medical profession is well aware of the importance of patient confidentiality. *State ex. rel. Kitzmiller v. Henning, 437 S.E.2d 452, 454.*

Wis. 1995 In medical malpractice suit, the court held that (1) subject to restrictions, defense counsel may engage in ex parte communications with plaintiff's treating physician if the communications do not involve disclosure of confidential information; (2) outside a judicial proceeding, defendant-physician may communicate ex parte with plaintiff's treating physician subject to a physician's duty of confidentiality; and (3) if defense counsel elicits confidential information from a treating physician during ex parte communications, the appropriate sanction is within the discretion of the court. The court expressly overruled *State ex rel. Klieger v. Alby*, 125 Wis. 2d 468, 373 N.W.2d 57 (Ct. App. 1985) and the cases applying it. The majority and concurring opinions referred to Principle IV and Opinion 5.05. *Steinberg v. Jensen, 194 Wis. 2d 440, 534 N.W.2d 361, 370, 377.*

Wis. App. 1999 Defendant who pled guilty to carrying a concealed weapon appealed on grounds that the police officer's search of the defendant was based on information obtained from the defendant's psychotherapist. The appellate court held that the defendant's statements made to his psychotherapist could be considered in evaluating the reasonableness of the search because the defendant posed a threat of danger. The court quoted Opinion 5.05, regarding confidentiality and noted the exception where safety is a concern. *State v. Agacki, 226 Wis. 2d 349, 595 N.W.2d 31, 37.*

Wis. App. 1994 In medical malpractice suit, defense counsel engaged in ex parte communications with plaintiff's consulting physicians. Plaintiff amended her complaint seeking punitive damages for breach of confidentiality. The court concluded that the rule of *State ex rel. Klieger v. Alby*, 125 Wis. 2d 468, 373 N.W.2d 57 (Ct. App. 1985), which prohibits ex parte communications that have the potential to breach physician-patient confidentiality, was violated and sanctions were required. The court referred to *Petrillo v. Syntax Labs., Inc.*, 148 Ill. App. 3d 581, 499 N.E.2d 952 (1986) and its use of Principle IV and Opinion 5.05. *Steinberg v. Jensen, 186 Wis. 2d 237, 519 N.W.2d 753, 761 n.9, rev'd, 194 Wis. 2d 440, 534 N.W.2d 361 (1995).*

Wis. Att'y Gen. 1987 Physicians may report cases of suspected child abuse or neglect when a patient discloses that he or she has abused a child in some manner. Where report is made in good faith, physicians are immune from any civil or criminal liability. Passing reference is made to Principle 9 (1957) [now Principle IV and Opinions 2.02 and 5.05] in support of this position. *Wisconsin Att'y Gen. Op. 10-87 (March 16, 1987) (LEXIS, States library, Wis. file).*

Journal 2011 Explores intimate partner violence (IPV) and various attempts to address it, such as mandatory reporting laws. Emphasizes the importance of distinguishing types of IPV and developing a multifaceted approach for responding to the needs of IPV victims. Cites Opinion 5.05. Hafemeister, *If All You Have Is a Hammer: Society's Ineffective Response to Intimate Partner Violence, 60 Cath. U. L. Rev. 919, 962 (2011).*

Journal 2011 Addresses why private Internet activity should always be protected by the warrant and probable cause requirements of the Fourth Amendment. Concludes that private Internet activity is exactly the type of activity that the courts and Congress have sought to protect from unreasonable searches and seizures by law enforcement. References Opinion 5.05. Mitter, *Deputizing Internet Service Providers: How the Government Avoids Fourth Amendment Protections, 67 N.Y.U. Ann. Surv. Am. L. 235, 273 (2011).*

Journal 2011 Considers the role of empirical evidence and moral principles in relation to the controversy surrounding attorney/client confidentiality. Concludes that rules of confidentiality should be revised to accommodate extreme situations where the lawyer has good reason to think that maintaining silence will cause serious undeserved harm to others. Further concludes that lawyers should not fear censure for coming forward in such situations. Cites Opinion 5.05. Morawetz, *Confidentiality and Common Sense: Insights From Philosophy, 48 San Diego L. Rev. 357, 373 (2011).*

Journal 2010 Discusses issues arising from the enactment of legislation by North Dakota involving a minor's reproductive rights. Explores ethical principles that govern physician's actions within the context of reproductive health. Concludes that, while a patient's expectation of confidentiality with a physician is critical, competing values come into play when the patient is a minor and parental involvement may be important. Provides practical guidance to address issues in this context. Quotes Opinions 2.01, 2.015, 5.055, 8.08, 8.115, 9.12, 10.01, 10.015, and 10.05. Cites Opinion 5.05, 5.055, 8.08, 8.11, 8.115, 9.12, and 10.05. Haas, *"Doctor, I'm Pregnant and Fifteen—I Can't Tell My Parents—Please Help Me": Minor Consent, Reproductive Rights, and Ethical Principles for Physicians, 86 N.D. L. Rev. 63, 70, 73, 75-78, 82, 84, 86-88, (2010).*

Journal 2010 Examines published resources within the medical and legal fields that focus on confidentiality and evaluates those resources to determine if they help clarify confidentiality issues. Further, discusses differences between these professions that may be hindrances when serving the same patient or client. Concludes that, while both professions guard against disclosure of patient/client communications, they also allow for disclosure in certain instances such as imminent death, harm, or injury. References Principle IV and cites Opinions 2.02, 2.23, 2.24, and 5.05. Johns, *Multidisciplinary Practice and Ethics Part II—Lawyers, Doctors, and Confidentiality, 6 NAELA J. 55, 57-65, 68 (2010).*

Journal 2010 Discusses the effects of using deidentified health information on privacy and considers the dangers of nonconsensual use of health information. Concludes deidentification of health information is a necessary though insufficient protection of privacy, and further research and regulations should be developed to demonstrate respect for individuals without unduly burdening research. Quotes Principle IV and Opinions 5.05 and 7.025. Rothstein, *Is Deidentification Sufficient to Protect Health Privacy in Research?* 10 Am. J. Bioethics 3, 5 (Sept. 2010).

Journal 2010 Explores how participation in online social networks may blur boundaries between personal and professional relationships for health care professionals and how such risks may be mitigated by use of network privacy and security settings. Suggests that health care institutions are likely to institute online social-networking policies for employees. Quotes Opinions 5.026, 5.027, 5.045, 5.046, 5.05, 5.059, 5.0591, 8.14, 9.08, and 9.123. Cites Opinions 5.026, 9.031, and 9.12. Terry, *Physicians and Patients Who "Friend" or "Tweet": Constructing a Legal Framework for Social Networking in a Highly Regulated Domain*, 43 Ind. L. Rev. 285, 314-16, 319, 334-36, 338 (2010).

Journal 2010 Examines legislative and judicial efforts to address hazards posed by drivers' use of cell phones and other communication technology with distracted driver laws. Concludes that the scope of a phone search under the automobile exception to verify suspected violations of such laws is limited to verifying when a message was sent or received. Cites Opinion 5.05. Williams, *The Trouble With Texting: The Future of Searches Under the Automobile Exception After Arizona v. Gant*, 4 Charleston L. Rev. 919, 929 (2010).

Journal 2009 Explains that, while the Restatement (Third) of Torts recognizes a mental health therapist's duty to warn foreseeable victims of risks posed by a patient, it takes no position regarding such a duty for physicians in other settings (eg, infectious diseases). Concludes while there is a basis to question this distinction, the issue is sufficiently complex and the considerations sufficiently balanced that the Restatement's position is justifiable. Cites Principles of Medical Ethics § 9 (1957) [now Opinion 5.05]. Cardi, *A Pluralistic Analysis of the Therapist/Physician Duty to Warn Third Parties*, 44 Wake Forest L. Rev. 877, 881 (2009).

Journal 2009 Discusses state open records statutes and the treatment of concealed carry permit records. Concludes concealed carry permit records should be disclosed to the public in order to achieve greater consistency in open records laws and to increase public safety. Quotes Opinion 5.05. Swanson, *The Right to Know: An Approach to Gun Licenses and Public Access to Government Records*, 56 UCLA L. Rev. 1579, 1594 (2009).

Journal 2009 Discusses the tension between duties of confidentiality and to protect third parties owed by mental health professionals to their patients and the public. Analyzes current Illinois law regarding these duties. Argues because Illinois law causes confusion regarding a professional's duty to disclose, inappropriately restricts the protected class, and leads to unnecessary breaches of confidentiality, clarification is necessary. Quotes Preamble and Opinion 5.05. Wood, *Protective Privilege Versus Public Peril: How Illinois Has Failed to Balance Patient Confidentiality With the Mental Health Professional's Duty to Protect the Public*, 29 N. Ill. U. L. Rev. 571, 581, 598 (2009).

Journal 2008 Discusses ex parte interviews with a treating physician in discovery before and after the HIPAA Privacy Rule and the issues facing physicians contacted for such interviews. Concludes courts and attorneys should work together to allow for efficient discovery while protecting physicians. Quotes Principles IV and VIII and Opinions 5.05 and 10.01. Burnette & Morning, *HIPAA and Ex Parte Interviews—the Beginning of the End?* 1 J. Health & Life Sci. L. 73, 100-01 (2008).

Journal 2008 Examines law governing the duty to warn a threatened individual. Proposes new criteria by which to evaluate whether a statement triggers a duty to warn, incorporating linguistic imperatives and professional standards. Quotes Opinion 5.05. Harmon, *Back from Wonderland: A Linguistic Approach to Duties Arising From Threats of Physical Violence*, 37 Cap. U. L. Rev. 27, 33 (2008).

Journal 2008 Argues a general physician-patient privilege is needed in West Virginia and outlines the manner in which the privilege could be adopted. Concludes that the privilege will allow physicians to maintain their fiduciary role, foster open communication between patient and physician, and encourage patients to freely seek medical treatment. Quotes Principle IV and Opinion 5.05. Johnson, *"I Will Not Divulge": How to Resolve the "Mass of Legal Confusion" Surrounding the Physician-Patient Relationship in West Virginia*, 110 W. Va. L. Rev. 1231, 1247 (2008).

Journal 2008 Examines prescription privacy and the sale of deidentified medical records. Suggests HIPAA must modernize its deidentification requirements to protect patient privacy amid technological advances in data mining. Quotes Opinion 5.05. Klocke, *Prescription Records for Sale: Privacy and Free Speech Issues Arising From the Sale of De-identified Medical Data*, 44 *Idaho L. Rev. 511, 518 (2008).*

Journal 2008 Examines the practicability and constitutionality of restrictions on drivers' licensing for the elderly. Concludes there are high-risk drivers in all age groups and licensing restrictions must not unfairly limit autonomy for the elderly. Cites Opinion 5.05. Mikel, *Drivers' Licenses and Age Limits: Imposition of Driving Restrictions on Elderly Drivers*, 9 *Marq. Elder's Advisor 359, 379 (2008).*

Journal 2008 Discusses privacy and disability laws concerning the mental health of college students. Concludes law and policy should be changed to promote student well-being while limiting liability for institutions. References Opinion 5.05. Pena, *Reevaluating Privacy and Disability Laws in the Wake of the Virginia Tech Tragedy: Considerations for Administrators and Lawmakers*, 87 *N. C. L. Rev. 305, 334 (2008).*

Journal 2008 Discusses student privacy and campus safety with respect to Family Education Rights and Privacy Act (FERPA) obligations and HIPAA regulations. Argues campus professionals should work together to effectively communicate pertinent student information to promote campus safety. Quotes Opinion 5.05 as it read before 2007 revision. Tribbensee, *Privacy and Confidentiality: Balancing Student Rights and Campus Safety*, 34 *J. C. & U. L. 393, 406-07 (2008).*

Journal 2007 Analyzes scientific, ethical, and legal issues raised in the exhumation and genetic analysis of historical figures. Concludes that biohistorical review boards should be created to generate guidelines for such research. Quotes Preamble and Opinion 2.08. Cites Opinions 2.079, 2.105, 5.05, 5.051, 5.075, 8.03, 8.031, 9.095, and 9.10. Paradise & Andrews, *Tales From the Crypt: Scientific, Ethical, and Legal Considerations for Biohistorical Analysis of Deceased Historical Figures*, 26 *Temp. J. Sci. Tech. & Envtl. L. 223, 287-88 (2007).*

Journal 2007 Examines relative vs absolute rights to confidentiality for military detainees considering the utilitarian need to protect the public at large. Concludes that evolving standards may favor individual rights to confidentiality, even from a utilitarian perspective. Quotes Opinions 1.02 and 5.05. References Principle III. Wynia, *Breaching Confidentiality to Protect the Public: Evolving Standards of Medical Confidentiality for Military Detainees*, 7 *Am. J. Bioethics, 1, 2 (Aug. 2007).*

Journal 2006 Analyzes the ethical and legal problems of confidentiality which arise in the context of genetic testing. Concludes that the disclosure of a patient's genetic disease to others is only allowable when the patient is a minor and the family has a right to know. Quotes Principle IV and References Principle 9 (1957) [now Principle IV and Opinion 5.05]. Denbo, *What Your Genes Know Affects Them: Should Patient Confidentiality Prevent Disclosure of Genetic Test Results to a Patient's Biological Relatives?* 43 *Am. Bus. L. J. 561, 572, 577 (2006).*

Journal 2006 Evaluates the influence that Justice Blackmun's experience at the Mayo Clinic had on his opinions related to medicine. Concludes that Blackmun's experience had less of an impact on his opinions than is traditionally assumed. Quotes Principle 9 (1957) [now Principle IV and Opinion 5.05]. Hunter, *Justice Blackmun, Abortion, and the Myth of Medical Independence*, 72 *Brooklyn L. Rev. 147, 190-91 (2006).*

Journal 2006 Examines a mental health professional's competing duties of confidentiality and reporting a patient's threats of violence. Suggests new legislation should clarify duty to report a threat. Quotes Preamble and Principles III, IV, and VIII. Cites Opinion 5.05. Mossman, *Critique of Pure Risk Assessment or, Kant Meets Tarasoff*, 75 *U. Cin. L. Rev. 523, 579 (2006).*

Journal 2006 Analyzes the privacy risks associated with introducing a system of electronic medical records. Concludes that cost and confidentiality concerns mandate that security must be built into the initial system. Cites Ch. I, Art. I, Sec. 2 (May 1847) [now Principle IV and Opinion 5.05]. Rothstein & Talbott, *Compelled Disclosure of Health Information: Protecting Against the Greatest Potential Threat to Privacy*, 295 *JAMA 2882, 2883 (2006).*

Journal 2006 Examines situations where physician-patient confidentiality may be breached to prevent violations of human rights. Suggests that new laws should be enacted to specify when a physician may testify about a violation of human rights. Quotes Principle IV and Opinion 5.05. Weissbrodt & Wilson, *Piercing the Confidentiality Veil: Physician Testimony in International Criminal Trials Against Perpetrators of Torture*, 15 *Minn. J. Int'l L. 43, 68, 68-69 (2006).*

Journal 2005 Reviews the lack of confidentiality in peer-run self-help programs. Concludes that new laws need to be enacted to protect participant confidentiality in such programs. References Opinion 5.05. Coleman, *Privilege and Confidentiality in 12-Step Self-Help Programs*, 26 J. Legal Med. 435, 441 (2005).

Journal 2005 Examines the argument that data privacy regulations violate the First Amendment. Concludes that neither privacy rights nor First Amendment free speech rights must be sacrificed in protecting data, and that balancing the two is a policy rather than a constitutional concern. Quotes Opinion 5.05. Richards, *Reconciling Data Privacy and the First Amendment*, 52 UCLA L. Rev. 1149, 1195 (2005).

Journal 2004 Argues that the intent of Congress to protect health information is clearly signaled in the language of HIPAA. Concludes that, despite this fact, a federal physician-patient privilege should be recognized, to ensure that gaps in the scope of available protection may be addressed. Quotes Opinion 5.05. Ruebner & Reis, *Hippocrates to HIPAA: A Foundation for a Federal Physician-Patient Privilege*, 77 Temp. L. Rev. 505, 572 (2004).

Journal 2004 Discusses the need for a greater understanding of and openness to religious values by the professions. Concludes that, although such openness is important, problems may arise when professional values and religious values clash. Quotes Opinion 5.05. References Principle v. Sullivan, *Naked Fitzies and Iron Cages: Individual Values, Professional Virtues, and the Struggle for Public Space*, 78 Tul. L. Rev. 1687, 1702, 1703 (2004).

Journal 2004 Argues that the privacy model rather than the property model is the most appropriate way to protect an individual's interest in genetic information. Concludes that privacy interests must nevertheless be balanced against other societal factors. References Principle IV and Opinion 5.05. Suter, *Disentangling Privacy From Property: Toward a Deeper Understanding of Genetic Privacy*, 72 Geo. Wash. L. Rev. 737, 787 (2004).

Journal 2003 Argues the legal profession must become meaningfully involved in efforts to address the causes and effects of domestic violence. Concludes that lawyers must do more in an effort to protect the interests of clients. Quotes Opinion 5.05. Burman, *Lawyers and Domestic Violence: Raising the Standard of Practice*, 9 Mich. J. Gender & L. 207, 254 (2003).

Journal 2003 Highlights HIPAA privacy issues that need to be monitored and have yet to be resolved. Concludes that HIPAA poses many challenges and it remains unclear whether HIPAA will increase privacy protection. Cites Opinions 5.05, 5.055, 5.057, 5.06, 5.07, 5.075, 5.08, and 5.09. Kutzko, Boyer, Thoman, & Scott, *HIPAA in Real Time: Practical Implications of the Federal Privacy Rule*, 51 Drake L. Rev. 403, 408 (2003).

Journal 2003 Considers the legal, medical, and ethical issues of physician-patient confidentiality in disclosure of paternity. Concludes that a balancing test should be applied to making determinations regarding disclosure of paternity. Quotes Principles I, IV, and V and Opinions 1.02, 5.055, and 10.01. Cites Principle II and Opinion 5.05. Richards & Wolf, *Medical Confidentiality and Disclosure of Paternity*, 48 S. D. L. Rev. 409, 411, 412, 413 (2003).

Journal 2003 Discusses legal principles governing electronic personal information and other digital media. Concludes that biometric security methods will become the standard for protecting private information. Quotes Opinion 5.05. Yang & Gorman, *What's Yours Is Mine: Protection and Security in a Digital World*, 36 Md. B. J. 24, 28-29 (Nov./Dec. 2003).

Journal 2002 Discusses issues regarding regulation of elderly drivers. Concludes that mandating physicians to report unfit elderly patients will protect the public and help resolve ethical and legal dilemmas. Quotes Opinions 1.02, 2.24, 5.05, and 10.01. Kane, *Driving Into the Sunset: A Proposal for Mandatory Reporting to the DMV by Physicians Treating Unsafe Elderly Drivers*, 25 U. Haw. L. Rev. 59, 59, 61, 62, 67, 69, 82, 83 (2002).

Journal 2002 Discusses legal and medical policies that protect confidentiality in the physician-patient relationship. Concludes that reducing the current level of privacy protection would jeopardize health care. Quotes Preamble and Opinions 2.136, 5.05, and 10.01. References Principles VIII and IX. Sciarrino, *Ferguson v. City of Charleston: "The Doctor Will See You Now, Be Sure to Bring Your Privacy Rights in With You!"* 12 Temp. Pol. & Civ. Rts. L. Rev. 197, 213, 215, 220, 221, 222 (2002).

Journal 2002 Discusses the lapse of Fourth Amendment protection in the collection of third-party records by the government. Concludes that a new paradigm is needed for regulating government collection of third-party information. Quotes Opinion 5.05. Solove, *Digital Dossiers and the Dissipation of Fourth Amendment Privacy, 75 S. Cal. L. Rev. 1083, 1155 (2002).*

Journal 2002 Considers issues of health information privacy in the electronic age. Concludes that protections afforded by the HIPAA privacy rules and common law will be increasingly important. Quotes Opinion 5.05. Winn, *Confidentiality in Cyberspace: The HIPAA Privacy Rules and the Common Law, 33 Rutgers L. J. 617, 622 (2002).*

Journal 2001 Examines ethical issues surrounding physician disclosure of information to attorneys. Observes that attorneys do not have an absolute right to interfere with the physician-patient relationship. Concludes that attorneys' efforts to obtain information may give rise to lawsuits for aiding and abetting the physician's breach of a fiduciary duty to preserve confidentiality. Quotes Opinion 5.05. Freeman, *Dealing With Doctors, 13 S. C. Law 11, 11 (July/Aug. 2001).*

Journal 2001 Explores the Uniform Mediation Act (UMA). Describes how certain exceptions to confidentiality in mediation arise from an inability to balance the means of confidentiality and the ends of self-determination. Concludes that, under the UMA, confidentiality does not promote self-determination. Quotes Opinion 5.05. Hughes, *The Uniform Mediation Act: To the Spoiled Go the Privileges, 85 Marq. L. Rev. 9, 26 (2001).*

Journal 2001 Compares the American system of patient confidentiality to the Austrian system. Discusses the debate between patients' rights and public safety. Concludes that the duty to warn third parties of dangerous patients should be discretionary instead of mandatory, except in cases of HIV seropositivity, which should involve mandatory disclosure to public health officials. Quotes Opinions 2.23, 5.05, and 5.06. Kenworthy, *The Austrian Psychotherapy Act: No Legal Duty to Warn, 11 Ind. Int'l & Comp. L. Rev. 469, 480-81, 485, 490, 496 (2001).*

Journal 2001 Considers whether or not it is ethical for physicians to prescribe, and pharmacists to dispense, syringes for use by injection drug users. Concludes that ethical considerations suggest such actions are permissible but not obligatory. Quotes Principle III and Opinion 1.02. References Opinion 5.05. Lazzarini, *An Analysis of Ethical Issues in Prescribing and Dispensing Syringes to Injection Drug Users, 11 Health Matrix 85, 107, 119 (2001).*

Journal 2001 Focuses on the case of *Weld v. CVS Pharmacy, Inc.* Examines whether an individual's privacy is invaded when pharmacies disclose prescription information about customers to aid other private organizations with implementation of marketing activities. Quotes Opinion 5.05. Schawbel, *Are You Taking Any Prescription Medication? A Case Comment on Weld v. CVS Pharmacy, Inc., 35 New Eng. L. Rev. 909, 957 (2001).*

Journal 2001 Evaluates current forms of cybermedicine and Internet resources that support it. Explores patient and regulatory concerns, including privacy issues, insurance reimbursement problems, licensure, and liability, which may thwart the growth of cybermedicine. Concludes that cybermedicine may facilitate delivery of cost-effective, quality medical care. Quotes Opinions 5.05, 6.02, and 6.03. Scott, *Cybermedicine and Virtual Pharmacies, 103 W. Va. L. Rev. 407, 441, 451 (2001).*

Journal 2001 Discusses the history of fetal abuse prosecution and the Medical University of South Carolina's Interagency Policy of Management of Substance Abuse During Pregnancy. Concludes that, although the *Ferguson v. City of Charleston* decision will continue to allow pregnant drug users to access prenatal care, it leaves open questions regarding the future of fetal abuse prosecutions. Quotes Opinion 5.05. Toll, *For My Doctor's Eyes Only: Ferguson v. City of Charleston, 33 Loy. U. Chi. L. J. 267, 305 (2001).*

Journal 2000 Explores confidentiality and discusses the legal standards pertaining to attorneys, physicians, and social workers. Concludes that the concept of confidentiality is the backbone of each profession and without privileged communications such professions would fail the American public. Quotes Opinion 5.05. Clark, *Confidential Communications in a Professional Context: Attorney, Physician, and Social Worker, 24 J. Legal Prof. 79, 92 (2000).*

Journal 2000 Describes possible solutions designed to improve postapproval regulation of prescription drugs so that fewer patients will suffer from adverse drug reactions. Concludes that the FDA along with physicians and clinical researchers should rethink the existing approach to monitoring of unexpected side effects. Quotes Principle V and Opinion 9.032. Cites Opinion 5.05. Noah, *Adverse Drug Reactions: Harnessing Experimental Data to Promote Patient Welfare, 49 Cath. U. L. Rev. 449, 477, 497-98 (2000).*

Journal 2000 Addresses the philosophical conflict between free speech and privacy. Examines the commercial speech doctrine and discusses the constitutional and human rights implications of use of private sector data. Cites Opinion 5.05. Singleton, *Privacy Versus the First Amendment: A Skeptical Approach,* 11 Fordham Intell. Prop. Media & Ent. L. J. 97, 122 (2000).

Journal 2000 Defines and explores current and future applications of telemedicine. Considers issues of cost, quality, access, and regulation. Concludes that telemedicine holds tremendous promise for improving the US health care system. Quotes Opinions 5.05 and 5.07. Volkert, *Telemedicine: Rx for the Future of Health Care,* 6 Mich. Telecomm. & Tech. L. Rev. 147, 214, 225 (2000).

Journal 1999 Explores changes in technology and the resulting impact on privacy of medical information. Observes that current federal and state laws inadequately protect medical information privacy and suggests that Congress needs to enact legislation addressing this issue. Quotes Opinion 5.05. References Opinions 7.02 and 7.05. Carter, *Health Information Privacy: Can Congress Protect Confidential Medical Information in the "Information Age"?* 25 Wm. Mitchell L. Rev. 223, 236, 273 (1999).

Journal 1999 Discusses the "ever-expanding" disclosure of confidential medical record information regarding patients. Emphasizes organizational problems relating to access and security in medical record systems. Argues in favor of stronger regulations limiting access to and use of information. Quotes Opinion 5.05. Hall, *Confidentiality as an Organizational Ethics Issue,* 10 J. Clinical Ethics 230, 232 (1999).

Journal 1999 Discusses the need for physicians to advocate on behalf of patients' rights in the context of health care delivery. Evaluates the nature and scope of the physician's role as advocate, noting that physicians cannot be expected to engage in attorney-like advocacy. Quotes Principles IV and VI, Fundamental Elements (2), (4), and (6) [now Opinion 10.01], Patient Responsibilities 5 [now Opinion 10.02], and Opinions 2.03, 2.07, 2.09, 2.16, 2.19, 3.06, 4.01, 4.04, 6.01, 7.02, 8.02, 8.03, 8.13, 8.132, 9.06, 9.07, and 9.131. Cites Opinions 5.05, 5.09, 7.01, 8.135, and 9.02. Sage, *Physicians as Advocates,* 35 Hous. L. Rev. 1529, 1537, 1541, 1542, 1552-53, 1554, 1556, 1557, 1559, 1561-62, 1564, 1571, 1574, 1576, 1580 (1999).

Journal 1999 Explores the increased use of physician-patient communication through e-mail. Analyzes current laws regarding medical privacy. Suggests that patients' communications to their physicians are part of their medical record and should be given the same protections. Quotes Opinions 5.05 and 5.07. Cites Opinions 5.04 and 5.06. Spielberg, *Online Without a Net: Physician-Patient Communication by Electronic Mail,* 25 Am. J. Law & Med. 267, 284-85 (1999).

Journal 1999 Explores Model Rules of Professional Conduct focusing on the attorney-client relationship. Compares confidentiality provisions in the Model Rules with the rules of confidentiality governing the medical profession. Observes that existing confidentiality rules are incomplete and ambiguous. Concludes that one remedy is to embrace a discretionary confidentiality rule. Quotes Opinion 5.05. Cites Principle IV and Opinion 5.07. Zer-Gutman, *Revising the Ethical Rules of Attorney-Client Confidentiality: Towards a New Discretionary Rule,* 45 Loy. L. Rev. 669, 683-84, 699, 709, 718 (1999).

Journal 1998 Describes the special nature of confidentiality in the relationship between the psychotherapist and patient. States that not many breach of confidentiality cases involve psychotherapists. Concludes that patients and psychotherapists must better understand their rights and responsibilities in this context. Quotes Opinion 5.05. Cites Opinions 5.06, 5.07, 5.08, and 5.09. Grabois, *The Liability of Psychotherapists for Breach of Confidentiality,* 12 J. Law & Health 39, 53-54 (1998).

Journal 1998 Explains risks involved with the use of electronic medical records. States that patients need to be aware of who has access to their medical records. Concludes that health care providers should equalize the risks and benefits related to the use of electronic medical records. Cites Opinion 5.05. References Opinion 5.07. Jurevic, *When Technology and Health Care Collide: Issues With Electronic Medical Records and Electronic Mail,* 66 UMKC L. Rev. 809, 819-20 (1998).

Journal 1998 Discusses issues of patient consent regarding disclosure of medical information. Points out that recent changes in the health care system have presented medical record privacy concerns. Discloses findings of a study regarding hospital consent forms and calls for more research to be conducted. Cites Principle IV and Opinion 5.05. Merz, Sankar, & Yoo, *Hospital Consent for Disclosure of Medical Records,* 26 J. Law Med. & Ethics 241, 248 (1998).

Journal 1998 Points out that most victims of elder abuse are socially isolated and thus few incidents of elder abuse are reported to authorities. Argues that current protections against elder abuse are inadequate. Suggests that the legal system and health professionals can make a difference in reducing elder abuse. Quotes Opinion 5.05. References Opinion 2.02. Moskowitz, *Saving Granny From the Wolf: Elder Abuse and Neglect—The Legal Framework*, 31 Conn. L. Rev. 77, 116, 120, 121, 122 (1998).

Journal 1998 Discusses issues of privacy concerning the collection and use of computerized pharmacy records by pharmaceutical companies. Concludes that federal legislation is needed to protect the privacy of prescription information. Quotes Opinion 5.05. Mowery, *A Patient's Right of Privacy in Computerized Pharmacy Records*, 66 U. Cin. L. Rev. 697, 717 (1998).

Journal 1998 Discusses the ramifications of physician license revocation for failing to pay child support. Points out that patients stand to lose access to trusted physicians and confidence in the health care system. Concludes that children need the most protection and that patients will have an easier time finding another physician than children will have finding another means for support. Quotes Opinion 5.05. Cites Opinions 9.02 and 9.06. Noyes, *Higher Penalties for Failing to Pay Child Support: A Look at Medical License Revocation*, 19 J. Legal Med. 127, 138 (1998).

Journal 1998 Explores the role of pharmacy benefits managers. Discusses the impact of pharmacy benefits managers on patients, consumers, and the medical field. Analyzes potential privacy problems stemming from pharmacy benefits managers. Cites Opinion 5.05. Rosoff, *The Changing Face of Pharmacy Benefits Management: Information Technology Pursues a Grand Mission*, 42 St. Louis U. L. J. 1, 25-26 (1998).

Journal 1998 Examines the use of e-mail in the physician-patient relationship. Focuses on privacy concerns stemming from the use of e-mail in the medical context. Suggests that physicians should discuss the implications of communicating through e-mail with their patients and should obtain informed consent prior to communicating in this manner. Cites Opinions 5.04, 5.05, 5.057, 5.07, 5.075, and 5.08. Spielberg, *On Call and Online: Sociohistorical, Legal, and Ethical Implications of E-mail for the Patient-Physician Relationship*, 280 JAMA 1353, 1356 (1998).

Journal 1998 Explores the increased use and benefits of telemedicine. Points out that there is inadequate protection of privacy rights regarding electronic medical information. Concludes that federal law does not uniformly address medical record privacy and that Missouri law lacks adequate specificity. Quotes Principle IV. References Opinion 5.05. Young, *Telemedicine: Patient Privacy Rights of Electronic Medical Records*, 66 UMKC L. Rev. 921, 926 (1998).

Journal 1997 Compares past ethical opinions to current opinions and notes the differences. Comments on the forces that have changed medical ethics through the years. Notes differing theories on the future course of medical ethics. Quotes Fundamental Elements (Preamble) and Opinions 5.05, 5.057, 7.01, 8.12, 9.12, and 9.131. Cites Fundamental Elements (5) and Opinions 8.115 and 8.13. Buchanan, *Medical Ethics at the Millennium: A Brief Retrospective*, 26 Colo. Law. 141, 142, 143, 144, 145 (1997).

Journal 1997 Describes the DNA profile and its use in the scientific community. Examines common misconceptions about the DNA profile. Considers implication of the DNA profile as a unique identifier in the context of community health information networks. Quotes Principle 9 (1957) [now Opinion 5.05]. Dahm, *Using DNA Profile as the Unique Patient Identifier in the Community Health Information Network: Legal Implications*, 15 J. Marshall J. Computer & Info. L. 227, 266, 275 (1997).

Journal 1997 Considers how breast cancer has given rise to numerous medical malpractice lawsuits. Discusses trial techniques and strategies for litigating these types of claims. Quotes Opinions 5.05 and 5.06. Hillerich, Ellerin, & Frieder, *Selecting and Presenting a Failure to Diagnose Breast Cancer Case*, 20 Am. J. Trial Advoc. 253, 271 (1996-97).

Journal 1997 Considers principles of confidentiality in the physician-patient relationship. Notes the current trend emphasizing public reporting obligations of physicians to protect members of society. Emphasizes need for balance between patient rights and societal interests. Quotes Principle IV and Opinion 5.05. References Preamble. Jozefowicz, *The Case Against Having Professional Privilege in the Physician-Patient Relationship*, 16 Med. & L. 385, 386-87, 391 (1997).

Journal 1997 Suggests that ex parte conferences between treating physicians and opposing counsel undermine the physician-patient relationship. Notes that there are no significant benefits within the fact-finding process that justify the conflicts of interest created. Concludes that ex parte conferences are unnecessary. Quotes Principle IV and Opinion 5.05. Kassel, *Counterpoint . . . Defense Counsel's Ex Parte Communication With Plaintiff's Doctors: A Bad One-Sided Deal,* 9 S. C. Law. 42, 43 (Sept./Oct. 1997).

Journal 1997 Discusses the practice of ex parte communications between treating physicians and their patients' legal adversaries without informing the patient or obtaining consent. Examines harms that may occur in these situations. Argues that Oklahoma needs to prohibit treating physicians from communicating ex parte with their patients' legal adversaries. Quotes Opinions 5.05, 5.07, 5.08, 8.02, 8.03, and 9.07. Cites Opinion 7.02. McNaughton & McNaughton, *Divided Loyalty: The Dilemma of the Treating Physician Advocate,* 22 Okla. City U. L. Rev. 1051, 1052, 1054, 1056, 1058, 1059, 1062 (1997).

Journal 1997 Considers Connecticut AIDS statute, which relates to testing and confidentiality of patient medical information. Discusses statutory construction of provisions of this law by the Connecticut Supreme Court in *Doe v. Marselle.* Quotes Opinion 5.05. Note, *A Case Study of New Textualism in State Courts: Doe v. Marselle and the Confidentiality of HIV-Related Information,* 30 Conn. L. Rev. 295, 297 (1997).

Journal 1997 Considers whether the physician-patient privilege should be extended to protect communications to alternative health practitioners. Suggests that these practitioners treat and diagnose patients within the meaning of the privilege. Advocates an extension of the privilege to recognize the importance of confidentiality. Quotes Opinion 5.05. Note, *Healer-Patient Privilege: Extending the Physician-Patient Privilege to Alternative Health Practitioners in California,* 48 Hastings L. J. 633, 657 (1997).

Journal 1996 Explains the benefits of high-tech access to patient information by pharmacists. Considers related issues of patient confidentiality. Advocates a pharmacist-patient privilege. Quotes Opinion 5.05. Berger, *Patient Confidentiality in a High Tech World,* 5 J. Pharmacy & L., 139, 141 (1996).

Journal 1996 Suggests that attorneys representing HIV-infected and sexually active adolescents face an ethical conflict between their duty of client confidentiality and the duty to protect third parties. Notes that attorneys failing to warn third parties may face liability. Concludes that clients should be informed of potential limitations on the right to confidentiality. Quotes Opinion 5.05. Katner, *The Ethical Dilemma Awaiting Counsel Who Represent Adolescents With HIV/AIDS: Criminal Law and Tort Suits Pressure Counsel to Breach the Confidentiality of the Clients' Medical Status,* 70 Tul. L. Rev. 2311, 2341 (1996).

Journal 1996 Discusses sexual abuse litigation in which accusers have recovered memories of molestation in psychotherapy sessions. Observes that, to successfully defend against such claims, it is necessary for the accused to have access to the clinical record. Posits that confidentiality problems can be eliminated with in camera record inspections. References Principle IV and Opinion 5.05. Loftus, Paddock, & Guernsey, *Patient-Psychotherapist Privilege: Access to Clinical Records in the Tangled Web of Repressed Memory Litigation,* 30 U. Rich L. Rev. 109, 127 (1996).

Journal 1996 Reviews two Washington State Supreme Court decisions in which subsequent treating physicians testified against their patients and on behalf of defendant physicians in malpractice litigation. Observes that these decisions erode the physician-patient privilege. Posits that the decisions are inconsistent with current medical ethics and proposes a statutory enactment as a solution. Quotes Opinion 5.05. Cites Principle 9 (1957) [now Principle IV]. Oppenheim, *Physicians as Experts Against Their Own Patients? What Happened to the Privilege?* 63 Def. Couns. J. 254, 257, 261 (1996).

Journal 1996 Considers prearraignment forensic evaluations. Notes the prohibition against use of such evaluations. Examines underlying ethical precepts. Observes that principles of beneficence are misapplied to forensic psychiatry in this context. Advocates a new ethical framework. Quotes Preamble. References Principle IV and Opinion 5.05. Ornish, Mills, & Ornish, *Prearraignment Forensic Evaluations: Toward a New Policy,* 24 Bull. Am. Acad. Psychiatry Law 453, 454, 469 (1996).

Journal 1996 Examines the psychiatrist-patient duty of confidentiality. Notes that Principles of Medical Ethics prohibit the disclosure of patient confidences and medical records. Observes that exceptions to this prohibition exist when required by law or to protect the community. Quotes Principle 9 (1957) [now Principle IV and Opinion 5.05]. Sadoff, *Ethical Obligations for the Psychiatrist: Confidentiality, Privilege, and Privacy in Psychiatric Treatment,* 29 Loy. L. A. L. Rev. 1709, 1710, 1711 (1996).

Journal 1995 Addresses presidential disability, its past impact on American government, and possible solutions to potential problems. Proposes enhancement of the role of the President's physician. Quotes Opinion 8.03. Cites Opinions 5.04 and 5.05. Abrams, *The Vulnerable President and the Twenty-Fifth Amendment, With Observations on Guidelines, a Health Commission, and the Role of the President's Physician, 30 Wake Forest L. Rev. 453, 466, 471 (1995).*

Journal 1995 Discusses the belief of health care providers that they have an ethical obligation to warn the partners of HIV-positive patients. Examines both the scope of a Massachusetts statute that prevents providers from releasing HIV test results of patients and possible defenses that providers may assert. Quotes Principle IV and Opinion 5.05. Friedland, *HIV Confidentiality and the Right to Warn—The Health Care Provider's Dilemma, 80 Mass. L. Rev. 3, 4 (March 1995).*

Journal 1995 Considers how the use of health care identification cards and medical record databases would threaten privacy rights. Concludes that federal legislation should be enacted to protect health care record privacy and prevent misuse of health care identification cards. Quotes Opinion 5.05. Minor, *Identity Cards and Databases in Health Care: The Need for Federal Privacy Protections, 28 Colum. J. L. & Soc. Probs. 253, 279 (1995).*

Journal 1995 Examines the impact of health care reform on physician-patient relationships. Discusses how reform may threaten the physician's fiduciary duty of loyalty by forcing physicians to make rationing decisions and giving physicians financial incentives to limit use of health care resources. Quotes Fundamental Elements (5) [now Opinion 10.0]. Cites Opinion 5.05. Orentlicher, *Health Care Reform and the Patient-Physician Relationship, 5 Health Matrix 141, 143, 148 (1995).*

Journal 1995 Analyzes the secular approach to the duty to treat HIV-infected individuals and the duty to warn those who are sexual partners of, or who share needles with, people infected with HIV. Observes that the secular approach leaves these issues unresolved but indicates that Jewish law compels physicians both to treat and to warn. Quotes Opinions 5.05 and 9.131. Shorr, *AIDS, Judaism, and the Limits of the Secular Society, 20 Second Opinion 23, 24, 27 (1995).*

Journal 1994 Considers whether an exception should be made to physician-patient confidentiality that would allow a physician to reveal parental medical history to a child. Concludes that such an exception would not completely erode physician-patient confidentiality. Quotes Principle IV, Fundamental Elements (4), and Opinion 5.05. Cites Principle I and Fundamental Elements (1). Friedland, *Physician-Patient Confidentiality: Time to Re-Examine a Venerable Concept in Light of Contemporary Society and Advances in Medicine, 15 J. Legal Med. 249, 257, 264, 276 (1994).*

Journal 1994 Explores the ethical issues involved in a multidisciplinary team working with children in legal proceedings. Focuses on the relationships between professionals and the conflicts that arise regarding disclosure of confidential information and forced disclosure of nonprivileged information. Quotes Principles III and IV, Fundamental Elements (4), and Opinions 1.02 (1992) and 5.07 (1992) [now Opinion 5.05]. Cites Opinions 2.02. Glynn, *Multidisciplinary Representation of Children: Conflicts Over Disclosures of Client Communications, 27 J. Marshall L. Rev. 617, 625, 626, 630-32, 637, 639, 643 (1994).*

Journal 1994 Compares Texas law with Illinois law on the issue of ex parte communications between defense counsel and the patient/plaintiff's physician in civil litigation. Argues that preservation of the physician-patient relationship requires prohibition of such contact. Quotes Principles II and IV and Opinion 5.05. Comment, *From the Land of Lincoln a Healing Rule: Proposed Texas Rule of Civil Procedure Prohibiting Ex Parte Contact Between Defense Counsel and a Plaintiff's Treating Physician, 25 Tex. Tech L. Rev. 1081, 1081, 1082 (1994).*

Journal 1994 Considers how computerized medical records might threaten patient confidentiality. Explores proposed legislation for computerized records and the potential need for new legal standards in this area. Cites Opinion 5.05. Field, *Overview: Computerized Medical Records Create New Legal and Business Confidentiality Problems, 11 HealthSpan 3, 4 (1994).*

Journal 1993 Discusses family privacy rights and considers the meaning of justice, self-respect, and the fundamental principles of physician ethics. Concludes that physicians have an ethical duty to intervene in domestic violence so long as such intervention does not breach confidentiality or violate patient autonomy. Quotes Principle IV and Opinion 5.05. References Opinions 8.14 and 9.131. Jecker, *Privacy Beliefs and the Violent Family: Extending the Ethical Argument for Physician Intervention, 269 JAMA 776, 778, 779 (1993).*

Journal 1993 Evaluates the legal issues surrounding AIDS and HIV. Examines various aspects of the law that would be relevant to a medical or health care lawyer. Quotes Opinion 5.05. Skiver & Hickey, *AIDS: Legal Issues 1992, 19 Ohio No. Univ. L. Rev. 839, 860 (1993).*

Journal 1991 Discusses current law protecting confidential genetic information obtained in the workplace and presents several safeguard mechanisms. Analyzes the legal grounds upon which various parties may access this information. References Opinion 5.05. Andrews & Jaeger, *Confidentiality of Genetic Information in the Workplace, XVII Am. J. Law & Med. 75, 78 (1991).*

Journal 1991 Examines the problem of AIDS in this country and the risk of HIV transmission via sexual assault. Concludes that state laws requiring HIV testing for sex offenders are necessary to preserve the rights of victims of sexual assault. Quotes Opinion 5.05. McGuire, *AIDS and the Sexual Offender: The Epidemic Now Poses New Threats to the Victim and the Criminal Justice System, 96 Dickinson L. Rev. 95, 109, 110 (1991).*

Journal 1991 Focuses on the case *Crist v. Moffatt,* where a court permitted ex parte interview of a plaintiff's physician only after the plaintiff signed a written authorization. Concludes that Crist was correctly decided, but warns against expanding the decision to the point of unduly restricting discovery. Quotes Opinion 5.05. Note, *Restricting Ex Parte Interviews With Nonparty Treating Physicians: Crist v. Moffatt, 69 No. Carolina L. Rev. 1381, 1391, 1392 (1991).*

Journal 1991 Discusses confidentiality with respect to a patient's HIV status. Notes how confidentiality may be lost in the hospital setting and emphasizes importance of heightened attention to this issue by institutional health care providers. Quotes Opinion 5.05. Obade, *Whisper Down the Lane: AIDS, Privacy, and the Hospital Grapevine, 2 J. Clinical Ethics 133, 133 (1991).*

Journal 1990 Discusses the legal and ethical considerations associated with genetic research, including recombinant DNA technology. Offers case examples illustrating issues raised by the application of this technology in the clinical setting. Quotes Opinion 5.05. Elsas, *A Clinical Approach to Legal and Ethical Problems in Human Genetics, 39 Emory L. J. 811, 816, 820 (1990).*

Journal 1990 Advocates physician liability for failure to warn third parties of the potential risk of being infected with HIV from the physician's patient. Concludes that there should be no liability for disclosure because public health concerns outweigh an individual patient's right to confidentiality. References Opinion 5.05. Note, *AIDS: Establishing a Physician's Duty to Warn, 21 Rutgers L. J. 645, 652 (1990).*

Journal 1989 Discusses the history of the physician-patient privilege up through changes implemented under the Ohio Tort Reform Act of 1987. Aspects of the physician-patient privilege that are most significantly affected by this Tort Reform Act are highlighted, with recommendations for further refinement of the privilege in Ohio. Quotes Principles II and IV and Opinion 5.05. Note, *The Ohio Physician-Patient Privilege: Modified, Revised, and Defined, 49 Ohio St. L. J. 1147, 1167 (1989).*

5.051 Confidentiality of Medical Information Postmortem

All medically related confidences disclosed by a patient to a physician and information contained within a deceased patient's medical record, including information entered postmortem, should be kept confidential to the greatest possible degree. However, the obligation to safeguard patient confidences is subject to certain exceptions that are ethically and legally justifiable because of overriding societal considerations (Opinion 5.05, "Confidentiality"). At their strongest, confidentiality protections after death would be equal to those in force during a patient's life. Thus, if information about a patient may be ethically disclosed during life, it likewise may be disclosed after the patient has died.

Disclosure of medical information postmortem for research and educational purposes is appropriate as long as confidentiality is maintained to the greatest possible degree by removing any individual identifiers. Otherwise, in determining whether to disclose identified information after the death of a patient, physicians should consider the following factors:

(1) The imminence of harm to identifiable individuals or the public health

(2) The potential benefit to at-risk individuals or the public health (eg, if a communicable or inherited disease is preventable or treatable)

(3) Any statement or directive made by the patient regarding postmortem disclosure

(4) The impact disclosure may have on the reputation of the deceased patient

(5) Personal gain for the physician that may unduly influence professional obligations of confidentiality

When a family member or other decision maker has given consent to an autopsy, physicians may disclose the results of the autopsy to the individual(s) who granted consent to the procedure. (IV)

Issued December 2000 based on the report "Confidentiality of Medical Information Postmortem," adopted June 2000. Updated December 2001 (*Arch Pathol Lab Med.* 2001;125:1189-1192).

Journal 2011 Examines current legal and ethical frameworks governing the return of a deceased research participant's individual research results to related family members, including Canadian, American, and French legislation. Concludes that there is a lack of international consensus and that additional ethical and professional guidelines are necessary. Quotes Opinion 5.051. Tasse, *The Return of Results of Deceased Research Participants*, 39 J. L. Med. & Ethics 621, 624-625 (2011).

Journal 2007 Analyzes scientific, ethical, and legal issues raised in the exhumation and genetic analysis of historical figures. Concludes that biohistorical review boards should be created to generate guidelines for such research. Quotes Preamble and Opinion 2.08. Cites Opinions 2.079, 2.105, 5.05, 5.051, 5.075, 8.03, 8.031, 9.095, and 9.10. Paradise & Andrews, *Tales From the Crypt: Scientific, Ethical, and Legal Considerations for Biohistorical Analysis of Deceased Historical Figures,* 26 Temp. J. Sci. Tech. & Envtl. L. 223, 287-88 (2007).

Journal 2004 Examines the requirements of the Privacy Rule regarding use and disclosure of a patient's identifiable health information in the context of research. Concludes that the Rule's burdensome administrative requirements may discourage research and thus outweigh any benefits for research subject autonomy. Quotes Principle VIII and Opinions 5.051, 8.031, and 10.015. Tovino, *The Use and Disclosure of Protected Health Information for Research Under the HIPAA Privacy Rule: Unrealized Patient Autonomy and Burdensome Government Regulation,* 49 S. D. L. Rev. 447, 496, 502 (2004).

Journal 2001 Analyzes postmortem patient confidentiality and proposes a framework for appropriate information disclosure. Concludes that, following death, decisions regarding disclosure of confidential information should be made on a case-by-case basis. Quotes Opinions 5.051 and 7.02. Berg, *Grave Secrets: Legal and Ethical Analysis of Postmortem Confidentiality,* 34 Conn. L. Rev. 81, 87, 117 (2001).

5.055 Confidential Care for Minors

Physicians who treat minors have an ethical duty to promote the autonomy of minor patients by involving them in the medical decision-making process to a degree commensurate with their abilities.

When minors request confidential services, physicians should encourage them to involve their parents. This includes making efforts to obtain the minors' reasons for not involving their parents and correcting misconceptions that may be motivating their objections.

Where the law does not require otherwise, physicians should permit a competent minor to consent to medical care and should not notify parents without the patient's consent. Depending on the seriousness of the decision, competence may be evaluated by physicians for most minors. When necessary, experts in adolescent medicine or child psychological development should be consulted. Use of the courts for competence determinations should be made only as a last resort.

When an immature minor requests contraceptive services, pregnancy-related care (including pregnancy testing, prenatal and postnatal care, and delivery services), or treatment for sexually transmitted disease, drug and alcohol abuse, or mental illness, physicians must recognize that requiring parental involvement may be counterproductive to the health of the patient. Physicians should encourage parental involvement in these situations. However, if the minor continues to object, his or her wishes ordinarily should be respected. If the physician is uncomfortable with providing services without parental involvement, and alternative confidential services are available, the minor may be referred to those services. In cases when the physician believes that without parental involvement and guidance the minor will face a serious health threat, and there is reason to believe that the parents will be helpful and understanding, disclosing the problem to the parents is ethically justified. When the physician does breach confidentiality to the parents, he or she must discuss the reasons for the breach with the minor prior to the disclosure.

For minors who are mature enough to be unaccompanied by their parents for their examination, confidentiality of information disclosed during an exam, interview, or in counseling should be maintained. Such information may be disclosed to parents when the patient consents to disclosure. Confidentiality may be justifiably breached in situations for which confidentiality for adults may be breached, according to Opinion 5.05, "Confidentiality." In addition, confidentiality for immature minors may be ethically breached when necessary to enable the parent to make an informed decision about treatment for the minor or when such a breach is necessary to avert serious harm to the minor. (IV)

Issued June 1994 based on the report "Confidential Care for Minors," adopted June 1992. Updated June 1996.

Journal 2010 Discusses issues arising from the enactment of legislation by North Dakota involving a minor's reproductive rights. Explores ethical principles that govern physician's actions within the context of reproductive health. Concludes that, while a patient's expectation of confidentiality with a physician is critical, competing values come into play when the patient is a minor and parental involvement may be important. Provides practical guidance to address issues in this context. Quotes Opinions 2.01, 2.015, 5.055, 8.08, 8.115, 9.12, 10.01, 10.015, and 10.05. Cites Opinion 5.05, 5.055, 8.08, 8.11, 8.115, 9.12, and 10.05. Haas, *"Doctor, I'm Pregnant and Fifteen—I Can't Tell My Parents—Please Help Me": Minor Consent, Reproductive Rights, and Ethical Principles for Physicians,* 86 N.D. L. Rev. 63, 70, 73, 75-78, 82, 84, 86-88, (2010).

Journal 2010 Discusses the importance of adolescent consent and confidentiality in providing quality health care to youth. Summarizes the relevant legal and ethical principles related to adolescent consent and confidentiality. Concludes the confidential care of minors is an integral component of routine adolescent care. Quotes Opinion 5.055. Berlan & Bravender, *Confidentiality, Consent and Caring for the Adolescent Patient,* 21 Current Opinion Pediatrics 450, 455 (2009).

Journal 2008 Discusses confidentiality rights of pediatric patients and the ethical considerations of physicians when establishing policies for managing patient confidentiality. Concludes that physicians must exercise discretion to protect the health interests of pediatric patients. Quotes Opinion 5.055. McGuire & Bruce, *Keeping Children's Secrets: Confidentiality in the Physician-Patient Relationship,* 8 Hous. J. Health L. & Pol'y 315, 332 (2008).

Journal 2006 Discusses the evolution of health law in Virginia. Concludes that the area of health law continues to expand, develop, and be refined. Cites Opinions 3.03, 3.08, 5.01, 5.015, 5.02, 5.04, 5.055, 6.02, 6.021, 6.03, 6.04, 7.03, 7.04, 7.05, 8.054, 8.08, 8.081, 8.085, 8.115, 8.12, 8.14, 8.145, 8.19, and 9.045. Guanzon, *Health Care Law, 41 U. Rich. L. Rev. 179, 199 (2006).*

Journal 2003 Highlights HIPAA privacy issues that need to be monitored and have yet to be resolved. Concludes that HIPAA poses many challenges and it remains unclear whether HIPAA will increase privacy protection. Cites Opinions 5.05, 5.055, 5.057, 5.06, 5.07, 5.075, 5.08, and 5.09. Kutzko, Boyer, Thoman, & Scott, *HIPAA in Real Time: Practical Implications of the Federal Privacy Rule, 51 Drake L. Rev. 403, 408 (2003).*

Journal 2003 Considers the legal, medical, and ethical issues of physician-patient confidentiality in disclosure of paternity. Concludes that a balancing test should be applied to making determinations regarding disclosure of paternity. Quotes Principles I, IV, and V and Opinions 1.02, 5.055, and 10.01. Cites Principle II and Opinion 5.05. Richards & Wolf, *Medical Confidentiality and Disclosure of Paternity, 48 S. D. L. Rev. 409, 411, 412, 413 (2003).*

The previous Opinion 5.057, "Confidentiality of HIV Status on Autopsy Reports," issued June 1994, was deleted in December 2004 and replaced by the current Opinion 5.051, "Confidentiality of Medical Information Postmortem."

5.059 Privacy in the Context of Health Care

In the context of health care, emphasis has been given to confidentiality, which is defined as information told in confidence or imparted in secret. However, physicians also should be mindful of patient privacy, which encompasses information that is concealed from others outside of the patient-physician relationship.

Physicians must seek to protect patient privacy in all of its forms, including (1) physical, which focuses on individuals and their personal spaces, (2) informational, which involves specific personal data, (3) decisional, which focuses on personal choices, and (4) associational, which refers to family or other intimate relations. Such respect for patient privacy is a fundamental expression of patient autonomy and is a prerequisite to building the trust that is at the core of the patient-physician relationship.

Privacy is not absolute, and must be balanced with the need for the efficient provision of medical care and the availability of resources. Physicians should be aware of and respect the special concerns of their patients regarding privacy. Patients should be informed of any significant infringement on their privacy of which they may otherwise be unaware. (I, IV)

Issued June 2002 based on the report "Privacy in the Context of Health Care," adopted December 2001.

Utah App. 2006 Following an automobile accident, plaintiff filed a personal injury suit against the driver. Plaintiff discovered that his treating physician had been subpoenaed by the driver's lawyer, had agreed to testify against plaintiff, and had engaged in ex parte communications with defense counsel. Plaintiff sued the physician. With apparent reference to Opinions 5.05 and 5.059 plaintiff relied in part on the AMA ethical principles to establish the standard of care. The court of appeals held that the physician could be liable for breach of the fiduciary duty of confidentiality as well as for intentional infliction of emotional distress. *Sorensen v. Barbuto, 143 P.3d 295, 299.*

Journal 2010 Explores how participation in online social networks may blur boundaries between personal and professional relationships for health care professionals and how such risks may be mitigated by use of network privacy and security settings. Suggests that health care institutions are likely to institute online social-networking policies for employees. Quotes Opinions 5.026, 5.027, 5.045, 5.046, 5.05, 5.059, 5.0591, 8.14, 9.08, and 9.123. Cites Opinions 5.026, 9.031, and 9.12. Terry, *Physicians and Patients Who "Friend" or "Tweet": Constructing a Legal Framework for Social Networking in a Highly Regulated Domain, 43 Ind. L. Rev. 285, 314-16, 319, 334-36, 338 (2010).*

Journal 2007 Explores solutions to the growing need for palliative care of prison inmates. Concludes that a partnership between community and correctional physicians is the optimal solution. References Opinion 5.059. Linder & Meyers, *"Don't Let Me Die in Prison"—Palliative Care for Prison Inmates, 298 JAMA 894, 898 (2007).*

5.0591 Patient Privacy and Outside Observers to the Clinical Encounter

Outside observers are individuals who are present during patient-physician encounters and are neither members of a health care team nor enrolled in an educational program for health professionals such as medical students.

Physicians are ethically and legally responsible for safeguarding patient privacy and, therefore, must inform outside observers about medical standards of confidentiality and require them to agree to these standards.

Outside observers may be present during the medical encounter only with the patient's explicit agreement. Physicians should avoid situations in which an outside observer's presence may negatively influence the medical interaction and compromise care. The presence of outside observers during encounters between physicians and patients who lack decision-making capacity should not be permitted, except under rare circumstances and with consent of the parent or legal guardian.

Physicians should not accept payment from outside observers because accepting such payment may undermine the patient-physician relationship. (I, IV, VIII)

Issued November 2005 based on the report "Patient Privacy and Outside Observers to the Clinical Encounter," adopted June 2005.

Journal 2010 Explores how participation in online social networks may blur boundaries between personal and professional relationships for health care professionals and how such risks may be mitigated by use of network privacy and security settings. Suggests that health care institutions are likely to institute online social-networking policies for employees. Quotes Opinions 5.026, 5.027, 5.045, 5.046, 5.05, 5.059, 5.0591, 8.14, 9.08, and 9.123. Cites Opinions 5.026, 9.031, and 9.12. Terry, *Physicians and Patients Who "Friend" or "Tweet": Constructing a Legal Framework for Social Networking in a Highly Regulated Domain, 43 Ind. L. Rev. 285, 314-16, 319, 334-36, 338 (2010).*

5.06 Confidentiality: Attorney-Physician Relation

The patient's history, diagnosis, treatment, and prognosis may be discussed with the patient's lawyer with the consent of the patient or the patient's lawful representative.

A physician may testify in court or before a worker's compensation board or the like in any personal injury or related case. (IV)

Issued prior to April 1977.

M.D. Pa. 1987 Plaintiff in a medical malpractice action sought to preclude his treating physicians from serving as defendant's expert witnesses at trial. The court held that defense counsel's failure to provide prior notice of ex parte communication with plaintiff's treating physicians barred their use as defense experts. Referring to *Petrillo v. Syntex Laboratories, Inc.*, 148 Ill. App. 3d 581, 499 N.E.2d 952 (1986), the court noted that the court there favorably cited Principle IV and Opinions 5.05, 5.06, and 5.07 (1984) in support of a public policy protecting confidentiality between physician and patient and against ex parte discussion. *Manion v. N.P.W. Medical Center of N.E. Pa., Inc., 676 F. Supp. 585, 591.*

Fla. App. 1995 The court considered the issue of the effect of § 455.241(2) of the Florida Statutes on right of defense in a medical malpractice action to engage in ex parte communications with plaintiff's nonparty treating physician. The court held that a 1988 amendment to § 455.241(2) negated the applicability of the statute to medical malpractice cases. The dissent, citing *Petrillo v. Syntex Laboratories, Inc.,* 148 Ill. App. 3d 581, 499 N.E.2d 952 (1986), quoted Principles II and IV and Opinions 5.05, 5.06, and 5.08 as strong public policy support for its position that ex parte communications should be barred altogether. *Castillo-Plaza v. Green, 655 So. 2d 197, 206 n.4.*

Ill. App. 1986 Defense attorney in product liability suit was held in contempt of court for conducting ex parte discussions with plaintiff-patient's treating physician without patient's consent and contrary to authorized methods of discovery. The court held that the strong public policy favoring physician-patient confidentiality articulated in Principles II and IV and Opinions 5.05, 5.06, 5.07, and 5.08 (1984) justified a rule against such ex parte discussions. Further, the court held that the public has the right to rely on physicians to faithfully execute their ethical obligations. *Petrillo v. Syntex Laboratories, Inc., 148 Ill. App. 3d 581, 499 N.E.2d 952, 957, 958, 959 cert. denied, 483 US 1007 (1987).*

Journal 2003 Highlights HIPAA privacy issues that need to be monitored and have yet to be resolved. Concludes that HIPAA poses many challenges and it remains unclear whether HIPAA will increase privacy protection. Cites Opinions 5.05, 5.055, 5.057, 5.06, 5.07, 5.075, 5.08, and 5.09. Kutzko, Boyer, Thoman, & Scott, *HIPAA in Real Time: Practical Implications of the Federal Privacy Rule, 51 Drake L. Rev. 403, 408 (2003).*

Journal 1999 Explores the increased use of physician-patient communication through e-mail. Analyzes current laws regarding medical privacy. Suggests that patients' communications to their physicians are part of their medical record and should be given the same protections. Quotes Opinions 5.05 and 5.07. Cites Opinions 5.04 and 5.06. Spielberg, *Online Without a Net: Physician-Patient Communication by Electronic Mail, 25 Am. J. Law & Med. 267, 284-85 (1999).*

Journal 1998 Describes the special nature of confidentiality in the relationship between the psychotherapist and patient. States that not many breach of confidentiality cases involve psychotherapists. Concludes that patients and psychotherapists must better understand their rights and responsibilities in this context. Quotes Opinion 5.05. Cites Opinions 5.06, 5.07, 5.08, and 5.09. Grabois, *The Liability of Psychotherapists for Breach of Confidentiality, 12 J. Law & Health 39, 53-54 (1998).*

Journal 1997 Considers how breast cancer has given rise to numerous medical malpractice lawsuits. Discusses trial techniques and strategies for litigating these types of claims. Quotes Opinions 5.05 and 5.06. Hillerich, Ellerin, & Frieder, *Selecting and Presenting a Failure to Diagnose Breast Cancer Case, 20 Am. J. Trial Advoc. 253, 271 (1996-97).*

Journal 1991 Discusses the case of *Crist v. Moffat,* which prohibits ex parte communications with a plaintiff's treating physician in North Carolina. Examines the physician-patient privilege and looks at various jurisdictions that permit and forbid ex parte communications. Quotes Principle IV and Opinion 5.06. Comment, *Shielding the Plaintiff and Physician: The Prohibition of Ex Parte Contacts With a Plaintiff's Treating Physician, 13 Campbell L. Rev. 233, 243, 248 (1991).*

Journal 1984 Observes that available ethical and legal guidelines are insufficient to aid physicians in addressing issues of patient privacy and confidentiality. Concludes that there is need for legislation in order to provide suitable guidance to physicians who fulfill an important role in protecting patient privacy. Cites 1982 Opinions 5.03 [now Opinion 5.04], 5.04, 5.05 [now Opinion 5.06], 5.06 [now Opinion 5.07], 5.07 [now Opinion 5.08], and 5.08 [now Opinion 5.09]. Gellman, *Prescribing Privacy: The Uncertain Role of the Physician in the Protection of Patient Privacy, 62 No. Carolina L. Rev. 255, 271 (1984).*

5.07 Confidentiality: Computers

The utmost effort and care must be taken to protect the confidentiality of all medical records, including computerized medical records.

The guidelines below are offered to assist physicians and computer service organizations in maintaining the confidentiality of information in medical records when that information is stored in computerized databases:

(1) Confidential medical information should be entered into the computer-based patient record only by authorized personnel. Additions to the record should be time and date stamped, and the person making the additions should be identified in the record.

(2) The patient and physician should be advised about the existence of computerized databases in which medical information concerning the patient is stored. Such information should be communicated to the physician and patient prior to the physician's release of the medical information to the entity or entities maintaining the computer databases. All individuals and organizations with some form of access to the computerized databases, and the level of access permitted, should be specifically identified in advance. Full disclosure of this information to the patient is necessary in obtaining informed consent to treatment. Patient data should be assigned a security level appropriate for the data's degree of sensitivity, which should be used to control who has access to the information.

(3) The physician and patient should be notified of the distribution of all reports reflecting identifiable patient data prior to distribution of the reports by the computer facility. There should be approval by the patient and notification of the physician prior to the release of patient-identifiable clinical and administrative data to individuals or organizations external to the medical care environment. Such information should not be released without the express permission of the patient.

(4) The dissemination of confidential medical data should be limited to only those individuals or agencies with a bona fide use for the data. Only the data necessary for the bona fide use should be released. Patient identifiers should be omitted when appropriate. Release of confidential medical information from the database should be confined to the specific purpose for which the information is requested and limited to the specific time frame requested. All such organizations or individuals should be advised that authorized release of data to them does not authorize their further release of the data to additional individuals or organizations, or subsequent use of the data for other purposes.

(5) Procedures for adding to or changing data on the computerized database should indicate individuals authorized to make changes, time periods in which changes take place, and those individuals who will be informed about changes in the data from the medical records.

(6) Procedures for purging the computerized database of archaic or inaccurate data should be established and the patient and physician should be notified before and after the data have been purged. There should be no mixing of a physician's computerized patient records with those of other computer service bureau clients. In addition, procedures should be developed to protect against inadvertent mixing of individual reports or segments thereof.

(7) The computerized medical database should be online to the computer terminal only when authorized computer programs requiring the medical data are being used. Individuals and organizations external to the clinical facility should not be provided online access to a computerized database containing identifiable data from medical records concerning patients. Access to the computerized database should be controlled through security

measures such as passwords, encryption (encoding) of information, and scannable badges or other user identification.

(8) Backup systems and other mechanisms should be in place to prevent data loss and downtime as a result of hardware or software failure.

(9) Security:

(a) Stringent security procedures should be in place to prevent unauthorized access to computer-based patient records. Personnel audit procedures should be developed to establish a record in the event of unauthorized disclosure of medical data. Terminated or former employees in the data processing environment should have no access to data from the medical records concerning patients.

(b) Upon termination of computer services for a physician, those computer files maintained for the physician should be physically turned over to the physician. They may be destroyed (erased) only if it is established that the physician has another copy (in some form). In the event of file erasure, the computer service bureau should verify in writing to the physician that the erasure has taken place. (IV)

Issued prior to April 1977. Updated June 1994 and June 1998.

M.D. Pa. 1987 Plaintiff in a medical malpractice action sought to preclude his treating physicians from serving as defendant's expert witnesses at trial. The court held that defense counsel's failure to provide prior notice of ex parte communication with plaintiff's treating physicians barred their use as defense experts. Referring to *Petrillo v. Syntex Laboratories, Inc.*, 148 Ill. App. 3d 581, 499 N.E.2d 952 (1986), the court noted that the court there favorably cited Principle IV and Opinions 5.05, 5.06, and 5.07 (1984) in support of a public policy protecting confidentiality between physician and patient and against ex parte discussion. *Manion v. N.P.W. Medical Center of N.E. Pa., Inc.*, 676 F.Supp. 585, 591.

Ill. App. 1986 Defense attorney in product liability suit was held in contempt of court for conducting ex parte discussions with plaintiff-patient's treating physician without patient's consent and contrary to authorized methods of discovery. The court held that the strong public policy favoring physician-patient confidentiality articulated in Principles II and IV and Opinions 5.05, 5.06, 5.07, and 5.08 (1984) justified a rule against such ex parte discussions. Further, the court held that the public has the right to rely on physicians to faithfully execute their ethical obligations. *Petrillo v. Syntex Laboratories, Inc.*, 148 Ill. App. 3d 581, 499 N.E.2d 952, 957, 958, 959, cert. denied 483 US 1007 (1987).

Pa. Super. 1988 Plaintiff-patient sued her physician for breach of confidentiality when physician conferred with defense counsel in plaintiff's malpractice suit against the hospital (physician's employer). In its majority opinion, the court cited Principle IV, commenting that it gave very little guidance to physicians but nonetheless was not violated by the physician. The court also noted Opinion 5.07 (1986) finding that the plaintiff's suit minimized her expectations of confidentiality. The dissent, however, interpreted these same provisions, along with Opinion 5.05 (1986), as protecting plaintiff's expectations of confidentiality. *Moses v. McWilliams*, 379 Pa. Super. 150, 549 A.2d 950, 956, 962 (dissent) appeal denied 521 Pa. 630, 558 A.2d 532 (1989).

Journal 2006 Examines the benefits and privacy concerns associated with the adoption of electronic medical records. Suggests the federal government should embrace HIPAA to simultaneously protect privacy and facilitate transition to the new system. Cites Opinion 5.07. McLaughlin, *Pandora's Box: Can HIPAA Still Protect Patient Privacy Under a National Health Care Information Network?* 42 Gonz. L. Rev. 29, 42 (2006).

Journal 2003 Highlights HIPAA privacy issues that need to be monitored and have yet to be resolved. Concludes that HIPAA poses many challenges and it remains unclear whether HIPAA will increase privacy protection. Cites Opinions 5.05, 5.055, 5.057, 5.06, 5.07, 5.075, 5.08, and 5.09. Kutzko, Boyer, Thoman, & Scott, *HIPAA in Real Time: Practical Implications of the Federal Privacy Rule*, 51 Drake L. Rev. 403, 408 (2003).

Journal 2000 Defines and explores current and future applications of telemedicine. Considers issues of cost, quality, access, and regulation. Concludes that telemedicine holds tremendous promise for improving the US health care system. Quotes Opinions 5.05 and 5.07. Volkert, *Telemedicine: Rx for the Future of Health Care*, 6 Mich. Telecomm. & Tech. L. Rev. 147, 214, 225 (2000).

Journal 1999 Explores the increased use of physician-patient communication through e-mail. Analyzes current laws regarding medical privacy. Suggests that patients' communications to their physicians are part of their medical record and should be given the same protections. Quotes Opinions 5.05 and 5.07. Cites Opinions 5.04 and 5.06. Spielberg, *Online Without a Net: Physician-Patient Communication by Electronic Mail*, 25 Am. J. Law & Med. 267, 284-85 (1999).

Journal 1999 Explores Model Rules of Professional Conduct focusing on the attorney-client relationship. Compares confidentiality provisions in the Model Rules with the rules of confidentiality governing the medical profession. Observes that existing confidentiality rules are incomplete and ambiguous. Concludes that one remedy is to embrace a discretionary confidentiality rule. Quotes Opinion 5.05. Cites Principle IV and Opinion 5.07. Zer-Gutman, *Revising the Ethical Rules of Attorney-Client Confidentiality: Towards a New Discretionary Rule*, 45 Loy. L. Rev. 669, 683-84, 699, 709, 718 (1999).

Journal 1998 Describes the special nature of confidentiality in the relationship between the psychotherapist and patient. States that not many breach of confidentiality cases involve psychotherapists. Concludes that patients and psychotherapists must better understand their rights and responsibilities in this context. Quotes Opinion 5.05. Cites Opinions 5.06, 5.07, 5.08, and 5.09. Grabois, *The Liability of Psychotherapists for Breach of Confidentiality*, 12 J. Law & Health 39, 53-54 (1998).

Journal 1998 Explains risks involved with the use of electronic medical records. States that patients need to be aware of who has access to their medical records. Concludes that health care providers should equalize the risks and benefits related to the use of electronic medical records. Cites Opinion 5.05. References Opinion 5.07. Jurevic, *When Technology and Health Care Collide: Issues With Electronic Medical Records and Electronic Mail*, 66 UMKC L. Rev. 809, 819-20 (1998).

Journal 1998 Examines the use of e-mail in the physician-patient relationship. Focuses on privacy concerns stemming from the use of e-mail in the medical context. Suggests that physicians should discuss the implications of communicating through e-mail with their patients and should obtain informed consent prior to communicating in this manner. Cites Opinions 5.04, 5.05, 5.057, 5.07, 5.075, and 5.08. Spielberg, *On Call and Online: Sociohistorical, Legal, and Ethical Implications of E-mail for the Patient-Physician Relationship*, 280 JAMA 1353, 1356 (1998).

Journal 1998 Examines the transition from paper medical records to electronic medical records. Identifies issues of confidentiality and privacy that arise as a result of the move to electronic medical records. Concludes that federal protection is needed to safeguard personal medical information. Quotes Principle IV and Opinions 5.07 and 5.075. Cites Opinion 8.061. Tsai, *Cheaper and Better: The Congressional Administrative Simplification Mandate Facilitates the Transition to Electronic Medical Records*, 19 J. Legal Med. 549, 570, 581 (1998).

Journal 1997 Discusses the practice of ex parte communications between treating physicians and their patients' legal adversaries without informing the patient or obtaining consent. Examines harms that may occur in these situations. Argues that Oklahoma needs to prohibit treating physicians from communicating ex parte with their patients' legal adversaries. Quotes Opinions 5.05, 5.07, 5.08, 8.02, 8.03, and 9.07. Cites Opinion 7.02. McNaughton & McNaughton, *Divided Loyalty: The Dilemma of the Treating Physician Advocate*, 22 Okla. City U. L. Rev. 1051, 1052, 1054, 1056, 1058, 1059, 1062 (1997).

Journal 1997 Examines the benefits of unconstrained access to personal medical information. Discusses drawbacks to full disclosure and absolute confidentiality of medical information. Advocates increased awareness of how medical data are used. Proposes guidelines for the best approach to regulation of health care data. Cites Opinion 5.07. Schwartz, *Privacy and the Economics of Personal Health Care Information*, 76 Tex. L. Rev. 1, 59 (1997).

Journal 1997 Considers new data-collection technology enabling collection, storage, and dissemination of data, including medical records information. Discusses the confidentiality problems triggered by increased utilization of computers in health care delivery. Quotes Opinion 5.07. Woodward, *Medical Record Confidentiality and Data Collection: Current Dilemmas*, 25 J. Law Med. & Ethics 88, 90, 95 (1997).

Journal 1995 Examines federal legislative proposals intended to protect confidentiality of computerized medical records. Concludes that proposed legislation will significantly undermine confidentiality. Cites Opinion 5.07. References Principle IV. Hoge, *Proposed Federal Legislation Jeopardizes Patient Privacy*, 23 Bull. Am. Acad. Psychiatry Law 495, 498, 500 (1995).

Journal 1993 Discusses the issues surrounding the confidentiality of electronic and computerized medical records. Concludes that any legal standard addressing this problem should balance the need to protect patient confidentiality with the practical constraints limiting ideal security. References Principle IV and Opinion 5.07. Waller & Fulton, *The Electronic Chart: Keeping It Confidential and Secure*, 26 J. Health & Hosp. L. 104, 105 (April 1993).

Journal 1984 Observes that available ethical and legal guidelines are insufficient to aid physicians in addressing issues of patient privacy and confidentiality. Concludes that there is need for legislation in order to provide suitable guidance to physicians who fulfill an important role in protecting patient privacy. Cites 1982 Opinions 5.03 [now Opinion 5.04], 5.04, 5.05 [now Opinion 5.06], 5.06 [now Opinion 5.07], 5.07 [now Opinion 5.08], and 5.08 [now Opinion 5.09]. Gellman, *Prescribing Privacy: The Uncertain Role of the Physician in the Protection of Patient Privacy*, 62 No. Carolina L. Rev. 255, 271 (1984).

5.075 Confidentiality: Disclosure of Records to Data Collection Companies

Data collection from computerized or other patient records for marketing purposes raises serious ethical concerns. In some cases, firms have sought to amass information on physicians' prescribing practices on behalf of pharmaceutical houses for marketing purposes. Often, physicians are offered incentives such as computer hardware and software packages in return for agreeing to such an arrangement. They may be told that data-collecting software does not capture patients' names.

These arrangements may violate principles of informed consent and patient confidentiality. Patients divulge information to their physicians only for purposes of diagnosis and treatment. If other uses are to be made of the information, patients must give their permission after being fully informed about the purpose of such disclosures. If permission is not obtained, physicians violate patient confidentiality by sharing specific and intimate information from patients' records with commercial interests.

Arrangements of this kind may also violate Opinion 8.061, "Gifts to Physicians From Industry."

Finally, these arrangements may harm the integrity of the patient-physician relationship. The trust that is fundamental to this relationship is based on the principle that the physicians are the agents first and foremost of their patients. (I, II, IV)

Issued June 1994. Updated June 1998.

Journal 2007 Analyzes scientific, ethical, and legal issues raised in the exhumation and genetic analysis of historical figures. Concludes that biohistorical review boards should be created to generate guidelines for such research. Quotes Preamble and Opinion 2.08. Cites Opinions 2.079, 2.105, 5.05, 5.051, 5.075, 8.03, 8.031, 9.095, and 9.10. Paradise & Andrews, *Tales From the Crypt: Scientific, Ethical, and Legal Considerations for Biohistorical Analysis of Deceased Historical Figures*, 26 Temp. J. Sci. Tech. & Envtl. L. 223, 287-88 (2007).

Journal 2003 Highlights HIPAA privacy issues that need to be monitored and have yet to be resolved. Concludes that HIPAA poses many challenges and it remains unclear whether HIPAA will increase privacy protection. Cites Opinions 5.05, 5.055, 5.057, 5.06, 5.07, 5.075, 5.08, and 5.09. Kutzko, Boyer, Thoman, & Scott, *HIPAA in Real Time: Practical Implications of the Federal Privacy Rule*, 51 Drake L. Rev. 403, 408 (2003).

Journal 1998 Examines the use of e-mail in the physician-patient relationship. Focuses on privacy concerns stemming from the use of e-mail in the medical context. Suggests that physicians should discuss the implications of communicating through e-mail with their patients and should obtain informed consent prior to communicating in this manner. Cites Opinions 5.04, 5.05, 5.057, 5.07, 5.075, and 5.08. Spielberg, *On Call and Online: Sociohistorical, Legal, and Ethical Implications of E-mail for the Patient-Physician Relationship*, 280 JAMA 1353, 1356 (1998).

Journal 1998 Examines the transition from paper medical records to electronic medical records. Identifies issues of confidentiality and privacy that arise as a result of the move to electronic medical records. Concludes that federal protection is needed to safeguard personal medical information. Quotes Principle IV and Opinions 5.07 and 5.075. Cites Opinion 8.061. Tsai, *Cheaper and Better: The Congressional Administrative Simplification Mandate Facilitates the Transition to Electronic Medical Records*, 19 J. Legal Med. 549, 570, 581 (1998).

5.08 Confidentiality: Insurance Company Representative

History, diagnosis, prognosis, and the like acquired during the physician-patient relationship may be disclosed to an insurance company representative only if the patient or a lawful representative has consented to the disclosure. A physician's responsibilities to patients are not limited to the actual practice of medicine. They also include the performance of some services ancillary to the practice of medicine. These services might include certification that the patient was under the physician's care and comment on the diagnosis and therapy in the particular case. See also Opinion 2.135, "Insurance Companies and Genetic Information." (IV)

Issued prior to April 1977.

N.D. Ohio 1965 Plaintiff-patient alleged that the defendant-malpractice insurer induced physician to reveal confidential information about plaintiff on pretext that plaintiff filed a malpractice suit. In denying defendant's motion for reconsideration of the court's earlier opinion, the court confirmed its holding that actions of a third party inducing a physician to divulge confidential information may result in liability to the patient. In so holding, the court quoted (with incorrect citation to Ch. II, Sec.1) Principles Ch. I, Sec.2 (1912), [now Principle IV and Opinion 5.08], to emphasize the medical profession's established views regarding confidentiality. *Hammonds v. Aetna Casualty & Sur. Co., 243 F. Supp. 793, 803.*

Fla. App. 1995 The court considered the issue of the effect of § 455.241(2) of the Florida Statutes on right of defense in a medical malpractice action to engage in ex parte communications with plaintiff's nonparty treating physician. The court held that a 1988 amendment to § 455.241(2) negated the applicability of the statute to medical malpractice cases. The dissent, citing *Petrillo v. Syntex Laboratories, Inc.*, 148 Ill. App. 3d 581, 499 N.E.2d 952 (1986), quoted Principles II and IV and Opinions 5.05, 5.06, and 5.08 as strong public policy support for its position that ex parte communications should be barred altogether. *Castillo-Plaza v. Green, 655 So. 2d 197, 206 n.4.*

Ill. App. 1986 Defense attorney in product liability suit was held in contempt of court for conducting ex parte discussions with plaintiff-patient's treating physician without patient's consent and contrary to authorized methods of discovery. The court held that the strong public policy favoring physician-patient confidentiality articulated in Principles II and IV and Opinions 5.05, 5.06, 5.07, and 5.08 (1984) justified a rule against such ex parte discussions. Further, the court held that the public has the right to rely on physicians to faithfully execute their ethical obligations. *Petrillo v. Syntex Laboratories, Inc.*, 148 Ill. App. 3d 581, 499 N.E.2d 952, 957, 958, 959, cert. denied, 483 US 1007 (1987).

Journal 2003 Highlights HIPAA privacy issues that need to be monitored and have yet to be resolved. Concludes that HIPAA poses many challenges and it remains unclear whether HIPAA will increase privacy protection. Cites Opinions 5.05, 5.055, 5.057, 5.06, 5.07, 5.075, 5.08, and 5.09. Kutzko, Boyer, Thoman, & Scott, *HIPAA in Real Time: Practical Implications of the Federal Privacy Rule*, 51 Drake L. Rev. 403, 408 (2003).

Journal 2001 Discusses same-sex marriages in the transgender community. Explores Defense of Marriage Act statutes. Considers whether same-sex transgender marriages can prevail against attacks brought under such statutes. Cites Opinions 2.132, 2.135, 2.137, 5.08, and 5.09. Frye & Meiselman, *Same-Sex Marriages Have Existed Legally in the United States for a Long Time Now*, 64 Alb. L. Rev. 1031, 1053 (2001).

Journal 2000 Evaluates transgender legal and political activity in the US. Discusses the International Bill of Gender Rights against the background of the Texas case, *Littleton v. Prange*. Cites Opinions 2.132, 2.135, 2.137, 5.08, and 5.09. Frye, *The International Bill of Gender Rights vs. the Cider House Rules: Transgenders Struggle With the Courts Over What Clothing They Are Allowed to Wear on the Job, Which Restroom They Are Allowed to Use on the Job, Their Right to Marry, and the Very Definition of Their Sex*, 7 Wm. & Mary J. Women & L. 133, 149 (2000).

Journal 1998 Describes the special nature of confidentiality in the relationship between the psychotherapist and patient. States that not many breach of confidentiality cases involve psychotherapists. Concludes that patients and psychotherapists must better understand their rights and responsibilities in this context. Quotes Opinion 5.05. Cites Opinions 5.06, 5.07, 5.08, and 5.09. Grabois, *The Liability of Psychotherapists for Breach of Confidentiality*, 12 J. Law & Health 39, 53-54 (1998).

Journal 1998 Examines the use of e-mail in the physician-patient relationship. Focuses on privacy concerns stemming from the use of e-mail in the medical context. Suggests that physicians should discuss the implications of communicating through e-mail with their patients and should obtain informed consent prior to communicating in this manner. Cites Opinions 5.04, 5.05, 5.057, 5.07, 5.075, and 5.08. Spielberg, *On Call and Online: Sociohistorical, Legal, and Ethical Implications of E-mail for the Patient-Physician Relationship*, 280 JAMA 1353, 1356 (1998).

Journal 1997 Discusses the practice of ex parte communications between treating physicians and their patients' legal adversaries without informing the patient or obtaining consent. Examines harms that may occur in these situations. Argues that Oklahoma needs to prohibit treating physicians from communicating ex parte with their patients' legal adversaries. Quotes Opinions 5.05, 5.07, 5.08, 8.02, 8.03, and 9.07. Cites Opinion 7.02. McNaughton & McNaughton, *Divided Loyalty: The Dilemma of the Treating Physician Advocate*, 22 Okla. City U. L. Rev. 1051, 1052, 1054, 1056, 1058, 1059, 1062 (1997).

Journal 1984 Observes that available ethical and legal guidelines are insufficient to aid physicians in addressing issues of patient privacy and confidentiality. Concludes that there is need for legislation in order to provide suitable guidance to physicians who fulfill an important role in protecting patient privacy. Cites 1982 Opinions 5.03 [now Opinion 5.04], 5.04, 5.05 [now Opinion 5.06], 5.06 [now Opinion 5.07], 5.07 [now Opinion 5.08], and 5.08 [now Opinion 5.09]. Gellman, *Prescribing Privacy: The Uncertain Role of the Physician in the Protection of Patient Privacy*, 62 No. Carolina L. Rev. 255, 271 (1984).

5.09   The previous Opinion 5.09, "Confidentiality: Physicians in Industry," issued July 1983, was deleted in June 2000 and combined with Opinion 5.09, "Confidentiality: Industry-Employed Physicians and Independent Medical Examiners."

5.09   Confidentiality: Industry-Employed Physicians and Independent Medical Examiners

Where a physician's services are limited to performing an isolated assessment of an individual's health or disability for an employer, business, or insurer, the information obtained by the physician as a result of such examinations is confidential and should not be communicated to a third party without the individual's prior written consent, unless required by law. If the individual authorized the release of medical information to an employer or a potential employer, the physician should release only that information which is reasonably relevant to the employer's decision regarding that individual's ability to perform the work required by the job.

When a physician renders treatment to an employee with a work-related illness or injury, the release of medical information to the employer as to the treatment provided may be subject to the provisions of worker's compensation laws. The physician must comply with the requirements of such laws, if applicable. However, the physician may not otherwise discuss the employee's health condition with the employer without the employee's consent or, in the event of the employee's incapacity, the appropriate proxy's consent.

Whenever statistical information about employees' health is released, all employee identities should be deleted. (IV)

Issued July 1983. Updated June 1994; updated June 1996; updated December 1999 based on the report "Patient-Physician Relationship in the Context of Work-Related and Independent Medical Examinations," adopted June 1999.

Mass. 1984 Employee sued employer for libel and invasion of privacy following disclosure of medical facts about employee to other employees. In part, claim involved disclosure of opinion about employee's mental state to his supervisor by physician retained by employer. Citing Principle 9 (1957) [now Principle IV and Opinions 5.05 and 5.09], the court held that a physician retained by an employer may disclose to the employer information concerning an employee if receipt of the information is reasonably necessary to serve a substantial and valid business interest of the employer. *Bratt v. International Business Mach. Corp., 392 Mass. 508, 467 N.E.2d 126, 137 n.23.*

N.Y. Sup. 2000 Physician brought wrongful discharge claim against corporate employer. The physician alleged she was discharged because she refused to reveal confidential medical information regarding employees. With apparent reference to Principle IV and Opinions 5.05 and 5.09, the affidavit filed by the physician claimed she had an ethical and legal duty to protect patient confidentiality. The court found termination of an employee at will based upon such grounds is sufficient to state a cause of action for breach of contract. The court ruled that obligations of good faith and fair dealing may be implied in a contract for the employment of a physician and that no physician should be placed in the position of choosing between retaining employment and violating ethical standards. *Horn v. New York Times, 186 Misc. 2d 469, 719 N.Y.S. 2d 471, 474.*

Journal 2003 Highlights HIPAA privacy issues that need to be monitored and have yet to be resolved. Concludes that HIPAA poses many challenges and it remains unclear whether HIPAA will increase privacy protection. Cites Opinions 5.05, 5.055, 5.057, 5.06, 5.07, 5.075, 5.08, and 5.09. Kutzko, Boyer, Thoman, & Scott, *HIPAA in Real Time: Practical Implications of the Federal Privacy Rule, 51 Drake L. Rev. 403, 408 (2003).*

Journal 2001 Discusses same-sex marriages in the transgender community. Explores Defense of Marriage Act statutes. Considers whether same-sex transgender marriages can prevail against attacks brought under such statutes. Cites Opinions 2.132, 2.135, 2.137, 5.08, and 5.09. Frye & Meiselman, *Same-Sex Marriages Have Existed Legally in the United States for a Long Time Now, 64 Alb. L. Rev. 1031, 1053 (2001).*

Journal 2000 Evaluates transgender legal and political activity in the US. Discusses the International Bill of Gender Rights against the background of the Texas case, *Littleton v. Prange.* Cites Opinions 2.132, 2.135, 2.137, 5.08, and 5.09. Frye, *The International Bill of Gender Rights vs. the Cider House Rules: Transgenders Struggle With the Courts Over What Clothing They Are Allowed to Wear on the Job, Which Restroom They Are Allowed to Use on the Job, Their Right to Marry, and the Very Definition of Their Sex, 7 Wm. & Mary J. Women & L. 133, 149 (2000).*

Journal 1999 Discusses the need for physicians to advocate on behalf of patients' rights in the context of health care delivery. Evaluates the nature and scope of the physician's role as advocate, noting that physicians cannot be expected to engage in attorney-like advocacy. Quotes Principles IV and VI, Fundamental Elements (2), (4), and (6) [now Opinion 10.01], Patient Responsibilities 5 [now Opinion 10.02], and Opinions 2.03, 2.07, 2.09, 2.16, 2.19, 3.06, 4.01, 4.04, 6.01, 7.02, 8.02, 8.03, 8.13, 8.132, 9.06, 9.07, and 9.131. Cites Opinions 5.05, 5.09, 7.01, 8.135, and

9.02. Sage, *Physicians as Advocates*, 35 Hous. L. Rev. 1529, 1537, 1541, 1542, 1552-53, 1554, 1556, 1557, 1559, 1561-62, 1564, 1571, 1574, 1576, 1580 (1999).

Journal 1998 Analyzes the decision in *Spaulding v. Zimmerman*. Discusses the issue of an attorney's obligation to disclose information to protect a third-party's health or safety. Includes in this discussion consideration of the duty of an "examining" physician to disclose such information to an examinee. Cites Opinion 5.09. Cramton & Knowles, *Professional Secrecy and Its Exceptions: Spaulding v. Zimmerman Revisited*, 83 Minn. L. Rev. 63, 98 (1998).

Journal 1998 Describes the special nature of confidentiality in the relationship between the psychotherapist and patient. States that not many breach of confidentiality cases involve psychotherapists. Concludes that patients and psychotherapists must better understand their rights and responsibilities in this context. Quotes Opinion 5.05. Cites Opinions 5.06, 5.07, 5.08, and 5.09. Grabois, *The Liability of Psychotherapists for Breach of Confidentiality*, 12 J. Law & Health 39, 53-54 (1998).

Journal 1991 Explores ethical problems unique to the field of forensic psychiatry. Presents the results of a survey of members of the American Academy of Psychiatry and the Law (AAPL), asking their opinions regarding proposed ethical guidelines. Quotes Opinions 1.02 and 5.09. Weinstock, Leong, & Silva, *Opinions by AAPL Forensic Psychiatrists on Controversial Ethical Guidelines: A Survey*, 19 Bull. Am. Acad. Psychiatry Law 237, 238 (1991).

Journal 1984 Observes that available ethical and legal guidelines are insufficient to aid physicians in addressing issues of patient privacy and confidentiality. Concludes that there is need for legislation in order to provide suitable guidance to physicians who fulfill an important role in protecting patient privacy. Cites 1982 Opinions 5.03 [now Opinion 5.04], 5.04, 5.05 [now Opinion 5.06], 5.06 [now Opinion 5.07], 5.07 [now Opinion 5.08], and 5.08 [now Opinion 5.09]. Gellman, *Prescribing Privacy: The Uncertain Role of the Physician in the Protection of Patient Privacy*, 62 No. Carolina L. Rev. 255, 271 (1984).

5.10 A Physician's Role Following a Breach of Electronic Health Information

When used with appropriate attention to security, electronic medical records (EMRs) promise numerous benefits for quality clinical care and health-related research. However, when a security breach occurs, patients may face physical, emotional, and dignitary harms.

Dedication to upholding trust in the patient-physician relationship, to preventing harms to patients, and to respecting patients' privacy and autonomy create responsibilities for individual physicians, medical practices, and health care institutions when patient information is inappropriately disclosed. The degree to which an individual physician has an ethical responsibility to address inappropriate disclosure depends in part on his or her awareness of the breach, relationship to the patient(s) affected, administrative authority with respect to the records, and authority to act on behalf of the practice or institution.

When there is reason to believe that patients' confidentiality has been compromised by a breach of the EMR, physicians should:

(1) Ensure that patients are promptly informed about the breach and potential for harm, either by disclosing directly (when the physician has administrative responsibility for the EMR), participating in efforts by the practice or health care institution to disclose, or ensuring that the practice or institution takes appropriate action to disclose.

(2) Follow ethically appropriate procedures for disclosure, which should at minimum include:

(a) carrying out the disclosure confidentially and within a time frame that provides patients ample opportunity to take steps to minimize potential adverse consequences; and

(b) describing what information was breached; how the breach happened; what the consequences may be; what corrective actions have been taken by the physician, practice, or institution; and what steps patients themselves might take to minimize adverse consequences.

(3) Support responses to security breaches that place the interests of patients above those of the physician, medical practice, or institution.

(4) To the extent possible, provide information to patients to enable them to mitigate potential adverse consequences of inappropriate disclosure of their personal health information, such as credit monitoring services or identity theft hotline. (IV, VIII)

Issued November 2009 based on the report "A Physician's Role Following a Breach of Electronic Health Information," adopted June 2009 (*J Clin Ethics*. Spring 2010).

6.00 **Opinions on Fees and Charges**

6.01 Contingent Physician Fees

If a physician's fee for medical service is contingent on the successful outcome of a claim, such as a malpractice or worker's compensation claim, there is the ever-present danger that the physician may become less of a healer and more of an advocate or partisan in the proceedings. Accordingly, a physician's fee for medical services should be based on the value of the service provided by the physician to the patient and not on the uncertain outcome of a contingency that does not in any way relate to the value of the medical service.

A physician's fee should not be made contingent on the successful outcome of medical treatment. Such arrangements are unethical because they imply that successful outcomes from treatment are guaranteed, thus creating unrealistic expectations of medicine and false promises to consumers. (VI)

Issued prior to April 1977. Updated June 1994.

Cal. App. 1992 Lower court held that a contingent fee agreement between plaintiff and a medical-legal consulting service violated public policy and was void. In reversing, appellate court referred to *Polo v. Gotchel* 225 N.J. Super. 492, 542 A.2d 947 (1987) and *Dupree v. Malpractice Research, Inc.*, 179 Mich. App. 254, 445 N.W.2d 498 (1989) which had relied on Opinion 8.04 (1984) [now Opinion 6.01] to hold that contingent fee consulting contracts were per se invalid. The court was unpersuaded by the reasoning of these decisions, stating that (1) the contingent fee agreement was with a company, not with a physician, and (2) the term "medical services" in the Opinion refers to patient treatment and not to consulting services provided in conjunction with the services of an attorney. *Ojeda v. Sharp Cabrillo Hosp.*, 8 Cal. App. 4th 1, 12, 13 n.11, 14, 10 Cal. Rptr. 2d 230, 237 n.11, 238.

Mich. App. 1989 Plaintiffs, who settled an underlying medical malpractice suit, sought to invalidate contingent fee contract with expert witness service. Plaintiffs had paid witness and report fees, travel costs, and other expenses in advance according to a fee schedule but objected to a charge of 20% of their recovery. The court, citing Opinion 8.04 (1984) [now Opinion 6.01], held that the contingent fee contract for expert witnesses was repugnant to the public policy of preserving the plaintiff's recovery and preventing the exaggeration of favorable testimony and would not be enforced. Further, the court refused to consider defendant's quantum meruit claim, since some fees had been paid in advance, and any further attempt to collect fees would fail to deter such contracts. *Dupree v. Malpractice Research, Inc.*, 179 Mich. App. 254, 445 N.W.2d 498, 501.

N.J. Super. 1987 Contingent fee agreement between plaintiff's attorney in a medical malpractice action and a medical-legal consulting service which linked plaintiff with potential expert witnesses violated public policy and was void. The court cited with approval Opinion 8.04 (1984) [now Opinion 6.01], which states that a physician's fees should not be based upon the outcome of litigation because of the risk that the physician may become more of an advocate than a healer. *Polo v. Gotchel*, 225 N.J. Super. 429, 542 A.2d 947, 948.

Tenn. 1998 Physician sued patient and patient's attorney for breach of contract after the patient settled a personal injury claim. Physician claimed that under contract, he was entitled to receive a contingency fee for services as the medical expert in the patient's case and contingency fees for medical services rendered. Alternatively, the physician claimed that he could recover under the theory of quantum meruit. The court held that the contingency fee both for the physician acting as a medical expert and for medical services violated public policy. The court quoted Opinions 6.01 and 9.07, stating that the Tennessee Board of Medical Examiners, that governs state medical licenses, had adopted the AMA's stance on contingency fees. The court also rejected the physician's argument that he should be allowed to recover under the theory of quantum meruit because the underlying contracts were void as against public policy. *Swafford v. Harris, 967 S.W.2d 319, 321-323.*

Journal 2011 Explains how to prepare for and take a physician's deposition for trial, including obtaining records and opinions and preserving answers. Cites Opinion 6.01. Radnor, *How to Prepare for and Take a Doctor's Deposition, 22 Prac. Litigator 40, 52 (May 2011).*

Journal 2009 Discusses financing assisted reproduction and adoption using specialty loans and the political and economic implications of such practices. Concludes parenthood loans could increase access to assisted reproduction and adoption for those otherwise unable to afford these services. Cites Opinion 6.01. Jacoby, *Show Me the Money: Making Markets in Forbidden Exchange: The Debt Financing of Parenthood, 72 Law & Contemp. Prob. 147, 156 (2009).*

Journal 2006 Examines ethical dilemmas physicians may face as providers of pay-for-performance medical care. Concludes that this strategy offers a benefit to patients as long as physicians uphold stringent ethical standards and work together to ensure optimum patient care. Cites Principles I, V, VIII, and IX and Opinions 2.035, 2.095, 6.01, 8.021, 8.03, 8.0501, 8.053, 8.054, and 8.121. Bostick, Sade, & McMahon, *Report of the Council on Ethical and Judicial Affairs: Physician Pay-for-Performance Programs, 3 Ind. Health L. Rev. 429, 430, 431, 432-33, 434, 435, 436 (2006).*

Journal 2006 Discusses health care reform in the interest of social justice. Concludes that such reform is feasible, but requires extensive planning and effort. References Opinion 6.01. Hyman, *Getting the Haves to Come Out Behind: Fixing the Distributive Injustices of American Health Care, 69 Law & Contemp. Probs. 265, 268-69 (2006).*

Journal 2006 Discusses the benefits and drawbacks to pay-for-performance medical care. Concludes that pay-for-performance may increase the quality of medical care if implemented correctly and with increased government support. Cites Opinion 6.01. Sage, *Pay For Performance: Will It Work in Theory? 3 Ind. Health L. Rev. 305, 308-09 (2006).*

Journal 2005 Argues that abolishing or weakening the tort liability system will not improve the quality of health care, but may diminish it. Concludes that a systems-based approach coupled with a liability system that encourages high quality care may improve health care delivery in the US. Quotes Opinion 8.12. References Opinion 6.01. Hyman & Silver, *The Poor State of Health Care Quality in the U.S.: Is Malpractice Liability Part of the Problem or Part of the Solution? 90 Cornell L. Rev. 893, 926, 965 (2005).*

Journal 2001 Considers result-based compensation arrangements for medical services. Focuses on a 1994 AMA amendment to Opinion 6.01 that prohibits payment of physicians contingent upon outcome. Concludes that such arrangements may be appropriate in some circumstances. Quotes Opinion 6.01. Hyman & Silver, *Just What the Patient Ordered: The Case for Result-Based Compensation Arrangements, 29 J. L. Med. & Ethics 170, 170 (2001).*

Journal 2001 Explains the design and potential benefits of result-based compensation arrangements for health care. Concludes that a more reliable and efficient health care delivery system is fostered by such arrangements. Quotes Opinion 6.01. References Opinions 9.121 and 9.122. Hyman & Silver, *You Get What You Pay For: Result-Based Compensation for Health Care, 58 Wash. & Lee L. Rev. 1427, 1459, 1460, 1461, 1481-82 (2001).*

Journal 2000 Considers the rules governing expert testimony. Explores professional ethical standards affecting expert witnesses and concludes that codes of ethics have not succeeded in eliminating biased expert testimony. Recommends creation of an organization to assist courts in obtaining reliable expert witness testimony. Quotes Principle III and Opinion 6.01. Cites Principles I, II, and V and Opinions 1.02 and 9.07. Murphy, *Expert Witnesses at Trial: Where Are the Ethics? 14 Geo. J. Legal Ethics 217, 231-32 (2000).*

Journal 1999 Discusses the need for physicians to advocate on behalf of patients' rights in the context of health care delivery. Evaluates the nature and scope of the physician's role as advocate, noting that physicians cannot be expected to engage in attorney-like advocacy. Quotes Principles IV and VI, Fundamental Elements (2), (4), and (6) [now Opinion 10.01], Patient Responsibilities 5 [now Opinion 10.02], and Opinions 2.03, 2.07, 2.09, 2.16, 2.19, 3.06, 4.01, 4.04, 6.01, 7.02, 8.02, 8.03, 8.13, 8.132, 9.06, 9.07, and 9.131. Cites Opinions 5.05, 5.09, 7.01, 8.135, and

9.02. Sage, *Physicians as Advocates*, 35 Hous. L. Rev. 1529, 1537, 1541, 1542, 1552-53, 1554, 1556, 1557, 1559, 1561-62, 1564, 1571, 1574, 1576, 1580 (1999).

Journal 1998 Examines mechanisms of oversight for expert witness testimony by medical, legal, legislative, and regulatory agencies. Points out that the amount of malpractice litigation will increase the need for medical expert witnesses. Concludes that improvements in this context must uphold principles of due process and be acceptable to the medical and legal communities. Cites Opinions 6.01, 8.04, and 9.07. McAbee, *Improper Expert Medical Testimony: Existing and Proposed Mechanisms of Oversight*, 19 J. Legal Med. 257, 265 (1998).

Journal 1991 Looks at the problem of high expert witness fees and lack of access to expert testimony by those who may need it. Proposes revamping the current system to allow certain types of contingent fee arrangements. Quotes Opinion 8.04 (1984) [now Opinion 6.01]. Note, *Contingent Expert Witness Fees: Access and Legitimacy*, 64 So. Cal. L. Rev. 1363, 1374, 1382 (1991).

Journal 1990 Examines conflicting court decisions that have addressed the appropriateness of medical-legal consulting services and their use of contingent fee arrangements. Concludes by discussing the need for a less troublesome solution to the problems plaintiffs face in malpractice and personal injury cases. Quotes Opinion 6.01. Cites Opinions 6.12 (1989) [now Opinion 6.05] and 9.07. Dillon, *Contingent Fees and Medical-Legal Consulting Services: Economical or Unethical?* 11 J. Legal Med. 93, 101, 111 (1990).

6.02   Fee Splitting

Payment by or to a physician solely for the referral of a patient is fee splitting and is unethical.

A physician may not accept payment of any kind, in any form, from any source, such as a pharmaceutical company or pharmacist, an optical company, or the manufacturer of medical appliances and devices, for prescribing or referring a patient to said source.

In each case, the payment violates the requirement to deal honestly with patients and colleagues. The patient relies upon the advice of the physician on matters of referral. All referrals and prescriptions must be based on the skill and quality of the physician to whom the patient has been referred or the quality and efficacy of the drug or product prescribed. (II)

Issued prior to April 1977. Updated June 1994.

Ill. App. 2004 Appellant physicians moved for a declaration that flat and percentage-based fees assessed by respondents for inclusion on a list of health care providers constituted fee-splitting and was a violation of state law. The trial court found that the percentage-based fee, but not the flat fee, violated the Illinois Medical Practice Act, but denied appellants recovery for past fees paid. The appellate court, quoting Opinion 6.02, found that both flat and percentage-based fees constituted fee-splitting and violated the Medical Practice Act, but still denied recovery for past fees paid. *Vine Street Clinic v. Healthlink, Inc.*, 353 Ill. App. 3d 929, 819 N.E.2d 363, 367.

Kan. App. 1985 Members of a medical partnership sought an injunction to enforce a covenant not to compete against defendant-physician, a former partner. Defendant asserted that the covenant was void as against public policy relying on Opinion 9.02 (1984). The court, however, ruled that the covenant was reasonable as defined by precedent and that it was bound to follow this precedent as opposed to the AMA's position regarding such covenants. Defendant further argued enforcement of the covenant was precluded because the partnership had violated ethical norms, apparently referring to Opinions 6.03 and 6.04 (1984) [now Opinions 6.02 and 6.03] which were part of partnership contract. The court held that defendant was estopped from complaining about the partnership's actions due to his own conduct. *Axtell Clinic v. Cranston*, No. 56,745 (Kan. Ct. App. June 20, 1985) (LEXIS, States Library, Kan. file).

Mass. 1955 Plaintiff-physician was charged under state licensing statute by defendant-board with conspiracy and fee-splitting. Both parties sought a declaratory judgment as to whether the defendant-board had jurisdiction to determine plaintiff's guilt or innocence. In holding that the board was qualified to determine if plaintiff's actions constituted gross misconduct under the statute, the court referred to Principles Ch. I, Secs. 1 and 6 (1947) [now Principle II and Opinion 6.02] delineating, in part, limitations on payment for medical services. These provisions, the court said, reflected the medical profession's understanding of its peculiar obligations. *Forziati v. Board of Registration in Medicine, 333 Mass. 125, 128 N.E.2d 789, 791.*

Mass. Super. 1998 Plaintiff-surgeon filed suit against a medical group practice claiming that the defendants reduced referrals to him because he declined to join the group. Plaintiff claimed that the decline harmed his surgical practice. He alleged that the group's practice of taking 10% of members' income constituted unethical and illegal kickbacks. The court held that the decline in referrals was not connected to plaintiff not being a member of the group. The court also found that the plaintiff had not presented evidence that the decline in referrals harmed his practice. Finally, the court found that the fees paid by members of the group practice were gatekeeper fees rather than referral fees. The court quoted Opinion 6.02, in support of its decision that the defendants' fees did not constitute fee splitting. Further, the court referenced Opinion 8.032 concluding that a self-referral was not necessarily unethical if disclosed to the patient. *Boman v. Southeast Medical Services Group, 1998 WL 1182063, 11-12.*

Journal 2010 Examines medical tourism and the referral-type fees foreign providers pay to brokers to bring patients from the United States. Concludes that while medical tourism is a viable option for uninsured or underinsured patients, disclosure of broker's fees would enhance competition and patient trust. Quotes Opinion 6.021, References Opinions 6.02 and 6.021. Spece, *Medical Tourism: Protecting Patients From Conflicts of Interest in Broker's Fees Paid by Foreign Providers*, 6 J. Health & Biomedical L. 1, 3, 19 (2010).

Journal 2007 Examines the effectiveness of banning conflicts of interest in order to promote ethical medical research. Concludes that regulation of research practice should be based on the overall nature of relationships rather than on purely financial issues. Cites Opinion 6.02. Sage, *Some Principles Require Principals: Why Banning "Conflicts Of Interest" Won't Solve Incentive Problems in Biomedical Research*, 85 Tex. L. Rev. 1413, 1458 (2007).

Journal 2006 Discusses the evolution of health law in Virginia. Concludes that the area of health law continues to expand, develop, and be refined. Cites Opinions 3.03, 3.08, 5.01, 5.015, 5.02, 5.04, 5.055, 6.02, 6.021, 6.03, 6.04, 7.03, 7.04, 7.05, 8.054, 8.08, 8.081, 8.085, 8.115, 8.12, 8.14, 8.145, 8.19, and 9.045. Guanzon, *Health Care Law*, 41 U. Rich. L. Rev. 179, 199 (2006).

Journal 2002 Suggests a reconceptualization for bioethics that integrates an analysis of the history of moral change. Concludes that bioethical textbooks should include discussion about the history of bioethics and medical ethics. Quotes Opinion 2.20. References Opinions 6.02, 6.03, 6.04 [now Opinion 8.06], and 8.032. Baker, *Bioethics and History*, 27 J. Med. & Phil. 447, 455, 469 (2002).

Journal 2001 Evaluates current forms of cybermedicine and Internet resources that support it. Explores patient and regulatory concerns, including privacy issues, insurance reimbursement problems, licensure, and liability, which may thwart the growth of cybermedicine. Concludes that cybermedicine may facilitate delivery of cost-effective, quality medical care. Quotes Opinions 5.05, 6.02, and 6.03. Scott, *Cybermedicine and Virtual Pharmacies*, 103 W. Va. L. Rev. 407, 441, 451 (2001).

Journal 1999 Provides a historical account of fee splitting and the corporate practice of medicine doctrine. Suggests that legislation on kickbacks should allow an exception for goods and services supplied at fair market value. Concludes that the legislature's approach to fee splitting should be revised to fit contemporary circumstances. References Opinion 6.02. Jacobs & Goodman, *Splitting Fees or Splitting Hairs? Fee Splitting and Health Care—The Florida Experience*, 8 Annals Health L. 239, 244 (1999).

Journal 1998 Explores aspects of trust in physician-patient relations. Discusses the transformation of the health care system and the need for regulation. Points out that too much involvement by politicians and legislators will put the health care system at risk. References Opinions 6.02 and 8.03. Mechanic, *The Functions and Limitations of Trust in the Provision of Medical Care*, 23 J. Health Pol. Pol'y & Law 661, 667 (1998).

Journal 1985 Initially describes how existing doctrines protect the value of autonomy in the context of the physician-patient relationship, then examines various problems in the current protective scheme. Concludes by recommending the creation of an independent articulable protected interest in patient autonomy. Quotes Principles II and IV. Cites Opinions 4.04 (1984) [now Opinions 8.03 and 8.032] and 6.03 (1984) [now Opinion 6.02]. Shultz, *From Informed Consent to Patient Choice: A New Protected Interest*, 95 Yale L. J. 219, 275 (1985).

6.021   Financial Incentives to Patients for Referrals

Physicians should not offer financial incentives or other valuable considerations to patients in exchange for recruitment of other patients. Such incentives can distort the information that patients provide to potential patients, thus distorting the expectations of potential patients and compromising the trust that is the foundation of the patient-physician relationship.

Issued December 2004 based on the report "Financial Incentives to Patients for Referrals," adopted June 2004.

Journal 2010 Examines medical tourism and the referral-type fees foreign providers pay to brokers to bring patients from the United States. Concludes that while medical tourism is a viable option for uninsured or underinsured patients, disclosure of broker's fees would enhance competition and patient trust. Quotes Opinion 6.021, References Opinions 6.02 and 6.021. Spece, *Medical Tourism: Protecting Patients From Conflicts of Interest in Broker's Fees Paid by Foreign Providers*, 6 J. Health & Biomedical L. 1, 3, 19 (2010).

Journal 2006 Discusses the evolution of health law in Virginia. Concludes that the area of health law continues to expand, develop, and be refined. Cites Opinions 3.03, 3.08, 5.01, 5.015, 5.02, 5.04, 5.055, 6.02, 6.021, 6.03, 6.04, 7.03, 7.04, 7.05, 8.054, 8.08, 8.081, 8.085, 8.115, 8.12, 8.14, 8.145, 8.19, and 9.045. Guanzon, *Health Care Law*, 41 U. Rich. L. Rev. 179, 199 (2006).

6.03   Fee Splitting: Referrals to Health Care Facilities

Clinics, laboratories, hospitals, or other health care facilities that compensate physicians for referral of patients are engaged in fee splitting, which is unethical.

Health care facilities should not compensate a physician who refers patients there for the physician's cognitive services in prescribing, monitoring, or revising the patient's course of treatment. Payment for these cognitive services is acceptable when it comes from patients, who are the beneficiaries of the physician's services, or from the patient's designated third-party payer.

Offering or accepting payment for referring patients to research studies (finder's fees) is also unethical. (II)

Issued prior to April 1977. Updated June 1994 and updated June 1996 based on the report "Finder's Fees: Payment for the Referral of Patients to Clinical Research Studies," adopted December 1994.

Kan. App. 1985 Members of a medical partnership sought an injunction to enforce a covenant not to compete against defendant-physician, a former partner. Defendant asserted that the covenant was void as against public policy relying on Opinion 9.02 (1984). The court, however, ruled that the covenant was reasonable as defined by precedent and that it was bound to follow this precedent as opposed to the AMA's position regarding such covenants. Defendant further argued enforcement of the covenant was precluded because the partnership had violated ethical norms, apparently referring to Opinions 6.03 and 6.04 (1984) [now Opinions 6.02 and 6.03] which were part of partnership contract. The court held that defendant was estopped from complaining about the partnership's actions due to his own conduct. *Axtell Clinic v. Cranston*, No. 56,745 (Kan. Ct. App. June 20, 1985) (LEXIS, States Library, Kan. file).

Journal 2006 Discusses the evolution of health law in Virginia. Concludes that the area of health law continues to expand, develop, and be refined. Cites Opinions 3.03, 3.08, 5.01, 5.015, 5.02, 5.04, 5.055, 6.02, 6.021, 6.03, 6.04, 7.03, 7.04, 7.05, 8.054, 8.08, 8.081, 8.085, 8.115, 8.12, 8.14, 8.145, 8.19, and 9.045. Guanzon, *Health Care Law*, 41 U. Rich. L. Rev. 179, 199 (2006).

Journal 2003 Discusses financial incentive programs for physicians who enroll patients in clinical trials. Concludes that more regulatory oversight is needed to protect research subjects and the integrity of the medical research process. Quotes Opinions 6.03 and 8.031. Lemmens & Miller, *The Human Subjects Trade: Ethical and Legal Issues Surrounding Recruitment Incentives*, 31 J. L. Med. & Ethics 398, 407 (2003).

Journal 2002 Suggests a reconceptualization for bioethics that integrates an analysis of the history of moral change. Concludes that bioethical textbooks should include discussion about the history of bioethics and medical ethics. Quotes Opinion 2.20. References Opinions 6.02, 6.03, 6.04 [now Opinion 8.06], and 8.032. Baker, *Bioethics and History*, 27 J. Med. & Phil. 447, 455, 469 (2002).

Journal 2001 Evaluates current forms of cybermedicine and Internet resources that support it. Explores patient and regulatory concerns, including privacy issues, insurance reimbursement problems, licensure, and liability, which may thwart the growth of cybermedicine. Concludes that cybermedicine may facilitate delivery of cost-effective, quality medical care. Quotes Opinions 5.05, 6.02, and 6.03. Scott, *Cybermedicine and Virtual Pharmacies*, 103 W. Va. L. Rev. 407, 441, 451 (2001).

6.04   "Fee Splitting: Drug or Device Prescription Rebates," issued March 1980, was deleted in June 2002 and combined with Opinion 8.07, "Gifts to Physicians: Offers of Indemnity" and Opinion 8.06, "Drugs and Devices: Prescribing," into the current Opinion 8.06, "Prescribing and Dispensing Drugs and Devices."

6.05   Fees for Medical Services

A physician should not charge or collect an illegal or excessive fee. For example, an illegal fee occurs when a physician accepts an assignment as full payment for services rendered to a Medicare patient and then bills the patient for an additional amount. A fee is excessive when after a review of the facts a person knowledgeable as to current charges made by physicians would be left with a definite and firm conviction that the fee is in excess of a reasonable fee. Factors to be considered as guides in determining the reasonableness of a fee include the following:

(1)   The difficulty and/or uniqueness of the services performed and the time, skill, and experience required

(2)   The fee customarily charged in the locality for similar physician services

(3)   The amount of the charges involved

(4)   The quality of performance

(5)   The experience, reputation, and ability of the physician in performing the kind of services involved (II)

Issued prior to April 1977. Updated June 1994.

Journal 1990 Examines conflicting court decisions that have addressed the appropriateness of medical-legal consulting services and their use of contingent fee arrangements. Concludes by discussing the need for a less troublesome solution to the problems plaintiffs face in malpractice and personal injury cases. Quotes Opinion 6.01. Cites Opinions 6.12 (1989) [now Opinion 6.05] and 9.07. Dillon, *Contingent Fees and Medical-Legal Consulting Services: Economical or Unethical?* 11 J. Legal Med. 93, 101, 111 (1990).

6.06   The previous Opinion 6.06, "Fees: Group Practice," issued in March 1981, was deleted in June 1994.

6.07   Insurance Form Completion Charges

The attending physician should complete without charge the appropriate "simplified" insurance claim form as a part of service to the patient to enable the patient to receive his or her benefits. A charge for more complex or multiple forms may be made in conformity with local custom. (II)

Issued prior to April 1977. Updated June 1994.

Journal 1992 Discusses the ethical and legal boundaries of medical treatment. Concludes that minor boundary violations occur frequently, but warns that if they become too frequent or serious, physicians risk substantial liability. Quotes Opinion 6.06 [sic] 6.07. Simon, *Treatment Boundary Violations: Clinical, Ethical, and Legal Considerations,* 20 Bull. Am. Acad. Psychiatry Law 269, 282 (1992).

6.08   Interest Charges and Finance Charges

Although harsh or commercial collection practices are discouraged in the practice of medicine, a physician who has experienced problems with delinquent accounts may properly choose to request that payment be made at the time of treatment or add interest or other reasonable charges to delinquent accounts. The patient must be notified in advance of the interest or other reasonable finance or service charges by such means as the posting of a notice in the physician's waiting room, the distribution of leaflets describing the office billing practices, and appropriate notations on the billing statement. The physician must comply with state and federal laws and regulations applicable to the imposition of such charges. Physicians are encouraged to review their accounting/collection policies to ensure that no patient's account is sent to collection without the physician's knowledge. Physicians who choose to add an interest or finance charge to accounts not paid within a reasonable time are encouraged to use compassion and discretion in hardship cases. (II)

Issued prior to April 1977. Updated June 1994.

Cal. App. 1968 Plaintiff-physician sought dissolution of a medical partnership with defendant's decedent, and also sought a larger percentage of the partnership receipts based upon an alleged oral agreement. Defendant cross-claimed to enjoin plaintiff from taking physical control of the partnership offices and patient records. The trial court enjoined plaintiff from treating previous patients, requiring that he return all medical records and pay defendant all fees received from patients he had treated during the time of dispute. The appellate court reversed insofar as the injunction prohibited the plaintiff from treating patient who desired to continue to receive his services or prevented access to medical records essential for this purpose, citing Opinions and Reports of the Judicial Council Sec. 7, Para. 16, Sec. 5, Para. 21 and Sec. 9 (1966) [now Opinions 6.08, 5.02, and 5.05] to support view that patients may not be regarded as the subject of ownership. *Jones v. Fakehany, 261 Cal. App. 2d 298, 67 Cal. Rptr. 810, 815, 816 n.1.*

Journal 2010 Describes how physicians act as bankers in financing fertility treatments for patients and how this significantly contributes to medical debt and bankruptcies. Proposes regulations which would address these issues within fertility markets. Quotes Opinion 6.08. Cites Opinion 2.055. Hawkins, *Doctors as Bankers: Evidence From Fertility Markets,* 84 Tul. L. Rev. 841, 848, 874 (2010).

Journal 2010 Examines competing methods of measuring the role of medical debt in bankruptcies. Concludes that court records alone reveal very little about the burden of medical bills on financially distressed families and ultimately diminish bankruptcy cases in which medical bills were particularly significant. References Opinion 6.08. Holman & Jacoby, *Managing Medical Bills on the Brink of Bankruptcy,* 10 Yale J. Health Pol'y, L. & Ethics 239, 255 (2010).

Journal 2008 Reviews current physician practices of collecting money from indebted patients. Concludes that physicians should continue to refrain from aggressive debt collection. Quotes Opinions 6.08 and 6.12. Hall & Schneider, *The Professional Ethics of Billing and Collections,* 300 JAMA 1806, 1807 (2008).

6.09   Laboratory Bill

When it is not possible for the laboratory bill to be sent directly to the patient, the referring physician's bill to the patient should indicate the actual charges for laboratory services, including the name of the laboratory, as well as any separate charges for the physician's own professional services. (II)

Issued prior to April 1977.

6.10   Services Provided by Multiple Physicians

Each physician engaged in the care of the patient is entitled to compensation commensurate with the value of the service he or she has personally rendered.

No physician should bill or be paid for a service which is not performed; mere referral does not constitute a professional service for which a professional charge should be made or for which a fee may be ethically paid or received.

When services are provided by more than one physician, each physician should submit his or her own bill to the patient and be compensated separately, if possible. A physician should not charge a markup, commission, or profit on the services rendered by others.

It is ethically permissible in certain circumstances, however, for a surgeon to engage other physicians to assist in the performance of a surgical procedure and to pay a reasonable amount for such assistance, provided the nature of the financial arrangement is made known to the patient. This principle applies regardless of whether the assisting physician is the referring physician. (II)

Issued prior to April 1977. Updated June 1994.

6.11   Competition

Competition between and among physicians and other health care practitioners on the basis of competitive factors such as quality of services, skill, experience, miscellaneous conveniences offered to patients, credit terms, fees charged, etc, is not only ethical but is encouraged. Ethical medical practice thrives best under free market conditions when prospective patients have adequate information and opportunity to choose freely between and among competing physicians and alternate systems of medical care. (VII)

Issued July 1983.

Ohio App. 1991 Medical corporation sought an injunction to enforce a covenant not to compete against defendant-physician. The lower court granted summary judgment based on a referee's report which concluded that, under Principle VI and Opinions 6.11, 9.02, and 9.06 (1989), restrictive covenants were per se unenforceable as a matter of public policy. While recognizing a strong public interest in allowing open access to health care, the appellate court in reversing held that Opinion 9.02, which applied specifically to restrictive covenants, only "discouraged" such covenants. *Ohio Urology, Inc. v. Poll,* 72 Ohio. *App.* 446, 450, 451, 594 N.E.2d 1027, 1030, 1031.

Journal 2006 Examines physician restrictive covenants. Concludes that under the current balancing test, courts should give considerable weight to the public interest in preserving the physician-patient relationship. Quotes Opinions 9.02 and 9.06. Cites Opinions 6.11, 8.11, 8.115, and 9.06. Malloy, *Physician Restrictive Covenants: The Neglect of Incumbent Patient Interests,* 41 *Wake Forest L. Rev.* 189, 207-08, 217, 218 (2006).

Journal 1998 Explores changes in the health care reimbursement system and the impact on the recovery of damages for medical expenses. Discusses the historical development of the collateral source rule. Suggests that the collateral source rule should not be applied to allow recovery for sums that were not actually paid for medical services. Cites Opinion 6.11. Beard, *The Impact of Changes in Health Care Provider Reimbursement Systems on the Recovery of Damages for Medical Expenses in Personal Injury Suits*, 21 Am. J. Trial Advoc. 453, 484 (1998).

Journal 1997 Examines noncompetition clauses in the medical field. Reviews policy concerns and historical and common-law analyses of agreements not to compete. Posits that the more commercialized the medical profession becomes, the more noncompetition clauses infringe upon the physician-patient relationship and patients' rights. Quotes Opinions 9.02 and 9.06. Cites Preamble and Opinion 6.11. Comment, *Noncompetition Clauses in Physician Employment Contracts in Oregon*, 76 Or. L. Rev. 195, 204-06 (1997).

Journal 1993 Discusses the controversies surrounding advertising in medicine and physician self-referral. Proposes adoption of the model of the physician as either professional or honest businessman. Quotes Opinion 6.11. Brody, *The Physician as Professional and the Physician as Honest Businessman*, 119 Arch. Otolaryngol. Head Neck Surg. 495, 496 (1993).

Journal 1991 Considers the question of whether physicians should provide medical treatment to those who come to them for second opinions. Concludes that each physician must individually decide whether to treat these patients. Quotes Opinions 6.11, 9.06, and 9.12. Cites Opinion 9.02. Ile, *Should Physicians Treat Patients Who Seek Second Opinions?* 266 JAMA 273, 274 (1991).

6.12   Forgiveness or Waiver of Insurance Copayments

Under the terms of many health insurance policies or programs, patients are made more conscious of the cost of their medical care through copayments. By imposing copayments for office visits and other medical services, insurers hope to discourage unnecessary health care. In some cases, financial hardship may deter patients from seeking necessary care if they would be responsible for a copayment for the care. Physicians commonly forgive or waive copayments to facilitate patient access to needed medical care. When a copayment is a barrier to needed care because of financial hardship, physicians should forgive or waive the copayment.

A number of clinics have advertised their willingness to provide detailed medical evaluations and accept the insurer's payment but waive the copayment for all patients. Cases have been reported in which some of these clinics have conducted excessive and unnecessary medical testing while certifying to insurers that the testing is medically necessary. Such fraudulent activity exacerbates the high cost of health care, violates Opinion 2.19, "Unnecessary Medical Services," and is unethical.

Physicians should be aware that forgiveness or waiver of copayments may violate the policies of some insurers, both public and private; other insurers may permit forgiveness or waiver if they are aware of the reasons for the forgiveness or waiver. Routine forgiveness or waiver of copayments may constitute fraud under state and federal law. Physicians should ensure that their policies on copayments are consistent with applicable law and with the requirements of their agreements with insurers. (II)

Issued June 1993.

Journal 2008 Argues waiver of patient coinsurance costs creates unfair competition among physicians and has negative economic consequences for those paying providers. Suggests close monitoring of waivers will reduce inflation of health care charges, diminish interference with the health plan insurer–network provider relationship, and discourage overutilization of medical services. Quotes Opinion 6.12. Cites Opinion 6.13. Bernstein & Seybert, *Everyone Pays the Price When Healthcare Providers Waive Patients' Co-insurance Obligations,* 21 Health Law. 20, 22 (Dec. 2008).

Journal 2008 Reviews current physician practices of collecting money from indebted patients. Concludes that physicians should continue to refrain from aggressive debt collection. Quotes Opinions 6.08 and 6.12. Hall & Schneider, *The Professional Ethics of Billing and Collections,* 300 JAMA 1806, 1807 (2008).

Journal 2005 Discusses legal and ethical problems associated with patient surcharges. Concludes that surcharges are necessary to combat rising malpractice insurance premiums and a declining payment environment. Cites Principle IX and Opinion 6.12. Landfair, *Transforming Physicians Into Business Savvy Entrepreneurs: Patient Surcharges Charge Onto the Scene of Physician Reimbursement,* 43 Duq. L. Rev. 257, 268, 269 (2005).

Journal 2000 Examines civil and criminal liability in connection with the practice of professional courtesy fee waivers and discounts. Discusses conflicts between the long-standing traditional practice of professional courtesy and a prudent and ethical course under current law. Quotes Opinion 6.12. Cites Opinion 6.13. Schmidt, *Professional Courtesy Discounts Under Siege—Part II,* 29 Colo. Law. 59, 62 (Jan. 2000).

6.13 Professional Courtesy

Professional courtesy refers to the provision of medical care to physician colleagues or their families free of charge or at a reduced rate. While professional courtesy is a long-standing tradition in the medical profession, it is not an ethical requirement. Physicians should use their own judgment in deciding whether to waive or reduce their fees when treating fellow physicians or their families. Physicians should be aware that accepting insurance payments while waiving patient copayments may violate Opinion 6.12, "Forgiveness or Waiver of Insurance Copayments." (II, IV)

Issued June 1994.

Journal 2008 Argues waiver of patient coinsurance costs creates unfair competition among physicians and has negative economic consequences for those paying providers. Suggests close monitoring of waivers will reduce inflation of health care charges, diminish interference with the health plan insurer–network provider relationship, and discourage overutilization of medical services. Quotes Opinion 6.12. Cites Opinion 6.13. Bernstein & Seybert, *Everyone Pays the Price When Healthcare Providers Waive Patients' Co-insurance Obligations,* 21 Health Law. 20, 22 (Dec. 2008).

Journal 2000 Examines civil and criminal liability in connection with the practice of professional courtesy fee waivers and discounts. Discusses conflicts between the long-standing traditional practice of professional courtesy and a prudent and ethical course under current law. Quotes Opinion 6.12. Cites Opinion 6.13. Schmidt, *Professional Courtesy Discounts Under Siege—Part II,* 29 Colo. Law. 59, 62 (Jan. 2000).

Opinions on Physician Records

7.00

7.01 Records of Physicians: Availability of Information to Other Physicians

The interest of the patient is paramount in the practice of medicine, and everything that can reasonably and lawfully be done to serve that interest must be done by all physicians who have served or are serving the patient. A physician who formerly treated a patient should not refuse for any reason to make records of that patient promptly available on request to another physician presently treating the patient. Proper authorization for the use of records must be granted by the patient. Medical reports should not be withheld because of an unpaid bill for medical services. (IV)

Issued prior to April 1977.

D. Colo. 2007 Plaintiff-inmate sued prison medical staff members claiming insufficient care and improper denial of outside care following an assault. The district court considered whether the plaintiff's Eighth Amendment right to receive adequate medical care had been violated. In support of his allegations, plaintiff attempted to show that in one instance a physician's recommendation for a second opinion was intentionally ignored. The court, quoting Opinion 7.01, found that the physician had merely transferred plaintiff's medical records to another physician upon request, consistent with his ethical obligation. The court held that plaintiff failed to show the required intent to disregard a substantial risk to his health. *Schaal v. Fender, 2007 WL 2461642, 7.*

N.D. Ill. 2010 Sister of deceased patient brought adversary proceeding against bankrupt physician to except from discharge debt stemming from physician's alleged breach of fiduciary duties. The bankruptcy court quotes Opinions 7.01 and 8.03 in finding that a fiduciary duty was established by nature of the physician-patient relationship that continued after patient's death. *In re Odeh, 431 B.R. 807, 814.*

Del. Super. 2002 Medical group sued physician for misappropriation of trade secrets and solicitation of patients while still employed with group. Group authorized physician to notify his patients of his departure. The physician used group's records and insurance data to send a mass-mail letter to about 900 patients. Appeals court held that the letter sent went beyond a notification and was instead a solicitation and that the group had not authorized him to use trade secrets to solicit patients. In so ruling the court quoted Opinions 7.01 and 7.03. *Total Care Physicians v. O'Hara, 2002 Del. Super. LEXIS 493, *19.*

Me. 1999 Physician appealed decision of the Board of Licensure in Medicine imposing a civil penalty for his failure to release medical records to patient's physicians. Physician argued that the board did not specify the ethical standards that his conduct violated. The court vacated the board's decision on the grounds that the physician was denied the opportunity to refute evidence of a violation of professional standards or to develop a defense predicated on those standards. The board, in defense of its decision, presented Opinions 7.01 and 7.02 to the court. The court, in vacating the decision, pointed out that the hearing record did not demonstrate which Opinions the board applied. Furthermore, the court, quoting Principle IV, stated that the physician had a responsibility to protect the patient's medical records. *Balian v. Board of Licensure in Medicine, 722 A.2d 364, 368.*

N.Y. Surr. 1968 Patients of a deceased physician filed an action seeking to obtain or copy records maintained by the decedent during his lifetime regarding them. The executor had refused to deliver the records by reason of a provision in the decedent's will directing that his "office records" be destroyed. Quoting Opinions and Reports of the Judicial Council, Sec. 9 Paras. 3, 4, 5, 6, and 7 (1966) [now Opinions 7.01, 7.02, 7.03, and 7.05], the court ruled that, while patient records are the property of the physician, it would be against public policy to permit their destruction. As a result, the court ordered the executor to make the records available to the patients' succeeding physicians at their request. *In re Culbertson's Will*, 57 Misc. 2d 391, 292 N.Y.S.2d 806, 808-10.

S.C. Att'y Gen. 1978 Citing Opinions 5.61, 5.62, and 5.63 (1977) [now Opinions 7.01, 7.02, and 7.03], state attorney general found that patient medical records are the property of the physician or hospital which compiled them and that patients have no ownership rights in them. Further, the opinion concludes that patients have a right to information contained in their records and the right to have records sent to another physician. Patients do not, however, have the right to unlimited direct access to their medical records. *South Carolina Att'y Gen. Op.*, 1978 S.C. AG LEXIS 806.

Journal 1999 Discusses the need for physicians to advocate on behalf of patients' rights in the context of health care delivery. Evaluates the nature and scope of the physician's role as advocate, noting that physicians cannot be expected to engage in attorney-like advocacy. Quotes Principles IV and VI, Fundamental Elements (2), (4), and (6) [now Opinion 10.01], Patient Responsibilities 5 [now Opinion 10.02], and Opinions 2.03, 2.07, 2.09, 2.16, 2.19, 3.06, 4.01, 4.04, 6.01, 7.02, 8.02, 8.03, 8.13, 8.132, 9.06, 9.07, and 9.131. Cites Opinions 5.05, 5.09, 7.01, 8.135, and 9.02. Sage, *Physicians as Advocates*, 35 Hous. L. Rev. 1529, 1537, 1541, 1542, 1552-53, 1554, 1556, 1557, 1559, 1561-62, 1564, 1571, 1574, 1576, 1580 (1999).

Journal 1997 Compares past ethical opinions to current opinions and notes the differences. Comments on the forces that have changed medical ethics through the years. Notes differing theories on the future course of medical ethics. Quotes Fundamental Elements (Preamble) and Opinions 5.05, 5.057, 7.01, 8.12, 9.12, and 9.131. Cites Fundamental Elements (5) and Opinions 8.115 and 8.13. Buchanan, *Medical Ethics at the Millennium: A Brief Retrospective*, 26 Colo. Law. 141, 142, 143, 144, 145 (1997).

7.02   Records of Physicians: Information and Patients

Notes made in treating a patient are primarily for the physician's own use and constitute his or her personal property. However, on request of the patient, a physician should provide a copy or a summary of the record to the patient or to another physician, an attorney, or other person designated by the patient.

Most states have enacted statutes that authorize patient access to medical records. These statutes vary in scope and mechanism for permitting patients to review or copy medical records. Access to mental health records, particularly, may be limited by statute or regulation. A physician should become familiar with the applicable laws, rules, or regulations on patient access to medical records.

The record is a confidential document involving the patient-physician relationship and should not be communicated to a third party without the patient's prior written consent, unless required by law or to protect the welfare of the individual or the community. Medical reports should not be withheld because of an unpaid bill for medical services. Physicians may charge a reasonable fee for copying medical records. (IV)

Issued prior to April 1977. Updated June 1994.

Me. 1999 Physician appealed decision of the Board of Licensure in Medicine imposing a civil penalty for his failure to release medical records to patient's physicians. Physician argued that the board did not specify the ethical standards that his conduct violated. The court vacated the board's decision on the grounds that the physician was denied the opportunity to refute evidence of a violation of professional standards or to develop a defense predicated on those standards. The board, in defense of its decision, presented Opinions 7.01 and 7.02 to the court. The court, in vacating the decision, pointed out that the hearing record did not demonstrate which Opinions the board applied. Furthermore, the court, quoting Principle IV, stated that the physician had a responsibility to protect the patient's medical records. *Balian v. Board of Licensure in Medicine, 722 A.2d 364, 368.*

N.Y. Surr. 1968 Patients of a deceased physician filed an action seeking to obtain or copy records maintained by the decedent during his lifetime regarding them. The executor had refused to deliver the records by reason of a provision in the decedent's will directing that his "office records" be destroyed. Quoting Opinions and Reports of the Judicial Council, Sec. 9 Paras. 3, 4, 5, 6, and 7 (1966) [now Opinions 7.01, 7.02, 7.03, and 7.05], the court ruled that, while patient records are the property of the physician, it would be against public policy to permit their destruction. As a result, the court ordered the executor to make the records available to the patients' succeeding physicians at their request. *In re Culbertson's Will, 57 Misc. 2d 391, 292 N.Y.S.2d 806, 808-10.*

S.C. Att'y Gen. 1978 Citing Opinions 5.61, 5.62, and 5.63 (1977) [now Opinions 7.01, 7.02, and 7.03], state attorney general found that patient medical records are the property of the physician or hospital which compiled them and that patients have no ownership rights in them. Further, the opinion concludes that patients have a right to information contained in their records and the right to have records sent to another physician. Patients do not, however, have the right to unlimited direct access to their medical records. *South Carolina Att'y Gen. Op., 1978 S.C. AG LEXIS 806.*

Tenn. App. 2007 Pursuant to a state statute, the Tennessee Board of Medical Examiners sought patient records from a physician. The physician refused the request. The court of appeals found that while patient privacy and a physician's right to practice were protected by substantive due process, these interests are balanced against the interest of the state in protecting the public health and welfare. Citing Opinion 7.02, the court found that the right to practice medicine freely was not infringed here because the statutory obligations were analogous to existing professional obligations. *McNiel v. Cooper, 241 S.W.3d 886, 897.*

Journal 2001 Analyzes postmortem patient confidentiality and proposes a framework for appropriate information disclosure. Concludes that, following death, decisions regarding disclosure of confidential information should be made on a case-by-case basis. Quotes Opinions 5.051 and 7.02. Berg, *Grave Secrets: Legal and Ethical Analysis of Postmortem Confidentiality, 34 Conn. L. Rev. 81, 87, 117 (2001).*

Journal 1999 Explores changes in technology and the resulting impact on privacy of medical information. Observes that current federal and state laws inadequately protect medical information privacy and suggests that Congress needs to enact legislation addressing this issue. Quotes Opinion 5.05. References Opinions 7.02 and 7.05. Carter, *Health Information Privacy: Can Congress Protect Confidential Medical Information in the "Information Age"? 25 Wm. Mitchell L. Rev. 223, 236, 273 (1999).*

Journal 1999 Discusses the need for physicians to advocate on behalf of patients' rights in the context of health care delivery. Evaluates the nature and scope of the physician's role as advocate, noting that physicians cannot be expected to engage in attorney-like advocacy. Quotes Principles IV and VI, Fundamental Elements (2), (4), and (6) [now Opinion 10.01], Patient Responsibilities 5 [now Opinion 10.02], and Opinions 2.03, 2.07, 2.09, 2.16, 2.19, 3.06, 4.01, 4.04, 6.01, 7.02, 8.02, 8.03, 8.13, 8.132, 9.06, 9.07, and 9.131. Cites Opinions 5.05, 5.09, 7.01, 8.135, and 9.02. Sage, *Physicians as Advocates, 35 Hous. L. Rev. 1529, 1537, 1541, 1542, 1552-53, 1554, 1556, 1557, 1559, 1561-62, 1564, 1571, 1574, 1576, 1580 (1999).*

Journal 1997 Discusses the practice of ex parte communications between treating physicians and their patients' legal adversaries without informing the patient or obtaining consent. Examines harms that may occur in these situations. Argues that Oklahoma needs to prohibit treating physicians from communicating ex parte with their patients' legal adversaries. Quotes Opinions 5.05, 5.07, 5.08, 8.02, 8.03, and 9.07. Cites Opinion 7.02. McNaughton & McNaughton, *Divided Loyalty: The Dilemma of the Treating Physician Advocate, 22 Okla. City U. L. Rev. 1051, 1052, 1054, 1056, 1058, 1059, 1062 (1997).*

7.025 Records of Physicians: Access by Nontreating Medical Staff

Physicians who use or receive information from medical records share in the responsibility for preserving patient confidentiality and should play an integral role in the designing of confidentiality safeguards in health care institutions. Physicians have a responsibility to be aware of the appropriate guidelines in their health care institution, as well as the applicable federal and state laws.

Informal case consultations that involve the disclosure of detailed medical information are appropriate in the absence of consent only if the patient cannot be identified from the information.

Only physicians or other health care professionals who are involved in managing the patient, including providing consultative, therapeutic, or diagnostic services, may access the patient's confidential medical information. All others must obtain explicit consent to access the information.

Monitoring user access to electronic or written medical information is an appropriate and desirable means for detecting breaches of confidentiality. Physicians should encourage the development and use of such monitoring systems.

This opinion focuses on the issue of access to medical records by medical staff not involved in the treatment or diagnosis of patients. It does not address the need to access medical records for clinical research, epidemiological research, quality assurance, or administrative purposes. (IV)

Issued December 1999 based on the report "Records of Physicians: Access by Nontreating Medical Staff," adopted June 1999.

Journal 2010 Discusses the effects of using deidentified health information on privacy and considers the dangers of nonconsensual use of health information. Concludes deidentification of health information is a necessary though insufficient protection of privacy, and further research and regulations should be developed to demonstrate respect for individuals without unduly burdening research. Quotes Principle IV and Opinions 5.05 and 7.025. Rothstein, *Is Deidentification Sufficient to Protect Health Privacy in Research?* 10 Am. J. Bioethics 3, 5 (Sept. 2010).

Journal 2003 Addresses the importance of medical record privacy for patients with HIV/AIDS. Concludes that US privacy laws afford patients less protection than privacy laws in the European Union. References Opinion 7.025. Gilbert, *Emerging Issues in Global AIDS Policy: Preserving Privacy,* 25 Whittier L. Rev. 273, 276 (2003).

7.03 Records of Physicians Upon Retirement or Departure From a Group

A patient's records may be necessary to the patient in the future not only for medical care, but also for employment, insurance, litigation, or other reasons. When a physician retires or dies, patients should be notified and urged to find a new physician and should be informed that upon authorization, records will be sent to the new physician. Records which may be of value to a patient and which are not forwarded to a new physician should be retained, either by the treating physician, another physician, or such other person lawfully permitted to act as a custodian of the records.

The patients of a physician who leaves a group practice should be notified that the physician is leaving the group. Patients of the physician should also be informed of the physician's new address and offered the opportunity to have their medical records forwarded to the departing physician at his or her new practice location. It is unethical to withhold such information upon request of a patient. If the responsibility for notifying patients falls to the departing physician rather than to the group, the group should not interfere with the discharge of these duties by withholding patient lists or other necessary information. (IV)

Issued prior to April 1977. Updated June 1994, June 1996, and February 2002.

N.D. Ill. 1996 A corporation which provided hair transplants brought suit against a physician group under contract to provide medical services to the corporation. The complaint alleged that the defendants had breached the contract in bad faith by attempting to start their own company, by hiring staff members away, and by threatening to enforce noncompetition covenants in their contracts should any physicians attempt to remain with the corporation. The court referred to Opinion 9.02 as explicitly discouraging the use of restrictive covenants in contracts with physicians. Additionally, with apparent reference to Opinion 7.03, the court noted that defendants had not sent notices advising patients of the departure of physicians from the corporation, or of the departing physicians' new practice locations. *Cleveland Hair Clinic, Inc. v. Puig,* 968 F. Supp. 1227, 1246.

Ark. App. 2003 Clinic appealed summary judgment for a medical group that hired two physicians previously practicing in the clinic. Clinic did not pay the physicians and had no noncompetition agreement with them. Physicians notified their patients of their departure. Clinic alleged the medical group solicited its patients by employing the physicians and using patient lists. Appeals court found the clinic failed to establish an employment relationship or rights to the records. The court held the physicians had a right to terminate their association with the clinic and that their patients had a right to follow them. Cites Opinion 7.03. *Springdale Diagnostic Clinic v. Northwest Physicians,* 2003 Ark. App. LEXIS 697, *13, n.1.

Del. Super. 2002 Medical group sued physician for misappropriation of trade secrets and solicitation of patients while still employed with group. Group authorized physician to notify his patients of his departure. The physician used group's records and insurance data to send a mass-mail letter to about 900 patients. Appeals court held that the letter sent went beyond a notification and was instead a solicitation and that the group had not authorized him to use trade secrets to solicit patients. In so ruling the court quoted Opinions 7.01 and 7.03. *Total Care Physicians v. O'Hara,* 2002 Del. Super. LEXIS 493, *19.

N.Y. Sup. 2006 Following termination from a medical group, a physician sought possession of her patients' original medical records. Her employment contract specified that the group would retain all original records and that the physician was entitled to copies. Plaintiff cited a state statute, as well as Opinions 7.03 and 7.04, arguing that a physician has a duty to personally maintain patient records. The court, while acknowledging the physician's duty in this regard, held there was no violation of the statute. There was no reason to believe the group would not safeguard the original records and comply with all statutory requirements. *Pullman v. Gormley,* 13 Misc.3d 1234(A), 831 N.Y.S.2d 356, 2006 WL 3232182, 3.

N.Y. Surr. 1968 Patients of a deceased physician filed an action seeking to obtain or copy records maintained by the decedent during his lifetime regarding them. The executor had refused to deliver the records by reason of a provision in the decedent's will directing that his "office records" be destroyed. Quoting Opinions and Reports of the Judicial Council, Sec. 9 Paras. 3, 4, 5, 6, and 7 (1966) [now Opinions 7.01, 7.02, 7.03, and 7.05], the court ruled that, while patient records are the property of the physician, it would be against public policy to permit their destruction. As a result, the court ordered the executor to make the records available to the patients' succeeding physicians at their request. *In re Culbertson's Will,* 57 Misc. 2d 391, 292 N.Y.S.2d 806, 808-10.

S.C. Att'y Gen. 1978 Citing Opinions 5.61, 5.62, and 5.63 (1977) [now Opinions 7.01, 7.02, and 7.03], state attorney general found that patient medical records are the property of the physician or hospital which compiled them and that patients have no ownership rights in them. Further, the opinion concludes that patients have a right to information contained in their records and the right to have records sent to another physician. Patients do not, however, have the right to unlimited direct access to their medical records. *South Carolina Att'y Gen. Op.,* 1978 S.C. AG LEXIS 806.

Journal 2006 Discusses the evolution of health law in Virginia. Concludes that the area of health law continues to expand, develop, and be refined. Cites Opinions 3.03, 3.08, 5.01, 5.015, 5.02, 5.04, 5.055, 6.02, 6.021, 6.03, 6.04, 7.03, 7.04, 7.05, 8.054, 8.08, 8.081, 8.085, 8.115, 8.12, 8.14, 8.145, 8.19, and 9.045. Guanzon, *Health Care Law,* 41 U. Rich. L. Rev. 179, 199 (2006).

7.04   Sale of a Medical Practice

A physician or the estate of a deceased physician may sell the elements that comprise his or her practice, such as furniture, fixtures, equipment, office leasehold, and goodwill. In the sale of a medical practice, the purchaser is buying not only furniture and fixtures, but also goodwill, ie, the opportunity to take over the patients of the seller. A patient's records may be necessary to the patient in the future not only for medical care, but also for employment, insurance, litigation, matriculation, or other reasons. Therefore, the transfer of records of patients is subject to the following:

(1) The physician (or the estate) must ensure that all medical records are transferred to another physician or entity who is held to the same standards of confidentiality and is lawfully permitted to act as custodian of the records.

(2) All active patients should be notified that the physician (or the estate) is transferring the practice to another physician or entity who will retain custody of their records and that at their written request, within a reasonable time as specified in the notice, the records (or copies) will be sent to another physician or entity of their choice.

(3) A reasonable charge may be made for the cost of locating, duplicating, and mailing records. (IV)

Issued July 1983. Updated June 2000.

N.Y. Sup. 2006 Following termination from a medical group, a physician sought possession of her patients' original medical records. Her employment contract specified that the group would retain all original records and that the physician was entitled to copies. Plaintiff cited a state statute, as well as Opinions 7.03 and 7.04, arguing that a physician has a duty to personally maintain patient records. The court, while acknowledging the physician's duty in this regard, held there was no violation of the statute. There was no reason to believe the group would not safeguard the original records and comply with all statutory requirements. *Pullman v. Gormley, 13 Misc.3d 1234(A), 831 N.Y.S.2d 356, 2006 WL 3232182, 3.*

N.Y. Surr. 1977 In a discovery proceeding, respondent-psychiatrist, who had treated some patients of deceased psychiatrist subsequent to his death, allegedly misappropriated decedent's patient records. Estate petitioned court for return of records and damages for injury to value of decedent's practice. Respondent sought dismissal of claim arguing that estate could not sell patient records. The court rejected respondent's request. In so ruling, the court noted that under Principle 9 (1957) [now Principle IV and Opinion 5.05] prohibiting physicians from revealing patient confidences, various guidelines had been issued regarding sale of a medical practice [now Opinion 7.04]. Whether respondent's actions had interferred with the estate's efforts to dispose of decedent's practice in keeping with these guidelines presented the court with factual issues for later resolution. *Estate of Finkle, 90 Misc. 2d 550, 395 N.Y.S.2d 343, 346.*

Journal 2006 Discusses the evolution of health law in Virginia. Concludes that the area of health law continues to expand, develop, and be refined. Cites Opinions 3.03, 3.08, 5.01, 5.015, 5.02, 5.04, 5.055, 6.02, 6.021, 6.03, 6.04, 7.03, 7.04, 7.05, 8.054, 8.08, 8.081, 8.085, 8.115, 8.12, 8.14, 8.145, 8.19, and 9.045. Guanzon, *Health Care Law, 41 U. Rich. L. Rev. 179, 199 (2006).*

Journal 2004 Discusses the practice of using an attorney retaining lien over a client's papers and argues that the practice should be abolished. Concludes that this practice is coercive and inconsistent with a lawyer's role as a fiduciary. Quotes Opinion 7.02. References Opinion 8.10. Leubsdorf, *Against Lawyer Retaining Liens, 72 Fordham L. Rev. 849, 864, 865 (2004).*

7.05 Retention of Medical Records

Physicians have an obligation to retain patient records which may reasonably be of value to a patient. The following guidelines are offered to assist physicians in meeting their ethical and legal obligations:

(1) Medical considerations are the primary basis for deciding how long to retain medical records. For example, operative notes and chemotherapy records should always be part of the patient's chart. In deciding whether to keep certain parts of the record, an appropriate criterion is whether a physician would want the information if he or she were seeing the patient for the first time.

(2) If a particular record no longer needs to be kept for medical reasons, the physician should check state laws to see if there is a requirement that records be kept for a minimum length of time. Most states will not have such a provision. If they do, it will be part of the statutory code or state licensing board.

(3) In all cases, medical records should be kept for at least as long as the length of time of the statute of limitations for medical malpractice claims. The statute of limitations may be three or more years, depending on the state law. State medical associations and insurance carriers are the best resources for this information.

(4) Whatever the statute of limitations, a physician should measure time from the last professional contact with the patient.

(5) If a patient is a minor, the statute of limitations for medical malpractice claims may not apply until the patient reaches the age of majority.

(6) Immunization records always must be kept.

(7) The records of any patient covered by Medicare or Medicaid must be kept at least five years.

(8) In order to preserve confidentiality when discarding old records, all documents should be destroyed.

(9) Before discarding old records, patients should be given an opportunity to claim the records or have them sent to another physician, if it is feasible to give them the opportunity. (IV, V)

Issued June 1994.

N.Y. Surr. 1968 Patients of a deceased physician filed an action seeking to obtain or copy records maintained by the decedent during his lifetime regarding them. The executor had refused to deliver the records by reason of a provision in the decedent's will directing that his "office records" be destroyed. Quoting Opinions and Reports of the Judicial Council, Sec. 9 Paras. 3, 4, 5, 6, and 7 (1966) [now Opinions 7.01, 7.02, 7.03, and 7.05], the court ruled that, while patient records are the property of the physician, it would be against public policy to permit their destruction. As a result, the court ordered the executor to make the records available to the patients' succeeding physicians at their request. *In re Culbertson's Will, 57 Misc. 2d 391, 292 N.Y.S.2d 806, 808-10.*

Tex. 1998 Plaintiff, whose daughter was injured at birth, sued physician for intentional spoliation of medical records pertinent to lawsuit against hospital. The Texas Supreme Court refused to recognize a separate cause of action for intentional or negligent spoliation of evidence by parties to litigation. The court stated that creating a new cause of action for spoliation would result in duplicative litigation. Concurring judge explained other remedies available to the plaintiff. Quoting Opinion 7.05, judge stated that the ethical duty to retain medical records could be treated as a legal duty. *Trevino v. Ortega, 41 Tex. Sup. Ct. J. 907, 969 S.W.2d 950, 955.*

Journal 2007 Highlights inconsistencies in applying judicial deference to medical ethics. Concludes that courts should afford greater deference to established medical ethics standards. Quotes Principle I and Opinions 2.06 and Ch. II, Art. I, Sec. 3 (May 1847) [now Opinion 5.02]. Cites Opinions 4.01 and 7.05. Lerman, *Second Opinion: Inconsistent Deference to Medical Ethics in Death Penalty Jurisprudence*, 95 Geo. L. J. 1941, 1945, 1974-75, 1976, 1977 (2007).

Journal 2007 Examines regulation of medical tourism and the outsourcing of medical goods and services. Concludes that little regulation currently exists, and that patient privacy is a foremost concern. Quotes Opinion 7.05. Terry, *Under-Regulated Health Care Phenomena in a Flat World: Medical Tourism and Outsourcing*, 29 W. New Eng. L. Rev. 421, 441 (2007).

Journal 2006 Discusses the evolution of health law in Virginia. Concludes that the area of health law continues to expand, develop, and be refined. Cites Opinions 3.03, 3.08, 5.01, 5.015, 5.02, 5.04, 5.055, 6.02, 6.021, 6.03, 6.04, 7.03, 7.04, 7.05, 8.054, 8.08, 8.081, 8.085, 8.115, 8.12, 8.14, 8.145, 8.19, and 9.045. Guanzon, *Health Care Law*, 41 U. Rich. L. Rev. 179, 199 (2006).

Journal 1999 Explores changes in technology and the resulting impact on privacy of medical information. Observes that current federal and state laws inadequately protect medical information privacy and suggests that Congress needs to enact legislation addressing this issue. Quotes Opinion 5.05. References Opinions 7.02 and 7.05. Carter, *Health Information Privacy: Can Congress Protect Confidential Medical Information in the "Information Age"?* 25 Wm. Mitchell L. Rev. 223, 236, 273 (1999).

8.00 Opinions on Practice Matters

8.01 Appointment Charges

A physician may charge a patient for a missed appointment or for one not cancelled 24 hours in advance if the patient is fully advised that the physician will make such a charge. (VI)

Issued prior to April 1977. Updated June 1994.

8.02   The previous Opinion 8.02, "Clinics," was deleted in June 1994.

8.02 Ethical Guidelines for Physicians in Administrative or Other Nonclinical Roles

The practice of medicine focuses primarily on diagnosis and treatment of disease and injury, but its concerns extend broadly to include human experiences related to health and illness. Throughout their formal education and their practice of medicine, physicians profess and are therefore held to standards of medical ethics and professionalism, such as those expressed in the AMA Code of Medical Ethics. Complying with these standards enables physicians to earn the trust of their patients and the general public. Trust is essential to successful healing relationships and, therefore, to the practice of medicine.

The ethical obligations of physicians are not suspended when a physician assumes a position that does not directly involve patient care. Rather, these obligations are binding on physicians in nonclinical roles to the extent that they rely on their medical training, experience, or perspective. When physicians make decisions in nonclinical roles, they should strive to protect the health of individuals and communities.

Issued June 1994 based on the report "Ethical Guidelines for Medical Consultants," adopted December 1992. Updated June 1998. Updated November 2007 based on the report "Physicians in Administrative or Other Non-clinical Roles," adopted June 2007.

Journal 2010 Reviews a book with case studies of controversial issues of bioethics, health law, and human rights. Concludes that, while in many areas bioethics relates to human rights issues, human rights issues not directly involving the conduct of health professionals or human health are not within the scope of expertise of bioethicist. Quotes Opinion 8.02. Rothstein, *Worst Case Bioethics: Death, Disaster, and Public Health, 31 J. Legal Med. 331, 333 (2010).*

Journal 2001 Examines issues relating to health care cost containment. Concludes that, if physicians are to meet the goals assigned to them in a cost-constrained health care system, then professional standards must be reevaluated and modified to afford meaningful guidance for clinical decision-making in the face of health care spending controls. Quotes Opinions 2.03, 2.09, 2.095, 8.032, and 9.04. Cites Opinions 8.02, 8.021, 8.051, and 8.13. Agrawal, *Resuscitating*

Professionalism: Self-regulation in the Medical Marketplace, 66 Mo. L. Rev. 341, 354, 355, 360, 361, 378, 388 (2001).

Journal 2001 Discusses the prohibition on nonlawyer ownership of legal service providers. Considers how ethical rules and standards governing physicians have been directed toward preserving independent judgment. Concludes that ethical conflicts created by abandoning the prohibition on nonlawyer ownership of legal service providers may be managed by following the medical ethics model. Quotes Principle VI and Opinions 2.03, 2.09, 8.02, 8.021, 8.03, 8.05, 8.051, 8.054, 8.13, and 8.132. Harris & Foran, *The Ethics of Middle-Class Access to Legal Services and What We Can Learn From the Medical Profession's Shift to a Corporate Paradigm, 70 Fordham L. Rev. 775, 817, 821, 822, 823, 824 (2001).*

Journal 1999 Discusses the need for physicians to advocate on behalf of patients' rights in the context of health care delivery. Evaluates the nature and scope of the physician's role as advocate, noting that physicians cannot be expected to engage in attorney-like advocacy. Quotes Principles IV and VI, Fundamental Elements (2), (4), and (6) [now Opinion 10.01], Patient Responsibilities 5 [now Opinion 10.02], and Opinions 2.03, 2.07, 2.09, 2.16, 2.19, 3.06, 4.01, 4.04, 6.01, 7.02, 8.02, 8.03, 8.13, 8.132, 9.06, 9.07, and 9.131. Cites Opinions 5.05, 5.09, 7.01, 8.135, and 9.02. Sage, *Physicians as Advocates, 35 Hous. L. Rev. 1529, 1537, 1541, 1542, 1552-53, 1554, 1556, 1557, 1559, 1561-62, 1564, 1571, 1574, 1576, 1580 (1999).*

Journal 1997 Discusses the practice of ex parte communications between treating physicians and their patients' legal adversaries without informing the patient or obtaining consent. Examines harms that may occur in these situations. Argues that Oklahoma needs to prohibit treating physicians from communicating ex parte with their patients' legal adversaries. Quotes Opinions 5.05, 5.07, 5.08, 8.02, 8.03, and 9.07. Cites Opinion 7.02. McNaughton & McNaughton, *Divided Loyalty: The Dilemma of the Treating Physician Advocate, 22 Okla. City U. L. Rev. 1051, 1052, 1054, 1056, 1058, 1059, 1062 (1997).*

8.021 Ethical Obligations of Medical Directors

Assuming a title or position that removes the physician from direct patient-physician relationships does not override professional ethical obligations. The term "medical directors," as used here, refers to physicians who are employed by third-party payers in the health care delivery system (ie, insurance companies, managed care organizations, self-insured employers) or by entities that perform medical appropriateness determinations on behalf of payers. These types of medical directors have specific functions, such as making coverage determinations, which go beyond mere administrative responsibility. The following stem from this understanding.

Whenever physicians employ professional knowledge and values gained through medical training and practice, and in so doing affect individual or group patient care, they are functioning within the professional sphere of physicians and must uphold ethical obligations, including those articulated by the AMA's *Code of Medical Ethics.*

Medical directors acting within the professional sphere, such as when making decisions regarding medical appropriateness, have an overriding ethical obligation to promote professional medical standards. Adherence to professional medical standards includes:

(1) Placing the interests of patients above other considerations, such as personal interests (eg, financial incentives) or employer business interests (eg, profit). This entails applying the plan parameters to each patient equally and engaging in neither discrimination nor favoritism.

(2) Using fair and just criteria when making care-related determinations. This entails contributing professional expertise to help craft plan guidelines

that ensure fair and equal consideration of all plan enrollees. In addition, medical directors should review plan policies and guidelines to ensure that decision-making mechanisms are objective, flexible, and consistent, and apply only ethically appropriate criteria, such as those identified by the Council in Opinion 2.03, "Allocation of Limited Medical Resources."

(3) Working toward achieving access to adequate medical services. This entails encouraging employers to provide services that would be considered part of an adequate level of health care, as articulated in Opinion 2.095, "The Provision of Adequate Health Care." (I, III, VII)

Issued December 1999 based on the report "Ethical Obligations of Medical Directors," adopted June 1999.

Journal 2006 Examines ethical dilemmas physicians may face as providers of pay-for-performance medical care. Concludes that this strategy offers a benefit to patients as long as physicians uphold stringent ethical standards and work together to ensure optimum patient care. Cites Principles I, V, VIII, and IX and Opinions 2.035, 2.095, 6.01, 8.021, 8.03, 8.0501, 8.053, 8.054, and 8.121. Bostick, Sade, & McMahon, *Report of the Council on Ethical and Judicial Affairs: Physician Pay-for-Performance Programs,* 3 Ind. Health L. Rev. 429, 430, 431, 432-33, 434, 435, 436 (2006).

Journal 2001 Examines issues relating to health care cost containment. Concludes that, if physicians are to meet the goals assigned to them in a cost-constrained health care system, then professional standards must be reevaluated and modified to afford meaningful guidance for clinical decision-making in the face of health care spending controls. Quotes Opinions 2.03, 2.09, 2.095, 8.032, and 9.04. Cites Opinions 8.02, 8.021, 8.051, and 8.13. Agrawal, *Resuscitating Professionalism: Self-regulation in the Medical Marketplace,* 66 Mo. L. Rev. 341, 354, 355, 360, 361, 378, 388 (2001).

Journal 2001 Discusses the prohibition on nonlawyer ownership of legal service providers. Considers how ethical rules and standards governing physicians have been directed toward preserving independent judgment. Concludes that ethical conflicts created by abandoning the prohibition on nonlawyer ownership of legal service providers may be managed by following the medical ethics model. Quotes Principle VI and Opinions 2.03, 2.09, 8.02, 8.021, 8.03, 8.05, 8.051, 8.054, 8.13, and 8.132. Harris & Foran, *The Ethics of Middle-Class Access to Legal Services and What We Can Learn From the Medical Profession's Shift to a Corporate Paradigm,* 70 Fordham L. Rev. 775, 817, 821, 822, 823, 824 (2001).

8.03 Conflicts of Interest: Guidelines

Under no circumstances may physicians place their own financial interests above the welfare of their patients. The primary objective of the medical profession is to render service to humanity; reward or financial gain is a subordinate consideration. For a physician to unnecessarily hospitalize a patient, prescribe a drug, or conduct diagnostic tests for the physician's financial benefit is unethical. If a conflict develops between the physician's financial interest and the physician's responsibilities to the patient, the conflict must be resolved to the patient's benefit. (II)

Issued July 1986. Updated June 1994.

7th Cir. 1984 Plaintiff brought medical malpractice suit against several physicians appointed to the Veterans Administration Department of Medicine and Surgery. The court held that strict control test for determining whether defendants ought to be considered employees or independent contractors under the Federal Tort Claims Act was not appropriate because the ethical obligation of a physician to a patient, evidenced by Principle 6 (1957) [now Opinions 8.03 and 8.05], required that independent judgment be exercised, preventing a physician from being strictly controlled by the Veterans Administration. *Quilico v. Kaplan,* 749 F.2d 480, 483-84.

10th Cir. 1983 Pursuant to the Federal Tort Claims Act, plaintiff sued the federal government for the negligence of a neurosurgeon, allegedly an employee of a Veteran's Administration (VA) hospital. Plaintiff argued that applying the traditional control test to determine a physician's employment status was inappropriate because physicians are bound by Principle 6 (1957) [now Opinions 8.03 and 8.05] requiring them to have free and complete exercise of [their] medical judgment and skill. . . . However, the court did not reach the merits of that argument because the contractual agreement between the neurosurgeon and the VA hospital was outside the parameters of an employer-employee relationship with the government, thus precluding plaintiff's claim. *Lurch v. United States, 719 F.2d 333, 337, cert. denied, 466 US 927 (1984).*

N.D. Ill. 2010 Sister of deceased patient brought adversary proceeding against bankrupt physician to except from discharge debt stemming from physician's alleged breach of fiduciary duties. The bankruptcy court quotes Opinions 7.01 and 8.03 in finding that a fiduciary duty was established by nature of the physician-patient relationship that continued after patient's death. *In re Odeh, 431 B.R. 807, 814.*

N.D. Ill. 2008 Administrator of the estate of patient filed suit under the Federal Tort Claims Act and state wrongful death act after patient died as a result of a mistake during surgery at Veteran's Administration (VA) hospital. Defendant physician moved to dismiss on the grounds that, as a federal employee, she was exempt from personal liability for services performed within the scope of her employment at the VA. The court cited earlier case quoting Principle 6 (1957) [now Opinions 8.03 and 8.05] and determining that, because physicians are free to choose whom to serve, they are not federal employees and the strict control test may not be appropriate. Finding issues of fact to resolve, the court denied the defendant's motion for summary judgment. *Monroe v. United States, 2008 U.S. Dist. LEXIS 22455, 9.*

Army Crim. App. 2004 Appellant, in a general court martial hearing, was found guilty of unpremeditated murder. The Court of Appeals for the Armed Forces set aside and remanded the judgment to the Army Court of Criminal Appeals to determine whether there was a conflict of interest in allowing mental health providers who had a prior psychotherapist-patient relationship with the appellant to serve on his sanity board. The court determined there was no conflict of interest. In making this determination, the court quoted Opinion 10.015 and cited Opinion 8.03 to analyze the aspects of the physician-patient relationship. *United States v. Best, 59 M.J. 886, 891 n. 8.*

Cal. App. 1967 Physician-stockholders of publicly owned pharmaceutical corporations and physicians whose medical partnerships owned and operated pharmacies challenged statutory prohibition of physician membership, proprietory interest, and co-ownership of pharmacies. The court quoted Principles Ch. I, Sec. 6 (1947) and a 1960 Judicial Council rule, later included in Opinions and Reports of the Judicial Council Sec. 7, Para. 38 (1965) [now Opinions 8.03, 8.032, and 8.06] in its discussion of the potential conflict of interest created by such ownership. The court held that the statute prohibited physician partnerships from directly owning pharmacies but did not apply to an individual physician or a partnership of physicians who own stock in a corporation which owns and operates a pharmacy. *Magan Medical Clinic v. California State Bd. of Medical Examiners, 249 Cal. App. 2d 124, 57 Cal. Rptr. 256, 262.*

Mich. Att'y Gen. 1977 State attorney general determined that, within limits, it was not illegal for physicians to refer patient specimens to clinical laboratories which they own or in which they have a financial interest. Opinion observes, however, that, under the Opinions and Reports of the Judicial Council Sec. 7, Paras. 21 and 22 (1972) [now Opinions 8.03 and 8.032] such referrals may be unethical. *Mich. Att'y Gen. Opinion No. 5229, 1977-78 Att'y. Gen. Op. 234.*

Miss. 2003 Patient's estate appealed summary judgment in favor of physician and hospital in wrongful death action. Supreme Court affirmed, holding that physician was a state employee and that purchase of liability insurance did not waive immunity. In examining physician's status, the court found that the exercise of professional judgment and discretion are not determinative of employment status. Quotes Principle 6 (1957) [now Opinions 8.03 and 8.05]. *Corey v. Skelton, 834 So.2d 681, 685.*

Miss. 2002 Plaintiff in malpractice action appealed grant of summary judgment in favor of neurosurgeon who allegedly performed a thoracic diskectomy on the wrong disk. A resident performed the patient's physical and wrote the majority of the chart notes. The Mississippi Supreme Court affirmed the lower court. The court held that as a state employee the physician was immune from liability and that his exercise of professional judgment in treating patients did not change his status and insurance did not waive immunity. Quotes Principle 6 (1957) [now Opinions 8.03 and 8.05]. *Clayton v. Harkey, 826 So.2d 1283, 1287.*

Miss. 2001 Patient filed suit asserting that a physician was negligent in performing surgery. The trial court granted the physician's summary judgment motion and held that the physician, employed by a state university medical center, was immune under state law. Finding genuine issues of fact, the state Supreme Court reversed and remanded the case for further proceedings. In a separate opinion, one justice quoted Principle 6 (1957) [now Opinions 8.03 and 8.05], in evaluating the degree of control exercised by the state over the physician. This justice, stressing that the physician exercised discretion in treating the patient independent of the state's control, found no basis to hold the physician an employee for immunity purposes. *Conley v. Warren, 797 So. 2d 881, 886.*

Miss. 2000 Beneficiaries of patient's estate appealed summary judgment in malpractice action for a physician on sovereign immunity grounds. The court reversed and remanded the case finding issues of fact to be resolved at trial. The majority set out a five-part test to determine the employment status of a physician working at a state health care facility, including the degree of control and direction exercised by the state over the physician. In a separate opinion one justice quoted Principle 6 (1957) [now Opinions 8.03 and 8.05], stating that, "A physician should not dispose of his services under terms or conditions which tend to interfere with or impair the free and complete exercise of his medical judgment and skill. . . ." This justice reasoned that the physician could not claim the state controlled his medical discretion or treatment of patients and thus was clearly not an employee entitled to immunity. *Miller v. Meeks, 762 So. 2d 302, 314.*

Miss. 2000 Patient brought a medical malpractice action against physicians after receiving treatment at a state university medical center. The jury returned a verdict against the physicians. The Mississippi Supreme Court reversed, finding that the physicians were immune from liability as state employees. In determining the status of the physicians, the court noted that the physicians retained a considerable amount of professional discretion in treating the patient, quoting Principle 6 (1957) [now Opinions 8.03 and 8.05]. However, this alone was not determinative, and in the court's view the physicians were state employees. *Sullivan v. Washington, 768 So. 2d 881, 885.*

Miss. App. 2003 Patient brought malpractice action against physicians working at a state university teaching hospital. Patient argued that the physicians were independent contractors and sovereign immunity did not apply. Appellate court, citing the Mississippi Supreme Court's decision in *Miller v. Mecks, 762 So.2d 302 (Miss. 2000)*, affirmed the trial court and held that sovereign immunity applied because the physicians were state employees. Quotes Principle 6 (1957) [now Opinions 8.03 and 8.05]. *Brown v. Warren, 858 So.2d 168, 175 (2003).*

Ohio Att'y Gen. 1999 State attorney general concluded that physicians who render opinions regarding the necessity of medical services for health insuring corporations are not engaged in the practice of medicine. Additionally, physicians who render opinions regarding medical necessity for appeals of adverse determinations do not fall under the regulatory, investigatory, or enforcement authority of the Ohio State Medical Board. Quoting Opinions 8.03, 8.11, and 8.13, the attorney general stated that physicians have an ethical duty to provide appropriate treatment for patients. *Ohio Att'y Gen. Op. No. 99-044, 1999 WL 692623.*

Journal 2009 Explores the nature of the physician-patient relationship and the impact of increased availability of medical information on patient autonomy and physician responsibility to exercise independent judgment. Concludes physicians must treat patients in accordance with their fiduciary obligation to use their own judgment when confronted with a patient demanding unnecessary medical services. Quotes Preamble, Principles I and VIII, and Opinions 2.035, 8.03, and 10.015. Hafemeister, *The Fiduciary Obligation of Physicians to "Just Say No" if an "Informed" Patient Demands Services That Are Not Medically Indicated, 39 Seton Hall L. Rev. 335, 372, 373, 374 (2009).*

Journal 2007 Analyzes scientific, ethical, and legal issues raised in the exhumation and genetic analysis of historical figures. Concludes that biohistorical review boards should be created to generate guidelines for such research. Quotes Preamble and Opinion 2.08. Cites Opinions 2.079, 2.105, 5.05, 5.051, 5.075, 8.03, 8.031, 9.095, and 9.10. Paradise & Andrews, *Tales From the Crypt: Scientific, Ethical, and Legal Considerations for Biohistorical Analysis of Deceased Historical Figures, 26 Temp. J. Sci. Tech. & Envtl. L. 223, 287-88 (2007).*

Journal 2006 Examines ethical dilemmas physicians may face as providers of pay-for-performance medical care. Concludes that this strategy offers a benefit to patients as long as physicians uphold stringent ethical standards and work together to ensure optimum patient care. Cites Principles I, V, VIII, and IX and Opinions 2.035, 2.095, 6.01, 8.021, 8.03, 8.0501, 8.053, 8.054, and 8.121. Bostick, Sade, & McMahon, *Report of the Council on Ethical and Judicial Affairs: Physician Pay-for-Performance Programs, 3 Ind. Health L. Rev. 429, 430, 431, 432-33, 434, 435, 436 (2006).*

Journal 2006 Discusses the prevalence and cause of physicians' failure to provide proper care. Concludes that patients should be able to sue their physicians for breach of fiduciary duty. Quotes Principle VIII and Opinion 8.03. Mehlman, *Dishonest Medical Mistakes*, 59 *Vand. L. Rev.* 1137, *1144 (2006).*

Journal 2003 Discusses the practice of gainsharing and argues that providing physicians and hospitals with certain financial incentives to reduce health costs may be of value in health care reform. Concludes with suggestions for how best to proceed in this difficult context. Quotes Opinion 2.03, 2.09, 4.04, and 8.03. References Opinion 8.13. Saver, *Squandering the Gain: Gainsharing and the Continuing Dilemma of Physician Financial Incentives*, 98 *Nw. U. L. Rev.* 145, *219, 221, 222 (2003).*

Journal 2003 Discusses conflicts of interest caused when managed care organizations provide financial incentives to physicians. Concludes that the focus of managed care is not well-suited for the doctor-patient relationship. Quotes Opinion 8.03. Cites Principle VII. References Opinion 8.051. Hall, *Bargaining With Hippocrates: Managed Care and the Doctor-Patient Relationship*, 54 *S. C. L. Rev.* 689, 696, 735 (2003).

Journal 2002 Examines how managed care has adversely affected information disclosure in the physician-patient relationship. Concludes that, unless courts expand applicability of principles of informed consent, patient self-determination and autonomy will continue to be undermined. Quotes Principle VIII and Opinions 8.03, 8.053, 8.054, and 8.08. Morris, *Dissing Disclosure: Just What the Doctor Ordered*, 44 *Ariz. L. Rev.* 313, 344, 349, 362, 363, 366 (2002).

Journal 2001 Considers conflicts of interest in clinical research and other types of medical practice. Compares the way in which doctors and lawyers address conflicts of interest in professional practice. Concludes that physicians are unaware of the need to create a meaningful conflict-of-interest doctrine for medical practice. Quotes Preamble, Principle IV, and Opinions 2.07, 8.03, 8.031, and 10.01. Moore, *What Doctors Can Learn From Lawyers About Conflicts of Interest*, 81 *B. U. L. Rev.* 445, 447, 449-50 (2001).

Journal 2001 Examines financial conflict of interest issues that arise in the context of clinical research. Concludes that open communication among stakeholders is necessary to resolve these issues. Quotes Opinions 8.03 and 8.031. Rose, *Financial Conflicts of Interest: How Are We Managing?* 8 *Wid. L. Symp. J.* 1, 24 (2001).

Journal 2000 Discusses patent law and policy. Examines whether or not those who practice medicine should be excused from patent laws because of the conflict that medical procedure patents create with respect to the practice of medicine. Concludes that Congress should repeal section 287(c) of the Patent Act. Quotes Principle V and Opinions 9.08 and 9.09. Cites Opinion 8.03. References Opinion 10.01. Ho, *Patents, Patients, and Public Policy: An Incomplete Intersection at 35 USC § 287(c)*, 33 *U. C. Davis L. Rev.* 601, 603, 623, 624, 625, 631 (2000).

Journal 2000 Examines issues relating to parental consent to circumcision. Identifies legal and ethical requirements for consent when medical professionals are treating adult patients. Analyzes the implications of those requirements for routine circumcision of infant males. Concludes that only when the male is an adult and capable of making decisions can circumcision be ethically and legally performed. Quotes Opinion 8.08. References Opinions 8.03 and 9.011. Svoboda, Van Howe, & Dwyer, *Informed Consent for Neonatal Circumcision: An Ethical and Legal Conundrum*, 17 *J. Contemp. Health L. & Pol'y* 61, 67, 73, 82 (2000).

Journal 1999 Asserts that patient autonomy is closely linked to patient-doctor discourse. Proposes a constitutional framework for evaluating how governmental regulations may interfere with such discourse. Concludes by emphasizing the importance of protecting the quality of doctor-patient discourse. Quotes Preamble and Opinion 8.03. Gatter, *Protecting Patient-Doctor Discourse: Informed Consent and Deliberative Autonomy*, 78 *Or. L. Rev.* 941, 956 (1999).

Journal 1999 Explores ethical and legal issues surrounding physician incentives in managed care. Concludes that successful ERISA claims for breach of fiduciary duty will hold managed care organizations accountable for controlling medical costs. Quotes Opinion 8.03. Marsh, *Sacrificing Patients for Profits: Physician Incentives to Limit Care and ERISA Fiduciary Duty*, 77 *Wash. U. L. Q.* 1323, 1332 (1999).

Journal 1999 Discusses the need for physicians to advocate on behalf of patients' rights in the context of health care delivery. Evaluates the nature and scope of the physician's role as advocate, noting that physicians cannot be expected to engage in attorney-like advocacy. Quotes Principles IV and VI, Fundamental Elements (2), (4), and (6) [now Opinion 10.01], Patient

Responsibilities 5 [now Opinion 10.02], and Opinions 2.03, 2.07, 2.09, 2.16, 2.19, 3.06, 4.01, 4.04, 6.01, 7.02, 8.02, 8.03, 8.13, 8.132, 9.06, 9.07, and 9.131. Cites Opinions 5.05, 5.09, 7.01, 8.135, and 9.02. Sage, *Physicians as Advocates*, 35 Hous. L. Rev. 1529, 1537, 1541, 1542, 1552-53, 1554, 1556, 1557, 1559, 1561-62, 1564, 1571, 1574, 1576, 1580 (1999).

Journal 1999 Explores the impact managed care organizations have had on health care. Explains that patients may not understand restrictions and incentives imposed by their managed care organizations when entering the program. Argues that such information should be disclosed at various times during the period of plan coverage. Cites Opinions 2.03, 8.03, 8.032, 8.051, 8.13, and 8.132. Wolf, *Toward a Systemic Theory of Informed Consent in Managed Care*, 35 Hous. L. Rev. 1631, 1641, 1658, 1661, 1662, 1679 (1999).

Journal 1998 Discusses conflicts of interest in the physician-patient relationship arising out of use of financial incentives by managed care organizations. Considers how such conflicts are dealt with in the attorney-client relationship. Suggests that a financial incentive should be legally denounced if it unreasonably interferes with a physician's duty to properly care for and treat patients. Quotes Preamble, Fundamental Elements (1) [now Opinion 10.01], and Opinions 4.04, 5.01, 8.03, 8.13, and 9.06. Cites Fundamental Elements (4) [now Opinion 10.01] and Opinions 2.07, 2.08, and 2.132. Hall, *Third-Party Payor Conflicts of Interest in Managed Care: A Proposal for Regulation Based on the Model Rules of Professional Conduct*, 29 Seton Hall L. Rev. 95, 96, 107, 108, 109, 110, 111, 112, 134, 135, 136 (1998).

Journal 1998 Discusses the physician's fiduciary duty to the patient. Explores the expansion of the "honest services" mail fraud statute to prosecute undisclosed fiduciary breaches. Concludes that the mail fraud statute may be used to prosecute physicians who fail to disclose financial incentives to their patients. Quotes Opinion 8.03. Cites Opinions 2.03 and 8.07 [now Opinion 8.06]. Jones, *Primum Non Nocere: The Expanding "Honest Services" Mail Fraud Statute and the Physician-Patient Fiduciary Relationship*, 51 Vand. L. Rev. 139, 161, 164 (1998).

Journal 1998 Explores aspects of trust in physician-patient relations. Discusses the transformation of the health care system and the need for regulation. Points out that too much involvement by politicians and legislators will put the health care system at risk. References Opinions 6.02 and 8.03. Mechanic, *The Functions and Limitations of Trust in the Provision of Medical Care*, 23 J. Health Pol. Pol'y & Law 661, 667 (1998).

Journal 1997 Discusses physician-patient trust in the managed care environment. Explores options for enhancing trustworthiness in this context. Quotes Opinion 8.03. Gray, *Trust and Trustworthy Care in the Managed Care Era*, 16 Health Affairs 34, 38, 47-48 (1997).

Journal 1997 Discusses the practice of ex parte communications between treating physicians and their patients' legal adversaries without informing the patient or obtaining consent. Examines harms that may occur in these situations. Argues that Oklahoma needs to prohibit treating physicians from communicating ex parte with their patients' legal adversaries. Quotes Opinions 5.05, 5.07, 5.08, 8.02, 8.03, and 9.07. Cites Opinion 7.02. McNaughton & McNaughton, *Divided Loyalty: The Dilemma of the Treating Physician Advocate*, 22 Okla. City U. L. Rev. 1051, 1052, 1054, 1056, 1058, 1059, 1062 (1997).

Journal 1995 Addresses presidential disability, its past impact on American government, and possible solutions to potential problems. Proposes enhancement of the role of the President's physician. Quotes Opinion 8.03. Cites Opinions 5.04 and 5.05. Abrams, *The Vulnerable President and the Twenty-Fifth Amendment, With Observations on Guidelines, a Health Commission, and the Role of the President's Physician*, 30 Wake Forest L. Rev. 453, 466, 471 (1995).

Journal 1994 Discusses the issue of whom physicians must serve first: themselves, their patients, insurers, or society. Focuses on risks arising out of provider economic arrangements and risks arising out of other individual physician characteristics. Quotes Opinions 8.03 and 9.13. Cites Opinion 8.15. Bobinski, *Autonomy and Privacy: Protecting Patients From Their Physicians*, 55 U. Pitt. L. Rev. 291, 302, 313 (1994).

Journal 1994 Observes that health care reform proposals present significant challenges to the role and ethics of attending physicians. Emphasizes that reform proposals must set forth the role envisioned for physicians and must articulate an acceptable ethical framework within which physicians may fulfill that role. Quotes Opinions 4.04, 9.121, and 9.122. Cites Opinions 2.03, 2.09, 5.01, and 8.03. Wolf, *Health Care Reform and the Future of Physician Ethics*, 24 Hastings Center Rep. 28, 32, 40 (March/April 1994).

Journal 1993 Discusses the problem of physicians withholding needed medical treatment from HIV-infected infants. Concludes that current law should be expanded to eliminate this discrimination. Quotes Opinions 2.09, 2.17, 2.20, 2.22, 4.04, and 8.03. Crossley, *Of Diagnoses and Discrimination: Discriminatory Nontreatment of Infants With HIV Infection,* 93 Columbia L. Rev. 1581, 1620, 1621 (1993).

Journal 1992 Examines issues related to the responsibility of HIV-infected health care workers to protect patients from infection, including mandatory testing, disclosure to coworkers and supervisors, and the degree to which the practice of an HIV-infected health care worker should be modified. Concludes that courts likely will impose a requirement to disclose HIV-positive status to patients when there is a substantial risk of HIV transmission. Quotes Opinions 8.03 (1989) [now Opinion 8.032] and 8.07 (1989) [now Opinion 8.03]. References Opinion 9.131. Lieberman & Derse, *HIV-Positive Health Care Workers and the Obligation to Disclose: Do Patients Have a Right to Know?* 13 J. Legal Med. 333, 353, 354 (1992).

Journal 1990 Explains how the federal Medicare and Medicaid Anti-Fraud and Abuse statute limits the ability of physicians to adapt investment and referral strategies to an increasingly competitive health care marketplace. Proposes giving regulatory power over physician investments back to the states, which are more able to recognize and exempt beneficial arrangements from otherwise restrictive statutory schemes. Cites Opinion 8.03. Comment, *Regulating Physician Investment and Referral Behavior in the Competitive Health Care Marketplace of the '90s—An Argument for Decentralization,* 65 Wash. L. Rev. 657, 658 (1990).

Journal 1990 Examines various cost-control mechanisms utilized by prepaid health plans and other managed care programs and considers the impact of such mechanisms on clinical decision making. Emphasis is placed on the possible existence of conflicts of interest on the part of health care providers in this context. Quotes Opinions 8.03 [now Opinions 8.03 and 8.032] and 8.13 [now Opinion 8.132]. Hirshfeld, *Defining Full and Fair Disclosure in Managed Care Contracts,* 60 The Citation 67, 70 (1990).

Journal 1990 Discusses efforts of third-party payers to control health care expenditures for beneficiaries. Concludes that financial incentives to limit care and other cost-control techniques should be disclosed and that the rationale for such disclosure is compelling. Quotes Opinions 2.03, 2.09, and 8.03 [now Opinions 8.03 and 8.032]. Cites Opinions 2.19, 4.04, and 4.06. Hirshfeld, *Should Third Party Payors of Health Care Services Disclose Cost Control Mechanisms to Potential Beneficiaries?* 14 Seton Hall Legis. J. 115, 130, 131, 144, 145, 146 (1990).

Journal 1989 Analyzes the Medicare and Medicaid Patient and Program Protection Act of 1987 and discusses the complexity of fraud and abuse issues that confront hospitals and health care providers who undertake financially attractive business arrangements. Concludes that the 1987 Act, along with its implementing regulations, can offer meaningful guidance in an area of uncertainty for the health care industry. Quotes Opinion 4.05 (1986) [now Opinion 8.03]. Comment, *Curing the Health Care Industry: Government Response to Medicare Fraud and Abuse,* 5 J. Contemp. Health L. & Pol'y 175, 189 (1989).

Journal 1985 Initially describes how existing doctrines protect the value of autonomy in the context of the physician-patient relationship, then examines various problems in the current protective scheme. Concludes by recommending the creation of an independent articulable protected interest in patient autonomy. Quotes Principles II and IV. Cites Opinions 4.04 (1984) [now Opinions 8.03 and 8.032] and 6.03 (1984) [now Opinion 6.02]. Shultz, *From Informed Consent to Patient Choice: A New Protected Interest,* 95 Yale L. J. 219, 275 (1985).

8.031 Conflicts of Interest: Biomedical Research

Avoidance of real or perceived conflicts of interest in clinical research is imperative if the medical community is to ensure objectivity and maintain individual and institutional integrity. All medical centers should develop specific guidelines for their clinical staff on conflicts of interest. These guidelines should include the following rules:

(1) Once a clinical investigator becomes involved in a research project for a company or knows that he or she might become involved, she or he, as an individual, cannot ethically buy or sell the company's stock until the

involvement ends and the results of the research are published or otherwise disseminated to the public;

(2) Any remuneration received by the researcher from the company whose product is being studied must be commensurate with the efforts of the researcher on behalf of the company; and

(3) Clinical investigators should disclose any material ties to companies whose products they are investigating, including financial ties, participation in educational activities supported by the companies, participation in other research projects funded by the companies, consulting arrangements, and any other ties. The disclosures should be made in writing to the medical center where the research is conducted, organizations that are funding the research, and journals that publish the results of the research. An explanatory statement that discloses conflicts of interest should accompany all published research. Other types of publications, such as a letters to the editor, should also include an explanatory statement that discloses any potential conflict of interest.

In addition, medical centers should form review committees to examine disclosures by clinical staff about financial associations with commercial corporations. (II, IV)

Issued March 1992 based on the report "Conflicts of Interest in Biomedical Research," adopted December 1989 (JAMA. 1990;263:2790-2793). Updated June 1999 based on the report "Conflicts of Interest: Biomedical Research," adopted December 1998.

Journal 2011 Reviews the responsible conduct of research (RCR) domains of publication practices and authorship, conflicts of interest, and research misconduct. Concludes that because the accuracy, completeness and value of the scientific record impacts the health of society, scientists are obligated to use the highest possible standards of research conduct. Quotes Principle VIII and Opinion 8.031. Horner & Minifie, *Research Ethics III: Publication Practices and Authorship, Conflicts of Interest, and Research Misconduct, 54 J. Speech, Language, & Hearing Res. S346, S351, S352 (2011).*

Journal 2008 Examines the ethical issues surrounding stem cell research. Concludes science, religion, and politics are all important in appropriately addressing the ethics of scientific innovation. Cites Opinion 8.031. Packer, *Embryonic Stem Cells, Intellectual Property, and Patents: Ethical Concerns, 37 Hofstra L. Rev. 487, 495 (2008).*

Journal 2007 Analyzes scientific, ethical, and legal issues raised in the exhumation and genetic analysis of historical figures. Concludes that biohistorical review boards should be created to generate guidelines for such research. Quotes Preamble and Opinion 2.08. Cites Opinions 2.079, 2.105, 5.05, 5.051, 5.075, 8.03, 8.031, 9.095, and 9.10. Paradise & Andrews, *Tales From the Crypt: Scientific, Ethical, and Legal Considerations for Biohistorical Analysis of Deceased Historical Figures, 26 Temp. J. Sci. Tech. & Envtl. L. 223, 287-88 (2007).*

Journal 2005 Discusses ethical, legal, and policy issues associated with treatment and research involving patients who are in a persistent vegetative or minimally conscious state. Concludes that patients in these states are at risk for therapeutic failures until physicians can more accurately determine which patients will benefit from treatment and accurately convey such information to families or surrogates. Quotes Principles VII and IX and Opinions 8.031, 8.0315, 9.065, 10.01, and 10.015. Tovino & Winslade, *A Primer on the Law and Ethics of Treatment, Research, and Public Policy in the Context of Severe Traumatic Brain Injury, 14 Ann. Health L. 1, 18, 38, 39, 40, 41 (2005).*

Journal 2004 Examines the requirements of the Privacy Rule regarding use and disclosure of a patient's identifiable health information in the context of research. Concludes that the Rule's burdensome administrative requirements may discourage research and thus outweigh any benefits for research subject autonomy. Quotes Principle VIII and Opinions 5.051, 8.031, and 10.015. Tovino, *The Use and Disclosure of Protected Health Information for Research Under the HIPAA*

Privacy Rule: Unrealized Patient Autonomy and Burdensome Government Regulation, 49 S. D. L. Rev. 447, 496, 502 (2004).

Journal 2003 Discusses financial incentive programs for physicians who enroll patients in clinical trials. Concludes that more regulatory oversight is needed to protect research subjects and the integrity of the medical research process. Quotes Opinion 6.03 and 8.031. Lemmens & Miller, *The Human Subjects Trade: Ethical and Legal Issues Surrounding Recruitment Incentives, 31 J. L. Med. & Ethics 398, 407 (2003).*

Journal 2002 Considers the implications of using pharmacogenomics in drug development and health care delivery. Emphasizes various legal, economic, and social issues. Concludes that these issues must be meaningfully addressed given the benefits of pharmacogenomics. Cites Opinion 8.031. Malinowski, *Law, Policy, and Market Implications of Genetic Profiling in Drug Development, 2 Hous. J. Health L. & Pol'y 31, 51 (2002).*

Journal 2002 Discusses ethical and legal issues involving acquisition of biological specimens by commercial biobanks. Sets forth areas of inquiry for institutional review boards in evaluating the propriety of research collaborations with commercial biobanks. Cites Opinion 8.031. Rothstein, *The Role of IRBs in Research Involving Commercial Biobanks, 30 J. Law Med. & Ethics 105, 106, 108 (2002).*

Journal 2001 Explores institutional conflicts of interest arising from the impact of biotechnology and the genetics revolution on clinical research. Concludes that federal oversight changes should be implemented in order to maintain the public's trust in health science. Quotes Opinion 8.031. Malinowski, *Conflicts of Interest in Clinical Research: Legal and Ethical Issues: Institutional Conflicts and Responsibilities in an Age of Academic-Industry Alliances, 8 Wid. L. Symp. J. 47, 70 (2001).*

Journal 2001 Considers conflicts of interest in clinical research and other types of medical practice. Compares the way in which doctors and lawyers address conflicts of interest in professional practice. Concludes that physicians are unaware of the need to create a meaningful conflict-of-interest doctrine for medical practice. Quotes Preamble, Principle IV, and Opinions 2.07, 8.03, 8.031, and 10.01. Moore, *What Doctors Can Learn From Lawyers About Conflicts of Interest, 81 B. U. L. Rev. 445, 447, 449-50 (2001).*

Journal 2001 Examines financial conflict of interest issues that arise in the context of clinical research. Concludes that open communication among stakeholders is necessary to resolve these issues. Quotes Opinions 8.03 and 8.031. Rose, *Financial Conflicts of Interest: How Are We Managing? 8 Wid. L. Symp. J. 1, 24 (2001).*

Journal 1996 Explores biotechnology advances made possible through cooperation between universities and industries. Observes that clinical investigators involved in company research are ethically prohibited from buying or selling company stock, until results are published. Concludes that cooperation in the biotechnology field will benefit society. Cites Opinion 8.031. Comment, *Alliances for the Future: Cultivating a Cooperative Environment for Biotech Success, 11 Berkeley Tech. L. J. 311, 344 (1996).*

Journal 1991 Considers whether patients should be permitted or required to pay for research in which they participate. Concludes that patient-funded research may be useful, so long as the potential for individual harm and abuse can be minimized. References Opinion 8.031. Morreim, *Patient-Funded Research: Paying the Piper or Protecting the Patient? 13 IRB 1, 2 (May/June 1991).*

Journal 1991 Discusses the ethical issues involved when physicians and scientists enroll patients in drug company–sponsored clinical trials in exchange for reimbursement. Concludes that financial arrangements between drug companies and scientists give the appearance and the opportunity for conflict of interest; thus physicians should be required to disclose funding sources to patients. References Opinion 8.031. Shimm & Spece, *Conflict of Interest and Informed Consent in Industry-Sponsored Clinical Trials, 12 J. Legal Med. 477, 481, 507, 510 (1991).*

8.0315 Managing Conflicts of Interest in the Conduct of Clinical Trials

As the biotechnology and pharmaceutical industries continue to expand research activities and funding of clinical trials, and as increasing numbers of physicians both within and outside academic health centers become involved in partnerships with industry to perform these activities, greater safeguards against conflicts of interest are needed to ensure the integrity of the research and to protect the welfare of human subjects. Physicians should be mindful of the conflicting roles of investigator and clinician and of the financial conflicts of interest that arise from incentives to conduct trials and to recruit subjects. In particular, physicians involved in clinical research should heed the following guidelines:

(1) Physicians should agree to participate as investigators in clinical trials only when it relates to their scope of practice and area of medical expertise. They should have adequate training in the conduct of research and should participate only in protocols which they are satisfied are scientifically sound.

(2) Physicians should be familiar with the ethics of research and should agree to participate in trials only if they are satisfied that an institutional review board has reviewed the protocol, that the research does not impose undue risks upon research subjects, and that the research conforms to government regulations.

(3) When a physician has treated or continues to treat a patient who is eligible to enroll as a subject in a clinical trial that the physician is conducting, the informed consent process must differentiate between the physician's roles as clinician and investigator. This is best achieved when someone other than the treating physician obtains the participant's informed consent to participate in the trial. This individual should be protected from the pressures of financial incentives, as described in the following section.

(4) Any financial compensation received from trial sponsors must be commensurate with the efforts of the physician performing the research. Financial compensation should be at fair market value and the rate of compensation per patient should not vary according to the volume of subjects enrolled by the physician, and should meet other existing legal requirements. Furthermore, according to Opinion 6.03, "Fee Splitting: Referral to Health Care Facilities," it is unethical for physicians to accept payment solely for referring patients to research studies.

(5) Physicians should ensure that protocols include provisions for the funding of subjects' medical care in the event of complications associated with the research. Also, a physician should not bill a third-party payer when he or she has received funds from a sponsor to cover the additional expenses related to conducting the trial.

(6) The nature and source of funding and financial incentives offered to the investigators must be disclosed to a potential participant as part of the informed consent process. Disclosure to participants also should include information on uncertainties that may exist regarding funding of treatment for possible complications that may arise during the course of the trial. Physicians should ensure that such disclosure is included in any written informed consent.

(7) When entering into a contract to perform research, physicians should ensure themselves that the presentation or publication of results will not be unduly delayed or otherwise obstructed by the sponsoring company. (II, V)

Issued June 2001 based on the report "Managing Conflicts of Interest in the Conduct of Clinical Trials," adopted December 2000 (JAMA. 2002;287:78-84).

Journal 2005 Discusses ethical, legal, and policy issues associated with treatment and research involving patients who are in a persistent vegetative or minimally conscious state. Concludes that patients in these states are at risk for therapeutic failures until physicians can more accurately determine which patients will benefit from treatment and accurately convey such information to families or surrogates. Quotes Principles VII and IX and Opinions 8.031, 8.0315, 9.065, 10.01, and 10.015. Tovino & Winslade, *A Primer on the Law and Ethics of Treatment, Research, and Public Policy in the Context of Severe Traumatic Brain Injury*, 14 Ann. Health L. 1, 18, 38, 39, 40, 41 (2005).

Journal 2004 Discusses the effect of state regulatory requirements on drug companies conducting clinical research. Concludes that, although FDA requirements are compelling, drug companies also must carefully consider applicable state regulations. Quotes Opinion 8.0315. Gibbs, *State Regulation of Pharmaceutical Clinical Trials*, 59 Food & Drug L. J. 265, 279 (2004).

Journal 2004 Evaluates weaknesses in institutional review board (IRB) protection of human subjects. Concludes that one vehicle for enhancing human subjects protection is to hold IRBs legally accountable for negligent conduct. Cites Opinions 2.071, 2.075, and 8.0315. Noah, *Bioethical Malpractice: Risk and Responsibility in Human Research*, 7 J. Health Care L. & Pol'y 175, 183, 235 (2004).

8.032   The previous Opinion 8.032, "Conflicts of Interest: Health Facility Ownership by a Physician," issued prior to 1977, was deleted and replaced by the current Opinion 8.0321, "Physicians' Self-referral."

8.0321 Physicians' Self-referral

Business arrangements among physicians in the health care marketplace have the potential to benefit patients by enhancing quality of care and access to health care services. However, these arrangements can also be ethically challenging when they create opportunities for self-referral in which patients' medical interests can be in tension with physicians' financial interests. Such arrangements can undermine a robust commitment to professionalism in medicine as well as trust in the profession.

In general, physicians should not refer patients to a health care facility that is outside their office practice and at which they do not directly provide care or services when they have a financial interest in that facility. Physicians who enter into legally permissible contractual relationships—including acquisition of ownership or investment interests in health facilities, products, or equipment; or contracts for service in group practices—are expected to uphold their responsibilities to patients first. When physicians enter into arrangements that provide opportunities for self-referral they must:

(1) Ensure that referrals are based on objective, medically relevant criteria.

(2) Ensure that the arrangement:

  (a) is structured to enhance access to appropriate, high quality health care services or products; and

  (b) within the constraints of applicable law:

    (i) does not require physician-owners/investors to make referrals to the entity or otherwise generate revenues as a condition of participation;

    (ii) does not prohibit physician-owners/investors from participating in or referring patients to competing facilities or services; and

      (iii) adheres to fair business practices vis-à-vis the medical professional community—for example, by ensuring that the arrangement does not prohibit investment by nonreferring physicians.

(3) Take steps to mitigate conflicts of interest, including:

    (a) ensuring that financial benefit is not dependent on the physician-owner/investor's volume of referrals for services or sales of products;

    (b) establishing mechanisms for utilization review to monitor referral practices; and

    (c) identifying or if possible making alternate arrangements for care of the patient when conflicts cannot be appropriately managed/mitigated.

(4) Disclose their financial interest in the facility, product, or equipment to patients; inform them of available alternatives for referral; and assure them that their ongoing care is not conditioned on accepting the recommended referral. (II, III, VIII)

Issued June 2009 based on the report "Physicians' Self-referral," adopted November 2008.

C.D. Ill. 1992 A contractual agreement between a clinic and hospital providing undisclosed financial incentives for referrals constituted a "business" aspect of the medical profession and was not exempt from state's Consumer Fraud Act. Reference is made to Council on Ethical Judicial Affairs, Conflicts of Interest Physician Ownership of Medical Facilities, 267 JAMA 2366 (1992) [now Opinion 8.032], which mandates that a physician disclose his financial interest to his patient when making a referral. *Gadson v. Newman, 807 F. Supp. 1412, 1416.*

E.D. N.Y. 1975 Medical laboratories sought injunction against city's award of exclusive contracts for Medicaid services. The court granted a preliminary injunction and held that the laboratories had a substantial probability of success on the merits of the claim that Medicaid recipients would be deprived of statutory right of free choice of providers. In balancing the equities, the court also noted that the contracts would create an ethical dilemma for physicians who are required to provide patients with free choice of ancillary services under Opinions and Reports of the Judicial Council Sec. 1, Paras. 6 and 14 (1971) [now Opinions 8.032, 8.06, and 9.06]. *Bay Ridge Diagnostic Laboratory, Inc. v. Dumpson, 400 F. Supp. 1104, 1109-10.*

E.D. Va. 1995 Claimants sustained personal injuries when ships collided. In an admiralty action, court had to determine the extent of probable injuries sustained by the claimants. The court observed that a treating physician had referred one of the claimants for tests to a facility in which the physician had a substantial ownership interest. In finding that these tests and procedures were unnecessary and unreasonable, the court quoted Opinion 8.032. *In re Capt. Wool, Inc., 1995 US Dist. LEXIS 20128.*

Cal. App. 1967 Physician-stockholders of publicly owned pharmaceutical corporations and physicians whose medical partnerships owned and operated pharmacies challenged statutory prohibition of physician membership, proprietory interest, and co-ownership of pharmacies. The court quoted Principles Ch. I, Sec. 6 (1947) and a 1960 Judicial Council rule, later included in Opinions and Reports of the Judicial Council Sec. 7, Para. 38 (1965) [now Opinions 8.03, 8.032, and 8.06] in its discussion of the potential conflict of interest created by such ownership. The court held that the statute prohibited physician partnerships from directly owning pharmacies, but did not apply to an individual physician or a partnership of physicians who own stock in a corporation which owns and operates a pharmacy. *Magan Medical Clinic v. California State Bd. of Medical Examiners, 249 Cal. App. 2d 124, 57 Cal. Rptr. 256, 262.*

Mass. Super. 1998 Plaintiff-surgeon filed suit against a medical group practice claiming that the defendants reduced referrals to him because he declined to join the group. Plaintiff claimed that the decline harmed his surgical practice. He alleged that the group's practice of taking 10% of members' income constituted unethical and illegal kickbacks. The court held that the decline in referrals was not connected to plaintiff not being a member of the group. The court also found that the plaintiff had not presented evidence that the decline in referrals harmed his practice. Finally, the court found that the fees paid by members of the group practice were gatekeeper fees rather than referral fees. The court quoted Opinion 6.02, in support of its decision that the defendants' fees did not constitute fee splitting. Further, the court referenced Opinion 8.032

concluding that a self-referral was not necessarily unethical if disclosed to the patient. *Boman v. Southeast Medical Services Group, 1998 WL 1182063, 11-12.*

Mich. Att'y Gen. 1977 State attorney general determined that, within limits, it was not illegal for physicians to refer patient specimens to clinical laboratories which they own or in which they have a financial interest. Opinion observes however that, under the Opinions and Reports of the Judicial Council Sec. 7, Paras. 21 and 22 (1972) [now Opinions 8.03 and 8.032], such referrals may be unethical. *Mich. Att'y Gen. Opinion No. 5229, 1977-78 Att'y. Gen. Op. 234.*

Journal 2006 Discusses physician and attorney financial interests in ancillary businesses. Concludes that such interests are permissible, but that patients and clients should not be referred to any business in which the professional has an interest. Cites Opinion 8.032. Falit, *Ancillary Service and Self-referral Arrangements in the Medical and Legal Professions: Do Current Ethical, Legislative, and Regulatory Policies Adequately Serve the Interests of Patients and Clients? 58 S. C. L. Rev. 371, 373-74 (2006).*

Journal 2006 Reviews legislation and case law governing conscience clauses for medical professionals. Concludes that conscientious objections to providing care should be permitted only when based on accepted principles of medical ethics. Quotes Opinion 2.18 (1986) [now Opinion 2.20]. References Opinion 8.032. Swartz, *"Conscience Clauses" or "Unconscionable Clauses": Personal Beliefs Versus Professional Responsibilities, 6 Yale J. Health Pol'y, L. & Ethics 269, 317, 347 (2006).*

Journal 2005 Analyzes federal and state laws that address concerns associated with physician self-referral. Concludes that additional restrictions are needed to prohibit physicians from referring patients to publicly or privately funded facilities in which physicians have a financial interest. Quotes Opinion 8.032. Bethard, *Physician Self-referral: Beyond Stark II, 43 Brandeis L. J. 465, 468 (2005).*

Journal 2004 Discusses the practice of "economic credentialing," offering an overview of recent legal activity with respect to this controversial practice. Concludes that, despite certain areas of potential risk, it would appear that hospitals may utilize economic criteria when making credentialing decisions. Cites Opinion 8.032. Cohen, *An Examination of the Right of Hospitals to Engage in Economic Credentialing, 77 Temp. L. Rev. 705, 741 (2004).*

Journal 2004 Examines the practice of "self-referral" and various problems associated with regulation of this practice. Concludes that regulatory emphasis should focus on limiting conflicts of interest, particularly as they may arise when physician investors self-refer to specialty hospitals. Quotes Opinion 8.032. Kwiecinski, *Limiting Conflicts of Interest Arising From Physician Investment in Specialty Hospitals, 88 Marq. L. Rev. 413, 414, 428 (2004).*

Journal 2002 Suggests a reconceptualization for bioethics that integrates an analysis of the history of moral change. Concludes that bioethical textbooks should include discussion about the history of bioethics and medical ethics. Quotes Opinion 2.20. References Opinions 6.02, 6.03, 6.04 [now Opinion 8.06], and 8.032. Baker, *Bioethics and History, 27 J. Med. & Phil. 447, 455, 469 (2002).*

Journal 2001 Examines issues relating to health care cost containment. Concludes that, if physicians are to meet the goals assigned to them in a cost-constrained health care system, then professional standards must be reevaluated and modified to afford meaningful guidance for clinical decision-making in the face of health care spending controls. Quotes Opinions 2.03, 2.09, 2.095, 8.032, and 9.04. Cites Opinions 8.02, 8.021, 8.051, and 8.13. Agrawal, *Resuscitating Professionalism: Self-regulation in the Medical Marketplace, 66 Mo. L. Rev. 341, 354, 355, 360, 361, 378, 388 (2001).*

Journal 2001 Considers ethical aspects of physician conflicts of interest in the context of human subjects research. Focuses on conflicts that are associated with clinical trials of new drugs and devices. Concludes by discussing the impact of these conflicts of interest on trust in the physician-patient relationship. References Principle IV and Opinion 8.032. Miller, *Trusting Doctors: Tricky Business When It Comes to Clinical Research, 81 B. U. L. Rev. 423, 427-28 (2001).*

Journal 2000 Examines physician value neutrality (PVN). Defines PVN as providing a foundation to suggest physicians must keep their values—religious, political, or otherwise—out of the patient-physician relationship. Concludes it is not clear how values can be removed from the patient-physician relationship without removing the very thing PVN supporters are trying to protect, the intrinsic value of persons. References Opinions 2.01, 2.02, 8.032, 8.05, 8.08, and

8.132. Beckwith & Peppin, *Physician Value Neutrality: A Critique, 28 J. L. Med. & Ethics 67, 72-73 (2000).*

Journal 2000 Examines justice in health care by focusing on concepts of access and allocation. Presents four principles for the just allocation of health care resources: improving health; informing patients about the manner in which resources are allocated in the context of managed care; affording patients an opportunity to consent to such allocation of resources; and minimization of conflicts of interest. References Opinion 8.032. Emanuel, *Justice and Managed Care: Four Principles for the Just Allocation of Health Care Resources, 30 Hastings Center Rep. 8, 16 (May/June 2000).*

Journal 2000 Explores the legal, ethical, social, and economic considerations associated with use of new genetic techniques in the prediction and diagnosis of Alzheimer disease. Outlines the potential responsibilities and liabilities of physicians in connection with use of these techniques. References Opinions 2.132, 2.139, and 8.032. Kapp, *Physicians' Legal Duties Regarding the Use of Genetic Tests to Predict and Diagnose Alzheimer Disease, 21 J. Legal Med. 445, 456-57, 465-66 (2000).*

Journal 2000 Compares the changes in physician roles in Japan and the US that exacerbate their conflicts of interest. Examines American physicians' dispensing practices and relations with pharmaceutical firms and hospital ownership. Concludes the US is reducing one of the main strengths it had in addressing physician conflicts: institutions of countervailing power and countervailing incentives. References Opinions 8.032 and 8.061. Rodwin & Okamoto, *Physicians' Conflicts of Interest in Japan and the United States: Lessons for the United States, 25 J. Health Pol. Pol'y & L. 343, 355, 358 (2000).*

Journal 1999 Discusses issues surrounding ambulatory surgical centers. Focuses on self-referral laws, the federal antikickback statute, and tax issues. Outlines legal requirements pertaining to ambulatory surgical centers. Cites Opinion 8.032. DeMuro, *A Review of Key Legal Requirements Affecting Ambulatory Surgical Centers, 11 Health Law. 1, 7 (1999).*

Journal 1999 Explores the increased push toward mandatory disclosure laws regarding financial incentives imposed by managed care organizations. Discusses current laws and ethical guidelines. Emphasizes that efforts to mandate disclosure force physicians to focus on the effects of imposed incentives and the essence of the physician-patient relationship. References Opinions 8.032, 8.13, and 8.132. Miller & Sage, *Disclosing Physician Financial Incentives, 281 JAMA 1424, 1425 (1999).*

Journal 1999 Discusses the practice of physicians using nonpublic information to invest in stocks. Provides guidelines on insider trading laws for physicians. Observes that insider trading damages the public perception of the medical profession. References Opinion 8.032. Prentice, *Clinical Trial Results, Physicians, and Insider Trading, 20 J. Legal Med. 195, 221 (1999).*

Journal 1999 Discusses the push to mandate disclosure in managed care programs. Explains the dangers of disclosing too much information. Provides objectives and goals for disclosure. Quotes Opinion 8.051. References Opinions 8.032 and 8.13. Sage, *Regulating Through Information: Disclosure Laws and American Health Care, 99 Colum. L. Rev. 1701, 1753, 1758, 1760 (1999).*

Journal 1999 Explores the impact managed care organizations have had on health care. Explains that patients may not understand restrictions and incentives imposed by their managed care organizations when entering the program. Argues that such information should be disclosed at various times during the period of plan coverage. Cites Opinions 2.03, 8.03, 8.032, 8.051, 8.13, and 8.132. Wolf, *Toward a Systemic Theory of Informed Consent in Managed Care, 35 Hous. L. Rev. 1631, 1641, 1658, 1661, 1662, 1679 (1999).*

Journal 1998 Discusses conflicts of interest in the physician-patient relationship arising out of use of financial incentives by managed care organizations. Considers how such conflicts are dealt with in the attorney-client relationship. Suggests that a financial incentive should be legally denounced if it unreasonably interferes with a physician's duty to properly care for and treat patients. Quotes Preamble, Fundamental Elements (1) [now Opinion 10.01] and Opinions 4.04, 5.01, 8.03, 8.13, and 9.06. Cites Fundamental Elements (4) [now Opinion 10.01] and Opinions 2.07, 2.08, and 2.132. Hall, *Third-Party Payor Conflicts of Interest in Managed Care: A Proposal for Regulation Based on the Model Rules of Professional Conduct, 29 Seton Hall L. Rev. 95, 96, 107, 108, 109, 110, 111, 112, 134, 135, 136 (1998).*

Journal 1997 Discusses the quality of neurological care and the ethical conflicts that are created by the drive to contain costs. Focuses on quality management and cost-containment programs and the conflicts created when neurologists attempt to reconcile the interests of patients and society. References Opinions 8.032 and 8.13. Bernat, *Quality of Neurological Care: Balancing Cost Control and Ethics*, 54 Arch. Neurol. 1341, 1343, 1345 (1997).

Journal 1995 Examines the metaphor of physicians as fiduciaries. Considers how the law holds physicians accountable in this regard. Quotes Preamble. Cites Opinion 8.03 (1986) [now Opinion 8.032]. Rodwin, *Strains in the Fiduciary Metaphor: Divided Physician Loyalties and Obligations in a Changing Health Care System*, XXI Am. J. Law & Med. 241, 246, 250 (1995).

Journal 1993 Argues that legislative efforts to curb or prohibit physician investment and self-referral are misdirected. Proposes a more effective solution to this problem: enforcement of existing laws. Quotes Opinion 8.032. Morreim, *Blessed Be the Tie That Binds? Antitrust Perils of Physician Investment and Self-referral*, 14 J. Legal Med. 359, 367, 374, 377, 394, 409 (1993).

Journal 1993 Examines financial conflicts of interest involving physicians. Discusses ways to identify conflicts and possible remedies. References Opinion 8.032. Thompson, *Understanding Financial Conflicts of Interest*, 329 New Eng. J. Med. 573 (1993).

Journal 1992 Discusses the safe harbor regulations under the Medicare and Medicaid Antikickback Statute, examines the Hanlester Network case, and describes the problem of physician self-referral. Concludes that a societal consensus is evolving against self-referral. References Opinion 8.032. Crane, *The Problem of Physician Self-referral Under the Medicare and Medicaid Antikickback Statute: The Hanlester Network Case and the Safe Harbor Regulation*, 268 JAMA 85, 89, 90 (1992).

Journal 1992 Analyzes the Medicare Antifraud Statute and the safe harbor regulations in light of recent criticisms. Concludes that the antifraud statute is an appropriate way to deal with fraud, but that other steps also should be taken. References Opinion 8.032. Farley, *The Medicare Antifraud Statute and Safe Harbor Regulations: Suggestions for Change*, 81 Georgetown L. J. 167, 184 (1992).

Journal 1992 Examines issues related to the responsibility of HIV-infected health care workers to protect patients from infection, including mandatory testing, disclosure to coworkers and supervisors, and the degree to which the practice of an HIV-infected health care worker should be modified. Concludes that courts likely will impose a requirement to disclose HIV-positive status to patients when there is a substantial risk of HIV transmission. Quotes Opinions 8.03 (1989) [now Opinion 8.032] and 8.07 (1989) [now Opinion 8.03]. References Opinion 9.131. Lieberman & Derse, *HIV-Positive Health Care Workers and the Obligation to Disclose: Do Patients Have a Right to Know?* 13 J. Legal Med. 333, 353, 354 (1992).

Journal 1992 Examines a memorandum issued by the chief counsel of the Internal Revenue Service, which clearly identified certain transactions that could jeopardize the tax exempt status of hospitals. Concludes that the memorandum provides valuable guidance for hospitals in spite of its shortcomings. References Opinion 8.032. Mancino, *New GCM Suggests Rules for Ventures Between Nonprofit Hospitals and Doctors*, 76 J. Taxation 164, 167 (1992).

Journal 1992 Analyzes the controversy over physician ownership of health care facilities. Considers a study of physician joint ventures in Florida and finds that current legislation prohibiting or restricting such arrangements is inadequate. Quotes Opinion 8.032. Mitchell & Scott, *Evidence on Complex Structures of Physician Joint Ventures*, 9 Yale J. Regulation 489, 503 (1992).

Journal 1992 Discusses the problem of physician joint ventures and examines their prevalence in Florida. Concludes that these arrangements may cause physicians to prioritize economic incentives over patients' medical needs. References Opinion 8.032. Mitchell & Scott, *New Evidence of the Prevalence and Scope of Physician Joint Ventures*, 268 JAMA 80, 84 (1992).

Journal 1992 Examines the issue of physician joint ventures in the context of physical therapy and rehabilitation services. Finds that facility utilization, patient cost, and physician profits were higher at joint venture facilities. References Opinion 8.032. Mitchell & Scott, *Physician Ownership of Physical Therapy Services: Effects on Charges, Utilization, Profits, and Service Characteristics*, 268 JAMA 2055, 2058 (1992).

Journal 1992 Presents results of a study indicating that joint ventures in radiation therapy increase the use and cost of these services and reduce access to care in inner-city and rural areas. Concludes that physician joint ventures have negative consequences and proposes that carefully crafted legislation be enacted to ban such arrangements. Quotes Opinion 8.032. Mitchell & Sunshine, *Consequences of Physicians' Ownership of Health Care Facilities—Joint Ventures in Radiation Therapy*, 327 New Eng. J. Med. 1497, 1500 (1992).

Journal 1992 Examines the debate regarding physician self-referral. Argues in favor of the AMA's statement in general, but urges an even stronger and more comprehensive position in this context. References Opinion 8.032. Relman, *"Self-referral"—What's at Stake? 327 New Eng. J. Med. 1522, 1524 (1992).*

Journal 1992 Explores the problem of physician self-referral and overuse of physician-owned facilities. Concludes that in cases studied, physician ownership of a facility increased the use and cost of services. Quotes Opinion 8.032. Swedlow, Johnson, Smithline, & Milstein, *Increased Costs and Rates of Use in the California Workers' Compensation System as a Result of Self-referral by Physicians, 327 New Eng. J. Med. 1502 (1992).*

Journal 1991 Looks at the physician as a fiduciary and the law governing fiduciary relationships. Concludes that fiduciary concepts are a valuable basis for establishing ethical and legal guidelines for physician behavior. Quotes Opinions 2.19, 8.03 (1989) [now Opinion 8.032], and 8.06. Healey & Dowling, *Controlling Conflicts of Interest in the Doctor-Patient Relationship: Lessons From Moore v. Regents of the University of California, 42 Mercer L. Rev. 989, 997, 998 (1991).*

Journal 1991 Discusses the issue of HIV-infected surgeons in light of the New Jersey case decision in *Behringer v. Medical Center*. Considers future developments. References Opinions 8.032 and 9.131. Orentlicher, *HIV-Infected Surgeons: Behringer v. Medical Center, 266 JAMA 1134, 1136 (1991).*

Journal 1990 Discusses efforts of third-party payers to control health care expenditures for beneficiaries. Concludes that financial incentives to limit care and other cost-control techniques should be disclosed and that the rationale for such disclosure is compelling. Quotes Opinions 2.03, 2.09, and 8.03 [now Opinions 8.03 and 8.032]. Cites Opinions 2.19, 4.04, and 4.06. Hirshfeld, *Should Third Party Payors of Health Care Services Disclose Cost Control Mechanisms to Potential Beneficiaries? 14 Seton Hall Legis. J. 115, 130, 131, 144, 145, 146 (1990).*

Journal 1990 Examines various cost-control mechanisms utilized by prepaid health plans and other managed care programs and considers the impact of such mechanisms on clinical decision making. Emphasis is placed on the possible existence of conflicts of interest on the part of health care providers in this context. Quotes Opinions 8.03 [now Opinions 8.03 and 8.032] and 8.13 [now Opinion 8.132]. Hirshfeld, *Defining Full and Fair Disclosure in Managed Care Contracts, 60 The Citation 67, 70 (1990).*

Journal 1990 Balances the "laissez-faire" concerns of individual freedom and personal choice with the "prohibitionists" desire to protect patients from poor quality care and unnecessary referrals. Concludes that civil remedies should be emphasized by extending the doctrines of "bad faith" and "breach of contract" into this arena. References Opinion 8.032. Morreim, *Physician Investment and Self-referral: Philosophical Analysis of a Contentious Debate, 15 J. Med. & Phil. 425, 428, 429, 430, 431 (1990).*

Journal 1985 Initially describes how existing doctrines protect the value of autonomy in the context of the physician-patient relationship, then examines various problems in the current protective scheme. Concludes by recommending the creation of an independent articulable protected interest in patient autonomy. Quotes Principles II and IV. Cites Opinions 4.04 (1984) [now Opinions 8.03 and 8.032] and 6.03 (1984) [now Opinion 6.02]. Shultz, *From Informed Consent to Patient Choice: A New Protected Interest, 95 Yale L. J. 219, 275 (1985).*

8.035   The previous Opinion 8.035, "Conflicts of Interest in Home Health Care," issued June 1994, was delated and replaced by the current Opinion 8.0321, "Physicians' Self-referral."

8.04 Consultation

Physicians should obtain consultation whenever they believe that it would be medically indicated in the care of the patient or when requested by the patient or the patient's representative. When a patient is referred to a consultant, the referring physician should provide a history of the case and such other information as the consultant may need, calling to the attention of the consultant any specific questions about which guidance is sought, and the consultant should advise the referring physician of the results of the consultant's examination and recommendations. (V)

Issued prior to April 1977. Updated June 1992 and June 1996.

D.S.C. 1968 Military dependent sued government physicians under Federal Tort Claims Act where child with acute abdominal pain was twice referred to naval hospital with diagnosis of possible appendicitis and twice sent home without treatment, eventually suffering ruptured appendix and serious complications. In finding for the plaintiff, the court quoted Principle 8 (1957) [now Principle V and Opinion 8.04] in considering whether the physicians had a duty to seek consultation in such a situation. *Steeves v. United States, 294 F. Supp. 446, 454.*

Wash. 1951 Plaintiff, a charitable, not-for-profit medical corporation, offered prepaid health care services to members and their families. Suit was filed against county medical society and others for damages and injunction for defendants' alleged efforts to monopolize prepaid medical care in area and unlawfully restrain competition by plaintiff and its physicians. Defendants alleged as affirmative defense that their efforts were designed to curb unethical prepaid contract practice by plaintiff. Court examined at length AMA's position regarding contract practice including Principles Ch. III, Art. VI, Secs. 3 and 4 (1947) [now Principle VI and Opinions 8.05 and 9.06] concluding nothing in plaintiff's practice violated the AMA's ethical guidelines. Further, quoting Principles Ch. III, Art. III, Sec.1 (1947) [now Opinion 8.04] dealing with consultations, court noted that defendants' efforts impeded plaintiff's physicians from obtaining consultations. Court concluded defendants' actions constituted unlawful, monopolistic behavior and issued an injunction, although it declined to award damages. *Group Health Coop. v. King County Medical Soc'y, 39 Wash. 2d 586, 237 P.2d 737, 744, 750-51, 759-60.*

Journal 1998 Examines mechanisms of oversight for expert witness testimony by medical, legal, legislative, and regulatory agencies. Points out that the amount of malpractice litigation will increase the need for medical expert witnesses. Concludes that improvements in this context must uphold principles of due process and be acceptable to the medical and legal communities. Cites Opinions 6.01, 8.04, and 9.07. McAbee, *Improper Expert Medical Testimony: Existing and Proposed Mechanisms of Oversight, 19 J. Legal Med. 257, 265 (1998).*

Journal 1994 Focuses on physicians' legal and ethical duties to pregnant women to provide medical information relevant to patient choice regarding abortion and to make referrals for services that physicians are unable or unwilling to perform. Concludes that medical educators, professional associations, women's groups, and state legislatures should address these issues. Cites Opinions 3.04 and 8.04. Law, *Silent No More: Physicians' Legal and Ethical Obligations to Patients Seeking Abortions, 21 N. Y. U. Rev. L. & Soc. Change 279, 289, 290, 300 (1994).*

8.041 Second Opinions

Physicians should recommend that a patient obtain a second opinion whenever they believe it would be helpful in the care of the patient. When recommending a second opinion, physicians should explain the reasons for the recommendation and inform their patients that patients are free to choose a second-opinion physician on their own or with the assistance of the first physician. Patients are also free to obtain second opinions on their own initiative, with or without their physician's knowledge.

With the patient's consent, the first physician should provide a history of the case and such other information as the second-opinion physician may need, including the recommendations about management. The second-opinion physician should maintain the confidentiality of the evaluation and should report to the first physician if the consent of the patient has been obtained.

After evaluating the patient, a second-opinion physician should provide the patient with a clear understanding of the opinion, whether or not it agrees with the recommendations of the first physician.

When a patient initiates a second opinion, it is inappropriate for the primary physician to terminate the patient-physician relationship solely because of the patient's decision to obtain a second opinion.

In some cases, patients may ask the second-opinion physician to provide the needed medical care. In general, second-opinion physicians are free to assume responsibility for the care of the patient. It is not unethical to enter into a patient-physician relationship with a patient who has been receiving care from another physician. By accepting second-opinion patients for treatment, physicians affirm the right of patients to have free choice in the selection of their physicians.

There are situations in which physicians may choose not to treat patients for whom they provide second opinions. Physicians may decide not to treat the patient in order to avoid any perceived conflict of interest or loss of objectivity in rendering the requested second opinion. However, the concern about conflicts of interest does not require physicians to decline to treat second-opinion patients. This inherent conflict in the practice of medicine is resolved by the responsible exercise of professional judgment.

Physicians may agree not to treat second-opinion patients as part of their arrangements with insurers or other third-party payers. Physicians who enter into such contractual agreements must honor their commitments.

Physicians must decide independently of their colleagues whether to treat second-opinion patients. Physicians may not establish an agreement or understanding among themselves that they will refuse to treat each others' patients when asked to provide a second opinion. Such agreements compromise the ability of patients to receive care from the physicians of their choice and are therefore not only unethical but also unlawful. (IV, V)

Issued June 1992. Updated June 1996.

Journal 2009 Discusses the judicial standard for reviewing physician noncompete covenants. Concludes courts should apply a strict standard to such covenants, rather than declare the covenants per se invalid. Quotes Principles IV and VII, Principles of Medical Ethics §5 (1957) [now Principle VI], Code of Medical Ethics Ch. II, Art. I §3 (1847) [now Opinion 5.02], Opinion 9.02, and Code of Medical Ethics Ch. II, Art. I §4 (1847) [now Opinion 9.09]. Cites Opinions 8.041, 8.115, 9.02, 9.06, 9.065, 9.067, 10.01, and 10.015. Koons, *Physician Employee Non-Compete Agreements on the Examining Table: The Need to Better Protect Patients' and the Public's Interests in Indiana*, 6 Ind. Health L. Rev. 253, 272-77, 280-81 (2009).

8.043 Ethical Implications of Surgical Comanagement

For the purpose of this report, the term "surgical comanagement" refers to the practice of allotting specific responsibilities of patient care to designated caregivers. The following guidelines stem from this understanding:

(1) Physicians should engage in comanagement arrangements only to assure the highest quality of care.

(2) When surgical comanagement arrangements are made between duly licensed physicians, their responsibilities should be delineated according to the scope of the physicians' expertise. Likewise, when physicians enter into surgical comanagement arrangements with allied health professionals, each caregiver's responsibility should correspond to his or her qualifications.

(3) Even though different caregivers will be responsible for rendering specific portions of the patient's care, a single physician should be ultimately
responsible for ensuring that the care is delivered in a coordinated and
appropriate manner. Other caregivers should support this obligation by
communicating with this physician.

(4) The treating physicians are responsible for ensuring that the patient
has consented not only to take part in the surgical comanagement
arrangement, but also to the services that will be provided within the
arrangement. In addition to disclosing medical facts to the patient, the
patient should also be informed of other significant aspects of the surgical
comanagement arrangement such as the credentials of the other caregivers,
the specific services each will provide, and the billing arrangement.

(5) Physicians should ensure that their surgical comanagement arrangements
do not violate the ethical or legal restrictions on self-referral.

(6) Referrals to another caregiver should be based only on that caregiver's
skill and ability to meet the patient's needs and not on expected further
referrals or other self-serving bases. Physicians who participate in surgical
comanagement arrangements must avoid such financial agreements as fee
splitting, which are both unethical and illegal.

Physicians who participate in surgical comanagement arrangements should
employ appropriate safeguards to ensure that confidential information is protected. (I, II, IV, V, VI)

Issued June 2000 based on the report "Ethical Implications of Surgical Co-Management,"
adopted December 1999.

8.045 Direct-to-Consumer Diagnostic Imaging Tests

Diagnostic imaging services that have not been scientifically validated for
screening purposes are being offered without prior referral by a personal
physician. Examples include total body scanning, electron beam computed
tomography (CT) for determining coronary artery calcification, spiral CT
for lung cancer screening, and CT colonography for colon cancer screening.
Physicians and relevant specialty societies should advocate for the conduct
of appropriate trials aimed at determining the predictive power of the tests,
and their sensitivity and specificity for target abnormalities. When adequate
data regarding a screening diagnostic imaging service become available, the
profession has a responsibility to develop suitable guidelines, as has been done
for mammography.

The following ethical guidelines apply to physicians providing screening
imaging services that have not been scientifically validated, without referral
from another physician:

(1) Performance of a diagnostic imaging test at the request of an individual is
justifiable only if, in the judgment of the physician, the potential benefits
of the service outweigh the risks.

(2) Once a physician agrees to perform the test, a patient-physician relation-
ship is established with all the obligations such a relationship entails.
(See Opinion 10.01, "Fundamental Elements of the Patient-Physician
Relationship" and Opinion 10.015, "The Patient-Physician Relationship").

In the absence of a referring physician who orders the test, the testing physician assumes responsibility for relevant clinical evaluation, as well as pretest and post-test counseling concerning the test, its results, and indicated follow-up. Post-test counseling may also be accomplished through referral to an appropriate physician who accepts the patient.

In obtaining the patient's informed consent (see Opinion 8.08, "Informed Consent"), the testing physician should discuss, in a manner the patient can understand, the usual elements of informed consent as well as:

(a) the inaccuracies inherent in the proposed test,

(b) the possibility of inconclusive results,

(c) false-positives or false-negatives, and

(d) circumstances which may require further assessment and additional costs.

(3) Physicians who hold financial interests in imaging facilities must not place those interests above the welfare of their patients, as stated in Opinions 8.03, "Conflicts of Interest: Guidelines" and 8.032, "Conflicts of Interest: Health Facility Ownership by a Physician."* Moreover, physicians who advertise diagnostic imaging services should ensure that advertisements are truthful and not misleading or deceptive. (I, II, V, VIII)

Issued November 2005 based on the report "Direct-to-Consumer Diagnostic Imaging Tests," adopted June 2005.

*Opinion 8.032, "Conflicts of Interest: Health Facility Ownership by a Physician," was replaced by the current Opinion 8.0321, "Physicians' Self-referral," June 2009.

8.047   Industry Representatives in Clinical Settings

Manufacturers of medical devices may facilitate their use through industry representatives who can play an important role in patient safety and quality of care by providing information about the proper use of the device or equipment as well as technical assistance to physicians.

Because of their obligation to protect their patients, physicians must strive to prevent industry representatives from breaching patient privacy and confidentiality, and seek to verify that they are properly credentialed and do not exceed the bounds of their training. Physicians may fulfill these obligations by satisfying themselves that the facility has suitable mechanisms in place to accomplish these functions.

Physicians or their designees must disclose to patients the anticipated presence and roles of industry representatives during clinical encounters, and obtain patients' approval. This requires neither disclosure of the representative's specific identity nor a formal informed consent process. (I, IV, V)

Issued November 2007 based on the report "Industry Representatives in Clinical Settings," adopted June 2007.

8.05   Contractual Relationships

The contractual relationships that physicians assume when they join or affiliate with group practices or agree to provide services to the patients of an insurance plan are varied.

Income arrangements may include hourly wages for physicians working part time, annual salaries for those working full time, and share of group income for physicians who are partners in groups that are somewhat autonomous and contract with plans to provide the required medical care. Arrangements also usually include a range of fringe benefits, such as paid vacations, insurance, and pension plans.

Physicians may work directly for plans or may be employed by the medical group or the hospital that has contracted with the plan to provide services. In the operation of such plans, physicians should not be subjected to lay interference in professional medical matters and their primary responsibility should be to the patients they serve. (VI)

Issued prior to April 1977. Updated June 1994 and June 1996.

1st Cir. 1984 Plaintiff-physicians sued defendant-insurer, alleging defendant's ban on balance billing practice violated antitrust law. That practice required defendant to pay the physicians treating defendant's insureds only if the physicians agreed not to make any additional charges to the insureds. In holding that defendant's billing practice did not violate antitrust law, the court noted in passing a 1954 law journal article that cited, with an incorrect reference, Principles Ch. III, Art. VI, Sec. 3 (1947) in arguing that selling services to third parties . . . might interfere with the absolute ethical obligation that a doctor owes to the patient. The specific concept treated by this Principle is no longer directly treated although Opinion 8.05 reflects similar concerns. *Kartell v. Blue Shield of Mass., Inc., 749 F.2d 922, 926, cert. denied, 471 US 1029 (1985).*

2d Cir. 1980 Federal Trade Commission ordered AMA and others to cease, with some exceptions, imposing restraints on advertising and contract practice by physicians, as well as on business relations between physicians and laypersons. Commission found restraints violated 15 USC § 45(a)(1). See 94 FTC 701 (1979). AMA petitioned for judicial review of Commission's order. Court reviewed order, noting specific ethical pronouncements of AMA which Commission found improper, including the following: restrictions upon advertising and solicitation, Principle 5 (1957) and Opinions and Reports of the Judicial Council Sec. 5, Para. 11 (1971) [now Opinion 5.02]; restrictions on contract practice, Principle 6 (1957) and Opinions and Reports of the Judicial Council Sec. 6, Paras. 3, 4, and 5 (1971) [now Opinion 8.05]; and restrictions on business organizations and relations with laypersons, Opinions and Reports of the Judicial Council Sec. 6, Paras. 14 and 15 (1971). Court rejected AMA's argument that its ethical rules did not provide impetus for local and state medical societies to act against physicians violating its rules. Further, court rejected AMA's position that liability should be precluded because of revisions in the Opinions in 1977 and the Principles in 1980. Specifically, the court found that removal of the ban on patient solicitation and changes reflected in Principles II and IV (1980) did not render Commission's order moot. The order was therefore enforced with modifications. Dissenting judge, referring to 1980 revisions in Principles and to Opinions and Reports of the Judicial Council 4.05 and 6.00 (1977) [now Opinions 5.02 and 8.05], concluded order should not be enforced on grounds of mootness. *American Medical Ass'n v. FTC, 638 F.2d 443, 446, 446 n.1, 448, 449, 449 n.5, 450, 451, 455-57, aff'd, 455 US 676 (1982).*

7th Cir. 1984 Plaintiff brought medical malpractice suit against several physicians appointed to the Veterans Administration Department of Medicine and Surgery. The court held that strict control test for determining whether defendants ought to be considered employees or independent contractors under the Federal Tort Claims Act was not appropriate because the ethical obligation of a physician to a patient, evidenced by Principle 6 (1957) [now Opinions 8.03 and 8.05], required that independent judgment be exercised, preventing a physician from being strictly controlled by the Veterans Administration. *Quilico v. Kaplan, 749 F.2d 480, 483-84.*

10th Cir. 1983 Pursuant to the Federal Tort Claims Act, plaintiff sued the federal government for the negligence of a neurosurgeon, allegedly an employee of a Veteran's Administration (VA) hospital. Plaintiff argued that applying the traditional control test to determine a physician's employment status was inappropriate because physicians are bound by Principle 6 (1957) [now Opinions 8.03 and 8.05] requiring them to have free and complete exercise of [their] medical judgment and skill. . . . However, the court did not reach the merits of that argument because the contractual agreement between the neurosurgeon and the VA hospital was outside the parameters of an employer-employee relationship with the government, thus precluding plaintiff's claim. *Lurch v. United States, 719 F.2d 333, 337, cert. denied, 466 US 927. (1984).*

D.C. Cir. 1942 Medical associations appealed conviction on charges of conspiracy to restrain trade or commerce where associations attempted to prevent competition by elimination of prepaid, low-cost medical and hospital care. Principles Ch. III, Art. VI, Secs. 2 and 3 [now Opinion 8.05] limiting contract practice had been used as a basis to discipline members of medical association employed by prepaid medical organization. The court held that the associations were subject to the Sherman Antitrust Act and that the evidence sustained the conviction. *American Medical Ass'n v. United States, 130 F.2d 233, 238-239 n.23, aff'd, 317 US 519 (1943).*

N.D. Ill. 2008 Administrator of the estate of patient filed suit under the Federal Tort Claims Act and state wrongful death act after patient died as a result of a mistake during surgery at Veteran's Administration hospital. Defendant physician moved to dismiss on the grounds that, as a federal employee, she was exempt from personal liability for services performed within the scope of her employment at the VA. The court cited earlier case quoting Principle 6 (1957) [now Opinions 8.03 and 8.05] and determining that, because physicians are free to choose whom to serve, they are not federal employees and the strict control test may not be appropriate. Finding issues of fact to resolve, the court denied the defendant's motion for summary judgment. *Monroe v. United States, 2008 U.S. Dist. LEXIS 22455, 9.*

Miss. 2003 Patient's estate appealed summary judgment in favor of physician and hospital in wrongful death action. Supreme Court affirmed, holding that physician was a state employee and that purchase of liability insurance did not waive immunity. In examining physician's status, the court found that the exercise of professional judgment and discretion are not determinative of employment status. Quotes Principle 6 (1957) [now Opinions 8.03 and 8.05]. *Corey v. Skelton, 834 So.2d 681, 685.*

Miss. 2002 Plaintiff in malpractice action appealed grant of summary judgment in favor of neurosurgeon who allegedly performed a thoracic diskectomy on the wrong disk. A resident performed the patient's physical and wrote the majority of the chart notes. The Mississippi Supreme Court affirmed the lower court. The court held that as a state employee the physician was immune from liability and that his exercise of professional judgment in treating patients did not change his status and insurance did not waive immunity. Quotes Principle 6 (1957) [now Opinions 8.03 and 8.05]. *Clayton v. Harkey, 826 So.2d 1283, 1287.*

Miss. 2001 Patient filed suit asserting that a physician was negligent in performing surgery. The trial court granted the physician's summary judgment motion and held that the physician, employed by a state university medical center, was immune under state law. Finding genuine issues of fact, the state Supreme Court reversed and remanded the case for further proceedings. In a separate opinion, one justice quoted Principle 6 (1957) [now Opinions 8.03 and 8.05], in evaluating the degree of control exercised by the state over the physician. This justice, stressing that the physician exercised discretion in treating the patient independent of the state's control, found no basis to hold the physician an employee for immunity purposes. *Conley v. Warren, 797 So. 2d 881, 886.*

Miss. 2000 Beneficiaries of patient's estate appealed summary judgment in malpractice action for a physician on sovereign immunity grounds. The court reversed and remanded the case finding issues of fact to be resolved at trial. The majority set out a five-part test to determine the employment status of a physician working at a state health care facility, including the degree of control and direction exercised by the state over the physician. In a separate opinion one justice quoted Principle 6 (1957) [now Opinions 8.03 and 8.05], stating that, "A physician should not dispose of his services under terms or conditions which tend to interfere with or impair the free and complete exercise of his medical judgment and skill. . . ." This justice reasoned that the physician could not claim the state controlled his medical discretion or treatment of patients and thus was clearly not an employee entitled to immunity. *Miller v. Meeks, 762 So. 2d 302, 314.*

Miss. 2000 Patient brought a medical malpractice action against physicians after receiving treatment at a state university medical center. The jury returned a verdict against the physicians. The Mississippi Supreme Court reversed, finding that the physicians were immune from liability as state employees. In determining the status of the physicians, the court noted that the physicians retained a considerable amount of professional discretion in treating the patient, quoting Principle 6 (1957) [now Opinions 8.03 and 8.05]. However, this alone was not determinative, and in the court's view the physicians were state employees. *Sullivan v. Washington, 768 So. 2d 881, 885.*

Miss. App. 2003 Patient brought malpractice action against physicians working at a state university teaching hospital. Patient argued that the physicians were independent contractors and sovereign immunity did not apply. Appellate court, citing the Mississippi Supreme Court's decision in *Miller v. Mecks*, 762 So.2d 302 (Miss. 2000), affirmed the trial court and held that sovereign immunity applied because the physicians were state employees. Quotes Principle 6 (1957) [now Opinions 8.03 and 8.05]. *Brown v. Warren*, 858 So.2d 168, 175 (2003).

Wash. 1951 Plaintiff, a charitable, not-for-profit medical corporation, offered prepaid health care services to members and their families. Suit was filed against county medical society and others for damages and injunction for defendants' alleged efforts to monopolize prepaid medical care in area and unlawfully restrain competition by plaintiff and its physicians. Defendants alleged as affirmative defense that their efforts were designed to curb unethical prepaid contract practice by plaintiff. Court examined at length AMA's position regarding contract practice including Principles Ch. III, Art. VI, Secs. 3 and 4 (1947) [now Principle VI and Opinions 8.05 and 9.06] concluding nothing in plaintiff's practice violated the AMA's ethical guidelines. Further, quoting Principles Ch. III, Art. III, Sec. 1 (1947) [now Opinion 8.04] dealing with consultations, court noted that defendants' efforts impeded plaintiff's physicians from obtaining consultations. Court concluded defendants' actions constituted unlawful, monopolistic behavior and issued an injunction, although it declined to award damages. *Group Health Coop. v. King County Medical Soc'y*, 39 Wash. 2d 586, 237 P.2d 737, 744, 750-51, 759-60.

Journal 2007 Reviews the legal and ethical problems surrounding concierge medical practice. Concludes that concierge medicine should remain restricted to a small class of wealthy individuals. Cites Opinions 8.05, 8.055, 8.115, 9.06, and 9.065. Carnahan, *Concierge Medicine: Legal and Ethical Issues*, 35 J. L. Med. & Ethics 211, 212-13 (2007).

Journal 2006 Examines external review systems used for adjudication of disputes between patients and managed care organizations. Concludes that external review systems do not satisfy constitutional due process requirements. Quotes Opinions and Reports of the Judicial Council Sec. 6, Para. 4 (1969) [now Opinion 8.05]. References Opinion 8.13. Hunter, *Managed Process, Due Care: Structures of Accountability in Health Care*, 6 Yale J. Health Pol'y L. & Ethics 93, 107, 113 (2006).

Journal 2004 Discusses the concept of medical necessity and its effect on the health care system. Concludes that issues regarding medical necessity must be dealt with to achieve meaningful health care reform. Quotes Opinion 8.05. Blanchard, *"Medical Necessity" Determinations—A Continuing Healthcare Policy Problem*, 37 J. Health L. 599, 620 (2004).

Journal 2001 Discusses the prohibition on nonlawyer ownership of legal service providers. Considers how ethical rules and standards governing physicians have been directed toward preserving independent judgment. Concludes that ethical conflicts created by abandoning the prohibition on nonlawyer ownership of legal service providers may be managed by following the medical ethics model. Quotes Principle VI and Opinions 2.03, 2.09, 8.02, 8.021, 8.03, 8.05, 8.051, 8.054, 8.13, and 8.132. Harris & Foran, *The Ethics of Middle-Class Access to Legal Services and What We Can Learn From the Medical Profession's Shift to a Corporate Paradigm*, 70 Fordham L. Rev. 775, 817, 821, 822, 823, 824 (2001).

Journal 2000 Examines physician value neutrality (PVN). Defines PVN as providing a foundation to suggest physicians must keep their values—religious, political, or otherwise—out of the patient-physician relationship. Concludes it is not clear how values can be removed from the patient-physician relationship without removing the very thing PVN supporters are trying to protect, the intrinsic value of persons. References Opinions 2.01, 2.02, 8.032, 8.05, 8.08, and 8.132. Beckwith & Peppin, *Physician Value Neutrality: A Critique*, 28 J. L. Med. & Ethics 67, 72-73 (2000).

Journal 1997 Discusses the practice of physician deselection by managed care organizations. Suggests that deselection harms the physician-patient relationship and creates a conflict of interest. Argues that solutions to deselection should consider effects on the patient rather than on the physician. Quotes Principle III. Cites Principle I and Opinions 8.05 and 8.13. Liner, *Physician Deselection: The Dynamics of a New Threat to the Physician-Patient Relationship*, 23 Am. J. Law & Med. 511, 513, 527 (1997).

8.0501 Professionalism and Contractual Relations

Physicians are free to enter into a wide range of contractual arrangements. However, physicians should not sign contracts containing provisions that may undermine their ethical obligation to advocate for patient welfare. Therefore, before entering into contractual agreements to provide services that directly or indirectly impact patient care, physicians should negotiate the removal of any terms, such as financial incentives or administrative conditions, that are known to compromise professional judgment or integrity. Particularly, when contractual compensation varies according to performance (see Opinion 8.054, "Financial Incentives and the Practice of Medicine"), physicians should beware of incentives that may adversely impact patient care. (VI, VIII)

Issued June 2004 based on the report "Professionalism and Contractual Relations," adopted December 2003.

1st. Cir. 2008 Trial court granted summary judgment for orthopedic surgeon in suit brought against manufacturer of orthopedic implant devices for breach of contract and violations of state consumer protection statutes. On appeal, the surgeon submitted an affidavit from a medical ethics expert that cited Opinion 8.0501, declaring that the payment of kickbacks from a medical device manufacturer to a physician is unethical. The appeals court held that the manufacturer breached the contract by halting royalty payments to the physician. *Jasty v. Wright Medical Technology, Inc.*, 528 F.3d 28, 38, n. 12.

Journal 2010 Examines legal and ethical issues confronting medical-legal partnerships, as well as the benefits and challenges of such partnerships. Concludes that as long as critical professional obligations are recognized and ethical boundaries are maintained, medical and legal professionals can collaborate without compromising professional duties or ethical goals. Quotes Opinion 8.0501. Boumil, Freitas, & Freitas, *Multidisciplinary Representation of Patients: The Potential for Ethical Issues and Professional Duty Conflicts in the Medical-Legal Partnership Model*, 13 J. Health Care L. & Pol'y 107, 124 (2010).

Journal 2006 Examines ethical dilemmas physicians may face as providers of pay-for-performance medical care. Concludes that this strategy offers a benefit to patients as long as physicians uphold stringent ethical standards and work together to ensure optimum patient care. Cites Principles I, V, VIII, and IX and Opinions 2.035, 2.095, 6.01, 8.021, 8.03, 8.0501, 8.053, 8.054, and 8.121. Bostick, Sade, & McMahon, *Report of the Council on Ethical and Judicial Affairs: Physician Pay-for-Performance Programs*, 3 Ind. Health L. Rev. 429, 430, 431, 432-33, 434, 435, 436 (2006).

8.051 Conflicts of Interest Under Capitation

The application of capitation to physicians' practices can result in the provision of cost-effective, quality medical care. It is important to note, however, that the potential for conflict exists under such systems. Physicians who contract with health care plans should attempt to minimize these conflicts and to ensure that capitation is applied in a manner consistent with patients' interests.

(1) Physicians have an obligation to evaluate a health plan's capitation payments prior to contracting with that plan to ensure that the quality of patient care is not threatened by inadequate rates of capitation. Physicians should advocate that capitation payments be calculated primarily on the basis of relevant medical factors, available outcomes data, the costs associated with involved providers, and consensus-oriented standards of necessary care. Furthermore, the predictable costs resulting from existing conditions of enrolled patients should be considered when determining the rate of capitation. Different populations of patients have different medical needs and the costs associated with those needs should be reflected in the

per-member per-month payment. Physicians should seek agreements with plans that provide sufficient financial resources for all care that is the physician's obligations to deliver and should refuse to sign agreements that fail in this regard.

(2) Physicians must not assume inordinate levels of financial risk and should therefore consider a number of factors when deciding whether or not to sign a provider agreement. The size of the plan and the time period over which the rate is figured should be considered by physicians evaluating a plan as well as in determinations of the per-member per-month payment. The capitation rate for large plans can be calculated more accurately than for smaller plans because of the mitigating influence of probability and the behavior of large systems. Similarly, length of time will influence the predictability of the cost of care. Therefore, physicians should advocate for capitation rates calculated for large plans over an extended period of time.

(3) Stop-loss plans can prevent the potential of catastrophic expenses from influencing physician behavior. Physicians should ensure that such arrangements are finalized prior to signing an agreement to provide services in a health plan.

(4) Physicians must be prepared to discuss with patients any financial arrangements which could impact patient care. Physicians should avoid reimbursement systems that, if disclosed to patients, could negatively affect the patient-physician relationship. (II, III, VI)

Issued December 1997 based on the report "The Ethical Implications of Capitation," adopted June 1997. Updated June 2002.

Journal 2003 Discusses conflicts of interest caused when managed care organizations provide financial incentives to physicians. Concludes that the focus of managed care is not well-suited for the doctor-patient relationship. Quotes Opinion 8.03. Cites Principle VII. References Opinion 8.051. Hall, *Bargaining With Hippocrates: Managed Care and the Doctor-Patient Relationship, 54 S. C. L. Rev. 689, 696, 735 (2003).*

Journal 2001 Discusses the prohibition on nonlawyer ownership of legal service providers. Considers how ethical rules and standards governing physicians have been directed toward preserving independent judgment. Concludes that ethical conflicts created by abandoning the prohibition on nonlawyer ownership of legal service providers may be managed by following the medical ethics model. Quotes Principle VI and Opinions 2.03, 2.09, 8.02, 8.021, 8.03, 8.05, 8.051, 8.054, 8.13, and 8.132. Harris & Foran, *The Ethics of Middle-Class Access to Legal Services and What We Can Learn From the Medical Profession's Shift to a Corporate Paradigm, 70 Fordham L. Rev. 775, 817, 821, 822, 823, 824 (2001).*

Journal 1999 Discusses the push to mandate disclosure in managed care programs. Explains the dangers of disclosing too much information. Provides objectives and goals for disclosure. Quotes Opinion 8.051. References Opinions 8.032 and 8.13. Sage, *Regulating Through Information: Disclosure Laws and American Health Care, 99 Colum. L. Rev. 1701, 1753, 1758, 1760 (1999).*

Journal 1999 Explores the impact managed care organizations have had on health care. Explains that patients may not understand restrictions and incentives imposed by their managed care organizations when entering the program. Argues that such information should be disclosed at various times during the period of plan coverage. Cites Opinions 2.03, 8.03, 8.032, 8.051, 8.13, and 8.132. Wolf, *Toward a Systemic Theory of Informed Consent in Managed Care, 35 Hous. L. Rev. 1631, 1641, 1658, 1661, 1662, 1679 (1999).*

8.052 Negotiating Discounts for Specialty Care

Patients are entitled to all the benefits outlined in their insurance plan. Therefore, it is unethical for a referring physician to restrict the referral options of patients who have chosen a plan that provides for access to an unlimited or broad selection of specialist physicians. It is also unethical to base the referral of these patients on a discount for the capitated patients in a primary care physician's practice. (II)

Issued December 1997 based on the report "Ethical Issues in Negotiating Discounts for Specialty Care," adopted June 1996.

8.053 The previous Opinion 8.053, "Restrictions on Disclosure in Managed Care Contracts," issued June 1998, was replaced by the current Opinion 8.053, "Restrictions on Disclosure in Health Care Plan Contracts."

8.053 Restrictions on Disclosure in Health Care Plan Contracts

Despite ethical requirements demanding full disclosure of treatment options regardless of limitations imposed by plan coverage, some health care plans include clauses in their employment contracts that directly inhibit the ability of physicians to keep their patients fully informed. These types of contract clauses erect inappropriate barriers to necessary communications between physicians and patients, labeled "gag clauses" by some observers. Restrictive clauses of this type impact the ability of physicians to provide information to their patients and to act effectively as a patient advocate. They also threaten to undermine individual and public trust in the profession of medicine.

(1) Health care plans have the right to protect proprietary information. However, physicians should oppose any such protection that inhibits them from disclosing relevant information to patients. For this reason, physicians should advocate for the elimination of contract clauses that could prevent them from raising or discussing matters relevant to patients' medical care.

(2) The right of patients to be informed of all pertinent medical information must be reaffirmed by the medical profession, and individual physicians must continue to uphold their ethical obligation to disclose such information.

(3) Physicians, individually or through their representative, should review their contracts carefully to ensure that they are able to fulfill their ethical obligations to patients. (II, III, VI)

Issued June 1998 based on the report "Restrictions on Disclosure in Managed Care Contracts," adopted June 1996. Updated June 2002.

S.D. Fla. 2001 Insured patients under health care plans sued managed care companies alleging improper nondisclosure of policies and procedures imposing restrictions on physicians' judgment as to appropriate medical treatment. The insureds sued under both the Racketeer Influenced and Corrupt Organizations Act (RICO) and the Employee Retirement Income Security Act (ERISA). The court, with one exception, dismissed without prejudice both the RICO and ERISA claims. Among the plaintiffs' arguments was that the defendants had included "gag clauses" in their physician contracts in violation of Opinion 8.053. *In Re Managed Care Litigation,* 150 F.Supp.2d 1330, 1335.

Journal 2006 Examines ethical dilemmas physicians may face as providers of pay-for-performance medical care. Concludes that this strategy offers a benefit to patients as long as physicians uphold stringent ethical standards and work together to ensure optimum patient care. Cites Principles I, V, VIII, and IX and Opinions 2.035, 2.095, 6.01, 8.021, 8.03, 8.0501, 8.053, 8.054, and 8.121. Bostick, Sade, & McMahon, *Report of the Council on Ethical and Judicial Affairs: Physician Pay-for-Performance Programs*, 3 Ind. Health L. Rev. 429, 430, 431, 432-33, 434, 435, 436 (2006).

Journal 2006 Discusses preemption of lawsuits against managed care organizations by the Employee Retirement Income Security Act of 1974 (ERISA). Proposes a "bifurcated legal regime" to decrease the protective scope of ERISA. Quotes Opinions 8.053 and 8.135. Madison, *ERISA and Liability for Provision of Medical Information*, 84 N. C. L. Rev. 471, 540 (2006).

Journal 2002 Examines how managed care has adversely affected information disclosure in the physician-patient relationship. Concludes that, unless courts expand applicability of principles of informed consent, patient self-determination and autonomy will continue to be undermined. Quotes Principle VIII and Opinions 8.03, 8.053, 8.054, and 8.08. Morris, *Dissing Disclosure: Just What the Doctor Ordered*, 44 Ariz. L. Rev. 313, 344, 349, 362, 363, 366 (2002).

8.054 Financial Incentives and the Practice of Medicine

In order to achieve the necessary goals of patient care and to protect the role of physicians as advocates for individual patients, the following statement is offered for the guidance of physicians:

(1) Although physicians have an obligation to consider the needs of broader patient populations within the context of the patient-physician relationship, their first duty must be to the individual patient. This obligation must override considerations of the reimbursement mechanism or specific financial incentives applied to a physician's clinical practice.

(2) Physicians, individually or through their representatives, should evaluate the financial incentives associated with participation in a health plan before contracting with that plan. The purpose of the evaluation is to ensure that the quality of patient care is not compromised by unrealistic expectations for utilization or by placing that physician's payments for care at excessive risk. In the process of making judgments about the ethical propriety of such reimbursement systems, physicians should refer to the following general guidelines:

(a) Monetary incentives may be judged in part on the basis of their size. Large incentives may create conflicts of interest that can in turn compromise clinical objectivity. While an obligation has been established to resolve financial conflicts of interest to the benefit of patients, it is important to recognize that sufficiently large incentives can create an untenable position for physicians.

(b) The proximity of large financial incentives to individual treatment decisions should be limited in order to prevent physicians' personal financial concerns from creating a conflict with their role as individual patient advocates. When the proximity of incentives cannot be mitigated, as in the case of fee-for-service payments, physicians must behave in accordance with prior Council recommendations limiting the potential for abuse. This includes the Council's prohibitions on fee-splitting arrangements, the provision of unnecessary services, unreasonable fees, and self-referral. For incentives that can be distanced from clinical decisions, physicians should consider the following factors in order to evaluate the correlation between individual act and monetary reward or penalty:

(i) In general, physicians should favor incentives that are applied across broad physician groups. This dilutes the effect any one physician can have on his or her financial situation through clinical recommendations, thus allowing physicians to provide those services they feel are necessary in each case. Simultaneously, however, physicians are encouraged by the incentive to practice efficiently.

(ii) The size of the patient pool considered in calculations of incentive payments will affect the proximity of financial motivations to individual treatment decisions. The laws of probability dictate that in large populations of patients, the overall level of utilization remains relatively stable and predictable. Physicians practicing in plans with large numbers of patients in a risk pool therefore have greater freedom to provide the care they feel is necessary based on the likelihood that the needs of other plan patients will balance out decisions to provide extensive care.

(iii) Physicians should advocate for the time period over which incentives are determined to be long enough to accommodate fluctuations in utilization resulting from the random distribution of patients and illnesses. For example, basing incentive payments on an annual analysis of resource utilization is preferable to basing them on monthly review.

(iv) Financial rewards or penalties that are triggered by specific points of utilization may create enormous incentives as a physician's practice approaches the established level. Therefore, physicians should advocate that incentives be calculated on a continuum of utilization rather than a bracketed system with tiers of widely varied bonuses or penalties.

(v) Physicians should ascertain that a stop-loss plan is in place to prevent the costs associated with unusual outliers from significantly impacting the reward or penalty offered to a physician.

(3) Physicians also should advocate for incentives that promote efficient practice, but are not be designed to realize cost savings beyond those attainable through efficiency. As a counterbalance to the focus on utilization reduction, physicians also should advocate for incentives based on quality of care and patient satisfaction.

(4) Patients must be informed of financial incentives that could impact the level or type of care they receive. Although this responsibility should be assumed by the health plan, physicians, individually or through their representatives, must be prepared to discuss with patients any financial arrangements that could impact patient care. Physicians should avoid reimbursement systems that, if disclosed to patients, could negatively affect the patient-physician relationship. (II, III)

Issued June 1998 based on the report "Financial Incentives and the Practice of Medicine," adopted December 1997. Updated June 2002

Journal 2008 Explores the tension experienced by health care professionals who provide care and compete in a market economy. Concludes if health care professions continue commercializing, providers must strive to maintain ethical standards and appropriate professional-patient relationships. Quotes Opinion 8.054. Peltier & Guisti, *Commerce and Care: The Irreconcilable Tension Between Selling and Caring*, 39 McGeorge L. Rev. 785, 794 (2008).

Journal 2006 Examines ethical dilemmas physicians may face as providers of pay-for-performance medical care. Concludes that this strategy offers a benefit to patients as long as physicians uphold stringent ethical standards and work together to ensure optimum patient care. Cites Principles I, V, VIII, and IX and Opinions 2.035, 2.095, 6.01, 8.021, 8.03, 8.0501, 8.053, 8.054, and 8.121. Bostick, Sade, & McMahon, *Report of the Council on Ethical and Judicial Affairs: Physician Pay-For-Performance Programs*, 3 Ind. Health L. Rev. 429, 430, 431, 432-33, 434, 435, 436 (2006).

Journal 2006 Discusses the evolution of health law in Virginia. Concludes that the area of health law continues to expand, develop, and be refined. Cites Opinions 3.03, 3.08, 5.01, 5.015, 5.02, 5.04, 5.055, 6.02, 6.021, 6.03, 6.04, 7.03, 7.04, 7.05, 8.054, 8.08, 8.081, 8.085, 8.115, 8.12, 8.14, 8.145, 8.19, and 9.045. Guanzon, *Health Care Law*, 41 U. Rich. L. Rev. 179, 199 (2006).

Journal 2005 Argues that in *Aetna v. Davila/Cigna v. Calad*, the Supreme Court missed an opportunity to overturn unjust ERISA policies. Concludes that the principle of complete ERISA preemption as articulated in these consolidated cases is unsatisfactory because it violates the separation of powers doctrine. Quotes Principle VIII. Cites Opinions 8.054, 8.13, 8.135, 9.123, 10.01, and 10.015. Nelson, *AETNA v. DAVILA/CIGNA v. CALAD: A Missed Opportunity*, 31 Wm. Mitchell L. Rev. 843, 847, 849, 850, 880 (2005).

Journal 2003 Reviews state laws designed to protect physicians acting as patient advocates in managed care organizations. Concludes that federal and state law must make it easier for physicians to challenge denials of or delays in patient care. Quotes Opinions 8.054, 8.13, and 10.01. Fentiman, *Patient Advocacy and Termination From Managed Care Organizations. Do State Laws Protecting Health Care Professional Advocacy Make Any Difference?* 82 Neb. L. Rev. 508, 515-16, 517-18 (2003).

Journal 2002 Examines how managed care has adversely affected information disclosure in the physician-patient relationship. Concludes that, unless courts expand applicability of principles of informed consent, patient self-determination and autonomy will continue to be undermined. Quotes Principle VIII and Opinions 8.03, 8.053, 8.054, and 8.08. Morris, *Dissing Disclosure: Just What the Doctor Ordered*, 44 Ariz. L. Rev. 313, 344, 349, 362, 363, 366 (2002).

Journal 2001 Discusses the prohibition on nonlawyer ownership of legal service providers. Considers how ethical rules and standards governing physicians have been directed toward preserving independent judgment. Concludes that ethical conflicts created by abandoning the prohibition on nonlawyer ownership of legal service providers may be managed by following the medical ethics model. Quotes Principle VI and Opinions 2.03, 2.09, 8.02, 8.021, 8.03, 8.05, 8.051, 8.054, 8.13, and 8.132. Harris & Foran, *The Ethics of Middle-Class Access to Legal Services and What We Can Learn From the Medical Profession's Shift to a Corporate Paradigm*, 70 Fordham L. Rev. 775, 817, 821, 822, 823, 824 (2001).

8.055 Retainer Practices

Individuals are free to select and supplement insurance for their health care on the basis of what appears to them to be an acceptable tradeoff between quality and cost. Retainer contracts, whereby physicians offer special services and amenities (such as longer visits, guaranteed availability by phone or pager, counseling for healthy lifestyles, and various other customized services) to patients who pay additional fees distinct from the cost of medical care, are consistent with pluralism in the delivery and financing of health care. However, they also raise ethical concerns that warrant careful attention, particularly if retainer practices become so widespread as to threaten access to care.

(1) When entering into a retainer contract, both parties must be clear about the terms of the relationship and must agree to them. Physicians must present the terms of the contract in an honest manner, and must not exert

undue pressure on patients to agree to the arrangement. If a physician has knowledge that the patient's health care insurance coverage will be compromised by the retainer contract, the information must be discussed with the patient before reaching an agreement on the terms of the retainer contract. Also, patients must be able to opt out of a retainer contract without undue inconveniences or financial penalties.

(2) Concern for quality of care the patient receives should be the physician's first consideration. However, it is important that a retainer contract not be promoted as a promise for more or better diagnostic and therapeutic services. Physicians must always ensure that medical care is provided only on the basis of scientific evidence, sound medical judgment, relevant professional guidelines, and concern for economic prudence. Physicians who engage in mixed practices, in which some patients have contracted for special services and amenities and others have not, must be particularly diligent to offer the same standard of diagnostic and therapeutic services to both categories of patients. All patients are entitled to courtesy, respect, dignity, responsiveness, and timely attention to their needs.

(3) In accord with medicine's ethical mandate to provide for continuity of care and the ethical imperative that physicians not abandon their patients, physicians converting their traditional practices into retainer practices must facilitate the transfer of their nonparticipating patients, particularly their sickest and most vulnerable ones, to other physicians. If no other physicians are available to care for nonretainer patients in the local community, the physician may be ethically obligated to continue caring for such patients.

(4) Physicians who enter into retainer contracts will usually receive reimbursement from their patients' health care plans for medical services. Physicians are ethically required to be honest in billing for reimbursement, and must observe relevant laws, rules, and contracts. It is desirable that retainer contracts separate clearly special services and amenities from reimbursable medical services. In the absence of such clarification, identification of reimbursable services should be determined on a case-by-case basis.

(5) Physicians have a professional obligation to provide care to those in need, regardless of ability to pay, particularly to those in need of urgent care. Physicians who engage in retainer practices should seek specific opportunities to fulfill this obligation. (I, II, VI, VIII, IX)

Issued December 2003 based on the report "Retainer Practices," adopted June 2003.

Journal 2008 Explores the legal, ethical, and policy implications of concierge medicine. Argues physicians engaged in concierge care must strive to meet ethical and legal standards, and take care to communicate clearly with patients about services and fees. Quotes Opinion 8.055. Cites Principles II and VI and Opinion 8.055. Portman & Romanow, *Concierge Medicine: Legal Issues, Ethical Dilemmas, and Policy Challenges,* 1 J. Health & Life Sci. L. 1, 4, 28-29 (2008).

Journal 2007 Reviews the legal and ethical problems surrounding concierge medical practice. Concludes that concierge medicine should remain restricted to a small class of wealthy individuals. Cites Opinions 8.05, 8.055, 8.115, 9.06, and 9.065. Carnahan, *Concierge Medicine: Legal and Ethical Issues,* 35 J. L. Med. & Ethics 211, 212-13 (2007).

Journal 2007 Analyzes current retainer care practices. Concludes that retainer care offers some benefits, but should be regulated to prevent patients who pay a retainer from receiving quicker access to care. References Opinion 8.055. Pasquale, *The Three Faces of Retainer Care: Crafting a Tailored Regulatory Response,* 7 Yale J. Health Pol'y L. & Ethics 39, 74 (2007).

Journal 2006 Explores the legal and ethical issues surrounding concierge medicine. Concludes that concierge medicine is best restricted to a small class of wealthy individuals. Quotes Principle IX and Opinion 8.055. Cites Principle VI and Opinions 8.055, 8.11, 8.115, 9.065, and 10.05. Carnahan, *Law, Medicine, and Wealth: Does Concierge Medicine Promote Health Care Choice, or Is It a Barrier to Access?* 17 Stan. L. & Pol'y Rev. 121, 149-50, 151, 152, 153-54 (2006).

Journal 2006 Discusses health care service fees and the Maryland "Hold Harmless" statute. Concludes that physicians may charge administrative fees for services not covered by insurance as long as they do not violate a statute or impede proper care. Quotes Opinions 4.01 and 8.055. Doherty & Freed, *User Fees in Health Care,* 39 Md. B. J. 5, 9 (April 2006).

Journal 2006 Evaluates legal implications of consumer-driven health care. Concludes that a system of consumer-driven health care is feasible and offers many benefits to patients. Quotes Opinions 8.055 and 9.065. Hall, *Paying for What You Get and Getting What You Pay For: Legal Responses to Consumer-Driven Health Care,* 69 Law & Contemp. Prob. 159, 165 (2006).

Journal 2005 Examines the practice of "boutique medicine" and considers legal and ethical implications. Concludes that boutique medical services would be ethical only if physicians used retainer money from their boutique clients to augment health care costs of the poor. Quotes Principles VII and IX and Opinion 8.055. Russano, *Is Boutique Medicine a New Threat to American Health Care or a Logical Way of Revitalizing the Doctor-Patient Relationship?* 17 Wash. U. J. L. & Pol'y 313, 331, 332 (2005).

8.056 Physician Pay-for-Performance Programs

Physician pay-for-performance (PFP) compensation arrangements should be designed to improve health care quality and patient safety by linking remuneration to measures of individual, group, or organizational performance. To uphold their ethical obligations, physicians who are involved with PFP programs must take appropriate measures to promote patients' well-being.

(1) Physicians who are involved in the design or implementation of PFP programs should advocate for:

    (a) incentives that are intended to promote health care quality and patient safety, and are not primarily intended to contain costs;

    (b) program flexibility that allows physicians to accommodate the varying needs of individual patients;

    (c) adjustment of performance measures by risk and case-mix in order to avoid discouraging the treatment of high-risk individuals and populations; and

    (d) processes to make practice guidelines and explanations of their intended purposes and the clinical findings upon which they are based available to participating physicians.

(2) Practicing physicians who participate in PFP programs while providing medical services to patients should:

    (a) maintain primary responsibility to their patients and provide competent medical care, regardless of financial incentives;

    (b) support access to care for all people and avoid selectively treating healthier patients for the purpose of bolstering their individual or group performance outcomes;

    (c) be aware of evidence-based practice guidelines and the findings upon which they are based;

    (d) always provide care that considers patients' individual needs and preferences, even if that care conflicts with applicable practice guidelines; and

(e) not participate in PFP programs that incorporate incentives that conflict with physicians' professional values or otherwise compromise physicians' abilities to advocate for the interests of individual patients. (I, II, VI, VIII, IX)

Issued June 2006 based on the report "Physician Pay-for-Performance Programs," adopted November 2005 (*Indiana Health Law Review*. 2006;3(2):421-37).

Journal 2006 Scrutinizes the benefits of pay-for-performance financial incentives. Concludes that such incentives will not alleviate the need for health insurance. Cites Opinion 6.01. References Opinion 8.056. Sage & Kalyan, *Horses or Unicorns: Can Paying for Performance Make Quality Competition Routine?* 31 *J. Health Pol. Pol'y & L. 531, 531-32, 554 (2006).*

8.06   The previous Opinion 8.06, "Drugs and Devices: Prescribing," issued prior to April 1977, was combined with Opinion 6.04, "Fee Splitting: Drug or Device Prescription Rebates," and Opinion 8.07, "Gifts to Physicians: Offers of Indemnity," into the current Opinion 8.06 in June 2002.

8.06   Prescribing and Dispensing Drugs and Devices

(1) Physicians should prescribe drugs, devices, and other treatments based solely upon medical considerations and patient need and reasonable expectations of the effectiveness of the drug, device, or other treatment for the particular patient.

(2) Physicians may not accept any kind of payment or compensation from a drug company or device manufacturer for prescribing its products. Furthermore, physicians should not be influenced in the prescribing of drugs, devices, or appliances by a direct or indirect financial interest in a firm or other supplier, regardless of whether the firm is a manufacturer, distributor, wholesaler, or repackager of the products involved.

(3) Physicians may own or operate a pharmacy, but generally may not refer their patients to the pharmacy. Exceptionally, a physician may refer patients to his or her pharmacy in accord with guidelines established in Opinion 8.032, "Conflicts of Interest: Health Facility Ownership by a Physician."* Physicians may dispense drugs within their office practices provided such dispensing primarily benefits the patient.

(4) In all instances, physicians should respect the patient's freedom of choice in selecting who will fill their prescriptions as they are in the choice of a physician and, therefore, have the right to have a prescription filled wherever they wish. (See Opinions 9.06, "Free Choice," and 8.03, "Conflicts of Interest: Guidelines.") Physicians should not urge patients to fill prescriptions from an establishment which has entered into a business or other preferential arrangement with the physician with respect to the filling of the physician's prescriptions.

(5) A third party's offer to indemnify a physician for lawsuits arising from the physician's prescription or use of the third party's drug, device, or other product introduces inappropriate incentives into medical decision making. Such offers, regardless of their limitations, therefore constitute unacceptable gifts. This does not address contractual assignments of liability

between employers or in research arrangements, nor does it address government indemnification plans.

(6) Patients have an ethically and legally recognized right to prompt access to the information contained in their individual medical records. Since a prescription is part of the patient's medical record, the patient is entitled to a copy of the physician's prescription for drugs or devices, including eyeglasses and contact lenses. Therefore, physicians should not discourage patients from requesting a written copy of a prescription. (II, III, IV, V)

Issued June 2002. This opinion is a consolidation of previous Opinions 6.04, "Fee Splitting: Drug or Device Prescription Rebates;" 8.06, "Drugs and Devices: Prescribing;" and 8.07, "Gifts to Physicians: Offers of Indemnity."

*Opinion 8.032, "Conflicts of Interest: Health Facility Ownership by a Physician," was replaced by the current Opinion 8.0321, "Physicians' Self-referral," June 2009.

E.D. N.Y. 1975 Medical laboratories sought injunction against city's award of exclusive contracts for Medicaid services. The court granted a preliminary injunction and held that the laboratories had a substantial probability of success on the merits of the claim that Medicaid recipients would be deprived of statutory right of free choice of providers. In balancing the equities, the court also noted that the contracts would create an ethical dilemma for physicians who are required to provide patients with free choice of ancillary services under Opinions and Reports of the Judicial Council Sec. 1, Paras. 6 and 14 (1971) [now Opinions 8.03, 8.06, and 9.06]. *Bay Ridge Diagnostic Laboratory, Inc. v. Dumpson, 400 F. Supp. 1104, 1109-10.*

Cal. App. 1967 Physician-stockholders of publicly owned pharmaceutical corporations and physicians whose medical partnerships owned and operated pharmacies challenged statutory prohibition of physician membership, proprietory interest, and co-ownership of pharmacies. The court quoted Principles Ch. I, Sec. 6 (1947) and a 1960 Judicial Council rule, later included in Opinions and Reports of the Judicial Council Sec. 7, Para. 38 (1965) [now Opinions 8.03, 8.032, and 8.06] in its discussion of the potential conflict of interest created by such ownership. The court held that the statute prohibited physician partnerships from directly owning pharmacies but did not apply to an individual physician or a partnership of physicians who own stock in a corporation which owns and operates a pharmacy. *Magan Medical Clinic v. California State Bd. of Medical Examiners, 249 Cal. App. 2d 124, 57 Cal. Rptr. 256, 262.*

Minn. App. 1997 Patients brought suit against physician for prescribing a growth hormone drug while receiving kickbacks, in violation of the physician-patient fiduciary duty and the Minnesota Consumer Fraud Act. The distributor of the drug induced physicians to refer patients for the drug. The court cited Opinion 8.06 for the proposition that patients are entitled to receive medical opinions and referrals which are not motivated by physician gain. The court found, however, that the complaint sounded in medical malpractice and declined to allow a new cause of action based on breach of a fiduciary duty. Because the malpractice limitations had expired and the patients had failed to allege sufficient injury under the Consumer Fraud Act, the court affirmed dismissal with prejudice. *D.A.B v. Brown, 570 N.W. 2d 168, 170.*

Ohio 1980 A physician, charged with violating the state medical licensing statute by distributing controlled substances without a proper license and writing prescriptions for narcotics in the name of one person when they were intended for another, challenged the state medical board's decision to suspend his license and place him on two years' probation. Under the statute, a physician could be disciplined for various activities including violation of any provision of a code of ethics of a national professional organization such as the AMA. The board found in part that the physician's actions violated Principles 4 and 7 (1957) [now Principles II and III and Opinions 8.06 and 9.04]. The trial court reversed, holding that the board had insufficient evidence for its decision, and the court of appeals affirmed. On appeal, the Supreme Court held that expert testimony was not required at a hearing before a medical licensing board because they were experts and could determine for themselves whether the Principles had been violated. *Arlen v. State, 61 Ohio St. 2d 168, 399 N.E.2d 1251, 1252, 1253-54.*

Mo. Att'y Gen. 1982 State attorney general, citing Opinion 8.06 (1982), concluded that a physician who requires a patient to accept drugs dispensed by the physician and refuses to provide the patient with a prescription for the patient's use elsewhere violates state antitrust law and has engaged in professional misconduct. A similar conclusion, again based in part on Opinion 8.06, was rendered regarding a physician who requires a patient to fill a prescription at a pharmacy in which the physician has a personal interest. *Missouri Att'y Gen. Op. No. 6 (July 8, 1982) (LEXIS, States library, Mo. file).*

Journal 2008 Analyzes off-label drug prescribing patterns, the limited market demand for post-approval clinical trials, and increased litigation targeted at financial relationships between physicians and pharmaceutical firms. Concludes issues in learning patterns in the medical profession and deficiencies in the production and dissemination of clinical knowledge must be addressed in the context of off-label prescribing. Cites Opinion 8.06. Johnson, *Polluting Medical Judgment? False Assumptions in the Pursuit of False Claims Regarding Off-Label Prescribing*, 9 Minn. J. L. Sci. & Tech. 61, 103 (2009).

Journal 2007 Explores regulation of the pharmacy benefit management industry. Concludes that current regulations are inadequate to prevent fraud and self-dealing, and that private sector regulation is the best solution. Cites Opinion 8.06. Garrett & Garis, *Leveling the Playing Field in the Pharmacy Benefit Management Industry*, 42 Val. U. L. Rev. 33, 64 (2007).

Journal 2006 Discusses the evolution of health law in Virginia. Concludes that the area of health law continues to expand, develop, and be refined. Cites Opinions 3.03, 3.08, 5.01, 5.015, 5.02, 5.04, 5.055, 6.02, 6.021, 6.03, 6.04 [now Opinion 8.06], 7.03, 7.04, 7.05, 8.054, 8.08, 8.081, 8.085, 8.115, 8.12, 8.14, 8.145, 8.19, and 9.045. Guanzon, *Health Care Law*, 41 U. Rich. L. Rev. 179, 199 (2006).

Journal 2006 Discusses regulation of complementary and alternative medicine. Concludes that only minimal regulation of these practices is required. References Principle 7 (1957) [now Opinion 8.06 and Opinion 8.062]. Lunstroth, *Voluntary Self-regulation of Complementary and Alternative Medicine Practitioners*, 70 Alb. L. Rev. 209, 243 (2006).

Journal 2002 Suggests a reconceptualization for bioethics that integrates an analysis of the history of moral change. Concludes that bioethical textbooks should include discussion about the history of bioethics and medical ethics. Quotes Opinion 2.20. References Opinions 6.02, 6.03, 6.04 [now Opinion 8.06], and 8.032. Baker, *Bioethics and History*, 27 J. Med. & Phil. 447, 455, 469 (2002).

Journal 2001 Explores how the *Pegram* case restricted the protection provided to HMOs by ERISA's state law preemption. Concludes that HMOs will be subject to increased litigation under two areas of state law—breach of statutory fiduciary duty and medical malpractice claims. Cites Opinion 8.06. McLean & Richards, *Managed Care Liability for Breach of Fiduciary Duty After Pegram v. Herdrich: The End of ERISA Preemption for State Law Liability for Medical Care Decision Making*, 53 Fla. L. Rev. 1, 38 (2001).

Journal 2001 Considers office dispensing of products within the dermatology practice. Examines related ethical issues. Concludes that the primary reasons patients buy products from their physicians are trust and knowledge, not convenience. Quotes Opinion 8.06. Ogbogu, Fleischer, Brodell, Bhalla, Draelos, & Feldman, *Physicians' and Patients' Perspectives on Office-Based Dispensing: The Central Role of the Physician-Patient Relationship*, 137 Arch. Dermatol. 151, 151 (2001).

Journal 2001 Explores the extent to which pediatricians should rely on their expertise when prescribing therapies and durable medical equipment for children with special health care needs. Emphasizes the importance of the pediatrician's role in this context and urges pediatricians to comply with pertinent AMA guidelines and relevant state and federal laws. Quotes Opinion 8.06. References Opinion 9.132. Sneed, May, & Stencel, *Physicians' Reliance on Specialists, Therapists, and Vendors When Prescribing Therapies and Durable Medical Equipment for Children With Special Health Care Needs*, 107 Pediatrics 1283, 1287, 1288, 1289 (2001).

Journal 1998 Discusses the physician's fiduciary duty to the patient. Explores the expansion of the "honest services" mail fraud statute to prosecute undisclosed fiduciary breaches. Concludes that the mail fraud statute may be used to prosecute physicians who fail to disclose financial incentives to their patients. Quotes Opinion 8.03. Cites Opinions 2.03 and 8.07 [now Opinion 8.06]. Jones, *Primum Non Nocere: The Expanding "Honest Services" Mail Fraud Statute and the Physician-Patient Fiduciary Relationship*, 51 Vand. L. Rev. 139, 161, 164 (1998).

Journal 1992 Surveys federal and state antikickback and antireferral statutes pertaining to drug and device marketing activities. Considers the effectiveness of regulatory safe harbors. Quotes Opinion 6.04 [now Opinion 8.06]. References Opinion 8.061. Kirschenbaum & Kuhlik, *Federal and State Laws Affecting Discounts, Rebates, and Other Marketing Practices for Drugs and Devices*, 47 Food & Drug L. J. 533, 560 (1992).

Journal 1991 Looks at the physician as a fiduciary and the law governing fiduciary relationships. Concludes that fiduciary concepts are a valuable basis for establishing ethical and legal guidelines for physician behavior. Quotes Opinions 2.19, 8.03 (1989) [now Opinion 8.032], and 8.06. Healey & Dowling, *Controlling Conflicts of Interest in the Doctor-Patient Relationship: Lessons From Moore v. Regents of the University of California*, 42 Mercer L. Rev. 989, 997, 998 (1991).

8.061 Gifts to Physicians From Industry

Many gifts given to physicians by companies in the pharmaceutical, device, and medical equipment industries serve an important and socially beneficial function. For example, companies have long provided funds for educational seminars and conferences. However, there has been growing concern about certain gifts from industry to physicians. Some gifts that reflect customary practices of industry may not be consistent with the Principles of Medical Ethics. To avoid the acceptance of inappropriate gifts, physicians should observe the following guidelines:

(1) Any gifts accepted by physicians individually should primarily entail a benefit to patients and should not be of substantial value. Accordingly, textbooks, modest meals, and other gifts are appropriate if they serve a genuine educational function. Cash payments should not be accepted. The use of drug samples for personal or family use is permissible as long as these practices do not interfere with patient access to drug samples. It would not be acceptable for nonretired physicians to request free pharmaceuticals for personal use or use by family members.

(2) Individual gifts of minimal value are permissible as long as the gifts are related to the physician's work (eg, pens and notepads).

(3) The Council on Ethical and Judicial Affairs defines a legitimate "conference" or "meeting" as any activity, held at an appropriate location, where (a) the gathering is primarily dedicated, in both time and effort, to promoting objective scientific and educational activities and discourse (one or more educational presentation(s) should be the highlight of the gathering), and (b) the main incentive for bringing attendees together is to further their knowledge on the topic(s) being presented. An appropriate disclosure of financial support or conflict of interest should be made.

(4) Subsidies to underwrite the costs of continuing medical education conferences or professional meetings can contribute to the improvement of patient care and therefore are permissible. Since the giving of a subsidy directly to a physician by a company's representative may create a relationship that could influence the use of the company's products, any subsidy should be accepted by the conference's sponsor who in turn can use the money to reduce the conference's registration fee. Payments to defray the costs of a conference should not be accepted directly from the company by the physicians attending the conference.

(5) Subsidies from industry should not be accepted directly or indirectly to pay for the costs of travel, lodging, or other personal expenses of physicians attending conferences or meetings, nor should subsidies be accepted to compensate for the physicians' time. Subsidies for hospitality should not be accepted outside of modest meals or social events held as a part of a conference or meeting. It is appropriate for faculty at conferences or meetings to

accept reasonable honoraria and to accept reimbursement for reasonable travel, lodging, and meal expenses. It is also appropriate for consultants who provide genuine services to receive reasonable compensation and to accept reimbursement for reasonable travel, lodging, and meal expenses. Token consulting or advisory arrangements cannot be used to justify the compensation of physicians for their time or their travel, lodging, and other out-of-pocket expenses.

(6) Scholarship or other special funds to permit medical students, residents, and fellows to attend carefully selected educational conferences may be permissible as long as the selection of students, residents, or fellows who will receive the funds is made by the academic or training institution. Carefully selected educational conferences are generally defined as the major educational, scientific, or policy-making meetings of national, regional, or specialty medical associations.

(7) No gifts should be accepted if there are strings attached. For example, physicians should not accept gifts if they are given in relation to the physician's prescribing practices. In addition, when companies underwrite medical conferences or lectures other than their own, responsibility for and control over the selection of content, faculty, educational methods, and materials should belong to the organizers of the conferences or lectures. (II)

Issued June 1992 based on the report "Gifts to Physicians From Industry," adopted December 1990 (JAMA. 1991;265:501). Updated June 1996 and June 1998.

Journal 2011 Compares how the US, France, and Japan oversee pharmaceutical industry–physician financial relationships. Concludes that reforms are needed in each nation, including an alternative to pharmaceutical industry funding for professional medical activities. References Opinion 8.061. Rodwin, *Reforming Pharmaceutical Industry-Physician Financial Relationships: Lessons From the United States, France, and Japan,* 39 J. L. Med. & Ethics 662, 664 (2011).

Journal 2010 Examines manufacturer-physician consulting arrangements and discusses the evolution of fair market valuation. Proposes a set of standards for calculating fair market value for physician services to ensure compliance with legal requirements. Quotes Opinion 8.061. Eaton & Reid, *Mirror, Mirror on the Wall: Evaluating Fair Market Value for Manufacturer-Physician Consulting Arrangements,* 65 Food & Drug L. J. 141, 147 (2010).

Journal 2010 Examines the economic basis of physician-industry relationships that result in conflicts of interest. Considers the measures taken by developed countries in response to such conflicts. Concludes by proposing an approach that comprehensively addresses problems caused by drug and device company marketing to physicians. Cites Opinion 8.061. Jost, *Confronting Conflict: Addressing Institutional Conflicts of Interest in Academic Medical Centers,* 36 Am. J. L. & Med. 326, 336 (2010).

Journal 2010 Examines conflicts of interest experienced by academic medical centers between scientific integrity and corporate interests. Discusses approaches to ensure that academic medical centers effectively manage these conflicts. Proposes comprehensive policies to provide ways to identify, manage, and address institutional conflicts of interest in academic medical centers. Cites Opinion 8.061. Liang & Mackey, *Confronting Conflict: Addressing Institutional Conflicts of Interest in Academic Medical Centers,* 36 Am. J. L. & Med. 136, 149 (2010).

Journal 2010 Discusses the importance of prescription medication, the factors that influence patient access to pharmaceuticals, and the potential for greater access to drugs with expiring patents. Concludes patent law reforms are unlikely to help patients afford medications in the near future, but that initiatives to concentrate the federal government's purchasing power could be effective in increasing access to pharmaceuticals. References Opinion 8.061. Tironi, *Pharmaceutical Pricing: A Review of Proposals to Improve Access and Affordability of Prescription Drugs,* 19 Ann. Health L. 311, 360 (2010).

Journal 2009 Examines the effects of pharmaceutical marketing on physicians' fiduciary duty to place patients' interest first. Concludes that because of the fiduciary duty owed to patients, physicians have a legal obligation to avoid inappropriate exposure to pharmaceutical marketing. Quotes and cites Opinion 8.061. Hafemeister & Bryan, *Beware Those Bearing Gifts: Physicians' Fiduciary Duty to Avoid Pharmaceutical Marketing*, 57 U. Kan. L. Rev. 491, 499,512, 529 (2009).

Journal 2009 Discusses conflict of interest between cardiothoracic surgeons and industry. Concludes that 13 ethical guidelines should be followed to avoid conflicts of interest. Cites Opinion 8.061. Mack & Sade, *Relations Between Cardiothoracic Surgeons and Industry*, 87 Ann. Thorac. Surg. 1334, 1335 (2009).

Journal 2009 Examines the uses and prescribing patterns for antipsychotic medications, legal claims under which product liability suits may be brought, and the marketing techniques used by pharmaceutical companies in an effort to convince physicians to prescribe their drugs. Concludes pharmaceutical companies must be incentivized to provide physicians with more information about their drugs so they can make appropriate prescribing decisions. References Opinion 8.061. Mossman & Steinberg, *Promoting, Prescribing, and Pushing Pills: Understanding the Lessons of Anti-Psychotic Drug Litigation*, 13 Mich. St. U. J. Med. & L. 263, 315-16 (2009).

Journal 2009 Explores the influence of pharmaceutical and medical device industry gift giving on physicians and discusses recent restrictions and prohibitions on gifting. Concludes that recent changes in industry gifting standards may not decrease overall spending on professional promotion and may not eliminate the benefit to industry. Quotes Opinion 8.061. Steinbrook, *Physician-Industry Relations—Will Fewer Gifts Make a Difference?* 360 New Eng. J. Med. 557, 558 (2009).

Journal 2008 Discusses the pharmaceutical industry's practice of gifting to physicians and the failure of both parties to prevent corruption. Concludes state statutes are the most effective method to control prescription corruption. Quotes Opinion 8.061. Mehta, *Why Self-regulation Does Not Work: Resolving Prescription Corruption Caused by Excessive Gift-Giving by Pharmaceutical Manufacturers*, 63 Food & Drug L. J. 799, 810-811 (2008).

Journal 2008 Examines expectations about hormone therapy and the controversy surrounding the treatment. Concludes patients and physicians must be more realistic in weighing hormone therapy's medical value while respecting patient choice. Apparent reference to Opinion 8.061. Schulkin, *Hormone Therapy, Dilemmas, Medical Decisions*, 36 J. L. Med. & Ethics 73, 82 (2008).

Journal 2008 Examines marketing practices commonly utilized by the pharmaceutical industry aimed at health care professionals and the legal, ethical, and legislative implications of such practices. Concludes health care providers and pharmaceutical vendors need to adopt policies to address legislative and regulatory changes, as well as the ethical issues stemming from their relationship. Quotes Opinion 8.061. Washlick & Welch, *Physician-Vendor Marketing and Financial Relationships Under Attack*, 2 J. Health & Life Sci. L. 151, 164, 178-81 (2008).

Journal 2007 Discusses liability of pharmaceutical companies for failure to provide package warnings with sample prescription drugs. Concludes that while the "learned intermediary" doctrine protects companies against tort liability, such protection should be eliminated. References Opinion 8.061. Poser, *Unlabeled Drug Samples and the Learned Intermediary: The Case for Drug Company Liability Without Preemption*, 62 Food Drug L. J. 653, 667 (2007).

Journal 2007 Analyzes the availability of data on pharmaceutical gifts to physicians in Vermont and Minnesota. Concludes that state laws requiring disclosure of industry gifts have not guaranteed easy access to this information. Cites Opinion 8.061. Ross, Lackner, Lurie, Gross, Wolfe, & Krumholz, *Pharmaceutical Company Payments to Physicians: Early Experiences With Disclosure Laws in Vermont and Minnesota*, 297 JAMA 1216, 1216 (2007).

Journal 2006 Discusses the dynamic of the patient-physician relationship. Concludes that truly shared decision-making is likely unattainable. References Opinion 8.061. Clayton, *The Web of Relations: Thinking About Physicians and Patients*, 6 Yale J. Health Pol'y, L. & Ethics 465, 473 (2006).

Journal 2006 Describes public dissatisfaction with self-regulation of pharmaceutical industry gifts to medical professionals, concluding that more regulatory restrictions may be needed. References Opinion 8.061. Dresser, *Pharmaceutical Company Gifts: From Voluntary Standards to Legal Demands*, 36 Hastings Center Rep. 8, 9 (May/June 2006).

Journal 2006 Considers regulation of pharmaceutical sales and marketing. Suggests that drug companies have an opportunity to modify their practices to better comply with new regulations. Quotes Opinion 8.061. Henderson & Cassady, *Drug Deals in 2006: Cutting Edge Legal and Regulatory Issues in the Pharmaceutical Industry*, 15 Ann. Health L. 107, 131-32 (2006).

Journal 2006 Discusses increased regulation of gifts by pharmaceutical companies to physicians. Concludes that attorneys must be aware of the increased regulation in order to best advise their clients. Quotes Opinion 8.061. Rickard & Fehn, *Recent Developments in Regulation of Pharmaceutical Marketing Practices*, 19 Health Lawyer 16, 17 (Dec. 2006).

Journal 2005 Examines the pharmaceutical industry's influence on the shape and quality of medical education and practice. Concludes that the industry's influence on medical practitioners and the consequences of that influence on the American health care system are in transition. Quotes Opinion 8.061. Kapp, *Drug Companies, Dollars, and the Shaping of American Medical Practice*, 29 S. Ill. U. L. J. 237, 249 (2005).

Journal 2005 Conducted a survey to measure medical students' attitudes about interactions with drug companies. Concludes that future research should focus on ways to limit drug company influence so that decisions to prescribe medication are based upon the patient's best interest. Cites 8.061. Sierles, Brodkey, Cleary, McCurdy, Mintz, Frank, Lynn, Chao, Morgenstern, Shore, & Woodard, *Medical Students' Exposure to and Attitudes About Drug Company Interactions: A National Survey*, 294 JAMA 1034, 1035 (2005).

Journal 2004 Examines the intermediary doctrine and its effect on pharmaceutical manufacturer liability. Concludes that a balancing test must be employed in each instance to determine whether the physician or the pharmaceutical company is in the best position to warn the patient of dangers. References Opinion 8.061. Calabro, *Breaking the Shield of the Learned Intermediary Doctrine: Placing the Blame Where It Belongs*, 25 Cardozo L. Rev. 2241, 2262, 2263 (2004).

Journal 2004 Discusses the effect of federal fraud and abuse laws on the relationship between physicians and the pharmaceutical industry. Concludes that federal regulation of conflicts of interest created by physicians' relationships with pharmaceutical companies likely will increase. Cites Opinion 8.061. Studdert, Mello, & Brennan, *Financial Conflicts of Interest in Physicians' Relationships With the Pharmaceutical Industry—Self-regulation in the Shadow of Federal Prosecution*, 351 New Eng. J. Med. 1891, 1900 (2004).

Journal 2004 Describes financial conflicts of interest that may arise when physicians conduct clinical trials in the private practice setting. Concludes that safeguards must be put in place to protect patients, preserve the physician-patient relationship, and uphold the integrity of the research process. Cites Opinion 8.061. Williams, *Managing Physician Financial Conflicts of Interest in Clinical Trials Conducted in the Private Practice Setting*, 59 Food & Drug L. J. 45, 67 (2004).

Journal 2000 Compares the changes in physician roles in Japan and the US that exacerbate their conflicts of interest. Examines American physicians' dispensing practices and relations with pharmaceutical firms and hospital ownership. Concludes the US is reducing one of the main strengths it had in addressing physician conflicts: institutions of countervailing power and countervailing incentives. References Opinions 8.032 and 8.061, Rodwin & Okamoto, *Physicians' Conflicts of Interest in Japan and the United States: Lessons for the United States*, 25 J. Health Pol. Pol'y & L. 343, 355, 358 (2000).

Journal 2000 Examines the practice of gift giving by the health care technology industry as incentives in the context of continuing medical education activities. Concludes that industry-wide standards must be developed governing interactions between physicians and representatives of health care technology industry companies. Cites Opinions 8.061 and 9.011. Tenery, *Interactions Between Physicians and the Health Care Technology Industry*, 283 JAMA 391, 393 (2000).

Journal 2000 Examines data from several studies evaluating conflicts of interest triggered by gifts given to physicians by the pharmaceutical industry. Concludes that the efficacy of professional society guidelines to control such conflicts is questionable and there should be more systematic policies to address these concerns. References Opinion 8.061. Wazana, *Physicians and the Pharmaceutical Industry: Is a Gift Ever Just a Gift?* 283 JAMA 373, 380 (2000).

Journal 1999 Focuses on the purposes and broad applicability of the Medicare antikickback law. Describes how the law pertains to prescription drug and medical device manufacturers. Provides suggestions for antikickback law reform. Quotes Opinion 8.061. Bulleit & Krause, *Kickbacks, Courtesies, or Cost-Effectiveness? Application of the Medicare Antikickback Law to the Marketing* *and Promotional Practices of Drug and Medical Device Manufacturers, 54 Food & Drug L. J. 279, 296 (1999).*

Journal 1999 Discusses the impact *Daubert v. Merrell Dow Pharmaceuticals, Inc.* has had on scientific expert testimony. Explains that the scientific approach of dealing with bias may be inappropriate for maintaining scientific objectivity in litigation. Provides a strategy to deal with conflicts of interest in this context. Quotes Opinion 9.07. Cites Opinion 8.061. Patterson, *Conflicts of Interest in Scientific Expert Testimony, 40 Wm. & Mary L. Rev. 1313, 1330, 1332, 1335, 1371 (1999).*

Journal 1998 Discusses the conflict of interest posed by managed care organizations offering financial incentives to physicians. Explains that the duty to disclose and professionalism are not adequate protections against conflicts of interest. Suggests that financial incentives should be carefully circumscribed and that managed care organizations should focus primarily on quality of care. References Opinion 8.061. Emanuel & Goldman, *Protecting Patient Welfare in Managed Care: Six Safeguards, 23 J. Health Pol. Pol'y & L. 635, 641 (1998).*

Journal 1998 Examines the transition from paper medical records to electronic medical records. Identifies issues of confidentiality and privacy that arise as a result of the move to electronic medical records. Concludes that federal protection is needed to safeguard personal medical information. Quotes Principle IV and Opinions 5.07 and 5.075. Cites Opinion 8.061. Tsai, *Cheaper and Better: The Congressional Administrative Simplification Mandate Facilitates the Transition to Electronic Medical Records, 19 J. Legal Med. 549, 570, 581 (1998).*

Journal 1997 Discusses the process for marketing new drugs, medical devices, or biologics. Considers issues such as whether insurers or payers will cover these products, how much each will cost, and whether marketing programs comply with government regulations. References Opinion 8.061. Reiss, *Commentary on Payment and Reimbursement Issues Affecting the Marketing of Drugs, Medical Devices, and Biologics, With Emphasis on the Anti-Kickback Statute and Stark II, 52 Food & Drug L. J. 99,107 (1997).*

Journal 1997 Explores the extent to which pharmaceutical drug samples are taken by physicians or other medical staff for personal use. Concludes that this practice is common and raises pertinent ethical issues. Quotes Opinion 8.061. Westfall, McCabe, & Nicholas, *Personal Use of Drug Samples by Physicians and Office Staff, 278 JAMA 141, 142 (1997).*

Journal 1994 Discusses the role of professional societies in establishing ethical guidelines for physicians in the context of using medical innovations and new technologies. Observes that these standards must be supplemented by additional external measures or incentives in order to be most effective. Cites Opinions 1.01, 1.02, 8.061, 9.04, and 9.131. Orentlicher, *The Influence of a Professional Organization on Physician Behavior, 57 Alb. L. Rev. 583, 592, 593, 594, 595, 596 (1994).*

Journal 1993 Examines how the Food and Drug Administration (FDA) regulates marketing of new medical devices and its authority to do so. Describes how these regulations differ from those governing drugs. References Opinion 8.061. Dennis, *Promotion of Devices: An Extension of FDA Drug Regulation or a New Frontier? 48 Food & Drug L. J. 87 (1993).*

Journal 1992 Surveys federal and state antikickback and antireferral statutes pertaining to drug and device marketing activities. Considers the effectiveness of regulatory safe harbors. Quotes Opinion 6.04 [now Opinion 8.06]. References Opinion 8.061. Kirschenbaum & Kuhlik, *Federal and State Laws Affecting Discounts, Rebates, and Other Marketing Practices for Drugs and Devices, 47 Food & Drug L. J. 533, 560 (1992).*

Journal 1992 Discusses the extent of the Food and Drug Administration's (FDA's) authority to regulate oral sales promotion of pharmaceuticals. Explores the debate over the extent of the FDA's power to regulate. References Opinion 8.061. Noah, *Death of a Salesman: To What Extent Can the FDA Regulate the Promotional Statements of Pharmaceutical Sales Representatives? 47 Food & Drug L. J. 309, 316 (1992).*

Journal 1992 Reviews concerns about commercial involvement in and funding of continuing medical education (CME). Discusses CME requirements, accumulation of CME credits, and changes in standards governing commercial sponsorship. References Opinions 8.061 and 9.011. Wentz, Osteen, & Cannon, *Continuing Medical Education: Unabated Debate, 268 JAMA 1118 (1992).*

Journal 1991 Examines legal, ethical, and economic concerns surrounding pharmaceutical company promotions. Concludes that pharmaceutical freebies can serve a positive role in health care if adequately regulated. Quotes Opinions 8.061 and 8.08. Note, *The Economic Wisdom of Regulating Pharmaceutical "Freebies,"* 1991 Duke L. J. 206, 216, 233, 234 (1991).

Journal 1991 Discusses commercial support of continuing medical education. Explains ethical guidelines for accepting such assistance and how those guidelines have changed. References Opinions 8.061 and 9.011. Wentz, Osteen, & Gannon, *Refocusing Support and Direction,* 266 JAMA 953 (1991).

Clarification of Opinion 8.061, "Gifts to Physicians From Industry"

Scope
Opinion 8.061, "Gifts to Physicians From Industry," is intended to provide ethical guidance to physicians. Other parties involved in the health care sector, including the pharmaceutical, devices, and medical equipment industries and related entities or business partners, should view the guidelines as indicative of standards of conduct for the medical profession. Ultimately, it is the responsibility of individual physicians to minimize conflicts of interest that may be at odds with the best interest of patients and to access the necessary information to inform medical recommendations.

The guidelines apply to all forms of gifts, whether they are offered in person, through intermediaries, or through the Internet. Similarly, limitations on subsidies for educational activities should apply regardless of the setting in which, or the medium through which, the educational activity is offered.

General Questions
(a) **Do the guidelines apply only to pharmaceutical, device, and equipment manufacturers?**

"Industry" includes all "proprietary health-related entities that might create a conflict of interest."

Guideline 1
Any gifts accepted by physicians individually should primarily entail a benefit to patients and should not be of substantial value. Accordingly, textbooks, modest meals, and other gifts are appropriate if they serve a genuine educational function. Cash payments should not be accepted. The use of drug samples for personal or family use is permissible as long as these practices do not interfere with patient access to drug samples. It would not be acceptable for nonretired physicians to request free pharmaceuticals for personal use or for use by family members.

(a) **May physicians accept Gram stain test kits, stethoscopes, or other diagnostic equipments?**

Diagnostic equipment primarily benefits the patient. Hence, such gifts are permissible as long as they are not of substantial value. In considering the value of the gift, the relevant measure is not the cost to the company of providing the gift. Rather, the relevant measure is the cost to the physician if the physician purchased the gift on the open market.

(b) **May companies invite physicians to a dinner with a speaker and donate $100 to a charity or medical school on behalf of the physician?**
There are positive aspects to the proposal. The donations would be used for a worthy cause, and the physicians would receive important information about patient care. There is a direct personal benefit to the physician as well, however. An organization that is important to the physician—and one that the physician might have ordinarily felt obligated to make a contribution to—receives financial support as a result of the physician's decision to attend the meeting. On balance, physicians should make their own judgment about these inducements. If the charity is predetermined without the physician's input, there would seem to be little problem with the arrangement.

(c) **May contributions to a professional society's general fund be accepted from industry?**
The guidelines are designed to deal with gifts from industry which affect, or could appear to affect, the judgment of individual practicing physicians. In general, a professional society should make its own judgment about gifts from industry to the society itself.

(d) **When companies invite physicians to a dinner with a speaker, what are the relevant guidelines?**
First, the dinner must be a modest meal. Second, the guideline does allow gifts that primarily benefit patients and that are not of substantial value. Accordingly, textbooks and other gifts that primarily benefit patient care and that have a value to the physician in the general range of $100 are permissible. When educational meetings occur in conjunction with a social event such as a meal, the educational component must have independent value, such as a presentation by an authoritative speaker other than a sales representative of the company. Also, the meal should be a modest one similar to what a physician routinely might have when dining at his or her own expense. In an office or hospital encounter with a company representative, it is permissible to accept a meal of nominal value, such as a sandwich or snack.

(e) **May physicians accept vouchers that reimburse them for uncompensated care they have provided?**
No. Such a voucher would result directly in increased income for the physician.

(f) **May physicians accumulate "points" by attending several educational or promotional meetings and then choose a gift from a catalogue of education options?**
This guideline permits gifts only if they are not of substantial value. If accumulation of points would result in physicians receiving a substantial gift by combining insubstantial gifts over a relatively short period of time, it would be inappropriate.

(g) **May physicians accept gift certificates for educational materials when attending promotional or educational events?**

The Council views gift certificates as a gray area which is not per se prohibited by the guidelines. Medical textbooks are explicitly approved as gifts under the guidelines. A gift certificate for educational materials, ie, for the selection by the physician from an exclusively medical textbook catalogue, would not seem to be materially different. The issue is whether the gift certificate gives the recipient such control as to make the certificate similar to cash. As with charitable donations, preselection by the sponsor removes any question. It is up to the individual physician to make the final judgment.

(h) **May physicians accept drug samples or other free pharmaceuticals for personal use or use by family members?**

The Council's guidelines permit personal or family use of free pharmaceuticals (i) in emergencies and other cases where the immediate use of a drug is indicated, (ii) on a trial basis to assess tolerance, and (iii) for the treatment of acute conditions requiring short courses of inexpensive therapy, as permitted by Opinion 8.19, "Self-treatment or Treatment of Immediate Family Members." It would not be acceptable for physicians to accept free pharmaceuticals for the long-term treatment of chronic conditions.

(i) **May companies invite physicians to a dinner with a speaker and offer them a large number of gifts from which to choose one?**

In general, the greater the freedom of choice given to the physician, the more the offer seems like cash. A large number of gifts presented to physicians who attend a dinner would therefore be inappropriate.

There is no precise way of deciding an appropriate upper limit on the amount of choice that is acceptable. However, it is important that a specific limit be chosen to ensure clarity in the guidelines. A limit of eight has been chosen because it permits flexibility but prevents undue freedom of choice. Each of the choices must have a value to the physicians of no more than $100.

(j) **May physicians charge for their time with industry representatives or otherwise receive material compensation for participation in a detail visit?**

Guideline 1 states that gifts in the form of cash payments should not be accepted. Also, Guideline 6 makes clear that, in the context of the industry-physician relationship, only physicians who provide genuine services may receive reasonable compensation. When considering the time a physician spends with an industry representative, it is the representative who offers a service, namely the presentation of information. The physician is a beneficiary of the service. Overall, these guidelines do not view that physicians should be compensated for the time spent participating in educational activities, nor for time spent receiving detail information from an industry representative.

Guideline 2

Individual gifts of minimal value are permissible as long as the gifts are related to the physician's work (eg, pens and notepads).

(a) **May physicians, individually or through their practice group, accept electronic equipment, such as handheld devices or computers, intended to facilitate their ability to receive detail information electronically?**
Although Guideline 2 recognizes that gifts related to a physician' s practice may be appropriate, it also makes clear that these gifts must remain of minimal value. It is not appropriate for physicians to accept expensive hardware or software equipment even though one purpose only may pertain to industry-related activities of a modest value.

Guideline 3

The Council on Ethical and Judicial Affairs defines a legitimate "conference" or "meeting" as any activity, held at an appropriate location, where (a) the gathering is primarily dedicated, in both time and effort, to promoting objective scientific and educational activities and discourse (one or more educational presentation(s) should be the highlight of the gathering), and (b) the main incentive for bringing attendees together is to further their knowledge on the topic(s) being presented. An appropriate disclosure of financial support or conflict of interest should be made.

Guideline 4

Subsidies to underwrite the costs of continuing medical education conferences or professional meetings can contribute to the improvement of patient care and therefore are permissible. Since the giving of a subsidy directly to a physician by a company's sales representative may create a relationship which could influence the use of the company's products, any subsidy should be accepted by the conference's sponsor who in turn can use the money to reduce the conference's registration fee. Payments to defray the costs of a conference should not be accepted directly from the company by the physicians attending the conference.

(a) **Are conference subsidies from the educational division of a company covered by the guidelines?**
Yes. When the Council says "any subsidy," it would not matter whether the subsidy comes from the sales division, the educational division, or some other section of the company.

(b) **May a company or its intermediary send physicians a check or voucher to offset the registration fee at a specific conference or a conference of the physician's choice?**
Physicians should not directly accept checks or certificates which would be used to offset registration fees. The gift of a reduced registration should be made across the board and through the accredited sponsor.

Guideline 5

Subsidies from industry should not be accepted directly or indirectly to pay for the costs of travel, lodging, or other personal expenses of physicians attending conferences or meetings, nor should subsidies be accepted to compensate for the physicians' time. Subsidies for hospitality should not be accepted outside of modest meals or social events held as a part of a conference or meeting. It is appropriate for faculty at conferences or meetings to accept reasonable honoraria and to accept reimbursement for reasonable travel, lodging, and meal expenses. It is also appropriate for consultants who provide genuine services to receive reasonable compensation and to accept reimbursement for reasonable travel, lodging, and meal expenses. Token consulting or advisory arrangements cannot be used to justify the compensation of physicians for their time or their travel, lodging, and other out-of-pocket expenses.

(a) **If a company invites physicians to visit its facilities for a tour or to become educated about one of its products, may the company pay travel expenses and honoraria?**
This question has come up in the context of a rehabilitation facility that wants physicians to know of its existence so that they may refer their patients to the facility. It has also come up in the context of surgical device or equipment manufacturers who want physicians to become familiar with their products.

In general, travel expenses should not be reimbursed, nor should honoraria be paid for the visiting physician's time since the presentations are analogous to a pharmaceutical company's educational or promotional meetings. The Council recognizes that medical devices, equipment, and other technologies may require, in some circumstances, special evaluation or training in proper usage which cannot practicably be provided except on site. Medical specialties are in a better position to advise physicians regarding the appropriateness of reimbursement with regard to these trips. In cases where the company insists on such visits as a means of protection from liability for improper usage, physicians and their specialties should make the judgment. In no case would honoraria be appropriate and any travel expenses should be only those strictly necessary.

(b) **If the company invites physicians to visit its facilities for review and comment on a product, to discuss their independent research projects, or to explore the potential for collaborative research, may the company pay travel expenses and an honorarium?**
If the physician is providing genuine services, reasonable compensation for time and travel expenses can be given. However, token advisory or consulting arrangements cannot be used to justify compensation.

(c) **May a company hold a sweepstakes for physicians in which five entrants receive a trip to the Virgin Islands or airfare to the medical meeting of their choice?**

No. The use of a sweepstakes or raffle to deliver a gift does not affect the permissibility of the gift. Since the sweepstakes is not open to the public, the guidelines apply in full force.

(d) **If a company convenes a group of physicians to recruit clinical investigators or convenes a group of clinical investigators for a meeting to discuss their results, may the company pay for their travel expenses?**
Expenses may be paid if the meetings serve a genuine research purpose. One guide to their propriety would be whether the National Institutes of Health (NIH) conducts similar meetings when it sponsors multicenter clinical trials. When travel subsidies are acceptable, the guidelines emphasize that they be used to pay only for "reasonable" expenses. The reasonableness of expenses would depend on a number of considerations. For example, meetings are likely to be problematic if overseas locations are used for exclusively domestic investigators. It would be inappropriate to pay for recreation or entertainment beyond the kind of modest hospitality described in this guideline.

(e) **How can a physician tell whether there is a "genuine research purpose"?**
A number of factors can be considered. Signs that a genuine research purpose exists include the facts that there are (1) a valid study protocol, (2) recruitment of physicians with appropriate qualifications or expertise, and (3) recruitment of an appropriate number of physicians in light of the number of study participants needed for statistical evaluation.

(f) **May a company compensate physicians for their time and travel expenses when they participate in focus groups?**
Yes. As long as the focus groups serve a genuine and exclusive research purpose and are not used for promotional purposes, physicians may be compensated for time and travel expenses. The number of physicians used in a particular focus group or in multiple focus groups should be an appropriate size to accomplish the research purpose, but no larger.

(g) **Do the restrictions on travel, lodging, and meals apply to educational programs run by medical schools, professional societies, or other accredited organizations which are funded by industry, or do they apply only to programs developed and run by industry?**
The restrictions apply to all conferences or meetings which are funded by industry. The Council drew no distinction on the basis of the organizer of the conference or meeting. The Council felt that the gift of travel expenses is too substantial even when the conference is run by a nonindustry sponsor. (Industry includes all "proprietary health-related entities that might create a conflict of interest.")

(h) **May company funds be used for travel expenses and honoraria for bona fide faculty at educational meetings?**
This guideline draws a distinction between attendees and faculty. As was stated, "[i]t is appropriate for faculty at conferences or meetings to accept

reasonable honoraria and to accept reimbursement for reasonable travel, lodging, and meal expenses."

Companies need to be mindful of the guidelines of the Accreditation Council on Continuing Medical Education. According to those guidelines, "[f]unds from a commercial source should be in the form of an educational grant made payable to the CME sponsor for the support of programming."

(i) **May travel expenses be reimbursed for physicians presenting a poster or a "free paper" at a scientific conference?**
Reimbursement may be accepted only by bona fide faculty. The presentation of a poster or a free paper does not by itself qualify a person as a member of the conference faculty for purposes of these guidelines.

(j) **When a professional association schedules a long-range planning meeting, is it appropriate for industry to subsidize the travel expenses of the meeting participants?**
The guidelines are designed to deal with gifts from industry which affect, or could appear to affect, the judgment of individual practicing physicians. In general, a professional society should make its own judgment about gifts from industry to the society itself.

(k) **May continuing medical education conferences be held in the Bahamas, Europe, or South America?**
There are no restrictions on the location of conferences as long as the attendees are paying their own travel expenses.

(l) **May travel expenses be accepted by physicians who are being trained as speakers or faculty for educational conferences and meetings?**
In general, no. If a physician is presenting as an independent expert at a CME event, both the training and its reimbursement raise questions about independence. In addition, the training is a gift because the physician's role is generally more analogous to that of an attendee than a participant. Speaker training sessions can be distinguished from meetings (see 5d) with leading researchers, sponsored by a company, designed primarily for an exchange of information about important developments or treatments, including the sponsor's own research, for which reimbursement for travel may be appropriate.

(m) **What kinds of social events during conferences and meetings may be subsidized by industry?**
Social events should satisfy three criteria. First, the value of the event to the physician should be modest. Second, the event should facilitate discussion among attendees and/or discussion between attendees and faculty. Third, the educational part of the conference should account for a substantial majority of the total time accounted for by the educational activities and social events together. Events that would be viewed (as in the succeeding question) as lavish or expensive should be avoided. But modest social activities that are not elaborate or unusual are permissible, eg, inexpensive

boat rides, barbecues, entertainment that draws on the local performers. In general, any such events which are a part of the conference program should be open to all registrants.

(n) **May a company rent an expensive entertainment complex for an evening during a medical conference and invite the physicians attending the conference?**
No. The guidelines permit only modest hospitality.

(o) **If physicians attending a conference engage in interactive exchange, may their travel expenses be paid by industry?**
No. Mere interactive exchange would not constitute genuine consulting services.

(p) **If a company schedules a conference and provides meals for the attendees that fall within the guidelines, may the company also pay for the costs of the meals for spouses?**
If a meal falls within the guidelines, then the physician's spouse may be included.

(q) **May companies donate funds to sponsor a professional society's charity golf tournament?**
Yes. But it is sensible if physicians who play in the tournament make some contribution themselves to the event.

(r) **If a company invites a group of consultants to a meeting and a consultant brings a spouse, may the company pay the costs of lodging or meals of the spouse? Does it matter if the meal is part of the program for the consultants?**
Since the costs of having a spouse share a hotel room or join a modest meal are nominal, it is permissible for the company to subsidize those costs. However, if the total subsidies become substantial, then they become unacceptable.

Guideline 6
Scholarship or other special funds to permit medical students, residents, and fellows to attend carefully selected educational conferences may be permissible as long as the selection of students, residents, or fellows who will receive the funds is made by the academic or training institution. Carefully selected educational conferences are generally defined as the major educational, scientific, or policy-making meetings of national, regional, or specialty medical associations.

(a) **When a company subsidizes the travel expenses of residents to an appropriately selected conference, may the residents receive the subsidy directly from the company?**
Funds for scholarships or other special funds should be given to the academic departments or the accredited sponsor of the conference. The

disbursement of funds can then be made by the departments or the conference sponsor.

(b) **What is meant by "carefully selected educational conferences?"**
The intent of Guideline 6 is to ensure that financial hardship does not prevent students, residents, and fellows from attending major educational conferences. For example, we did not want to deny cardiology fellows the opportunity to attend the annual scientific meeting of the American College of Cardiology or orthopedic surgery residents the opportunity to attend the annual scientific meeting of the American Academy of Orthopaedic Surgeons. However, it was not the intent of the guideline to permit reimbursement of travel expenses in other circumstances, such as when conferences or symposia are designed specifically for students, residents, or fellows. Funds are limited to travel and lodging expanses for attendance at major educational, scientific, or policy-making meetings of national, regional, or specialty medical associations.

Guideline 7
No gifts should be accepted if there are strings attached. For example, physicians should not accept gifts if they are given in relation to the physician's prescribing practices. In addition, when companies underwrite medical conferences or lectures other than their own, responsibility for and control over the selection of content, faculty, educational methods, and materials should belong to the organizers of the conferences or lectures.

(a) **May companies send their top prescribers, purchasers, or referrers on cruises?**
No. There can be no link between prescribing or referring patterns and gifts. In addition, travel expenses, including cruises, are not permissible.

(b) **May the funding company itself develop the complete educational program that is sponsored by an accredited continuing medical education sponsor?**
No. The funding company may finance the development of the program through its grant to the sponsor, but the accredited sponsor must have responsibility and control over the content and faculty of conferences, meetings, or lectures. Neither the funding company nor an independent consulting firm should develop the complete educational program for approval by the accredited sponsor.

(c) **How much input may a funding company have in the development of a conference, meeting, or lectures?**
The guidelines of the Accreditation Council on Continuing Medical Education on commercial support of continuing medical education address this question.

Issued 1992. Updated December 2000, June 2002, (Food and Drug Law Journal, 2001;56(1):27-40), and June 2004.

8.062   Sale of Non–Health-Related Goods From Physicians' Offices

The sale of non–health-related goods by physicians presents a conflict of interest and threatens to erode the primary obligation of physicians to serve the interests of their patients before their own. Furthermore, this activity risks placing undue pressure on the patient and risks demeaning the practice of medicine.

Physicians should not sell non–health-related goods from their offices or other treatment settings, with the exception noted below.

Physicians may sell low-cost non–health-related goods from their offices for the benefit of community organizations, provided that (1) the goods in question are low cost; (2) the physician takes no share in profit from their sale; (3) such sales are not a regular part of the physician's business; (4) sales are conducted in a dignified manner; and (5) sales are conducted in such a way as to assure that patients are not pressured into making purchases. (I, II)

Issued June 1998 based on the report "Sale of Non–Health-Related Goods From Physicians' Offices," adopted December 1997 (JAMA. 1998;280(6):563).

N.Y. Sup. 2009 Physician moved to dismiss patient's claim for breach of fiduciary duty. Patient claimed that but for a physician-patient relationship with the physician, he would not have invested in the physician's new company. The court quoted Opinion 8.062 in determining that physician's conduct was objectionable, but nonetheless granted the motion to dismiss. *Otto v. Melman, 2009 WL 4348827, 4.*

Journal 2006 Discusses regulation of complementary and alternative medicine. Concludes that only minimal regulation of these practices is required. References Principle 7 (1957) [now Opinion 8.06 and Opinion 8.062]. Lunstroth, *Voluntary Self-regulation of Complementary and Alternative Medicine Practitioners, 70 Alb. L. Rev. 209, 243 (2006).*

Journal 2002 Examines the ethical aspects of e-medicine. Concludes that, although e-medicine has benefits, physicians must understand its impact on the physician-patient relationship. Cites Opinions 8.062 and 8.063. Berg, *Ethics and E-Medicine, 46 St. Louis U. L. J. 61, 66 (2002)*

Clarification of Opinions 8.062, Sale of Non–Health-Related Goods From Physicians' Offices, and 8.063, Sale of Health-Related Goods From Physicians' Offices

Do the guidelines discussing the sale of health-related products (8.063) and the sale of non–health-related goods (8.062) apply to physicians' practice Web sites?
Yes. The physician who provides or sells products to patients must follow the above guidelines regardless of whether the products are provided in the physician's office or through a practice Web site.

Adopted December 2000 as "Addendum III: Council on Ethical and Judicial Affairs Clarification on Sale of Products from Physicians' Offices (E-8.062 and E-8.063)."

8.063   Sale of Health-Related Products From Physicians' Offices

"Health-related products" are any products that, according to the manufacturer or distributor, benefit health. "Selling" refers to the activity of dispensing items that are provided from the physician's office in exchange for money and also includes the activity of endorsing a product that the patient may order or purchase elsewhere that results in direct remuneration for the physician. This Opinion does not apply to the sale of prescription items which is already addressed in Opinion 8.06, "Prescribing and Dispensing Drugs and Devices."

Physicians who engage in in-office sales practices should be aware of the related guidelines presented in Opinion 8.062, "Sale of Non–Health-Related Goods from Physicians' Offices"; Opinion 8.06, "Prescribing and Dispensing Drugs and Devices"; Opinion 8.032, "Conflicts of Interest: Health Facility Ownership by a Physician";* Opinion 3.01, "Nonscientific Practitioners"; Opinion 8.20, "Invalid Medical Treatment"; as well as the reports from which these opinions are extracted.

In-office sale of health-related products by physicians presents a financial conflict of interest, risks placing undue pressure on the patient, and threatens to erode patient trust and undermine the primary obligation of physicians to serve the interests of their patients before their own.

(1) Physicians who choose to sell health-related products from their offices should not sell any health-related products whose claims of benefit lack scientific validity. When judging the efficacy of a product, physicians should rely on peer-reviewed literature and other unbiased scientific sources that review evidence in a sound, systematic, and reliable fashion.

(2) Because of the risk of patient exploitation and the potential to demean the profession of medicine, physicians who choose to sell health-related products from their offices must take steps to minimize their financial conflicts of interest. The following guidelines apply:

(a) In general, physicians should limit sales to products that serve the immediate and pressing needs of their patients. For example, if traveling to the closest pharmacy would in some way jeopardize the welfare of the patient (eg, forcing a patient with a broken leg to travel to a local pharmacy for crutches), then it may be appropriate to provide the product from the physician's office. These conditions are explained in more detail in the Council's Opinion 8.06, "Prescribing and Dispensing Drugs and Devices," and are analogous to situations that constitute exceptions to the permissibility of self-referral.

(b) Physicians may distribute other health-related products to their patients free of charge or at cost, in order to make useful products readily available to their patients. When health-related products are offered free or at cost, it helps to ensure removal of the elements of personal gain and financial conflicts of interest that may interfere, or appear to interfere, with the physician's independent medical judgment.

(3) Physicians must disclose fully the nature of their financial arrangement with a manufacturer or supplier to sell health-related products. Disclosure includes informing patients of financial interests as well as about the availability of the product or other equivalent products elsewhere. Disclosure can be accomplished through face-to-face communication or by posting an easily understandable written notification in a prominent location that is accessible by all patients in the office. In addition, physicians should, upon request, provide patients with understandable literature that relies on scientific standards in addressing the risks, benefits, and limits of knowledge regarding the health-related product.

(4) Physicians should not participate in exclusive distributorships of health-related products which are available only through physicians' offices. Physicians should encourage manufacturers to make products of established benefit more fairly and more widely accessible to patients than exclusive distribution mechanisms allow. (II)

Issued December 1999 based on the report "Sale of Health-Related Products From Physicians' Offices," adopted June 1999.

*Opinion 8.032, "Conflicts of Interest: Health Facility Ownership by a Physician," was replaced by the current Opinion 8.0321, "Physicians' Self-referral," June 2009.

Journal 2006 Reviews the regulation of dietary supplement manufacturing and labeling. Concludes that the FDA may have adequate authority to regulate dietary supplements. Quotes Opinion 8.063. Noah, *A Drug by Any Other Name. . . ? Paradoxes in Dietary Supplement Risk Regulation, 17 Stan. L. & Pol'y Rev. 165, 192 (2006).*

Journal 2002 Examines the ethical aspects of e-medicine. Concludes that, although e-medicine has benefits, physicians must understand its impact on the physician-patient relationship. Cites Opinions 8.062 and 8.063. Berg, *Ethics and E-Medicine, 46 St. Louis U. L. J. 61, 66 (2002).*

Clarification of Opinions 8.062, Sale of Non–Health-Related Goods From Physicians' Offices, and 8.063, Sale of Health-Related Goods From Physicians' Offices

Do the guidelines discussing the sale of health-related products (8.063) and the sale of non–health-related goods (8.062) apply to physicians' practice Web sites?

Yes. The physician who provides or sells products to patients must follow the above guidelines regardless of whether the products are provided in the physician's office or through a practice Web site.

Adopted December 2000 as "Addendum III: Council on Ethical and Judicial Affairs Clarification on Sale of Products from Physicians' Offices (E-8.062 and E-8.063)."

8.07 "Gifts to Physicians: Offers of Indemnity," issued June 1992, was deleted in June 2002 and combined with Opinion 6.04, "Fee Splitting: Drug or Device Prescription Rebates" and Opinion 8.06, "Drugs and Devices: Prescribing" into the current Opinion 8.06, "Prescribing and Dispensing Drugs and Devices."

8.07 Expedited Partner Therapy

Expedited partner therapy (EPT) is the practice of treating the sex partners of patients with sexually transmitted diseases via patient-delivered partner therapy without the partner receiving a medical evaluation or professional prevention counseling. While this practice is presently recommended by the Centers for Disease Control and Prevention for use in very limited circumstances (for gonorrhea or chlamydial infection in heterosexual men and women), EPT may be recommended for additional applications in the future.

Although EPT has been demonstrated to be effective at reducing the burden of certain diseases, it also has ethical implications. EPT potentially abrogates the standard informed consent process, compromises continuity of care for patients' partners, encroaches upon the privacy of patients and their partners, increases the possibility of harm by a medical or allergic reaction, leaves other diseases or complications undiagnosed, and may violate state practice laws. The following guidelines are offered for use in establishing whether EPT is appropriate:

(1) Physicians should determine the need for EPT by engaging in open discussions with patients to ascertain their partners' abilities to access medical services. Only if the physician reasonably believes that a patient's partner(s) will be unwilling or unable to seek treatment within the context of a traditional patient-physician relationship should the use of EPT be considered.

(2) Prior to initiating EPT, physicians are advised to seek the guidance of public health officials, as well as determine the legal status of EPT in their state.

(3) If the physician chooses to initiate EPT, he or she must provide patients with appropriate instructions regarding EPT and its accompanying medications and answers to any questions that they may have.

(4) Physicians must provide patients with educational material to share with their partners that encourages the partners to consult a physician as a preferred alternative to EPT, and that discloses the risk of potential adverse drug reactions and the possibility of dangerous interactions between the patient-delivered therapy and other medications that the partner may be taking. The partner should also be informed that he or she may be affected by other sexually transmitted diseases (STDs) that may be left untreated by the delivered medicine.

(5) The treating physician should also make reasonable efforts to refer a patient's partner(s) to appropriate health care professionals. (VII)

Issued November 2008 based on the report "Expedited Partner Therapy," adopted June 2008.

8.08 Informed Consent

The patient's right of self-decision can be effectively exercised only if the patient possesses enough information to enable an informed choice. The patient should make his or her own determination about treatment. The physician's obligation is to present the medical facts accurately to the patient or to the individual responsible for the patient's care and to make recommendations for management in accordance with good medical practice. The physician has an ethical obligation to help the patient make choices from among the therapeutic alternatives consistent with good medical practice. Informed consent is a basic policy in both ethics and law that physicians must honor, unless the patient is unconscious or otherwise incapable of consenting and harm from failure to treat is imminent. In special circumstances, it may be appropriate to postpone disclosure of information (see Opinion E-8.122, "Withholding Information from Patients").

Physicians should sensitively and respectfully disclose all relevant medical information to patients. The quantity and specificity of this information should be tailored to meet the preferences and needs of individual patients. Physicians need not communicate all information at one time, but should assess the amount of information that patients are capable of receiving at a given time and present the remainder when appropriate. (I, II, V, VIII)

Issued March 1981. Updated November 2006, based on the report "Withholding Information From Patients (Therapeutic Privilege)," adopted June 2006.

7th Cir. 2002 Prosecutors appealed order enjoining enforcement of informed consent provisions of Indiana abortion statute on the grounds that they unconstitutionally created an undue burden. Court of Appeals reversed and held injunction was an abuse of discretion. The court found the statute was substantively identical to a law upheld in previous decisions. Further, the court held that the state was entitled to have the law evaluated on the basis of actual experience. Dissenting judge quoted Opinion 8.08 regarding need for patient to be capable of giving informed consent. *A Woman's Choice-East Side Women's Clinic v. Newman*, 305 F.3d 684, 716.

Alaska 2002 Patient brought malpractice and informed consent claims against physician. In part, patient alleged physician's failure to appropriately advise her regarding her abdominal pain after surgery led to permanent injuries. Trial court entered judgment for physician. On appeal, Alaska Supreme Court remanded the informed consent claim, holding that the jury instruction should have reflected a "reasonable patient" standard. Quotes Opinion 8.08. *Marsingill v. O'Malley*, 58 P.3d 495, 499, 504-05.

Ga. App. 2000 Plaintiff alleged failure on the part of a dentist to inform him of the risks of root canal in a malpractice action. The appeals court noted that state case law did not recognize the informed consent doctrine. In evaluating this precedent, the court quoted Opinion 8.08 and Fundamental Element (1) [now Opinion 10.01]. The court stated that the AMA *Code of Medical Ethics* should be understood to reflect the standard of care of the medical profession on the issue of informed consent. While the court ruled in favor of the dentist, it prospectively recognized the doctrine of informed consent. *Ketchup v. Howard*, 247 Ga. App. 54, 543 S.E.2d 371, 376, 377.

Ind. 1992 Plaintiffs filed suit against physician after medical review panel found no evidence that physician committed malpractice in performing a bladder suspension and cryosurgery that resulted in plaintiff's cervix adhering to wall of her vagina. The trial court granted summary judgment for the defendant but appellate court reversed in part holding that the informed consent claim did not require expert medical testimony. The state Supreme Court affirmed the summary judgment, determining that the reasonably prudent physician standard applied in informed consent cases. In support of its decision, the court quoted Opinion 8.08, regarding informed consent. The court also held that expert medical testimony was required for plaintiff's informed consent claim because the standard of care for the procedure performed was not common knowledge for lay persons. *Culbertson v. Mernitz*, 602 N.E.2d 98, 103, 106.

Ind. App. 1999 Patient brought malpractice suit against surgeon, claiming that he would not have consented to surgery if the surgeon had disclosed that he would perform only a fusion for the patient's back, rather than the recommended procedure. The trial court granted summary judgment. The appellate court reversed, and held that a plaintiff is not required to introduce expert testimony to establish the standard of care or the causation elements in an informed consent action when lay people can understand that a failure to meet the standard of care occurred. The court cited *Culbertson v. Mernitz*, 602 N.E.2d 98 (Ind. 1992), where the Indiana Supreme Court quoted Opinion 8.08, regarding informed consent. *Bowman v. Beghin*, 713 N.E.2d 913, 916.

N.J. 2007 After consultation with her physician, plaintiff signed a consent form and had an abortion. Plaintiff was later diagnosed with an incomplete abortion which, she alleged, alerted her to the fact that the procedure resulted in the death of a human being. She sued her physician for negligent infliction of emotional distress and failure to obtain informed consent. Summary judgment was granted for the physician and plaintiff appealed. The Supreme Court of New Jersey, quoting Opinion 8.08, considered whether a reasonable patient would find the information regarding whether a human being was killed, material in giving consent. Finding that there is no consensus that a "human being" is killed during an abortion, that a fetus has not been deemed to be a person under the Constitution, and that the question is a value judgment, the court found no duty for a physician to provide such information. *Acuna v. Turkish*, 192 N.J. 399, 930 A.2d 416, 425.

N.J. 1999 Patient sued surgeon for lack of informed consent and malpractice on grounds that the surgeon decided to treat patient's hip fracture with bed rest rather than utilizing other alternatives. The trial court held that the patient could not sustain a claim for lack of informed consent. The New Jersey Supreme Court held that the informed consent requirement extends to noninvasive procedures. The court quoted Opinion 8.08 regarding a patient's right to be fully informed of medically reasonable treatments. *Matthies v. Mastromonaco*, 160 N.J. 26, 733 A.2d 456, 463.

N.Y. Fam. 2006 During proceedings regarding a foster child, an issue was raised contesting the legality of the County Department of Human Services' procedures for administering drugs to children. The mother's consent for prescribing medication to the child was obtained by a case-worker, without direct consultation with a physician and with no explanation of side effects. The court cited Opinions 8.08, 8.081, 8.11, and 10.01 in determining the physician's duty to honor the decision of the parent/surrogate. The mother's consent was invalidated and she was given an opportunity to consult with a physician. *Matter of Lyle A., 14 Misc. 3d 842, 830 N.Y.S.2d 486, 492, 494.*

W. Va. 1995 West Virginia Board of Medicine received a complaint from patient that physician was using depossession treatment. The hearing examiner in part found that there had been a lack of informed consent for such treatment. The Board changed the examiner's report and added sanctions. In doing so, it quoted Opinion 8.08. On appeal, the circuit court reversed, finding the Board's order arbitrary and an abuse of discretion. The appellate court agreed that the Board abused its discretion, but remanded the case for consideration of the issue of informed consent for depossession treatment. *Modi v. West Virginia Board of Medicine, 465 S.E.2d230,236.*

Journal 2011 Discusses the doctrine of informed consent and the influence of physician groups on the dissemination of information to patients. Concludes the doctrine of informed consent should be expanded by the courts, rather than continuing to allow professional professional societies to dictate provider guidelines for obtaining informed consent. Quotes Opinions 8.08, 10.01, and 10.015. References Opinion 2.065. Ginsberg, *Informed Consent: No Longer Just What the Doctor Ordered? The "Contributions" of Medical Associations and Courts to a More Patient Friendly Doctrine, 15 Mich. St. J. Med. & Law 17, 23, 24, 25, 26, 46 (2011).*

Journal 2011 Argues that autonomy should be compromised for the welfare of certain research subjects who would benefit from the particular medical research. Concludes that although autonomy is sometimes sacrificed for welfare, it should go even further to prefer subject groups with the greatest risk/benefit ratio. Quotes Opinion 8.08. Stein & Savulescu, *Welfare Versus Autonomy in Human Subjects Research, 38 Fla. St. U. L. Rev. 303, 332 (2011).*

Journal 2010 Examines a prisoner's substantive due process right under the Fourteenth Amendment to receive sufficient information to make an informed decision on whether to consent to or refuse medical treatment. Concludes that the doctrinal grounds for this claimed right are weak and that public policy considerations counsel against it. Quotes Opinion 8.08. Gatter, *A Prisoner's Constitutional Right to Medical Information: Doctrinally Flawed and a Threat to State Informed Consent Law, 45 Wake Forest L. Rev. 1025, 1062 (2010).*

Journal 2010 Discusses issues arising from the enactment of legislation by North Dakota involving a minor's reproductive rights. Explores ethical principles that govern physician's actions within the context of reproductive health. Concludes that, while a patient's expectation of confidentiality with a physician is critical, competing values come into play when the patient is a minor and parental involvement may be important. Provides practical guidance to address issues in this context. Quotes Opinions 2.01, 2.015, 5.055, 8.08, 8.115, 9.12, 10.01, 10.015, and 10.05. Cites Opinion 5.05, 5.055, 8.08, 8.11, 8.115, 9.12, and 10.05. Haas, *"Doctor, I'm Pregnant and Fifteen—I Can't Tell My Parents—Please Help Me": Minor Consent, Reproductive Rights, and Ethical Principles for Physicians, 86 N.D. L. Rev. 63, 70, 73, 75-78, 82, 84, 86-88 (2010).*

Journal 2010 Analyzes the practice of coerced sterilization of HIV-positive women to prevent transmission of the virus to offspring and discusses current litigation challenging such sterilization as a rights violation. Concludes forced sterilization is a major problem in Latin America and Africa, and the human rights community must work closely with the medical community to ensure patients are making informed medical decisions. Cites Opinion 8.08. Nair, *Litigating Against the Forced Sterilization of HIV-Positive Women: Recent Developments in Chile and Nambia, 23 Harv. Hum. Rts. J. 223, 226 (2010).*

Journal 2009 Discusses the availability and scope of the doctrine of informed consent in Georgia, citing *Doreika v. Blotner* as an important pending case in which the Georgia Supreme Court will review the doctrine. Concludes *Doreika* should be affirmed to provide full recognition of a patient's rights to self-determination and bodily integrity in Georgia. Cites Opinions 8.08 and 8.15. Leppert, *Doreika v. Blotner: Affirming Ketchup Against Judicial Mustard, 60 Mercer L. Rev. 807, 817, 820 (2009).*

Journal 2009 Argues race-based genetic biomedical research is necessary because of the significant impact of race and ethnicity on various aspects of life. Concludes law and policy should promote socially responsible race-based genetic research to gain more meaningful and applicable scientific knowledge. Quotes Opinion 8.08. Malinowski, *Dealing With the Realities of Race and Ethnicity: A Bioethics-Centered Argument in Favor of Race-Based Genetics Research, 45 Hous. L. Rev. 1415, 1463 (2009).*

Journal 2009 Compares the tort law doctrine of informed consent to abortion law's approach to informed consent. Discusses woman-protective reasoning as the cause of divergence between the two bodies of law. Concludes abortion law lacks confidence in women's decision-making capabilities and that lawmakers should recognize abortion law's approach to informed consent is contrary to other patient health care decision-making and denies women equal treatment. References Opinion 8.08. Manian, *The Irrational Woman: Informed Consent and Abortion Decision-Making, 16 Duke J. Gender L. & Pol'y 223, 241 (2009).*

Journal 2009 Argues First Amendment rights of physicians are being violated by government control and imposition of ideology through statutes, using South Dakota's informed consent to abortion statute as an example. Concludes statutes endorsing a particular ideology damage the physician-patient relationship and infringe upon physician First Amendment rights. References Code of Ethics Art. I(4) (1847) [now Opinion 8.08]. Robbins, *Open Your Mouth and Say "Ideology": Physicians and the First Amendment, 12 U. Pa. J. Const. L. 155, 159 (2009).*

Journal 2009 Discusses potential liability of a medical device or pharmaceutical company due to its representative's presence in the treatment room, including privacy claims and claims based on the representative's acts or omissions. Concludes companies must be aware of such liability risks and train their representatives accordingly. Quotes Opinion 8.08. Summerhill & Chandler, *Company Representatives in the Operating & Treatment Room: How to Navigate the Ever-Expanding Theories of Liability for Medical Device & Pharmaceutical Companies, 12 DePaul J. Health Care L. 253, 258-259 (2009).*

Journal 2008 Reviews procedural guidelines for fine-needle aspiration of the thyroid gland. Concludes, in part, that particular attention must be paid to the informed consent process to ensure patients undergoing such procedures appropriately understand procedure risks and benefits. References Opinion 8.08. Cibas, Alexander, Benson, Patricio de Agustín, Doherty, Faquin, Middleton, Miller, Raab, White, & Mandel, *Indications for Thyroid FNA and Pre-FNA Requirements: A Synopsis of the National Cancer Institute Thyroid Fine-Needle Aspiration State of the Science Conference, 36 Diagnostic Cytopathology 390, 394 (2008).*

Journal 2008 Considers the utility of physician apologies for medical error and legal protection for physicians who apologize for mistakes. Concludes physicians must openly communicate with their patients and apologize for medical errors to strengthen the health care community. Quotes Opinions 8.08, 8.12, 10.01, and 10.015. References Opinion 8.12. Ebert, *Attorneys, Tell Your Clients to Say They're Sorry: Apologies in the Health Care Industry, 5 Ind. Health L. Rev. 337, 340-41, 344 (2008).*

Journal 2008 Argues the Alaska Supreme Court erroneously extended the physician's informed consent duty to disclose to situations in which the physician had no opportunity to evaluate the patient. Concludes *Marsingill v. O'Malley* requires physicians to inconvenience patients or bear unreasonable risk. Quotes Opinion 8.08. Hutchinson, *Marsingill v. O'Malley: The Duty to Disclose Becomes the Duty to Divine, 25 Alaska L. Rev. 241, 252 (2008).*

Journal 2008 Explores issues regarding treatment decisions for incapacitated patients. Concludes patient decision-making capacity should be tested in many situations to ensure the treatment decisions made are those the patient would make if competent. Cites Opinion 8.08. Vars, *Illusory Consent: When an Incapacitated Patient Agrees to Treatment, 87 Or. L. Rev. 353, 359 (2008).*

Journal 2007 Discusses the evolution of informed consent doctrine. Concludes that, in context of research, informed consent exceptions should be substantially narrowed. Quotes Ch. I, Art. I, Sec. 4 (May 1847) [now Opinion 8.082] and Ch. I, Art. I, Sec. 1 (May 1847) [now Principles I and VIII]. References Opinions 2.08 and 8.08. Grimm, *Informed Consent for All! No Exceptions, 37 N. M. L. Rev. 39, 39, 61 (2007).*

Journal 2007 Discusses patients' right to refuse medical treatment and the corresponding duties of health care professionals. Concludes that detailed, carefully prepared advance directives are necessary to fulfill patients' wishes. Quotes Ch. II (1940) [now Opinions 8.08 and 8.082] and Opinions 2.035, 2.037, 2.20, 2.225, 8.081, and 10.015. Cites Opinions 9.11 and 9.115. Stamatakis, *Beyond Advance Directives: Personal Autonomy and the Right to Refuse Life-Sustaining Medical Treatment, 47 N. H. B. J. 20, 29-30 (2007).*

Journal 2007 Examines statutes giving pharmacists the right to refuse dispensing of emergency contraceptives. Concludes that a woman should be allowed to bring a wrongful conception claim against a pharmacist who refuses her medication. References Opinion 8.08. Weisser, *Abolishing the Pharmacist's Veto: An Argument in Support of a Wrongful Conception Cause of Action Against Pharmacists Who Refuse to Provide Emergency Contraception, 80 S. Cal. L. Rev. 865, 881-81 (2007).*

Journal 2006 Reviews the concept of therapeutic privilege. Concludes that the practice creates conflict between physician obligations under the concepts of autonomy and beneficence. Recommends that physicians maximize communication with patients by providing all pertinent information in the context of patient preferences. Cites Opinions 8.08, 8.081, 8.121, and 10.015. References Chap. I, Art. I, Sec. 4 (May 1847) [premise deleted from Code]. Bostick, Sade, McMahon, & Benjamin, *Report of the American Medical Association Council on Ethical and Judicial Affairs: Withholding Information From Patients: Rethinking the Propriety of "Therapeutic Privilege," 17 J. Clinical Ethics 302, 303 (Winter 2006).*

Journal 2006 Discusses the evolution of health law in Virginia. Concludes that the area of health law continues to expand, develop, and be refined. Cites Opinions 3.03, 3.08, 5.01, 5.015, 5.02, 5.04, 5.055, 6.02, 6.021, 6.03, 6.04, 7.03, 7.04, 7.05, 8.054, 8.08, 8.081, 8.085, 8.115, 8.12, 8.14, 8.145, 8.19, and 9.045. Guanzon, *Health Care Law, 41 U. Rich. L. Rev. 179, 199 (2006).*

Journal 2005 Speculates on the issues raised if the US government were to force drug addicts to take pharmaceuticals designed to prevent reaction to illegal drug. Concludes that such a policy violates multiple constitutional rights as well as the ethical principles underlying informed consent. Quotes Opinion 8.08. Boire, *Neurocops: The Politics of Prohibition and the Future of Enforcing Social Policy From Inside the Body, 19 J. L. & Health 215, 237 (2005)*

Journal 2005 Evaluates informed consent in the practice of teaching medical students by having them perform unnecessary procedures on hospital patients. Concludes that consent must be obtained in all cases. Cites Opinion 8.08. Oberman, *Panel Discussion American Association of Law Schools Panel: Panel on the Use of Patients for Teaching Purposes Without Their Knowledge or Consent, 8 J. Health Care L. & Pol'y 210, 210 (2005).*

Journal 2004 Examines whether performing genital reconstruction surgery on intersexed children to prevent psychological harm is necessary. Concludes that courts around the world should prohibit medically unnecessary genital reconstruction surgery during childhood. Quotes Opinion 8.08. Haas, *Who Will Make Room for the Intersexed? 30 Am. J. L. & Med. 41, 63 (2004).*

Journal 2003 Discusses whether, and how, legal rights may be waived. Concludes that, in addressing these questions, emphasis should be placed on concepts of autonomy and voluntariness. Cites Opinion 8.08. Berg, *Understanding Waiver, 40 Hous. L. Rev. 281, 329 (2003).*

Journal 2003 Examines the manner in which psychiatrists participate in the criminal justice system. Concludes that, in some situations, this participation may violate principles of medical ethics. Cites Opinions 2.06 and 8.08. Dolin, *A Healer or an Executioner? The Proper Role of a Psychiatrist in a Criminal Justice System, 17 J. L. & Health 169, 206, 213-14 (2003).*

Journal 2003 Evaluates patient autonomy in the physician-patient relationship. Concludes that it may be time to reject its dominance in favor of requiring physicians to provide patients with the maximum benefit of their expertise without imposing authority in areas beyond that expertise. Quotes Opinion 8.08. Dworkin, *Getting What We Should From Doctors: Rethinking Patient Autonomy and the Doctor-Patient Relationship, 13 Health Matrix 235, 240 (2003).*

Journal 2003 Argues that affirmative measures should be taken by the Air Force to ensure access to abortion services. Concludes that regulatory changes will reduce barriers to access. Quotes Opinion 10.01. Cites Opinion 8.08. Wilde, *Air Force Women's Access to Abortion Services and the Erosion of 10 USC § 1093, 9 Wm. & Mary J. Women & L. 351, 371 (2003).*

Journal 2002 Examines how managed care has adversely affected information disclosure in the physician-patient relationship. Concludes that, unless courts expand applicability of principles of informed consent, patient self-determination and autonomy will continue to be undermined. Quotes Principle VIII and Opinions 8.03, 8.053, 8.054, and 8.08. Morris, *Dissing Disclosure: Just What the Doctor Ordered, 44 Ariz. L. Rev. 313, 344, 349, 362, 363, 366 (2002).*

Journal 2002 Considers the dilemma of informed consent in the context of prescribing psychotropic medication to patients with mental illness and mental retardation. Recognizes the need for substituted decision-making in certain situations. Concludes that legislation would help address this issue. Quotes Preamble, Principles I, III, IV, VIII, and IX, and Opinion 8.08. O'Sullivan & Borcherding, *Informed Consent for Medication in Persons With Mental Retardation and Mental Illness,* 12 Health Matrix 63, 75, 86, 87, 88 (2002).

Journal 2002 Analyzes the role of prognostication in physician-patient communication. Concludes that the patient-physician model of shared decision-making offers the best hope for reestablishing prognostication. Quotes Principles Ch. I, Art. I, Sec. 2 and 4 (1846) [now Principle IV and Opinions 8.12 and 10.01]. Cites Opinion 8.08. Rich, *Prognostication in Clinical Medicine: Prophecy or Professional Responsibility?* 23 J. Legal Med. 297, 299, 318, 327 (2002).

Journal 2000 Examines physician value neutrality (PVN). Defines PVN as providing a foundation to suggest physicians must keep their values—religious, political, or otherwise—out of the patient-physician relationship. Concludes it is not clear how values can be removed from the patient-physician relationship without removing the very thing PVN supporters are trying to protect, the intrinsic value of persons. References Opinions 2.01, 2.02, 8.032, 8.05, 8.08, and 8.132. Beckwith & Peppin, *Physician Value Neutrality: A Critique,* 28 J. L. Med. & Ethics 67, 72-73 (2000).

Journal 2000 Explores the US Supreme Court's use of the First Amendment's viewpoint neutrality mandate. Concludes that viewpoint discrimination should be applied to limit government censorship of private speech in nonpublic forums and selective subsidy programs. Quotes Opinion 8.08. Casarez, *Public Forums, Selective Subsidies, and Shifting Standards of Viewpoint Discrimination,* 64 Alb. L. Rev. 501, 558 (2000).

Journal 2000 Considers the objective of the informed consent doctrine. Concludes that, in practice, the doctrine falls short of its intended purpose. Quotes Opinion 8.08. Kurtz, *The Law of Informed Consent: From "Doctor Is Right" to "Patient Has Rights,"* 50 Syracuse L. Rev. 1243, 1245 (2000).

Journal 2000 Describes the fiduciary aspects of the physician-patient relationship. Explores the conflicts that may occur between physicians and pregnant women in the health care setting. Proposes legal strategies to address these conflicts. Quotes Opinions 8.08 and 10.01. References Opinion 8.13. Oberman, *Mothers and Doctors' Orders: Unmasking the Doctor's Fiduciary Role in Maternal-Fetal Conflicts,* 94 Nw. U. L. Rev. 451, 456, 462, 493 (2000).

Journal 2000 Examines issues relating to parental consent to circumcision. Identifies legal and ethical requirements for consent when medical professionals are treating adult patients. Analyzes the implications of those requirements for routine circumcision of infant males. Concludes that only when the male is an adult and capable of making decisions can circumcision be ethically and legally performed. Quotes Opinion 8.08. References Opinions 8.03 and 9.011. Svoboda, Van Howe, & Dwyer, *Informed Consent for Neonatal Circumcision: An Ethical and Legal Conundrum,* 17 J. Contemp. Health L. & Pol'y 61, 67, 73, 82 (2000).

Journal 2000 Discusses traditional medical ethics and the physician's duty to benefit patients. Concludes that, in the 21st century, physicians will no longer be expected to determine on their own what will benefit their patients. Quotes Principle II and Opinion 8.08. Veatch, *Doctor Does Not Know Best: Why in the New Century Physicians Must Stop Trying to Benefit Patients,* 25 J. Med. & Phil. 701, 710, 711 (2000).

Journal 2000 Discusses the development and history of the ethical doctrine of informed consent. Examines the current state of the law in Pennsylvania and concludes it does not adequately fulfill the goals of ethical and legal doctrines. Quotes Principle IV and Opinion 10.01. References Opinion 8.08. Warren, *Pennsylvania Medical Informed Consent Law: A Call to Protect Patient Autonomy Rights by Abandoning the Battery Approach,* 38 Duq. L. Rev. 917, 925 (2000).

Journal 1999 Observes that, under statute and common law, the doctrine of informed consent in Pennsylvania does not apply in situations involving nonsurgical procedures. Argues that state law should be expanded to include a duty to obtain informed consent in these situations. Quotes Opinion 8.08. Durst, *Cutting Through Pennsylvania's Medical Informed Consent Statute: A Reasonable Interpretation Abolishing the Surgical Requirement,* 104 Dick. L. Rev. 197, 225 (1999).

Journal 1998 Discusses legal aspects of physician-assisted suicide. Identifies acceptable end-of-life choices and compares them to physician-assisted suicide. Points out that physician-assisted suicide has the potential for abuse and that safeguards have not been implemented to protect people from that risk. Quotes Opinion 2.211. Cites Opinions 2.20 and 8.08. Mitchell, *Physician-Assisted Suicide: A Survey of the Issues Surrounding Legalization,* 74 N. D. L. Rev. 341, 349 (1998).

Journal 1998 Discusses current abortion malpractice claims. Describes three general types of malpractice causes of action. Argues that specialized procreative torts should be implemented to adequately protect a woman's procreative autonomy. Quotes Opinion 8.08. Northern, *Procreative Torts: Enhancing the Common-Law Protection for Reproductive Autonomy*, 1998 U. Ill. L. Rev. 489, 525 (1998).

Journal 1998 Explains the connection and differences between bioethics and the law. States that the distinction between ethics and law is that ethics places additional emphasis on moral ideals. References Opinions 8.08 and 8.115. Sullivan & Reynolds, *Where Law and Bioethics Meet . . . and Where They Don't*, 75 U. Det. Mercy L. Rev. 607, 612 (1998).

Journal 1997 Examines the evolution of the Indiana health care system. Discusses developments in Indiana jurisprudence regarding the physician-patient relationship. Explores various challenges facing the relationship and recognizes the need for legal rules to help address these challenges. Quotes Opinion 8.08. Cites Opinions 2.20, 9.06, and 9.12. Kinney & Selby, *History and Jurisprudence of the Physician-Patient Relationship in Indiana*, 30 Ind. L. Rev. 263, 269, 272, 276 (1997).

Journal 1997 Explores the meaning of cardiopulmonary resuscitation and legal issues involving do-not-resuscitate (DNR) orders. Considers problems created by DNR orders in operating rooms in light of patients' rights. Concludes that hospitals must adopt clear policies for their surgical teams to follow. Quotes Opinion 8.08. References Opinion 2.22. Lonchyna, *To Resuscitate or Not . . . In the Operating Room: The Need for Hospital Policies for Surgeons Regarding DNR Orders*, 6 Annals Health L. 209, 215, 217 (1997).

Journal 1996 Examines the constitutional implications of government-subsidized speech. Proposes two key characterization questions that should be answered when undertaking legal analysis. Observes, among other things, that potential ethical conflicts may exist when governmental subsidies are utilized to control the discourse between physicians and their patients. Quotes Opinion 8.08. Post, *Subsidized Speech*, 106 Yale L. J. 151, 173 (1996).

Journal 1996 Discusses new abortion legislation in Utah. Notes that patient consent must be obtained in accordance with AMA ethical standards, requiring physicians to provide all relevant data. Concludes that new laws require more detailed and comprehensive information be given to women. Quotes Opinion 8.08. Schnibbe, *Recent Legislative Developments in Utah Law: Family Law*, 1996 Utah L. Rev. 1335, 1394 (1996).

Journal 1996 Considers the ethical requirement for physicians to receive informed consent from patients before beginning treatment. Reviews the case of *Jacobson v. Massachusetts*, discussing its impact on informed consent and vaccination policy in the US. Quotes Fundamental Elements (2). References Opinion 8.08. Severyn, *Jacobson v. Massachusetts: Impact on Informed Consent and Vaccine Policy*, 5 J. Pharmacy & L. 249, 253, 274 (1996).

Journal 1995 Observes that physicians are unable to obtain informed consent because they cannot guess which treatment alternatives will best serve an individual patient's interests. Suggests that this situation would be improved if patients were paired with physicians who share their personal values. Quotes Opinion 8.08. Veatch, *Abandoning Informed Consent*, 25 Hastings Center Rep. 5, 6 (March/April 1995).

Journal 1994 Discusses how physicians historically have taken too much license with patients' bodies and placed greater value on longevity than on quality of life. Suggests that greater emphasis should be given to physician disclosure obligations in order to improve the quality of patient consent. Quotes Opinion 8.07 (1981) [now Opinion 8.08]. Katz, *Informed Consent: Must It Remain a Fairy Tale?* 10 J. Contemp. Health L. & Pol'y 69, 80 (1994).

Journal 1994 Reviews the evolution of the physician-patient relationship, with attention to patient autonomy. Examines the changing health care delivery environment. Quotes Preamble, Principles I, II, III, IV, V, and VI, Fundamental Elements (1) and (2), and Opinions 1.02 and 8.07 (1981) [now Opinion 8.08]. Cites Opinion 1.01. Szczygiel, *Beyond Informed Consent*, 21 Ohio N. U. L. Rev. 171, 217, 218, 220, 225, 226, 256 (1994).

Journal 1993 Considers how patient self-determination may be affected by cardiopulmonary resuscitation and do-not-resuscitate policies. Opposes a "futility" exception to informed consent as being violative of a physician's fiduciary duties to patients. Cites Opinion 8.07 (1986) [now Opinion 8.08]. References Opinion 2.22. Boozang, *Death Wish: Resuscitating Self-determination for the Critically Ill*, 35 Ariz. L. Rev. 23, 24, 28, 52 (1993).

Journal 1993 Discusses physicians' duty to disclose medical treatment alternatives to patients that are not readily available. Proposes that based on the historical development and legal requirements of the informed consent doctrine, physicians should be required to inform patients of non–readily available alternatives or face liability for breach of such obligation. Quotes Principles I, II, III, IV, and V and Opinion 8.08. Note, *Informed Choice: Physicians' Duty to Disclose Nonreadily Available Alternatives, 43 Case W. Res. L. Rev. 491, 491, 498-499, 508, 509 (1993).*

Journal 1993 Examines the case of *Rust v. Sullivan,* in which the Supreme Court sustained regulations barring abortion counseling and referral at federally funded clinics. Criticizes the Court's deference to the executive branch and its failure to classify the regulations as violative of constitutional rights to free speech. Quotes Opinion 8.08. Note, *Rust on the Constitution: Politics and Gag Rules, 37 How. L. J. 83, 96 (1993).*

Journal 1993 Critiques the Supreme Court's decision in *Rust v. Sullivan,* which upheld regulations prohibiting employees of Title X–funded clinics from discussing abortions with patients. Advocates an affirmative government obligation to provide abortion counseling to Title X patients. Cites Opinion 8.08. Roberts, *Rust v. Sullivan and the Control of Knowledge, 61 Geo. Wash. L. Rev. 587, 641 (1993).*

Journal 1993 Discusses legal attempts to control reproduction by HIV-positive women. Suggests that controls will not achieve the goal of lessening children's suffering, but will discourage HIV-positive women from seeking health care services. Quotes Opinion 8.08. Sangree, *Control of Childbearing by HIV-Positive Women: Some Responses to Emerging Legal Policies, 41 Buff. L. Rev. 309, 362 (1993).*

Journal 1992 Examines the constitutionality of certain restrictions on speech in federally funded programs. Advocates greater First Amendment protections in these situations. Quotes Opinion 8.08. Cole, *Beyond Unconstitutional Conditions: Charting Spheres of Neutrality in Government-Funded Speech, 67 N. Y. U. L. Rev. 675, 744 (1992).*

Journal 1992 Discusses the problem of protecting the privacy and confidentiality of public figures in light of contemporary tabloid journalism. Argues that current tort law does not adequately address this problem and advocates a new cause of action based on breach of confidentiality. Quotes Opinion 8.08. Harvey, *Confidentiality: A Measured Response to the Failure of Privacy, 140 Univ. Pa. L. Rev. 2385, 2454 (1992).*

Journal 1992 Analyzes the case of *Rust v. Sullivan* in which the US Supreme Court let stand regulations restricting abortion counseling in federally funded clinics. Concludes that *Rust* limits this right by expanding government powers. Cites Opinion 8.08. Note, *Constitutional Law—Judicial Deference—Supreme Court Will Defer to "Reasonable" Abortion Restrictions, 14 Univ. Ark. Little Rock 557, 573 (1992).*

Journal 1992 Discusses limitations on abortion counseling in federally funded clinics in light of the US Supreme Court decision in *Rust v. Sullivan.* Concludes that the *Rust* decision improperly limits freedom of speech. Cites Opinion 8.08. Note, *The Policy Against Federal Funding for Abortions Extends Into the Realm of Free Speech After Rust v. Sullivan, 19 Pepperdine L. Rev. 637, 681 (1992).*

Journal 1991 Discusses the manner in which a changing economy and an evolving health care system require society to expand its understanding of the physician-patient relationship. Concludes that open patient-physician discussion about available medical services and costs may become part of the standard of care. References Opinions 8.08 and 8.12. Morreim, *Economic Disclosure and Economic Advocacy: New Duties in the Medical Standard of Care, 12 J. Legal Med. 275, 306 (1991).*

Journal 1991 Considers how administrative restrictions on abortion counseling in Title X–funded clinics were affected by the Supreme Court's decision in *Rust v. Sullivan.* Concludes that *Rust* expands the powers of administrative agencies and narrows First Amendment free speech rights and Fifth Amendment due process rights. Cites Opinion 8.08. Note, *Administrative Agencies Get Their Way Over Constitutional Rights in Rust v. Sullivan, 28 Willamette L. Rev. 173, 193 (1991).*

Journal 1991 Examines legal, ethical, and economic concerns surrounding pharmaceutical company promotions. Concludes that pharmaceutical freebies can serve a positive role in health care if adequately regulated. Quotes Opinions 8.061 and 8.08. Note, *The Economic Wisdom of Regulating Pharmaceutical "Freebies," 1991 Duke L. J. 206, 216, 233, 234 (1991).*

Journal 1990 Examines Minnesota's "Crack Baby" law as a response to the increasing problem of drug abuse. Concludes that Minnesota's "Crack Baby" law endangers basic constitutional rights of women. Quotes Opinion 8.07 (1986) [now Opinion 8.08]. Johnson, *Minnesota's "Crack Baby" Law: Weapon of War or Link in a Chain? 8 Law & Ineq. 485, 494, 495, 496 (1990).*

Journal 1983 Discusses both moral and legal dilemmas in the use of placebos in treating patients. Concludes that, while arguments against placebo therapy are noble, a complete ban of placebo therapy is impractical and undesirable. Quotes Opinions 8.07 (1982) [now Opinion 8.08] and 8.11 (1982) [now Opinion 8.12]. Kapp, *Placebo Therapy and the Law: Prescribe With Care, 8 Am. J. Law & Med. 371, 391 (1983).*

8.081 Surrogate Decision Making

Competent adults may formulate, in advance, preferences regarding a course of treatment in the event that injury or illness causes severe impairment or loss of decision-making capacity. These preferences generally should be honored by the health care team out of respect for patient autonomy. Patients may establish an advance directive by documenting their treatment preferences and goals in a living will or by designating a health care proxy (durable power of attorney for health care) to make health care decisions on their behalf.

In some instances, a patient with diminished or impaired decision-making capacity can participate in various aspects of health care decision making. The attending physician should promote the autonomy of such individuals by involving them to a degree commensurate with their capabilities.

If a patient lacks the capacity to make a health care decision, a reasonable effort should be made to identify a prior written expression of values such as a pertinent living will or a health care proxy. When reasonable efforts have failed to uncover relevant documentation, physicians should consult state law. Physicians should be aware that under special circumstances (for example, reproductive decisions for individuals who are incompetent), state laws may specify court intervention. In the absence of state law specifying either appropriate surrogate decision makers or a process to identify them, the patient's family, domestic partner, or close friend should become the surrogate decision maker. When there is no family, domestic partner, or close friend, persons who have some relevant knowledge of the patient should participate in the decision-making process. In all other instances, a physician may wish to consult an ethics committee to aid in identifying a surrogate decision maker or to facilitate sound decision making.

When there is evidence of the patient's preferences and values, decisions concerning the patient's care should be made by substituted judgment. This entails considering the patient's advance directive (if any), the patient's views about life and how it should be lived, how the patient has constructed his or her identity or life story, and the patient's attitudes toward sickness, suffering, and certain medical procedures.

If there is no reasonable basis on which to interpret how a patient would have decided, the decision should be based on the best interests of the patient, or the outcome that would best promote the patient's well-being. Factors that should be considered when weighing the harms and benefits of various treatment options include the pain and suffering associated with treatment, the degree of and potential for benefit, and any impairments that may result from treatment. Any quality-of-life considerations should be measured as the worth to the individual whose course of treatment is in question, and not as a measure of social worth. One way to ensure that a decision using the best interest standard is not inappropriately influenced by the surrogate's own values is to determine the course of treatment that most reasonable persons would choose for themselves in similar circumstances.

Physicians should recognize the proxy or surrogate as an extension of the patient, entitled to the same respect as the competent patient. Physicians should provide advice, guidance, and support; explain that decisions should be based on substituted judgment when possible and otherwise on the best interest principle; and offer relevant medical information as well as medical opinions in a timely manner. In addition to the physician, other hospital staff or ethics committees are often helpful to providing support for the decision makers.

In general, physicians should respect decisions that are made by the appropriately designated surrogate and based on the standard of substituted judgment or best interest. In cases where there is a dispute among family members, physicians should work to resolve the conflict through mediation. Physicians or an ethics committee should try to uncover the reasons that underlie the disagreement and present information that will facilitate decision making. When a physician believes that a decision is clearly not what the patient would have decided, could not be reasonably judged to be within the patient's best interests, or primarily serves the interest of a surrogate or a third party, an ethics committee should be consulted before requesting court intervention.

Physicians should encourage their patients to document their treatment preferences or to appoint a health care proxy with whom they can discuss their values regarding health care and treatment in advance. Because documented advance directives are often not available in emergency situations, physicians should emphasize to patients the importance of discussing treatment preferences with individuals who are likely to act as their surrogates. (I, III, VIII)

Issued December 2001 based on the report "Surrogate Decision Making," adopted June 2001; updated December 2004.

N.Y. Fam. 2006 During proceedings regarding a foster child, an issue was raised contesting the legality of the County Department of Human Services' procedures for administering drugs to children. The mother's consent for prescribing medication to the child was obtained by a caseworker, without direct consultation with a physician and with no explanation of side effects. The court cited Opinions 8.08, 8.081, 8.11, and 10.01 in determining the physician's duty to honor the decision of the parent/surrogate. The mother's consent was invalidated and she was given an opportunity to consult with a physician. *Matter of Lyle A., 14 Misc. 3d 842, 830 N.Y.S.2d 486, 492, 494.*

Journal 2010 Discusses conflicts between surrogates and health care professionals in the context of "futile" care for patients. Further, discusses how "surrogate selection" laws may be used to replace a surrogate demanding inappropriately aggressive end-of-life treatment. Concludes that while surrogate selection has resolved some futility issues, an increase in independent ethics committees would be beneficial in dispelling other major issues. Quotes and cites Opinions 2.20 and 8.081. Pope, *Surrogate Selection: An Increasingly Viable, but Limited, Solution to Intractable Futility Disputes, 3 St. Louis U. J. Health L. & Pol'y 183, 207, 208, 211-214, 224, 228 (2010).*

Journal 2009 Examines the question of when a physician should seek a court order to override a surrogate decision maker's authority. Concludes that such an order should be sought only if the surrogate choices do not accurately reflect the wishes of the patient. Quotes Opinion 8.081. D'Amico, Krasna, Krasna, & Sade, *No Heroic Measures: How Soon Is Too Soon to Stop? 87 Ann. Thorac. Surg. 11, 17 (2009).*

Journal 2007 Discusses patients' right to refuse medical treatment and the corresponding duties of health care professionals. Concludes that detailed, carefully prepared advance directives are necessary to fulfill patients' wishes. Quotes Ch. II (1940) [now Opinions 8.08 and 8.082] and Opinions 2.035, 2.037, 2.20, 2.225, 8.081, and 10.015. Cites Opinions 9.11 and 9.115. Stamatakis, *Beyond Advance Directives: Personal Autonomy and the Right to Refuse Life-Sustaining Medical Treatment, 47 N. H. B. J. 20, 29-30 (2007).*

Journal 2006 Reviews the concept of therapeutic privilege. Concludes that the practice creates conflict between physician obligations under the concepts of autonomy and beneficence. Recommends that physicians maximize communication with patients by providing all pertinent information in the context of patient preferences. Cites Opinions 8.08, 8.081, 8.121, and 10.015. References Chap. I, Art. I, Sec. 4 (May 1847) [premise deleted from Code]. Bostick, Sade, McMahon, & Benjamin, *Report of the American Medical Association Council on Ethical and Judicial Affairs: Withholding Information From Patients: Rethinking the Propriety of "Therapeutic Privilege," 17 J. Clinical Ethics 302, 303 (Winter 2006).*

Journal 2006 Discusses the evolution of health law in Virginia. Concludes that the area of health law continues to expand, develop, and be refined. Cites Opinions 3.03, 3.08, 5.01, 5.015, 5.02, 5.04, 5.055, 6.02, 6.021, 6.03, 6.04, 7.03, 7.04, 7.05, 8.054, 8.08, 8.081, 8.085, 8.115, 8.12, 8.14, 8.145, 8.19, and 9.045. Guanzon, *Health Care Law, 41 U. Rich. L. Rev. 179, 199 (2006).*

Journal 2004 Discusses the law in Tennessee regarding surrogate decision-making. Concludes that recent legislation passed in Tennessee will assist those who care for incapacitated patients. Cites Opinions 2.035, 8.081, and 8.115. Wampler, *To Be or Not to Be in Tennessee: Deciding Surrogate Issues, 34 U. Mem. L. Rev. 333, 365 (2004).*

8.082   Withholding Information From Patients

The practice of withholding pertinent medical information from patients in the belief that disclosure is medically contraindicated is known as "therapeutic privilege." It creates a conflict between the physician's obligations to promote patients' welfare and respect for their autonomy by communicating truthfully. Therapeutic privilege does not refer to withholding medical information in emergency situations, or reporting medical errors (see E-8.08, "Informed Consent," and E-8.121, "Ethical Responsibility to Study and Prevent Error and Harm").

Withholding medical information from patients without their knowledge or consent is ethically unacceptable. Physicians should encourage patients to specify their preferences regarding communication of their medical information, preferably before the information becomes available. Moreover, physicians should honor patient requests not to be informed of certain medical information or to convey the information to a designated proxy, provided these requests appear to genuinely represent the patient's own wishes.

All information need not be communicated to the patient immediately or all at once; physicians should assess the amount of information a patient is capable of receiving at a given time, delaying the remainder to a later, more suitable time, and should tailor disclosure to meet patients' needs and expectations in light of their preferences.

Physicians may consider delaying disclosure only if early communication is clearly contraindicated. Physicians should continue to monitor the patient carefully and offer complete disclosure when the patient is able to decide whether or not to receive this information. This should be done according to a definite plan, so that disclosure is not permanently delayed. Consultation with patients' families, colleagues, or an ethics committee may help in assessing the balance of benefits and harms associated with delayed disclosure. In all circumstances, physicians should communicate with patients sensitively and respectfully. (I, III, V, VIII)

Issued November 2006 based on the report "Withholding Information From Patients (Therapeutic Privilege)," adopted June 2006.

Journal 2007 Analyzes problems with the current medical malpractice system. Concludes that Hillary Clinton's proposed National Medical Error and Compensation (MEDiC) Act of 2005 would be effective in facilitating physician apologies, reducing incidence of medical errors, and improving resolution of malpractice disputes. Quotes Opinion 8.12. References Opinion 8.082. Geckeler, *The Clinton-Obama Approach to Medical Malpractice Reform: Reviving the Most Meaningful Features of Alternative Dispute Resolution, 8 Pepp. Disp. Resol. L. J. 171, 193 (2007).*

Journal 2007 Discusses the evolution of informed consent doctrine. Concludes that, in context of research, informed consent exceptions should be substantially narrowed. Quotes Ch. I, Art. I, Sec. 4 (May 1847) [now Opinion 8.082] and Ch. I, Art. I, Sec. 1 (May 1847) [now Principles I and VIII]. References Opinions 2.08 and 8.08. Grimm, *Informed Consent for All! No Exceptions, 37 N. M. L. Rev. 39, 39, 61 (2007).*

Journal 2007 Discusses patients' right to refuse medical treatment and the corresponding duties of health care professionals. Concludes that detailed, carefully prepared advance directives are necessary to fulfill patients' wishes. Quotes Ch. II (1940) [now Opinions 8.08 and 8.082] and Opinions 2.035, 2.037, 2.20, 2.225, 8.081, and 10.015. Cites Opinions 9.11 and 9.115. Stamatakis, *Beyond Advance Directives: Personal Autonomy and the Right to Refuse Life-Sustaining Medical Treatment, 47 N. H. B. J. 20, 29-30 (2007).*

Journal 2007 Argues for informed consent in the process of child adoption. Concludes that prospective parents have a right to be informed of any general increases in prevalence of learning or developmental problems among adopted children. Cites Opinion 8.082. Wertheimer, *Of Apples and Trees: Adoption and Informed Consent, 25 QLR 601, 618 (2007).*

Journal 2006 Explores the possibility of "Medicare-led malpractice reform." Concludes that such reform may be successful if beneficiaries are given the proper incentives and the option of opting out. References Opinion 8.082. Kinney & Sage, *Resolving Medical Malpractice Claims in the Medicare Program: Can It Be Done? 12 Conn. Ins. L. J. 77, 105 (2006).*

8.083 Placebo Use in Clinical Practice

A placebo is a substance provided to a patient that the physician believes has no specific pharmacological effect upon the condition being treated. In the clinical setting, the use of a placebo without the patient's knowledge may undermine trust, compromise the patient-physician relationship, and result in medical harm to the patient.

Physicians may use placebos for diagnosis or treatment only if the patient is informed of and agrees to its use. A placebo may still be effective if the patient knows it will be used but cannot identify it and does not know the precise timing of its use. A physician should enlist the patient's cooperation by explaining that a better understanding of the medical condition could be achieved by evaluating the effects of different medications, including the placebo. The physician need neither identify the placebo nor seek specific consent before its administration. In this way, the physician respects the patient's autonomy and fosters a trusting relationship, while the patient still may benefit from the placebo effect.

A placebo must not be given merely to mollify a difficult patient, because doing so serves the convenience of the physician more than it promotes the patient's welfare. Physicians can avoid using a placebo, yet produce a placebo-like effect through the skillful use of reassurance and encouragement. In this way, the physician builds respect and trust, promotes the patient-physician relationship, and improves health outcomes (I, II, VIII).

Issued June 2007 based on the report "Placebo Use in Clinical Practice," adopted November 2006.

Journal 2011 Compares academic psychiatrist patterns of placebo use with physicians in other specialties to evaluate physician attitudes and beliefs toward placebos. Concludes psychiatrists are less likely to report that placebos have no clinical benefit and suggests greater discussion is needed to optimally incorporate placebos into medical practice. Quotes Opinion 8.083. Raz, Campbell, Guindi, Holcraft, Déry, & Cukier, *Placebos in Clinical Practice: Comparing Attitudes, Beliefs, and Patterns of Use Between Academic Psychiatrists and Nonpsychiatrists, 56 Can. J. Psychiatry 199 (2011).*

Journal 2009 Proposes an ethical approach for the administration of opioid therapy in treatment of chronic nonmalignant pain. Concludes that bioethical principles can guide a treatment plan, but that widespread consensus is still needed on rules for ethical treatment. Cites Opinion 8.083. Novy, Ritter, & McNeill, *A Primer of Ethical Issues Involving Opioid Therapy for Chronic Nonmalignant Pain in a Multidisciplinary Setting, 10 Pain Med. 356, 360 (2009).*

8.085 Waiver of Informed Consent for Research in Emergency Situations

The current state of emergency medicine and research has resulted in the application of standard treatments that often have not been scientifically evaluated for safety and effectiveness and may render unsatisfactory outcomes. Given the insufficiency of standard treatment alternatives, it is appropriate, in certain situations and with special safeguards, to provide experimental treatments without obtaining the informed consent of the subject. However, in order to protect the rights and welfare of the subjects, several conditions must be met:

(1) This type of research is limited to emergency, life-threatening situations, and may involve only experimental treatments that are ready for trials involving human subjects.

(2) The subject must lack the capacity to give informed consent for participation in the research.

(3) The window of opportunity for intervention must be so narrow as to make obtaining surrogate consent unfeasible.

(4) Obtaining prospective informed consent for the protocol must not be feasible (ie, the life-threatening emergency situation could not have been anticipated).

(5) The experimental treatment must have a realistic probability of benefit equal to or greater than standard care.

(6) The risks associated with the research should be reasonable in light of the critical nature of the conditions and the risks associated with standard treatment.

(7) Where informed consent is waived, subjects or their representatives must be informed as soon as possible about inclusion in the study and asked to consent to further participation. Subjects, or their representatives, may choose to discontinue participation at any time after being fully informed about the possible consequences. Additionally, if the patient dies while participating in the research protocol, the patient's family or representative must be informed that the patient was involved in an experimental protocol.

(8) Community input should be sought prior to approval of the protocol, and public disclosure should be made of study results. Fair randomization of research subjects should be given thorough consideration. Moreover, an independent data monitoring board should be established to oversee the ongoing trial. (I, V)

Issued December 1997 based on the report "Waiver of Informed Consent for Research in Emergency Situations," adopted June 1997.

Journal 2006 Discusses the evolution of health law in Virginia. Concludes that the area of health law continues to expand, develop, and be refined. Cites Opinions 3.03, 3.08, 5.01, 5.015, 5.02, 5.04, 5.055, 6.02, 6.021, 6.03, 6.04, 7.03, 7.04, 7.05, 8.054, 8.08, 8.081, 8.085, 8.115, 8.12, 8.14, 8.145, 8.19, and 9.045. Guanzon, *Health Care Law, 41 U. Rich. L. Rev. 179, 199 (2006).*

8.087 Medical Student Involvement in Patient Care

(1) Patients and the public benefit from the integrated care that is provided by health care teams that include medical students. Patients should be informed of the identity and training status of individuals involved in their care and all health care professionals share the responsibility for properly identifying themselves. Students and their supervisors should refrain from using terms that may be confusing when describing the training status of students.

(2) Patients are free to choose from whom they receive treatment. When medical students are involved in the care of patients, health care professionals should relate the benefits of medical student participation to patients and should ensure that they are willing to permit such participation. Generally, attending physicians are best suited to fulfill this responsibility.

(3) In instances where the patient will be temporarily incapacitated (eg, anesthetized) and where student involvement is anticipated, involvement should be discussed before the procedure is undertaken whenever possible. Similarly, in instances where a patient may not have the capacity to make decisions, student involvement should be discussed with the surrogate decision-maker involved in the care of the patient whenever possible. (V, VII)

Issued June 2001 based on the report "Medical Student Involvement in Patient Care," adopted December 2000 (*J Clin Ethics.* 2001;12:111-115).

Journal 2008 Discusses the problem of using patients for medical education purposes without patient consent. Concludes that new rules are needed to clarify when anesthetized, deceased, and conscious patients may be used for medical student training. Cites Opinion 8.087. Wilson, *"Unauthorized Practice": Regulating the Use of Anesthetized, Recently Deceased, and Conscious Patients in Medical Teaching, 44 Idaho L. Rev. 423, 424 (2008).*

Journal 2004 Discusses the practice of allowing medical students to perform pelvic examinations on female patients under anesthesia without obtaining consent. Concludes that physicians should obtain consent for this procedure as female patients have a right to control what is done to their body. Cites Opinion 8.087. Duncan, Luginbill, Richardson, & Wilson, *Using Tort Law to Secure Patient Dignity, 40 Trial 42, 46 (Oct. 2004).*

8.088 Resident Physicians' Involvement in Patient Care

Residents and fellows have dual roles as trainees and caregivers. First and foremost, they are physicians and therefore should always regard the interests of patients as paramount. To facilitate both patient care and educational goals, physicians involved in the training of residents and fellows should ensure that the health care delivery environment is respectful of the learning process as well as the patient's welfare and dignity.

(1) In accordance with graduate medical education standards such as those promulgated by the Accreditation Council for Graduate Medical Education (ACGME), training must be structured to provide residents and fellows with appropriate faculty supervision and availability of faculty consultants, and with graduated responsibility relative to level of training and expertise.

(2) Residents' and fellows' interactions with patients must be based on honesty. Accordingly, residents and fellows should clearly identify themselves as members of a team that is supervised by the attending physician.

(3) If a patient refuses care from a resident or fellow, the attending physician should be notified. If after discussion, a patient does not want to participate in training, the physician may exclude residents or fellows from that patient's care or, if appropriate, transfer the patient's care to another physician or nonteaching service or to another health care facility.

(4) Residents and fellows should participate fully in established mechanisms for error reporting and analysis in their training programs and hospital systems. They should cooperate with attending physicians in the communication of errors to patients. (See Opinion 8.121, "Ethical Responsibility to Study and Prevent Error and Harm.")

(5) Residents and fellows are obligated, as are all physicians, to monitor their own health and level of alertness so that these factors do not compromise their ability to care for patients safely. (See Opinion 9.0305, "Physician Health and Wellness.") Residents and fellows should recognize that providing patient care beyond time permitted by their programs (for example, "moonlighting") might be potentially harmful to themselves and patients. Other activities that interfere with adequate rest during off-hours might be similarly harmful.

(6) Residency and fellowship programs must offer means to resolve educational or patient care conflicts that can arise in the course of training. All parties involved in such conflicts must continue to regard patient welfare as the first priority. Conflict resolution should not be punitive, but should aim at assisting residents and fellows to complete their training successfully. When necessary, higher administrative authorities or the relevant residency review committee (RRC) should be involved, as articulated in ACGME guidelines. (I, II, V, VIII)

Issued November 2005 based on the report "Resident Physicians' Involvement in Patient Care," adopted June 2005.

8.09 Laboratory Services

(1) A physician should not misrepresent or aid in the misrepresentation of laboratory services performed and supervised by a nonphysician as the physician's professional services. Such situations could involve a laboratory owned by a physician who directs and manages its financial and business

affairs with no professional medical services being provided; laboratory work being performed by technicians and directly supervised by a medical technologist with no participation by the physician; or the physician's name being used in connection with the laboratory so as to create the appearance that it is owned, operated, and supervised by a physician when this is not so.

(2) If a laboratory is owned, operated, and supervised by a nonphysician in accordance with state law and performs tests exclusively for physicians who receive the results and make their own medical interpretations, the following considerations would apply:

The physician's ethical responsibility is to provide patients with high quality services. This includes services that the physician performs personally and those that are delegated to others. A physician should not utilize the services of any laboratory, irrespective of whether it is operated by a physician or nonphysician, unless she or he has the utmost confidence in the quality of its services. A physician must always assume personal responsibility for the best interests of his or her patients. Medical judgment based upon inferior laboratory work is likewise inferior. Medical considerations, not cost, must be paramount when the physician chooses a laboratory. The physician who disregards quality as the primary criterion or who chooses a laboratory solely because it provides low-cost laboratory services on which the patient is charged a profit is not acting in the best interests of the patient. However, if reliable, quality laboratory services are available at lower cost, the patient should have the benefit of the savings. As a professional, the physician is entitled to fair compensation for his or her services. A physician should not charge a markup, commission, or profit on the services rendered by others. A markup is an excessive charge that exploits patients if it is nothing more than a tacked on amount for a service already provided and accounted for by the laboratory. A physician may make an acquisition charge or processing charge. The patient should be notified of any such charge in advance. (I, II, III, IV, V)

Issued prior to April 1977. Updated June 1994.

Journal 2007 Examines the ethical obligations of a corporate health lawyer. Concludes that the ethical health lawyer must balance obligations to the client with obligations to patients and the public. Quotes Opinion 8.09. Weeks, *Loopholes: Opportunity, Responsibility, or Liability?* 35 J. L. Med. & Ethics 320, 322 (2007).

8.095 Reporting Clinical Test Results: General Guidelines

To alleviate patients' anxieties, physicians should report clinical test results to patients within a reasonable time frame. Since many variables contribute to the urgency of a particular situation, physicians should use their best professional judgment when determining what length of time is reasonable for the particular situation at hand. Anticipated delays should be explained to patients at the time of testing.

Physicians should adopt a consistent reporting policy that accommodates the demands of their practice while at the same time being considerate of patients' anxieties. The reporting policy should be disclosed to patients, for instance when tests are administered, so patients know what to expect. Reporting policies should take into consideration under what circumstances (eg, all results, only abnormal results) and by whom (eg, the laboratory or the physician) test results are appropriately reported to the patient. Any anticipated inconsistencies should be disclosed to patients as soon as they are discovered.

Physicians should provide test results in language understandable to the patient and in the manner deemed most appropriate by the physician. Any information gathered from test results that would be necessary for patients to make intelligent medical decisions and give informed consent on future medical treatments must be disclosed to them.

Physicians should take all appropriate precautions to ensure the confidentiality of test results. Such precautions may include, but are not limited to, not leaving test results on an answering machine, on voice mail, or with a third party unless previously given permission to do so by the patient, not delivering test results via electronic mail, and not sending test results through the mail in any form other than a sealed envelope. (II, IV, V)

Issued December 1998 based on the report "Reporting Clinical Test Results: General Guidelines," adopted June 1998.

8.10   Lien Laws

In states where there are lien laws, a physician may file a lien as a means of assuring payment of his or her fee provided the fee is fixed in amount and not contingent on the amount of settlement of the patient's claim against a third party. (I, VI)

Issued prior to April 1977.

Journal 2004 Discusses the practice of using an attorney retaining lien over a client's papers and argues that the practice should be abolished. Concludes that this practice is coercive and inconsistent with a lawyer's role as a fiduciary. Quotes Opinion 7.02. References Opinion 8.10. Leubsdorf, *Against Lawyer Retaining Liens*, 72 Fordham L. Rev. 849, 864, 865 (2004).

8.11   Neglect of Patient

Physicians are free to choose whom they will serve. The physician should, however, respond to the best of his or her ability in cases of emergency where first aid treatment is essential. Once having undertaken a case, the physician should not neglect the patient. (I, VI)

Issued prior to April 1977. Updated June 1996.

Ariz. 1965 Physician appealed denial of medical license which was based on alleged violations of local medical society rules and Principles 3, 5, and 10 (1957) [now Principles III and VII and Opinions 3.01, 8.11, and 9.06]. Alleged violations included treating a patient without first obtaining a prior treating physician's permission, inadequate patient care, performing operations without hospital privileges, and signing the medical record of a deceased patient who had been treated by interns. The court held that the evidence failed to show any clear violation of the Principles and that a local medical society had no right to prescribe a code of ethics for state licensing purposes. *Arizona State Bd. of Medical Examiners v. Clark*, 97 Ariz. 205, 398 P.2d 908, 914-915, 915 n.3.

Ariz. App. 1980 Malpractice suit against a paid on-call physician for refusal to treat decedent resulting in delay in treatment. The court quoted Principle 5 (1957) [now Principle VI and Opinion 8.11] as establishing an ethical duty to provide emergency care. However, court distinguished any such ethical obligation from its holding that physician had a contractual duty to treat emergency patients to the best of his ability. *Hiser v. Randolph, 126 Ariz. 608, 617 P.2d 774, 776 n.1, 777, 778.*

Cal. App. 1978 Surviving spouse sued physicians who were on emergency surgical call panel for malpractice where patient died during surgery. Although defendants claimed immunity under state Good Samaritan statute, the court held the statute inapplicable since the legislative purpose was to encourage physicians to render care on an irregular basis to unattended persons discovered by chance at the scene of an emergency. In so holding, the court noted that Principle 5 (1957) [now Principle VI and Opinions 8.11 and 9.06] imposed an ethical duty to render emergency medical care. *Colby v. Schwartz, 78 Cal. App. 3d 885, 144 Cal. Rptr. 624, 627 n.2.*

Ill. App. 1997 Physician was found to be in civil contempt for violating a covenant not to compete by performing administrative functions from his home office. The trial court ordered the physician to desist from practicing medicine within the restricted area. The appellate court, in reversing, found that although the language of the agreement was ambiguous, it could be construed to prohibit the physician from practicing medicine. However, the court found that the practice of medicine does not include activities which are administrative or managerial in nature. Further, the court, quoting from Opinion 8.11, found that physicians have a legal and ethical duty to care for their patients, and may not neglect patients once they begin treatment. The court held that a finding of contempt for violating an agreement not to compete cannot be supported where physicians do not examine patients, but merely address medically related questions by phone. *Bloomington Urological Associates v. Scaglia, 292 Ill. App. 3d, 793, 686 N.E. 2d 389, 394.*

Ky. App. 1989 Malpractice suit was initiated against physician for failure to treat plaintiff's brother where defendant had repeatedly rebuffed plaintiff's request for emergency assistance and told him to get in line or sign in. Plaintiff removed his brother to another hospital where he subsequently died of heart attack. Plaintiff argued that defendant was under a duty to treat based upon, inter alia, the AMA Code of Ethics [apparently Principle VI and Opinion 8.11]. The court rejected the argument, finding that a breach of ethical standards may establish grounds for professional discipline, but not a civil cause of action, and held that defendant was under no legal duty to treat. *Noble v. Sartori, 1989 Ky. App. LEXIS 67.*

N.Y. Fam. 2006 During proceedings regarding a foster child, an issue was raised contesting the legality of the County Department of Human Services' procedures for administering drugs to children. The mother's consent for prescribing medication to the child was obtained by a caseworker, without direct consultation with a physician and with no explanation of side effects. The court cited Opinions 8.08, 8.081, 8.11, and 10.01 in determining the physician's duty to honor the decision of the parent/surrogate. The mother's consent was invalidated and she was given an opportunity to consult with a physician. *Matter of Lyle A., 14 Misc. 3d 842, 830 N.Y.S.2d 486,492,494.*

Ohio Att'y Gen. 1999 State attorney general concluded that physicians who render opinions regarding the necessity of medical services for health insuring corporations are not engaged in the practice of medicine. Additionally, physicians who render opinions regarding medical necessity for appeals of adverse determinations do not fall under the regulatory, investigatory, or enforcement authority of the Ohio State Medical Board. Quoting Opinions 8.03, 8.11, and 8.13, the attorney general stated that physicians have an ethical duty to provide appropriate treatment for patients. *Ohio Att'y Gen. Op. No. 99-044, 1999 WL 692623.*

Journal 2010 Discusses issues arising from the enactment of legislation by North Dakota involving a minor's reproductive rights. Explores ethical principles that govern physician's actions within the context of reproductive health. Concludes that, while a patient's expectation of confidentiality with a physician is critical, competing values come into play when the patient is a minor and parental involvement may be important. Provides practical guidance to address issues in this context. Quotes Opinions 2.01, 2.015, 5.055, 8.08, 8.115, 9.12, 10.01, 10.015, and 10.05. Cites Opinion 5.05, 5.055, 8.08, 8.11, 8.115, 9.12, and 10.05. Haas, *"Doctor, I'm Pregnant and Fifteen—I Can't Tell My Parents—Please Help Me": Minor Consent, Reproductive Rights, and Ethical Principles for Physicians, 86 N.D. L. Rev. 63, 70, 73, 75-78, 82, 84, 86-88, (2010).*

Journal 2006 Explores the legal and ethical issues surrounding concierge medicine. Concludes that concierge medicine is best restricted to a small class of wealthy individuals. Quotes Principle IX and Opinion 8.055. Cites Principle VI and Opinions 8.055, 8.11, 8.115, 9.065, and 10.05. Carnahan, *Law, Medicine, and Wealth: Does Concierge Medicine Promote Health Care Choice, or Is It a Barrier to Access? 17 Stan. L. & Pol'y Rev. 121, 149-50, 151, 152, 153-54 (2006).*

Journal 2006 Examines physician restrictive covenants. Concludes that under the current balancing test, courts should give considerable weight to the public interest in preserving the physician-patient relationship. Quotes Opinions 9.02 and 9.06. Cites Opinions 6.11, 8.11, 8.115, and 9.06. Malloy, *Physician Restrictive Covenants: The Neglect of Incumbent Patient Interests, 41 Wake Forest L. Rev. 189, 207-08, 217, 218 (2006).*

Journal 1999 Discusses potential conflicts between a criminal defense attorney's religious beliefs and representation of the client. Explores theories that would allow an attorney to put religious beliefs over the client's interest. Offers analogies within the physician-patient relationship. Concludes that a defense attorney is bound by duty and must set aside conflicting religious beliefs. Quotes Principle VI and Opinions 8.11, 9.06, and 9.12. Reza, *Religion and the Public Defender, 26 Fordham Urb. L. J. 1051, 1062, 1063 (1999).*

Journal 1998 Explains when a surrogate is required to make health care decisions. Discusses limitations of a surrogate's authority. Emphasizes that the health care provider must recognize that ultimate decision-making regarding care first belongs to the patient, and then to the surrogate. Quotes Opinion 2.035. Cites Opinion 8.11. References Opinion 2.22. O'Neill, *Surrogate Health Care Decisions for Adults in Illinois—Answers to the Legal Questions That Health Care Providers Face on a Daily Basis, 29 Loy. Univ. Chi. L. J. 411, 445, 448 (1998).*

Journal 1995 Argues that nonabandonment should be a core physician obligation. Suggests that if nonabandonment is better incorporated into medical ethics, medicine will become more humanized and responsive to everyday physician-patient problems. Quotes Opinion 8.10 (1986) [now Opinion 8.11]. Quill & Cassel, *Nonabandonment: A Central Obligation for Physicians, 10 Trends in Health Care, Law & Ethics 25, 27 (Winter/Spring 1995).*

Journal 1995 Offers relevant historical perspectives and provides comprehensive ethical and legal discussion of physician-assisted suicide and euthanasia. Highlights important legislative developments, including the Oregon Death with Dignity Act, and analyzes significant judicial opinions. Quotes Principles III, IV, and VI and Opinions 2.21 and 9.12. Cites Opinions 2.20 and 8.11. Stone & Winslade, *Physician-Assisted Suicide and Euthanasia in the United States: Legal and Ethical Observations, 16 J. Legal Med. 481, 483, 490, 497, 498, 499 (1995).*

Journal 1993 Explores the idea of reverse informed consent, which would impose a duty on patients to inform health care professionals of their infectious status. Concludes that such a duty is justified. Quotes Principles IV and VI and Opinions 8.11 and 9.131. Oddi, *Reverse Informed Consent: The Unreasonably Dangerous Patient, 46 Vand. L. Rev. 1417, 1449, 1463, 1465, 1479 (1993).*

Journal 1988 Discusses the question of whether health professionals are obligated to subject themselves to the risks that attend treating patients with communicable diseases, particularly AIDS. Examines the ethical pronouncements and codes of the nursing and medical professions in this respect, noting that the most recent statements of professional values imply the existence of an obligation to treat HIV-infectious patients. Quotes Opinion 8.10 (1986) [now Opinion 8.11] and Principle VI. Cites Opinion 9.11 (1986) [now Opinion 9.12]. Freedman, *Health Professions, Codes, and the Right to Refuse to Treat HIV-Infectious Patients, 18 Hastings Center Rep. 20 (Supp.), 23, 24 (April/May 1988).*

Journal 1987 Concludes that a policy or practice of active voluntary euthanasia is not desirable, linking a moral prohibition against active voluntary euthanasia to the moral prohibition against physicians actively participating in capital punishment. In place of any practice of active voluntary euthanasia, recommends increased use of hospices, greater emphasis on training physicians to care for the dying patient, and further research aimed at producing symptomatic relief in dying patients. Cites Opinions 2.06, 8.10 (1986) [now Opinion 8.11], and 9.06. Shewmon, *Active Voluntary Euthanasia: A Needless Pandora's Box, 3 Issues in Law and Med. 219, 220, 222, 243 (1987).*

Journal 1986 Examines common law and statutory law applicable to patient dumping, and emphasizes the antidumping provisions of COBRA. Weaknesses in this federal legislative scheme are highlighted and recommendations for strengthening the statute and maximizing access to emergency medical care are offered. Quotes Principle VI and Opinion 8.10 (1986) [now Opinion 8.11]. Note, *Preventing Patient Dumping: Sharpening the COBRA's Fangs, 61 N. Y. U. L. Rev. 1186, 1189-90 (1986).*

8.115 Termination of the Physician-Patient Relationship

Physicians have an obligation to support continuity of care for their patients. While physicians have the option of withdrawing from a case, they cannot do so without giving notice to the patient, the relatives, or responsible friends sufficiently long in advance of withdrawal to permit another medical attendant to be secured. (I, VI)

Issued June 1996 (formerly included in Opinion 8.11, "Neglect of Patients").

Ill. 2006 Physicians appealed a grant of preliminary injunction enforcing restrictive covenants in their employment contracts. Quoting Opinions 9.02, 9.06, and 10.01 and referencing Opinion 8.115, the Illinois Supreme Court gave thorough consideration to the AMA's position on restrictive covenants. While acknowledging the ethical problems associated with such contracts, the court found the covenants reasonable in scope. The decision to ban restrictive covenants, the court reasoned, was best left to the legislature. *Mohanty v. St. John Heart Clinic, S.C., 225 Ill.2d 52, 866 N.E.2d 85, 94, 106-07, 107-08.*

Mass. Super. 1993 Plaintiff sought to enjoin defendant-physician from contacting patients that defendant treated while employed with plaintiff. The court denied the injunction, noting that under Opinion 8.11 [now Opinion 8.115] defendant has a duty to notify his patients before withdrawing from a case and an injunction would force defendant to choose between violating professional ethics and violating a court order. *Plastic Surgical Servs. of New England, P.C. v. Hall, 1993 WL 818637.*

Wis. App. 2007 Plaintiff brought action for medical abandonment against his physician. The physician had cancelled an elective surgery and terminated the relationship with the patient after the plaintiff sued the surgical center employing the physician. The circuit court granted summary judgment for the physician finding plaintiff's claim unsupported by expert testimony. With apparent reference to Opinions 8.115 and 10.01, the plaintiff argued that AMA ethics opinions supported his claim. The appeals court held, however, that expert testimony was required to prove the appropriate standard of care. *Casperson v. N.E. Wis. Ctr. for Surgery & Rehab of Hand, Ltd., 2007 WL 1191782, 3.*

Journal 2010 Examines instances where physicians assert a right to refuse to participate in certain activities deemed immoral based upon claims of conscience. Concludes that this right may be limited by various factors, such as the risk of patient harm. Further concludes that through the informed consent process and other means, physicians can properly accommodate patient care needs and their right of conscience. Cites Opinion 8.115. Antommaria, *Conscientious Objection in Clinical Practice: Notice, Informed Consent, Referral, and Emergency Treatment, 9 Ave Maria L. Rev. 81, 98 (2010).*

Journal 2010 Discusses issues arising from the enactment of legislation by North Dakota involving a minor's reproductive rights. Explores ethical principles that govern physician's actions within the context of reproductive health. Concludes that, while a patient's expectation of confidentiality with a physician is critical, competing values come into play when the patient is a minor and parental involvement may be important. Provides practical guidance to address issues in this context. Quotes Opinions 2.01, 2.015, 5.055, 8.08, 8.115, 9.12, 10.01, 10.015, and 10.05. Cites Opinion 5.05, 5.055, 8.08, 8.11, 8.115, 9.12, and 10.05. Haas, *"Doctor, I'm Pregnant and Fifteen—I Can't Tell My Parents—Please Help Me": Minor Consent, Reproductive Rights, and Ethical Principles for Physicians, 86 N.D. L. Rev. 63, 70, 73, 75-78, 82, 84, 86-88 (2010).*

Journal 2009 Discusses the judicial standard for reviewing physician noncompete covenants. Concludes courts should apply a strict standard to such covenants, rather than declare the covenants per se invalid. Quotes Principles IV and VII, Principles of Medical Ethics §5 (1957) [now Principle VI], Code of Medical Ethics Ch. II, Art. I §3 (1847) [now Opinion 5.02], Opinion 9.02, and Code of Medical Ethics Ch. II, Art. I §4 (1847) [now Opinion 9.09]. Cites Opinions 8.041, 8.115, 9.02, 9.06, 9.065, 9.067, 10.01, and 10.015. Koons, *Physician Employee Non-Compete*

Agreements on the Examining Table: The Need to Better Protect Patients' and the Public's Interests in Indiana, 6 Ind. Health L. Rev. 253, 272-77, 280-81 (2009).

Journal 2008 Examines patient-provider conflicts in end-of-life care and the use of dispute resolution mechanisms. Concludes dispute resolution processes are needed to aid interaction among the various participants in the health care system to prevent injustice to patients. Cites Opinion 8.115. Antommaria, *How Can I Give Her IV Antibiotics at Home When I Have Three Other Children to Care For? Using Dispute System Design to Address Patient Provider Conflicts in Health Care, 29 Hamline J. Pub. L. & Pol'y 273, 275 (2008).*

Journal 2008 Explores the ethical issues associated with writing prescriptions for family members and acquaintances. Concludes that informal treatment often compromises the quality of care, and that a referral to an objective provider is the best choice. Quotes Opinion 8.19. Cites Opinion 8.115. Ares, *An Uncommon Skin Condition Illustrates the Need for Caution When Prescribing for Friends, 20 J. Am. Acad. of Nurse Prac. 389, 390 (2008).*

Journal 2007 Reviews the legal and ethical problems surrounding concierge medical practice. Concludes that concierge medicine should remain restricted to a small class of wealthy individuals. Cites Opinions 8.05, 8.055, 8.115, 9.06, and 9.065. Carnahan, *Concierge Medicine: Legal and Ethical Issues, 35 J. L. Med. & Ethics 211, 212-13 (2007).*

Journal 2007 Compares laws of client abandonment with those of patient abandonment by physicians. Concludes that physicians should be required to show good cause to justify abandonment. Quotes Ch. II, Art. I, Sec. 5 (1903) [now Preamble]. References Opinion 8.115. LeBlanc, *Abandoning Patients and Clients: Where Medicine Can Learn From Law, 1 Charleston L. Rev. 237, 237-38, 256 (2007).*

Journal 2006 Explores the legal and ethical issues surrounding concierge medicine. Concludes that concierge medicine is best restricted to a small class of wealthy individuals. Quotes Principle IX and Opinion 8.055. Cites Principle VI and Opinions 8.055, 8.11, 8.115, 9.065, and 10.05. Carnahan, *Law, Medicine, and Wealth: Does Concierge Medicine Promote Health Care Choice, or Is It a Barrier to Access? 17 Stan. L. & Pol'y Rev. 121, 149-50, 151, 152, 153-54 (2006).*

Journal 2006 Discusses the evolution of health law in Virginia. Concludes that the area of health law continues to expand, develop, and be refined. Cites Opinions 3.03, 3.08, 5.01, 5.015, 5.02, 5.04, 5.055, 6.02, 6.021, 6.03, 6.04, 7.03, 7.04, 7.05, 8.054, 8.08, 8.081, 8.085, 8.115, 8.12, 8.14, 8.145, 8.19, and 9.045. Guanzon, *Health Care Law, 41 U. Rich. L. Rev. 179, 199 (2006).*

Journal 2006 Examines the efficacy of informed consent when a physician acts both as a researcher and care provider. Concludes that a patient cannot give truly informed consent in such cases. Cites Opinions 8.115 and 10.015. Lenrow, *The Treating Physician as Researcher: Is Assuming This Dual Role a Violation of the Nuremberg Code? 25 Temp. J. Sci. Tech. & Envtl. L. 15, 42-43 (2006).*

Journal 2006 Examines physician restrictive covenants. Concludes that under the current balancing test, courts should give considerable weight to the public interest in preserving the physician-patient relationship. Quotes Opinions 9.02 and 9.06. Cites Opinions 6.11, 8.11, 8.115, and 9.06. Malloy, *Physician Restrictive Covenants: The Neglect of Incumbent Patient Interests, 41 Wake Forest L. Rev. 189, 207-08, 217, 218 (2006).*

Journal 2004 Discusses the law in Tennessee regarding surrogate decision-making. Concludes that recent legislation passed in Tennessee will assist those who care for incapacitated patients. Cites Opinions 2.035, 8.081, and 8.115. Wampler, *To Be or Not to Be in Tennessee: Deciding Surrogate Issues, 34 U. Mem. L. Rev. 333, 365 (2004).*

Journal 1998 Explains the connection and differences between bioethics and the law. States that the distinction between ethics and law is that ethics places additional emphasis on moral ideals. References Opinions 8.08 and 8.115. Sullivan & Reynolds, *Where Law and Bioethics Meet . . . and Where They Don't, 75 U. Det. Mercy L. Rev. 607, 612 (1998).*

Journal 1997 Compares past ethical opinions to current opinions and notes the differences. Comments on the forces that have changed medical ethics through the years. Notes differing theories on the future course of medical ethics. Quotes Fundamental Elements (Preamble) and Opinions 5.05, 5.057, 7.01, 8.12, 9.12, and 9.131. Cites Fundamental Elements (5) and Opinions 8.115 and 8.13. Buchanan, *Medical Ethics at the Millennium: A Brief Retrospective, 26 Colo. Law. 141, 142, 143, 144, 145 (1997).*

8.12 Patient Information

It is a fundamental ethical requirement that a physician should at all times deal honestly and openly with patients. Patients have a right to know their past and present medical status and to be free of any mistaken beliefs concerning their conditions. Situations occasionally occur in which a patient suffers significant medical complications that may have resulted from the physician's mistake or judgment. In these situations, the physician is ethically required to inform the patient of all the facts necessary to ensure understanding of what has occurred. Only through full disclosure is a patient able to make informed decisions regarding future medical care.

Ethical responsibility includes informing patients of changes in their diagnoses resulting from retrospective review of test results or any other information. This obligation holds even though the patient's medical treatment or therapeutic options may not be altered by the new information.

Concern regarding legal liability which might result following truthful disclosure should not affect the physician's honesty with a patient. (I, II, III, IV)

Issued March 1981. Updated June 1994.

7th Cir. 2011 Plaintiffs brought suit against physicians employed by federally funded health care facilities, alleging medical malpractice. Affirming, the court held that information conveyed by hospital to parents was not sufficient for parents to know there was malpractice-related cause to child's injuries and a reasonable person, when informed of the child's injuries had been caused by infection that had been transmitted during birth, would not have searched for potential causes. The concurrence cites Opinion 8.12 in describing the physicians' responsibilities to the plaintiffs. *Arroyo v. United States, 656 F.3d 663, 678.*

Minn. 1970 Defendant-physician appealed order to answer interrogatories, claiming that a medical malpractice plaintiff is prohibited from compelling expert testimony from a defendant to prove a charge of malpractice without calling other medical witnesses. In holding that a defendant could be compelled to provide expert medical opinion in response to interrogatories, the court quoted Principle 1 (1957) [now Principle II and Opinion 8.12] for the proposition that physicians owe a duty of disclosure to their patients. *Anderson v. Florence, 288 Minn. 351, 181 N.W.2d 873, 880, 880 n.7.*

Journal 2011 Explains how the Padilla opinion provides guidance on scope far beyond its dialogue on clarity. Concludes that defense attorneys must advise noncitizen clients as specifically as research allows to adequately inform them about the immigration consequences of contemplated criminal dispositions. Cites Opinion 8.12. Nash, *Considering the Scope of Advisal Duties Under Padilla, 33 Cardozo L. Rev. 549, 550 (2011).*

Journal 2011 Examines the impact of the Patient Protection and Affordable Care Act on medical liability and the controversy over the need for federal medical liability reforms, including a damage cap. Concludes that further studies are needed regarding liability reforms and the Affordable Care Act. References Opinion 8.12. Nelson, Becker, & Morrisey, *Medical Liability and Health Care Reform, 21 Health Matrix 443, 510 (2011).*

Journal 2011 Discusses current research and initiatives regarding physician apologies and the possibility of amending the Federal Rules of Evidence to exclude admission of physician apologies. Concludes that physician apologies and general admissions of fault should be protected under Fed. R. Evid. 409. Quotes Opinion 8.12. Pearlmutter, *Physician Apologies and General Admissions of Fault: Amending the Federal Rules of Evidence, 72 Ohio St. L. J. 687, 713 (2011).*

Journal 2011 Analyzes opinion of Supreme Court of Ohio in *Ward v. Summa Health System* addressing statutory physician-patient privilege and whether it precludes discovery of relevant medical information from a physician regarding his or her own medical condition. Concludes that in holding that it does not court reached the proper result. Quotes Opinion 8.12. Searl, *Ward v. Summa Health System, 37 Ohio N.U. L. Rev. 879, 887-888 (2011).*

Journal 2011 Examines and analyzes medical apology programs. Argues that such programs allow for the manipulation of injured patients as a means to persuade them not to pursue monetary damages. Suggests changes in design for medical apology programs. Quotes Opinion 8.12. Teninbaum, *How Medical Apology Programs Harm Patients*, 15 *Chap. L. Rev.* 307, 310 (2011).

Journal 2009 Discusses the importance of disclosure for establishing trust in the physician-patient relationship and the infrequency of disclosure in the American health care industry. Concludes physicians should be required to disclose mistakes to their patients, and the law should impose tort liability on physicians who fail to disclose. Quotes Opinion 8.12. Bourne, *Medical Malpractice: Should Courts Force Doctors to Confess Their Own Negligence to Their Patients?* 61 *Ark. L. Rev.* 621, 629 (2009).

Journal 2009 Explores the jurisprudential foundation of the fiduciary duty physicians owe their patients and discusses the failure of physicians to disclose to patients errors and other emergent medical risks. Concludes law should recognize the physician's duty to disclose such risks by enforcing a cause of action for breach of that duty. Quotes Principles III and VIII and Opinions 8.12, 10.015, and 10.02. References Opinion 8.12. Hafemeister, *Lean on Me: A Physician's Fiduciary Duty to Disclose an Emergent Medical Risk to the Patient*, 86 *Wash. U. L. Rev.* 1167, 1172-1173, 1178, 1182, 1185, 1188, 1209 (2009).

Journal 2009 Discusses the absence of tort liability for medical malpractice in New Zealand, and the newly created patient right to health care services of an appropriate standard. Concludes New Zealand's statutory code and Health and Disability Commissioner Act allow for clear rulings without invoking tort law. Cites Opinion 8.12. Sladden & Graydon, *Liability for Medical Malpractice—Recent New Zealand Developments*, 28 *Med. & L.* 301, 310 (2009).

Journal 2008 Considers the utility of physician apologies for medical error and legal protection for physicians who apologize for mistakes. Concludes physicians must openly communicate with their patients and apologize for medical errors to strengthen the health care community. Quotes Opinions 8.08, 8.12, 10.01, and 10.015. References Opinion 8.12. Ebert, *Attorneys, Tell Your Clients to Say They're Sorry: Apologies in the Health Care Industry*, 5 *Ind. Health L. Rev.* 337, 340-41, 344 (2008).

Journal 2008 Explores the fiduciary relationship between physicians and patients, professional and ethical obligations of both physicians and lawyers, and the implications for conflict resolution in health care. Concludes physicians must put patient interests above their own and lawyers must work to discern clients' best interests and support client welfare. Quotes Principle VIII and Opinions 8.12 and 10.015. Cites Principles I and II and Opinions 10.01 and 10.015. Scott, *Doctors as Advocates, Lawyers as Healers*, 29 *Hamline J. Pub. L. Pol'y*, 331, 340-41, 347, 371 (2008).

Journal 2007 Analyzes problems with the current medical malpractice system. Concludes that Hillary Clinton's proposed National Medical Error and Compensation (MEDiC) Act of 2005 would be effective in facilitating physician apologies, reducing incidence of medical errors, and improving resolution of malpractice disputes. Quotes Opinion 8.12. References Opinion 8.082. Geckeler, *The Clinton-Obama Approach to Medical Malpractice Reform: Reviving the Most Meaningful Features of Alternative Dispute Resolution*, 8 *Pepp. Disp. Resol. L. J.* 171, 193 (2007).

Journal 2007 Examines barriers to reporting of medical errors in professional journals. Concludes that legal protection should be provided for error reporting and that medical journals could serve as a suitable forum for disclosure. Quotes Opinion 8.12. Murphy, Stee, McEvoy, & Oshiro, J. *Reporting of Medical Errors*, 131 *Chest* 890, 892 (2007).

Journal 2007 Argues that issuance of apologies from physicians who commit medical errors will diminish the number of malpractice suits brought. Concludes that patients desire apologies in the case of medical errors and are less likely to sue when they are given. Cites Principles I, II, III, and IV and Opinion 8.12. Tabler, *Should Physicians Apologize for Medical Errors?* 19 *Health Lawyer* 23, 23 (Jan. 2007).

Journal 2006 Reviews the arguments made in Thomas Baker's book *The Medical Malpractice Myth*. Concludes that Baker's book provides the kind of useful dialogue which will lead to positive reform of the malpractice system. Quotes Opinion 8.12. Coombs, *The Medical Malpractice Myth*, 27 *J. Legal Med.* 243, 249-50 (2006).

Journal 2006 Discusses the evolution of health law in Virginia. Concludes that the area of health law continues to expand, develop, and be refined. Cites Opinions 3.03, 3.08, 5.01, 5.015, 5.02, 5.04, 5.055, 6.02, 6.021, 6.03, 6.04, 7.03, 7.04, 7.05, 8.054, 8.08, 8.081, 8.085, 8.115, 8.12, 8.14, 8.145, 8.19, and 9.045. Guanzon, *Health Care Law*, 41 *U. Rich. L. Rev.* 179, 199 (2006).

Journal 2006 Discusses tort liability for medical malpractice. Concludes that both physicians and attorneys should support a legal system which promotes patient safety. Quotes Opinions 8.12 and 10.015. Pegalis, *A Proposal to Use Common Ground That Exists Between the Medical and Legal Professions to Promote a Culture of Safety*, 51 N. Y. L. Sch. L. Rev. 1057, 1070, 1073 (2006).

Journal 2006 Reviews law and policy regulating the reporting of medical errors. Concludes that federal health programs will play a significant role in shaping future policies. Quotes Opinion 8.12. Sage, Zivin, & Chase, *Bridging the Relational-Regulatory Gap*, 59 Vand. L. Rev. 1263, 1284 (2006).

Journal 2006 Examines tort reform and the application of principles of restorative justice. Concludes that a "healing-centered framework" serves the best interest of patients and health care providers. Cites Opinion 8.12. Todres, *Toward Healing and Restoration for All: Reframing Medical Malpractice Reform*, 39 Conn. L. Rev. 667, 728-29 (2006).

Journal 2006 Discusses an attorney's role in advising health care professionals on disclosure of medical errors. Concludes attorneys should always encourage full disclosure to prevent harm to the patient. Quotes Opinion 8.12. Winslade & McKinney, *The Ethical Health Lawyer: To Tell or Not to Tell: Disclosing Medical Error*, 34 J. L. Med. & Ethics 813, 814 (2006).

Journal 2005 Considers tort liability reforms that focus on compensating injured patients fairly and quickly while increasing patient safety. Concludes that the current system is ineffective, and that nontort alternatives should be implemented to achieve these goals. Quotes Opinion 8.12. Bovbjerg & Tancredi, *Liability Reform Should Make Patients Safer: "Avoidable Classes of Events" Are a Key Improvement*, 33 J. L. Med. & Ethics 478, 482 (2005).

Journal 2005 Argues that abolishing or weakening the tort liability system will not improve the quality of health care, but may diminish it. Concludes that a systems-based approach coupled with a liability system that encourages high quality care may improve health care delivery in the US. Quotes Opinion 8.12. References Opinion 6.01. Hyman & Silver, *The Poor State of Health Care Quality in the U.S.: Is Malpractice Liability Part of the Problem or Part of the Solution?* 90 Cornell L. Rev. 893, 926, 965 (2005).

Journal 2004 Argues that reduction of medical errors will reduce the number of medical malpractice lawsuits and insurance premiums while stabilizing health care access and costs. Concludes that short-term liability reform, open communication, and the integration of patients as partners in system improvement are necessary. References Opinion 8.12. Liang & Ren, *Medical Liability Insurance and Damage Caps: Getting Beyond Band Aids to Substantive Systems Treatment to Improve Quality and Safety in Healthcare*, 30 Am. J. L. & Med. 501, 534 (2004).

Journal 2002 Discusses therapeutic jurisprudence and the importance of trust in the structure of health care law. Concludes that understanding trust provides tools to formulate responses to new ethical, legal, and policy challenges. Quotes Principle Ch. I, Art. I, Sec. 4 (May 1847) [now Principle II and Opinion 8.12]. Hall, *Law, Medicine, and Trust*, 55 Stan. L. Rev. 463, 471 (2002).

Journal 2002 Advocates in favor of disclosure of information regarding a physician's clinical experience when obtaining informed consent. Concludes that the physician's experience is material and patients who inquire should be given this information. Quotes Principle Ch. I, Art. I, Sec. 4 (May 1847) [now Principle II and Opinion 8.12]. Iheukwumere, *Doctor, Are You Experienced? The Relevance of Disclosure of Physician Experience to a Valid Informed Consent*, 18 J. Contemp. Health L. & Pol'y 373, 376-77 (2002).

Journal 2002 Examines various interpretations of JCAHO standards regarding informing patients about medical errors. Concludes that further clarification is needed regarding reportable events. Quotes Opinion 8.12. LeGros & Pinkall, *The New JCAHO Patient Safety Standards and the Disclosure of Unanticipated Outcomes*, 35 J. Health L. 189, 203 (2002).

Journal 2002 Analyzes the role of prognostication in physician-patient communication. Concludes that the patient-physician model of shared decision-making offers the best hope for reestablishing prognostication. Quotes Principles Ch. I, Art. I, Sec. 2 and 4 (1846) [now Principle IV and Opinions 8.12 and 10.01]. Cites Opinion 8.08. Rich, *Prognostication in Clinical Medicine: Prophecy or Professional Responsibility?* 23 J. Legal Med. 297, 299, 318, 327 (2002).

Journal 2001 Discusses whether or not the medical profession needs a policy on honesty. Reviews ethical codes and concludes they fail to offer physicians With meaningful guidance about what constitutes "the truth" and when and how to disclose it. Quotes Principle II and

Opinions 8.12 and 10.01. DeVita, *Honestly, Do We Need a Policy on Truth?* 11 Kennedy Inst. Ethics J. 157, 158 (2001).

Journal 2001 Examines the duty of physicians and medical students to disclose physician mistakes. Concludes that students develop professionally by recognizing personal ethical standards and determining how to manage conflicting priorities. Quotes Opinion 8.12. Wusthoff, *Medical Mistakes and Disclosure: The Role of the Medical Student*, 286 JAMA 1080, 1080 (2001).

Journal 2000 Examines the lost chance doctrine in medical malpractice cases. Reviews Texas law by evaluating the cases of *Kramer v. Lewisville Mem'l Hosp.* and *Park Place Hosp. v. Estate of Milo.* Examines the distinction between affirmative acts and omissions. Discusses the limitations and pitfalls of both cases. Quotes Opinion 8.12. Perdue & Binion, *A License to Kill: The Unintended (?) Consequence of Milo on Kramer*, 41 S. Tex. L. Rev. 293, 309 (2000).

Journal 1997 Compares past ethical opinions to current opinions and notes the differences. Comments on the forces that have changed medical ethics through the years. Notes differing theories on the future course of medical ethics. Quotes Fundamental Elements (Preamble) and Opinions 5.05, 5.057, 7.01, 8.12, 9.12, and 9.131. Cites Fundamental Elements (5) and Opinions 8.115 and 8.13. Buchanan, *Medical Ethics at the Millennium: A Brief Retrospective*, 26 Colo. Law. 141, 142, 143, 144, 145 (1997).

Journal 1996 Presents clinical problem-solving scenarios. Notes the AMA's instruction that physicians deal openly and honestly with patients. Considers the physician's role as educator and counselor. Opines that physicians must ensure that patients have the ability to make informed decisions. Quotes Opinion 8.12. Sirmon & Kreisberg, *The Invisible Patient*, 334 New Eng. J. Med. 908, 910, 911 (1996).

Journal 1991 Discusses the manner in which a changing economy and an evolving health care system require society to expand its understanding of the physician-patient relationship. Concludes that open physician-patient discussion about available medical services and costs may become part of the standard of care. References Opinions 8.08 and 8.12. Morreim, *Economic Disclosure and Economic Advocacy: New Duties in the Medical Standard of Care*, 12 J. Legal Med. 275, 306 (1991).

Journal 1983 Discusses both moral and legal dilemmas in the use of placebos in treating patients. Concludes that, while arguments against placebo therapy are noble, a complete ban of placebo therapy is impractical and undesirable. Quotes Opinions 8.07 (1982) [now Opinion 8.08] and 8.11 (1982) [now Opinion 8.12]. Kapp, *Placebo Therapy and the Law: Prescribe With Care*, 8 Am. J. Law & Med. 371, 391 (1983).

8.121 Ethical Responsibility to Study and Prevent Error and Harm

In the context of health care, an error is an unintended act or omission, or a flawed system or plan, that harms or has the potential to harm a patient. Patient safety can be enhanced by studying the circumstances surrounding health care errors. This can best be achieved through a legally protected review process, which is essential for reducing health care errors and preventing patient harm.

(1) Because they are uniquely positioned to have a comprehensive view of the care patients receive, physicians must strive to ensure patient safety and should play a central role in identifying, reducing, and preventing health care errors. This responsibility exists even in the absence of a patient-physician relationship.

(2) Physicians should participate in the development of reporting mechanisms that emphasize education and systems change, thereby providing a substantive opportunity for all members of the health care team to learn. Specifically, physicians should work with other relevant health care professionals to:

(a) Establish and participate fully in an effective, confidential, and protected error-reporting mechanism

(b) Develop means for objective review and analysis of reports regarding errors, and to conduct appropriate investigations into the causes of harm to a patient

(c) Ensure that the investigation of causes of harm, and the review and study of error reports result in preventive measures that are conveyed to all relevant individuals

(d) Identify and promptly report impaired and/or incompetent colleagues so that rehabilitation, retraining, or disciplinary action can occur in order to prevent harm to patients

(3) Physicians must offer professional and compassionate concern toward patients who have been harmed, regardless of whether the harm was caused by a health care error. An expression of concern need not be an admission of responsibility. When patient harm has been caused by an error, physicians should offer a general explanation regarding the nature of the error and the measures being taken to prevent similar occurrences in the future. Such communication is fundamental to the trust that underlies the patient-physician relationship, and may help reduce the risk of liability.

(4) Physicians have a responsibility to provide for continuity of care to patients who may have been harmed during the course of their health care. If, because of the harm suffered under the care of a physician, a patient loses trust in that physician, the obligation may best be fulfilled by facilitating the transfer of the patient to the care of another physician.

(5) Physicians should seek changes to the current legal system to ensure that all errors in health care can be safely and securely reported and studied as a learning experience for all participants in the health care system, without threat of discoverability, legal liability, or punitive action. (I, II, III, IV, VIII)

Issued December 2003 based on the report "Ethical Responsibility to Study and Prevent Error and Harm in the Provision of Health Care," adopted June 2003.

Journal 2009 Argues it is inappropriate to create an evidentiary exclusion for medical apologies in an attempt to improve physician-patient communication. Concludes that the exclusion for medical apologies will allow lawyers to have greater involvement in the communications between physicians and patients, and will decrease the openness and efficacy of that communication. Quotes Opinion 8.121. Jesson & Knapp, *My Lawyer Told Me to Say I'm Sorry: Lawyers, Doctors, and Medical Apologies*, 35 Wm. Mitchell L. Rev. 1410, 1420 (2009).

Journal 2009 Explores the value of incident reports and their use for hospital quality assurance research. Discusses the relationship between incident reports and confidentiality statutes. Concludes incident reports should be used strictly as research aids in alerting hospitals to their own shortcomings and that greater legal protection is needed for providers to freely report errors and improve care. Quotes Opinion 8.121. Mikk, *Making the Plaintiff's Bar Earn Its Keep: Rethinking the Hospital Incident Report*, 53 N. Y. L. Sch. L. Rev. 133, 156 (2009).

Journal 2008 Examines ethical issues related to broadcasting cardiothoracic surgeries for educational and media purposes. Concludes that seven ethical guidelines should be followed to ensure patient safety. Quotes Principle VIII and Opinion 8.121. Sade, *Broadcast of Surgical Procedures as a Teaching Instrument in Cardiothoracic Surgery*, 86 Ann. Thorac. Surg. 357, 359 (2008).

Journal 2006 Reviews the concept of therapeutic privilege. Concludes that the practice creates conflict between physician obligations under the concepts of autonomy and beneficence. Recommends that physicians maximize communication with patients by providing all pertinent information in the context of patient preferences. Cites Opinions 8.08, 8.081, 8.121, and 10.015. References Chap. I, Art. I, Sec. 4 (May 1847) [premise deleted from Code]. Bostick, Sade, McMahon, & Benjamin, *Report of the American Medical Association Council on Ethical and Judicial Affairs: Withholding Information From Patients: Rethinking the Propriety of "Therapeutic Privilege,"* 17 J. Clinical Ethics 302, 303 (Winter 2006).

Journal 2006 Examines ethical dilemmas physicians may face as providers of pay-for-performance medical care. Concludes that this strategy offers a benefit to patients as long as physicians uphold stringent ethical standards and work together to ensure optimum patient care. Cites Principles I, V, VIII, and IX and Opinions 2.035, 2.095, 6.01, 8.021, 8.03, 8.0501, 8.053, 8.054, and 8.121. Bostick, Sade, & McMahon, *Report of the Council on Ethical and Judicial Affairs: Physician Pay-for-Performance Programs,* 3 Ind. Health L. Rev. 429, 430, 431, 432-33, 434, 435, 436 (2006).

8.13   The previous Opinion 8.13, "Referral of Patients: Disclosure of Limitations," was changed to Opinion 8.132, "Referral of Patients: Disclosure of Limitations," in June 1996.

8.13   Managed Care

The expansion of managed care has brought a variety of changes to medicine including new and different reimbursement systems for physicians with complex referral restrictions and benefits packages for patients. Some of these changes have raised concerns that a physician's ability to practice ethical medicine will be adversely affected by the modifications in the system. In response to these concerns, the following points were developed to provide physicians with general guidelines that will assist them in fulfilling their ethical responsibilities to patients given the changes heralded by managed care.

(1) The duty of patient advocacy is a fundamental element of the patient-physician relationship that should not be altered by the system of health care delivery. Physicians must continue to place the interests of their patients first.

(2) When health care plans place restrictions on the care that physicians in the plan may provide to their patients, physicians should insist that the following principles be followed:

    (a) Any broad allocation guidelines that restrict care and choices—which go beyond the cost/benefit judgments made by physicians as a part of their normal professional responsibilities—should be established at a policy-making level so that individual physicians are not asked to engage in bedside rationing.

    (b) Regardless of any allocation guidelines or gatekeeper directives, physicians must advocate for any care they believe will materially benefit their patients.

    (c) Physicians should be given an active role in contributing their expertise to any allocation process and should advocate for guidelines that are sensitive to differences among patients. Health care plans should create structures similar to hospital medical staffs that allow physicians to have meaningful input into the plan's development of allocation guidelines. Guidelines for allocating health care should be reviewed on a regular basis and updated to reflect advances in medical knowledge and changes in relative costs.

(d) Adequate appellate mechanisms for both patients and physicians should be in place to address disputes regarding medically necessary care. In some circumstances, physicians have an obligation to initiate appeals on behalf of their patients. Cases may arise in which a health plan has an allocation guideline that is generally fair but in particular circumstances results in unfair denials of care, ie, denial of care that, in the physician's judgment, would materially benefit the patient. In such cases, the physician's duty as patient advocate requires that the physician challenge the denial and argue for the provision of treatment in the specific case. Cases may also arise when a health plan has an allocation guideline that is generally unfair in its operations. In such cases, the physician's duty as patient advocate requires not only a challenge to any denials of treatment from the guideline, but also advocacy at the health plan's policy-making level to seek an elimination or modification of the guideline. Physicians should assist patients who wish to seek additional, appropriate care outside the plan when the physician believes the care is in the patient's best interests.

(e) Health care plans must adhere to the requirement of informed consent that patients be given full disclosure of material information. Full disclosure requires that health care plans inform potential subscribers of limitations or restrictions on the benefits package when they are considering entering the plan.

(f) Physicians also should continue to promote full disclosure to patients enrolled in health care plans. The physician's obligation to disclose treatment alternatives to patients is not altered by any limitations in the coverage provided by the patient's health care plan. Full disclosure includes informing patients of all of their treatment options, even those that may not be covered under the terms of the health care plan. Patients may then determine whether an appeal is appropriate, or whether they wish to seek care outside the plan for treatment alternatives that are not covered.

(g) Physicians should not participate in any plan that encourages or requires care below minimum professional standards.

(3) When physicians are employed or reimbursed by health care plans that offer financial incentives to limit care, serious potential conflicts are created between the physicians' personal financial interests and the needs of their patients. Efforts to contain health care costs should not place patient welfare at risk. Thus, physicians should accept only those financial incentives that promote the cost-effective delivery of health care and not the withholding of medically necessary care.

(a) Physicians should insist that any incentives to limit care must be disclosed fully to patients by plan administrators upon enrollment and at least annually thereafter.

(b) Physicians should advocate that limits be placed on the magnitude of fee withholds, bonuses, and other financial incentives to limit care and that incentive payments be calculated according to the performance of a sizable group of physicians rather than on an individual basis.

   (c) Physicians should advocate that health care plans or other groups develop financial incentives based on quality of care. Such incentives should complement those based on the quantity of services used.

(4) Physicians should encourage both that patients be aware of the benefits and limitations of their health care coverage and that they exercise their autonomy by public participation in the formulation of benefits packages and by prudent selection of health care coverage that best suits their needs. (I, II, III, V)

Issued June 1996 based on the report "Ethical Issues in Managed Care," adopted June 1994 (*JAMA.* 1995;273:330-335). Updated June 2002.

D. N. J. 1999 Patient sued her managed care organization alleging that she suffered injuries due to failure to obtain timely approval for a nonmember physician to perform her back surgery. The plaintiff apparently relied on Opinion 8.13 to show that the defendant had a duty to advocate for her in seeking prompt approval for her surgery. The court, however, stated that the plaintiff's reference to the Opinion failed to establish such a duty because the Code of Medical Ethics does not have the force of law. *Pryzbowski v. US Health Care, Inc.,* 64 F. Supp. 2d 361, 370.

S.D.N.Y. 1997 Employee brought suit against a health maintenance organization (HMO) under contract with her employer to provide health benefits. The suit alleged various theories of liability ranging from breach of implied contract to breach of fiduciary duties. Employee sought redress pursuant to the civil enforcement provisions of the Employee Retirement Income Security Act of 1974. The court granted HMO's motion to dismiss all claims except for the breach of fiduciary duty stemming from HMO's alleged policy of restricting the disclosure of noncovered treatments. The court quoted report of AMA Council on Ethical and Judicial Affairs [now Opinion 8.13] in holding that physicians have an ethical duty to fully disclose treatment options to patients regardless of whether treatment occurs in a managed care environment. *Weiss v. Cigna Healthcare, Inc.,* 972 F. Supp. 748, 751-52.

Mass. Super. 2004 Defendants filed a motion for partial summary judgment in an action alleging they were liable for not disclosing their financial interests in an experimental program that the decedent participated in. The court denied the defendants' motion, referencing Opinion 8.13 in stating physicians should disclose financial incentives and restrictions placed on them by their HMO. *Darke v. Estate of Isner,* 2004 WL 1325635, 3.

Ohio Att'y Gen. 1999 State attorney general concluded that physicians who render opinions regarding the necessity of medical services for health insuring corporations are not engaged in the practice of medicine. Additionally, physicians who render opinions regarding medical necessity for appeals of adverse determinations do not fall under the regulatory, investigatory, or enforcement authority of the Ohio State Medical Board. Quoting Opinions 8.03, 8.11, and 8.13, the attorney general stated that physicians have an ethical duty to provide appropriate treatment for patients. *Ohio Att'y Gen. Op. No. 99-044, 1999 WL 692623.*

Journal 2006 Examines the process of physician deselection and the protections afforded to physicians. Concludes that physicians should be able to make a legal challenge to a dismissal made without cause. Quotes Opinion 8.13. Coppolo, *Not Just a Minimum Income Policy for Physicians: The Need for Good Faith and Fair Dealing in Physician Deselection Disputes,* 48 Wm and Mary L. Rev. 677, 686 (2006).

Journal 2006 Examines external review systems used for adjudication of disputes between patients and managed care organizations. Concludes that external review systems do not satisfy constitutional due process requirements. Quotes Opinions and Reports of the Judicial Council Sec. 6, Para. 4 (1969) [now Opinion 8.05]. References Opinion 8.13. Hunter, *Managed Process, Due Care: Structures of Accountability in Health Care,* 6 Yale J. Health Pol'y L. & Ethics 93, 107, 113 (2006).

Journal 2006 Argues for an alternative framework by which health ethics, policy, and law can address equitable distribution of health care. Concludes that a new paradigm would lead to a more efficient and compassionate system. References Opinions 2.22 and 8.13. Ruger, *Health, Capability, and Justice: Toward a New Paradigm of Health Ethics, Policy and Law,* 15 Cornell J. L. & Pub. Pol'y 403, 425, 465 (2006).

Journal 2006 Considers the role of informed consent and patient autonomy as a central tenet of bioethics. Concludes that the field should focus most strongly on serving the practical needs and desires of patients. References Opinion 8.13. Schneider, *After Autonomy, 41 Wake Forest L. Rev. 411, 429-30 (2006).*

Journal 2006 Critiques the Uniform Health-Care Decisions Act. Concludes that the Act poses dangers to disabled patients, and proposes safeguards against such dangers. References Opinion 8.13. Stith, *The Semblance of Autonomy: Treatment of Persons With Disabilities Under the Uniform Health-Care Decisions Act, 22 Issues L. & Med. 39, 63-64 (2006).*

Journal 2005 Argues that in *Aetna v. Davila/Cigna v. Calad*, the Supreme Court missed an opportunity to overturn unjust ERISA policies. Concludes that the principle of complete ERISA preemption as articulated in these consolidated cases is unsatisfactory because it violates the separation of powers doctrine. Quotes Principle VIII. Cites Opinions 8.054, 8.13, 8.135, 9.123, 10.01, and 10.015. Nelson, *AETNA v. DAVILA/CIGNA v. CALAD: A Missed Opportunity, 31 Wm. Mitchell L. Rev. 843, 847, 849, 850, 880 (2005).*

Journal 2003 Reviews state laws designed to protect physicians acting as patient advocates in managed care organizations. Concludes that federal and state law must make it easier for physicians to challenge denials of or delays in patient care. Quotes Opinions 8.054, 8.13, and 10.01. Fentiman, *Patient Advocacy and Termination From Managed Care Organizations. Do State Laws Protecting Health Care Professional Advocacy Make Any Difference? 82 Neb. L. Rev. 508, 515-16, 517-18 (2003).*

Journal 2002 Observes that changes in the health professions challenge certain assumptions about professional ethics. Concludes that these long-standing assumptions must be re-examined. Cites Opinion 2.161. References Opinion 8.13. Kelley, *The Meanings of Professional Life: Teaching Across the Health Professions, 27 J. Med. & Phil. 475, 485, 490, 491 (2002).*

Journal 2002 Considers whether physicians should be required to disclose information regarding financial incentives received from patients' HMOs. Concludes that physicians should not be required to disclose these incentives. References Opinion 8.13. Reuland, *Health Maintenance Organizations and Physician Financial Incentive Plans: Should Physician Disclosure Be Mandatory? 27 Iowa J. Corp. L. 293, 312 (2002).*

Journal 2002 Examines whether managed care organizations should be obligated to disclose physician financial incentives that may limit patient care. Concludes that mandatory disclosure is in the best interest of patients and physicians. Quotes Opinions 2.03 and 8.13. Talesh, *Breaking the Learned Helplessness of Patients: Why MCOs Should Be Required to Disclose Financial Incentives, 26 Law & Psychol. Rev. 49, 60-61, 63 (2002).*

Journal 2001 Examines issues relating to health care cost containment. Concludes that, if physicians are to meet the goals assigned to them in a cost-constrained health care system, then professional standards must be reevaluated and modified to afford meaningful guidance for clinical decision-making in the face of health care spending controls. Quotes Opinions 2.03, 2.09, 2.095, 8.032, and 9.04. Cites Opinions 8.02, 8.021, 8.051, and 8.13. Agrawal, *Resuscitating Professionalism: Self-regulation in the Medical Marketplace, 66 Mo. L. Rev. 341, 354, 355, 360, 361, 378, 388 (2001).*

Journal 2001 Examines the doctrine of informed consent with respect to nontraditional issues, such as a physician's duty to disclose personal information. Concludes there must be a balance that will accommodate the needs of both the patient and the physician. References Opinion 8.13. Hanson, *Informed Consent and the Scope of a Physician's Duty of Disclosure, 77 N. D. L. Rev. 71, 89, 91 (2001).*

Journal 2001 Discusses the prohibition on nonlawyer ownership of legal service providers. Considers how ethical rules and standards governing physicians have been directed toward preserving independent judgment. Concludes that ethical conflicts created by abandoning the prohibition on nonlawyer ownership of legal service providers may be managed by following the medical ethics model. Quotes Principle VI and Opinions 2.03, 2.09, 8.02, 8.021, 8.03, 8.05, 8.051, 8.054, 8.13, and 8.132. Harris & Foran, *The Ethics of Middle-Class Access to Legal Services and What We Can Learn From the Medical Profession's Shift to a Corporate Paradigm, 70 Fordham L. Rev. 775, 817, 821, 822, 823, 824 (2001).*

Journal 2000 Discusses and evaluates different systems for addressing consumer concerns about managed health care. Asserts that current legal systems for identifying and resolving consumer concerns are not understood by most consumers and are not accessible by many, especially the uninsured. Concludes that several immediate steps are realistic for moving toward reform. Cites Principle VI. References Opinions 8.13 and 9.065. Kinney, *Tapping and Resolving Consumer Concerns About Health Care*, 26 Am. J. Law & Med. 335, 337, 375 (2000).

Journal 2000 Reviews the case of *Corporate Health Insurance, Inc. v. Texas Dept. of Insurance* and discusses its impact on HMO liability in Texas. Considers the conflicts of interest managed care imposes upon physicians. Concludes that, without national amendments to the scope of ERISA, HMOs are not compelled to provide quality health care. References Opinion 8.13. Lockhart, *The Safest Care Is to Deny Care: Implications of Corporate Health Insurance, Inc. v. Texas Department of Insurance on HMO Liability in Texas*, 41 S. Tex. L. Rev. 621, 628, 634 (2000).

Journal 2000 Describes the fiduciary aspects of the physician-patient relationship. Explores the conflicts that may occur between physicians and pregnant women in the health care setting. Proposes legal strategies to address these conflicts. Quotes Opinions 8.08 and 10.01. References Opinion 8.13. Oberman, *Mothers and Doctors' Orders: Unmasking the Doctor's Fiduciary Role in Maternal-Fetal Conflicts*, 94 Nw. U. L. Rev. 451, 456, 462, 493 (2000).

Journal 1999 Describes the gag clause debate in managed care and analyzes the types of incentives that might limit physician-patient communication. Concludes that, to protect patient access to information about treatment options and their health plans, antigag legislation must be coupled with a thorough examination of the extent to which financial incentives will be permitted to impact managed health care delivery. Quotes Opinion 8.13. Krause, *The Brief Life of the Gag Clause: Why Antigag Clause Legislation Isn't Enough*, 67 Tenn. L. Rev. 1, 4, 43 (1999).

Journal 1999 Describes the development of managed care organizations. Examines professional associations' statements regarding managed care organizations. Argues that physicians and managed care organizations should be viewed as economically disciplined, moral cofiduciaries for patients. References Opinion 8.13. McCullough, *A Basic Concept in the Clinical Ethics of Managed Care: Physicians and Institutions as Economically Disciplined Moral Co-Fiduciaries of Populations of Patients*, 24 J. Med. Phil. 77, 82-83, 87, 89, 91, 96 (1999).

Journal 1999 Explores the increased push toward mandatory disclosure laws regarding financial incentives imposed by managed care organizations. Discusses current laws and ethical guidelines. Emphasizes that efforts to mandate disclosure force physicians to focus on the effects of imposed incentives and the essence of the physician-patient relationship. References Opinions 8.032, 8.13, and 8.132. Miller & Sage, *Disclosing Physician Financial Incentives*, 281 JAMA 1424, 1425 (1999).

Journal 1999 Discusses the need for physicians to advocate on behalf of patients' rights in the context of health care delivery. Evaluates the nature and scope of the physician's role as advocate, noting that physicians cannot be expected to engage in attorney-like advocacy. Quotes Principles IV and VI, Fundamental Elements (2), (4), and (6) [now Opinion 10.01], Patient Responsibilities 5 [now Opinion 10.02], and Opinions 2.03, 2.07, 2.09, 2.16, 2.19, 3.06, 4.01, 4.04, 6.01, 7.02, 8.02, 8.03, 8.13, 8.132, 9.06, 9.07, and 9.131. Cites Opinions 5.05, 5.09, 7.01, 8.135, and 9.02. Sage, *Physicians as Advocates*, 35 Hous. L. Rev. 1529, 1537, 1541, 1542, 1552-53, 1554, 1556, 1557, 1559, 1561-62, 1564, 1571, 1574, 1576, 1580 (1999).

Journal 1999 Discusses the push to mandate disclosure in managed care programs. Explains the dangers of disclosing too much information. Provides objectives and goals for disclosure. Quotes Opinion 8.051. References Opinions 8.032 and 8.13. Sage, *Regulating Through Information: Disclosure Laws and American Health Care*, 99 Colum. L. Rev. 1701, 1753, 1758, 1760 (1999).

Journal 1999 Argues that the benefits of managed care organizations are outweighed by the resulting changes in the physician's role as advocate. Characterizes the traditional notion of physician advocacy. States that recent changes in the law regarding communication in managed care organizations have shifted the matter more toward patient self-advocacy. Quotes Opinion 8.13. Spielman, *Managed Care Regulation and the Physician-Advocate*, 47 Drake L. Rev. 713, 717, 719 (1999).

Journal 1999 Discusses financial incentives offered to physicians by managed care organizations. Argues that evidence of financial incentives should be admissible in medical malpractice cases. Quotes Opinion 8.13. References Opinion 8.132. Sugarman & Yarashus, *Admissibility of Managed Care Financial Incentives in Medical Malpractice Cases*, 34 Tort & Ins. L. J. 735, 743, 746, 759 (1999).

Journal 1999 Explores the impact managed care organizations have had on health care. Explains that patients may not understand restrictions and incentives imposed by their managed care organizations when entering the program. Argues that such information should be disclosed at various times during the period of plan coverage. Cites Opinions 2.03, 8.03, 8.032, 8.051, 8.13, and 8.132. Wolf, *Toward a Systemic Theory of Informed Consent in Managed Care*, 35 Hous. L. Rev. 1631, 1641, 1658, 1661, 1662, 1679 (1999).

Journal 1998 Analyzes Hall's book *Making Medical Spending Decisions: The Law, Ethics and Economics of Rationing Mechanisms*. Discusses cost-based rationing for medical services and physician bedside rationing. Concludes that patients should be informed in advance when their physician may receive financial incentives for withholding care. Quotes Opinion 8.13. Agrawal, *Chicago Hope Meets the Chicago School*, 96 Mich. L. Rev. 1793, 1804 (1998).

Journal 1998 Discusses changes in the health care system. Explains why patients need more power in the managed care system. Suggests that patients should use class action suits as a method to assert power over managed care organizations. References Opinions 8.13 and 8.132. Cerminara, *The Class Action Suit as a Method of Patient Empowerment in the Managed Care Setting*, 24 Am. J. Law & Med. 7, 16, 17, 23 (1998).

Journal 1998 Discusses conflicts of interest in the physician-patient relationship arising out of use of financial incentives by managed care organizations. Considers how such conflicts are dealt with in the attorney-client relationship. Suggests that a financial incentive should be legally denounced if it unreasonably interferes with a physician's duty to properly care for and treat patients. Quotes Preamble, Fundamental Elements (1) [now Opinion 10.01], and Opinions 4.04, 5.01, 8.03, 8.13, and 9.06. Cites Fundamental Elements (4) [now Opinion 10.01] and Opinions 2.07, 2.08, and 2.132. Hall, *Third-Party Payor Conflicts of Interest in Managed Care: A Proposal for Regulation Based on the Model Rules of Professional Conduct*, 29 Seton Hall L. Rev. 95, 96, 107, 108, 109, 110, 111, 112, 134, 135, 136 (1998).

Journal 1998 Asserts that managed care organizations assume fiduciary obligations by exercising discretionary control over the administration of an ERISA plan. Argues that ERISA requires managed care organizations and physicians to disclose financial incentives intended to influence physician decision-making. References Opinions 8.13 and 8.132. Johnson, *ERISA Doctor in the House? The Duty to Disclose Physician Incentives to Limit Health Care*, 82 Minn. L. Rev. 1631, 1639, 1649, 1655 (1998).

Journal 1998 Discusses changes in the health care system. Analyzes conflicts of interest arising from the practice of capitation. Argues that physicians should refuse to sign contracts with health care plans offering incentives that may present a temptation to undertreat patients. References Opinion 8.13. Kassirer, *Managing Care—Should We Adopt a New Ethic?* 339 New Eng. J. Med. 397 (1998).

Journal 1998 Expresses concern about the impact of managed care cost-containment practices on the physician-patient relationship. Advocates the need for disclosure of information about these practices to patients. Evaluates and recommends a Maryland law that requires such disclosure. Cites Opinion 8.13. Khanna, Silverman, & Schwartz, *Disclosure of Operating Practices by Managed-Care Organizations to Consumers of Healthcare: Obligations of Informed Consent*, 9 J. Clinical Ethics 291, 293, 296 (1998).

Journal 1998 Discusses quality and safety concerns arising under managed care systems. Explores benefits and detriments of the proposed patients' bill of rights. Advocates legislation to provide safeguards from cost-containment mechanisms utilized by managed care programs. Quotes Opinion 8.13. Misocky, *The Patients' Bill of Rights: Managed Care Under Siege*, 15 J. Contemp. Health L. & Pol'y 57, 73 (1998).

Journal 1998 Explores clinical freedom and the Hippocratic Oath. Discusses issues of patient trust and confidence. Suggests that a sense of confidence will not be present if managerial priorities are dominant factors in resource allocation. References Opinion 8.13. Newdick, *Public Health Ethics and Clinical Freedom*, 14 J. Contemp. Health L. & Pol'y 335, 336, 339, 356, 359, 361 (1998).

Journal 1998 Discusses communication conflicts between physicians and managed care organizations. Describes legal responses to gag provisions imposed by managed care organizations. Assesses the impact of gag practices on physician-patient communication. Quotes Opinion 8.13. Spielman, *After the Gag Episode: Physician Communication in Managed Care Organizations*, 22 Seton Hall Legis. J. 437, 453, 461, 463 (1998).

Journal 1998 Argues that health maintenance organizations (HMOs) do not have an incentive to act reasonably because they are not held accountable under tort law. Points out that the duty to act reasonably is imposed on most of society in order to deter negligence. Advocates imposing the same duty on HMOs. References Opinion 8.13. Wertheimer, *Ockham's Scalpel: A Return to a Reasonableness Standard, 43 Vill. L. Rev. 321, 327 (1998).*

Journal 1997 Discusses the quality of neurological care and the ethical conflicts that are created by the drive to contain costs. Focuses on quality management and cost-containment programs and the conflicts created when neurologists attempt to reconcile the interests of patients and society. References Opinions 8.032 and 8.13. Bernat, *Quality of Neurological Care: Balancing Cost Control and Ethics, 54 Arch. Neurol. 1341, 1343, 1345 (1997).*

Journal 1997 Compares past ethical opinions to current opinions and notes the differences. Comments on the forces that have changed medical ethics through the years. Notes differing theories on the future course of medical ethics. Quotes Fundamental Elements (Preamble) and Opinions 5.05, 5.057, 7.01, 8.12, 9.12, and 9.131. Cites Fundamental Elements (5) and Opinions 8.115 and 8.13. Buchanan, *Medical Ethics at the Millennium: A Brief Retrospective, 26 Colo. Law. 141, 142, 143, 144, 145 (1997).*

Journal 1997 Examines the use of gag clauses in the managed care setting. Explores the conflict of interest between physicians' loyalty to HMOs and their duty to patients. Questions whether patients can give informed consent based on inadequate information. Emphasizes the need for more comprehensive regulation. Quotes Opinion 8.13. Comment, *Physician Gag Clauses—The Hypocrisy of the Hippocratic Oath, 21 So. Ill. U. L. J. 313, 318, 320 (1997).*

Journal 1997 Reviews the conflict between the economics of managed care and physicians' ethical obligations to patients. Questions whether a patient may give informed consent to treatment without knowledge of all available alternatives. Offers a proposal for disclosure of managed care cost-containment mechanisms and incentives to patients. Quotes Opinion 8.13. Hall, *A Theory of Economic Informed Consent, 31 Ga. L. Rev. 511, 521, 524-25 (1997).*

Journal 1997 Posits that cost-containment schemes in managed care systems have eroded the fiduciary duty physicians owe patients. Notes that managed care organizations (MCOs) are prohibiting patients from trusting and relying on physicians. Concludes that patients must seek quality assurance from sources other than their physicians. Quotes Opinions 2.03, 2.09, and 8.13. Jacobi, *Patients at a Loss: Protecting Health Care Consumers Through Data Driven Quality Assurance, 45 U. Kan. L. Rev. 705, 720, 721, 759 (1997).*

Journal 1997 Explores the responsibilities imposed on physicians by managed care and capitation. Notes that physicians are called on to act as gatekeepers, controlling access to specialty services and tests. Considers whether primary care physicians in capitated groups are satisfied with the quality of care they provide. References Opinion 8.13. Kerr, Hays, Mittman, Siu, Leake, & Brook, *Primary Care Physicians' Satisfaction With Quality of Care in California Capitated Medical Groups, 278 JAMA 308, 312 (1997).*

Journal 1997 Discusses the practice of physician deselection by managed care organizations. Suggests that deselection harms the physician-patient relationship and creates a conflict of interest. Argues that solutions to deselection should consider effects on the patient rather than on the physician. Quotes Principle III. Cites Principle I and Opinions 8.05 and 8.13. Liner, *Physician Deselection: The Dynamics of a New Threat to the Physician-Patient Relationship, 23 Am. J. Law & Med. 511, 513, 527 (1997).*

Journal 1997 Examines national health care reform and managed care. Notes that state regulatory policies in this context evidence common concerns. Suggests ways in which the government can promote patient and physician rights. References Opinion 8.13. Miller, *Managed Care Regulation: In the Laboratory of the States, 278 JAMA 1102, 1104, 1108-09 (1997).*

Journal 1997 Discusses physician frustration with managed care plans caused by gag clauses and cost-containment mechanisms. Reviews the development of managed care organizations and federal attempts at limiting the use of gag clauses. Concludes that gag clauses are inherently flawed and compromise quality health care. Quotes Principles II and V, Fundamental Elements (1), and Opinion 8.13. Note, *Physicians, Bound and Gagged: Federal Attempts to Combat Managed Care's Use of Gag Clauses, 21 Seton Hall Legis. J. 567, 601-02 (1997).*

Journal 1997 Describes gag provisions in managed care contracts. Explains the context in which gag provisions may undermine the physician-patient relationship, as well as the conflicts of interest they may create. Proposes legislation to address these problems. Quotes Opinion 8.13. Note, *Stop Gagging Physicians! 7 Health Matrix 187, 193, 200, 208-09 (1997).*

Journal 1997 Examines the need for change in interpretation of state laws under the saving clause of the Employment Retirement Income Security Act. Discusses any willing provider laws and concludes that they should receive saving clause protection. References Opinion 8.13. Pittman, *Any Willing Provider Laws and ERISA's Saving Clause: A New Solution for an Old Problem, 64 Tenn. L. Rev. 409, 416 (1997).*

Journal 1997 Discusses the need for balance between business ethics and medical ethics in the context of managed care. Explores two models for integrating ethics and managed care. Proposes the adoption of a collective responsibility model to improve quality of care. Quotes Principles I, II, III, IV, and V. Cites Preamble. References Opinion 8.13. Regan, *Regulating the Business of Medicine: Models for Integrating Ethics and Managed Care, 30 Colum. J. L. & Soc. Probs. 635, 651, 656, 657 (1997).*

Journal 1997 Examines utilization review in the managed care context. Discusses a survey of third-party utilization review firms, noting practices that advance and undermine adherence to important professional norms. Quotes Opinion 9.031. References Opinion 8.13. Schlesinger, Gray, & Perreira, *Medical Professionalism Under Managed Care: The Pros and Cons of Utilization Review, 16 Health Affairs 106, 119, 120, 124 (1997).*

Journal 1996 Discusses the use of practice guidelines to improve medical care quality and to aid in decreasing health care costs. Evaluates pertinent ethical considerations. Concludes that, when used appropriately, guidelines have clinical value. References Opinion 8.13. Berger & Rosner, *The Ethics of Practice Guidelines, 156 Arch. Intern. Med. 2051, 2053, 2056 (1996).*

Journal 1996 Considers the economic implications for physicians brought about by the change from traditional fee-for-service care to capitation. Discusses capitation payments in the American health care system. Alludes to pertinent ethical issues. References Opinion 8.13. Bodenheimer & Grumbach, *Capitation or Decapitation: Keeping Your Head in Changing Times, 276 JAMA 1025, 1031 (1996).*

Journal 1996 Examines the business of health care and the ethical implications of managed care. Describes incentives that affect the delivery of health care. Suggests that a redistribution of excess revenues would help both patients and nonprofit hospitals coexist with managed care. Quotes Opinion 8.13. Bond, *Diverse and Perverse Incentives in Managed Care: Where Will the Pendulum Stop? 1 Widener L. Symp. J. 141, 151, 154 (1996).*

Journal 1996 Discusses the trend toward health care reform. Focuses on benefits and problems posed by managed mental health care. Posits that the moral problems of managed mental health care, including quality concerns, are curable. Concludes that managed mental health care may prove superior to fee-for-service care. References Opinion 8.13. Boyle, *Managed Care in Mental Health: A Cure, or a Cure Worse Than the Disease? 40 St. Louis U. L. J. 437, 448 (1996).*

Journal 1996 Discusses the threat managed health care poses to patients and physicians. Explores direct incentives given to physicians by managed care organizations and the impact these incentives have on physician behavior. Proposes possible methods for dealing with the problems that such incentives create. References Opinion 8.13. Greely, *Direct Financial Incentives in Managed Care: Unanswered Questions, 6 Health Matrix 53, 81 (1996).*

Journal 1996 Discusses the change from fee-for-service health care financing to managed care. Notes that cost-containment mechanisms modify physicians' behaviors and patients' access to health care. Emphasizes that physicians must remain committed to following ethical guidelines. References Opinion 8.13. Hammes & Webster, *Professional Ethics and Managed Care in Dermatology, 132 Arch. Dermatol. 1070, 1072, 1073 (1996).*

Journal 1996 Discusses workers' compensation and the medical care provided to injured employees. Examines the effect of managed care on workers' compensation. Advocates focusing on prevention of injuries and quality of care. References Opinion 8.13. Hashimoto, *The Future Role of Managed Care and Capitation in Workers' Compensation, XXII Am. J. Law & Med. 233, 258, 259 (1996).*

Journal 1996 Considers challenges to the psychiatrist-patient relationship that are triggered by managed care cost-containment methodologies. Offers guidance to psychiatrists for addressing these challenges. References Opinions 2.095, 8.13, and 8.132. Hoge, *APA Resource Document: I. The Professional Responsibilities of Psychiatrists in Evolving Health Care Systems, 24 Bull. Am. Acad. Psychiatry Law 393, 405 (1996).*

Journal 1996 Discusses the problems managed care raises within the framework of the physician-patient relationship. Considers issues specific to psychiatry. Advocates legal regulation to improve upon and bring structural change to managed care systems. Cites Opinion 8.13. Hoge, *APA Resource Document: II. Regulatory Guidelines for Protecting the Interests of Psychiatric Patients in Emerging Health Care Systems*, 24 Bull. Am. Acad. Psychiatry Law 407, 412, 418 (1996).

Journal 1996 Considers procedural issues relative to patient protection in the context of capitated health care plans. Examines regulations governing capitated health plans and consumer protection issues. Offers suggestions regarding policy making, rate setting, dispute resolution, and judicial review. References Opinion 8.13. Kinney, *Procedural Protections for Patients in Capitated Health Plans*, XXII Am. J. Law & Med. 301, 319-20 (1996).

Journal 1996 Explains the conflict between managed care, which focuses on controlling costs, and traditional health care values, which focus on patient autonomy. Proposes a solution to this conflict requiring that patients incur certain economic consequences in obtaining health care and that managed care organizations disclose resource management techniques. References Opinion 8.13. Morreim, *Diverse and Perverse Incentives of Managed Care: Bringing Patients Into Alignment*, 1 Widener L. Symp. J. 89, 129 (1996).

Journal 1996 Discusses efforts to reduce health care costs. Considers whether personal financial incentives given to physicians decrease level of care given to patients. Suggests that, while financial incentives may create ethical concerns, they serve an important function by containing costs. Concludes that efforts to eliminate them completely are misguided. References Opinion 8.13. Orentlicher, *Paying Physicians More to Do Less: Financial Incentives to Limit Care*, 30 U. Rich. L. Rev. 155, 167 (1996).

In June 1996, Opinion 8.13, "Referral of Patients: Disclosure of Limitations," was renumbered as Opinion 8.132, "Referral of Patients: Disclosure of Limitations."

8.132 Referral of Patients: Disclosure of Limitations

Physicians should always make referral decisions based on the best interests of their patients, regardless of the financing and delivery mechanisms or contractual agreements between patients, health care practitioners and institutions, and third-party payers. When physicians agree to provide treatment, they assume an ethical obligation to treat their patients to the best of their ability. If a physician knows that a patient's health care plan or other agreement does not cover referral to a noncontracting medical specialist or to a facility that the physician believes to be in the patient's best interest, the physician should so inform the patient to permit the patient to decide whether to accept the outside referral.

Physicians must not deny their patients access to appropriate medical services based upon the promise of personal financial reward, or the avoidance of financial penalties. Because patients must have the necessary information to make informed decisions about their care, physicians have an obligation to disclose medically appropriate treatment alternatives. Physicians should also promote an effective program to monitor and improve the quality of the patient care services within their practice settings.

Physicians must ensure disclosure of any financial incentives that may limit appropriate diagnostic and therapeutic alternatives that are offered to patients or that may limit patients' overall access to care. This obligation may be satisfied if the health care plan or other agreement makes adequate disclosure to enrolled patients. (II, IV)

Issued June 1986. Updated June 1994 based on the report "Financial Incentives to Limit Care: Ethical Implications for HMO's and IPA," adopted June 1990. Updated June 2002. Updated November 2007 based on the report "Opinion E-8.132, 'Referral of Patients: Disclosure of Limitations,' Amendment," adopted June 2007.

Ill. App. 1999 Administrator of estate brought suit against physician and health maintenance organization (HMO). The suit alleged medical negligence and breach of a fiduciary duty to deceased for the physician's failure to disclose contract with the HMO that created incentives to minimize diagnostic tests and specialist referrals. The court quoted Opinion 8.132, stating that, while a violation of professional ethics does not in itself establish a breach of the legal standard of care, it is relevant in determining whether such a breach occurred. *Neade v. Portes, 303 Ill. App.3d 799, 710 N.E. 2d 418, 427.*

Journal 2002 Explores how courts have attempted to provide relief when managed care organizations cause harm. Concludes that the judiciary has evidenced respect for the legislative process in this context. Quotes Opinion 8.132. Spector, *Managed Healthcare Liability Issues, 32 Cumb. L. Rev. 311, 335-36 (2002).*

Journal 2001 Discusses the prohibition on nonlawyer ownership of legal service providers. Considers how ethical rules and standards governing physicians have been directed toward preserving independent judgment. Concludes that ethical conflicts created by abandoning the prohibition on nonlawyer ownership of legal service providers may be managed by following the medical ethics model. Quotes Principle VI and Opinions 2.03, 2.09, 8.02, 8.021, 8.03, 8.05, 8.051, 8.054, 8.13, and 8.132. Harris & Foran, *The Ethics of Middle-Class Access to Legal Services and What We Can Learn From the Medical Profession's Shift to a Corporate Paradigm, 70 Fordham L. Rev. 775, 817, 821, 822, 823, 824 (2001).*

Journal 2001 Examines the changing duties of health care providers to disclose managed care financial incentives to patients. Concludes that managed care organizations, not physicians, should be obligated to make such disclosures. Quotes Opinion 8.132. Kurfirst, *The Duty to Disclose HMO Physician Incentives, 13 (3) Health Law. 18, 18, 22 (2001).*

Journal 2001 Examines patient attitudes toward physician compensation models. Concludes that most wealthier, well-educated, Caucasian patients are the least satisfied with capitation. References Opinion 8.132. Pereira & Pearson, *Patient Attitudes Toward Physician Financial Incentives, 161 Arch. Intern. Med. 1313, 1316, 1317 (2001).*

Journal 2001 Examines the concept of fiduciary duty in the managed care context. Considers potential liability of health plans and providers for breach of this duty. Reviews the US Supreme Court decision in *Pegram v. Herdrich.* Concludes that *Pegram* left many unanswered questions concerning ERISA's fiduciary requirements for health plans and providers. Quotes Opinion 8.132. Rosoff, *Breach of Fiduciary Duty Lawsuits Against MCOs, 22 J. Legal Med. 55, 65 (2001).*

Journal 2000 Examines physician value neutrality (PVN). Defines PVN as providing a foundation to suggest physicians must keep their values—religious, political, or otherwise—out of the patient-physician relationship. Concludes it is not clear how values can be removed from the patient-physician relationship without removing the very thing PVN supporters are trying to protect, the intrinsic value of persons. References Opinions 2.01, 2.02, 8.032, 8.05, 8.08, and 8.132. Beckwith & Peppin, *Physician Value Neutrality: A Critique, 28 J. L. Med. & Ethics 67, 72-73 (2000).*

Journal 2000 Examines the fiduciary nature of the physician-patient relationship. Explores crucial policy implications of the *Neade v. Portes* decision. Concludes that policy makers, not courts, should address whether physician involvement in managed care plans fundamentally implies a profit motive. Quotes Opinion 8.132. Potter, *Failure to Disclose HMO Incentives and the Breach of Fiduciary Duty: Is a New Cause of Action Against Physicians the Best Solution? 34 USF. L. Rev. 733, 753 (2000).*

Journal 1999 Considers the viability of a legal cause of action for negligent referral in the physician-patient relationship. Examines differences between the legal and medical professions and discusses variations in the applicable standards of care. Cites Opinion 8.132. Martin, *Legal Malpractice: Negligent Referral as a Cause of Action, 29 Cumb. L. Rev. 679, 686 (1999).*

Journal 1999 Explores the increased push toward mandatory disclosure laws regarding financial incentives imposed by managed care organizations. Discusses current laws and ethical guidelines. Emphasizes that efforts to mandate disclosure force physicians to focus on the effects of imposed incentives and the essence of the physician-patient relationship. References Opinions 8.032, 8.13, and 8.132. Miller & Sage, *Disclosing Physician Financial Incentives*, 281 JAMA 1424, 1425 (1999).

Journal 1999 Discusses the need for physicians to advocate on behalf of patients' rights in the context of health care delivery. Evaluates the nature and scope of the physician's role as advocate, noting that physicians cannot be expected to engage in attorney-like advocacy. Quotes Principles IV and VI, Fundamental Elements (2), (4), and (6) [now Opinion 10.01], Patient Responsibilities 5 [now Opinion 10.02], and Opinions 2.03, 2.07, 2.09, 2.16, 2.19, 3.06, 4.01, 4.04, 6.01, 7.02, 8.02, 8.03, 8.13, 8.132, 9.06, 9.07, and 9.131. Cites Opinions 5.05, 5.09, 7.01, 8.135, and 9.02. Sage, *Physicians as Advocates*, 35 Hous. L. Rev. 1529, 1537, 1541, 1542, 1552-53, 1554, 1556, 1557, 1559, 1561-62, 1564, 1571, 1574, 1576, 1580 (1999).

Journal 1999 Discusses financial incentives offered to physicians by managed care organizations. Argues that evidence of financial incentives should be admissible in medical malpractice cases. Quotes Opinion 8.13. References Opinion 8.132. Sugarman & Yarashus, *Admissibility of Managed Care Financial Incentives in Medical Malpractice Cases*, 34 Tort & Ins. L. J. 735, 743, 746, 759 (1999).

Journal 1999 Explores the impact managed care organizations have had on health care. Explains that patients may not understand restrictions and incentives imposed by their managed care organizations when entering the program. Argues that such information should be disclosed at various times during the period of plan coverage. Cites Opinions 2.03, 8.03, 8.032, 8.051, 8.13, and 8.132. Wolf, *Toward a Systemic Theory of Informed Consent in Managed Care*, 35 Hous. L. Rev. 1631, 1641, 1658, 1661, 1662, 1679 (1999).

Journal 1998 Discusses changes in the health care system. Explains why patients need more power in the managed care system. Suggests that patients should use class action suits as a method to assert power over managed care organizations. References Opinions 8.13 and 8.132. Cerminara, *The Class Action Suit as a Method of Patient Empowerment in the Managed Care Setting*, 24 Am. J. Law & Med. 7, 16, 17, 23 (1998).

Journal 1998 Asserts that managed care organizations assume fiduciary obligations by exercising discretionary control over the administration of an ERISA plan. Argues that ERISA requires managed care organizations and physicians to disclose financial incentives intended to influence physician decision-making. References Opinions 8.13 and 8.132. Johnson, *ERISA Doctor in the House? The Duty to Disclose Physician Incentives to Limit Health Care*, 82 Minn. L. Rev. 1631, 1639, 1649, 1655 (1998).

Journal 1996 Considers challenges to the psychiatrist-patient relationship that are triggered by managed care cost-containment methodologies. Offers guidance to psychiatrists for addressing these challenges. References Opinions 2.095, 8.13, and 8.132. Hoge, *APA Resource Document: I. The Professional Responsibilities of Psychiatrists in Evolving Health Care Systems*, 24 Bull. Am. Acad. Psychiatry Law 393, 405 (1996).

Journal 1990 Examines various cost-control mechanisms utilized by prepaid health plans and other managed care programs and considers the impact of such mechanisms on clinical decision making. Emphasis is placed on the possible existence of conflicts of interest on the part of health care providers in this context. Quotes Opinions 8.03 and 8.13 [now Opinion 8.132]. Hirshfeld, *Defining Full and Fair Disclosure in Managed Care Contracts*, 60 The Citation 67, 70 (1990).

8.135   The previous Opinion 8.135, "Managed Care Cost Containment Involving Prescription Drugs," issued June 1996, was replaced by the current Opinion 8.135, "Cost Containment Involving Prescription Drugs in Health Care Plans."

8.135   **Cost Containment Involving Prescription Drugs in Health Care Plans**

When health care plans, whether publicly or privately financed, establish drug formulary systems, physicians are obligated to advocate for formularies that meet the medical needs of their patients.

(1) Physicians should maintain awareness of plan decisions about drug selection by staying informed, where appropriate, about pharmacy and therapeutics (P&T) committee actions and by ongoing personal review of formulary composition. P&T committee members should include independent physician representatives. Mechanisms should be established for ongoing peer review of formulary policy. Physicians who perceive inappropriate influences on formulary development should notify the proper regulatory authorities.

(2) When scientifically based evidence is available, physicians are ethically required to advocate for changes to the formulary that would benefit the patient. Physicians also should advocate for exceptions to the formulary on a case-by-case basis when justified by the health care needs of particular patients. Mechanisms to appeal formulary exclusions should be established. Other cost-containment mechanisms, including prescription caps and prior authorization, should not unduly burden physicians or patients in accessing optimal drug therapy. Quality improvement rather than cost containment should be the primary determinant for formulary exclusions. In order to be cost efficient, however, physicians should select the lowest cost medication of equal efficacy for their patients.

(3) Physicians should advocate that limits be placed on the extent to which health care plans use incentives or pressures to lower prescription drug costs. Financial incentives are permissible when they promote cost-effectiveness, not when they require withholding medically necessary care. Physicians should not be made to feel that they jeopardize their compensation or participation in a health care plan if they prescribe drugs that are necessary for their patients but that may also be costly. There should be limits on the magnitude of financial incentives, which should be calculated according to the practices of a sizeable group of physicians rather than on an individual basis, and incentives based on quality of care rather than cost of care should be used. Prescriptions should not be changed without the physician's knowledge and authorization. This affords the physician the opportunity to discuss the change with the patient.

(4) Physicians should encourage health care plans to develop mechanisms to educate and assist physicians in cost-effective prescribing practices, including the availability of clinical pharmacists. Such initiatives are preferable to financial incentives or pressures by health care plans or hospitals, which can be ethically problematic.

(5) Physicians should advocate that methods to limit prescription drug costs within health care plans in which they participate be disclosed to patients. In particular, they should encourage health care plans to inform patients upon enrollment concerning:
   (a) the existence of formularies
   (b) provisions for cases in which the physician prescribes a drug that is not included in the formulary
   (c) incentives or other mechanisms used to encourage formulary compliance by physicians
   (d) relationships with pharmaceutical benefit management companies or pharmaceutical companies that could influence the composition of the formulary

If physicians exhaust all avenues to secure a formulary exception for a significantly advantageous drug, they are still obligated to disclose the option of the more beneficial drug to the patient, so that the patient can consider whether to obtain the medication out-of-plan. Under circumstances in which the health care program will not subsidize the drug, physicians should help patients by identifying alternative forms of financial assistance, such as those available through pharmaceutical companies' assistance programs. (III)

Issued June 1996 based on the report "Managed Care Cost Containment Involving Prescription Drugs," adopted June 1995 (*Food and Drug Law Journal.* 1998;53:25-34); updated June 2002.

Cal. App. 2002 State agency appealed a writ of mandamus requiring it to approve managed care plan's proposed amendment to discontinue coverage of sexual dysfunction prescription drugs. Agency based its authority to disapprove on a statute empowering it to regulate health plan prescription drug coverage. California Court of Appeals affirmed. The court held that the agency exceeded its statutory authority. References Opinion 8.135 regarding managed care drug formulary systems. *Kaiser Foundation Health Plan, Inc. v. Zingale, 99 Cal. App. 4th 1018, 121 Cal. Rptr. 2d 741, 746.*

Journal 2006 Discusses preemption of lawsuits against managed care organizations by the Employee Retirement Income Security Act of 1974 (ERISA). Proposes a "bifurcated legal regime" to decrease the protective scope of ERISA. Quotes Opinions 8.053 and 8.135. Madison, *ERISA and Liability for Provision of Medical Information, 84 N. C. L. Rev. 471, 540 (2006).*

Journal 2005 Argues that in *Aetna v. Davila/Cigna v. Calad,* the Supreme Court missed an opportunity to overturn unjust ERISA policies. Concludes that the principle of complete ERISA preemption as articulated in these consolidated cases is unsatisfactory because it violates the separation of powers doctrine. Quotes Principle VIII. Cites Opinions 8.054, 8.13, 8.135, 9.123, 10.01, and 10.015. Nelson, *AETNA v. DAVILA/CIGNA v. CALAD: A Missed Opportunity, 31 Wm. Mitchell L. Rev. 843, 847, 849, 850, 880 (2005).*

Journal 2000 Describes the American formulary system and the economic efficiencies that can be realized when physicians comply. Describes how the formulary system fits into and underlies health care electronic data interchange. Concludes that congressional action is needed to fully extend the formulary system to Medicaid programs in all 50 states. References Opinion 8.135. Buckles, *Electronic Formulary Management and Medicaid: Maximizing Economic Efficiency and Quality of Care in the Age of Electronic Prescribing, 11 U. Fla. J. L. & Pub. Pol'y 179, 182-83 (2000).*

Journal 1999 Discusses the need for physicians to advocate on behalf of patients' rights in the context of health care delivery. Evaluates the nature and scope of the physician's role as advocate, noting that physicians cannot be expected to engage in attorney-like advocacy. Quotes Principles IV and VI, Fundamental Elements (2), (4), and (6) [now Opinion 10.01], Patient Responsibilities 5 [now Opinion 10.02], and Opinions 2.03, 2.07, 2.09, 2.16, 2.19, 3.06, 4.01, 4.04, 6.01, 7.02, 8.02, 8.03, 8.13, 8.132, 9.06, 9.07, and 9.131. Cites Opinions 5.05, 5.09, 7.01, 8.135, and 9.02. Sage, *Physicians as Advocates, 35 Hous. L. Rev. 1529, 1537, 1541, 1542, 1552-53, 1554, 1556, 1557, 1559, 1561-62, 1564, 1571, 1574, 1576, 1580 (1999).*

8.137   The previous Opinion 8.137, "Restrictions on Disclosure in Managed Care Contracts," issued June 1997, was deleted in June 2000 and combined with Opinion 8.053, "Restrictions on Disclosure in Managed Care Contracts."

8.14   Sexual Misconduct in the Practice of Medicine

Sexual contact that occurs concurrent with the patient-physician relationship constitutes sexual misconduct. Sexual or romantic interactions between physicians and patients detract from the goals of the physician-patient relationship, may exploit the vulnerability of the patient, may obscure the physician's objective judgment concerning the patient's health care, and ultimately may be detrimental to the patient's well-being.

If a physician has reason to believe that nonsexual contact with a patient may be perceived as or may lead to sexual contact, then he or she should avoid the nonsexual contact. At a minimum, a physician's ethical duties include terminating the physician-patient relationship before initiating a dating, romantic, or sexual relationship with a patient.

Sexual or romantic relationships between a physician and a former patient may be unduly influenced by the previous physician-patient relationship. Sexual or romantic relationships with former patients are unethical if the physician uses or exploits trust, knowledge, emotions, or influence derived from the previous professional relationship. (I, II, IV)

Issued December 1989. Updated March 1992 based on the report "Sexual Misconduct in the Practice of Medicine," adopted December 1990 (JAMA. 1991;266:2741-2745).

S.D. N.Y. 1999 Physician brought a 42 USC § 1983 claim seeking to enjoin the state board from revoking his license to practice medicine. The charges against the physician included allegations of engaging in sexual relations with patients. The board quoted Opinion 8.14 as a basis for its conclusion that engaging in sexual relations with patients is an ethical violation. The court held that, in order to enjoin the board, the physician had to show a substantial likelihood of success on the merits. Further, the court found that abstention was appropriate because the physician's case was pending administrative appeal. Finally, the court held that the statute that prohibited the stay of a license revocation pending appeal complied with due process. *Selkin v. State Board for Professional Medical Conduct, 63 F. Supp. 2d 397, 399-400.*

Cal. 1995 Patient sued ultrasound technician, who sexually assaulted her, and hospital for professional negligence, battery, and intentional and negligent infliction of emotional distress. In differentiating between the physician-patient relationship and the technician-patient relationship, the court cited AMA Council on Ethical and Judicial Affairs, Sexual Misconduct in the Practice of Medicine, 266 JAMA 2741 (1991) [now Opinion 8.14]. Finding that the technician's acts did not arise from any events or conditions of his employment, the court held that the hospital was not liable under respondeat superior. *Lisa M. v. Henry Mayo Newhall Memorial Hosp., 12 Cal. 4th 291, 907 P.2d 358, 48 Cal. Rptr. 2d 510, 517.*

Cal. App. 1992 Physician who had sexual relationship with patient brought a mandamus action challenging discipline imposed by medical board. The court concluded that a sexual relationship between physician and patient was alone an insufficient basis for discipline. An expert witness, referring to Opinion 8.14, testified that it is unethical for a physician to have a sexual relationship with a patient. However, focusing on the applicable state statute, the court found the relationship must affect the functions and duties of a physician to be a basis for discipline. *Gromis v. Medical Board, 8 Cal. App. 4th 589, 10 Cal. Rptr. 2d 452, 455 n.3, reh'g denied, 1992 Cal. App. LEXIS 1047, and review denied, 1992 Cal. LEXIS 5101.*

Ga. 2007 A physician who applied to the Georgia bar appealed a denial of his application by the Board to Determine Bar Fitness. The Georgia Supreme Court reviewed for abuse of discretion. In making its decision, the Board had considered that the physician had violated Opinion 8.14 by engaging in sexual relations with a patient and lost his medical license as a result. Based on this and other circumstances, the court held that the Board properly concluded the applicant lacked moral fitness. *In re Baska, 281 Ga. 676, 641 S.E.2d 533, 534.*

Md. App. 2003 Physician appealed decision upholding state board's order to revoke his medical license for unprofessional conduct. The physician engaged in consensual sexual relationships with several of his patients at places and times other than when medical care was given. Appeals court affirmed the board's ruling and held that the conduct occurred within the practice of medicine. Quotes Opinion 8.14. *Finucan v. Maryland State Board of Physicians Quality Assurance, 151 Md. App. 399, 827 A.2d 176, 181-82.*

Md. App. 1992 Patient's husband sought damages from defendant psychiatrist because of the sexual relationship initiated during treatment of the patient by the defendant. Although the court held that the plaintiff in this case could not recover damages in tort for disruption of a marriage, it cited favorably Opinion 8.14 (1989) for its declaration that "sexual misconduct in the practice of medicine" is unethical. *Homer v. Long, 90 Md. App. 1, 3 n.1 , 599 A.2d 1193, 1193 n.1.*

Mass. 2005 Massachusetts Board of Registration in Medicine revoked the license of appellant physician for engaging in inappropriate sexual conduct with a patient. The administrative magistrate cited Opinion 8.14 in making her determination that a sexual relationship with a patient was professional misconduct. The court affirmed the board's ruling, finding that sufficient evidence existed to find professional misconduct by the appellant arising out of a sexual relationship with his patient. *Weinberg v. Board of Registration in Medicine, 443 Mass. 679, 824 N.E.2d 38, 42.*

Mass. App. 2003 Patient appealed summary judgment in suit against physician's estate for harm caused by their two-year consensual sexual affair. Once the affair began, the physician stopped treating the patient. The patient alleged malpractice, breach of fiduciary duty, intentional infliction of emotional distress, and unfair or deceptive practices. Appellate court upheld summary judgment. In analyzing the fiduciary duty claim, the court quoted Opinion 8.14. *Korper v. Weinstein, 57 Mass. App. 433, 783 N.E.2d 877, 881, n. 9.*

Mont. 2005 A psychiatrist had sexual relations with a patient. Following a hearing, the Montana Board of Medical Examiners revoked the psychiatrist's license, despite a recommendation by the hearing examiner for a 90-day suspension. With apparent reference to Opinion 8.14, one of the board members posited at the hearing that the psychiatrist had violated the code of medical ethics. The psychiatrist sought judicial review. The Supreme Court of Montana found that the board's decision was proper, that the penalty was consistent with findings of fact, and was not arbitrary or capricious. *Munn v. Montana Board of Medical Examiners, 329 Mont. 401, 124 P.3d 1123, 1126.*

N.Y. 2002 Surgical resident sexually assaulted patient while she was in recovery room. Patient sued hospital for negligence and vicarious liability. Trial court denied hospital's motion for summary judgment, but intermediate appellate court granted motion. New York Court of Appeals modified the ruling. It held that patient's vicarious liability claim failed because the misconduct was not in furtherance of hospital business or in the scope of the resident's employment. The court found, however, a sufficient basis for a negligence claim. References Opinion 8.14. *N.X. v. Cabrini Medical Center, 97 N.Y 2d 247, 765 N.E 2d 844, 847, n.2, 739 N.Y.S.2d 348.*

N.Y. Sup. 1998 Physician was convicted of sodomizing a patient and falsifying her records. He appealed in part on grounds that the prosecutor had introduced evidence regarding his sexual relationship with another patient in violation of a pretrial ruling. The court reversed the convictions and remanded the case for a new trial. The dissent cited Opinion 8.14, stating that the physician's sexual relationship with another patient violated ethical standards. Furthermore, the dissent argued that evidence of such a relationship was relevant to the case at hand. *People v. Griffin, 242 A.D.2d 70, 671 N.Y.S. 2d 34, 39.*

Ohio 1991 State medical board revoked license of physician who had consensual sexual relations with his patient. The court upheld the board's ruling that this violated Principles I, II, and IV. Dissenting judge, citing AMA Council on Ethical and Judicial Affairs, Sexual Misconduct in the Practice of Medicine, 266 JAMA 2741 [now Opinion 8.14], argued that until 1991, the AMA did not clearly deem sexual contact with a patient unethical. *Pons v. Ohio State Medical Bd., 66 Ohio St. 3d 619, 623, 625, 614 N.E.2d 748, 752, 753.*

Wash. App. 2006 A physician treated an elderly patient prior to her death. The patient's son-in-law later brought a malpractice suit alleging that the physician had sexual relations with his wife and that a sexual relationship existed between himself and the physician. In opposing a motion for summary judgment, the plaintiff filed an affidavit from a physician. With apparent reference to Opinion 8.14, the affidavit stated the defendant had violated the AMA Code of Medical Ethics and thereby, breached her duty of care. The trial court acknowledged that the AMA Code helped establish such a duty, but granted summary judgment. Plaintiff's claims were found to be deficient because he failed to set forth any facts that would prove the alleged sexual relationship with the physician. On appeal, the court affirmed. *Prestrud v. Blanco, 2006 WL 1633707, 2.*

Journal 2010 Explores how participation in online social networks may blur boundaries between personal and professional relationships for health care professionals and how such risks may be mitigated by use of network privacy and security settings. Suggests that health care institutions are likely to institute online social-networking policies for employees. Quotes Opinions 5.026, 5.027, 5.045, 5.046, 5.05, 5.059, 5.0591, 8.14, 9.08, and 9.123. Cites Opinions 5.026, 9.031, and 9.12. Terry, *Physicians and Patients Who "Friend" or "Tweet": Constructing a Legal Framework for Social Networking in a Highly Regulated Domain, 43 Ind. L. Rev. 285, 314-16, 319, 334-36, 338 (2010).*

Journal 2009 Discusses the willful blindness doctrine with respect to physicians charged with drug trafficking after prescribing to patients who resell drugs. Concludes there is a distinction between knowledge and willful blindness, and an actor who is morally justified in choosing to be blind should not be prosecuted under a statute requiring knowledge. Quotes Opinion 8.14. Hellman, *Prosecuting Doctors for Trusting Patients*, 16 Geo. Mason L. Rev. 701, 712 (2009).

Journal 2008 Argues that organ donation from a patient to his or her physician is unethical. Concludes that this practice would be exploitative to the patient and undermine public trust in the medical profession. Cites Opinions 8.14, 10.017, and 10.018. Steinberg & Pomfret, *A Novel Boundary Issue: Should a Patient Be an Organ Donor for Their Physician?* 34 J. Med. Ethics 772, 772 (2008).

Journal 2006 Discusses the evolution of health law in Virginia. Concludes that the area of health law continues to expand, develop, and be refined. Cites Opinions 3.03, 3.08, 5.01, 5.015, 5.02, 5.04, 5.055, 6.02, 6.021, 6.03, 6.04, 7.03, 7.04, 7.05, 8.054, 8.08, 8.081, 8.085, 8.115, 8.12, 8.14, 8.145, 8.19, and 9.045. Guanzon, *Health Care Law*, 41 U. Rich. L. Rev. 179, 199 (2006).

Journal 2006 Considers prisoners' rights to expression of sexuality and the state's legitimate interest in regulating that expression. Concludes that states should encourage healthy expressions of sexuality while protecting the goals of the Prison Rape Elimination Act. Cites Opinions 3.08, 8.14, 8.145, and 10.015. Smith, *Rethinking Prison Sex: Self-expression and Safety*, 15 Colum. J. Gender & L. 185, 202 (2006).

Journal 2004 Examines the relationship between administrative law and health law. Concludes that administrative law and health law will continue to be intertwined and that this relationship may provide benefits in the context of health care delivery. Cites Opinion 8.14. Jost, *Health Law and Administrative Law: A Marriage Most Convenient*, 49 St. Louis U. L. J. 1, 20 (2004).

Journal 2004 Analyzes various issues relating to the role of mental health professionals in capital punishment in light of Albert Bandura's model of "mechanisms of moral disengagement." Concludes that facilitating participation of mental health professionals in executions creates conflicts with the humanistic norms of the profession. Quotes Preamble and Opinions 1.01, 1.02, 2.06, 2.067, 2.20, 2.21, 2.211, and 8.14. Judges, *The Role of Mental Health Professionals in Capital Punishment: An Exercise in Moral Disengagement*, 41 Hous. L. Rev. 515, 562, 568, 569, 570, 571-72, 581, 586, 588, 598 (2004).

Journal 2003 Highlights the inadequacies of Washington tort law with respect to holding employers of sexually exploitative therapists accountable. Concludes that courts should premise employer liability on the foreseeability of transference. References Opinion 8.14. Allen, *The Foreseeability of Transference: Extending Employer Liability Under Washington Law for Therapist Sexual Exploitation of Patients*, 78 Wash. L. Rev. 525, 531 (2003).

Journal 2001 Explores changes in common law and statutory law that have promoted the marginalization of chastity. Considers rules governing the professions. Concludes with a legal agenda intended to help restore the social value of chastity. References Opinion 8.14. Rodes, *On Law and Chastity*, 76 Notre Dame L. Rev. 643, 675 (2001).

Journal 2000 Evaluates consensual sexual relationships between patients and physicians. Emphasis is placed on whether, and in what situation, a sexual relationship may constitute medical malpractice. Concludes that people should learn to take responsibility for their actions and that certain limitations should be placed on recovery for malpractice. References Opinion 8.14. Puglise, *"Calling Dr. Love": The Physician-Patient Sexual Relationship as Grounds for Medical Malpractice—Society Pays While the Doctor and Patient Play*, 14 J. L. & Health 321, 324-25, 349 (2000).

Journal 1999 Examines countertransference in professional relationships. Observes how the resulting power imbalance may give rise to the potential for sexual exploitation. Concludes by offering strategies for identifying and addressing emotional interference in the lawyer/client relationship. Cites Opinion 8.14. Silver, *Love, Hate, and Other Emotional Interference in the Lawyer/Client Relationship*, 6 Clinical L. Rev. 259, 266 (1999).

Journal 1998 Provides policy reasons why attorney-client sexual relations should be prohibited. Urges states to codify rules precluding such conduct during representation. Explains that such rules would pass constitutional scrutiny. Cites Opinion 8.14. Awad, *Attorney-Client Sexual Relations*, 22 J. Legal. Prof. 131, 190 (1998).

Journal 1998 Discusses types of discipline taken against physicians for sexual offenses. Points out that some physicians still may be permitted to practice medicine despite the commission of sexual misconduct. Proposes ways that might increase the chance that sex-related offenses will be reported. Quotes Opinion 8.14. Dehlendorf & Wolfe, *Physicians Disciplined for Sex-Related Offenses*, 279 JAMA 1883 (1998).

Journal 1997 Examines the balance needed between clinical objectivity and physician-patient bonding. Discusses personal boundaries and methods of coping with transgressions by both physicians and patients. Advocates a focus on communication with patients to allow physicians to maintain both an empathetic and objective relationship. References Opinion 8.14. Farber, Novack, & O'Brien, *Love, Boundaries, and the Physician-Patient Relationship*, 157 Arch. Intern. Med. 2291, 2292, 2293, 2294 (1997).

Journal 1996 Discusses the ethical implications of sexual misconduct in the medical field. Examines the current civil and criminal tools used to curb physician-patient misconduct. Notes the inadequacy of physician reporting. Proposes a statutory approach to discipline physicians who abuse their fiduciary duties. Quotes Principle II. References Opinion 8.14. Note, *Sexual Conduct Within the Physician-Patient Relationship: A Statutory Framework for Disciplining This Breach of Fiduciary Duty*, 1 Widener L. Symp. J. 501, 507 (1996).

Journal 1994 Explores the negative consequences of physician-patient sexual relationships. Suggests that sexual contact be prohibited during the physician-patient relationship and for a period of time thereafter. Quotes Opinion 8.14. Appelbaum, Jorgenson, & Sutherland, *Sexual Relationships Between Physicians and Patients*, 154 Arch. Intern. Med. 2561, 2561 (1994).

Journal 1993 Examines the potential problems created by attorney-client sexual relations and the need for ethical guidelines. Examines ethical rules being debated in various states and proposes a model rule. References Opinion 8.14. Davis & Grimaldi, *Sexual Confusion: Attorney-Client Sex and the Need for a Clear Ethical Rule*, 7 Notre Dame J. Law, Ethics, & Pub. Pol. 57, 61 (1993).

Journal 1993 Discusses family privacy rights and considers the meaning of justice, self-respect, and the fundamental principles of physician ethics. Concludes that physicians have an ethical duty to intervene in domestic violence so long as such intervention does not breach confidentiality or violate patient autonomy. Quotes Principle IV and Opinion 5.05. References Opinions 8.14 and 9.131. Jecker, *Privacy Beliefs and the Violent Family: Extending the Ethical Argument for Physician Intervention*, 269 JAMA 776, 778, 779 (1993).

Journal 1993 Discusses the potential impact on health care practitioners of the AMA's prohibition against sexual relations between physicians and patients. Focuses on how the prohibition will influence disciplinary actions. Cites Opinion 8.14. Johnson, *Judicial Review of Disciplinary Action for Sexual Misconduct in the Practice of Medicine*, 270 JAMA 1596 (1993).

Journal 1993 Discusses potential problems caused by attorney-client sexual relations and examines various means to check such conduct. Proposes a new rule that would prohibit attorney-client sexual relations. References Opinion 8.14. Livingston, *When Libido Subverts Credo: Regulation of Attorney-Client Sexual Relations*, 62 Fordham L. Rev. 5, 55 (1993).

Journal 1993 Discusses the problems physicians may encounter by exposing the errant colleague, such as harm to the reporting physician's reputation and the fear of litigation. States that problems involving physician competency and unethical behavior should be investigated, and that physicians should take personal responsibility for reporting problems they observe. References Principle II and Opinions 8.14 and 9.031. Morreim, *Am I My Brother's Warden? Responding to the Unethical or Incompetent Colleague*, 23 Hastings Center Rep. 19, 23 (May/June 1993).

Journal 1993 Discusses the medical profession's ethical prohibition on physician-patient sexual contact. Concludes that legislatures and courts should give greater weight to the ethical code when defining standards of conduct for physician-patient sexual contact. Quotes Opinion 8.14. Note, *Physician-Patient Sexual Contact: The Battle Between the State and the Medical Profession*, 50 Wash. & Lee L. Rev. 1725, 1725-26, 1734, 1752 (1993).

Journal 1992 Discusses the problem of sex in the attorney-client relationship and compares this to that of the physician-patient. Proposes an explicit ban on sexual involvement between attorneys and their clients and advocates promulgation of a "bright line" rule. References Opinion 8.14. Goldberg, *Sex and the Attorney-Client Relationship: An Argument for a Prophylactic Rule*, 26 Akron L. Rev. 45 (1992).

Journal 1992 Examines the similarities and differences between the physician-patient and lawyer-client relationships regarding the problems associated with sexual relations. Advocates a rebuttable presumption that sexual contact between attorneys and clients is wrongful. Cites Opinion 8.14. Gutheil, Jorgenson, & Sutherland, *Prohibiting Lawyer-Client Sex*, 20 *Bull. Am. Acad. Psychiatry Law* 365 (1992).

Journal 1992 Finds that state medical boards increasingly rely upon psychiatric testimony in cases of alleged sexual abuse by physicians. Proposes that states adopt clear standards governing the admissibility of psychiatric testimony in administrative hearings. Quotes Opinion 8.14. Hyams, *Expert Psychiatric Evidence in Sexual Misconduct Cases Before State Medical Boards*, XVIII *Am. J. Law & Med.* 171, 173, 174 (1992).

8.145 Sexual or Romantic Relations Between Physicians and Key Third-Parties

Patients are often accompanied by third-parties who play an integral role in the patient-physician relationship. The physician interacts and communicates with these individuals and often is in a position to offer them information, advice, and emotional support. The more deeply involved the individual is in the clinical encounter and in medical decision making, the more troubling sexual or romantic contact with the physician would be. This is especially true for the individual whose decisions directly impact on the health and welfare of the patient. Key third-parties include, but are not limited to, spouses or partners, parents, guardians, and proxies.

Physicians should refrain from sexual or romantic interactions with key third-parties when it is based on the use or exploitation of trust, knowledge, influence, or emotions derived from a professional relationship. The following factors should be considered when considering whether a relationship is appropriate: the nature of the patient's medical problem, the length of the professional relationship, the degree of the third-party's emotional dependence on the physician, and the importance of the clinical encounter to the third-party and the patient. (I, II)

Issued December 1998 based on the report "Sexual or Romantic Relations Between Physicians and Key Third-Parties," adopted June 1998.

Journal 2007 Addresses physician liability for an extramarital affair with a patient's spouse. Concludes that such an affair should be regarded as a breach of a fiduciary duty. Quotes Preamble, Principles I, II, and VIII, and Opinions 8.145, 9.04, 9.123, and 10.015. Demaine, *"Playing Doctor" With the Patient's Spouse: Alternative Conceptions of Health Professional Liability*, 14 *Va. J. Soc. Pol'y & L.* 308, 325, 330-31, 331-32 (2007).

Journal 2006 Discusses the evolution of health law in Virginia. Concludes that the area of health law continues to expand, develop, and be refined. Cites Opinions 3.03, 3.08, 5.01, 5.015, 5.02, 5.04, 5.055, 6.02, 6.021, 6.03, 6.04, 7.03, 7.04, 7.05, 8.054, 8.08, 8.081, 8.085, 8.115, 8.12, 8.14, 8.145, 8.19, and 9.045. Guanzon, *Health Care Law*, 41 *U. Rich. L. Rev.* 179, 199 (2006).

Journal 2006 Considers prisoners' rights to expression of sexuality and the state's legitimate interest in regulating that expression. Concludes that states should encourage healthy expressions of sexuality while protecting the goals of the Prison Rape Elimination Act. Cites Opinions 3.08, 8.14, 8.145, and 10.015. Smith, *Rethinking Prison Sex: Self-expression and Safety*, 15 *Colum. J. Gender & L.* 185, 202 (2006).

8.15 Substance Abuse

It is unethical for a physician to practice medicine while under the influence of a controlled substance, alcohol, or other chemical agents which impair the ability to practice medicine. (I)

Issued December 1986.

Journal 1994 Discusses the issue of whom physicians must serve first: themselves, their patients, insurers, or society. Focuses on risks arising out of provider economic arrangements and risks arising out of other individual physician characteristics. Quotes Opinions 8.03 and 9.13. Cites Opinion 8.15. Bobinski, *Autonomy and Privacy: Protecting Patients From Their Physicians*, 55 U. Pitt. L. Rev. 291, 302, 313 (1994).

8.16 Substitution of Surgeon Without Patient's Knowledge or Consent

A surgeon who allows a substitute to operate on his or her patient without the patient's knowledge and consent is deceitful. The patient is entitled to choose his or her own physician and should be permitted to acquiesce to or refuse the substitution.

The surgeon's obligation to the patient requires the surgeon to perform the surgical operation: (1) within the scope of authority granted by the consent to the operation; (2) in accordance with the terms of the contractual relationship; (3) with complete disclosure of facts relevant to the need and the performance of the operation; and (4) utilizing best skill.

It should be noted that it is the operating surgeon to whom the patient grants consent to perform the operation. The patient is entitled to the services of the particular surgeon with whom he or she contracts. The operating surgeon, in accepting the patient, is obligated to utilize his or her personal talents in the performance of the operation to the extent required by the agreement creating the physician-patient relationship. The surgeon cannot properly delegate to another the duties which he or she is required to perform personally.

Under the normal and customary arrangement with patients, and with reference to the usual form of consent to operation, the operating surgeon is obligated to perform the operation but may be assisted by residents or other surgeons. With the consent of the patient, it is not unethical for the operating surgeon to delegate the performance of certain aspects of the operation to the assistant provided this is done under the surgeon's participatory supervision, ie, the surgeon must scrub. If a resident or other physician is to perform the operation under nonparticipatory supervision, it is necessary to make a full disclosure of this fact to the patient, and this should be evidenced by an appropriate statement contained in the consent. Under these circumstances, it is the resident or other physician who becomes the operating surgeon. (I, II, IV, V)

Issued prior to April 1977. Updated June 1994.

Ala. 1985 Patient sued physicians alleging fraud and conspiracy to commit fraud. The court clarified its previous holding in the case (461 So. 2d 775) that a new trial was ordered only on fraud and conspiracy to commit fraud theories. The court also noted that the trier of fact would need to decide whether the Current Opinions of the Judicial Council of the AMA pamphlet was properly excluded under the learned treatise doctrine and whether, if properly authenticated, it might be admissible at a new trial as to the issue of whether ghost surgery, condemned by Opinion 8.12 (1984) [now Opinion 8.16], constitutes fraud. *McMurray v. Johnson, 481 So. 2d 887, 889.*

Md. 2000 Plaintiff scheduled surgery with the defendant physician. During surgery, a resident mistakenly dissected the common bile duct. Plaintiff sued for negligence and breach of contract, alleging that defendant had agreed personally to perform all incisions. The circuit court dismissed the contract claim as subsumed by the negligence claim. While the Court of Appeals of Maryland found a contractual relationship does exist between a physician and patient, citing Opinions 8.12 (1982) [now Opinion 8.16] and 8.16, the court nonetheless held for the physician because the jury had found he never made the alleged promise. *Dingle v. Belin*, 358 Md. 354, 749 A.2d 157, 168.

Md. App. 1999 Patient sued hospital and the surgeon named in consent form for negligence and breach of contract. The plaintiff claimed that the defendants breached their contract when a resident performed surgery, rather than the surgeon authorized by the plaintiff. The trial court dismissed the breach of contract claim and entered judgment upon the jury verdict for the defendants. The appeals court cited Opinion 8.12 (1982) [now Opinion 8.16], stating that it is unethical and deceitful for another surgeon to perform an operation without the patient's knowledge or consent. *Belin v. Dingle*, 127 Md. App. 68, 732 A.2d 301, 302-03, 307.

N.J. 1983 Patient who consented to surgery by one surgeon, but was actually operated on by another, sued both surgeons. Pursuant to state law, patient submitted case to malpractice panel which found no basis to patient's claims and jury returned verdict for defendant surgeons. In holding that failure to permit plaintiff to show possible bias of panel doctor and to impeach the testimony constituted reversible error, the court quoted Opinion 8.12 (1982) [now Opinion 8.16] indicating that substitution of one surgeon for another without patient consent is a deceit and deviates from standard medical care, constituting the violation of a legal obligation as well as a tenet of the medical profession. *Perna v. Pirozzi*, 92 N.J. 446, 457 A.2d 431, 434, 440, n.3.

N.J. Super. 1991 Two physicians were sued by a patient claiming that one of the physician-surgeons had committed "ghost surgery" battery. The court acknowledged the rule in *Perna v. Pirozzi*, 92 N.J. 446, 457 A.2d 431 (1983). The court there, taking judicial notice of the standard of care set out by Opinion 8.12 (1982) [now Opinion 8.16], held that an intent to injure is not required to establish battery when a medical procedure is performed by a "substitute" physician. However, the court here held that the plaintiff had failed to establish by competent medical opinion that one of the physicians was an unauthorized operating surgeon. Furthermore, the court stated that to hold otherwise would create a punitive damage claim based on a patient's lay opinion concerning the proper role of an authorized surgeon in team surgery. *Monturi v. Englewood Hosp.*, 246 N.J. Super. 547, 552, 588 A.2d 408, 410, 411.

N.J. Super. 1982 In a medical malpractice suit against a surgeon for negligence and for allowing a different surgeon to operate on plaintiff without plaintiff's express consent, the court noted Opinions and Reports of the Judicial Council Sec. 1, Para. 5 (1969) [now Opinion 8.16] as quoted in 209 JAMA 947-48 (1969) that it is fraudulent and deceitful for a surgeon to allow another surgeon to operate on a patient without that patient's consent. The court ultimately concluded that the doctrine of informed consent is a theory of professional liability independent from malpractice, and thus was not relevant to the case at bar. *Perna v. Pirozzi*, 182 N.J. Super. 510, 442 A.2d 1016, 1019, rev'd, 92 N.J. 446, 457 A.2d 431 (1983).

Okla. App. 1974 Owner of a bull sued veterinarian for malpractice and failure to disclose possible adverse reactions to penicillin. The appellate court held that the veterinarian was liable for damages to the plaintiff resulting from the death of the bull. In so holding, the court noted Opinions and Reports of the Judicial Council Sec. 1, Para. 5 (1969) [now Opinion 8.16] which, inter alia, requires a surgeon to make a complete disclosure of all facts relevant to the operation to be performed. *Hull v. Tate*, No. 46443 (Okla. Ct. App. April 16, 1974) (LEXIS, States library, Okla. file), rev'd, No. 46443 (Okla. Sup. Ct. Oct. 29, 1974) (LEXIS, States library, Okla. file).

Pa. Super. 1998 Parents of child who died during a catheterization procedure sued the pediatrician, cardiologist, and the hospital on various theories including battery. In referring to an earlier decision, the court quoted Opinion 8.12 (1982) [now Opinion 8.16], in support of a patient's right to consent to a specific physician to perform a medical procedure. The court held that the jury should have decided whether the parents consented for the pediatrician instead of the cardiologist, to perform the procedure. *Taylor v. Albert Einstein Medical Ctr.*, 723 A.2d 1027, 1036.

Pa. Super. 1996 Physician told patient he would perform necessary surgery. As a result of the surgery, patient developed a drop foot which would drag whenever he walked. The patient later discovered that his treating physician did not appear for or participate in his surgery. When the hospital was unable to reach the physician, it contacted his office where another physician instructed the hospital to perform the surgery with a third physician. All of this was done without patient's consent and was not disclosed after recovery. Patient sued the physician for failure to perform the surgery and for directing or permitting a third party to perform the surgery. The court quoted from Opinion 8.12 (1982) [now Opinion 8.16] which provides that the patient is entitled to choose his or her physician and should be permitted to acquiesce in or refuse to accept any substitutions. *Grabowski v. Quigley, 454 Pa. Super. 27, 684 A.2d 610, 617.*

Journal 2006 Evaluates standard of care rules for medical residents. Proposes a minimum standard equivalent to that of a general practitioner and an appropriate standard of care for residents who fully disclose their status. Quotes Opinions 8.12 (1982) [now Opinion 8.16] and Opinion 8.16. King, *The Standard of Care for Residents and Other Medical School Graduates in Training*, 55 Am. U. L. Rev. 683, 727 (2006).

Journal 2006 Reviews informed consent law. Concludes that physicians in certain jurisdictions may be required to disclose their level of experience. Quotes Opinion 8.12 (1982) [now Opinion 8.16]. Wiltbank, *Informed Consent and Physician Inexperience: A Prescription for Liability?* 42 Willamette L. Rev. 563, 570 (2006).

Journal 1996 Considers how practice guidelines may be used in malpractice litigation as inculpatory or exculpatory evidence. Concludes that use of guidelines as inculpatory evidence should not be eliminated until there is evidence of undesirable effects. Quotes Opinion 8.16. Hyams, Shapiro, & Brennan, *Medical Practice Guidelines in Malpractice Litigation: An Early Retrospective*, 21 J. Health Pol. Pol'y & L. 289, 298 (1996).

Journal 1996 Discusses tort liability in cases of substitution of surgeons without patient consent. Explores whether substitutions are a battery thereby allowing recovery, regardless of outcome. Concludes that ghost surgery should not automatically constitute a battery but that courts should allow recovery for infliction of emotional distress stemming from the substitution. Quotes Opinion 8.12 (1982) [now Opinion 8.16]. Lundmark, *Surgery by an Unauthorized Surgeon as a Battery*, 10 J. L. & Health 287, 293 (1996).

8.17   Use of Restraints

All individuals have a fundamental right to be free from unreasonable bodily restraint. Physical and chemical restraints should therefore be used only in the best interest of the patient and in accordance with the following guidelines:

(1) The use of restraints, except in emergencies, may be implemented only upon the explicit order of a physician, in conformance with reasonable professional judgment.

(2) Judgment should be exercised in issuing pro re nata (PRN) orders for the use of physical or chemical restraints, and the implementation of such orders should be frequently reviewed and documented by the physician.

(3) The use of restraints should not be punitive, nor should they be used for convenience or as an alternative to reasonable staffing.

(4) Restraints should be used only in accordance with appropriate clinical indications.

(5) As with all therapeutic interventions, informed consent by the patient or surrogate decision maker is a key element in the application of physical and chemical restraints, and should be incorporated into institutional policy.

(6) In certain limited situations, it may be appropriate to restrain a patient involuntarily. For example, restraints may be needed for the safety of the patient or others in the area. When restraints are used involuntarily, the restraints should be removed when they are no longer needed. (I, IV)

Issued March 1992 based on the report "Guidelines for the Use of Restraints in Long-Term Care Facilities," adopted June 1989.

8.18 Informing Families of a Patient's Death

Disclosing the death of a patient to the patient's family is a duty which goes to the very heart of the patient-physician relationship and should not be readily delegated to others by the attending physician. The emotional needs of the family and the integrity of the physician-patient relationship must at all times be given foremost consideration.

Physicians in residency training may be asked to participate in the communication of information about a patient's death, if that request is commensurate with the physician's prior training or experience and previous close personal relationship with the family.

It would not be appropriate for the attending physician or resident to request that a medical student notify family members of a patient's death. Medical students should be trained in issues of death and dying, and should be encouraged to accompany attending physicians when news of a patient's death is conveyed to the family members. (I, IV)

Issued March 1992 based on the report "Informing Families of a Patient's Death: Guidelines for the Involvement of Medical Students," adopted December 1989. Updated June 1994.

Journal 1995 Examines four essential principles of bioethics—patient autonomy, nonmaleficence, beneficence, and justice—and describes the application of these in clinical settings according to bioethical norms and AMA opinions. Concludes that such an approach promotes compassionate medical caregiving and that laws should reflect these values. Quotes Opinions 2.01 and 8.18. References Opinion 2.211. Cohen, *Toward a Bioethics of Compassion*, 28 Ind. L. Rev. 667, 673, 681-82, 683 (1995).

8.181 Performing Procedures on the Newly Deceased for Training Purposes

Physicians should work to develop institutional policies that address the practice of performing procedures on the newly deceased for purposes of training. Any such policy should ensure that the interests of all the parties involved are respected under established and clear ethical guidelines. Such policies should consider rights of patients and their families, benefits to trainees and society, as well as potential harm to the ethical sensitivities of trainees, and risks to staff, the institution, and the profession associated with performing procedures on the newly deceased without consent. The following considerations should be addressed before medical trainees perform procedures on the newly deceased:

(1) The teaching of lifesaving skills should be the culmination of a structured training sequence, rather than relying on random opportunities. Training should be performed under close supervision, in a manner and environment that takes into account the wishes and values of all involved parties.

(2) Physicians should inquire whether the deceased individual had expressed preferences regarding handling of the body or procedures performed after death. In the absence of previously expressed preferences, physicians should obtain permission from the family before performing such procedures. When reasonable efforts to discover previously expressed preferences of the deceased or to find someone with authority to grant permission for the procedure have failed, physicians must not perform procedures for training purposes on the newly deceased patient.

In the event postmortem procedures are undertaken on the newly deceased, they must be recorded in the medical record. (I, V)

Issued December 2001, based on the report, "Performing Procedures on the Newly Deceased for Training Purposes," adopted June 2001 (Acad Med. 2002;77:1212-1216).

Journal 2008 Argues preservation of individuals who die of uncontrolled cardiac death is authorized by the Uniform Anatomical Gift Act and does not violate the rights of family members. Concludes that organ donor population should be expanded to include individuals who die uncontrolled cardiac deaths to increase the number of organs available for transplant. Cites Opinions 2.157 and 8.181. Bonnie, Wright, & Dineen, *Legal Authority to Preserve Organs in Cases of Uncontrolled Cardiac Death: Preserving Family Choice, 36 J. L. Med. & Ethics 741, 743 (2008).*

Journal 2004 Questions whether newly dead patients may suffer any legal harm when resuscitation training procedures are performed on them without consent. Concludes that performing these procedures without proper consent is illegal. Cites Opinion 8.181. Sperling, *Breaking Through the Silence: Illegality of Performing Resuscitation Procedures on the "Newly-Dead," 13 Ann. Health L. 393, 394, 396, 401, 425 (2004).*

Journal 2003 Analyzes the effect of Virginia law and court decisions on administrative law. Discusses one provision of law that incorporates the AMA's nonbinding ban on nonconsensual use of newly dead patients as training subjects. References Opinion 8.181. Kibler, *Administrative Law, 38 U. Rich. L. Rev. 39, 47 (2003).*

8.19   Self-treatment or Treatment of Immediate Family Members

Physicians generally should not treat themselves or members of their immediate families. Professional objectivity may be compromised when an immediate family member or the physician is the patient; the physician's personal feelings may unduly influence his or her professional medical judgment, thereby interfering with the care being delivered. Physicians may fail to probe sensitive areas when taking the medical history or may fail to perform intimate parts of the physical examination. Similarly, patients may feel uncomfortable disclosing sensitive information or undergoing an intimate examination when the physician is an immediate family member. This discomfort is particularly the case when the patient is a minor child, and sensitive or intimate care should especially be avoided for such patients. When treating themselves or immediate family members, physicians may be inclined to treat problems that are beyond their expertise or training. If tensions develop in a physician's professional relationship with a family member, perhaps as a result of a negative medical outcome, such difficulties may be carried over into the family member's personal relationship with the physician.

Concerns regarding patient autonomy and informed consent are also relevant when physicians attempt to treat members of their immediate family. Family members may be reluctant to state their preference for another physician or decline a recommendation for fear of offending the physician. In particular, minor children will generally not feel free to refuse care from their parents. Likewise, physicians may feel obligated to provide care to immediate family members even if they feel uncomfortable providing care.

It would not always be inappropriate to undertake self-treatment or treatment of immediate family members. In emergency settings or isolated settings where there is no other qualified physician available, physicians should not hesitate to treat themselves or family members until another physician becomes available. In addition, while physicians should not serve as a primary or regular care provider for immediate family members, there are situations in which routine care is acceptable for short-term, minor problems.

Except in emergencies, it is not appropriate for physicians to write prescriptions for controlled substances for themselves or immediate family members. (I, II, IV)

Issued June 1993.

Journal 2008 Explores the ethical issues associated with writing prescriptions for family members and acquaintances. Concludes that informal treatment often compromises the quality of care, and that a referral to an objective provider is the best choice. Quotes Opinion 8.19. Cites Opinion 8.115. Ares, *An Uncommon Skin Condition Illustrates the Need for Caution When Prescribing for Friends*, 20 J. Am. Acad. of Nurse Prac. 389, 390 (2008).

Journal 2008 Explores the role of an attorney and the attorney's obligation to provide dispassionate counsel and to avoid emotional conflicts. Concludes the American Bar Association Model Rules of Professional Conduct should be amended to prohibit attorney representation of persons with whom the attorney has a significant emotional relationship. Quotes Opinion 8.19. Buhai, *Emotional Conflicts: Impaired Dispassionate Representation of Family Members*, 21 Geo. J. Legal Ethics 1159, 1191-92 (2008).

Journal 2007 Questions whether it is ethical for a physician to provide medical care to a family member. Concludes that providing such care becomes increasingly problematic as the likelihood of complications increases. Quotes Principle VI and Opinion 8.19. Oberheu, Jones, & Sade, *A Surgeon Operates on His Son: Wisdom or Hubris?* 84 Ann. Thorac. Surg. 723, 725, 726 (2007).

Journal 2006 Discusses the evolution of health law in Virginia. Concludes that the area of health law continues to expand, develop, and be refined. Cites Opinions 3.03, 3.08, 5.01, 5.015, 5.02, 5.04, 5.055, 6.02, 6.021, 6.03, 6.04, 7.03, 7.04, 7.05, 8.054, 8.08, 8.081, 8.085, 8.115, 8.12, 8.14, 8.145, 8.19, and 9.045. Guanzon, *Health Care Law*, 41 U. Rich. L. Rev. 179, 199 (2006).

8.191 Peers as Patients

The opportunity to care for a fellow physician is a privilege and may represent a gratifying experience and serve as a show of respect or competence. In emergencies or isolated or rural settings when options for care by other physicians are limited or where there is no other qualified physician available, physicians should not hesitate to treat peers. There are, however, a number of ethical considerations to weigh before undertaking the care of a colleague.

(1) Physicians who provide care to a peer should be alerted to the possibility that their professional relationship with the patient may affect their ability to exercise objective professional judgment and make unbiased treatment recommendations. They must also recognize that the physician-patient may be reluctant to disclose sensitive information or permit an intimate examination.

(2) Physicians providing care to a professional colleague have an obligation to respect informational and physical privacy of physician-patients as they would for any patient. Treating physicians should consider, and possibly discuss with the physician-patient, how to respond appropriately to the inquiries about the physician-patient's medical care from other physicians or medical staff. Treating physicians should also recognize that special measures may be required to ensure that the physician-patient's physical privacy is respected.

(3) Physicians providing care to a colleague should respect the physician-patient's right to participate in informed decision-making. Treating physicians should make no assumptions about the physician-patient's knowledge about her or his medical condition and should provide information to enable the physician-patient to make voluntary, fully informed decisions about care.

(4) Physicians-in-training and medical students face unique challenges when asked to provide or participate in care for peers given the circumstances of their roles in medical schools and residency programs. Except in emergency situations or when other care is not available, physicians-in-training should not be required to care for fellow trainees, faculty members, or attending physicians if they are reluctant to do so. (VI)

Issued November 2008 based on the report "Peers as Patients," adopted June 2008.

8.20 Invalid Medical Treatment

The following general guidelines are offered to serve physicians when they are called upon to decide among treatments:

(1) Treatments which have no medical indication and offer no possible benefit to the patient should not be used (Opinion 2.035, "Futile Care").

(2) Treatments which have been determined scientifically to be invalid should not be used (Opinion 3.01, "Nonscientific Practitioners").

(3) Among the treatments that are scientifically valid, medically indicated, and offer a reasonable chance of benefit for patients, some are regulated or prohibited by law; physicians should comply with these laws. If physicians disagree with such laws, they should seek to change them.

(4) Among the various treatments that are scientifically valid, medically indicated, legal, and offer a reasonable chance of benefit for patients, the decision of which treatment to use should be made between the physician and patient. (I, III, IV)

Issued June 1998 based on the report "Invalid Medical Treatment," adopted December 1997.

8.21 Use of Chaperones During Physical Exams

From the standpoint of ethics and prudence, the protocol of having chaperones available on a consistent basis for patient examinations is recommended. Physicians aim to respect the patient's dignity and to make a positive effort to secure a comfortable and considerate atmosphere for the patient; such actions include the provision of appropriate gowns, private facilities for undressing, sensitive use of draping, and clear explanations on various components of the physical examination. A policy that patients are free to make a request for a chaperone should be established in each health care setting. This policy should be communicated to patients, either by means of a well-displayed notice or preferably through a conversation initiated by the intake nurse or the physician. The request by a patient to have a chaperone should be honored.

An authorized health professional should serve as a chaperone whenever possible. In their practices, physicians should establish clear expectations about respecting patient privacy and confidentiality to which chaperones must adhere.

If a chaperone is to be provided, a separate opportunity for private conversation between the patient and the physician should be allowed. The physician should keep inquiries and history-taking, especially those of a sensitive nature, to a minimum during the course of the chaperoned examination. (I, IV)

Issued December 1998 based on the report "Use of Chaperones During Physical Exams," adopted June 1998.

9.00 Opinions on Professional Rights and Responsibilities

9.01 Accreditation

Physicians who engage in activities that involve the accreditation, approval, or certification of institutions, facilities, and programs that provide patient care or medical education or certify the attainment of specialized professional competence have the ethical responsibility to apply standards that are relevant, fair, reasonable, and nondiscriminatory. The accreditation of institutions and facilities that provide patient care should be based upon standards that focus upon the quality of patient care achieved. Standards used in the accreditation of patient care and medical education, or the certification of specialized professional attainment should not be adopted or used as a means of economic regulation. (II, IV, VII)

Issued December 1982.

9.011 Continuing Medical Education

Physicians should strive to further their medical education throughout their careers, for only by participating in continuing medical education (CME) can they continue to serve patients to the best of their abilities and live up to professional standards of excellence. Fulfillment of mandatory state CME requirements does not necessarily fulfill the physician's ethical obligation to maintain his or her medical expertise.

Attendees. Guidelines for physicians attending a CME conference or activity are as follows:
(1) The physician choosing among CME activities should assess their educational value and select only those activities which are of high quality and appropriate for the physician's educational needs. When selecting formal CME activities, the physician should, at a minimum, choose only those activities that (a) are offered by sponsors accredited by the Accreditation Council for Continuing Medical Education (ACCME), the American Academy of Family Physicians (AAFP), or a state medical society; (b) contain information on subjects relevant to the physician's needs; (c) are responsibly conducted by qualified faculty; (d) conform to Opinion 8.061, "Gifts to Physicians From Industry."

(2) The educational value of the CME conference or activity must be the primary consideration in the physician's decision to attend or participate. Though amenities unrelated to the educational purpose of the activity may play a role in the physician's decision to participate, this role should be secondary to the educational content of the conference.

(3) Physicians should claim credit commensurate with only the actual time spent attending a CME activity or in studying a CME enduring material.

(4) Attending promotional activities put on by industry or their designees is not unethical as long as the conference conforms to Opinion 8.061, "Gifts to Physicians From Industry," and is clearly identified as promotional to all participants.

Faculty. Guidelines for physicians serving as presenters, moderators, or other faculty at a CME conference are as follows:

(1) Physicians serving as presenters, moderators, or other faculty at a CME conference should ensure that (a) research findings and therapeutic recommendations are based on scientifically accurate, up-to-date information and are presented in a balanced, objective manner; (b) the content of their presentation is not modified or influenced by representatives of industry or other financial contributors, and they do not employ materials whose content is shaped by industry. Faculty may, however, use scientific data generated from industry-sponsored research, and they may also accept technical assistance from industry in preparing slides or other presentation materials, as long as this assistance is of only nominal monetary value and the company has no input in the actual content of the material.

(2) When invited to present at non-CME activities that are primarily promotional, faculty should avoid participation unless the activity is clearly identified as promotional in its program announcements and other advertising.

(3) All conflicts of interest or biases, such as a financial connection to a particular commercial firm or product, should be disclosed by faculty members to the activity's sponsor and to the audience. Faculty may accept reasonable honoraria and reimbursement for expenses in accordance with Opinion 8.061, "Gifts to Physicians From Industry."

Sponsors. Guidelines for physicians involved in the sponsorship of CME activities are as follows:

(1) Physicians involved in the sponsorship of CME activities should ensure that (a) the program is balanced, with faculty members presenting a broad range of scientifically supportable viewpoints related to the topic at hand; (b) representatives of industry or other financial contributors do not exert control over the choice of moderators, presenters, or other faculty, or modify the content of faculty presentations. Funding from industry or others may be accepted in accordance with Opinion 8.061, "Gifts to Physicians From Industry."

(2) Sponsors should not promote CME activities in a way that encourages attendees to violate the guidelines of the Council on Ethical and Judicial Affairs, including Opinion 8.061, "Gifts to Physicians From Industry," or

the principles established for the AMA's Physician Recognition Award. CME activities should be developed and promoted consistent with guideline 2 for attendees.

(3) Any non-CME activity that is primarily promotional must be identified as such to faculty and participants, both in its advertising and at the conference itself.

(4) The entity presenting the program should not profit unfairly or charge a fee which is excessive for the content and length of the program.

(5) The program, content, duration, and ancillary activities should be consistent with the ideals of the AMA CME program. (I, V)

Issued December 1993. Updated June 1996.

Journal 2000 Examines legal and ethical issues bearing upon pain management. Asserts that health care professionals have a legal and ethical duty to relieve pain and suffering of patients whenever possible. Suggests that this duty is legally enforceable. Quotes Principle V and Opinions 2.20 and 9.011. Rich, *A Prescription for the Pain: The Emerging Standard of Care for Pain Management*, 26 Wm. Mitchell L. Rev. 1, 35-36, 85 (2000).

Journal 2000 Examines issues relating to parental consent to circumcision. Identifies legal and ethical requirements for consent when medical professionals are treating adult patients. Analyzes the implications of those requirements for routine circumcision of infant males. Concludes that only when the male is an adult and capable of making decisions can circumcision be ethically and legally performed. Quotes Opinion 8.08. References Opinions 8.03 and 9.011. Svoboda, Van Howe, & Dwyer, *Informed Consent for Neonatal Circumcision: An Ethical and Legal Conundrum*, 17 J. Contemp. Health L. & Pol'y 61, 67, 73, 82 (2000).

Journal 2000 Examines the practice of gift giving by the health care technology industry as incentives in the context of continuing medical education activities. Concludes that industry-wide standards must be developed governing interactions between physicians and representatives of health care technology industry companies. Cites Opinions 8.061 and 9.011. Tenery, *Interactions Between Physicians and the Health Care Technology Industry*, 283 JAMA 391, 393 (2000).

Journal 1992 Reviews concerns about commercial involvement in and funding of continuing medical education. Discusses CME requirements, accumulation of CME credits, and changes in standards governing commercial sponsorship. References Opinions 8.061 and 9.011. Wentz, Osteen, & Cannon, *Continuing Medical Education: Unabated Debate*, 268 JAMA 1118 (1992).

Journal 1991 Discusses commercial support of continuing medical education. Explains ethical guidelines for accepting such assistance and how those guidelines have changed. References Opinions 8.061 and 9.011. Wentz, Osteen, & Gannon, *Refocusing Support and Direction*, 266 JAMA 953 (1991).

9.0115 Financial Relationships With Industry in Continuing Medical Education

In an environment of rapidly changing information and emerging technology, physicians must maintain the knowledge, skills, and values central to a healing profession. They must protect the independence and commitment to fidelity and service that define the medical profession.

Financial or in-kind support from pharmaceutical, biotechnology or medical device companies that have a direct interest in physicians' recommendations creates conditions in which external interests could influence the availability and/or content of continuing medical education (CME). Financial relationships between such sources and individual physicians who organize CME, teach in CME, or have other roles in continuing professional education can carry similar potential to influence CME in undesired ways.

CME that is independent of funding or in-kind support from sources that have financial interests in physicians' recommendations promotes confidence in the independence and integrity of professional education, as does CME in which organizers, teachers, and others involved in educating physicians do not have financial relationships with industry that could influence their participation. When possible, CME should be provided without such support or the participation of individuals who have financial interests in the educational subject matter.

In some circumstances, support from industry or participation by individuals who have financial interests in the subject matter may be needed to enable access to appropriate, high-quality CME. In these circumstances, physician-learners should be confident that vigorous efforts will be made to maintain the independence and integrity of educational activities.

Individually and collectively physicians must ensure that the profession independently defines the goals of physician education, determines educational needs, and sets its own priorities for CME. Physicians who attend CME activities should expect that, in addition to complying with all applicable professional standards for accreditation and certification, their colleagues who organize, teach, or have other roles in CME will:

(a) be transparent about financial relationships that could potentially influence educational activities.

(b) provide the information physician-learners need to make critical judgments about an educational activity, including:

   (i) the source(s) and nature of commercial support for the activity; and/or

   (ii) the source(s) and nature of any individual financial relationships with industry related to the subject matter of the activity; and

   (iii) what steps have been taken to mitigate the potential influence of financial relationships.

(c) protect the independence of educational activities by:

   (i) ensuring independent, prospective assessment of educational needs and priorities;

   (ii) adhering to a transparent process for prospectively determining when industry support is needed;

   (iii) giving preference in selecting faculty or content developers to similarly qualified experts who do not have financial interests in the educational subject matter;

   (iv) ensuring a transparent process for making decisions about participation by physicians who may have a financial interest in the educational subject matter;

   (v) permitting individuals who have a substantial financial interest in the educational subject matter to participate in CME only when their participation is central to the success of the educational activity; the activity meets a demonstrated need in the professional community; and the source, nature, and magnitude of the individual's specific financial interest is disclosed; and

   (vi) taking steps to mitigate potential influence commensurate with the nature of the financial interest(s) at issue, such as prospective peer review. (I, V)

Issued November 2011 based on the report "Financial Relationships With Industry in Continuing Medical Education," adopted June 2011.

9.012 Physicians' Political Communications With Patients and Their Families

Physicians enjoy the rights and privileges of free political speech shared by all Americans. It is laudable for physicians to run for political office; to lobby for political positions, parties, or candidates; and in every other way to exercise the full scope of their political rights as citizens. These rights may be exercised individually or through involvement with organizations such as professional societies and political action committees.

In addition, physicians have a responsibility to work for the reform of, and to press for the proper administration of, laws that are related to health care. Physicians should keep themselves well-informed as to current political questions regarding needed and proposed changes to laws concerning such issues as access to health care, quality of health care services, scope of medical research, and promotion of public health.

It is natural that in fulfilling these political responsibilities, physicians will express their views to patients or their families. However, communications by telephone or other modalities with patients and their families about political matters must be conducted with the utmost sensitivity to patients' vulnerability and desire for privacy. Conversations about political matters are not appropriate at times when patients or families are emotionally pressured by significant medical circumstances. Physicians are best able to judge both the intrusiveness of the discussion and the patient's level of comfort. In general, when conversation with the patient or family concerning social, civic, or recreational matters is acceptable, discussion of items of political import may be appropriate.

Under no circumstances should physicians allow their differences with patients or their families about political matters to interfere with the delivery of high-quality professional care. (I, VII)

Issued June 1999 based on the report "Physicians' Political Communications With Patients and Their Families," adopted December 1998.

Journal 2009 Considers a physician's role in educating patients about health care reform. Concludes that reform would be aided by educating patients on all aspects of the health care system. Quotes Opinion 10.015. Cites Opinion 9.012. Abemayor, *United We Stand, Divided We Fall*, 135 Arch. Otolaryngol. Head Neck Surg. 432, 432, 433 (2009).

9.02   The previous Opinion 9.02, "Agreements Restricting the Practice of Medicine," was deleted in June 1998 and replaced with the current Opinion 9.02, "Restrictive Covenants and the Practice of Medicine."

9.02 Restrictive Covenants and the Practice of Medicine

Covenants not-to-compete restrict competition, disrupt continuity of care, and potentially deprive the public of medical services. The Council on Ethical and Judicial Affairs discourages any agreement which restricts the right of a physician to practice medicine for a specified period of time or in a specified area upon termination of an employment, a partnership, or a corporate agreement. Restrictive covenants are unethical if they are excessive in geographic scope or duration in the circumstances presented, or if they fail to make reasonable accommodation of patients' choice of physician. (VI, VII)

Issued prior to April 1977. Updated June 1994 and June 1998.

N.D. Ill. 1996 A corporation which provided hair transplants brought suit against a physician group under contract to provide medical services to the corporation. The complaint alleged that the defendants had breached the contract in bad faith by attempting to start their own company, by hiring staff members away, and by threatening to enforce noncompetition covenants in their contracts should any physicians attempt to remain with the corporation. The court referred to Opinion 9.02 as explicitly discouraging the use of restrictive covenants in contracts with physicians. Additionally, with apparent reference to Opinion 7.03, the court noted that defendants had not sent notices advising patients of the departure of physicians from the corporation, or of the departing physicians' new practice locations. *Cleveland Hair Clinic, Inc. v. Puig, 968 F. Supp. 1227, 1246.*

Ariz. 1999 Medical practice sought to enforce a restrictive covenant with defendant-physician. The trial court denied the plaintiff's request for a preliminary injunction and found that the restrictive covenant was unenforceable. The Arizona Supreme Court held that covenants not to compete between physicians will be strictly construed for reasonableness. Under this analysis, the court found that the restrictive covenant was unreasonable, overbroad, and unenforceable. The court quoted Opinions 9.02 and 9.06, recognizing that the AMA discourages restrictive covenants and supports free choice and competition. *Valley Medical Specialists v. Farber, 194 Ariz. 363, 982 P.2d 1277, 1282.*

Ariz. App. 1989 Plaintiff, an orthopaedic surgeon formerly employed by defendant, appealed a lower court's grant of a preliminary injunction which enforced the restrictive covenant in plaintiff's employment contract with defendant. Plaintiff asserted that Opinion 9.02 discouraged the use of such restrictive covenants and thus the covenant at issue should be declared per se unenforceable. The appellate court declined to make that declaration, noting that not all restrictive covenants are contrary to public policy and that the lower court had appropriately modified the terms of the covenant. *Phoenix Orthopaedic Surgeons, Ltd. v. Peairs, 164 Ariz. 54, 60, 790 P.2d 752, 758.*

Ga. 1988 Following termination of employment contract between the employer, a provider of psychiatric services, and a physician, the employer filed suit seeking an injunction to enforce a covenant not to compete. Supreme Court, without opinion, upheld trial court's order granting an injunction. Dissenting judge, quoting Opinion 9.02 (1986) reasoned that restrictive covenants in such physician employment agreements are "illegal per se as against public policy irrespective of whether the covenant is reasonable." *Shankman v. Coastal Psychiatric Assocs., 258 Ga. 294, 295, 368 S.E.2d 753, 754 (dissent).*

Ill. 2006 Physicians appealed a grant of preliminary injunction enforcing restrictive covenants in their employment contracts. Quoting Opinions 9.02, 9.06, and 10.01 and referencing Opinion 8.115, the Illinois Supreme Court gave thorough consideration to the AMA's position on restrictive covenants. While acknowledging the ethical problems associated with such contracts, the court found the covenants reasonable in scope. The decision to ban restrictive covenants, the court reasoned, was best left to the legislature. *Mohanty v. St. John Heart Clinic, S.C., 225 Ill.2d 52, 866 N.E.2d 85, 94, 106-07, 107-08.*

Ill. App. 2002 Ophthalmologist terminated employment contract with an eye clinic and intentionally practiced in an area prohibited by a noncompetition clause in the contract. The Illinois Appellate Court, while noting that under Opinion 9.02 (1986) noncompetition agreements are "discouraged," held that such agreements are enforceable in the medical profession in Illinois. *Prairie Eye Center v. Butler, 329 Ill. App. 3d 293, 768 N.E.2d 414, 420.*

Ill. App. 2000 Physician challenged trial court's decision upholding noncompete clause in the physician's employment contract with a health care provider. The appellate court reversed the decision, quoting Opinions 9.02 (1986) and 9.06 (1982). The court stated that the AMA disfavors the use of any restrictive employment or partnership agreements among physicians and emphasized the fact that such agreements are not in the public interest. The court also noted that patients might suffer if such agreements are upheld. *Carter-Shields v. Alton Health Institute,* *317 Ill. App. 3d 260, 739 N.E.2d 569, 576-77, vacated 201 Ill. 2d 441, 777 N.E.2d 948 (2002).*

Ind. 2008 Professional corporation brought suit against a podiatrist it formerly employed to enforce noncompetition restriction of employment contract. The court quoted Opinion 9.02 with respect to the enforceability of such covenants. The court held that noncompetition agreements between a physician and a medical group are not per se void as against public policy and are enforceable so long as they are reasonable. *Cent. Ind. Podiatry, P.C. v. Krueger, 882 N.E.2d 723, 728, n. 4.*

Ind. App. 1987 Medical corporation sued physician who was former employee at will pursuant to covenant not to compete in employment contract seeking an injunction or liquidated damages. Court upheld covenant against physician's claim that enforcement was inappropriate where he had been terminated without good cause. Concurring judge, citing Opinion 9.02 (1986), expressed view that such covenants should be unenforceable as against public policy. *Gomez v. Chua Medical Corp., 510 N.E.2d 191, 197.*

Kan. 2005 Appellee surgeons sought a restraining order and injunction prohibiting enforcement of covenants not to compete in their employment contracts on the grounds that Opinion 9.02 prohibits such covenants, making them void as against public policy. The Kansas Supreme Court held that neither Opinion 9.02 nor Kansas case law makes restrictive covenants unenforceable per se. Restrictive covenants are unenforceable only if they are excessive in geographic scope and duration or fail to make reasonable accommodations for the patient's choice of physician. *Idbeis v. Wichita Surgical Specialists, 279 Kan. 755, 112 P.2d 81, 87, 88.*

Kan. App. 1985 Members of a medical partnership sought an injunction to enforce a covenant not to compete against defendant-physician, a former partner. Defendant asserted that the covenant was void as against public policy relying on Opinion 9.02 (1984). The court however ruled that the covenant was reasonable as defined by precedent and that it was bound to follow this precedent as opposed to the AMA's position regarding such covenants. Defendant further argued enforcement of the covenant was precluded because the partnership had violated ethical norms, apparently referring to Opinions 6.03 and 6.04 (1984) [now Opinions 6.02 and 6.03] which were part of partnership contract. The court held defendant was estopped from complaining about the partnership's actions due to his own conduct. *Axtell Clinic v. Cranston, No. 56,745 (Kan. Ct. App. June 20, 1985) (LEXIS, States Library, Ka. file).*

Mich. App. 2006 Physician signed an employment contract with a restrictive covenant and liquidated damages provision. When the physician resigned and violated the covenant, the employer brought an action seeking payment of liquidated damages. The physician counterclaimed, alleging the restrictive covenant was unreasonable and void on both statutory and public policy grounds. On appeal, the physician argued that the covenant was unreasonable in light of Opinion 9.02. The appeals court reasoned that the employer had a valid interest in retaining patients in the area and that the covenant was not unreasonable. *St. Clair Medical, P.C. v. Borgiel, 270 Mich.App. 260, 715 N.W.2d 914, 920-21.*

Minn. 1983 Dispute arose between physician and clinic concerning covenant not to compete contained in employment contract entered into by physician after commencement of employment. Physician challenged enforceability of covenant due to lack of consideration to support it. The court agreed with physician and denied enforcement. In so ruling court did not reach issue of whether such covenants, in the context of medical practice, are against public policy. The court however noted that under Opinion 9.01 (1982) [now Opinion 9.02] the AMA discourages such restrictive covenants. *Freeman v. Duluth Clinic, 334 N.W.2d 626, 631.*

N.J. 2005 Appellant hospital filed suit in superior court to enforce a covenant not to compete against respondent, a neurosurgeon. The court refused to enforce the covenant and found for the respondent. On appeal, the appellate division reversed. It found that Opinion 9.02 and case law support the conclusion that restrictive covenants are unenforceable only when they are unreasonable in scope and duration or do not make reasonable accommodations for the patient's choice of physician. Quoting Opinion 9.02, the Supreme Court of New Jersey agreed that physician restrictive covenants are not unenforceable per se, but reversed the appellate division because the geographic restriction of the covenant was injurious to the public. *Community Hosp. Group Inc. v. More, 183 N.J. 36, 869 A.2d 884, 896.*

N.J. 1978 Plaintiff and defendant, both physicians, had entered into an employment contract which included in its terms a restrictive covenant provision. When defendant failed to abide by the covenant upon termination of the employment contract, plaintiff sued to enforce the covenant. In affirming the lower court's decision to enforce the restrictive covenant, the appellate court quoted Opinion 4.63 (1977) [now Opinion 9.02] and stated that, although it hesitated to give weight to the rules of private organizations, even if it followed the Opinion the decision to uphold the covenant would be proper. *Karlin v. Weinberg, 77 N.J. 408, 390 A.2d 1161, 1168 n.6.*

N.J. Super. 2004 Respondent physician appealed dismissal of complaint, arguing that restrictive covenants are void per se as a matter of public policy and that the court should not follow prior case law. The trial court quoted Opinion 9.02 and compared it to the previous opinion on restrictive covenants to determine that the AMA is currently more hostile toward restrictive covenants than it had been previously. The court noted that it must apply precedent and enforce the restrictive covenant. If any change is to be made in the law, it must be made by the New Jersey Supreme Court. The appeals court agreed and affirmed. *Pierson v. Med. Health Ctrs., 2004 WL 1416265, 3.*

N.J. Super. 2003 Hospital filed suit to enforce a covenant not to compete against respondent neurosurgeon. The court refused to enforce the covenant and found for the respondent. In reversing, the appellate division found the respondent's argument that the restrictive covenant should be unenforceable based on Opinion 9.02, unpersuasive. The appellate division stated that AMA ethical standards and case law support the conclusion that restrictive covenants are unenforceable only when they are unreasonable in scope and duration or do not make reasonable accommodations for the patient's choice of physician. *Community Hosp. Group Inc. v. More, 365 N.J. Super. 84, 838 A.2d 472, 488.*

N.J. Super. 1977 Plaintiff, a dermatologist who had previously employed defendant-dermatologist, sued to enforce a postemployment restrictive covenant signed by defendant. In holding the covenant enforceable, the court noted Opinion 4.63 (1977) [now Opinion 9.02] which at the time stated there was "no ethical proscription" against entering into a restrictive covenant if its terms are reasonable. Note that Opinion 9.02 now "discourages" such restrictive agreements. *Karlin v. Weinberg, 148 N.J. Super. 243, 372 A.2d 616, 618, aff'd, 77 N.J. 408, 390 A.2d 1161 (1978).*

N.Y. Sup. 2007 Plaintiff, an otolaryngologist, signed an employment contract with defendant, which included a covenant not to compete, restricting practice within 30 miles of defendant's offices for a period of three years. Plaintiff resigned and defendant sought enforcement. Citing Opinion 9.02, plaintiff argued that the contract was unreasonable in scope and unnecessary to protect any legitimate business interest of defendant. The court disagreed, noting that Opinion 9.02 merely discourages such agreements and does not prohibit them. The noncompete agreement was held reasonable, in both temporal and geographic scope, to protect the legitimate business interests of defendant's goodwill and patient base. Although it was overbroad in prohibiting the general practice of medicine, partial enforcement was appropriate to prohibit practice of otolaryngology. *Awwad v. Capital Region Otolaryngology Head & Neck Group, 2007 N.Y. Misc. LEXIS 8593, 19.*

N.Y. Sup. 2005 Plaintiff health center moved for an injunction to stop defendant physician and former employee from opening up a pediatric practice within 10 miles of the health center. The court, citing Opinion 9.02, stated that the AMA does not hold that restrictive covenants are unethical and unenforceable per se and that court should not utilize the AMA's position to impose an outright ban on physician restrictive covenants. The court found that the plaintiff had not shown that the defendant would use unfair means to compete, and therefore the plaintiff was not entitled to the protection of the restrictive covenant. *Oak Orchard Cmty. Health Ctr. v. Blasco, 8 Misc. 3d 927, 800 N.Y.S.2d. 277, 281, n. 3.*

N.C. App. 2006 Physicians entered an employment contract that included a noncompetition clause, as well as a clause stating the contract would be void if it did not comply with the AMA Code of Medical Ethics. In an action challenging the enforceability of the noncompete agreement, the physicians argued the provision violated Opinion 9.02 and was void under either the contractual terms or on public policy grounds. The court concluded the noncompete agreement was not per se against public policy and that the clause requiring compliance with the AMA Code was intended solely to address concerns regarding physician autonomy. *Calhoun v. WHA Medical Clinic, PLLC, 178 N.C.App. 585, 632 S.E.2d 563, 568.*

Ohio App. 1991 Medical corporation sought an injunction to enforce a covenant not to compete against defendant-physician. The lower court granted summary judgment based on a referee's report which concluded that, under Principle VI and Opinions 6.11, 9.02, and 9.06 (1989), restrictive covenants were per se unenforceable as a matter of public policy. While recognizing a strong public interest in allowing open access to health care, the appellate court in reversing held that Opinion 9.02, which applied specifically to restrictive covenants, only "discouraged" such covenants. *Ohio Urology, Inc. v. Poll, 72 Ohio. App. 446, 450, 451, 594 N.E.2d 1027, 1030, 1031.*

Tenn. 2005 Respondent, a private medical practice, filed suit to enforce a noncompetition covenant contained in a physician's employment contract. The trial court found that the covenant was enforceable and the court of appeals affirmed. The Tennessee Supreme Court reversed. Quoting Opinions 9.02 and 9.06 it found that such covenants are not enforceable because they violate public policy. *Murfreesboro Med. Clinic v. Udom, 166 S.W.3d 674, 679, 684, 685.*

Journal 2010 Discusses the background and policies of traditional noncompete agreements and evaluates the arguments underlying the use of restrictive covenants in the health care field. Concludes that enforcing physician noncompete clauses ultimately hurts patients, and that courts should create an exception regarding such clauses similar to that for attorney noncompete clauses. Quotes Opinion 9.06. Cites Opinion 9.02. Klimkina, *Are Noncompete Contracts Between Physicians Bad Medicine? Advocating in the Affirmative by Drawing a Public Policy Parallel to the Legal Profession, 98 Ky. L. J. 131, 147-148 (2010).*

Journal 2009 Discusses the judicial standard for reviewing physician noncompete covenants. Concludes courts should apply a strict standard to such covenants, rather than declare the covenants per se invalid. Quotes Principles IV and VII, Principles of Medical Ethics §5 (1957) [now Principle VI], Code of Medical Ethics Ch. II, Art. I §3 (1847) [now Opinion 5.02], Opinion 9.02, and Code of Medical Ethics Ch. II, Art. I §4 (1847) [now Opinion 9.09]. Cites Opinions 8.041, 8.115, 9.02, 9.06, 9.065, 9.067, 10.01, and 10.015. Koons, *Physician Employee Non-Compete Agreements on the Examining Table: The Need to Better Protect Patients' and the Public's Interests in Indiana, 6 Ind. Health L. Rev. 253, 272-77, 280-81 (2009).*

Journal 2009 Examines the economic impact of specialty hospitals on general hospitals and discusses efforts of general hospitals to remove competition. Concludes that specialty hospitals are not responsible for ensuring the economic viability of general hospitals and that general hospitals should focus on bolstering their own resources, rather than on eliminating competition from specialty hospitals. Quotes Opinion 9.02. Steinbuch, *Placing Profits Above Hippocrates: The Hypocrisy of General Service Hospitals, 31 U. Ark. Little Rock L. Rev. 505, 512 (2009).*

Journal 2008 Examines for-profit medical specialty groups and their impact on competition for specialty services. Concludes for-profit medical groups must not be allowed to eliminate competition to garner higher profits until a market for affordable health care services is established. Cites Opinion 9.02. Kinney, *The Corporate Transformation of Medical Specialty Care: The Exemplary Case of Neonatology, 36 J. L. Med. & Ethics 790, 791 (2008).*

Journal 2008 Discusses covenants not to compete and Kentucky cases dealing with physician noncompetition agreements. Concludes Kentucky should enact legislation permitting reasonable noncompetition agreements ancillary to sale of practice contracts to increase patient choice of physician. Quotes Principle VIII and Opinion 9.02. Naiser, *Physician Noncompetition Agreements in Kentucky: The Past Discounting of Public Interests and a Proposed Solution, 47 U. Louisville L. Rev. 195, 195, 200 (2008).*

Journal 2007 Examines the role of the medical profession in participating in state-sanctioned lethal injection. Concludes that any participation is unethical because it causes harm and undermines trust. Cites Opinion 2.06. References Opinions 2.211 and 9.02. Black & Sade, *Lethal Injection and Physicians: State Law vs Medical Ethics, 298 JAMA 2779, 2780, 2781 (2007).*

Journal 2007 Discusses the enforceability of medical noncompete agreements in Michigan. Concludes that such agreements are likely enforceable, but may be invalidated based on local availability of medical services. Quotes Opinion 9.02. Quick, *Contract Law: Physician, Meet Thy Covenant: Noncompete Agreements in the Medical Profession, 86 Mich. Bar J. 22, 23 (2007).*

Journal 2006 Explores the use of "no-hire" clauses in the field of health care. Concludes that enforcement of such clauses should be determined on the basis of reasonableness. Cites Opinion 9.02. Basanta, *"No-Hire" Clauses in Healthcare Sector Contracts: Their Use and Enforceability, 39 J. Health L. 451, 453 (2006).*

Journal 2006 Reviews the Tennessee Supreme Court decision banning physician covenants not to compete. Concludes the policy decisions discussed by the court are vital in deciding if and when to enforce covenants not to compete. References Opinion 9.02. Belville, *Most Covenants*

Not to Compete Against Physicians Are No Longer Enforceable in Tennessee, 7 Transactions 419, 434 (2006).

Journal 2006 Discusses the Tennessee Supreme Court decision prohibiting physician non-compete agreements. Suggests the court should have adopted a standard of reasonableness for noncompete agreements. Quotes Opinion 9.02. Cites Opinion 9.06. Carr, *Contracts—Murfreesboro Medical Clinic, P.A. v. Udom: Physician Noncompete Agreements Go Under the Knife: The Tennessee Supreme Court Rejects Physician Noncompete Agreements, 36 U. Mem. L. Rev. 1115, 1128, 1131 (2006).*

Journal 2006 Examines physician restrictive covenants. Concludes that under the current balancing test, courts should give considerable weight to the public interest in preserving the physician-patient relationship. Quotes Opinions 9.02 and 9.06. Cites Opinions 6.11, 8.11, 8.115, and 9.06. Malloy, *Physician Restrictive Covenants: The Neglect of Incumbent Patient Interests, 41 Wake Forest L. Rev. 189, 207-08, 217, 218 (2006).*

Journal 2006 Discusses noncompete agreements in surgeon employment contracts. Concludes that covenants not to compete should be unenforceable per se against surgeons. Quotes Opinions 9.02 and 9.06. Wyatt, *Buy Out or Get Out: Why Covenants Not to Compete in Surgeon Employment Contracts Are Truly Bad Medicine, 45 Washburn L. J. 715, 720 (2006).*

Journal 2005 Discusses the ban of physician noncompetition covenants by the Tennessee Supreme Court. Concludes that new contractual terms will need to be drafted to balance employer and employee interests in the medical profession. Quotes Opinion 9.06. References Opinion 9.02. Schuler, *Knock Out? Supreme Court Deals a Blow to Non-Competes for Docs, but This Fight Is Not Over, 41 Tenn. B.J. 16, 19 (Dec. 2005).*

Journal 2003 Discusses conflicting Illinois case law regarding medical restrictive covenants. Concludes the Illinois Supreme Court should validate medical restrictive covenants that protect a business interest. Quotes Opinion 9.02. Gimbel & Zaremski, *Medical Restrictive Covenants in Illinois: At the Crossroads of Carter-Shields and Prairie Eye Center, 12 Annals Health L. 1, 12 (2003).*

Journal 2003 Highlights the legal and ethical concerns surrounding use of noncompetition clauses. Concludes that physicians should carefully evaluate these clauses given their likely enforceability. Quotes Opinions 9.02, 9.06, 10.01, and 10.015. Loeser, *The Legal, Ethical, and Practical Implications of Noncompetition Clauses: What Physicians Should Know Before They Sign, 31 J. L. Med. & Ethics 283, 286, 287, 290 (2003).*

Journal 2000 Examines strikingly different approaches to enforcement of reasonable contractual restraints on competition in the medical and legal fields. Observes that most recent cases find the public harm caused by noncompetition agreements to be generally insufficient to deny enforcement. Quotes Opinion 9.02. Wilcox, *Enforcing Lawyer Non-Competition Agreements While Maintaining the Profession: The Role of Conflict of Interest Principles, 84 Minn. L. Rev. 915, 966 (2000).*

Journal 1999 Discusses the need for physicians to advocate on behalf of patients' rights in the context of health care delivery. Evaluates the nature and scope of the physician's role as advocate, noting that physicians cannot be expected to engage in attorney-like advocacy. Quotes Principles IV and VI, Fundamental Elements (2), (4), and (6) [now Opinion 10.01], Patient Responsibilities 5 [now Opinion 10.02], and Opinions 2.03, 2.07, 2.09, 2.16, 2.19, 3.06, 4.01, 4.04, 6.01, 7.02, 8.02, 8.03, 8.13, 8.132, 9.06, 9.07, and 9.131. Cites Opinions 5.05, 5.09, 7.01, 8.135, and 9.02. Sage, *Physicians as Advocates, 35 Hous. L. Rev. 1529, 1537, 1541, 1542, 1552-53, 1554, 1556, 1557, 1559, 1561-62, 1564, 1571, 1574, 1576, 1580 (1999).*

Journal 1998 Discusses the ramifications of physician license revocation for failing to pay child support. Points out that patients stand to lose access to trusted physicians and confidence in the health care system. Concludes that children need the most protection and that patients will have an easier time finding another physician than children will have finding another means for support. Quotes Opinion 5.05. Cites Opinions 9.02 and 9.06. Noyes, *Higher Penalties for Failing to Pay Child Support: A Look at Medical License Revocation, 19 J. Legal Med. 127, 138 (1998).*

Journal 1997 Examines noncompetition clauses in the medical field. Reviews policy concerns and historical and common-law analyses of agreements not to compete. Posits that, the more commercialized the medical profession becomes, the more noncompetition clauses infringe upon the physician-patient relationship and patients' rights. Quotes Opinions 9.02 and 9.06.

Cites Preamble and Opinion 6.11. Comment, *Noncompetition Clauses in Physician Employment Contracts in Oregon*, 76 Or. L. Rev. 195, 204-06 (1997).

Journal 1997 Examines the judicial assessment of restrictive covenants within the legal and medical fields. Observes that courts tend to uphold physician, but not attorney, restrictive covenants. Concludes that covenants in medical practice should be treated in a manner similar to those in legal practice. Opinion 9.02. Levy, *Because Judges Went to Law School, Not Medical School: Restrictive Covenants in the Practices of Law and Medicine*, 30 J. Health & Hosp. L. 89, 92, 101 (1997).

Journal 1995 Analyzes South Carolina judicial treatment of covenants not to compete and liquidated damages provisions. Considers approaches in other jurisdictions and proposes guidelines for drafting contractual agreements. Quotes Opinion 9.06. Cites Opinion 9.01 (1982) [now Opinion 9.02]. Note, *Covenants Not to Compete and Liquidated Damages Clauses: Diagnosis and Treatment for Physicians*, 46 S. C. L. Rev. 505, 514 (1995).

Journal 1991 Considers the question of whether physicians should provide medical treatment to those who come to them for second opinions. Concludes that each physician must individually decide whether to treat these patients. Quotes Opinions 6.11, 9.06, and 9.12. Cites Opinion 9.02. Ile, *Should Physicians Treat Patients Who Seek Second Opinions?* 266 JAMA 273, 274 (1991).

Journal 1982 Discusses the legal status of restrictive covenants in employment contracts against the background of the AMA's position discouraging such agreements as not serving the public interest. Observes that courts generally have upheld restrictive covenants if the limits are reasonable. Cites Opinion 9.01 (1982) [now Opinion 9.02]. Cooper, *Restrictive Covenants*, 248 JAMA 3091, 3091 (1982).

9.021 Covenants Not-to-Compete for Physicians-in-Training

It is unethical for a teaching institution to seek a noncompetition guarantee in return for fulfilling its educational obligations. Physicians-in-training (residents in programs approved by the Accreditation Council for Graduate Medical Education [ACGME], fellows in ACGME-approved fellowship programs, and fellows in programs approved by one of the American Board of Medical Specialties specialty boards) should not be asked to sign covenants not-to-compete as a condition of their entry into any residency or fellowship program. (III, IV, VI)

Issued December 1997 based on the report "Covenants Not-to-Compete for Physicians-in-Training," adopted June 1997 (JAMA. 1997;278:530).

9.025 Advocacy for Change in Law and Policy

Physicians may participate in individual acts, grassroots activities, or legally permissible collective action to advocate for change, as provided for in the AMA's Principles of Medical Ethics. Whenever engaging in advocacy efforts, physicians must ensure that the health of patients is not jeopardized and that patient care is not compromised.

Formal unionization of physicians, including physicians-in-training, may tie physicians' obligations to the interests of workers who may not share physicians' primary and overriding commitment to patients. Physicians should not form workplace alliances with those who do not share these ethical priorities.

Strikes and other collective action may reduce access to care, eliminate or delay necessary care, and interfere with continuity of care. Each of these consequences raises ethical concerns. Physicians should refrain from the use of the strike as a bargaining tactic. In rare circumstances, individual or grassroots actions, such as brief limitations of personal availability, may be appropriate as a means of calling attention to needed changes in patient care. Physicians are cautioned that some actions may put them or their organizations at risk of violating antitrust laws. Consultation with legal counsel is advised.

Physicians and physicians-in-training should press for needed reforms through the use of informational campaigns, nondisruptive public demonstrations, lobbying and publicity campaigns, and collective negotiation, or other options that do not jeopardize the health of patients or compromise patient care.

Physicians are free to decide whether participation in advocacy activities is in patients' best interests. Colleagues should not unduly influence or pressure them to participate nor should they punish them, overtly or covertly, for deciding whether or not to participate. (I, III, VI)

Issued December 1998 based on the report "Collective Action and Patient Advocacy," adopted June 1998. Updated June 2005 based on the report "Amendment to Opinion 9.025, 'Collective Action and Patient Advocacy,'" adopted December 2004.

Journal 2006 Examines medical resident labor rights. Concludes that hospitals should allow residents to unionize. References Opinion 9.025. Geiger, *The Ailing Labor Rights of Medical Residents: Curable Ill or a Lost Cause?* 8 U. Pa. J. Lab. & Emp. L. 523, 538 (2006)

Journal 2005 Discusses physician responses to the medical malpractice liability crisis. Concludes that certain responses may violate ethical obligations that physicians owe to their patients and to society as a whole. Cites Opinions 9.025 and 10.015. References Principle VIII. Kachalia, Choudhry, & Studdert, *Physician Responses to the Malpractice Crisis: From Defense to Offense*, 33 J. L. Med. & Ethics 416, 419, 421, 424 (2005).

Journal 2004 Examines whether unionization is a feasible solution to the commodification of the professional work force. Concludes that unionization is a tool used to protect the class status and livelihood of professional employees and that the law should support such efforts. References Opinion 9.025. Crain, *The Transformation of the Professional Workforce*, 79 Chi.-Kent L. Rev. 543, 582 (2004).

Journal 1999 Considers the growing interest on the part of physicians to unionize and engage in collective bargaining. Discusses how legislatures and the courts may affect the evolution of physician unions. Analyzes potential benefits and detriments of unionization. References Opinion 9.025. Phan, *Physician Unionization: The Impact on the Medical Profession*, 20 J. Legal Med. 115, 136, 137 (1999).

9.03 Civil Rights and Professional Responsibility

Opportunities in medical society activities or membership, medical education and training, employment, and all other aspects of professional endeavors should not be denied to any duly licensed physician because of race, color, religion, creed, ethnic affiliation, national origin, sex, sexual orientation, gender identity, age, or handicap. (IV)

Issued prior to April 1977. Updated June 1994 and June 2008 based on the report "Modification of Ethics Policy to Ensure Inclusion for Transgender Physicians, Medical Students, and Patients," adopted November 2007.

Journal 1996 Examines possible legal avenues for addressing claims of employment discrimination based upon sexual orientation. Concludes that lesbians and gay men need greater employment protection and an explicit statutory cause of action. Quotes Opinion 9.03. Gilmore, *Employment Protection for Lesbians and Gay Men*, 6 L. & Sex. 83, 95 (1996).

9.0305 Physician Health and Wellness

To preserve the quality of their performance, physicians have a responsibility to maintain their health and wellness, construed broadly as preventing or treating acute or chronic diseases, including mental illness, disabilities, and occupational stress. When health or wellness is compromised, so may the safety and effectiveness of the medical care be provided. When failing physical or mental health reaches the point of interfering with a physician's ability to engage safely in professional activities, the physician is said to be impaired.

In addition to maintaining healthy lifestyle habits, every physician should have a personal physician whose objectivity is not compromised. Physicians whose health or wellness is compromised should take measures to mitigate the problem, seek appropriate help as necessary, and engage in an honest self-assessment of their ability to continue practicing.

Those physicians caring for colleagues should not disclose without the physician-patient's consent any aspects of their medical care, except as required by law, by ethical and professional obligation (Opinion 9.031, "Reporting Impaired, Incompetent, or Unethical Colleagues"), or when essential to protect patients from harm. Under such circumstances, only the minimum amount of information required by law or to preserve patient safety should be disclosed.

The medical profession has an obligation to ensure that its members are able to provide safe and effective care. This obligation is discharged by:

- promoting health and wellness among physicians;
- supporting peers in identifying physicians in need of help;
- intervening promptly when the health or wellness of a colleague appears to have become compromised, including the offer of encouragement, coverage, or referral to a physician health program;
- establishing physician health programs that provide a supportive environment to maintain and restore health and wellness;
- establishing mechanisms to assure that impaired physicians promptly cease practice;
- assisting recovered colleagues when they resume patient care;
- reporting impaired physicians who continue to practice, despite reasonable offers of assistance, to appropriate bodies as required by law and/or ethical obligations. This may entail reporting to the licensing authority. (I, II)

Issued June 2004 based on the report "Physician Health and Wellness," adopted December 2003.

9.031 Reporting Impaired, Incompetent, or Unethical Colleagues

Physicians have an ethical obligation to report impaired, incompetent, and/or unethical colleagues in accordance with the legal requirements in each state and assisted by the following guidelines:

Impairment. Physicians' responsibilities to colleagues who are impaired by a condition that interferes with their ability to engage safely in professional activities include timely intervention to ensure that these colleagues cease practicing and receive appropriate assistance from a physician health program (see Opinion 9.0305, "Physician Health and Wellness"). Ethically and legally, it may be necessary to report an impaired physician who continues to practice despite reasonable offers of assistance and referral to a hospital or state physician health program. The duty to report under such circumstances, which stems from physicians' obligation to protect patients against harm, may entail reporting to the licensing authority.

Incompetence. Initial reports of incompetence should be made to the appropriate clinical authority who would be empowered to assess the potential impact on patient welfare and to facilitate remedial action. The hospital peer-review body should be notified where appropriate. Incompetence that poses an immediate threat to the health and safety of patients should be reported directly to the state licensing board. Incompetence of physicians without a hospital affiliation should be reported to the local or state medical society and/or the state licensing or disciplinary board.

Unethical conduct. With the exception of incompetence or impairment, unethical behavior should be reported in accordance with the following guidelines and, considering, as necessary, the right to privacy of any patients involved:

Unethical conduct that threatens patient care or welfare should be reported to the appropriate authority for a particular clinical service. Unethical conduct that violates state licensing provisions should be reported to the state licensing board. It is appropriate to report unethical conduct that potentially violates criminal statutes to law enforcement authorities. All other unethical conduct should be reported to the local or state professional medical organization.

When the inappropriate conduct of a physician continues despite the initial report(s), the reporting physician should report to a higher or additional authority. The person or body receiving the initial report should notify the reporting physician when appropriate action has been taken. Physicians who receive reports of inappropriate behavior, including reports submitted anonymously, have an ethical duty to critically, objectively, and confidentially evaluate the reported information and assure that identified deficiencies are either remedied or further reported to a higher or additional authority. Information regarding reports or investigations of impairment, or of incompetent or unethical behavior should be held in confidence until the matter is resolved. (II)

Issued March 1992 based on the report "Reporting Impaired, Incompetent, or Unethical Colleagues," adopted December 1991 (*J Miss St Med Assoc.* 1992;33:176-177); updated June 1994; updated June 1996; and updated June 2004, based on the report "Physician Health and Wellness," adopted December 2003.

7th Cir. 2009 Plaintiff, a surgeon and resident of New Jersey, brought a defamation action against defendant, a surgeon and resident of New York, in federal district court in Illinois. The suit was based upon a letter sent by the defendant to a professional organization based in Chicago complaining about the plaintiff's testimony against the defendant in a malpractice action. The district judge dismissed the suit for improper venue and plaintiff appealed. The appeals court cited Opinion 9.031 in noting that a physician has a duty to notify the proper public or private authorities of unprofessional conduct by a fellow professional. The court held that New Jersey law governed the defamation action. *Kamelgard v. Macura, 585 F.3d 334, 338.*

D. Vt. 2004 Defendants filed a motion for summary judgment in physician's suit alleging, among other claims, defamation. The court granted the motion citing Opinion 9.031, holding that the

AMA's Code of Medical Ethics required the defendants to report the plaintiff, given questions about his ability to practice medicine. *Agee v. Grunert, 349 F. Supp.2d 838, 843, 844.*

Ga. App. 1998 An emergency room physician sued another physician who examined a patient one day after the plaintiff, for libel and unfair business practices stemming from letters the second physician wrote regarding the emergency room physician's treatment of the patient. The court affirmed the trial court's grant of summary judgment on grounds that the concerns addressed in the letters were protected by a conditional privilege and that the plaintiff had not proved that the defendant wrote the letters with malice. The court quoted Opinion 9.031, as imposing a duty to report the plaintiff's treatment of the patient. Furthermore, the court noted that according to the Opinion, the defendant was neither required to address the problem with the offending physician first, nor required to confine her concerns to peer review groups. *Dominy v. Shumpert, 235 Ga. App. 500, 510 S.E.2d 81, 85-86.*

Mich. App. 1968 Physician was properly dismissed from hospital staff for violating Principle 4 (1957) [now Principle II and Opinion 9.031] when on numerous occasions physician vilified other physicians, swore and screamed in the hospital, and quarreled with staff and hospital visitors. *Anderson v. Bd. of Trustees of Caro Community Hosp., 10 Mich. App. 348, 159 N.W.2d 347, 348-50.*

Journal 2010 Explores how participation in online social networks may blur boundaries between personal and professional relationships for health care professionals and how such risks may be mitigated by use of network privacy and security settings. Suggests that health care institutions are likely to institute online social-networking policies for employees. Quotes Opinions 5.026, 5.027, 5.045, 5.046, 5.05, 5.059, 5.0591, 8.14, 9.08, and 9.123. Cites Opinions 5.026, 9.031, and 9.12. Terry, *Physicians and Patients Who "Friend" or "Tweet": Constructing a Legal Framework for Social Networking in a Highly Regulated Domain,* 43 Ind. L. Rev. 285, 314-16, 319, 334-36, 338 (2010).

Journal 2004 Discusses application of the Americans with Disabilities Act in the professional disciplinary context. Concludes that medical and legal professionals who are unfit are being disciplined not because they are disabled, but primarily because of misconduct. Quotes Opinion 9.031. Walker, *Protecting the Public: The Impact of the Americans with Disabilities Act on Licensure Considerations Involving Mentally Impaired Medical and Legal Professionals,* 25 J. Legal Med. 441, 454 (2004).

Journal 1993 Discusses the problems physicians may encounter by exposing an errant colleague, such as harm to the reporting physician's reputation and the fear of litigation. States that problems involving physician competency and unethical behavior should be investigated, and that physicians should take personal responsibility for reporting problems they observe. References Principle II and Opinions 8.14 and 9.031. Morreim, *Am I My Brother's Warden? Responding to the Unethical or Incompetent Colleague,* 23 Hastings Center Rep. 19, 23 (May/June 1993).

9.032 Reporting Adverse Drug or Device Events

A physician who suspects the occurrence of an adverse reaction to a drug or medical device has an obligation to communicate that information to the broader medical community, (eg, through submitting a report or letter to a medical journal or informing the manufacturer of the suspect drug or device). In the case of a serious adverse event, the event should be reported to the Food and Drug Administration (FDA). Spontaneous reports of adverse events are irreplaceable as a source of valuable information about drugs and medical devices, particularly their rare or delayed effects, as well as their safety in vulnerable patient populations. Although premarketing and mandated post-marketing studies provide basic safeguards for the public health, they suffer from inherent deficiencies that limit their ability to detect rare or unexpected consequences of drug or medical device use. Physicians who prescribe and monitor the use of drugs and medical devices constitute the group best able to observe and communicate information about resulting adverse events.

Serious adverse events, such as those resulting in death, hospitalization, or medical or surgical intervention, are the most important to report and are the only adverse events for which the FDA desires a report. Certainty, or even reasonable likelihood, of a causal relationship between the drug or medical device and the serious adverse event will rarely exist and is not required before reporting the event to the FDA. Suspicion of such a relationship is sufficient to give rise to an obligation to participate in the reporting system. (I, V, VII)

Issued June 1993 based on the report "Reporting Adverse Drug and Medical Device Events," adopted June 1993. Updated June 1994 (*Food & Drug L. J.* 1994;49:359-366).

Journal 2002 Challenges the general use of special informed consent disclosure rules in experimental therapy. Discusses the lack of a bright-line distinction between standard and experimental interventions. Concludes that focus should be placed on the distinctiveness of experimentation. Quotes Opinion 2.07. References Opinion 9.032. Noah, *Informed Consent and the Elusive Dichotomy Between Standard and Experimental Therapy*, 28 Am. J. L. & Med. 361, 394, 395 (2002).

Journal 2000 Describes possible solutions designed to improve postapproval regulation of prescription drugs so that fewer patients will suffer from adverse drug reactions. Concludes that the FDA along with physicians and clinical researchers should rethink the existing approach to monitoring of unexpected side effects. Quotes Principle V and Opinion 9.032. Cites Opinion 5.05. Noah, *Adverse Drug Reactions: Harnessing Experimental Data to Promote Patient Welfare*, 49 Cath. U. L. Rev. 449, 477, 497-98 (2000).

Journal 2000 Evaluates the regulatory framework governing prescription drugs. Considers problems faced by elderly patients when taking FDA-approved medications. Concludes that, in order to optimize patient safety, the existing regulatory system must undergo important structural changes. Quotes Principle V and Opinion 9.032. Noah & Brushwood, *Adverse Drug Reactions in Elderly Patients: Alternative Approaches to Postmarket Surveillance*, 33 J. Health L. 383, 400, 445 (2000).

Journal 1999 Discusses the duty of manufacturers to discover potential adverse drug interactions with new drugs. Suggests that a manufacturer's duty to warn about adverse drug interactions may be the future subject of products liability lawsuits. References Opinion 9.032. McCormick, *Pharmaceutical Manufacturer's Duty to Warn of Adverse Drug Interactions*, 66 Def. Couns. J. 59, 61 (1999).

Journal 1993 Explains MedWatch, an FDA program designed to facilitate the reporting of adverse events associated with the use of FDA-approved drugs and medical devices. Emphasizes that physicians are best able to provide such information. Quotes Opinion 9.032. Rheinstein, *MedWatch: The FDA Medical Products Reporting Program*, 48 Am. Fam. Physician 636, 636 (1993).

9.035   Gender Discrimination in the Medical Profession

Physician leaders in medical schools and other medical institutions should take immediate steps to increase the number of women in leadership positions as such positions become open. There is already a large enough pool of female physicians to provide strong candidates for such positions. Also, adjustments should be made to ensure that all physicians are equitably compensated for their work. Women and men in the same specialty with the same experience and doing the same work should be paid the same compensation.

Physicians in the workplace should actively develop the following: (1) retraining or other programs which facilitate the re-entry of physicians who take time away from their careers to have a family; (2) on-site child care services for dependent children; and (3) policies providing job security for physicians who are temporarily not in practice due to pregnancy or family obligations.

Physicians in the academic medical setting should strive to promote the following: (1) extension of tenure decisions through "stop the clock" programs, relaxation of the seven-year rule, or part-time appointments that would give faculty members longer to achieve standards for promotion and tenure; (2) more reasonable guidelines regarding the appropriate quantity and timing of published material needed for promotion or tenure that would emphasize quality over quantity and that would encourage the pursuit of careers based on individual talent rather than tenure standards that undervalue teaching ability and overvalue research; and (3) fair distribution of teaching, clinical, research, administrative responsibilities, and access to tenure tracks between men and women. Also, physicians in academic institutions should consider formally structuring the mentoring process, possibly matching students or faculty with advisors through a fair and visible system.

Where such policies do not exist or have not been followed, all medical workplaces and institutions should create strict policies to deal with sexual harassment. Grievance committees should have broad representation of both sexes and other groups. Such committees should have the power to enforce harassment policies and be accessible to those persons they are meant to serve.

Grantors of research funds and editors of scientific or medical journals should consider blind peer review of grant proposals and articles for publication to help prevent bias. However, grantors and editors will be able to consider the author's identity and give it appropriate weight. (II, VII)

Issued June 1994 based on the report "Gender Discrimination in the Medical Profession," adopted June 1993 (*Women's Health Issues*. 1994;4:1-11).

Journal 2000 Reports on a study conducted to evaluate issues relating to the advancement of women through the ranks of surgery and academic medicine. Concludes that many of the obstacles women face in this context appear to be based upon subtle, even unconscious, societal attitudes and behaviors. References Opinion 9.035. Colletti, Mulholland, & Sonnad, *Perceived Obstacles to Career Success for Women in Academic Surgery*, 135 Arch. Surg. 972, 976 (2000).

Journal 1996 Considers the pharmaceutical industry's failure to test products on female subjects. Comments on the potential for harm. Notes legal difficulties women experience when attempting to prove a drug was not adequately tested. Posits that litigation can affect the behavior of pharmaceutical companies. References Opinion 9.035. Comment, *Tort Reform to Ensure the Inclusion of Fertile Women in Early Phases of Commercial Drug Research*, 3 U. Chi. L. Sch. Roundtable 355, 359 (1996).

9.037 Signing Bonuses to Attract Graduates of US Medical Schools

Signing bonuses or compensation should not be offered or denied to a resident based on the country where the resident attended or graduated from medical school. (II, III, IV, VI)

Issued June 2000 based on the report "Signing Bonuses to Attract Graduates of US Medical Schools," adopted December 1999.

9.04 Discipline and Medicine

Incompetence, corruption, or dishonest or unethical conduct on the part of members of the medical profession is reprehensible. In addition to posing a real or potential threat to patients, such conduct undermines the public's confidence in the profession. A physician should expose, without fear or loss of favor, incompetent or corrupt, dishonest, or unethical conduct on the part of members of the profession. Questions of such conduct should be reported and reviewed in accordance with Opinion 9.031, "Reporting Impaired, Incompetent, or Unethical Colleagues."

Violation of governmental laws may subject the physician to civil or criminal liability. Expulsion from membership is the maximum penalty that may be imposed by a medical society upon a physician who violates the ethical standards involving a breach of moral duty or principle. However, medical societies have a civic and professional obligation to report to the appropriate governmental body or state board of medical examiners credible evidence that may come to their attention involving the alleged criminal conduct of any physician relating to the practice of medicine.

Although a physician charged with allegedly illegal conduct may be acquitted or exonerated in civil or criminal proceedings, this does not discharge a medical society from its obligation to initiate a disciplinary proceeding against a member with reference to the same conduct where there is credible evidence tending to establish unethical conduct.

The Council cannot pass judgment in advance on a situation that may later come before it on appeal. The Council cannot be an attorney for a society or a member thereof and later judge in the same factual situation. The local medical society has the initial obligation of determining all the facts and whether or not disciplinary action is indicated. Questions asking for a review of a proposed course of action or an evaluation of an existing factual situation should be presented to the appropriate official of the physician's local society. (II, III, VII)

Issued prior to April 1977. Updated June 1994.

Cal. App. 1956 Physician-petitioner sought mandamus against local medical association whose bylaws provided for the expulsion of any member who violated the Principles. Petitioner had been expelled under the provision and the expulsion was affirmed by the AMA's Judicial Council. The initial grounds for expulsion was alleged violation of Principles Ch. III, Art. IV, Sec.4 (1947) [now Opinions 9.04 and 9.07] for disparaging statements regarding another physician in a report used in judicial proceedings. In holding that application of the provision to petitioner was contrary to public policy, the court noted that the physician's statements had been made at the request of a civil litigant and enjoyed a statutory testimonial privilege. Further, the court found that the AMA's right to formulate ethical principles did not extend to defining the duties of witnesses. Expulsion was also based on petitioner's critical comments about other physicians overheard by their patients in violation of Principles Ch. III, Art. IV, Sec.1 (1947) [now Principle II and Opinion 9.04]. The court found application of this Principle under the circumstances reasonable and not contrary to public policy. *Bernstein v. Alameda-Contra Costa Medical Ass'n*, 139 Cal. App. 2d 241, 293 P.2d 862, 863, 863 nn.1, 2, 865 nn.4, 6, 866, 866 n.8, 867.

Ohio 1980 A physician, charged with violating the state medical licensing statute by distributing controlled substances without a proper license and writing prescriptions for narcotics in the name of one person when they were intended for another, challenged the state medical board's decision to suspend his license and place him on two years' probation. Under the statute, a physician could be disciplined for various activities including violation of any provision of a code of ethics of a national professional organization such as the AMA. The board found in part that the physician's actions violated Principles 4 and 7 (1957) [now Principles II and III and Opinions 8.06 and 9.04]. The trial court reversed, holding that the board had insufficient evidence for its decision, and the court of appeals affirmed. On appeal, the Supreme Court held that expert testimony was not required at a hearing before a medical licensing board because they were experts and could determine for themselves whether the Principles had been violated. *Arlen v. State*, 61 Ohio St. 2d 168, 399 N.E.2d 1251, 1252, 1253-54.

Journal 2007 Addresses physician liability for an extramarital affair with a patient's spouse. Concludes that such an affair should be regarded as a breach of a fiduciary duty. Quotes Preamble, Principles I, II, and VIII, and Opinions 8.145, 9.04, 9.123, and 10.015. Demaine, *"Playing Doctor" With the Patient's Spouse: Alternative Conceptions of Health Professional Liability,* 14 Va. J. Soc. Pol'y & L. 308, 325, 330-31, 331-32 (2007).

Journal 2001 Examines issues relating to health care cost containment. Concludes that, if physicians are to meet the goals assigned to them in a cost-constrained health care system, then professional standards must be reevaluated and modified to afford meaningful guidance for clinical decision-making in the face of health care spending controls. Quotes Opinions 2.03, 2.09, 2.095, 8.032, and 9.04. Cites Opinions 8.02, 8.021, 8.051, and 8.13. Agrawal, *Resuscitating Professionalism: Self-regulation in the Medical Marketplace,* 66 Mo. L. Rev. 341, 354, 355, 360, 361, 378, 388 (2001).

Journal 1994 Discusses the role of professional societies in establishing ethical guidelines for physicians in the context of using medical innovations and new technologies. Observes that these standards must be supplemented by additional external measures or incentives in order to be most effective. Cites Opinions 1.01, 1.02, 8.061, 9.04, and 9.131. Orentlicher, *The Influence of a Professional Organization on Physician Behavior,* 57 Alb. L. Rev. 583, 592, 593, 594, 595, 596 (1994).

9.045 Physicians With Disruptive Behavior

This Opinion is limited to the conduct of individual physicians and does not refer to physicians acting as a collective, which is considered separately in Opinion 9.025, "Collective Action and Patient Advocacy."*

(1) Personal conduct, whether verbal or physical, that negatively affects or that potentially may negatively affect patient care constitutes disruptive behavior. (This includes but is not limited to conduct that interferes with one's ability to work with other members of the health care team.) However, criticism that is offered in good faith with the aim of improving patient care should not be construed as disruptive behavior.

(2) Each medical staff should develop and adopt bylaw provisions or policies for intervening in situations where a physician's behavior is identified as disruptive. The medical staff bylaw provisions or policies should contain procedural safeguards that protect due process. Physicians exhibiting disruptive behavior should be referred to a medical staff wellness—or equivalent—committee.

(3) In developing policies that address physicians with disruptive behavior, attention should be paid to the following elements:

   (a) Clearly stating principal objectives in terms that ensure high standards of patient care and promote a professional practice and work environment.

   (b) Describing the behavior or types of behavior that will prompt intervention.

   (c) Providing a channel through which disruptive behavior can be reported and appropriately recorded. A single incident may not be sufficient for action, but each individual report may help identify a pattern that requires intervention.

   (d) Establishing a process to review or verify reports of disruptive behavior.

   (e) Establishing a process to notify a physician whose behavior is disruptive that a report has been made, and providing the physician with an opportunity to respond to the report.

(f) Including means of monitoring whether a physician's disruptive conduct improves after intervention.

(g) Providing for evaluative and corrective actions that are commensurate with the behavior, such as self-correction and structured rehabilitation. Suspension of responsibilities or privileges should be a mechanism of final resort. Additionally, institutions should consider whether the reporting requirements of Opinion 9.031, "Reporting Impaired, Incompetent, or Unethical Colleagues," apply in particular cases.

(h) Identifying which individuals will be involved in the various stages of the process, from reviewing reports to notifying physicians and monitoring conduct after intervention.

(i) Providing clear guidelines for the protection of confidentiality.

(j) Ensuring that individuals who report physicians with disruptive behavior are duly protected. (I, II, VIII)

Issued December 2000 based on the report "Physicians With Disruptive Behavior," adopted June 2000.

*Opinion 9.025, "Collection Action and Patient Advocacy," was updated and replaced by the current Opinion 9.025, "Advocacy for Changes in Law and Policy," June 2005.

Journal 2010 Observes that miscommunicated, misunderstood, and forgotten information among physicians, nurses, and other hospital staff leads to serious patient injury. Concludes that to assess if a client's injury resulted from a miscommunication among hospital staff, attorneys must examine hospital policies and procedures, medical ethics, and communications technology in relation to information sharing. Quotes Opinions 3.02 and 9.045. Cohen, Dicecco, & Levin, *Failure to Communicate: When It Comes to Hospital Patient Care, Communication Between Doctor and Nurse Should Be Seamless. If It's Not, Patients Suffer. Here's How to Find Out if a Miscommunication Is at the Core of Your Client's Case*, 46 Trial 38, 40-41 (May 2010).

Journal 2009 Discusses the appropriateness of immunity in the institutional peer-review process in the context of a competitive market for physician services. Concludes that while the peer-review process performs an essential function for ensuring patient safety and quality care, reforms are needed to avoid abuses and ensure the process is conducted effectively. Cites Opinion 9.045. Kinney, *Hospital Peer Review of Physicians: Does Statutory Immunity Increase Risk of Unwarranted Professional Injury?* 13 Mich. St. U. J. Med. & L. 57, 78 (2009).

Journal 2006 Analyzes dismissals of disruptive physicians from hospitals and the role of a whistleblower defense. Proposes hospitals should be granted a greater presumption of validity in dismissals made according to their bylaws. Quotes Opinion 9.045. Erwin, *Analyzing the Disruptive Physician: How State and Federal Courts Should Handle Whistleblower Cases Brought by Disruptive Physicians*, 44 Duq. L. Rev. 275, 276 (2006).

Journal 2006 Discusses the evolution of health law in Virginia. Concludes that the area of health law continues to expand, develop, and be refined. Cites Opinions 3.03, 3.08, 5.01, 5.015, 5.02, 5.04, 5.055, 6.02, 6.021, 6.03, 6.04, 7.03, 7.04, 7.05, 8.054, 8.08, 8.081, 8.085, 8.115, 8.12, 8.14, 8.145, 8.19, and 9.045. Guanzon, *Health Care Law*, 41 U. Rich. L. Rev. 179, 199 (2006).

9.05 Due Process

The basic principles of a fair and objective hearing should always be accorded to the physician or medical student whose professional conduct is being reviewed. The fundamental aspects of a fair hearing are a listing of specific charges, adequate notice of the right of a hearing, the opportunity to be present and to rebut the evidence, and the opportunity to present a defense. These principles apply when the hearing body is a medical society tribunal, medical staff committee, or other similar body composed of peers. The composition of committees sitting in judgment of medical students, residents, or fellows should include a significant number of persons at a similar level of training.

These principles of fair play apply in all disciplinary hearings and in any other type of hearing in which the reputation, professional status, or livelihood of the physician or medical student may be negatively impacted.

All physicians and medical students are urged to observe diligently these fundamental safeguards of due process whenever they are called upon to serve on a committee which will pass judgment on a peer. All medical societies and institutions are urged to review their constitutions and bylaws and/or policies to make sure that these instruments provide for such procedural safeguards. (II, III, VII)

Issued prior to April 1977. Updated June 1994.

Ill. App. 1979 Physician sued professional association of orthopaedic surgeons after it denied his application for membership. Plaintiff claimed he was not fully informed of the basis of denial, received no notice or opportunity to attend the hearing in which his application was considered, and was neither allowed to hear adverse evidence nor present a defense. Since the association's bylaws required adherence to the Principles, including Opinion 6.18 (1977) [now Opinion 9.05], which demanded that due process be afforded a physician whose conduct is being reviewed, plaintiff alleged that the association had violated its own procedures in the application process. The court held that the applicant did not have a right to have his application considered according to the association's bylaws and could not obtain judicial review without a showing of economic necessity. *Treister v. American Academy of Orthopaedic Surgeons*, 78 Ill. App. 3d 746, 396 N.E.2d 1225, 1228, 1232, 1238.

Va. App. 2003 Physician appealed board of medicine's license probation order for unprofessional conduct. Board found the physician's pattern of inappropriate advances toward medical students violated medical ethical standards. Appellate court reversed, holding that the evidence was insufficient to support Board's finding, since the ethical standards by which the physician should be adjudicated were not established by competent evidence. Quotes Opinions 3.08 and 9.05. *Goad v. Virginia Board of Medicine*, 40 Va. App. 621, 580 S.E.2d 494, 498, n.7, 499, n.9.

Journal 2006 Considers licensing and disciplinary procedures of medical boards. Concludes that the standard of proof for a finding of unprofessional conduct should be heightened from a preponderance of the evidence to clear and convincing evidence. Cites Opinion 9.05. Spece & Marchalonis, *Sound Constitutional Analysis, Moral Principle, and Wise Policy Judgment Require a Clear and Convincing Evidence Standard of Proof in Physician Disciplinary Proceedings*, 3 Ind. Health L. Rev. 107, 109 (2006).

Journal 1984 Discusses litigation by physicians in situations where medical staff privileges have been denied, curtailed, or revoked. Offers an analysis of the relevant legal theories and practice considerations that form part of hospital privilege antitrust litigation but concludes that litigation based on the Sherman Act—the predominant antitrust legislative scheme—in this context generally has been unsuccessful due to stringent requirements of proof. Cites Opinion 9.04 (1982) [now Opinion 9.05]. Tabor, *The Battle for Hospital Privileges*, 251 JAMA 1602, 1602 (1984).

Journal 1983 Describes special problems that may confront family physicians in the context of applying for hospital privileges. Offers a recommended approach to the application process which encourages physicians to document areas of residency training; become familiar with the hospital policies, guidelines, and procedures involved in applying for privileges; and solicit the support of staff physicians. Quotes Opinion 9.04 (1981) [now Opinion 9.05]. Pugno, *Hospital Privileges for Family Physicians: Rights, Rationale, and Resources*, 17 J. Fam. Practice 77, 79 (1983).).

9.055 Disputes Between Medical Supervisors and Trainees

Clear policies for handling complaints from medical students, resident physicians, and other staff should be established. These policies should include adequate provisions for protecting the confidentiality of complainants whenever possible. Confidentiality of complainants should be protected when doing so does not hinder the subject's ability to respond to the complaint. Access to employment and evaluation files should be carefully monitored to remove the possibility of tampering. Resident physicians should be permitted access to their employment files and also the right to copy the contents thereof, within the provisions of applicable federal and state laws.

Medical students, resident physicians, and other staff should refuse to participate in patient care ordered by their supervisors in those rare cases in which they believe the orders reflect serious errors in clinical or ethical judgment, or physician impairment, that could result in a threat of imminent harm to the patient or to others. In these rare cases, the complainant may withdraw from the care ordered by the supervisor, provided withdrawal does not itself threaten the patient's immediate welfare. The complainant should communicate his or her concerns to the physician issuing the orders and, if necessary, to the appropriate persons for mediating such disputes. Mechanisms for resolving these disputes, which require immediate resolution, should be in place. Third-party mediators of such disputes may include the chief of staff of the involved service, the chief resident, a designated member of the institutional grievance committee, or, in large institutions, an institutional ombudsperson largely outside of the established hospital staff hierarchy.

Retaliatory or punitive actions against those who raise complaints are unethical and are a legitimate cause for filing a grievance with the appropriate institutional committee. (II, III, VII)

Issued June 1994 based on the report "Disputes Between Medical Supervisors and Trainees," adopted December 1993 (*JAMA.* 1994;272:1861-1865).

Journal 1997 Discusses professionalism among attorneys. Emphasizes the need for individual accountability. Concludes that the rules of professional conduct should be modified to hold lawyers responsible for their actions. Quotes Opinion 9.055. Rice, *The Superior Orders Defense in Legal Ethics: Sending the Wrong Message to Young Lawyers,* 32 Wake Forest L. Rev. 887, 908-09 (1997).

Journal 1995 Examines the rights of health care professionals to refuse to participate in patient care on the basis of conscientious objection. Suggests steps that health care facilities may take when dealing with health care professionals who object to participating in patient care. Quotes Principles I and VI and Opinions 1.02, 2.035, and 9.055. Dellinger & Vickery, *When Staff Object to Participating in Care,* 28 J. Health & Hospital Law 269, 272, 276 (1995).

9.06 Free Choice

Free choice of physicians is the right of every individual. One may select and change at will one's physicians, or one may choose a medical care plan such as that provided by a closed panel or group practice or health maintenance or service organization. The individual's freedom to select a preferred system of health care and free competition among physicians and alternative systems of care are prerequisites of ethical practice and optimal patient care.

In choosing to subscribe to a health maintenance or service organization or in choosing or accepting treatment in a particular hospital, the patient is thereby accepting limitations upon free choice of medical services.

The need of an individual for emergency treatment in cases of accident or sudden illness may, as a practical matter, preclude free choice of a physician, particularly where there is loss of consciousness.

Although the concept of free choice assures that an individual can generally choose a physician, likewise a physician may decline to accept that individual as a patient. In selecting the physician of choice, the patient may sometimes be obliged to pay for medical services which might otherwise be paid by a third party. (VI)

Issued prior to April 1977.

E.D. N.Y. 1975 Medical laboratories sought injunction against city's award of exclusive contracts for Medicaid services. The court granted a preliminary injunction and held that the laboratories had a substantial probability of success on the merits of the claim that Medicaid recipients would be deprived of statutory right of free choice of providers. In balancing the equities, the court also noted that the contracts would create an ethical dilemma for physicians who are required to provide patients with free choice of ancillary services under Opinions and Reports of the Judicial Council Sec. 1, Paras. 6 and 14 (1971) [now Opinions 8.03, 8.06, and 9.06]. *Bay Ridge Diagnostic Laboratory, Inc. v. Dumpson, 400 F. Supp. 1104, 1109-10.*

Ariz. 1999 Medical practice sought to enforce a restrictive covenant with defendant-physician. The trial court denied the plaintiff's request for a preliminary injunction and found that the restrictive covenant was unenforceable. The Arizona Supreme Court held that covenants not to compete between physicians will be strictly construed for reasonableness. Under this analysis, the court found that the restrictive covenant was unreasonable, overbroad, and unenforceable. The court quoted Opinions 9.02 and 9.06, recognizing that the AMA discourages restrictive covenants and supports free choice and competition. *Valley Medical Specialists v. Farber, 194 Ariz. 363, 982 P.2d 1277, 1282.*

Ariz. 1965 Physician appealed denial of medical license which was based on alleged violations of local medical society rules and Principles 3, 5, and 10 (1957) [now Principles III and VII and Opinions 3.01, 8.11, and 9.06]. Alleged violations included treating a patient without first obtaining a prior treating physician's permission, inadequate patient care, performing operations without hospital privileges, and signing the medical record of a deceased patient who had been treated by interns. The court held that the evidence failed to show any clear violation of the Principles and that a local medical society had no right to prescribe a code of ethics for state licensing purposes. *Arizona State Bd. of Medical Examiners v. Clark, 97 Ariz. 205, 398 P.2d 908, 914-915, 915 n.3.*

Cal. App. 1978 Surviving spouse sued physicians who were on emergency surgical call panel for malpractice where patient died during surgery. Although defendants claimed immunity under state Good Samaritan statute, the court held the statute inapplicable since the legislative purpose was to encourage physicians to render care on an irregular basis to unattended persons discovered by chance at the scene of an emergency. In so holding, the court noted that Principle 5 (1957) [now Principle VI and Opinions 8.11 and 9.06] imposed an ethical duty to render emergency medical care. *Colby v. Schwartz, 78 Cal. App. 3d 885, 144 Cal. Rptr. 624, 627 n.2.*

Ill. 2006 Physicians appealed a grant of preliminary injunction enforcing restrictive covenants in their employment contracts. Quoting Opinions 9.02, 9.06, and 10.01 and referencing Opinion 8.115, the Illinois Supreme Court gave thorough consideration to the AMA's position on restrictive covenants. While acknowledging the ethical problems associated with such contracts, the court found the covenants reasonable in scope. The decision to ban restrictive covenants, the court reasoned, was best left to the legislature. *Mohanty v. St. John Heart Clinic, S.C., 225 Ill.2d 52, 866 N.E.2d 85, 94, 106-07, 107-08.*

Ill. App. 2000 Physician challenged trial court's decision upholding noncompete clause in the physician's employment contract with a health care provider. The appellate court reversed the decision, quoting Opinions 9.02 (1986) and 9.06 (1982). The court stated that the AMA disfavors the use of any restrictive employment or partnership agreements among physicians and emphasized the fact that such agreements are not in the public interest. The court also noted that patients might suffer if such agreements are upheld. *Carter-Shields v. Alton Health Institute, 317 Ill. App. 3d 260, 739 N.E.2d 569, 576-77, vacated 201 Ill. 2d 441, 777 N.E.2d 948 (2002).*

Ohio App. 1991 Medical corporation sought an injunction to enforce a covenant not to compete against defendant-physician. The lower court granted summary judgment based on a referee's report which concluded that, under Principle VI and Opinions 6.11, 9.02, and 9.06 (1989) restrictive covenants were per se unenforceable as a matter of public policy. While recognizing a strong public interest in allowing open access to health care, the appellate court in reversing held that Opinion 9.02, which applied specifically to restrictive covenants, only "discouraged" such covenants. *Ohio Urology, Inc. v. Poll, 72 Ohio. App. 446, 450, 451, 594 N.E.2d 1027, 1030, 1031.*

Tenn. 2005 Respondent, a private medical practice, filed suit to enforce a noncompetition covenant contained in a physician's employment contract. The trial court found that the covenant was enforceable and the court of appeals affirmed. The Tennessee Supreme Court reversed. Quoting Opinions 9.02 and 9.06 it found that such covenants are not enforceable because they violate public policy. *Murfreesboro Med. Clinic v. Udom, 166 S.W.3d 674, 679, 684, 685.*

Wash. 1951 Plaintiff, a charitable, not-for-profit medical corporation, offered prepaid health care services to members and their families. Suit was filed against county medical society and others for damages and injunction for defendants' alleged efforts to monopolize prepaid medical care in area and unlawfully restrain competition by plaintiff and its physicians. Defendants alleged as affirmative defense that their efforts were designed to curb unethical prepaid contract practice by plaintiff. Court examined at length AMA's position regarding contract practice including Principles Ch. III, Art. VI, Secs. 3 and 4 (1947) [now Principle VI and Opinions 8.05 and 9.06] concluding nothing in plaintiff's practice violated the AMA's ethical guidelines. Further, quoting Principles Ch. III, Art. III, Sec.1 (1947) [now Opinion 8.04] dealing with consultations, court noted that defendants' efforts impeded plaintiff's physicians from obtaining consultations. Court concluded that defendants' actions constituted unlawful, monopolistic behavior and issued an injunction, although it declined to award damages. *Group Health Coop. v. King County Medical Soc'y, 39 Wash. 2d 586, 237 P.2d 737, 744, 750-51, 759-60.*

Journal 2011 Examines the Patient Protection and Affordable Care Act and its impact on patient access to physician services. Also considers the possibility that physicians might be required to provide services to all patients as a condition to practice. Concludes that regulations that try to conscript physician services would be practically ineffective, legally dubious, and unwise public policy. Quotes Opinion 9.06 and 10.015. Cites Opinion 2.09. Kapp, *Conscripted Physician Services and the Public's Health, 39 J. L. Med. & Ethics 414, 414, 418 (2011).*

Journal 2010 Discusses the background and policies of traditional noncompete agreements and evaluates the arguments underlying the use of restrictive covenants in the health care field. Concludes that enforcing physician noncompete clauses ultimately hurts patients, and that courts should create an exception regarding such clauses similar to that for attorney noncompete clauses. Quotes Opinion 9.06. Cites Opinion 9.02. Klimkina, *Are Noncompete Contracts Between Physicians Bad Medicine? Advocating in the Affirmative by Drawing a Public Policy Parallel to the Legal Profession, 98 Ky. L. J. 131, 147-148 (2010).*

Journal 2009 Examines the role of physicians during natural and man-made disasters. Concludes hospitals must make plans to define disaster response procedures that shift responsibility for survival from the physician to the community. Quotes Code of Ethics, Ch. III, Art. I §1 (1847) [now Opinion 9.067], Principle 5 (1957) [now Principle VI], Principle VI, and Opinions 2.23, 9.067, and 9.131. Cites Opinions 9.06, 9.067, and 9.12. Ahronheim, *Service by Health Care Providers in a Public Health Emergency: The Physician's Duty and the Law, 12 J. Health Care L. & Pol'y 195, 209-11, 215, 225 (2009).*

Journal 2009 Discusses the judicial standard for reviewing physician noncompete covenants. Concludes courts should apply a strict standard to such covenants, rather than declare the covenants per se invalid. Quotes Principles IV and VII, Principles of Medical Ethics §5 (1957) [now Principle VI], Code of Medical Ethics Ch. II, Art. I §3 (1847) [now Opinion 5.02], Opinion 9.02, and Code of Medical Ethics Ch. II, Art. I §4 (1847) [now Opinion 9.09]. Cites Opinions 8.041, 8.115, 9.02, 9.06, 9.065, 9.067, 10.01, and 10.015. Koons, *Physician Employee Non-Compete Agreements on the Examining Table: The Need to Better Protect Patients' and the Public's Interests in Indiana, 6 Ind. Health L. Rev. 253, 272-77, 280-81 (2009).*

Journal 2007 Reviews the legal and ethical problems surrounding concierge medical practice. Concludes that concierge medicine should remain restricted to a small class of wealthy individuals. Cites Opinions 8.05, 8.055, 8.115, 9.06, and 9.065. Carnahan, *Concierge Medicine: Legal and Ethical Issues, 35 J. L. Med. & Ethics 211, 212-13 (2007).*

Journal 2006 Discusses the Tennessee Supreme Court decision prohibiting physician noncompete agreements. Suggests the court should have adopted a standard of reasonableness for noncompete agreements. Quotes Opinion 9.02. Cites Opinion 9.06. Carr, *Contracts— Murfreesboro Medical Clinic, P.A. v. Udom: Physician Noncompete Agreements Go Under the Knife:*

The Tennessee Supreme Court Rejects Physician Noncompete Agreements, 36 U. Mem. L. Rev. 1115, 1128, 1131 (2006).

Journal 2006 Examines physician restrictive covenants. Concludes that under the current balancing test, courts should give considerable weight to the public interest in preserving the physician-patient relationship. Quotes Opinions 9.02 and 9.06. Cites Opinions 6.11, 8.11, 8.115, and 9.06. Malloy, *Physician Restrictive Covenants: The Neglect of Incumbent Patient Interests, 41 Wake Forest L. Rev. 189, 207-08, 217, 218 (2006).*

Journal 2006 Discusses noncompete agreements in surgeon employment contracts. Concludes that covenants not to compete should be unenforceable per se against surgeons. Quotes Opinions 9.02 and 9.06. Wyatt, *Buy Out or Get Out: Why Covenants Not to Compete in Surgeon Employment Contracts Are Truly Bad Medicine, 45 Washburn L. J. 715, 720 (2006).*

Journal 2005 Discusses the ban of physician noncompetition covenants by the Tennessee Supreme Court. Concludes that new contractual terms will need to be drafted to balance employer and employee interests in the medical profession. Quotes Opinion 9.06. References Opinion 9.02. Schuler, *Knock Out? Supreme Court Deals a Blow to Non-Competes for Docs, but This Fight Is Not Over, 41 Tenn. B. J. 16, 19 (Dec. 2005).*

Journal 2003 Highlights the legal and ethical concerns surrounding use of noncompetition clauses. Concludes that physicians should carefully evaluate these clauses given their likely enforceability. Quotes Opinions 9.02, 9.06, 10.01, and 10.015. Loeser, *The Legal, Ethical, and Practical Implications of Noncompetition Clauses: What Physicians Should Know Before They Sign, 31 J. L. Med. & Ethics 283, 286, 287, 290 (2003).*

Journal 1999 Discusses potential conflicts between a criminal defense attorney's religious beliefs and representation of the client. Explores theories that would allow an attorney to put religious beliefs over the client's interest. Offers analogies within the physician-patient relationship. Concludes that a defense attorney is bound by duty and must set aside conflicting religious beliefs. Quotes Principle VI and Opinions 8.11, 9.06, and 9.12. Reza, *Religion and the Public Defender, 26 Fordham Urb. L. J. 1051, 1062, 1063 (1999).*

Journal 1999 Discusses the need for physicians to advocate on behalf of patients' rights in the context of health care delivery. Evaluates the nature and scope of the physician's role as advocate, noting that physicians cannot be expected to engage in attorney-like advocacy. Quotes Principles IV and VI, Fundamental Elements (2), (4), and (6) [now Opinion 10.01], Patient Responsibilities 5 [now Opinion 10.02], and Opinions 2.03, 2.07, 2.09, 2.16, 2.19, 3.06, 4.01, 4.04, 6.01, 7.02, 8.02, 8.03, 8.13, 8.132, 9.06, 9.07, and 9.131. Cites Opinions 5.05, 5.09, 7.01, 8.135, and 9.02. Sage, *Physicians as Advocates, 35 Hous. L. Rev. 1529, 1537, 1541, 1542, 1552-53, 1554, 1556, 1557, 1559, 1561-62, 1564, 1571, 1574, 1576, 1580 (1999).*

Journal 1998 Discusses conflicts of interest in the physician-patient relationship arising out of use of financial incentives by managed care organizations. Considers how such conflicts are dealt with in the attorney-client relationship. Suggests that a financial incentive should be legally denounced if it unreasonably interferes with a physician's duty to properly care for and treat patients. Quotes Preamble, Fundamental Elements (1) [now Opinion 10.01], and Opinions 4.04, 5.01, 8.03, 8.13, and 9.06. Cites Fundamental Elements (4) [now Opinion 10.01] and Opinions 2.07, 2.08, and 2.132. Hall, *Third-Party Payor Conflicts of Interest in Managed Care: A Proposal for Regulation Based on the Model Rules of Professional Conduct, 29 Seton Hall L. Rev. 95, 96, 107, 108, 109, 110, 111, 112, 134, 135, 136 (1998).*

Journal 1998 Discusses the ramifications of physician license revocation for failing to pay child support. Points out that patients stand to lose access to trusted physicians and confidence in the health care system. Concludes that children need the most protection and that patients will have an easier time finding another physician than children will have finding another means for support. Quotes Opinion 5.05. Cites Opinions 9.02 and 9.06. Noyes, *Higher Penalties for Failing to Pay Child Support: A Look at Medical License Revocation, 19 J. Legal Med. 127, 138 (1998).*

Journal 1997 Examines noncompetition clauses in the medical field. Reviews policy concerns and historical and common-law analyses of agreements not to compete. Posits that, the more commercialized the medical profession becomes, the more noncompetition clauses infringe upon the physician-patient relationship and patients' rights. Quotes Opinions 9.02 and 9.06. Cites Preamble and Opinion 6.11. Comment, *Noncompetition Clauses in Physician Employment Contracts in Oregon, 76 Or. L. Rev. 195, 204-06 (1997).*

Journal 1997 Examines the evolution of the Indiana health care system. Discusses developments in Indiana jurisprudence regarding the physician-patient relationship. Explores various challenges facing the relationship and recognizes the need for legal rules to help address these challenges. Quotes Opinion 8.08. Cites Opinions 2.20, 9.06, and 9.12. Kinney & Selby, *History and Jurisprudence of the Physician-Patient Relationship in Indiana*, 30 Ind. L. Rev. 263, 269, 272, 276 (1997).

Journal 1995 Analyzes South Carolina judicial treatment of covenants not to compete and liquidated damages provisions. Considers approaches in other jurisdictions and proposes guidelines for drafting contractual agreements. Quotes Opinion 9.06. Cites Opinion 9.01 (1982) [now Opinion 9.02]. Note, *Covenants Not to Compete and Liquidated Damages Clauses: Diagnosis and Treatment for Physicians*, 46 S. C. L. Rev. 505, 514 (1995).

Journal 1991 Considers the question of whether physicians should provide medical treatment to those who come to them for second opinions. Concludes that each physician must individually decide whether to treat these patients. Quotes Opinions 6.11, 9.06, and 9.12. Cites Opinion 9.02. Ile, *Should Physicians Treat Patients Who Seek Second Opinions?* 266 JAMA 273, 274 (1991).

Journal 1987 Concludes that a policy or practice of active voluntary euthanasia is not desirable, linking a moral prohibition against active voluntary euthanasia to the moral prohibition against physicians actively participating in capital punishment. In place of any practice of active voluntary euthanasia, recommends increased use of hospices, greater emphasis on training physicians to care for the dying patient, and further research aimed at producing symptomatic relief in dying patients. Cites Opinions 2.06, 8.10 (1986) [now Opinion 8.11], and 9.06. Shewmon, *Active Voluntary Euthanasia: A Needless Pandora's Box*, 3 Issues in Law and Med. 219, 220, 222, 243 (1987).

9.065 Caring for the Poor

Each physician has an obligation to share in providing care to the indigent. The measure of what constitutes an appropriate contribution may vary with circumstances such as community characteristics, geographic location, the nature of the physician's practice and specialty, and other conditions. All physicians should work to ensure that the needs of the poor in their communities are met. Caring for the poor should be a regular part of the physician's practice schedule.

In the poorest communities, it may not be possible to meet the needs of the indigent for physicians' services by relying solely on local physicians. The local physicians should be able to turn for assistance to their colleagues in prosperous communities, particularly those in close proximity.

Physicians are meeting their obligation, and are encouraged to continue to do so, in a number of ways such as seeing indigent patients in their offices at no cost or at reduced cost, serving at freestanding or hospital clinics that treat the poor, and participating in government programs that provide health care to the poor. Physicians can also volunteer their services at weekend clinics for the poor and at shelters for battered women or the homeless.

In addition to meeting their obligation to care for the indigent, physicians can devote their energy, knowledge, and prestige to designing and lobbying at all levels for better programs to provide care for the poor. (I, VII)

Issued June 1994 based on the report "Caring for the Poor," adopted December 1992 (JAMA. 1993;269:2533-2537).

Journal 2011 Analyzes the ability of Medicaid patients to access subspecialty care in Connecticut based on a questionnaire directed towards physicians. Concludes reform in Medicaid reimbursement, changes in licensing requirements, new rules for participation in Medicaid, and greater regulation of community service could help equalize Medicaid patients' access to subspecialty care. Quotes Opinions 2.095 and 9.065. Grewal, Sofair, Guevara, &

Manthous, *Medicaid Patients' Access to Subspecialty Care in Connecticut*, 75 Conn. Med. 489, 490 (2011).

Journal 2011 Examines the medical-legal partnership (MLP) and its impact on legal services, health care delivery, and public policy. Concludes MLPs provide a unique opportunity to reach vulnerable populations and build advocacy capacity among all health care professionals by addressing health concerns with legal solutions as part of regular care. Quotes Opinion 9.065. Tames, Cotter, Melendez, Scudder, & Colvin, *Medical-Legal Partnership: Evolution or Revolution*, 45 Clearinghouse Rev. 124, 127 (2011).

Journal 2009 Discusses the judicial standard for reviewing physician noncompete covenants. Concludes courts should apply a strict standard to such covenants, rather than declare the covenants per se invalid. Quotes Principles IV and VII, Principles of Medical Ethics §5 (1957) [now Principle VI], Code of Medical Ethics Ch. II, Art. I §3 (1847) [now Opinion 5.02], Opinion 9.02, and Code of Medical Ethics Ch. II, Art. I §4 (1847) [now Opinion 9.09]. Cites Opinions 8.041, 8.115, 9.02, 9.06, 9.065, 9.067, 10.01, and 10.015. Koons, *Physician Employee Non-Compete Agreements on the Examining Table: The Need to Better Protect Patients' and the Public's Interests in Indiana*, 6 Ind. Health L. Rev. 253, 272-77, 280-81 (2009).

Journal 2008 Explores interdisciplinary training for law and medical students to advance broad social goals. Concludes partnerships in legal and medical education are useful for training effective practitioners in both fields and for increasing cooperation between physicians and lawyers to better serve the community. Quotes Opinion 9.065. Tyler, *Allies Not Adversaries: Teaching Collaboration to the Next Generation of Doctors and Lawyers to Address Social Inequality*, 11 J. Health Care L. & Pol'y 249, 259-60 (2008).

Journal 2007 Reviews the legal and ethical problems surrounding concierge medical practice. Concludes that concierge medicine should remain restricted to a small class of wealthy individuals. Cites Opinions 8.05, 8.055, 8.115, 9.06, and 9.065. Carnahan, *Concierge Medicine: Legal and Ethical Issues*, 35 J. L. Med. & Ethics 211, 212-13 (2007).

Journal 2007 Reviews Deborah Rhode's analysis of pro bono obligations of lawyers from her book, *Pro Bono in Principle and in Practice: Public Service and the Professions*. Concludes that a mandatory pro bono requirement is a better solution than an incentive-based system. Quotes Opinion 10.01. References Opinion 9.065. Lininger, *From Park Place to Community Chest: Rethinking Lawyers' Monopoly*, 101 Nw. U. L. Rev. 1343, 1349 (2007).

Journal 2006 Explores the legal and ethical issues surrounding concierge medicine. Concludes that concierge medicine is best restricted to a small class of wealthy individuals. Quotes Principle IX and Opinion 8.055. Cites Principle VI and Opinions 8.055, 8.11, 8.115, 9.065, and 10.05. Carnahan, *Law, Medicine, and Wealth: Does Concierge Medicine Promote Health Care Choice, or Is It a Barrier to Access?* 17 Stan. L. & Pol'y Rev. 121, 149-50, 151, 152, 153-54 (2006).

Journal 2006 Evaluates hospital-based charity health care programs. Concludes that improvements to these programs will benefit both patients and business for the hospital. References Opinion 9.065. Elliott, *The Charity Care Crisis—Where Does the Money Go?* 8 J. Health Care Compliance. 11, 13 (September/October 2006).

Journal 2006 Evaluates legal implications of consumer-driven health care. Concludes that a system of consumer-driven health care is feasible and offers many benefits to patients. Quotes Opinions 8.055 and 9.065. Hall, *Paying for What You Get and Getting What You Pay For: Legal Responses to Consumer-Driven Health Care*, 69 Law & Contemp. Prob. 159, 165 (2006).

Journal 2006 Discusses the role of EMTALA in mandating care for the uninsured. Concludes EMTALA is inadequate and Congress should take steps toward establishing a program for universal health care. Quotes Principle IX, Ch. II, Art. V, Sec. 9 (May 1847) [now Opinion 9.065], and Ch. III, Art. I, Sec. 3 (May 1847) [now Opinion 9.065]. Hermer, *The Scapegoat: EMTALA and Emergency Department Overcrowding*, 14 J. L. & Pol'y 695, 713-14 (2006).

Journal 2005 Argues that it is in the best interest of the public to ensure that all have access to the legal system. Concludes that government funding must be available in Wyoming to increase the availability of legal services to those in need. References Opinion 9.065. Burman, *Wyoming Attorneys' Pro Bono "Obligation,"* 5 Wyo. L. Rev. 421, 428 (2005).

Journal 2005 Discusses ethical, legal, and policy issues associated with treatment and research involving patients who are in a persistent vegetative or minimally conscious state. Concludes that patients in these states are at risk for therapeutic failures until physicians can more accurately determine which patients will benefit from treatment and accurately convey such information to families or surrogates. Quotes Principles VII and IX and Opinions 8.031, 8.0315, 9.065, 10.01, and 10.015. Tovino & Winslade, *A Primer on the Law and Ethics of Treatment, Research, and Public Policy in the Context of Severe Traumatic Brain Injury, 14 Ann. Health L. 1, 18, 38, 39, 40, 41 (2005).*

Journal 2000 Discusses and evaluates different systems for addressing consumer concerns about managed health care. Asserts that current legal systems for identifying and resolving consumer concerns are not understood by most consumers and are not accessible by many, especially the uninsured. Concludes that several immediate steps are realistic for moving toward reform. Cites Principle VI. References Opinions 8.13 and 9.065. Kinney, *Tapping and Resolving Consumer Concerns About Health Care, 26 Am. J. Law & Med. 335, 337, 375 (2000).*

Journal 2000 Evaluates recent Texas legislation that affords immunity to health care professionals who provide free health care services to the poor. Concludes that such legislation creates a dual standard of care, requiring indigent patients to forfeit their legal rights in exchange for health care. Quotes Opinion 10.01. References Opinion 9.065. Pulido, *Immunity of Volunteer Health Care Providers in Texas: Bartering Legal Rights for Free Medical Care, 2 Scholar: St. Mary's L. Rev. Minority Issues 323, 330 (2000).*

Journal 1999 Discusses regulatory concerns regarding genetic technology. Provides ideas on how society might regulate genetic enhancements. Argues that a variety of means of regulation need to be utilized to govern genetic technology. Quotes Opinion 2.11. Cites Opinion 9.065. References Opinion 2.138. Mehlman, *How Will We Regulate Genetic Enhancement? 34 Wake Forest L. Rev. 671, 693-94, 695 (1999).*

Journal 1997 Considers the current approach to health care in the US. Examines financing mechanisms, and suggests that reform could be effected through a decentralized, community-based approach. Proposes use of volunteer systems in which medical personnel would care for certain patients free of charge or at reduced rates. Quotes Fundamental Elements (6) [now Opinion 10.01]. References Opinion 9.065. Solomon & Asaro, *Community-Based Health Care: A Legal and Policy Analysis, 24 Fordham Urb. L. J. 235, 276-77 (1997).*

Journal 1996 Describes the problem of lack of access to medical care by the indigent. Recognizes the commitment of the medical profession to providing care for indigent patients. Observes that state initiatives that provide physicians tort immunity in exchange for volunteer service can improve access to care by the indigent. Quotes Fundamental Elements (6) [now Opinion 10.01]. References Opinion 9.065. Comment, *Statutory Immunity for Volunteer Physicians: A Vehicle for Reaffirmation of the Doctor's Beneficent Duties—Absent the Rights Talk, 1 Widener L. Symp. J. 425, 448, 449 (1996).*

9.0651 Financial Barriers to Health Care Access

Health care is a fundamental human good because it affects our opportunity to pursue life goals, reduces our pain and suffering, helps prevent premature loss of life, and provides information needed to plan for our lives. As professionals, physicians individually and collectively have an ethical responsibility to ensure that all persons have access to needed care regardless of their economic means. In view of this obligation:

(1) Individual physicians should take steps to promote access to care for individual patients.

(2) Individual physicians should help patients obtain needed care through public or charitable programs when patients cannot do so themselves.

(3) Physicians, individually and collectively through their professional organizations and institutions, should participate in the political process as advocates for patients (or support those who do) so as to diminish financial obstacles to access health care.

(4) The medical profession must work to ensure that societal decisions about the distribution of health resources safeguard the interests of all patients and promote access to health services.

(5) All stakeholders in health care, including physicians, health facilities, health insurers, professional medical societies, and public policymakers must work together to ensure sufficient access to appropriate health care for all people. (VI, IX)

Issued November 2009 based on the report "Financial Barriers to Health Care Access," adopted June 2009.

9.067 Physician Obligation in Disaster Preparedness and Response

National, regional, and local responses to epidemics, terrorist attacks, and other disasters require extensive involvement of physicians. Because of their commitment to care for the sick and injured, individual physicians have an obligation to provide urgent medical care during disasters. This ethical obligation holds even in the face of greater than usual risks to their own safety, health, or life. The physician workforce, however, is not an unlimited resource; therefore, when participating in disaster responses, physicians should balance immediate benefits to individual patients with ability to care for patients in the future.

In preparing for epidemics, terrorist attacks, and other disasters, physicians as a profession must provide medical expertise and work with others to develop public health policies that are designed to improve the effectiveness and availability of medical care during such events. These policies must be based on sound science and respect for patients. Physicians also must advocate for and, when appropriate, participate in the conduct of ethically sound biomedical research to inform these policy decisions. Moreover, individual physicians should take appropriate advance measures to ensure their ability to provide medical services at the time of disasters, including the acquisition and maintenance of relevant knowledge. (I, V, VI, VII, VIII)

Issued December 2004 based on the report "Physician Obligation in Disaster Preparedness and Response," adopted June 2004.

Journal 2010 Addresses whether health care workers should receive priority in treatment during an influenza epidemic. Using distributive justice principles and practical considerations, concludes that health care workers should not get priority treatment in such an epidemic and that medical utility should be the sole criterion in determining any treatment priority. Quotes Opinion 2.03. Cites Opinion 9.067. Rothstein, *Should Health Care Providers Get Treatment Priority in an Influenza Pandemic?* 38 J. L. Med. & Ethics 412, 413, 415 (2010).

Journal 2009 Examines the role of physicians during natural and man-made disasters. Concludes hospitals must make plans to define disaster response procedures that shift responsibility for survival from the physician to the community. Quotes Code of Ethics, Ch. III, Art. I §1 (1847) [now Opinion 9.067], Principle 5 (1957) [now Principle VI], Principle VI, and Opinions 2.23, 9.067, and 9.131. Cites Opinions 9.06, 9.067, and 9.12. Ahronheim, *Service by Health Care Providers in a Public Health Emergency: The Physician's Duty and the Law*, 12 J. Health Care L. & Pol'y 195, 209-11, 215, 225 (2009).

Journal 2009 Discusses the impact of pandemic influenza on customary legal standards of care imposed by state and federal regulatory authorities and the tort system. Concludes alternative standards of care should be developed in preparation for pandemic influenza to ensure health care providers are equipped to slow the spread of disease while caring for the sick. Quotes Opinion 9.067. Kinney, McCabe, Gilbert, & Shisler, *Altered Standards of Care for Health Care Providers in the Pandemic Influenza*, 6 Ind. Health L. Rev. 1, 14 (2009).

Journal 2009 Discusses the judicial standard for reviewing physician noncompete covenants. Concludes courts should apply a strict standard to such covenants, rather than declare the covenants per se invalid. Quotes Principles IV and VII, Principles of Medical Ethics §5 (1957) [now Principle VI], Code of Medical Ethics Ch. II, Art. I §3 (1847) [now Opinion 5.02], Opinion 9.02, and Code of Medical Ethics Ch. II, Art. I §4 (1847) [now Opinion 9.09]. Cites Opinions 8.041, 8.115, 9.02, 9.06, 9.065, 9.067, 10.01, and 10.015. Koons, *Physician Employee Non-Compete Agreements on the Examining Table: The Need to Better Protect Patients' and the Public's Interests in Indiana,* 6 Ind. Health L. Rev. 253, 272-77, 280-81 (2009).

Journal 2008 Examines the legal obligations of health care professionals during pandemics and discusses penalties imposed for refusing to do such work during a pandemic. Concludes policy makers should institute mechanisms to encourage professionals voluntarily to work during a pandemic. Quotes Opinions 9.067 and 9.131. Coleman, *Beyond the Call of Duty: Compelling Health Care Professionals to Work During an Influenza Pandemic,* 94 Iowa L. Rev. 1, 12 (2008).

Journal 2008 Examines the ethical reasons why physicians choose to provide treatment in disaster situations, even at great risk to themselves. Concludes that individual values play a substantial role in such decision making. Quotes Preamble, Opinion 9.131, and Ch. III, Art. 1, Sec. 1 (1847) [now Opinions 2.25 and 9.067]. Iserson, Heine, Larkin, Moskop, Baruch, & Aswegan, *Fight or Flight: The Ethics of Emergency Physician Disaster Response,* 51 Annals of Emergency Med. 345, 346-47 (2008).

Journal 2008 Discusses the duty of physicians to participate in pandemic care. Concludes that the extent of personal risk a physician is obligated to take has a limit, although the limit has yet to be clearly defined. Quotes Ch. III, Art. I, Sec. 1 (1847) [now Opinions 2.25 and 9.067]. Meerschaert, *Physicians' Duty to Participate in Pandemic Care,* 300 JAMA 284, 284 (2008).

Journal 2007 Examines physicians' duty to treat victims of highly infectious diseases during an epidemic. Concludes that no clear duty exists, and that if physicians are compelled to provide care by law they must be afforded sufficient due process to protect their property interests in their medical licenses. Quotes Ch. III, Art. I, Sec. I (May 1847) [now Opinions 2.25 and 9.067] and Opinion 9.131. References Principle 10 (1957) [now Principle VII]. Schwartz, *Doubtful Duty: Physicians' Legal Obligation to Treat During an Epidemic,* 60 Stan. L. Rev. 657, 662, 663 (2007).

Journal 2007 Speculates on the availability of funding for hospitals confronted with an infectious disease pandemic. Concludes that new legislation is required to ensure adequate funding for hospitals in such a situation. Quotes Ch. III, Art. I, Sec. 1 (May 1847) [now Opinions 2.25 and 9.067]. Williams, *Fluconomics: Preserving Our Hospital Infrastructure During and After a Pandemic,* 7 Yale J. Health Pol'y L. & Ethics 99, 115 (2007).

9.07   The previous Opinion 9.07, "Medical Testimony," issued June 1986, was replaced by the current Opinion 9.07, "Medical Testimony." (I, III, IV, V)

9.07 Medical Testimony

In various legal and administrative proceedings, medical evidence is critical. As citizens and as professionals with specialized knowledge and experience, physicians have an obligation to assist in the administration of justice.

When a legal claim pertains to a patient the physician has treated, the physician must hold the patient's medical interests paramount, including the confidentiality of the patient's health information, unless the physician is authorized or legally compelled to disclose the information.

Physicians who serve as fact witnesses must deliver honest testimony. This requires that they engage in continuous self-examination to ensure that their testimony represents the facts of the case. When treating physicians are called upon to testify in matters that could adversely impact their patients' medical interests, they should decline to testify unless the patient consents or unless ordered to do so by legally constituted authority. If, as a result of legal proceedings, the patient and the physician are placed in adversarial positions it may be appropriate for a treating physician to transfer the care of the patient to another physician.

When physicians choose to provide expert testimony, they should have recent and substantive experience or knowledge in the area in which they testify, and be committed to evaluating cases objectively and to providing an independent opinion. Their testimony should reflect current scientific thought and standards of care that have gained acceptance among peers in the relevant field. If a medical witness knowingly provides testimony based on a theory not widely accepted in the profession, the witness should characterize the theory as such. Also, testimony pertinent to a standard of care must consider standards that prevailed at the time the event under review occurred.

All physicians must accurately represent their qualifications and must testify honestly.

Physician testimony must not be influenced by financial compensation; for example, it is unethical for a physician to accept compensation that is contingent upon the outcome of litigation.

Organized medicine, including state and specialty societies, and medical licensing boards can help maintain high standards for medical witnesses by assessing claims of false or misleading testimony and issuing disciplinary sanctions as appropriate. (II and VII)

Issued December 2004 based on the report "Medical Testimony," adopted June 2004.

M.D. Pa. 1947 Motion for new trial in malpractice action following verdict for defendant-physicians. Patient had been treated surgically for tube-ovarian abscess, had profuse postoperative bleeding, and died of infection secondary to ruptured ectopic pregnancy. Plaintiff moved for a new trial on grounds that an officer of a local medical society persuaded plaintiff's expert not to testify. Although it denied the motion on other grounds, the court criticized the officer's conduct, noting that it was contrary to Principles Ch. 1, Sec. 7 (1947) [now Opinion 9.07], but refused to impute the impropriety to the defendants. *McHugh v. Audet, 72 F. Supp. 394, 404.*

Fed. Cl. 2010 Plaintiffs alleged that a vaccine administered by the defendant-physician caused injuries. In denying compensation to one of plaintiffs' experts, the court quotes Opinion 9.07 stating that physicians providing expert testimony should have recent and substantive experience in the area in question, and their testimony should reflect current scientific standards of care. The court found that a gene mutation in the plaintiff-patient more likely than not caused her injury and denied compensation. *Stone v. Secretary of the Department of Health and Human Services, 2010 WL 3790297, 8.*

Fed. Cl. 2007 Petitioners alleged their children's deafness was caused by vaccines. They sought compensation under the National Vaccine Injury Compensation Program. The court determined that petitioners' expert, a physician, lacked credibility and failed to present convincing evidence. The court questioned the expert's evidentiary presentation, his experience, and his education in the field. Citing Opinion 9.07, the court found that the physician went beyond his role as an expert and became an advocate for the family. The court held the petitioners were not entitled to compensation under the Program. *Hopkins v. Sec. of Dept. of Health and Human Services, 2007 WL 2454038, 6.*

Fed. Cl. 2006 Plaintiff filed suit under the National Childhood Vaccine Injury Act of 1986, claiming hepatitis B vaccination caused her transverse myelitis. Medical literature was inconclusive as to whether the vaccine could cause such injury. Medical experts testified for both parties and the court found in favor of plaintiff. Quoting Opinion 9.07, the court rebuked defendant's medical experts for their coercive efforts in threatening to undermine the reputation of plaintiff's expert witness. *Stevens v. Sec. of Dept. of Health and Human Services, 2006 WL 659525, 7-8.*

Fed. Cl. 2005 Petitioner filed suit under the National Vaccine Injury Compensation Program, alleging that his son suffered neurological injuries as a result of a tetanus toxoid vaccine. The court quoted Opinion 9.07 in determining that one of petitioner's expert witnesses gave testimony that departed from acceptable medical principles and was unsupported. The court concluded that the petitioner had not met the burden of proof and was not entitled to compensation. *Kelley v. Sec. of Dept. of Health and Human Services,* 2005 WL 1125671, 7.

Fed. Cl. 2004 Petitioner filed suit for injuries allegedly sustained after receiving a vaccination. The court found that petitioner had not shown by a preponderance of the evidence that she had suffered injury or that if she had, that the vaccination could cause the alleged injury. The court quoted Opinion 9.07 in holding that the petitioner did not present medical expert witnesses qualified to give testimony in the field of neurology. *Falksen v. Sec. of the Dept. of Health and Human Services,* 2004 WL 785056, 10.

Fed. Cl. 2003 Special master dismissed plaintiffs' allegation that, following a measles, mumps, rubella (MMR) vaccination, their infant son sustained acute encephalopathy. The special master, quoting Opinion 9.07, determined that plaintiffs' expert witness, a geneticist and obstetrician, was not qualified to testify about the effect of the MMR vaccine. *Weiss v. Sec. of the Dept. of Health and Human Services,* 2003 U.S. Claims LEXIS 359 n.1.

Cal. App. 1956 Physician-petitioner sought mandamus against local medical association whose bylaws provided for the expulsion of any member who violated the Principles. Petitioner had been expelled under the provision and the expulsion was affirmed by the AMA's Judicial Council. The initial grounds for expulsion was alleged violation of Principles, Ch. III, Art. IV, Sec. 4 (1947) [now Opinions 9.04 and 9.07] for disparaging statements regarding another physician in a report used in judicial proceedings. In holding that application of the provision to petitioner was contrary to public policy, the court noted that the physician's statements had been made at the request of a civil litigant and enjoyed a statutory testimonial privilege. Further, the court found that the AMA's right to formulate ethical principles did not extend to defining the duties of witnesses. Expulsion was also based on petitioner's critical comments about other physicians overheard by their patients in violation of Principles, Ch. III, Art. IV, Sec. 1 (1947) [now Principle II and Opinion 9.04]. The court found application of this Principle under the circumstances reasonable and not contrary to public policy. *Bernstein v. Alameda-Contra Costa Medical Ass'n,* 139 Cal. App. 2d 241, 293 P.2d 862, 863, 863 nn.1, 2, 865 nn.4, 6, 866, 866 n.8, 867.

N.J. 1995 Plaintiffs sued physician and manufacturer claiming that DPT shot administered to their daughter caused her to suffer seizures. Plaintiffs consulted pediatric neurologists, none of whom found a connection between the DPT vaccine and seizures. Court concluded that the videotaped depositions of two of the neurologists could be introduced by defendants because plaintiffs had waived all patient-physician privileges on this issue by bringing suit and because the neurologists did not examine the child in anticipation of litigation. The court cited Opinion 9.07 to support view that physicians have an obligation to assist in the administration of justice. *Stigliano v. Connaught Labs., Inc.,* 140 N. J. 305, 658 A.2d 715, 720-21.

Wash. 1994 In a medical malpractice action against her former physician, plaintiff waived her physician-patient privilege with all physicians who had provided her care or treatment. In an ex parte interview, plaintiff's treating physician opined that defendant's conduct was not negligent. The defense listed the treating physician as an expert witness and plaintiff objected. The court concluded that waiver of the physician-patient privilege extends to all knowledge of the plaintiff's physicians. In holding that a patient cannot insist on physician confidentiality after bringing a civil proceeding, the court quoted Opinion 9.07. *Carson v. Fine,* 123 Wash. 2d 206, 867 P.2d 610, 618.

Journal 2010 Discusses the movement to adjudicate medical malpractice claims in special health courts. Concludes that the psychosocial development of physicians, combined with the position of authority granted to the medical industry within health courts, will result in an antipatient, pro–medical industry bias in medical malpractice claims within such courts. Cites Opinion 9.07. Farrow, *The Anti-Patient Psychology of Health Courts: Prescriptions From a Lawyer-Physician,* 36 Am. J. L. & Med. 188, 219 (2010).

Journal 2008 Discusses the effect of *Crawford* and *Davis* on out-of-court statements made to medical personnel and the application of the Sixth Amendment Confrontation Clause to such statements. Concludes courts, when making a confrontation determination, must consider the intent of the declarant and the circumstances that influence the content of the declarant's statement. Quotes Opinion 9.07. Cites Opinion 2.02. Gordon, *Is There an Accuser in the House? Evaluating Statements Made to Physicians and Other Medical Personnel in the Wake of Crawford v. Washington and Davis v. Washington,* 38 N. M. L. Rev. 529, 529 (2008).

Journal 2008 Discusses the importance of experts and sources of experts for low-income parties. Concludes aid is necessary for improving the quality of experts and for increasing access to experts for low-income parties. References Opinion 9.07. Wiseman, *Pro Bono Publico: The Growing Need for Expert Aid*, 60 S. C. L. Rev. 493, 530 (2008).

Journal 2007 Considers the benefits, in medical malpractice cases, of using a panel of expert judges as the trier of fact. Concludes that the risks of such a system outweigh the benefits. Quotes Opinion 9.07. Chow, *Health Courts: An Extreme Makeover of Medical Malpractice With Potentially Fatal Complications*, 7 Yale J. Health Pol'y L. & Ethics 387, 399 (2007).

Journal 2006 Reviews regulation of physician expert witnesses by the medical profession. Concludes that members of the profession are the proper authorities to police and discipline medical experts. Quotes Opinion 9.07. Turner, *Going After the "Hired Guns": Is Improper Expert Witness Testimony Unprofessional Conduct or the Negligent Practice of Medicine?* 33 Pepp. L. Rev. 275, 304 (2006).

Journal 2003 Uses public policy arguments to support a preponderance standard for medical license revocations in situations involving false testimony by a medical expert witness. Concludes that medical licensing boards can more effectively protect the public by using a preponderance standard. Quotes Principles II, III, and IV and Opinions 1.02 and 9.07. Widmer, *South Dakota Should Follow Public Policy and Switch to the Preponderance Standard for Medical License Revocation After In Re the Medical License of Dr. Reuben Setliff, M.D.*, 48 S. D. L. Rev. 388, 396-97, 402 (2003).

Journal 2002 Examines the role and responsibilities of forensic bioethicists. Concludes that a professional code of conduct and other internal guidelines are needed to ensure professionalism in forensic bioethics. Quotes Opinion 9.07. Spielman, *Professionalism in Forensic Bioethics*, 30 J. L. Med. & Ethics 420, 425, 427, 436 (2002).

Journal 2000 Considers the rules governing expert testimony. Explores professional ethical standards affecting expert witnesses and concludes that codes of ethics have not succeeded in eliminating biased expert testimony. Recommends creation of an organization to assist courts in obtaining reliable expert witness testimony. Quotes Principle III and Opinion 6.01. Cites Principles I, II, and V and Opinions 1.02 and 9.07. Murphy, *Expert Witnesses at Trial: Where Are the Ethics?* 14 Geo. J. Legal Ethics 217, 231-32 (2000).

Journal 1999 Describes historical and present views regarding medical diagnosis. Discusses pressures physicians face that may affect the diagnostic process. Suggests that legal institutions can reduce these pressures, which will enhance the physician-patient therapeutic relationship. Quotes Principle II and Opinion 9.07. Noah, *Pigeonholing Illness: Medical Diagnosis as a Legal Construct*, 50 Hastings L. J. 241, 301, 302 (1999).

Journal 1999 Discusses the impact *Daubert v. Merrell Dow Pharmaceuticals, Inc.* has had on scientific expert testimony. Explains that the scientific approach of dealing with bias may be inappropriate for maintaining scientific objectivity in litigation. Provides a strategy to deal with conflicts of interest in this context. Quotes Opinion 9.07. Cites Opinion 8.061. Patterson, *Conflicts of Interest in Scientific Expert Testimony*, 40 Wm. & Mary L. Rev. 1313, 1330, 1332, 1335, 1371 (1999).

Journal 1999 Discusses the need for physicians to advocate on behalf of patients' rights in the context of health care delivery. Evaluates the nature and scope of the physician's role as advocate, noting that physicians cannot be expected to engage in attorney-like advocacy. Quotes Principles IV and VI, Fundamental Elements (2), (4), and (6) [now Opinion 10.01], Patient Responsibilities 5 [now Opinion 10.02], and Opinions 2.03, 2.07, 2.09, 2.16, 2.19, 3.06, 4.01, 4.04, 6.01, 7.02, 8.02, 8.03, 8.13, 8.132, 9.06, 9.07, and 9.131. Cites Opinions 5.05, 5.09, 7.01, 8.135, and 9.02. Sage, *Physicians as Advocates*, 35 Hous. L. Rev. 1529, 1537, 1541, 1542, 1552-53, 1554, 1556, 1557, 1559, 1561-62, 1564, 1571, 1574, 1576, 1580 (1999).

Journal 1998 Examines mechanisms of oversight for expert witness testimony by medical, legal, legislative, and regulatory agencies. Points out that the amount of malpractice litigation will increase the need for medical expert witnesses. Concludes that improvements in this context must uphold principles of due process and be acceptable to the medical and legal communities. Cites Opinions 6.01, 8.04, and 9.07. McAbee, *Improper Expert Medical Testimony: Existing and Proposed Mechanisms of Oversight*, 19 J. Legal Med. 257, 265 (1998).

Journal 1997 Reports on a study of physician attitudes regarding expert witnesses. Notes that a majority of physicians believe that medical expert testimony should be subject to peer review and, when appropriate, medical licensing board discipline. Quotes Principles II and VI and Opinion 9.07. Eitel, Hegeman, & Evans, *Medicine on Trial: Physicians' Attitudes About Expert Medical Witnesses*, 18 J. Legal Med. 345, 355, 358 (1997).

Journal 1997 Discusses the practice of ex parte communications between treating physicians and their patients' legal adversaries without informing the patient or obtaining consent. Examines harms that may occur in these situations. Argues that Oklahoma needs to prohibit treating physicians from communicating ex parte with their patients' legal adversaries. Quotes Opinions 5.05, 5.07, 5.08, 8.02, 8.03, and 9.07. Cites Opinion 7.02. McNaughton & McNaughton, *Divided Loyalty: The Dilemma of the Treating Physician Advocate*, 22 Okla. City U. L. Rev. 1051, 1052, 1054, 1056, 1058, 1059, 1062 (1997).

Journal 1994 Establishes guidelines for members of the American Academy of Pediatrics who are expert witnesses in medical liability cases. Emphasizes knowledge of the area of medicine involved, impartial testimony, evaluations based on generally accepted standards, and the duty to distinguish between malpractice and maloccurrence. Quotes Opinion 9.07. Cohn, Berger, Holzman, Lockhart, Reuben, Robertson, & Selbst, *Guidelines for Expert Witness Testimony in Medical Liability Cases*, 94 Pediatrics 755, 756 (1994).

Journal 1993 Discusses controversies surrounding how medical-legal consulting services and expert witnesses may be compensated. Examines relevant ethical guidelines in evaluating whether it is acceptable for a physician to be paid a flat fee for expert services rendered on behalf of a consulting business that receives a contingent fee. Quotes Opinion 9.07. Devlin, *Medical-Legal Consulting Services and Expert Witnesses: Payment Controversies*, 9 Medical Practice Management 141 (Nov./Dec. 1993).

Journal 1990 Considers the proper role of the expert witness in the realm of toxic tort litigation. Examines evidentiary rules regarding the admission of scientific evidence and considers various ways to solve testimonial problems. Quotes Opinion 9.07. Bernstein, *Out of the Frying Pan and Into the Fire: The Expert Witness Problem in Toxic Tort Litigation*, 10 Rev. Litigation 117, 143 (1990).

Journal 1990 Examines conflicting court decisions that have addressed the appropriateness of medical-legal consulting services and their use of contingent fee arrangements. Concludes by discussing the need for a less troublesome solution to the problems plaintiffs face in malpractice and personal injury cases. Quotes Opinion 6.01. Cites Opinions 6.12 (1989) [now Opinion 6.05] and 9.07. Dillon, *Contingent Fees and Medical-Legal Consulting Services: Economical or Unethical?* 11 J. Legal Med. 93, 101, 111 (1990).

9.08   New Medical Procedures

In the ethical tradition expressed by Hippocrates and continuously affirmed thereafter, the role of the physician has been that of a healer who serves patients, a teacher who imparts knowledge of skills and techniques to colleagues, and a student who constantly seeks to keep abreast of new medical knowledge.

Physicians have an obligation to share their knowledge and skills and to report the results of clinical and laboratory research. Both positive and negative studies should be included even though they may not support the author's hypothesis. This tradition enhances patient care, leads to the early evaluation of new technologies, and permits the rapid dissemination of improved techniques.

The intentional withholding of new medical knowledge, skills, and techniques from colleagues for reasons of personal gain is detrimental to the medical profession and to society and is to be condemned.

Prompt presentation before scientific organizations and timely publication of clinical and laboratory research in scientific journals are essential elements in the foundation of good medical care. (I, II, V, VII)

Issued December 1984. Updated June 1994.

Journal 2011 Examines patentable subject matter exclusion standards in light of the Supreme Court's decision in Bilski v. Kappos, as well as recent lower court eligibility decisions involving medical and biotechnological inventions. Argues for a greater degree of understanding and consensus regarding the degree of creativity in the applications of newly identified, fundamental knowledge to support patent rights for such inventions. Quotes Opinion 9.08. Sarnoff, *Patent Eligible Medical and Biotechnology Inventions After Bilski, Prometheus, and Myriad, 19 Tex. Intell. Prop. L. J. 393, 407 (2011).*

Journal 2010 Analyzes the federal courts' treatment of process patents and the mental steps associated with them. Concludes that medical diagnostic techniques have properly emerged from recent subject matter challenges as a viable candidate for patentability, despite the historical resistance to give protection to process patent claims incorporating mental steps. Quotes Opinion 9.08. Pessagno, *Prometheus and Bilski: Pushing the Bounds of Patentable Subject Matter in Medical Diagnostic Techniques With the Machine-or-Transformation Test, 36 Am. J. L. & Med. 619, 620 (2010).*

Journal 2010 Explores how participation in online social networks may blur boundaries between personal and professional relationships for health care professionals and how such risks may be mitigated by use of network privacy and security settings. Suggests that health care institutions are likely to institute online social-networking policies for employees. Quotes Opinions 5.026, 5.027, 5.045, 5.046, 5.05, 5.059, 5.0591, 8.14, 9.08, and 9.123. Cites Opinions 5.026, 9.031, and 9.12. Terry, *Physicians and Patients Who "Friend" or "Tweet": Constructing a Legal Framework for Social Networking in a Highly Regulated Domain, 43 Ind. L. Rev. 285, 314-16, 319, 334-36, 338 (2010).*

Journal 2009 Argues against the federal Physician Immunity Statute protecting physicians from infringement liability in certain situations involving patented medical procedures. Concludes the fundamental principles of the patent system can accommodate advances in biotechnology. Quotes Opinion 9.09. References Opinion 9.08. Rundle, *The Physician's Immunity Statute: A Botched Operation or a Model Procedure? 34 J. Corp. L. 943, 947 (2009).*

Journal 2008 Examines natural principles and relationships and the patentability of medical and diagnostic processes. Concludes patent laws should be strictly upheld to incentivize disclosure of medical innovations. Quotes Opinion 9.08. Anderson, *Distinguishing Patentable Process Claims From Unpatentable Laws of Nature in the Medical Technology Field, 59 Ala. L. Rev. 1203, 1216 (2008).*

Journal 2008 Discusses whether the current patent system fulfills the interests of incentivizing innovation in the medical device industry while making the devices available at a reasonable cost. Concludes a reform of the system to include an alternative compensation regimen is necessary to balance ethical and economic interests. Quotes Opinion 9.08. Nugent, *Patenting Medical Devices: The Economic Implications of Ethically Motivated Reform, 17 Ann. Health L. 135, 160 (2008).*

Journal 2002 Evaluates the application of biomedical knowledge in clinical practice. Concludes that serious inadequacies exist in the current practice of evidence-based medicine. Quotes Principle V and Opinion 9.08. References Opinion 9.095. Noah, *Medicine's Epistemology: Mapping the Haphazard Diffusion of Knowledge in the Biomedical Community, 44 Ariz. L. Rev. 373, 404, 447, 448 (2002).*

Journal 2000 Discusses patent law and policy. Examines whether or not those who practice medicine should be excused from patent laws because of the conflict that medical procedure patents create with respect to the practice of medicine. Concludes that Congress should repeal section 287(c) of the Patent Act. Quotes Principle V and Opinions 9.08 and 9.09. Cites Opinion 8.03. References Opinion 10.01. Ho, *Patents, Patients, and Public Policy: An Incomplete Intersection at 35 USC § 287(c), 33 U.C. Davis L. Rev. 601, 603, 623, 624, 625, 631 (2000).*

Journal 2000 Discusses the issues affecting the patentability of surgical procedures. Notes the ethical considerations involved in patenting surgical procedures versus surgical devices. Suggests each patent regimen should strike a balance by weighing all the ethical factors considered important to society. Quotes Opinion 9.09. References Opinion 9.08 and Opinion 9.095. Martin, *Patentability of Methods of Medical Treatment: A Comparative Study, 82 J. Pat. & Trademark Off. Soc'y 381, 383-84, 388, 423 (2000).*

Journal 1999 Discusses congressional amendment of the US patent code, which relieved health care providers from liability for medical procedure patent infringement. Explores the debate surrounding medical procedure patents and concludes that the enforcability of such patents should be reevaluated. Quotes Opinions 9.08 and 9.09. Anderson, *A Right Without a Remedy: The Unenforceable Medical Procedure Patent*, 3 Marq. Intell. Prop. L. Rev. 117, 132, 140 (1999).

Journal 1999 Describes historical and ethical considerations regarding medical patents. Points out that patenting medical procedures adversely affects the reputation of physicians in the eyes of the public. Argues that new laws need to be enacted to prevent abuse of the medical patent system. Quotes Opinion 9.08. Packer, *Ethics and Medical Patents*, 117 Arch. Ophthalmol. 824, 825 (1999).

Journal 1998 Rejects arguments to ban or permit unrestricted patenting of medical and surgical procedures. Explores arguments for and against patenting of medical and surgical procedures. Proposes a compromise position. Quotes Opinions 9.08 and 9.095. Wear, Coles, Szczygiel, McEvoy, & Pegels, *Patenting Medical and Surgical Techniques: An Ethical-Legal Analysis*, 23 J. Med. Phil. 75, 76, 87 (1998).

Journal 1997 Explores the debate enveloping the patenting of medical procedures. Examines the beneficial and detrimental aspects of a ban on medical patents and pertinent ethical and economical factors. Suggests that allowing patents exacts too great a toll on society and science. Quotes Opinion 9.08. References Opinion 9.095. Judge, *Issues Surrounding the Patenting of Medical Procedures*, 13 Santa Clara Computer & High Tech. L. J. 181, 202-03 (1997).

Journal 1997 Examines the controversy surrounding the patenting of medical procedures. Concludes that patenting medical procedures has a negative effect on the physician-patient relationship and the medical profession. Quotes Opinion 9.095. References Opinions 9.08 and 9.09. Note, *Patenting Medical Procedures: A Search for a Compromise Between Ethics and Economics*, 18 Cardozo L. Rev. 1527, 1544, 1547, 1554 (1997).

Journal 1996 Examines the current status of medical procedure patents and discusses the statutory and case law requirements for obtaining a patent. Considers the ethical implications of patenting medical procedures. Argues against a legislative ban on such patents. Quotes Opinions 9.08, 9.09, and 9.095. Garris, *The Case for Patenting Medical Procedures*, XXII Am. J. Law & Med. 85, 93, 94-95 (1996).

Journal 1996 Explores the current rules for patenting medical procedures. Discusses the AMA's position that medical procedure patents are unethical. Concludes that a failure to grant patents will deter the development of new medical procedures. Erroneously quotes Opinion 9.08 (see Opinion 9.095). Lafferty, *Statutory and Ethical Barriers in the Patenting of Medical and Surgical Procedures*, 29 J. Marshall L. Rev. 891, 912 (1996).

Journal 1995 Explores the debates and commentaries regarding patenting medical instruments and processes. Concludes that current patent law fails to address the ethical concerns of physicians and their patients. Quotes Principles of Medical Ethics XI (1971) [now Principle VII] and Principle II (1971) [now Opinion 9.095] and Opinions 9.08 and 9.09. Reisman, *Physicians and Surgeons as Inventors: Reconciling Medical Process Patents and Medical Ethics*, 10 High Tech. L. J. 355, 356, 368-70, 385 (1995).

9.09   Patent for Surgical or Diagnostic Instrument

A physician may patent a surgical or diagnostic instrument he or she has discovered or developed. The laws governing patents are based on the sound doctrine that one is entitled to protect one's discovery. (V, VII)

Issued prior to April 1977.

Journal 2009 Discusses the judicial standard for reviewing physician noncompete covenants. Concludes courts should apply a strict standard to such covenants, rather than declare the covenants per se invalid. Quotes Principles IV and VII, Principles of Medical Ethics §5 (1957) [now Principle VI], Code of Medical Ethics Ch. II, Art. I §3 (1847) [now Opinion 5.02], Opinion 9.02, and Code of Medical Ethics Ch. II, Art. I §4 (1847) [now Opinion 9.09]. Cites Opinions 8.041, 8.115, 9.02, 9.06, 9.065, 9.067, 10.01, and 10.015. Koons, *Physician Employee Non-Compete Agreements on the Examining Table: The Need to Better Protect Patients' and the Public's Interests in Indiana*, 6 Ind. Health L. Rev. 253, 272-77, 280-81 (2009).

Journal 2009 Argues against the federal Physician Immunity Statute protecting physicians from infringement liability in certain situations involving patented medical procedures. Concludes the fundamental principles of the patent system can accommodate advances in biotechnology. Quotes Opinion 9.09. References Opinion 9.08. Rundle, *The Physician's Immunity Statute: A Botched Operation or a Model Procedure?* 34 J. Corp. L. 943, 947 (2009).

Journal 2000 Discusses patent law and policy. Examines whether or not those who practice medicine should be excused from patent laws because of the conflict that medical procedure patents create with respect to the practice of medicine. Concludes that Congress should repeal section 287(c) of the Patent Act. Quotes Principle V and Opinions 9.08 and 9.09. Cites Opinion 8.03. References Opinion 10.01. Ho, *Patents, Patients, and Public Policy: An Incomplete Intersection at 35 USC § 287(c),* 33 U.C. Davis L. Rev. 601, 603, 623, 624, 625, 631 (2000).

Journal 2000 Discusses the issues affecting the patentability of surgical procedures. Notes the ethical considerations involved in patenting surgical procedures versus surgical devices. Suggests each patent regimen should strike a balance by weighing all the ethical factors considered important to society. Quotes Opinion 9.09. References Opinion 9.08 and Opinion 9.095. Martin, *Patentability of Methods of Medical Treatment: A Comparative Study,* 82 J. Pat. & Trademark Off. Soc'y 381, 383-84, 388, 423 (2000).

Journal 1999 Discusses congressional amendment of the US patent code, which relieved health care providers from liability for medical procedure patent infringement. Explores the debate surrounding medical procedure patents and concludes that the enforcability of such patents should be reevaluated. Quotes Opinions 9.08 and 9.09. Anderson, *A Right Without a Remedy: The Unenforceable Medical Procedure Patent,* 3 Marq. Intell. Prop. L. Rev. 117, 132, 140 (1999).

Journal 1997 Examines the controversy surrounding the patenting of medical procedures. Concludes that patenting medical procedures has a negative effect on the physician-patient relationship and the medical profession. Quotes Opinion 9.095. References Opinions 9.08 and 9.09. Note, *Patenting Medical Procedures: A Search for a Compromise Between Ethics and Economics,* 18 Cardozo L. Rev. 1527, 1544, 1547, 1554 (1997).

Journal 1996 Examines the current status of medical procedure patents and discusses the statutory and case law requirements for obtaining a patent. Considers the ethical implications of patenting medical procedures. Argues against a legislative ban on such patents. Quotes Opinions 9.08, 9.09, and 9.095. Garris, *The Case for Patenting Medical Procedures,* XXII Am. J. Law & Med. 85, 93, 94-95 (1996).

Journal 1995 Explores the debates and commentaries regarding patenting medical instruments and processes. Concludes that current patent law fails to address the ethical concerns of physicians and their patients. Quotes Principles of Medical Ethics §10 (1971) [now Principle VII] and Principle II (1971) [now Opinion 9.095] and Opinions 9.08 and 9.09. Reisman, *Physicians and Surgeons as Inventors: Reconciling Medical Process Patents and Medical Ethics,* 10 High Tech. L. J. 355, 356, 368-70, 385 (1995).

Journal 1990 Explains how medical patents have developed into widely accepted legal instruments that receive broad respect from the courts. Questions the lack of Congressional expansion of patent protection in the field of biotechnology and suggests that Congress should begin expanding protection in this area. References Opinion 9.09. Noonan, *Patenting Medical Technology,* 11 J. Legal Med. 263, 268 (1990).

9.095 The Use of Patents and Other Means to Limit Availability of Medical Procedures

Physicians have ethical responsibilities not only to learn from but also, when possible, to contribute to the total store of scientific knowledge. Physicians should strive to advance medical science and make their achievements known through publication or other means of disseminating such information. This encourages physicians to innovate and to share ensuing advances.

The use of patents, trade secrets, confidentiality agreements, or other means to limit the availability of medical procedures places significant limitation on the dissemination of medical knowledge, and is therefore unethical. (V, VII)

Report: Issued June 1996 based on the report "Ethical Issues in the Patenting of Medical Procedures," adopted June 1995 (*Food & Drug Law J.* 1998;53:341-357). Updated June 2008 based on the report "Trademarks, Patents, Copyrights, and Other Legal Restrictions on Medical Procedures," adopted November 2007.

Journal 2011 Discusses the science surrounding gene patents, including ethical, business, and policy concerns, and examines the history of patent law relating to genes. Concludes with a discussion of *Association for Molecular Pathology v. U. S. Patent and Trademark Office* and the future of gene patents. Quotes Opinion 9.095. Liddle, *Gene Patents: The Controversy and the Law in the Wake of Myriad, 44 Suffolk U. L. Rev. 683, 686 (2011).*

Journal 2007 Discusses how a dissenting Supreme Court opinion in the case of *Metabolite Laboratories, Inc. v. Laboratory Corp. of America Holdings* will affect the scope of patentable material. Concludes that despite the court's holding that certiorari was improvidently granted, the dissent's espousal of a new standard of patentability is likely to be extremely influential in future cases. References Opinion 9.095. Ho, *Lessons From Laboratory Corp. of America Holdings v. Metabolite Laboratories, Inc., 23 Santa Clara Computer & High Tech. L. J. 463, 482 (2007).*

Journal 2007 Argues that current US policy providing patent protection immunity to health care professionals violates the TRIPS agreement. Proposes a TRIPS-compliant compulsory licensing scheme to protect both economic and ethical interests in the patenting of medical procedures. References Opinion 9.095. Melvin, *An Unacceptable Exception: The Ramifications of Physician Immunity From Medical Procedure Patent Infringement Liability, 91 Minn. L. Rev. 1088, 1090 (2007).*

Journal 2007 Analyzes scientific, ethical, and legal issues raised in the exhumation and genetic analysis of historical figures. Concludes that biohistorical review boards should be created to generate guidelines for such research. Quotes Preamble and Opinion 2.08. Cites Opinions 2.079, 2.105, 5.05, 5.051, 5.075, 8.03, 8.031, 9.095, and 9.10. Paradise & Andrews, *Tales From the Crypt: Scientific, Ethical, and Legal Considerations for Biohistorical Analysis of Deceased Historical Figures, 26 Temp. J. Sci. Tech. & Envtl. L. 223, 287-88 (2007).*

Journal 2006 Examines competing interests arising in the granting of medical patents. Concludes that the law must restrict the granting of patents to the extent necessary to protect patient access to new procedures. Cites Opinion 9.095. Kesselheim & Mello, *Medical-Process Patents—Monopolizing the Delivery of Health Care, 355 New Eng. J. Med. 2036, 2036 (2006).*

Journal 2006 Examines the ethical use of patents. Proposes patent law reform to better serve societal interests. References Opinion 9.095. Washko, *Should Ethics Play a Special Role in Patent Law? 19 Geo. J. Legal Ethics 1027, 1029 (2006).*

Journal 2005 Examines the *Open Source Yoga Unity* lawsuit, raising the issue of whether Bikram Yoga can be copyrighted. Concludes that, by defining Bikram Yoga narrowly, it is subject to little or no copyright protection. Quotes Opinion 9.095. Susman, *Your Karma Ran Over My Dogma: Bikram Yoga and the (Im)Possibilities of Copyrighting Yoga, 25 Loy. L.A. Ent. L. Rev. 245, 272 (2005).*

Journal 2003 Discusses the US "patents first" policy and its impact on the field of biotechnology. Concludes it is poor policy to grant patents on morally controversial biotechnological subject matter before first examining whether the subject matter is patentable. Quotes Opinion 9.095. Bagley, *Patent First, Ask Questions Later: Morality and Biotechnology in Patent Law, 45 Wm. & Mary L. Rev. 469, 500 (2003).*

Journal 2003 Examines financial conflicts of interest that arise in the context of university-based human research. Concludes that federal regulations should replace traditional models of self-regulation to meaningfully protect human subjects. References Opinion 9.095. Jordan, *Financial Conflicts of Interest in Human Subjects Research: Proposals for a More Effective Regulatory Scheme, 60 Wash. & Lee L. Rev. 15, 23 (2003).*

Journal 2002 Examines various concerns regarding gene patents and discusses other policy alternatives. Concludes that policymakers are exploring alternatives to ensure that gene patents will benefit society. Quotes Opinion 2.08. Cites Opinion 9.095. Andrews, *The Gene Patent Dilemma: Balancing Commercial Incentives With Health Needs, 2 Hous. J. Health L. & Pol'y 65, 74, 104 (2002).*

Journal 2002 Evaluates the application of biomedical knowledge in clinical practice. Concludes that serious inadequacies exist in the current practice of evidence-based medicine. Quotes

Principle V and Opinion 9.08. References Opinion 9.095. Noah, *Medicine's Epistemology: Mapping the Haphazard Diffusion of Knowledge in the Biomedical Community*, 44 Ariz. L. Rev. 373, 404, 447, 448 (2002).

Journal 2000 Discusses the issues affecting the patentability of surgical procedures. Notes the ethical considerations involved in patenting surgical procedures versus surgical devices. Suggests each patent regimen should strike a balance by weighing all the ethical factors considered important to society. Quotes Opinion 9.09. References Opinion 9.08 and Opinion 9.095. Martin, *Patentability of Methods of Medical Treatment: A Comparative Study*, 82 J. Pat. & Trademark Off. Soc'y 381, 383-84, 388, 423 (2000).

Journal 1998 Rejects arguments to ban or permit unrestricted patenting of medical and surgical procedures. Explores arguments for and against patenting of medical and surgical procedures. Proposes a compromise position. Quotes Opinions 9.08 and 9.095. Wear, Coles, Szczygiel, McEvoy, & Pegels, *Patenting Medical and Surgical Techniques: An Ethical-Legal Analysis*, 23 J. Med. Phil. 75, 76, 87 (1998).

Journal 1997 Explores the debate enveloping the patenting of medical procedures. Examines the beneficial and detrimental aspects of a ban on medical patents and pertinent ethical and economical factors. Suggests that allowing patents exacts too great a toll on society and science. Quotes Opinion 9.08. References Opinion 9.095. Judge, *Issues Surrounding the Patenting of Medical Procedures*, 13 Santa Clara Computer & High Tech. L. J. 181, 202-03 (1997).

Journal 1997 Considers the issues surrounding medical procedure patents. Reviews the adoption of federal legislation granting patent infringement immunity to physicians while performing medical or surgical procedures. Discusses the medical community's position favoring immunity. Concludes that such a law sets a dangerous precedent. References Opinion 9.095. Lee, *35 USC § 287(c)—The Physician Immunity Statute*, 79 J. Pat. & Trademark Off. Soc'y 701, 702-04 (1997).

Journal 1997 Examines the controversy surrounding the patenting of medical procedures. Concludes that patenting medical procedures has a negative effect on the physician-patient relationship and the medical profession. Quotes Opinion 9.095. References Opinions 9.08 and 9.09. Note, *Patenting Medical Procedures: A Search for a Compromise Between Ethics and Economics*, 18 Cardozo L. Rev. 1527, 1544, 1547, 1554 (1997).

Journal 1997 Discusses federal patent legislation that protects physicians from liability for patent infringements. Describes legal and medical opinions on the matter. Notes that the legislation was passed in response to concerns regarding health care costs and patients' interests. Proposes that Congress reconsider the legislation. References Opinion 9.095. Note, *The New Patent Infringement Liability Exception for Medical Procedures*, 23 J. Legis. 265, 268 (1997).

Journal 1996 Examines the current status of medical procedure patents and discusses the statutory and case law requirements for obtaining a patent. Considers the ethical implications of patenting medical procedures. Argues against a legislative ban on such patents. Quotes Opinions 9.08, 9.09, and 9.095. Garris, *The Case for Patenting Medical Procedures*, XXII Am. J. Law & Med. 85, 93, 94-95 (1996).

Journal 1996 Explores the current rules for patenting medical procedures. Discusses the AMA's position that medical procedure patents are unethical. Concludes that a failure to grant patents will deter the development of new medical procedures. Erroneously quotes Opinion 9.08 (see Opinion 9.095). Lafferty, *Statutory and Ethical Barriers in the Patenting of Medical and Surgical Procedures*, 29 J. Marshall L. Rev. 891, 912 (1996).

Journal 1996 Discusses possible effects of a 1996 legislative enactment that was designed to limit the remedies for infringements on patented medical activities. Describes the legislative history of this enactment and notes the AMA's position against patenting of medical and surgical procedures. References Opinion 9.095. Mossinghoff, *Remedies Under Patents on Medical and Surgical Procedures*, 78 J. Pat. & Trademark Off. Soc'y 789, 790 (1996).

Journal 1995 Explores the debates and commentaries regarding patenting medical instruments and processes. Concludes that current patent law fails to address the ethical concerns of physicians and their patients. Quotes Principles of Medical Ethics §10 (1971) [now Principle VII] and Principle II (1971) [now Opinion 9.095] and Opinions 9.08 and 9.09. Reisman, *Physicians and Surgeons as Inventors: Reconciling Medical Process Patents and Medical Ethics*, 10 High Tech. L. J. 355, 356, 368-70, 385 (1995).

9.10　Peer Review

Medical society ethics committees, hospital credentials and utilization committees, and other forms of peer review have been long established by organized medicine to scrutinize physicians' professional conduct. At least to some extent, each of these types of peer review can be said to impinge upon the absolute professional freedom of physicians. They are, nonetheless, recognized and accepted. They are necessary, and committees performing such work act ethically as long as principles of due process (Opinion 9.05, "Due Process") are observed. They balance the physician's right to exercise medical judgment freely with the obligation to do so wisely and temperately. (II, III, VII)

Issued prior to April 1977. Updated June 1994.

Journal 2011 Discusses the far-reaching effects of 2005 Illinois medical liability reform legislation. Explains how the 2010 Illinois Supreme Court decision in *Lebron v. Gottlieb* invalidated many beneficial aspects of this legislation. Quotes Opinion 10.015. Cites Opinion 9.10. Nelson, Swanson, & Buckley, *Lebron v. Gottlieb Memorial Hospital: Capping Medical Practice Reform in Illinois*, 20 Annals Health L. 1, 7, 11 (Winter 2011).

Journal 2007 Analyzes scientific, ethical, and legal issues raised in the exhumation and genetic analysis of historical figures. Concludes that biohistorical review boards should be created to generate guidelines for such research. Quotes Preamble and Opinion 2.08. Cites Opinions 2.079, 2.105, 5.05, 5.051, 5.075, 8.03, 8.031, 9.095, and 9.10. Paradise & Andrews, *Tales From the Crypt: Scientific, Ethical, and Legal Considerations for Biohistorical Analysis of Deceased Historical Figures*, 26 Temp. J. Sci. Tech. & Envtl. L. 223, 287-88 (2007).

Journal 2006 Discusses the efficacy of peer-review programs in preventing medical malpractice. Concludes that peer review is effective and that confidentiality of peer review must remain protected by law. Quotes Opinion 4.07. Cites Opinions 4.07 and 9.10. Moore, Pichert, Hickson, Federspiel, & Blackford, *Rethinking Peer Review: Detecting and Addressing Medical Malpractice Claims Risk*, 59 Vand. L. Rev. 1175, 1144 (2006).

9.11　The previous Opinion 9.11, "Physician Impairment," issued December 1986, was deleted in June 1994.

9.11　Ethics Committees in Health Care Institutions

The following guidelines have been developed to aid in the establishment and functioning of ethics committees in hospitals and other health care institutions that may choose to form such committees.

(1)　Ethics committees in health care institutions should be educational and advisory in purpose. Generally, the function of the ethics committee should be to consider and assist in resolving unusual, complicated ethical problems involving issues that affect the care and treatment of patients within the health care institution. Recommendations of the ethics committee should impose no obligation for acceptance on the part of the institution, its governing board, medical staff, attending physician, or other persons. However, it should be expected that the recommendations of a dedicated ethics committee will receive serious consideration by decision makers.

(2)　The size of the committee should be consistent with the needs of the institution but not so large as to be unwieldy. Committee members should be selected on the basis of their concern for the welfare of the sick and infirm, their interest in ethical matters, and their reputation in the community and among their peers for integrity and mature judgment. Experience as a member of hospital or medical society committees concerned with ethical conduct or quality assurance should be considered in selecting ethics committee members. Committee members should not have other responsibilities that are likely to prove incompatible with their duties as members of the ethics committee. Preferably, a majority of the committee should consist of physicians, nurses, and other health care providers. In hospitals, medical staff bylaws should delineate the functions of the committee, general qualifications for membership, and manner of selection of members, in accordance with these guidelines.

(3) The functions of the ethics committee should be confined exclusively to ethical matters. The Code of Medical Ethics of the American Medical Association is recommended for the guidance of ethics committees in making their own recommendations. The matters to be considered by the committee should consist of ethical subjects that a majority of its members may choose to discuss on its own initiative, matters referred to it by the executive committee of the organized medical staff or by the governing board of the institution, or appropriate requests from patients, families, or health care providers.

(4) In denominational health care institutions or those operated by religious orders, the recommendations of the ethics committee may be anticipated to be consistent with published religious tenets and principles. Where particular religious beliefs are to be taken into consideration in the committee's recommendations, this fact should be publicized to physicians, patients, and others concerned with the committee's recommendations.

(5) In its deliberations and communication of recommendations, the procedures followed by the ethics committee should comply with institutional and ethical policies for preserving the confidentiality of information regarding patients.

(6) Committee members should be prepared to meet on short notice and to render their recommendations in a timely and prompt fashion in accordance with the demands of the situation and the issues involved. (II, IV, VII)

Issued June 1994 based on the report "Guidelines for Ethics Committees in Health Care Institutions," adopted December 1984 (JAMA. 1985;253:2698-2699).

Journal 2009 Examines the decision-making function of health care ethics committees (HECs) and their role in the adjudication of treatment disputes. Concludes the adjudicatory authority of HECs should be relocated to a multi-institutional HEC to prevent a single institution's HEC from having control in the adjudication of its own dispute. Quotes Opinions 9.11 and 9.115. Cites Opinion 9.115. Pope, *Multi-Institutional Healthcare Ethics Committees: The Procedurally Fair Internal Dispute Resolution Mechanism*, 31 Campbell L. Rev. 257, 276, 300, 312 (2009).

Journal 2007 Discusses patients' right to refuse medical treatment and the corresponding duties of health care professionals. Concludes that detailed, carefully prepared advance directives are necessary to fulfill patients' wishes. Quotes Ch. II (1940) [now Opinions 8.08 and 8.082] and Opinions 2.035, 2.037, 2.20, 2.225, 8.081, and 10.015. Cites Opinions 9.11 and 9.115. Stamatakis, *Beyond Advance Directives: Personal Autonomy and the Right to Refuse Life-Sustaining Medical Treatment*, 47 N. H. B. J. 20, 29-30 (2007).

Journal 2005 Discusses ethical issues that arise when attorneys serve on hospital ethics committees or as ethics consultants. Concludes that, despite certain potential hazards, attorneys may fairly participate in these important roles. Quotes Opinion 9.11. McQuire, Majumder, & Cheney, *The Ethical Health Lawyer, 33 J. L. Med. & Ethics 603, 604 (2005).*

Journal 2004 Compares formal and informal education in ethics for medical and law students. Concludes that law students would benefit from additional informal ethics education strategies while medical students would benefit from additional formal approaches. Cites Opinion 9.11. References Preamble. Egan, Parsi, & Ramirez, *Comparing Ethics Education in Medicine and Law: Combining the Best of Both Worlds, 13 Annals Health L. 303, 316, 323 (2004).*

Journal 2002 Discusses the role of clinical ethicists and their potential legal liability as a result of participating in case consultations. Concludes that clinical ethicists can limit their liability by acting primarily as mediators or facilitators. Quotes Opinion 9.11. Sontag, *Are Clinical Ethics Consultants in Danger? An Analysis of the Potential Legal Liability of Individual Clinical Ethicists, 151 U. Pa. L. Rev. 667, 679 (2002).*

9.115 Ethics Consultations

Ethics consultations may be called to clarify ethical issues without reference to a particular case, facilitate discussion of an ethical dilemma in a particular case, or resolve an ethical dispute. The consultation mechanism may be through an ethics committee, a subset of the committee, individual consultants, or consultation teams. The following guidelines are offered with respect to these services:

(1) All hospitals and other health care institutions should provide access to ethics consultation services. Health care facilities without ethics committees or consultation services should develop flexible, efficient mechanisms of ethics review that divide the burden of committee functioning among collaborating health care facilities.

(2) Institutions offering ethics consultation services must appreciate the complexity of the task, recognizing the potential for harm as well as benefit, and act responsibly. This includes true institutional support for the service.

(3) Ethics consultation services require a serious investment of time and effort by the individuals involved. Members should include either individuals with extensive formal training and experience in clinical ethics or individuals who have made a substantial commitment over several years to gain sufficient knowledge, skills, and understanding of the complexity of clinical ethics. A wide variety of background training is preferable, including such fields as philosophy, religion, medicine, and law.

(4) Explicit structural standards should be developed and consistently followed. These should include developing a clear description of the consultation service's role and determining which types of cases will be addressed, how the cases will be referred to the service, whether the service will provide recommendations or simply function as a forum for discussion, and whether recommendations are binding or advisory.

(5) Explicit procedural standards should be developed and consistently followed. These should include establishing who must be involved in the consultation process and how notification, informed consent, confidentiality, and case write-ups will be handled.

(6) In general, patient and staff informed consent may be presumed for ethics consultation. However, patients and families should be given the

opportunity not to participate in discussions either formally, through the institutional process, or informally.

(7) In those cases where the patient or family has chosen not to participate in the consultation process, the final recommendations of the consultant(s) should be tempered.

(8) In general, ethics consultation services, like social services, should be financed by the institution.

(9) A consultation service should be careful not to take on more than it can handle, ie, the complexity of the role should correspond to the level of sophistication of the service and the resources it has available. As a result, some services may offer only information and education, others a forum for discussion but not advice, others might serve a mediation role, and some might handle even administrative or organizational ethics issues. (IV, V)

Issued June 1998 based on the report "Ethics Consultations," adopted December 1997.

Journal 2009 Examines the decision-making function of health care ethics committees (HECs) and their role in the adjudication of treatment disputes. Concludes the adjudicatory authority of HECs should be relocated to a multi-institutional HEC to prevent a single institution's HEC from having control in the adjudication of its own dispute. Quotes Opinions 9.11 and 9.115. Cites Opinion 9.115. Pope, *Multi-Institutional Healthcare Ethics Committees: The Procedurally Fair Internal Dispute Resolution Mechanism,* 31 Campbell L. Rev. 257, 276, 300, 312 (2009).

Journal 2007 Discusses patients' right to refuse medical treatment and the corresponding duties of health care professionals. Concludes that detailed, carefully prepared advance directives are necessary to fulfill patients' wishes. Quotes Ch. II (1940) [now Opinions 8.08 and 8.082] and Opinions 2.035, 2.037, 2.20, 2.225, 8.081, and 10.015. Cites Opinions 9.11 and 9.115. Stamatakis, *Beyond Advance Directives: Personal Autonomy and the Right to Refuse Life-Sustaining Medical Treatment,* 47 N. H. B. J. 20, 29-30 (2007).

Journal 2006 Examines US and UK terminal illness jurisprudence. Proposes new legislation should be drafted to allow for palliative care when curative treatments are no longer appropriate. Cites Opinions 2.037 and 9.115. Feldhammer, *Medical Torture: End of Life Decision-Making in the United Kingdom and United States,* 14 Cardozo J. Int'l & Comp. L. 511, 514-15, 532 (2006).

9.12   Patient-Physician Relationship: Respect for Law and Human Rights

The creation of the patient-physician relationship is contractual in nature. Generally, both the physician and the patient are free to enter into or decline the relationship. A physician may decline to undertake the care of a patient whose medical condition is not within the physician's current competence. However, physicians who offer their services to the public may not decline to accept patients because of race, color, religion, national origin, sexual orientation, gender identity, or any other basis that would constitute invidious discrimination. Furthermore, physicians who are obligated under pre-existing contractual arrangements may not decline to accept patients as provided by those arrangements. (I, III, V, VI)

Issued July 1986. Updated June 1994. Updated June 2008 based on the report "Patient-Physician Relationship: Respect for Law and Human Rights," adopted November 2007.

N.Y. Sup. 1993 Plaintiff brought malpractice action against attending physician, resident, and hospital alleging that they caused premature birth and cerebral palsy of twin daughters. Plaintiff, pregnant and complaining of abdominal pains, was admitted to hospital by attending physician. She was also examined by resident. Despite indication of polyhydramnios, an increase of amniotic fluid creating a risk of premature delivery, attending physician released plaintiff from hospital. Resident and hospital moved for summary judgment on grounds that neither had provided independent treatment for plaintiff. They also relied on the principle that if a hospital properly follows attending physician's orders, it cannot be held responsible for the physician's actions in caring for patients. The court affirmed denial of motion for summary judgment stating that a question of fact existed as to whether plaintiff's release from hospital was so contrary to normal practice that resident physician should have inquired into situation. Quoting Opinion 9.12, the dissent argued that the motion for summary judgment should be granted because the attending physician makes medical decisions regarding the patient and neither hospital nor its residents should interfere. *Somoza v. St. Vincent's Hosp. & Med. Ctr. of New York*, 192 A.D.2d 429, 596 N.Y.S.2d 789, 793.

Journal 2010 Discusses issues arising from the enactment of legislation by North Dakota involving a minor's reproductive rights. Explores ethical principles that govern physician's actions within the context of reproductive health. Concludes that, while a patient's expectation of confidentiality with a physician is critical, competing values come into play when the patient is a minor and parental involvement may be important. Provides practical guidance to address issues in this context. Quotes Opinions 2.01, 2.015, 5.055, 8.08, 8.115, 9.12, 10.01, 10.015, and 10.05. Cites Opinion 5.05, 5.055, 8.08, 8.11, 8.115, 9.12, and 10.05. Haas, *"Doctor, I'm Pregnant and Fifteen—I Can't Tell My Parents—Please Help Me": Minor Consent, Reproductive Rights, and Ethical Principles for Physicians*, 86 N.D. L. Rev. 63, 70, 73, 75-78, 82, 84, 86-88 (2010).

Journal 2010 Explores how participation in online social networks may blur boundaries between personal and professional relationships for health care professionals and how such risks may be mitigated by use of network privacy and security settings. Suggests that health care institutions are likely to institute online social-networking policies for employees. Quotes Opinions 5.026, 5.027, 5.045, 5.046, 5.05, 5.059, 5.0591, 8.14, 9.08, and 9.123. Cites Opinions 5.026, 9.031, and 9.12. Terry, *Physicians and Patients Who "Friend" or "Tweet": Constructing a Legal Framework for Social Networking in a Highly Regulated Domain*, 43 Ind. L. Rev. 285, 314-16, 319, 334-36, 338 (2010).

Journal 2009 Examines the role of physicians during natural and man-made disasters. Concludes hospitals must make plans to define disaster response procedures that shift responsibility for survival from the physician to the community. Quotes Code of Ethics, Ch. III, Art. I §1 (1847) [now Opinion 9.067], Principle 5 (1957) [now Principle VI], Principle VI, and Opinions 2.23, 9.067, and 9.131. Cites Opinions 9.06, 9.067, and 9.12. Ahronheim, *Service by Health Care Providers in a Public Health Emergency: The Physician's Duty and the Law*, 12 J. Health Care L. & Pol'y 195, 209-11, 215, 225 (2009).

Journal 2008 Explores potential limitations on access to assisted reproductive technologies and possible negative implications of such barriers. Concludes individuals seeking to utilize third-party reproductive services should enjoy reproductive rights equal with those reproducing through natural means. Quotes Opinion 9.12. Daar, *Accessing Reproductive Technologies: Invisible Barriers, Indelible Harms*, 23 Berkeley J. Gender L. & Just. 18, 44, 61 (2008).

Journal 2008 Discusses forms of emergency contraception and whether pharmacists have a common law duty to dispense Plan B. Concludes that, while pharmacists do not currently have a duty to dispense Plan B, courts might impose that duty in the future. Quotes Opinion 9.12. Spreng, *Pharmacists and the "Duty" to Dispense Emergency Contraceptives*, 23 Issues L. & Med. 215, 253 (2008).

Journal 2007 Discusses laws and policies affecting the rights of homosexuals. Concludes that gays should be legally protected from violence and harassment, but that the government should stop short of condoning homosexuality. Quotes Opinion 9.12. Dent, *Civil Rights for Whom? Gay Rights Versus Religious Freedom*, 95 Ky. L. J. 553, 569 (2007).

Journal 2001 Discusses Internet auction technology and its application to health care services and products. Examines the medical industry's reaction to the emergence of surgery auction sites. Raises questions regarding the practice of online surgery auctions. Quotes Opinion 9.12. Caveney, *Going, Going, Gone . . . The Opportunities and Legal Pitfalls of Online Surgical Auctions*, 103 W. Va. L. Rev. 591, 607 (2001).

Journal 1999 Discusses potential conflicts between a criminal defense attorney's religious beliefs and representation of the client. Explores theories that would allow an attorney to put religious beliefs over the client's interest. Offers analogies within the physician-patient relationship. Concludes that a defense attorney is bound by duty and must set aside conflicting religious beliefs. Quotes Principle VI and Opinions 8.11, 9.06, and 9.12. Reza, *Religion and the Public Defender*, 26 Fordham Urb. L. J. 1051, 1062, 1063 (1999).

Journal 1998 Explores the increasing use of psychotherapy treatment via the Internet. Examines legal issues arising from Internet psychotherapy. Asserts that regulations need to be implemented to protect consumers. Quotes Opinion 9.12. Pergament, *Internet Psychotherapy: Current Status and Future Regulation, 8 Health Matrix 233, 253 (1998).*

Journal 1998 Discusses whether attorneys should be able to discriminate through the selection or handling of a client or potential client's case. Points out that standards for other professions prohibit discrimination. Concludes that attorneys should be prohibited from discriminating in selecting clients, but may use discretion regarding strategies to be used. Quotes Opinion 9.12. Stonefield, *Lawyer Discrimination Against Clients: Outright Rejection—No; Limitations on Issues and Arguments—Yes, 20 W. New Eng. L. Rev. 103, 112 (1998).*

Journal 1997 Compares past ethical opinions to current opinions and notes the differences. Comments on the forces that have changed medical ethics through the years. Notes differing theories on the future course of medical ethics. Quotes Fundamental Elements (Preamble) and Opinions 5.05, 5.057, 7.01, 8.12, 9.12, and 9.131. Cites Fundamental Elements (5) and Opinions 8.115 and 8.13. Buchanan, *Medical Ethics at the Millennium: A Brief Retrospective, 26 Colo. Law. 141, 142, 143, 144, 145 (1997).*

Journal 1997 Examines the evolution of the Indiana health care system. Discusses developments in Indiana jurisprudence regarding the physician-patient relationship. Explores various challenges facing the relationship and recognizes the need for legal rules to help address these challenges. Quotes Opinion 8.08. Cites Opinions 2.20, 9.06, and 9.12. Kinney & Selby, *History and Jurisprudence of the Physician-Patient Relationship in Indiana, 30 Ind. L. Rev. 263, 269, 272, 276 (1997).*

Journal 1995 Offers relevant historical perspectives and provides comprehensive ethical and legal discussion of physician-assisted suicide and euthanasia. Highlights important legislative developments, including the Oregon Death with Dignity Act, and analyzes significant judicial opinions. Quotes Principles III, IV, and VI and Opinions 2.21 and 9.12. Cites Opinions 2.20 and 8.11. Stone & Winslade, *Physician-Assisted Suicide and Euthanasia in the United States: Legal and Ethical Observations, 16 J. Legal Med. 481, 483, 490, 497, 498, 499 (1995).*

Journal 1994 Explores how the Americans with Disabilities Act has created, through federal civil rights mechanisms, a legal duty to treat HIV-infected patients. Discusses previous attempts to create a professional obligation to treat patients with AIDS. Quotes Principle VI and Opinion 9.131. Cites Opinion 9.12. Halevy & Brody, *Acquired Immunodeficiency Syndrome and the Americans with Disabilities Act: A Legal Duty to Treat, 96 Am. J. Med. 282, 283, 284 (1994).*

Journal 1993 Explores the traditional view that lawyers have unfettered discretion to select clients and New York's antidiscrimination disciplinary rule, statutes, and case law. Concludes that the legal profession should prohibit invidious or improper discrimination. Quotes Principle VI and Opinions 9.12 and 9.131. Begg, *Revoking the Lawyers' License to Discriminate in New York: The Demise of a Traditional Professional Prerogative, 7 Geo. J. Legal Ethics 275, 298, 299 (1993).*

Journal 1991 Considers the question of whether physicians should provide medical treatment to those who come to them for second opinions. Concludes that each physician must individually decide whether to treat these patients. Quotes Opinions 6.11, 9.06, and 9.12. Cites Opinion 9.02. Ile, *Should Physicians Treat Patients Who Seek Second Opinions? 266 JAMA 273, 274 (1991).*

Journal 1991 Discusses the problem of noncompliant patients and whether a physician may deny treatment to these individuals. Concludes that physicians are not relieved of their duty to treat noncompliant patients, especially because these patients may not be able to adequately control their behavior. Cites Principle VI and Opinion 9.12. Orentlicher, *Denying Treatment to the Noncompliant Patient, 265 JAMA 1579, 1581 (1991).*

Journal 1988 Observes that the view of medicine as a profession committed to the sick conflicts with the apparent position of the AMA, that a physician is free to choose his or her patients. (See Principle VI.) Concludes that physicians have a duty to treat AIDS patients and must be ready to assume certain levels of risk in fulfilling the duty. References Opinion 9.12. Emanuel, *Do Physicians Have an Obligation to Treat Patients With AIDS? 318 New Eng. J. Med. 1686, 1687 (1988).*

Journal 1988 Discusses the question of whether health professionals are obligated to subject themselves to the risks that attend treating patients with communicable diseases, particularly AIDS. Examines the ethical pronouncements and codes of the nursing and medical professions in this respect, noting that the most recent statements of professional values imply the existence of an obligation to treat HIV-infectious patients. Quotes Opinion 8.10 (1986) [now Opinion 8.11] and Principle VI. Cites Opinion 9.11 (1986) [now Opinion 9.12]. Freedman, *Health Professions, Codes, and the Right to Refuse to Treat HIV-Infectious Patients*, 18 Hastings Center Rep. 20 (Supp.), 23, 24 (April/May 1988).

9.121   The previous Opinion 9.121, "Racial Disparities in Health Care," issued March 1992, was replaced by the current Opinion 9.121, "Racial and Ethnic Health Care Disparities."

9.121   Racial and Ethnic Health Care Disparities

Differences in treatment that are not directly attributable to variances in clinical needs or patient preferences constitute disparities in health care. Among racial and ethnic minority populations, such disparities may contribute to health outcomes that are considerably worse than those of majority populations. This represents a significant challenge for physicians who ethically are called upon to serve patients without regard to medically irrelevant personal characteristics. The following guidelines are intended to help reduce racial and ethnic disparities in health care.

(1) Physicians must strive to offer the same quality of care to all their patients irrespective of personal characteristics such as race or ethnicity. The provision of care should be customized to meet patient needs and preferences.

(2) Physicians must learn to recognize racial and ethnic health care disparities and should examine their own practices to ensure that inappropriate considerations do not affect clinical judgment.

(3) Physicians should work to eliminate biased behavior toward patients by other health care professionals and staff who come into contact with patients. Inappropriate discrimination toward any patient or group of patients must not be permitted.

(4) Participatory decision making should be encouraged with all patients. This requires trust, which in turn requires effective communication. Physicians should seek to gain greater understanding of cultural or ethnic characteristics that can influence patients' health care decisions. Physicians should not rely upon stereotypes; they should customize care to meet the needs and preferences of individual patients.

(5) Physicians should recognize and take into account linguistic factors that affect patients' understanding of medical information. In particular, language barriers should be minimized so that information is exchanged in a manner that both parties can understand.

(6) Increasing the diversity of the physician workforce may be an important step in reducing racial and ethnic health care disparities. Physicians should therefore participate in efforts to encourage diversity in the profession.

(7) Physicians should help increase awareness of health care disparities by engaging in open and broad discussions about the issue in medical school curricula, in medical journals, at professional conferences, and as part of professional peer-review activities. Research should continue to investigate health care disparities, including the development of quality measures. (I, VII, VIII, IX)

Issued March 1992 based on the report "Black-White Disparities in Health Care," adopted December 1989 (JAMA. 1990;263:2344-2346). Updated June 1994 and November 2005 based on the report "Racial and Ethnic Health Care Disparities," adopted June 2005.

Journal 2006 Analyzes racial and ethnic disparities in health care. Concludes that greater political attention must be given to research in this area. References Opinion 9.121. Gamble & Stone, *U.S. Policy on Health Inequities: The Interplay of Politics and Research,* 31 J. Health Pol. Pol'y & L. 93, 105-06 (2006).

Journal 2006 Analyzes methods of measuring racial and ethnic disparities in health care. Concludes that calculating the disparity reduction profile and disparity index together provides a useful measure of change in disparity over time. References Opinion 9.121. Gibbs, Nsiah-Jefferson, McHugh, Trivedi, & Prothrow-Stith, *Reducing Racial and Ethnic Health Disparities: Exploring an Outcome-Oriented Agenda for Research and Policy,* 31 J. Health Pol. Pol'y & L. 185, 216 (2006).

Journal 2004 Examines how one-on-one social interactions may trigger racially biased conduct. Concludes that by affirmatively altering the nature of such interactions, discriminatory conduct may be thwarted. References Opinion 9.121. Wang, *Race as Proxy: Situational Racism and Self-fulfilling Stereotypes,* 53 DePaul L. Rev. 1013, 1082-83 (2004).

Journal 2003 Addresses physician bias in health care. Concludes that existing legal responses to biased medical decisions are inadequate and further development is needed. Quotes Opinions 9.121 and 9.122. Crossley, *Infected Judgment: Legal Responses to Physician Bias,* 48 Vill. L. Rev. 195, 239, 297 (2003).

Journal 2003 Examines the history of medical research involving racial and ethnic minorities. Concludes that medical researchers must ensure the inclusion of racial and ethnic minorities in clinical trials whenever it is scientifically appropriate. References Opinion 9.121. Noah, *The Participation of Underrepresented Minorities in Clinical Research,* 29 Am. J. Law & Med. 221, 223 (2003).

Journal 2002 Considers how to evaluate the performance of Medicare managed care plans in serving ethnic minorities. Concludes that additional monitoring could help reduce existing disparities. References Opinion 9.121. Langwell & Moser, *Strategies for Medicare Health Plans Serving Racial and Ethnic Minorities,* 23 Health Care Financing Rev. 131, 134, 146 (2002).

Journal 2002 Examines how implicit cognitive biases of physicians may contribute to racial disparities in medical care. Considers legal safeguards that may address these disparities. Concludes that Congress must take affirmative steps to help remedy this problem. References Opinion 9.121. Shin, *Redressing Wounds: Finding a Legal Framework to Remedy Racial Disparities in Medical Care,* 90 Cal. L. Rev. 2047, 2056, 2057, 2100 (2002).

Journal 2001 Addresses racial and ethnic disparities in medical care. Concludes that the law plays a vital role in ending racial disparities in medical treatment through the enforcement of civil rights legislation. Quotes Opinion 9.121. Bowser, *Eliminating Racial and Ethnic Disparities in Medical Care,* 30 Brief 24, 25 (Summer 2001).

Journal 2001 Provides a comprehensive theoretical approach and policy recommendations to address racial profiling in health care. Concludes that medicine needs to rethink research and treatment in light of disparities based on race. Quotes Opinion 9.121. Bowser, *Racial Profiling in Health Care: An Institutional Analysis of Medical Treatment Disparities,* 7 Mich. J. Race & L. 79, 119 (2001).

Journal 2001 Explains the design and potential benefits of result-based compensation arrangements for health care. Concludes that a more reliable and efficient health care delivery system is fostered by such arrangements. Quotes Opinion 6.01. References Opinions 9.121 and 9.122. Hyman & Silver, *You Get What You Pay For: Result-Based Compensation for Health Care,* 58 Wash. & Lee L. Rev. 1427, 1459, 1460, 1461, 1481-82 (2001).

Journal 2001 Examines racial and ethnic inequalities in health care. Explains civil rights enforcement strategies and limitations. Concludes by proposing a comprehensive systematic approach, including regulatory and market-based incentives, to decrease racial and ethnic disparities in health care. References Opinion 9.121. Watson, *Race, Ethnicity and Quality of Care: Inequalities and Incentives,* 27 Am. J. L. & Med. 203, 206 (2001).

Journal 1997 Considers the use of race and gender to assess health care status and medical needs. Discusses the lack of consideration that Asian American women receive in the health care agenda. Proposes an examination of factors such as race, gender, and class status to provide a better understanding of the health needs of this group. References Opinions 9.121 and 9.122. Ikemoto, *The Fuzzy Logic of Race and Gender in the Mismeasure of Asian American Women's Health Needs,* 65 U. Cin. L. Rev. 799, 800, 804, 810 (1997).

Journal 1994 Observes that health care reform proposals present significant challenges to the role and ethics of attending physicians. Emphasizes that reform proposals must set forth the role envisioned for physicians and must articulate an acceptable ethical framework within which physicians may fulfill that role. Quotes Opinions 4.04, 9.121, and 9.122. Cites Opinions 2.03, 2.09, 5.01, and 8.03. Wolf, *Health Care Reform and the Future of Physician Ethics,* 24 Hastings Center Rep. 28, 32, 40 (March/April 1994).

Journal 1993 Presents findings by the Council on graduate medical education regarding access to health care. Recommends that more emphasis be placed on primary care, the physician workforce be redistributed to increase the number of physicians in rural and inner city areas, and that there be more racial and ethnic diversity in the medical profession. References Opinion 9.121. Rivo & Satcher, *Improving Access to Health Care Through Physician Workforce Reform,* 270 JAMA 1074, 1075 (1993).

Journal 1992 Discusses the impact of physicians' values on end-of-life decision making for patients. Examines how and why physician values may become dominant. References Opinions 2.20, 2.22, and 9.121. Orentlicher, *The Illusion of Patient Choice in End-of-Life Decisions,* 267 JAMA 2101, 2102 (1992).

Journal 1991 Describes the attributes of women who self-report pelvic inflammatory disease (PID). Presents the results of a study that examined these attributes, noting that risk factors were consistent with prior studies. References Opinion 9.121. Aral, Mosher, & Cates, *Self-reported Pelvic Inflammatory Disease in the United States, 1988,* 266 JAMA 2570, 2573 (1991).

Journal 1991 Compares the health conditions of blacks in South Africa with those in the US. Concludes that policy changes to address the health problems of South African blacks are also needed in this country. References Opinion 9.121. Brooks, Smith, & Anderson, *Medical Apartheid: An American Perspective,* 266 JAMA 2746, 2748 (1991).

Journal 1991 Discusses the lack of health care among the poor and uninsured. Notes the traditional role of physician as advocate for the poor and prescribes a method by which physicians may act as spokespersons for underserved populations. References Opinion 9.121. Kleinman, *Health Care in Crisis: A Proposed Role for the Individual Physician as Advocate,* 265 JAMA 1991 (1991).

9.122 Gender Disparities in Health Care

A patient's gender plays an appropriate role in medical decision making when biological differences between the sexes are considered. However, some data suggest that gender bias may be playing a role in medical decision making. Social attitudes, including stereotypes, prejudices, and other evaluations based on gender role expectations, may play themselves out in a variety of subtle ways. Physicians must ensure that gender is not used inappropriately as a consideration in clinical decision making. Physicians should examine their practices and attitudes for influence of social or cultural biases which could be inadvertently affecting the delivery of medical care.

Research on health problems that affect both genders should include male and female subjects, and results of medical research done solely on males should not be generalized to females without evidence that results apply to both sexes. Medicine and society in general should ensure that resources for medical research should be distributed in a manner which promotes the health of both sexes to the greatest extent possible. (I, IV)

Issued March 1992 based on the report "Gender Disparities in Clinical Decision Making," adopted December 1990 (JAMA. 1991;266:559-562). Updated June 1994.

Journal 2003 Addresses physician bias in health care. Concludes that existing legal responses to biased medical decisions are inadequate and further development is needed. Quotes Opinions 9.121 and 9.122. Crossley, *Infected Judgment: Legal Responses to Physician Bias*, 48 Vill. L. Rev. 195, 239, 297 (2003).

Journal 2002 Analyzes gender disparities in the context of access to health care, insurance, treatment, and outcomes. Concludes that women are likely to encounter an unconscious bias in treatment or in the design of health care systems. References Opinion 9.122. Bobinski & Epps, *Women, Poverty, Access to Health Care, and the Perils of Symbolic Reform*, 5 J. Gender, Race & Just. 233, 238 (2002).

Journal 2001 Explains the design and potential benefits of result-based compensation arrangements for health care. Concludes that a more reliable and efficient health care delivery system is fostered by such arrangements. Quotes Opinion 6.01. References Opinions 9.121 and 9.122. Hyman & Silver, *You Get What You Pay For: Result-Based Compensation for Health Care*, 58 Wash. & Lee L. Rev. 1427, 1459, 1460, 1461, 1481-82 (2001).

Journal 2001 Examines the effects of sex and race on asthma care. Concludes that, in a group of well-educated and insured asthma patients, consistency of care varied in relationship to a patient's race and sex. References Opinion 9.122. Krishnan, Diette, Skinner, Clark, Steinwachs, & Wu, *Race and Sex Differences in Consistency of Care With National Asthma Guidelines in Managed Care Organizations*, 161 Arch. Intern. Med. 1660, 1660 (2001).

Journal 2001 Examines the woman-child stereotype and its connection to feminist goals. Concludes that the stereotype presents serious social and legal implications. References Opinion 9.122. Preston, *Baby Spice: Lost Between Feminine and Feminist*, 9 Am. U. J. Gender Soc. Pol'y & L. 541, 590 (2001).

Journal 2000 Describes mandatory prelitigation panels under the Utah Health Care Malpractice Act. Considers constitutional challenges to such panels. Concludes that prelitigation panels are an impediment to resolution of medical malpractice claims and should be eliminated. References Opinion 9.122. Brann, *Utah's Medical Malpractice Prelitigation Panel: Exploring State Constitutional Arguments Against a Nonbinding Inadmissible Procedure*, 2000 Utah L. Rev. 359, 399-400 (2000).

Journal 2000 Discusses racial disparities in health care. Supports development of national strategies to eliminate racial inequities in medical care. Concludes that strong political leadership and effective interdisciplinary research are needed to achieve this important goal. References Opinion 9.122. Williams & Rucker, *Understanding and Addressing Racial Disparities in Health Care*, 21 Health Care Fin. Rev. 75, 88 (2000).

Journal 1999 Discusses a study that evaluated the impact of gender differences on outcomes of hospitalized patients treated for infection. Concludes that gender may not be predictive of mortality. References Opinion 9.122. Crabtree, Pelletier, Gleason, Pruett, & Sawyer, *Gender-Dependent Differences in Outcome After the Treatment of Infection in Hospitalized Patients*, 282 JAMA 2143, 2148 (1999).

Journal 1997 Considers the use of race and gender to assess health care status and medical needs. Discusses the lack of consideration that Asian American women receive in the health care agenda. Proposes an examination of factors such as race, gender, and class status to provide a better understanding of the health needs of this group. References Opinions 9.121 and 9.122. Ikemoto, *The Fuzzy Logic of Race and Gender in the Mismeasure of Asian American Women's Health Needs*, 65 U. Cin. L. Rev. 799, 800, 804, 810 (1997).

Journal 1996 Considers the impact the doctrine of informed consent may have on the rate at which hysterectomy operations are performed. Discusses how stereotypes affect the quality of medical treatment women receive. Focuses on how informed consent may benefit the health and autonomy of women. References Opinion 9.122. Napoli, *The Doctrine of Informed Consent and Women: The Achievement of Equal Value and Equal Exercise of Autonomy*, 4 J. Gender & L. 335, 336 (1996).

Journal 1994 Observes that health care reform proposals present significant challenges to the role and ethics of attending physicians. Emphasizes that reform proposals must set forth the role envisioned for physicians and must articulate an acceptable ethical framework within which physicians may fulfill that role. Quotes Opinions 4.04, 9.121, and 9.122. Cites Opinions 2.03, 2.09, 5.01, and 8.03. Wolf, *Health Care Reform and the Future of Physician Ethics*, 24 Hastings Center Rep. 28, 32, 40 (March/April 1994).

Journal 1993 Discusses the underrepresentation of women in clinical trials and its medical relevance. Examines the extent to which women are underrepresented. Considers barriers to their participation and proposes ways to include women in clinical investigations. References Opinion 9.122. Bennett, *Inclusion of Women in Clinical Trials—Policies for Population Subgroups*, 329 New Eng. J. Med. 288, 289 (1993).

Journal 1993 Explains how the role of women in clinical trials has evolved historically. Examines specific current concerns related to women's involvement in clinical studies and how these concerns might be resolved. References Opinion 9.122. Merkatz, *Women in Clinical Trials: An Introduction*, 48 Food & Drug L. J. 161, 163 (1993).

Journal 1992 Investigates the exclusion of women and minorities from medical research study groups. Concludes that this problem illustrates the extent to which bias is still present in contemporary medicine and science. References Opinion 9.122. Dresser, *Wanted: Single, White Male for Medical Research*, 22 Hastings Center Rep. 24, 28 (Jan./Feb. 1992).

Journal 1992 Presents the results of a gender study analyzing the differences in quality of care for elderly patients hospitalized with one of four diseases. Concludes that study results are positive but notes that concerns regarding gender discrimination are not entirely eliminated. References Opinion 9.122. Pearson, Kahn, Harrison, Rubenstein, Rogers, Brook, & Keeler, *Differences in Quality of Care for Hospitalized Elderly Men and Women*, 268 JAMA 1883 (1992).

Journal 1992 Analyzes the impact of gender and age on hospital admissions for acute asthma attacks. Presents results of a study that looked at age and gender as factors affecting admissions and length of hospital stay. Concludes that biological distinctions between the sexes may play a role in the disease. References Opinion 9.122. Skobeloff, Spivey, St. Clair, & Schoffstall, *The Influence of Age and Sex on Asthma Admissions*, 268 JAMA. 3437, 3439, 3440 (1992).

9.123   Disrespect and Derogatory Conduct in the Patient-Physician Relationship

The relationship between patients and physicians is based on trust and should serve to promote patients' well-being while respecting their dignity and rights. Trust can be established and maintained only when there is mutual respect.

Derogatory language or actions on the part of physicians can cause psychological harm to those they target. Also, such language or actions can cause reluctance in members of targeted groups to seek or to trust medical care and thus create an environment that strains relationships among patients, physicians, and the health care team. Therefore, any such conduct is profoundly antithetical to the Principles of Medical Ethics.

Patients who use derogatory language or otherwise act in a prejudicial manner toward physicians, other health care professionals, or others in the health care setting seriously undermine the integrity of the patient-physician relationship. Such behavior, if unmodified, may constitute sufficient justification for the physician to arrange for the transfer of care. (I, II, VI, IX)

Issued December 2003 based on the report "Disrespect and Derogatory Conduct in the Patient-Physician Relationship," adopted June 2003.

Journal 2010 Explores how participation in online social networks may blur boundaries between personal and professional relationships for health care professionals and how such risks may be mitigated by use of network privacy and security settings. Suggests that health care institutions are likely to institute online social-networking policies for employees. Quotes Opinions 5.026, 5.027, 5.045, 5.046, 5.05, 5.059, 5.0591, 8.14, 9.08, and 9.123. Cites Opinions 5.026, 9.031, and 9.12. Terry, *Physicians and Patients Who "Friend" or "Tweet": Constructing a Legal Framework for Social Networking in a Highly Regulated Domain*, 43 Ind. L. Rev. 285, 314-16, 319, 334-36, 338 (2010).

Journal 2007 Addresses physician liability for an extramarital affair with a patient's spouse. Concludes that such an affair should be regarded as a breach of a fiduciary duty. Quotes Preamble, Principles I, II, and VIII, and Opinions 8.145, 9.04, 9.123, and 10.015. Demaine,

"Playing Doctor" With the Patient's Spouse: Alternative Conceptions of Health Professional Liability, 14 Va. J. Soc. Pol'y & L. 308, 325, 330-31, 331-32 (2007).

Journal 2005 Argues that in *Aetna v. Davila/Cigna v. Calad,* the Supreme Court missed an opportunity to overturn unjust ERISA policies. Concludes that the principle of complete ERISA preemption as articulated in these consolidated cases is unsatisfactory because it violates the separation of powers doctrine. Quotes Principle VIII. Cites Opinions 8.054, 8.13, 8.135, 9.123, 10.01, and 10.015. Nelson, *AETNA v. DAVILA/CIGNA v. CALAD: A Missed Opportunity,* 31 Wm. Mitchell L. Rev. 843, 847, 849, 850, 880 (2005).

9.124 Professionalism in the Use of Social Media

The Internet has created the ability for medical students and physicians to communicate and share information quickly and to reach millions of people easily. Participating in social networking and other similar Internet opportunities can support physicians' personal expression, enable individual physicians to have a professional presence online, foster collegiality and camaraderie within the profession, and provide opportunity to widely disseminate public health messages and other health communication. Social networks, blogs, and other forms of communication online also create new challenges to the patient-physician relationship. Physicians should weigh a number of considerations when maintaining a presence online:

(a) Physicians should be cognizant of standards of patient privacy and confidentiality that must be maintained in all environments, including online, and must refrain from posting identifiable patient information online.

(b) When using the Internet for social networking, physicians should use privacy settings to safeguard personal information and content to the extent possible, but should realize that privacy settings are not absolute and that once on the Internet, content is likely there permanently. Thus, physicians should routinely monitor their own Internet presence to ensure that the personal and professional information on their own sites and, to the extent possible, content posted about them by others, is accurate and appropriate.

(c) If they interact with patients on the Internet, physicians must maintain appropriate boundaries of the patient-physician relationship in accordance with professional ethical guidelines just, as they would in any other context.

(d) To maintain appropriate professional boundaries physicians should consider separating personal and professional content online.

(e) When physicians see content posted by colleagues that appears unprofessional they have a responsibility to bring that content to the attention of the individual, so that he or she can remove it and/or take other appropriate actions. If the behavior significantly violates professional norms and the individual does not take appropriate action to resolve the situation, the physician should report the matter to appropriate authorities.

(f) Physicians must recognize that actions online and content posted may negatively affect their reputations among patients and colleagues, may have consequences for their medical careers (particularly for physicians-in-training and medical students), and can undermine public trust in the medical profession. (I, II, IV)

Issued June 2011 based on the report "Professionalism in the Use of Social Media," adopted November 2010.

9.13 Physicians and Infectious Diseases

A physician who knows that he or she has an infectious disease, which if contracted by the patient would pose a significant risk to the patient, should not engage in any activity that creates a significant risk of transmission of that disease to the patient. The precautions taken to prevent the transmission of a contagious disease to a patient should be appropriate to the seriousness of the disease and must be particularly stringent in the case of a disease that is potentially fatal. (I, IV)

Issued August 1989. Updated June 1996 and June 1999.

Md. 1993 Patients sued hospital and physician alleging that an operating surgeon has a duty to disclose his or her HIV-infected status. Quoting Opinions 9.13 and 9.131 (1992) for the proposition that a seropositive physician should not engage in activity that would create a risk of transmission of the disease to his or her patients, the court held that it could not say as a matter of law that an HIV-infected physician did not have a duty to warn patients of his condition or refrain from operating on them. *Faya v. Almaraz, 329 Md. 435, 449, 450, 620 A.2d 327, 334.*

Minn. App. 1993 Patients sued HIV-positive physician alleging negligent infliction of emotional distress. Trial court granted summary judgment holding that plaintiffs had failed to produce evidence sufficient to show "actual exposure" to the AIDS virus. The appellate court, in an unpublished opinion, held that the plaintiffs need only show that they were in the "zone of danger" of contracting HIV. The court referred to *Faya v. Almaraz, 329 Md. 435, 449, 620 A.2d 327, 334* (1993) which had quoted Opinions 9.13 and 9.131 for the proposition that a physician who has an infectious disease should not engage in any activity that creates a risk of transmission of that disease to the patient. *K.A.C. v. Benson, 1993 Minn. App. LEXIS 1201.*

N.J. Super. 1991 Physician's estate sued hospital alleging that it violated state law against discrimination by restricting the physician's surgery privileges and requiring him to inform patients of his HIV-infected status before performing invasive procedures. The defendant hospital was also alleged to have breached its duty to maintain confidentiality of his seropositive diagnosis. The court held that the hospital had not discriminated against the physician since the hospital had relied on ethical and professional standards, including a report of the Council on Ethical and Judicial Affairs of the AMA dealing with the issue of AIDS [now Opinions 9.13 and 9.131]. However, the hospital was held to have breached its fiduciary duty to maintain the confidentiality of the physician's medical records. Referring to *McIntosh v. Milano, 168 N.J. Super. 466, 403 A.2d 500* (1979) which had quoted AMA Principles of Medical Ethics sec. 9 (1957) [now Principle IV and Opinion 5.05] in applying the "duty to warn" exception, the court noted that the disclosure in this case went far beyond the medical personnel directly involved in the treatment of the physician and those patients entitled to informed consent. *Estate of Behringer v. Medical Ctr., 249 N.J. Super. 597, 614, 633, 592 A.2d 1251, 1259, 1268.*

Journal 2000 Explores issues involving HIV-infected physicians and patients. Examines ethical and policy considerations and the Americans with Disabilities Act. Concludes that infected patients have the right to be treated, but infected physicians are not always afforded equal protection. Quotes Opinions 9.13 and 9.131. Halevy, *AIDS, Surgery, and the Americans with Disabilities Act, 135 Arch. Surg. 51, 52, 53 (2000).*

Journal 2000 Examines the effect of HIV/AIDS on the relationship between the general public and health care professionals (HCPs). Discusses the importance of creating an environment in which HIV-positive patients do not fear disclosing their HIV status. Discusses policies and guidelines that address methods to prevent transmission of HIV from HCPs to patients. Quotes Opinion 2.23. References Opinions 9.13 and 9.131. Rediger, *Living in a World With HIV: Balancing Privacy, Privilege and the Right to Know Between Patients and Health Care Professionals, 21 Hamline J. Pub. L. & Pol'y 443, 456-57, 461, 472 (2000).*

Journal 1997 Opines that physicians infected with HIV have an ethical and legal duty to disclose their status to patients before beginning invasive procedures. Suggests that the doctrine of informed consent and medical ethics guidelines require disclosure. Disagrees With public policy arguments favoring nondisclosure. References Opinions 9.13 and 9.131. Iheukwumere, *HIV-Positive Medical Practitioners: Legal and Ethical Obligations to Disclose, 71 St. John's L. Rev. 715, 732-34 (1997).*

Journal 1996 Discusses the doctrine of informed consent and its purpose. Posits that, due to patients' rights of self-determination, and the deadly nature of AIDS, physicians are morally and legally obligated to disclose their HIV status to patients where risk of transmission exists. Quotes Opinion 9.13. Note, *Torts: Defining the Duty Imposed on Physicians by the Doctrine of Informed Consent*, 22 Wm. Mitchell L. Rev. 149, 160 (1996).

Journal 1994 Examines the scope of a physician's duty to reveal HIV status to a patient before performing invasive procedures. Discusses applicable case law and advocates use of comprehensive and objective scientific data in evaluating potential liability in cases where physicians fail to disclose HIV status to patients. Quotes Opinions 9.13 and 9.131. Beane, *AIDS Crisis and the Health Care Community: Public Concerns Triggering Questionable Private Rights of Action for Emotional Harms and Legislative Response*, 45 Mercer L. Rev. 633, 669 (1994).

Journal 1994 Discusses the issue of whom physicians must serve first: themselves, their patients, insurers, or society. Focuses on risks arising out of provider economic arrangements and risks arising out of other individual physician characteristics. Quotes Opinions 8.03 and 9.13. Cites Opinion 8.15. Bobinski, *Autonomy and Privacy: Protecting Patients from Their Physicians*, 55 U. Pitt. L. Rev. 291, 302, 313 (1994).

Journal 1994 Analyzes problems in proving emotional distress claims based on the fear of contracting AIDS, such as proof of exposure and injury, reasonableness of fear, and proof of negligence. Proposes that courts follow evidentiary and public policy standards developed in other phobia cases. Quotes Opinions 9.13 and 9.131. Comment, *AIDSphobia: Forcing Courts to Face New Areas of Compensation for Fear of a Deadly Disease*, 39 Vill. L. Rev. 241, 277 (1994).

Journal 1994 Examines the responsibilities of real estate brokers to disclose a seller's AIDS status in light of a potential buyer's right to know all material facts affecting property value. Concludes that a seller's AIDS status is a material fact that a real estate broker must disclose. Quotes Opinions 9.13 and 9.131. Hartog, *The Psychological Impact of AIDS on Real Property and a Real Estate Broker's Duty to Disclose*, 36 Ariz. L. Rev. 757, 772 (1994).

Journal 1993 Provides an overview of the doctrine of informed consent and evaluates the disclosure obligations of HIV-positive health care professionals. Concludes that in developing coherent guidelines for informed consent in this context, the best approach is to have a public determination of what level of risk is tolerable. Cites Opinion 9.13. Nodzenski, *HIV-Infected Health Care Professionals and Informed Consent*, 2 S. Cal. Interdisciplinary L. J. 299, 327 (1993).

9.131   HIV-Infected Patients and Physicians

A physician may not ethically refuse to treat a patient whose condition is within the physician's current realm of competence solely because the patient is seropositive for HIV. Persons who are seropositive should not be subjected to discrimination based on fear or prejudice.

When physicians are unable to provide the services required by an HIV-infected patient, they should make appropriate referrals to those physicians or facilities equipped to provide such services.

A physician who knows that he or she is seropositive should not engage in any activity that creates a significant risk of transmission of the disease to others. A physician who has HIV disease or who is seropositive should consult colleagues as to which activities the physician can pursue without creating a risk to patients. (I, II, IV)

Issued March 1992 based on the report "Ethical Issues in the Growing AIDS Crisis," adopted December 1987 (JAMA. 1988;259:1360-1361). Updated June 1996 and June 1998.

Md. 1993 Patients sued hospital and physician alleging that an operating surgeon has a duty to disclose his or her HIV-infected status. Quoting Opinions 9.13 and 9.131 (1992) for the proposition that a seropositive physician should not engage in activity that would create a risk of transmission of the disease to his or her patients, the court held that it could not say as a matter of law that an HIV-infected physician did not have a duty to warn patients of his condition or refrain from operating on them. *Faya v. Almaraz, 329 Md. 435, 449, 450, 620 A.2d 327, 334.*

Md. App. 1996 Members of patient's family sued physician, hospital, and laboratory for negligence in failing to inform the patient and his family of patient's human immunodeficiency virus (HIV)-positive status. The patient was discharged from the hospital prior to receipt of test results. The patient's family provided home health care, and in so doing came into contact with the patient's bodily secretions. The family all tested negative for HIV. The court noted that the common law duty of care owed by a health care provider to diagnose, evaluate, and treat a patient ordinarily flows only to the patient, not to third parties. However, courts have recognized a duty to third parties in limited circumstances, mostly involving situations in which the patient has, or is thought to have, a communicable disease or otherwise presents a clear danger to a specific person. The court noted, with apparent reference to Opinion 9.131, that the AMA has urged that infected physicians should not engage in activity that creates a risk of transmission and therefore physicians have a duty to disclose their HIV-positive status prior to invasive surgery. However, in the instant case, the court held that no duty to inform third parties of a patient's HIV status could exist because such a duty would constitute a wholly unwarranted invasion of the patient's privacy. *Lemon v. Stewart, 111 Md. App. 511, 523, 682 A.2d 1177, 1182.*

Minn. App. 1993 Patients sued HIV-positive physician alleging negligent infliction of emotional distress. Trial court granted summary judgment holding that plaintiffs had failed to produce evidence sufficient to show "actual exposure" to the AIDS virus. The appellate court, in an unpublished opinion, held that the plaintiffs need only show that they were in the "zone of danger" of contracting HIV. The court referred to *Faya v. Almaraz*, 329 Md. 435, 449, 620 A.2d 327, 334 (1993) which had quoted Opinions 9.13 and 9.131 for the proposition that a physician who has an infectious disease should not engage in any activity that creates a risk of transmission of that disease to the patient. *K.A.C. v. Benson, 1993 Minn. App. LEXIS 1201.*

N.J. Super. 1991 Physician's estate sued hospital alleging that it violated state law against discrimination by restricting the physician's surgery privileges and requiring him to inform patients of his HIV-infected status before performing invasive procedures. The defendant hospital was also alleged to have breached its duty to maintain confidentiality of his seropositive diagnosis. The court held that the hospital had not discriminated against the physician since the hospital had relied on ethical and professional standards, including a report of the Council on Ethical and Judicial Affairs of the AMA dealing with the issue of AIDS [now Opinions 9.13 and 9.131]. However, the hospital was held to have breached its fiduciary duty to maintain the confidentiality of the physician's medical records. Referring to *McIntosh v. Milano*, 168 N.J. Super. 466, 403 A.2d 500 (1979) which had quoted AMA Principles of Medical Ethics sec. 9 (1957) [now Principle IV and Opinion 5.05] in applying the "duty to warn" exception, the court noted that the disclosure in this case went far beyond the medical personnel directly involved in the treatment of the physician and those patients entitled to informed consent. *Estate of Behringer v. Medical Ctr., 249 N.J. Super. 597, 614, 633, 592 A.2d 1251, 1259, 1268.*

N.Y. 1996 Two dentists were found guilty of unlawful discriminatory practice, in violation of the state human rights law, for refusing to treat patients who were known or suspected of having human immunodeficiency virus (HIV). On appeal the court affirmed the verdict and noted that both the American Dental Association and the AMA, in Opinion 9.131, have adopted the position that it is unethical to refuse to treat an HIV-positive patient solely because of that diagnosis. In clarifying its holding, the court noted that the decision does not interfere with the provider's ability to prescribe treatment or refer patients elsewhere, provided it is done for a legitimate nondiscriminatory reason. *Cahill v. Rosa, 89 N.Y.2d 14, 24, 674 N.E.2d 274, 278, 651 N.Y.S.2d 344, 348.*

Pa. Super. 1991 HIV-infected physician appealed order of lower court authorizing hospitals to disclose the physician's identity to the limited class of those patients whose contact with the physician involved intrusive procedures. Appellate court held that the hospitals met their burden of proving a compelling need under the state's confidentiality act. The court cited to AMA Council on Ethical and Judicial Affairs, Ethical Issues Involved in the Growing AIDS Crisis, 259 JAMA 1360, 1361 (March 4, 1988) [now Opinion 9.131] stating that medical professionals have an obligation to their patients to provide safe and adequate health care. *In re Milton S. Hershey Medical Ctr., 407 Pa. Super. 565, 575, 582 n.18, 595 A.2d 1290, 1295, 1300 n.18.*

Journal 2009 Examines the role of physicians during natural and man-made disasters. Concludes hospitals must make plans to define disaster response procedures that shift responsibility for survival from the physician to the community. Quotes Code of Ethics, Ch. III, Art. I §1 (1847) [now Opinion 9.067], Principle 5 (1957) [now Principle VI], Principle VI, and Opinions 2.23, 9.067, and 9.131. Cites Opinions 9.06, 9.067, and 9.12. Ahronheim, *Service by Health Care Providers in a*

Public Health Emergency: The Physician's Duty and the Law, 12 J. Health Care L. & Pol'y 195, 209-11, 215, 225 (2009).

Journal 2008 Examines the legal obligations of health care professionals during pandemics and discusses penalties imposed for refusing to do such work during a pandemic. Concludes policy makers should institute mechanisms to encourage professionals voluntarily to work during a pandemic. Quotes Opinions 9.067 and 9.131. Coleman, *Beyond the Call of Duty: Compelling Health Care Professionals to Work During an Influenza Pandemic,* 94 Iowa L. Rev. 1, 12 (2008).

Journal 2008 Discusses procedural guidelines for treating HIV-positive patients seeking cosmetic surgery for lipodystrophy syndrome. Concludes that this patient group is increasing in number, and that physicians could risk violating legal and ethical rules by refusing to provide treatment. Quotes Principle II and Opinion 9.131. Davison, Reisman, Pellegrino, Larson, Dermody, & Hutchison, *Perioperative Guidelines for Elective Surgery in the Human Immunodeficiency Virus–Positive Patient,* 121 Plastic and Reconstructive Surgery 1831, 1838 (2008).

Journal 2008 Examines the ethical reasons why physicians choose to provide treatment in disaster situations, even at great risk to themselves. Concludes that individual values play a substantial role in such decision making. Quotes Preamble, Opinion 9.131, and Ch. III, Art. 1, Sec. 1 (1847) [now Opinions 2.25 and 9.067]. Iserson, Heine, Larkin, Moskop, Baruch, & Aswegan, *Fight or Flight: The Ethics of Emergency Physician Disaster Response,* 51 Annals of Emergency Med. 345, 346-47 (2008).

Journal 2008 Analyzes three studies measuring HIV discrimination in health care services in Los Angeles County. Concludes stronger antidiscrimination policies are needed in the health care industry to protect individuals with HIV, and advises health care workers receive additional education and training about legal issues and treatment of HIV-positive patients. Quotes Opinion 9.131. Sears, *HIV Discrimination in Health Care Services in Los Angeles County: The Results of Three Testing Studies,* 15 Wash. & Lee J. Civil Rts. & Soc. Just. 85, 88 (2008).

Journal 2007 Examines physicians' duty to treat victims of highly infectious diseases during an epidemic. Concludes that no clear duty exists, and that if physicians are compelled to provide care by law they must be afforded sufficient due process to protect their property interests in their medical licenses. Quotes Ch. III, Art. I, Sec. I (May 1847) [now Opinions 2.25 and 9.067] and Opinion 9.131. References Principle 10 (1957) [now Principle VII]. Schwartz, *Doubtful Duty: Physicians' Legal Obligation to Treat During an Epidemic,* 60 Stan. L. Rev. 657, 662, 663 (2007).

Journal 2004 Discusses physical and other risks that may adversely affect the welfare of offspring of assisted reproductive technology (ART). Concludes that children born with the use of ART essentially suffer no harm because they would not have otherwise been born. Moreover, physicians who have moral reservations about using ART should not be obligated to do so. Quotes Opinion 9.131. Robertson, *Procreative Liberty and Harm to Offspring in Assisted Reproduction,* 30 Am. J. L. & Med. 7, 22 (2004).

Journal 2002 Provides ethical arguments in favor of transplantation in HIV-infected patients. Concludes that preventing such transplants is unethical and discriminatory. References Opinions 2.16 and 9.131. Halpern, Ubel, & Caplan, *Solid-Organ Transplantation in HIV-Infected Patients,* 347 New Eng. J. Med. 284, 287 (2002).

Journal 2000 Explores issues involving HIV-infected physicians and patients. Examines ethical and policy considerations and the Americans with Disabilities Act. Concludes that infected patients have the right to be treated, but infected physicians are not always afforded equal protection. Quotes Opinions 9.13 and 9.131. Halevy, *AIDS, Surgery, and the Americans with Disabilities Act,* 135 Arch. Surg. 51, 52, 53 (2000).

Journal 2000 Explores issues associated with wrongful transmission of HIV-AIDS within the family. Proposes possible legal avenues for compensating injured spouses and children. Concludes the current law in the area must be critically evaluated. Quotes Opinion 9.131. LeDoux, *Interspousal Liability and the Wrongful Transmission of HIV-AIDS: An Argument for Broadening Legal Avenues for the Injured Spouse and Further Expanding Children's Rights to Sue Their Parents,* 34 New Eng. L. Rev. 392, 411 (2000).

Journal 2000 Examines the effect of HIV/AIDS on the relationship between the general public and health care professionals (HCPs). Discusses the importance of creating an environment in which HIV-positive patients do not fear disclosing their HIV status. Discusses policies and guidelines that address methods to prevent transmission of HIV from HCPs to patients. Quotes Opinion 2.23. References Opinions 9.13 and 9.131. Rediger, *Living in a World With HIV: Balancing*

Privacy, Privilege and the Right to Know Between Patients and Health Care Professionals, 21 Hamline J. Pub. L. & Pol'y 443, 456-57, 461, 472 (2000).

Journal 2000 Examines current laws prohibiting discrimination in the context of access to health care, placing emphasis on people with HIV/AIDS. Considers the implications of *Bragdon v. Abbott.* Concludes that everyone should be entitled to health care in the absence of an acceptable justification for its denial. Quotes Preamble, Principle VI, and Opinion 9.131. Shepherd, *HIV, the ADA, and the Duty to Treat, 37 Hous. L. Rev. 1055, 1061, 1083-84 (2000).*

Journal 1999 Discusses the need for physicians to advocate on behalf of patients' rights in the context of health care delivery. Evaluates the nature and scope of the physician's role as advocate, noting that physicians cannot be expected to engage in attorney-like advocacy. Quotes Principles IV and VI, Fundamental Elements (2), (4), and (6) [now Opinion 10.01], Patient Responsibilities 5 [now Opinion 10.02], and Opinions 2.03, 2.07, 2.09, 2.16, 2.19, 3.06, 4.01, 4.04, 6.01, 7.02, 8.02, 8.03, 8.13, 8.132, 9.06, 9.07, and 9.131. Cites Opinions 5.05, 5.09, 7.01, 8.135, and 9.02. Sage, *Physicians as Advocates, 35 Hous. L. Rev. 1529, 1537, 1541, 1542, 1552-53, 1554, 1556, 1557, 1559, 1561-62, 1564, 1571, 1574, 1576, 1580 (1999).*

Journal 1999 Discusses whether health care professionals have the right to refuse to treat patients under common law and federal statutes and regulations. Explores the impact of the Americans with Disabilities Act and the US Supreme Court decision in *Bragdon v. Abbott* on the duties of health care professionals in the context of providing treatment to HIV-positive patients. Quotes Principle VI and Opinions 2.23 and 9.131. White, *Health Care Professionals and Treatment of HIV-Positive Patients, 20 J. Legal Med. 67, 86 (1999).*

Journal 1998 Examines two lines of cases stemming from the Americans with Disabilities Act. Discusses cases where courts have permitted discrimination claims against HIV-infected health care professionals, but conversely, have rejected discrimination claims against HIV-positive patients. Concludes that the diverging approaches may be attributed to a nonreciprocal assumption of risk. Cites Opinion 9.131. Bobinski, *Patients and Providers in the Courts: Fractures in the Americans with Disabilities Act, 61 Alb. L. Rev. 785, 790, 806 (1998).*

Journal 1998 Discusses provider secrets that may increase treatment risks for patients. Encourages greater disclosure of information to patients, including a physician's experience with and performance of a procedure. References Opinion 9.131. Furrow, *Doctor's Dirty Little Secrets: The Dark Side of Medical Privacy, 37 Washburn L. Rev. 283, 290 (1998).*

Journal 1998 Reflects on the *Bragdon v. Abbott* decision, which held that individuals infected with HIV are entitled to protection against discrimination under antidiscrimination law. Discusses HIV discrimination and application of the Americans with Disabilities Act to those infected with HIV. Cites Opinion 9.131. Parmet, *The Supreme Court Confronts HIV: Reflections on Bragdon v. Abbott, 26 J. Law Med. & Ethics 225 (1998).*

Journal 1997 Compares past ethical opinions to current opinions and notes the differences. Comments on the forces that have changed medical ethics through the years. Notes differing theories on the future course of medical ethics. Quotes Fundamental Elements (Preamble) [now Opinion 10.01] and Opinions 5.05, 5.057, 7.01, 8.12, 9.12, and 9.131. Cites Fundamental Elements (5) [now Opinion 10.01] and Opinions 8.115 and 8.13. Buchanan, *Medical Ethics at the Millennium: A Brief Retrospective, 26 Colo. Law. 141, 142, 143, 144, 145 (1997).*

Journal 1997 Opines that physicians infected with HIV have an ethical and legal duty to disclose their status to patients before beginning invasive procedures. Suggests that the doctrine of informed consent and medical ethics guidelines require disclosure. Disagrees with public policy arguments favoring nondisclosure. References Opinions 9.13 and 9.131. Iheukwumere, *HIV-Positive Medical Practitioners: Legal and Ethical Obligations to Disclose, 71 St. John's L. Rev. 715, 732-34 (1997).*

Journal 1996 Considers the extent of discrimination against HIV-infected patients in the dental setting. Reviews approaches to solving the problem of discrimination in this context. Concludes that legal intervention may aid in ending nontreatment based on discrimination. Quotes Opinion 9.131. Burris, *Dental Discrimination Against the HIV-Infected: Empirical Data, Law and Public Policy, 13 Yale J. On Reg. 1, 41 (1996).*

Journal 1996 Considers the extreme risk to patients where physicians and surgeons infected with HIV perform invasive medical procedures. Advocates civil litigation and liability in situations where HIV-infected physicians refuse testing but perform invasive procedures on patients who are uninformed. References Opinion 9.131. Closen, *HIV-AIDS, Infected Surgeons and Dentists,* *and the Medical Profession's Betrayal of Its Responsibility to Patients, 41 N. Y. L. Sch. L. Rev. 57, 65, 71-72, 129 (1996).*

Journal 1996 Explores whether patients have a duty to disclose their HIV status to treating physicians. Suggests that recognizing such a duty may subject patients to a lower standard of care and provide a disincentive to be tested. Concludes that courts should not impose a duty to disclose on patients. Quotes Principle 9 (1957) [now Principle IV] and Opinion 9.131. DeNatale & Parrish, *Health Care Workers' Ability to Recover in Tort for Transmission or Fear of Transmission of HIV From a Patient, 36 Santa Clara L. Rev. 751, 782-83, 787 (1996).*

Journal 1995 Analyzes the secular approach to the duty to treat HIV-infected individuals and the duty to warn those who are sexual partners of, or who share needles with, people infected with HIV. Observes that the secular approach leaves these issues unresolved, but indicates that Jewish law compels physicians both to treat and to warn. Quotes Opinions 5.05 and 9.131. Shorr, *AIDS, Judaism, and the Limits of the Secular Society, 20 Second Opinion 23, 24, 27 (1995).*

Journal 1994 Examines the scope of a physician's duty to reveal HIV status to a patient before performing invasive procedures. Discusses applicable case law and advocates use of comprehensive and objective scientific data in evaluating potential liability in cases where physicians fail to disclose HIV status to patients. Quotes Opinions 9.13 and 9.131. Beane, *AIDS Crisis and the Health Care Community: Public Concerns Triggering Questionable Private Rights of Action for Emotional Harms and Legislative Response, 45 Mercer L. Rev. 633, 669 (1994).*

Journal 1994 Considers how the Americans with Disabilities Act (ADA) has affected health care providers. Illustrates various legal issues arising under the ADA by analyzing cases involving patients and health care providers with AIDS. Quotes Opinion 9.131. Benesch, *Disability Discrimination in the Health Care Workplace, 9 Trends in Health Care, Law & Ethics 45, 46 (Summer 1994).*

Journal 1994 Analyzes problems in proving emotional distress claims based on the fear of contracting AIDS, such as proof of exposure and injury, reasonableness of fear, and proof of negligence. Proposes that courts follow evidentiary and public policy standards developed in other phobia cases. Quotes Opinions 9.13 and 9.131. Comment, *AIDSphobia: Forcing Courts to Face New Areas of Compensation for Fear of a Deadly Disease, 39 Vill. L. Rev. 241, 277 (1994).*

Journal 1994 Explores how the Americans with Disabilities Act has created, through federal civil rights mechanisms, a legal duty to treat HIV-infected patients. Discusses previous attempts to create a professional obligation to treat patients with AIDS. Quotes Principle VI and Opinion 9.131. Cites Opinion 9.12. Halevy & Brody, *Acquired Immunodeficiency Syndrome and the Americans with Disabilities Act: A Legal Duty to Treat, 96 Am. J. Med. 282, 283, 284 (1994).*

Journal 1994 Examines the responsibilities of real estate brokers to disclose a seller's AIDS status in light of a potential buyer's right to know all material facts affecting property value. Concludes that a seller's AIDS status is a material fact that a real estate broker must disclose. Quotes Opinions 9.13 and 9.131. Hartog, *The Psychological Impact of AIDS on Real Property and a Real Estate Broker's Duty to Disclose, 36 Ariz. L. Rev. 757, 772 (1994).*

Journal 1994 Discusses obligation of HIV-infected health professionals to inform patients of their serological status. Discusses common law and regulatory developments that appear to favor patients' rights to know their health professional's serological status before consenting to treatment. Quotes Opinion 9.131. LeBlang, *Obligations of HIV-Infected Health Professionals to Inform Patients of Their Serological Status: Evolving Theories of Liability, 27 J. Marshall L. Rev. 317, 318 (1994).*

Journal 1994 Analyzes competing privacy and public health interests as they relate to HIV transmission in the dentist-patient relationship. Proposes a statute and possible dental association policies to minimize the risk of HIV transmission. Quotes Opinion 9.131. Note, *HIV and Dentistry, 29 Val. U. L. Rev. 297, 317 (1994).*

Journal 1994 Discusses the role of professional societies in establishing ethical guidelines for physicians in the context of using medical innovations and new technologies. Observes that these standards must be supplemented by additional external measures or incentives in order to be most effective. Cites Opinions 1.01, 1.02, 8.061, 9.04, and 9.131. Orentlicher, *The Influence of a Professional Organization on Physician Behavior, 57 Alb. L. Rev. 583, 592, 593, 594, 595, 596 (1994).*

Journal 1993 Explores the traditional view that lawyers have unfettered discretion to select clients and New York's antidiscrimination disciplinary rule, statutes, and case law. Concludes that the legal profession should prohibit invidious or improper discrimination. Quotes Principle VI and Opinions 9.12 and 9.131. Begg, *Revoking the Lawyers' License to Discriminate in New York: The Demise of a Traditional Professional Prerogative*, 7 Geo. J. Legal Ethics 275, 298, 299 (1993).

Journal 1993 Addresses both patient rights under California consent and confidentiality laws relating to AIDS and prohibitions on unreasonable searches and seizures under the US Constitution. Concludes that any health care worker who can document an exposure to blood or body fluids should have the option of compelling a nonconsenting patient to be tested for HIV. Quotes Principle VI and Opinion 9.131. Comment, *Nonconsensual HIV Testing in the Health Care Setting: The Case for Extending the Occupational Protections of California Proposition 96 to Health Care Workers*, 26 Loy. L.A. L. Rev. 1251, 1269 (1993).

Journal 1993 Discusses family privacy rights and considers the meaning of justice, self-respect, and the fundamental principles of physician ethics. Concludes that physicians have an ethical duty to intervene in domestic violence so long as such intervention does not breach confidentiality or violate patient autonomy. Quotes Principle IV and Opinion 5.05. References Opinions 8.14 and 9.131. Jecker, *Privacy Beliefs and the Violent Family: Extending the Ethical Argument for Physician Intervention*, 269 JAMA 776, 778, 779 (1993).

Journal 1993 Examines the law regarding HIV testing for health care workers with particular emphasis on risk determination, mandatory testing, and duty to warn patients. Proposes that CDC guidelines be reformed to more closely match evolving common law. References Opinion 9.131. Johnson, *HIV Testing of Health Care Workers: Conflict Between the Common Law and the Centers for Disease Control*, 42 Am. Univ. L. Rev. 479, 518 (1993).

Journal 1993 Explores the idea of reverse informed consent, which would impose a duty on patients to inform health care professionals of their infectious status. Concludes that such a duty is justified. Quotes Principles IV and VI and Opinions 8.11 and 9.131. Oddi, *Reverse Informed Consent: The Unreasonably Dangerous Patient*, 46 Vand. L. Rev. 1417, 1449, 1463, 1465, 1479 (1993).

Journal 1992 Discusses the problem of discrimination based on HIV status, particularly among women and children. Examines medical and public health issues involving HIV. Cites Principle VII. References Opinion 9.131. Gittler & Rennart, *HIV Infection Among Women and Children and Antidiscrimination Laws: An Overview*, 77 Iowa L. Rev. 1313, 1363 (1992).

Journal 1992 Examines issues related to HIV-infected health care workers protecting patients from infection, including mandatory testing, disclosure to coworkers and supervisors, and the degree to which the practice of an HIV-infected health care worker should be modified. Concludes that courts likely will impose a requirement to disclose HIV-positive status to patients when there is a substantial risk of HIV transmission. Quotes Opinions 8.03 (1989) [now Opinion 8.032] and 8.07 (1989) [now Opinion 8.03]. References Opinion 9.131. Lieberman & Derse, *HIV-Positive Health Care Workers and the Obligation to Disclose: Do Patients Have a Right to Know?* 13 J. Legal Med. 333, 353, 354 (1992).

Journal 1992 Claims that a number of teaching hospitals deny emergency care to the impoverished. Concludes that medical educators must instill more altruistic values in their students. References Opinion 9.131. Miles, *What Are We Teaching About Indigent Patients?* 268 JAMA 2561, 2562 (1992).

Journal 1992 Argues that the ADA and other laws prohibiting discrimination will not alone solve discrimination against HIV-infected patients and the resulting lack of access to health care. Proposes additional steps to augment antidiscrimination laws including implementing protections for health care workers against accidental transmission and adequately funding health care needs of AIDS patients. References Opinion 9.131. Note, *The Americans with Disabilities Act: Magic Bullet or Band-Aid for Patients and Health Care Workers Infected With the Human Immunodeficiency Virus?* 57 Brooklyn L. Rev. 1277, 1279, 1305 (1992).

Journal 1991 Considers important issues of HIV testing of patients and health care workers, prevention of HIV transmission, and costs that attend accidental transmission. Proposes that hospitals develop comprehensive policies to address these issues. Quotes Opinion 9.131. Brennan, *Transmission of the Human Immunodeficiency Virus in the Health Care Setting–Time for Action*, 324 New Eng. J. Med. 1504, 1505, 1506 (1991).

Journal 1991 Considers whether physicians have an obligation to provide medical care to HIV-infected patients. Examines various sources for such a duty, including a moral obligation not to discriminate and a social responsibility to provide access to health care. Quotes Opinion 9.131. Cites Principle VI. Daniels, *Duty to Treat or Right to Refuse? 21 Hastings Center Rep. 36, 37, 42 (March/April 1991)*.

Journal 1991 Looks at two mandatory AIDS testing schemes and whether they serve the public interest. Concludes that mandatory HIV testing does not further legitimate public health concerns, except in the area of sexual assault. Quotes Opinion 9.131. Eisenstat, *An Analysis of the Rationality of Mandatory Testing for the HIV Antibody: Balancing the Governmental Public Health Interests With the Individual's Privacy Interest, 52 Univ. Pittsburgh L. Rev. 327, 347 (1991)*.

Journal 1991 Finds that a majority of dentists do not believe CDC report and feel that dentist-to-patient HIV transmission is unlikely. Also finds, however, that most dentists believe HIV-infected practitioners should modify their practice and that patients should be informed if their dentist is HIV-positive. References Opinion 9.131. Gerbert, Bleecker, Miyasaki, & Maguire, *Possible Health Care Professional-to-Patient HIV Transmission: Dentists' Reactions to a Centers for Disease Control Report, 265 JAMA 1845, 1846, 1847 (1991)*.

Journal 1991 Examines the extent to which physicians provide primary care to AIDS patients and various barriers that stand in the way. Presents the results of a survey indicating that many physicians are responding professionally to the AIDS crisis but that attitudinal barriers block some physicians from providing care. References Opinion 9.131. Gerbert, Maguire, Bleecker, Coates, & McPhee, *Primary Care Physicians and AIDS: Attitudinal and Structural Barriers to Care, 266 JAMA 2837, 2838 (1991)*.

Journal 1991 Examines why HIV-infected individuals have difficulty receiving medical care from private physicians. Presents a Virginia community's response to this problem, which is based on a voluntary rotating referral system using a pool of primary care physicians. References Opinion 9.131. Green, Haggerty, & Hale, *Community-Based Plan for Treating Human Immunodeficiency Virus–Infected Individuals Sponsored by Local Medical Societies and an Acquired Immunodeficiency Syndrome Service Organization, 151 Arch. Intern. Med. 2061, 2064 (1991)*.

Journal 1991 Discusses the issue of HIV-infected surgeons in light of the New Jersey case decision in *Behringer v. Medical Center*. Summarizes the case and presents its implications. Considers future developments. References Opinions 8.032 and 9.131. Orentlicher, *HIV-Infected Surgeons: Behringer v. Medical Center, 266 JAMA 1134, 1136 (1991)*.

Journal 1990 Suggests that hospitals should focus on infection control in general, rather than HIV transmission in particular. Concludes that HIV-infected health care workers should be allowed to continue working as long as they take prudent measures to avoid the risk of transmission. References Opinion 9.131. Barnes, Rango, Burke, & Chiarello, *The HIV-Infected Health Care Professional: Employment Policies and Public Health, 18 Law Med. & Health Care 311, 314, 315 (1990)*.

Journal 1990 Discusses ways in which physicians attempt to avoid malpractice liability, including use of written contracts and refusal to see certain types of patients. Concludes that this behavior is undesirable and that more positive steps can be taken to eliminate much of the tension between physicians, patients, and lawyers. Quotes Opinion 9.131. Comment, *Physician Retaliation: Can the Physician-Patient Relationship Be Protected? 94 Dickinson L. Rev. 965, 986 (1990)*.

Journal 1990 Analyzes the major issues involved in mandatory AIDS testing. Concludes that forced testing is inappropriate and that resources could be used better in other ways. References Opinion 9.131. Field, *Testing for AIDS: Uses and Abuses, XVI Am. J. Law & Med. 34, 50 (1990)*.

Journal 1990 Examines patients' fears about AIDS, their knowledge about transmission of the disease, and their perceived risk of HIV transmission by health care workers. Recommends that physicians actively work to educate the public. References Opinion 9.131. Marshall, O'Keefe, Fisher, Caruso, & Surdukowski, *Patients' Fear of Contracting the Acquired Immune Deficiency Syndrome From Physicians, 150 Arch. Intern. Med. 1501, 1505 (1990)*.

Journal 1990 Examines the risk of HIV transmission from surgeon to patient. Concludes that the risk of HIV transmission is extremely low. References Opinion 9.131. Mishu, Schaffner, Horan, Wood, Hutcheson, & McNabb, *A Surgeon With AIDS: Lack of Evidence of Transmission to Patients, 264 JAMA 467 (1990)*.

Journal 1990 Considers the propriety of HIV testing for hospital patients prior to nonemergency surgery. Concludes that testing of patients should be permitted so long as it is not done with the intent, nor the effect, of discriminating against individual patients. Quotes Principle VI and Opinion 9.131. Naccasha, *The Permissibility of Routine AIDS Testing in the Health Care Context*, 5 *Notre Dame J. L. Ethics & Pub. Pol'y*, 223, 241 (1990).

Journal 1989 Discusses the legal and ethical challenges that AIDS poses for health care providers. Proposes that health care providers actively participate in preventing HIV infection, providing care for HIV-infected individuals, and fighting AIDS and its associated stigma. Quotes Principle VI and Opinion 9.131. Forrester, *AIDS: The Responsibility to Care*, 34 *Vill. L. Rev.* 799, 811 (1989).

9.132 Health Care Fraud and Abuse

The following guidelines encourage physicians to play a key role in identifying and preventing fraud:

(1) Physicians must renew their commitment to Principle II of the American Medical Association's Principles of Medical Ethics which states that "a physician shall deal honestly with patients and colleagues, and strive to expose those physicians deficient in character, competence, or who engage in fraud or deception."

(2) Physicians should make no intentional misrepresentations to increase the level of payment they receive or to secure noncovered health benefits for their patients. (II)

Issued June 1998 based on the report "Health Care Fraud and Abuse," adopted December 1997 (*J. Okla. St. Med. Assoc.* 1998;91:408-409).

Journal 2001 Explores the extent to which pediatricians should rely on their expertise when prescribing therapies and durable medical equipment for children with special health care needs. Emphasizes the importance of the pediatrician's role in this context and urges pediatricians to comply with pertinent AMA guidelines and relevant state and federal laws. Quotes Opinion 8.06. References Opinion 9.132. Sneed, May, & Stencel, *Physicians' Reliance on Specialists, Therapists, and Vendors When Prescribing Therapies and Durable Medical Equipment for Children With Special Health Care Needs*, 107 *Pediatrics* 1283, 1287, 1288, 1289 (2001).

9.133 Routine Universal Immunization of Physicians for Vaccine-Preventable Diseases

As professionals committed to promoting the welfare of individual patients and the health of the public and to safeguarding their own and their colleagues' well-being, physicians have an ethical responsibility to take appropriate measures to prevent the spread of infectious disease in health care settings. Conscientious participation in routine infection control practices, such as hand washing and respiratory precautions is a basic expectation of the profession. In some situations, however, routine infection control is not sufficient to protect the interests of patients, the public, and fellow health care workers.

In the context of a highly transmissible disease that poses significant medical risk for vulnerable patients or colleagues, or threatens the availability of the health care workforce, particularly a disease that has potential to become epidemic or pandemic, and for which there is an available, safe, and effective vaccine, physicians have an obligation to:

(a) Accept immunization absent a recognized medical, religious, or philosophic reason to not be immunized.

(b) Accept a decision of the medical staff leadership or health care institution, or other appropriate authority to adjust practice activities if not immunized (eg, wear masks or refrain from direct patient care). It may be appropriate in some circumstances to inform patients about immunization status. (I, II)

Issued June 2011 based on the report "Routine Universal Immunization of Physicians for Vaccine-Preventable Disease," adopted November 2010.

9.14 Quality

As professionals dedicated to promoting the well-being of patients, physicians individually and collectively share the obligation to ensure that the care patients receive is safe, effective, patient centered, timely, efficient, and equitable.

While responsibility for quality of care does not rest solely with physicians, their role is essential. Individually and collectively, physicians should actively engage in efforts to improve the quality of health care by:

(1) Keeping current with best care practices and maintaining professional competence.

(2) Holding themselves accountable to patients, families, and fellow health care professionals for communicating effectively and coordinating care appropriately.

(3) Monitoring the quality of care they deliver as individual practitioners—eg, through personal case review and critical self-reflection, peer review, and use of other quality improvement tools.

(4) Demonstrating a commitment to develop, implement, and disseminate appropriate, well-defined quality and performance improvement measures in their daily practice.

(5) Participating in educational, certification, and quality improvement activities that are well designed and consistent with the core values of the medical profession. (I, V, VII, VIII)

Issued November 2009 based on the report "Quality," adopted June 2009.

10.00 Opinions on the Patient-Physician Relationship

10.01 Fundamental Elements of the Patient-Physician Relationship

From ancient times, physicians have recognized that the health and well-being of patients depends upon a collaborative effort between physician and patient. Patients share with physicians the responsibility for their own health care. The patient-physician relationship is of greatest benefit to patients when they bring medical problems to the attention of their physicians in a timely fashion, provide information about their medical condition to the best of their ability, and work with their physicians in a mutually respectful alliance. Physicians can best contribute to this alliance by serving as their patients' advocate and by fostering these rights:

(1) The patient has the right to receive information from physicians and to discuss the benefits, risks, and costs of appropriate treatment alternatives. Patients should receive guidance from their physicians as to the optimal course of action. Patients are also entitled to obtain copies or summaries of their medical records, to have their questions answered, to be advised of potential conflicts of interest that their physicians might have, and to receive independent professional opinions.

(2) The patient has the right to make decisions regarding the health care that is recommended by his or her physician. Accordingly, patients may accept or refuse any recommended medical treatment.

(3) The patient has the right to courtesy, respect, dignity, responsiveness, and timely attention to his or her needs.

(4) The patient has the right to confidentiality. The physician should not reveal confidential communications or information without the consent of the patient, unless provided for by law or by the need to protect the welfare of the individual or the public interest.

(5) The patient has the right to continuity of health care. The physician has an obligation to cooperate in the coordination of medically indicated care with other health care providers treating the patient. The physician may not discontinue treatment of a patient as long as further treatment is medically indicated, without giving the patient reasonable assistance and sufficient opportunity to make alternative arrangements for care.

(6) The patient has a basic right to have available adequate health care. Physicians, along with the rest of society, should continue to work toward this goal. Fulfillment of this right is dependent on society providing

resources so that no patient is deprived of necessary care because of an inability to pay for the care. Physicians should continue their traditional assumption of a part of the responsibility for the medical care of those who cannot afford essential health care. Physicians should advocate for patients in dealing with third parties when appropriate. (I, IV, V, VIII, IX)

Issued June 1992 based on the report "Fundamental Elements of the Patient-Physician Relationship," adopted June 1990 (JAMA. 1990;262:3133). Updated 1993.

Colo. App. 1999 Physician filed suit seeking reinstatement, compensatory damages, and an opportunity to respond to the reasons for termination. The defendants claimed that the contract with the physician provided for termination without cause. The trial court granted the defendants' motion for summary judgment. The appellate court affirmed, holding that the termination clause allowed either party to terminate the contract without cause. In a separate dissenting opinion, judge stated that termination without cause significantly impacts the physician-patient relationship and referenced Fundamental Elements (5) [now Opinion 10.01], regarding the continuity of this relationship. *Grossman v. Columbine Medical Group, Inc., 1999 WL 1024015, 4-5.*

Ga. App. 2000 Plaintiff alleged failure on the part of a dentist to inform him of the risks of root canal in a malpractice action. The appeals court noted that state case law did not recognize the informed consent doctrine. In evaluating this precedent, the court quoted Opinion 8.08 and Fundamental Element (1) [now Opinion 10.01]. The court stated that the AMA Code of Medical Ethics should be understood to reflect the standard of care of the medical profession on the issue of informed consent. While the court ruled in favor of the dentist, it prospectively recognized the doctrine of informed consent. *Ketchup v. Howard, 247 Ga. App. 54, 543 S.E.2d 371, 376, 377.*

Ill. 2006 Physicians appealed a grant of preliminary injunction enforcing restrictive covenants in their employment contracts. Quoting Opinions 9.02, 9.06, and 10.01 and referencing Opinion 8.115, the Illinois Supreme Court gave thorough consideration to the AMA's position on restrictive covenants. While acknowledging the ethical problems associated with such contracts, the court found the covenants reasonable in scope. The decision to ban restrictive covenants, the court reasoned, was best left to the legislature. *Mohanty v. St. John Heart Clinic, S.C., 225 Ill.2d 52, 866 N.E.2d 85, 94, 106-07, 107-08.*

N.Y. Fam. 2006 During proceedings regarding a foster child, an issue was raised contesting the legality of the county department of human services' procedures for administering drugs to children. The mother's consent for prescribing medication to the child was obtained by a caseworker, without direct consultation with a physician and with no explanation of side effects. The court cited Opinions 8.08, 8.081, 8.11, and 10.01 in determining the physician's duty to honor the decision of the parent/surrogate. The mother's consent was invalidated and she was given an opportunity to consult with a physician. *Matter of Lyle A., 14 Misc. 3d 842, 830 N.Y.S.2d 486, 492, 494.*

Tenn. App. 1998 Plaintiff challenged the constitutionality of various sections of state abortion statute. Among the provisions at issue was one requiring that a woman be "orally informed by her attending physician" as to specified information regarding the abortion. The court stated that the information requirement and physician counseling provision did not unduly burden a woman's right to an abortion. Physicians who supported this portion of the statute quoted Fundamental Element (1) [now Opinion 10.01], regarding a physician's duty to counsel a patient about the best treatments available. *Planned Parenthood of Middle Tennessee v. Sundquist, 1998 WL 467110, 33.*

Wis. App. 2007 Plaintiff brought action for medical abandonment against his physician. The physician had cancelled an elective surgery and terminated the relationship with the patient after the plaintiff sued the surgical center employing the physician. The circuit court granted summary judgment for the physician finding plaintiff's claim unsupported by expert testimony. With apparent reference to Opinions 8.115 and 10.01, the plaintiff argued that AMA ethics opinions supported his claim. The appeals court held, however, that expert testimony was required to prove the appropriate standard of care. *Casperson v. N.E. Wis. Ctr. for Surgery & Rehab of Hand, Ltd., 2007 WL 1191782, 3.*

Journal 2011 Describes off-label uses of prescription drugs and the associated risks and harms. Argues that such use should be restricted unless supported by high-quality evidence of efficacy and safety. Cites Opinions 10.01 and 10.015. Coleman & Rosoff, *The Case for Legal Regulation of Physicians' Off-Label Prescribing*, 86 Notre Dame L. Rev. 649, 679 (2011).

Journal 2011 Discusses the doctrine of informed consent and the influence of physician groups on the dissemination of information to patients. Concludes the doctrine of informed consent should be expanded by the courts, rather than continuing to allow professional societies to dictate provider guidelines for obtaining informed consent. Quotes Opinions 8.08, 10.01, and 10.015. References Opinion 2.065. Ginsberg, *Informed Consent: No Longer Just What the Doctor Ordered? The "Contributions" of Medical Associations and Courts to a More Patient Friendly Doctrine*, 15 Mich. St. J. Med. & Law 17, 23, 24, 25, 26, 46 (2011).

Journal 2011 Examines when constitutionally protected rights include a right to spend or give money to trigger them. Concludes that laws that restrict spending money on certain goods used to "speak," that are not distributed to the public via the market, are laws that protect the legislature's choice to remove that particular good from the market rather than laws that restrict speech. Cites Opinion 10.01. Hellman, *Money Talks But It Isn't Speech*, 95 Minn. L. Rev. 953, 1002 (2011).

Journal 2011 Examines the protection of a woman's autonomy in the context of reproductive choices including abortion. Argues that, when faced with such choices, women are not currently provided with balanced and comprehensive information necessary to promote autonomy. Concludes that the law should recognize the complexity involved in reproductive choices and provide an appropriate framework for women to make such choices in their own best interests. Cites Opinions 10.01 and 10.02. Laufer-Ukeles, *Reproductive Choices and Informed Consent: Fetal Interests, Women's Identity, and Relational Autonomy*, 37 Am. J. L. & Med. 567, 575 (2011).

Journal 2011 Examines the use of antibiotic prophylaxis for Lyme disease to prevent anaplasmosis from deer tick bites in patients in the upper Midwest. Concludes single-dose antibiotic prophylaxis is an appropriate response to bites, although an alternative recommendation of more aggressive antibiotic therapy following a bite may also be appropriate if patient is informed and such treatment is consistent with patient goals and values. References Opinions 10.01 and 10.02. Maloney, *The Management of Ixodes scapularis Bites in the Upper Midwest*, 110 World Med. J. 78, 80 (2011).

Journal 2011 Reviews the use and current regulation of medical marijuana to alleviate pain in terminally ill patients. Focusing on patient autonomy, concludes that patients should have access to medical marijuana in controlled doses under controlled conditions. Quotes Principle III and Opinions 10.01, 10.015, and 10.02. References Principle VIII. Pfeifer, *Smoking Gun: The Moral and Legal Struggle for Medical Marijuana*, 27 Touro L. Rev. 339, 340-41, 345-346 (2011).

Journal 2010 Assesses the legal environment underlying the identification, accommodation, response, and treatment of mental illnesses and behavioral conditions within the population during and after major emergencies. Concludes that diagnostic and treatment protocols need to be altered by modifying laws regulating psychotropic medications, compelled treatment of nonadherent persons, and assisted therapies during such emergencies. Cites Opinion 10.01. Corcoran, Hodge & Rutkow, *A Hidden Epidemic: Assessing the Legal Environment Underlying Mental and Behavioral Health Conditions in Emergencies*, 4 St. Louis U. J. Health L. & Pol'y 33, 68 (2010).

Journal 2010 Argues that a precise definition of death is needed to counteract the focus on reducing medical costs and increasing organ supplies for transplantations. Concludes that allowing dying patients more autonomy to determine conditions for organ donation will foster an atmosphere of trust in which more people will be willing to donate earlier in the dying process. Quotes Opinion 2.157. Cites Opinion 10.01. Fry-Revere, Ray, & Reher, *Death: A New Legal Perspective*, 27 J. Contemp. Health L. & Pol'y 1, 11, 50, 53 (2010).

Journal 2010 Discusses issues arising from the enactment of legislation by North Dakota involving a minor's reproductive rights. Explores ethical principles that govern physician's actions within the context of reproductive health. Concludes that, while a patient's expectation of confidentiality with a physician is critical, competing values come into play when the patient is a minor and parental involvement may be important. Provides practical guidance to address issues in this context. Quotes Opinions 2.01, 2.015, 5.055, 8.08, 8.115, 9.12, 10.01, 10.015, and 10.05. Cites Opinion 5.05, 5.055, 8.08, 8.11, 8.115, 9.12, and 10.05. Haas, *"Doctor, I'm Pregnant and Fifteen—I Can't Tell My Parents—Please Help Me": Minor Consent, Reproductive Rights, and Ethical Principles for Physicians*, 86 N.D. L. Rev. 63, 70, 73, 75-78, 82, 84, 86-88, (2010).

Journal 2009 Discusses the judicial standard for reviewing physician noncompete covenants. Concludes courts should apply a strict standard to such covenants, rather than declare the covenants per se invalid. Quotes Principles IV and VII, Principles of Medical Ethics §5 (1957) [now Principle VI], Code of Medical Ethics Ch. II, Art. I §3 (1847) [now Opinion 5.02], Opinion 9.02, and Code of Medical Ethics Ch. II, Art. I §4 (1847) [now Opinion 9.09]. Cites Opinions 8.041, 8.115, 9.02, 9.06, 9.065, 9.067, 10.01, and 10.015. Koons, *Physician Employee Non-Compete Agreements on the Examining Table: The Need to Better Protect Patients' and the Public's Interests in Indiana*, 6 Ind. Health L. Rev. 253, 272-77, 280-81 (2009).

Journal 2008 Discusses ex parte interviews with a treating physician in discovery before and after the HIPAA Privacy Rule and the issues facing physicians contacted for such interviews. Concludes courts and attorneys should work together to allow for efficient discovery while protecting physicians. Quotes Principles IV and VIII and Opinions 5.05 and 10.01. Burnette & Morning, *HIPAA and Ex Parte Interviews—The Beginning of the End?* 1 J. Health & Life Sci. L. 73, 100-01 (2008).

Journal 2008 Reviews the obligation of a physician to provide a referral for the termination of a pregnancy, when the treating physician objects to the procedure on ethical grounds. Concludes that the physician has an ethical duty to inform the patient of other providers who can offer competent care. Cites Opinion 10.01. Chervenak & McCullough, *The Ethics of Direct and Indirect Referral for Termination of Pregnancy*, 199 Am. J. Obstet. Gynecol. 232.e1, 232.e1 (2008).

Journal 2008 Considers the utility of physician apologies for medical error and legal protection for physicians who apologize for mistakes. Concludes physicians must openly communicate with their patients and apologize for medical errors to strengthen the health care community. Quotes Opinions 8.08, 8.12, 10.01, and 10.015. References Opinion 8.12. Ebert, *Attorneys, Tell Your Clients to Say They're Sorry: Apologies in the Health Care Industry*, 5 Ind. Health L. Rev. 337, 340-41, 344 (2008).

Journal 2008 Explores the fiduciary relationship between physicians and patients, professional and ethical obligations of both physicians and lawyers, and the implications for conflict resolution in health care. Concludes physicians must put patient interests above their own and lawyers must work to discern clients' best interests and support client welfare. Quotes Principle VIII and Opinions 8.12 and 10.015. Cites Principles I and II and Opinions 10.01 and 10.015. Scott, *Doctors as Advocates, Lawyers as Healers*, 29 Hamline J. Pub. L. Pol'y 331, 340-41, 347, 371 (2008).

Journal 2007 Reviews Deborah Rhode's analysis of pro bono obligations of lawyers from her book, *Pro Bono in Principle and in Practice: Public Service and the Professions*. Concludes that a mandatory pro bono requirement is a better solution than an incentive-based system. Quotes Opinion 10.01. References Opinion 9.065. Lininger, *From Park Place to Community Chest: Rethinking Lawyers' Monopoly*, 101 Nw. U. L. Rev. 1343, 1349 (2007).

Journal 2007 Considers relevant policy issues surrounding prenatal torts. Concludes that North Carolina should allow bringing of claims for prenatal, postconception malpractice. Quotes Opinion 10.01. McEntire, *Compensating Post-Conception Prenatal Medical Malpractice While Respecting Life: A Recommendation to North Carolina Legislators*, 29 Campbell L. Rev. 761, 763 (2007).

Journal 2006 Analyzes cases where a patient's right to refuse care conflicts with the physician's obligation to protect that patient's well-being. Concludes health care providers should seek a compromise that best promotes both patient autonomy and well-being. Quotes Principle IV and Ch. I, Art. II, Sec. 6 (May 1847) [now Opinion 10.01]. Carrese, *Refusal of Care: Patients' Well-being and Physicians' Ethical Obligations*, 296 JAMA 691, 692, 693 (2006).

Journal 2006 Reviews informed consent doctrine in the context of consumer-driven health care. Concludes that consumer-driven health care should not be undermined by arguments about patient competence to make health care decisions. References Opinion 10.01. Kapp, *Patient Autonomy in the Age of Consumer-Driven Health Care: Informed Consent and Informed Choice*, 2 J. Health & Biomedical L. 1, 5 (2006).

Journal 2005 Discusses standard of care issues surrounding physicians using complementary and alternative medicine (CAM). Concludes that a prudent physician standard should apply to physicians practicing CAM. Quotes Opinion 10.01. Cites Opinion 10.02. Kallmyer, *A Chimera in Every Sense: Standard of Care for Physicians Practicing Complementary and Alternative Medicine*, 2 Ind. Health L. Rev. 225, 229, 231 (2005).

Journal 2005 Argues that in *Aetna v. Davila/Cigna v. Calad*, the Supreme Court missed an opportunity to overturn unjust ERISA policies. Concludes that the principle of complete ERISA preemption as articulated in these consolidated cases is unsatisfactory because it violates the separation of powers doctrine. Quotes Principle VIII. Cites Opinions 8.054, 8.13, 8.135, 9.123, 10.01, and 10.015. Nelson, *AETNA v. DAVILA/CIGNA v. CALAD: A Missed Opportunity, 31 Wm. Mitchell L. Rev. 843, 847, 849, 850, 880 (2005).*

Journal 2005 Discusses ethical, legal, and policy issues associated with treatment and research involving patients who are in a persistent vegetative or minimally conscious state. Concludes that patients in these states are at risk for therapeutic failures until physicians can more accurately determine which patients will benefit from treatment and accurately convey such information to families or surrogates. Quotes Principles VII and IX and Opinions 8.031, 8.0315, 9.065, 10.01, and 10.015. Tovino & Winslade, *A Primer on the Law and Ethics of Treatment, Research, and Public Policy in the Context of Severe Traumatic Brain Injury, 14 Ann. Health L. 1, 18, 38, 39, 40, 41 (2005).*

Journal 2004 Discusses medical errors in various health care settings and offers an ethical framework to support immediate implementation of proposed solutions. Concludes that federal and state legislators must place priority on developing policies that will help reduce the number of medical errors. Quotes Opinion 10.01. Clark, *Medication Errors in Family Practice, in Hospitals and After Discharge From the Hospital: An Ethical Analysis, 32 J. L. Med & Ethics 349, 354 (2004).*

Journal 2004 Analyzes Maryland's Drug Addiction at Birth Act, which was passed to help health care professionals deal with drug-exposed infants. Concludes that more effective legislation could be enacted to educate health care providers regarding treatment of infants with prenatal drug exposure. Quotes Opinion 10.01. Reese & Burry, *Evaluating Maryland's Response to Drug-Exposed Babies, 10 Psychol. Pub. Pol'y & L. 343, 353 (2004).*

Journal 2003 Reviews state laws designed to protect physicians acting as patient advocates in managed care organizations. Concludes that federal and state law must make it easier for physicians to challenge denials of or delays in patient care. Quotes Opinions 8.054, 8.13, and 10.01. Fentiman, *Patient Advocacy and Termination From Managed Care Organizations. Do State Laws Protecting Health Care Professional Advocacy Make Any Difference? 82 Neb. L. Rev. 508, 515-16, 517-18 (2003).*

Journal 2003 Highlights the legal and ethical concerns surrounding use of noncompetition clauses. Concludes that physicians should carefully evaluate these clauses given their likely enforceability. Quotes Opinions 9.02, 9.06, 10.01, and 10.015. Loeser, *The Legal, Ethical, and Practical Implications of Noncompetition Clauses: What Physicians Should Know Before They Sign, 31 J. L. Med. & Ethics 283, 286, 287, 290 (2003).*

Journal 2003 Considers the legal, medical, and ethical issues of physician-patient confidentiality in disclosure of paternity. Concludes that a balancing test should be applied to making determinations regarding disclosure of paternity. Quotes Principles I, IV, and V and Opinions 1.02, 5.055, and 10.01. Cites Principle II and Opinion 5.05. Richards & Wolf, *Medical Confidentiality and Disclosure of Paternity, 48 S. D. L. Rev. 409, 411, 412, 413 (2003).*

Journal 2003 Evaluates medical necessity decisions in managed care, with emphasis on therapeutic effectiveness. Concludes that, in order to be effective, review procedures and policies governing medical necessity determinations must be improved. Quotes Opinion 10.01. Sage, *Managed Care's Crimea: Medical Necessity, Therapeutic Benefit, and the Goals of Administrative Process in Health Insurance, 53 Duke L. J. 597, 634 (2003).*

Journal 2003 Argues that affirmative measures should be taken by the Air Force to ensure access to abortion services. Concludes that regulatory changes will reduce barriers to access. Quotes Opinion 10.01. Cites Opinion 8.08. Wilde, *Air Force Women's Access to Abortion Services and the Erosion of 10 USC § 1093, 9 Wm. & Mary J. Women & L. 351, 371 (2003).*

Journal 2003 Discusses potential liability of mental health care providers who administer court-ordered treatment to patients. Concludes that providers should treat these patients as much like voluntary patients as possible. References Opinion 10.01. Wilde, *The Liability of Alaska Mental Health Providers for Mandated Treatment, 20 Alaska L. Rev. 271, 276 (2003).*

Journal 2002 Argues for a more comprehensive approach in the management and treatment of intersex children. Emphasizes the importance of informed decision-making by parents and children. Quotes Opinion 10.01. Hermer, *Paradigms Revised: Intersex Children, Bioethics & the Law, 11 Annals Health L. 195, 221 (2002).*

Journal 2002 Discusses issues regarding regulation of elderly drivers. Concludes that mandating physicians to report unfit elderly patients will protect the public and help resolve ethical and legal dilemmas. Quotes Opinions 1.02, 2.24, 5.05, and 10.01. Kane, *Driving Into the Sunset: A Proposal for Mandatory Reporting to the DMV by Physicians Treating Unsafe Elderly Drivers*, 25 U. Haw. L. Rev. 59, 59, 61, 62, 67, 69, 82, 83 (2002).

Journal 2002 Reviews how changes in the health care delivery system underscore the importance of information in patient empowerment. Concludes that patients should use information to take charge of their health care. Quotes Principle V and Opinion 10.02. Cites Opinion 10.01. Kane, *Information Is the Key to Patient Empowerment*, 11 Annals Health L. 25, 29-30, 44 (2002).

Journal 2002 Considers the ethical and legal issues regarding breach of confidentiality in situations where a patient is pregnant and uses teratogenic substances. Concludes that a breach of confidentiality causes damage to the physician-patient relationship. Quotes Principle IV and Opinion 10.01. Plambeck, *Divided Loyalties: Legal and Bioethical Considerations of Physician-Pregnant Patient Confidentiality and Prenatal Drug Abuse*, 23 J. Legal Med. 1, 8, 25 (2002).

Journal 2002 Analyzes the role of prognostication in physician-patient communication. Concludes that the patient-physician model of shared decision-making offers the best hope for reestablishing prognostication. Quotes Principles Ch. I, Art. I, Sec. 2 and 4 (1846) [now Principle IV and Opinions 8.12 and 10.01]. Cites Opinion 8.08. Rich, *Prognostication in Clinical Medicine: Prophecy or Professional Responsibility?* 23 J. Legal Med. 297, 299, 318, 327 (2002).

Journal 2002 Discusses legal and medical policies that protect confidentiality in the physician-patient relationship. Concludes that reducing the current level of privacy protection would jeopardize health care. Quotes Preamble and Opinions 2.136, 5.05, and 10.01. References Principles VIII and IX. Sciarrino, *Ferguson v. City of Charleston: "The Doctor Will See You Now, Be Sure to Bring Your Privacy Rights in With You!"* 12 Temp. Pol. & Civ. Rts. L. Rev. 197, 213, 215, 220, 221, 222 (2002).

Journal 2001 Explores the ethical and legal dilemmas associated with doctors and lawyers providing advice over the Internet. Concludes the law must ensure that cyberprofessionals comply with ethical and legal duties to their clients and their professions. Quotes Opinion 10.01. Deady, *Cyberadvice: The Ethical Implications of Giving Professional Advice Over the Internet*, 14 Geo. J. Legal Ethics 891, 905 (2001).

Journal 2001 Discusses whether or not the medical profession needs a policy on honesty. Reviews ethical codes and concludes they fail to offer physicians with meaningful guidance about what constitutes "the truth" and when and how to disclose it. Quotes Principle II and Opinions 8.12 and 10.01. DeVita, *Honestly, Do We Need a Policy on Truth?* 11 Kennedy Inst. Ethics J. 157, 158 (2001).

Journal 2001 Discusses issues surrounding the privacy of genetic information. Considers the social, ethical, and legal responses to problems that arise in this context. Concludes with a unique view of privacy that would protect the right of individuals not to know genetic information about themselves. Quotes Principle IV and Opinion 10.01. Laurie, *Challenging Medical-Legal Norms: The Role of Autonomy, Confidentiality, and Privacy in Protecting Individual and Familial Group Rights in Genetic Information*, 22 J. Legal Med. 1, 24 (2001).

Journal 2001 Considers conflicts of interest in clinical research and other types of medical practice. Compares the way in which doctors and lawyers address conflicts of interest in professional practice. Concludes that physicians are unaware of the need to create a meaningful conflict-of-interest doctrine for medical practice. Quotes Preamble, Principle IV, and Opinions 2.07, 8.03, 8.031, and 10.01. Moore, *What Doctors Can Learn From Lawyers About Conflicts of Interest*, 81 B. U. L. Rev. 445, 447, 449-50 (2001).

Journal 2001 Compares ongoing efforts to control reproduction and to control drug abuse with a view toward finding more effective solutions in both areas. Concludes that a coherent approach will build stronger coalitions in support of drug policy reform and reproductive freedom. Quotes Opinion 10.01. Paltrow, *The War on Drugs and the War on Abortion: Some Initial Thoughts on the Connections, Intersections and the Effects*, 28 S.U. L. Rev. 201, 219 (2001).

Journal 2001 Considers how much information regarding the adverse effects of medication physicians should disclose to patients. Concludes that most patients want complete information. Quotes Opinion 10.01. Ziegler, Mosier, Buenaver, & Okuyemi, *How Much Information About Adverse Effects of Medication Do Patients Want From Physicians?* 161 Arch. Intern. Med. 706, 710 (2001).

Journal 2000 Introduces the debate surrounding the benefits and dangers of diagnosing and treating patients over the Internet and explores the issue of how cybermedicine will change the traditional physician-patient relationship. Concludes cybermedicine is the future of medical care, and the physician-patient relationship will have to change to accommodate the predicted online medical boom. Quotes Opinion 10.01. Gelein, *Are Online Consultations a Prescription for Trouble? The Uncharted Waters of Cybermedicine*, 66 Brook. L. Rev. 209, 239 (2000).

Journal 2000 Discusses patent law and policy. Examines whether or not those who practice medicine should be excused from patent laws because of the conflict that medical procedure patents create with respect to the practice of medicine. Concludes that Congress should repeal section 287(c) of the Patent Act. Quotes Principle V and Opinions 9.08 and 9.09. Cites Opinion 8.03. References Opinion 10.01. Ho, *Patents, Patients, and Public Policy: An Incomplete Intersection at 35 USC § 287(c)*, 33 U.C. Davis L. Rev. 601, 603, 623, 624, 625, 631 (2000).

Journal 2000 Describes the fiduciary aspects of the physician-patient relationship. Explores the conflicts that may occur between physicians and pregnant women in the health care setting. Proposes legal strategies to address these conflicts. Quotes Opinions 8.08 and 10.01. References Opinion 8.13. Oberman, *Mothers and Doctors' Orders: Unmasking the Doctor's Fiduciary Role in Maternal-Fetal Conflicts*, 94 Nw. U. L. Rev. 451, 456, 462, 493 (2000).

Journal 2000 Evaluates recent Texas legislation that affords immunity to health care professionals who provide free health care services to the poor. Concludes that such legislation creates a dual standard of care, requiring indigent patients to forfeit their legal rights in exchange for health care. Quotes Opinion 10.01. References Opinion 9.065. Pulido, *Immunity of Volunteer Health Care Providers in Texas: Bartering Legal Rights for Free Medical Care*, 2 Scholar: St. Mary's L. Rev. Minority Issues 323, 330 (2000).

Journal 2000 Considers the topic of physician liability for genetic malpractice. Explores how new genetic technologies may affect the medical and legal communities. Concludes by observing that the legal system is not prepared to address the wave of litigation that may grow out of emerging genetic technologies. Quotes Opinion 10.01. Reutenauer, *Medical Malpractice Liability in the Era of Genetic Susceptibility Testing*, 19 QLR 539, 571 (2000).

Journal 2000 Discusses managed care in terms of problems, responses, and accomplishments. Demonstrates how a physician union's collective bargaining process can benefit patients and physicians in addressing problems with managed care. Concludes that barriers preventing such unions should be removed. Quotes Principles VI and VII and Opinion 10.01. Rugg, *An Old Solution to a New Problem: Physician Unions Take the Edge Off Managed Care*, 34 Colum. J. L. & Soc. Probs. 1, 41 (2000).

Journal 2000 Examines ethical and legal issues regarding medical privacy. Discusses authorized and unauthorized uses of information contained in medical records and identifies who may access these records. Analyzes the ethical balance between patient privacy and societal benefits derived from sacrificing it. Concludes privacy is very important to maintaining a full and open physician-patient relationship. Quotes Opinion 10.01. Scott, *Is Too Much Privacy Bad for Your Health? An Introduction to the Law, Ethics, and HIPAA Rule on Medical Privacy*, 17 Ga. St. U. L. Rev. 481, 494 (2000).

Journal 2000 Discusses the development and history of the ethical doctrine of informed consent. Examines the current state of the law in Pennsylvania and concludes it does not adequately fulfill the goals of ethical and legal doctrines. Quotes Principle IV and Opinion 10.01. References Opinion 8.08. Warren, *Pennsylvania Medical Informed Consent Law: A Call to Protect Patient Autonomy Rights by Abandoning the Battery Approach*, 38 Duq. L. Rev. 917, 925 (2000).

Journal 1999 Examines reporting of AIDS and HIV under Texas law. Discusses limitations on a physician's ability to warn potentially at-risk third parties. Concludes that Texas law should be changed to place a duty upon physicians to notify at-risk third parties of a patient's HIV-positive status. Quotes Principle IV and Opinion 10.01. Acosta, *The Texas Communicable Disease Prevention and Control Act: Are We Offering Enough Protection to Those Who Need It Most?* 36 Hous. L. Rev. 1819, 1822, 1830, 1831 (1999).

Journal 1999 Discusses the need for physicians to advocate on behalf of patients' rights in the context of health care delivery. Evaluates the nature and scope of the physician's role as advocate, noting that physicians cannot be expected to engage in attorney-like advocacy. Quotes Principles IV and VI, Fundamental Elements (2), (4), and (6) [now Opinion 10.01], Patient Responsibilities 5 [now Opinion 10.02], and Opinions 2.03, 2.07, 2.09, 2.16, 2.19, 3.06, 4.01, 4.04, 6.01, 7.02, 8.02, 8.03, 8.13, 8.132, 9.06, 9.07, and 9.131. Cites Opinions 5.05, 5.09, 7.01, 8.135, and

9.02. Sage, *Physicians as Advocates, 35 Hous. L. Rev. 1529, 1537, 1541, 1542, 1552-53, 1554, 1556, 1557, 1559, 1561-62, 1564, 1571, 1574, 1576, 1580 (1999).*

Journal 1998 Discusses conflicts of interest in the physician-patient relationship arising out of use of financial incentives by managed care organizations. Considers how such conflicts are dealt with in the attorney-client relationship. Suggests that a financial incentive should be legally denounced if it unreasonably interferes with a physician's duty to properly care for and treat patients. Quotes Preamble, Fundamental Elements (1) [now Opinion 10.01], and Opinions 4.04, 5.01, 8.03, 8.13, and 9.06. Cites Fundamental Elements (4) [now Opinion 10.01] and Opinions 2.07, 2.08, and 2.132. Hall, *Third-Party Payor Conflicts of Interest in Managed Care: A Proposal for Regulation Based on the Model Rules of Professional Conduct, 29 Seton Hall L. Rev. 95, 96, 107, 108, 109, 110, 111, 112, 134, 135, 136 (1998).*

Journal 1997 Compares past ethical opinions to current opinions and notes the differences. Comments on the forces that have changed medical ethics through the years. Notes differing theories on the future course of medical ethics. Quotes Fundamental Elements (Preamble) and Opinions 5.05, 5.057, 7.01, 8.12, 9.12, and 9.131. Cites Fundamental Elements (5) [now Opinion 10.01] and Opinions 8.115 and 8.13. Buchanan, *Medical Ethics at the Millennium: A Brief Retrospective, 26 Colo. Law. 141, 142, 143, 144, 145 (1997).*

Journal 1997 Reviews ethical issues raised by genetic research. Explores the duty a physician may have to reveal the genetic diseases found in patients to their relatives. Considers case law and statutory law, and concludes that a limited duty to disclose exists. Quotes Fundamental Elements (4) [now Opinion 10.01]. Deftos, *Genomic Torts: The Law of the Future—The Duty of Physicians to Disclose the Presence of a Genetic Disease to the Relatives of Their Patients With the Disease, 32 USF. L. Rev. 105, 130 (1997).*

Journal 1997 Discusses physician frustration with managed care plans caused by gag clauses and cost-containment mechanisms. Reviews the development of managed care organizations and federal attempts at limiting the use of gag clauses. Concludes that gag clauses are inherently flawed and compromise quality health care. Quotes Principles II and V, Fundamental Elements (1) [now Opinion 10.01], and Opinion 8.13. Note, *Physicians, Bound and Gagged: Federal Attempts to Combat Managed Care's Use of Gag Clauses, 21 Seton Hall Legis. J. 567, 601-02 (1997).*

Journal 1997 Considers the current approach to health care in the US. Examines financing mechanisms, and suggests that reform could be effected through a decentralized, community-based approach. Proposes use of volunteer systems in which medical personnel would care for certain patients free of charge or at reduced rates. Quotes Fundamental Elements (6) [now Opinion 10.01]. References Opinion 9.065. Solomon & Asaro, *Community-Based Health Care: A Legal and Policy Analysis, 24 Fordham Urb. L. J. 235, 276-77 (1997).*

Journal 1996 Describes the problem of lack of access to medical care by the indigent. Recognizes the commitment of the medical profession to providing care for indigent patients. Observes that state initiatives that provide physicians tort immunity in exchange for volunteer service can improve access to care by the indigent. Quotes Fundamental Elements (6) [now Opinion 10.01]. References Opinion 9.065. Comment, *Statutory Immunity for Volunteer Physicians: A Vehicle for Reaffirmation of the Doctor's Beneficent Duties—Absent the Rights Talk, 1 Widener L. Symp. J. 425, 448, 449 (1996).*

Journal 1996 Considers the ethical requirement for physicians to receive informed consent from patients before beginning treatment. Reviews the case of *Jacobson v. Massachusetts,* discussing its impact on informed consent and vaccination policy in the US. Quotes Fundamental Elements (2) [now Opinion 10.01]. References Opinion 8.08. Severyn, *Jacobson v. Massachusetts: Impact on Informed Consent and Vaccine Policy, 5 J. Pharmacy & L. 249, 253, 274 (1996).*

Journal 1996 Examines medically futile treatment in light of legislative enactments in Virginia and Maryland. Observes that the futility debate arises when requests for life-prolonging treatment are viewed as medically inappropriate by health care providers. Concludes that, while the ethical integrity of the medical profession justifies some legal recognition of futility, such recognition must be limited by respect for patient autonomy. References Fundamental Elements (5) [now Opinion 10.01]. Shiner, *Medical Futility: A Futile Concept? 53 Wash. & Lee L. Rev. 803, 834 (1996).*

Journal 1995 Examines the impact of health care reform on physician-patient relationships. Discusses how reform may threaten the physician's fiduciary duty of loyalty by forcing physicians to make rationing decisions and giving physicians financial incentives to limit use of health care resources. Quotes Fundamental Elements (5) [now Opinion 10.01]. Cites Opinion 5.05.

Orentlicher, *Health Care Reform and the Patient-Physician Relationship*, 5 Health Matrix 141, 143, 148 (1995).

Journal 1994 Considers whether an exception should be made to physician-patient confidentiality that would allow a physician to reveal parental medical history to a child. Concludes that such an exception would not completely erode physician-patient confidentiality. Quotes Principles IV, Fundamental Elements (4) [now Opinion 10.01], and Opinion 5.05. Cites Principle I and Fundamental Elements (1). Friedland, *Physician-Patient Confidentiality: Time to Re-Examine a Venerable Concept in Light of Contemporary Society and Advances in Medicine*, 15 J. Legal Med. 249, 257, 264, 276 (1994).

Journal 1994 Explores the ethical issues involved in a multidisciplinary team working with children in legal proceedings. Focuses on the relationships between professionals and the conflicts that arise regarding disclosure of confidential information and forced disclosure of nonprivileged information. Quotes Principles III and IV, Fundamental Elements (4) [now Opinion 10.01], and Opinions 1.02 (1992) and 5.07 (1992) [now Opinion 5.05]. Cites Opinions 2.02. Glynn, *Multidisciplinary Representation of Children: Conflicts Over Disclosures of Client Communications*, 27 J. Marshall L. Rev. 617, 625, 626, 630-32, 637, 639, 643 (1994).

Journal 1994 Discusses physician-patient confidentiality and the exception that permits breach of a patient's confidence if required by law. Argues that this is always a legitimate exception to the confidentiality rule. Quotes Principle IV and Fundamental Elements (4) [now Opinion 10.01]. McConnell, *Confidentiality and the Law*, 20 J. Med. Ethics 47, 47 (1994).

Journal 1994 Reviews the evolution of the physician-patient relationship, with attention to the changing health care delivery environment. Quotes Preamble, Principles I, II, III, IV, V, and VI, Fundamental Elements (1) and (2) [now Opinion 10.01], and Opinions 1.02 and 8.07 (1981) [now Opinion 8.08]. Cites Opinion 1.01. Szczygiel, *Beyond Informed Consent*, 21 Ohio N. U. L. Rev. 171, 217, 218, 220, 225, 226, 256 (1994).

Journal 1994 Discusses the importance of confidentiality in the physician-patient relationship and under what circumstances patient information may be released. Examines unique considerations that apply when a physician provides medical care to a minor or an HIV-infected individual. Quotes Principle IV and Fundamental Elements (4) [now Opinion 10.01]. Weiner & Wettstein, *Confidentiality of Patient-Related Information*, 112 Arch. Ophthalmology 1032, 1033 (1994).

Journal 1993 Analyzes the implications of giving patients and their families an absolute right to control medical treatment. Argues that courts should refrain from ordering physicians to treat patients when physicians believe that treatment would be ineffective. Quotes Fundamental Elements (5) [now Opinion 10.01] and Opinions 2.11 (1982) [now Opinion 2.20] and 2.18 (1986) [now Opinion 2.20]. Comment, *Beyond Autonomy: Judicial Restraint and the Legal Limits Necessary to Uphold the Hippocratic Tradition and Preserve the Ethical Integrity of the Medical Profession*, 9 J. Contemp. Health L. & Pol'y 451, 467, 468 (1993).

10.015 The Patient-Physician Relationship

The practice of medicine, and its embodiment in the clinical encounter between a patient and a physician, is fundamentally a moral activity that arises from the imperative to care for patients and to alleviate suffering.

A patient-physician relationship exists when a physician serves a patient's medical needs, generally by mutual consent between physician and patient (or surrogate). In some instances the agreement is implied, such as in emergency care or when physicians provide services at the request of the treating physician. In rare instances, treatment without consent may be provided under court order (see Opinion 2.065, "Court-Initiated Medical Treatments in Criminal Cases"). Nevertheless, the physician's obligations to the patient remain intact.

The relationship between patient and physician is based on trust and gives rise to physicians' ethical obligations to place patients' welfare above their own self-interest and above obligations to other groups, and to advocate for their patients' welfare.

Within the patient-physician relationship, a physician is ethically required to use sound medical judgment, holding the best interests of the patient as paramount. (I, II, VI, VIII)

Issued December 2001 based on the report "The Patient-Physician Relationship," adopted June 2001.

Minn. App. 2005 Minnesota Board of Medical Practice revoked the license of appellant, finding that appellant carried on an inappropriate sexual relationship with a patient. Quoting Opinion 10.015, the appeals court determined that the individual whom the appellant was treating fell within the definition of patient, and therefore, appellant's sexual relationship with the patient was a violation of the Minnesota Medical Practice Act, justifying the revocation of his license. *In re Woolley, 2005 WL 2077475, 6.*

Army Crim. App. 2004 Appellant, in a general court martial hearing, was found guilty of unpremeditated murder. The Court of Appeals for the Armed Forces set aside and remanded the judgment to the Army Court of Criminal Appeals to determine whether there was a conflict of interest in allowing mental health providers who had a prior psychotherapist-patient relationship with the appellant to serve on his sanity board. The court determined there was no conflict of interest. In making this determination, the court quoted Opinion 10.015 and cited Opinion 8.03 to analyze the aspects of the physician-patient relationship. *United States v. Best, 59 M.J. 886, 891 n. 8.*

Journal 2011 Reviews the issues surrounding the use of the Internet for medical consultations, as well as current guidelines and regulations. Concludes that, although online medical consultations may be cost-effective, the risks of liability outweigh the benefits. References Opinion 10.015. Bailey, *The Legal, Financial, and Ethical Implications of Online Medical Consultations, 16 J. Tech. L. & Pol'y 53, 95 (2011).*

Journal 2011 Describes off-label uses of prescription drugs and the associated risks and harms. Argues that such use should be restricted unless supported by high-quality evidence of efficacy and safety. Cites Opinions 10.01 and 10.015. Coleman & Rosoff, *The Case for Legal Regulation of Physicians' Off-Label Prescribing, 86 Notre Dame L. Rev. 649, 679 (2011).*

Journal 2011 Discusses the doctrine of informed consent and the influence of physician groups on the dissemination of information to patients. Concludes the doctrine of informed consent should be expanded by the courts, rather than continuing to allow professional societies to dictate provider guidelines for obtaining informed consent. Quotes Opinions 8.08, 10.01, and 10.015. References Opinion 2.065. Ginsberg, *Informed Consent: No Longer Just What the Doctor Ordered? The "Contributions" of Medical Associations and Courts to a More Patient Friendly Doctrine, 15 Mich. St. J. Med. & Law 17, 23, 24, 25, 26, 46 (2011).*

Journal 2011 Examines the Patient Protection and Affordable Care Act and its impact on patient access to physician services. Also considers the possibility that physicians might be required to provide services to all patients as a condition to practice. Concludes that regulations that try to conscript physician services would be practically ineffective, legally dubious, and unwise public policy. Quotes Opinions 9.06 and 10.015. Cites Opinion 2.09. Kapp, *Conscripted Physician Services and the Public's Health, 39 J. L. Med. & Ethics 414, 414, 418 (2011).*

Journal 2011 Discusses the far-reaching effects of 2005 Illinois medical liability reform legislation. Explains how the 2010 Illinois Supreme Court decision in *Lebron v. Gottlieb* invalidated many beneficial aspects of this legislation. Quotes Opinion 10.015. Cites Opinion 9.10. Nelson, Swanson, & Buckley, *Lebron v. Gottlieb Memorial Hospital: Capping Medical Practice Reform in Illinois, 20 Annals Health L. 1, 7, 11 (Winter 2011).*

Journal 2011 Reviews the use and current regulation of medical marijuana to alleviate pain in terminally ill patients. Focusing on patient autonomy, concludes that patients should have access to medical marijuana in controlled doses under controlled conditions. Quotes Principle III and Opinions 10.01, 10.015, and 10.02. References Principle VIII. Pfeifer, *Smoking Gun: The Moral and Legal Struggle for Medical Marijuana, 27 Touro L. Rev. 339, 340-41, 345-346 (2011).*

Journal 2010 Examines manufacturer-physician consulting arrangements and discusses the evolution of fair market valuation. Proposes a set of standards for calculating fair market value for physician services to ensure compliance with legal requirements. Quotes Opinion 8.061.

Eaton & Reid, *Mirror, Mirror on the Wall: Evaluating Fair Market Value for Manufacturer-Physician Consulting Arrangements*, 65 Food & Drug L. J. 141, 147 (2010).

Journal 2010 Discusses issues arising from the enactment of legislation by North Dakota involving a minor's reproductive rights. Explores ethical principles that govern physician's actions within the context of reproductive health. Concludes that, while a patient's expectation of confidentiality with a physician is critical, competing values come into play when the patient is a minor and parental involvement may be important. Provides practical guidance to address issues in this context. Quotes Opinions 2.01, 2.015, 5.055, 8.08, 8.115, 9.12, 10.01, 10.015, and 10.05. Cites Opinion 5.05, 5.055, 8.08, 8.11, 8.115, 9.12, and 10.05. Haas, *"Doctor, I'm Pregnant and Fifteen—I Can't Tell My Parents—Please Help Me": Minor Consent, Reproductive Rights, and Ethical Principles for Physicians*, 86 N.D. L. Rev. 63, 70, 73, 75-78, 82, 84, 86-88, (2010).

Journal 2010 Argues that it is ethically improper for medical practitioners to use their position of influence arising from superior scientific knowledge to impose their moral preferences on patients. Concludes physicians need education about their professional and legal obligations so they may protect their ability to participate in, or refuse participation in, particular services while ensuring the patient is not harmed. Quotes Opinion 10.015. Morrison & Allokotte, *Duty First: Towards Patient-Centered Care and Limitations on the Right to Refuse for Moral, Religious or Ethical Reasons*, 9 Ave Maria L. Rev. 141, 168 (2010).

Journal 2010 Argues that physicians are more likely to avoid improperly prescribing controlled substances if put on notice of the additional criminal liability they face in the event of a patient's death. Concludes that physicians who have caused a patient's death by administering illegal and lethal doses should be charged under various sections of the Controlled Substances Act as well as with involuntary manslaughter. Quotes Opinion 10.015. Nunziato, *Preventing Prescription Drug Overdose in the Twenty-First Century: Is the Controlled Substances Act Enough?* 38 Hofstra L. Rev. 1261, 1277 (2010).

Journal 2010 Examines disciplinary functions of state medical licensing boards and identifies fundamental principles underlying their authority. Concludes that medical boards have lost sight of the primary goal of protecting patients and suggests that they renew their focus, prioritizing disciplinary actions taken on the basis of competence. Quotes Opinion 10.015. Sawicki, *Character, Competence, and the Principles of Medical Discipline*, 13 J. Health Care L. & Pol'y 285, 291 (2010).

Journal 2009 Considers a physician's role in educating patients about health care reform. Concludes that reform would be aided by educating patients on all aspects of the health care system. Quotes Opinion 10.015. Cites Opinion 9.012. Abemayor, *United We Stand, Divided We Fall*, 135 Arch. Otolaryngol. Head Neck Surg. 432, 432, 433 (2009).

Journal 2009 Explores the jurisprudential foundation of the fiduciary duty physicians owe their patients and discusses the failure of physicians to disclose to patients errors and other emergent medical risks. Concludes law should recognize the physician's duty to disclose such risks by enforcing a cause of action for breach of that duty. Quotes Principles III and VIII and Opinions 8.12, 10.015, and 10.02. References Opinion 8.12. Hafemeister, *Lean on Me: A Physician's Fiduciary Duty to Disclose an Emergent Medical Risk to the Patient*, 86 Wash. U. L. Rev. 1167, 1172-1173, 1178, 1182, 1185, 1188, 1209 (2009).

Journal 2009 Explores the nature of the physician-patient relationship and the impact of increased availability of medical information on patient autonomy and physician responsibility to exercise independent judgment. Concludes physicians must treat patients in accordance with their fiduciary obligation to use their own judgment when confronted with a patient demanding unnecessary medical services. Quotes Preamble, Principles I and VIII, and Opinions 2.035, 8.03 and 10.015. Hafemeister, *The Fiduciary Obligation of Physicians to "Just Say No" if an "Informed" Patient Demands Services That Are Not Medically Indicated*, 39 Seton Hall L. Rev. 335, 372, 373, 374 (2009).

Journal 2009 Discusses the judicial standard for reviewing physician noncompete covenants. Concludes courts should apply a strict standard to such covenants, rather than declare the covenants per se invalid. Quotes Principles IV and VII, Principles of Medical Ethics §5 (1957) [now Principle VI], Code of Medical Ethics Ch. II, Art. I §3 (1847) [now Opinion 5.02], Opinion 9.02, and Code of Medical Ethics Ch. II, Art. I §4 (1847) [now Opinion 9.09]. Cites Opinions 8.041, 8.115, 9.02, 9.06, 9.065, 9.067, 10.01, and 10.015. Koons, *Physician Employee Non-Compete Agreements on the Examining Table: The Need to Better Protect Patients' and the Public's Interests in Indiana*, 6 Ind. Health L. Rev. 253, 272-77, 280-81 (2009).

Journal 2008 Considers the utility of physician apologies for medical error and legal protection for physicians who apologize for mistakes. Concludes physicians must openly communicate with their patients and apologize for medical errors to strengthen the health care community. Quotes Opinions 8.08, 8.12, 10.01, and 10.015. References Opinion 8.12. Ebert, *Attorneys, Tell Your Clients to Say They're Sorry: Apologies in the Health Care Industry*, 5 Ind. Health L. Rev. 337, 340-41, 344 (2008).

Journal 2008 Studies the likelihood and causes of physicians discharging patients. Concludes that physicians should be educated about the ethical and legal consequences of discharging patients for reasons other than dangerous or illegal behavior. References Opinion 10.015. Farber, Jordan, Silverstein, Collier, Weiner, & Boyer, *Primary Care Physicians' Decisions About Discharging Patients From Their Practices*, 23 J. of General Internal Med. 283, 283 (2008).

Journal 2008 Discusses FDA advisory opinion preempting failure-to-warn claims brought against pharmaceutical companies and examines ethical problems throughout pharmaceutical industry. Concludes that litigation is an important check on the industry, encouraging quality research and safe medications. Quotes Opinion 10.015. Martin, *Hugs and Drugs: Research Ethics, Conflict of Interest, and Why the FDA's Attempt to Preempt Pharma Failure-to-Warn Claims Is a Dangerous Prescription*, 6 Ave Maria L. Rev. 587, 621 (2008).

Journal 2008 Examines the medical malpractice system and the reasons why patients sue. Argues that lack of effective communication between physician and patient is the underlying cause of litigation. Concludes voluntary mediation of claims may decrease medical malpractice litigation if attorneys, health professionals, and the federal government encourage use of mediation. Quotes Opinion 10.015. Meruelo, *The Need to Understand Why Patients Sue and a Proposal for a Specific Model of Mediation*, 29 J. Legal Med. 285, 290 (2008).

Journal 2008 Argues that as a matter of public health, physicians must control antibiotic administration to combat antibiotic resistance. Concludes that despite limited incentives for antibiotic conservation, physicians must acknowledge their important role in mitigating the public health threat of antibiotic resistance. Quotes Principles VII and VIII and Opinions 2.09 and 10.015. Cites Opinion 2.03. Saver, *In Tepid Defense of Population Health: Physicians and Antibiotic Resistance*, 34 Am. J. L. & Med. 431, 457 (2008).

Journal 2008 Explores the fiduciary relationship between physicians and patients, professional and ethical obligations of both physicians and lawyers, and the implications for conflict resolution in health care. Concludes physicians must put patient interests above their own and lawyers must work to discern clients' best interests and support client welfare. Quotes Principle VIII and Opinions 8.12 and 10.015. Cites Principles I and II and Opinions 10.01 and 10.015. Scott, *Doctors as Advocates, Lawyers as Healers*, 29 Hamline J. Pub. L. Pol'y, 331, 340-41, 347, 371 (2008).

Journal 2007 Addresses physician liability for an extramarital affair with a patient's spouse. Concludes that such an affair should be regarded as a breach of a fiduciary duty. Quotes Preamble, Principles I, II, and VIII, and Opinions 8.145, 9.04, 9.123, and 10.015. Demaine, *"Playing Doctor" With the Patient's Spouse: Alternative Conceptions of Health Professional Liability*, 14 Va. J. Soc. Pol'y & L. 308, 325, 330-31, 331-32 (2007).

Journal 2007 Examines the history and effectiveness of medical malpractice screening panels. Concludes that screening panels are ineffective, then proposes an alternative dispute resolution model. Quotes Opinion 10.015. Kaufman, *The Demise of Medical Malpractice Screening Panels and Alternative Solutions Based on Trust and Honesty*, 28 J. Legal Med. 247, 250 (2007).

Journal 2007 Discusses patients' right to refuse medical treatment and the corresponding duties of health care professionals. Concludes that detailed, carefully prepared advance directives are necessary to fulfill patients' wishes. Quotes Ch. II (1940) [now Opinions 8.08 and 8.082] and Opinions 2.035, 2.037, 2.20, 2.225, 8.081, and 10.015. Cites Opinions 9.11 and 9.115. Stamatakis, *Beyond Advance Directives: Personal Autonomy and the Right to Refuse Life-Sustaining Medical Treatment*, 47 N. H. B. J. 20, 29-30 (2007).

Journal 2006 Reviews the concept of therapeutic privilege. Concludes that the practice creates conflict between physician obligations under the concepts of autonomy and beneficence. Recommends that physicians maximize communication with patients by providing all pertinent information in the context of patient preferences. Cites Opinions 8.08, 8.081, 8.121, and 10.015. References Chap. I, Art. I, Sec. 4 (May 1847) [premise deleted from Code]. Bostick, Sade, McMahon, & Benjamin, *Report of the American Medical Association Council on Ethical and Judicial Affairs: Withholding Information From Patients: Rethinking the Propriety of "Therapeutic Privilege,"* 17 J. Clinical Ethics 302, 303 (Winter 2006).

Journal 2006 Examines the efficacy of informed consent when a physician acts both as a researcher and care provider. Concludes that a patient cannot give truly informed consent in such cases. Cites Opinions 8.115 and 10.015. Lenrow, *The Treating Physician as Researcher: Is Assuming This Dual Role a Violation of the Nuremberg Code? 25 Temp. J. Sci. Tech. & Envtl. L. 15, 42-43 (2006).*

Journal 2006 Discusses tort liability for medical malpractice. Concludes that both physicians and attorneys should support a legal system which promotes patient safety. Quotes Opinions 8.12 and 10.015. Pegalis, *A Proposal to Use Common Ground That Exists Between the Medical and Legal Professions to Promote a Culture of Safety, 51 N. Y. L. Sch. L. Rev. 1057, 1070, 1073 (2006).*

Journal 2006 Examines the practice by physicians of billing a malpractice surcharge. Concludes that such practice is unethical and constitutes a breach of fiduciary duty. Quotes Opinions 10.015 and 10.018. Peterson, *The Malpractice Surcharge: A Simple Answer to Rising Malpractice Rates or a Greater Threat to Quality Patient Care? 27 J. Legal Med. 87, 96, 97-98 (2006).*

Journal 2006 Considers prisoners' rights to expression of sexuality and the state's legitimate interest in regulating that expression. Concludes that states should encourage healthy expressions of sexuality while protecting the goals of the Prison Rape Elimination Act. Cites Opinions 3.08, 8.14, 8.145, and 10.015. Smith, *Rethinking Prison Sex: Self-expression and Safety, 15 Colum. J. Gender & L. 185, 202 (2006).*

Journal 2005 Discusses physician responses to the medical malpractice liability crisis. Concludes that certain responses may violate ethical obligations that physicians owe to their patients and to society as a whole. Cites Opinions 9.025 and 10.015. References Principle VIII. Kachalia, Choudhry, & Studdert, *Physician Responses to the Malpractice Crisis: From Defense to Offense, 33 J. L. Med. & Ethics 416, 419, 421, 424 (2005).*

Journal 2005 Argues that in *Aetna v. Davila/Cigna v. Calad*, the Supreme Court missed an opportunity to overturn unjust ERISA policies. Concludes that the principle of complete ERISA preemption as articulated in these consolidated cases is unsatisfactory because it violates the separation of powers doctrine. Quotes Principle VIII. Cites Opinions 8.054, 8.13, 8.135, 9.123, 10.01, and 10.015. Nelson, *AETNA v. DAVILA/CIGNA v. CALAD: A Missed Opportunity, 31 Wm. Mitchell L. Rev. 843, 847, 849, 850, 880 (2005).*

Journal 2005 Discusses ethical, legal, and policy issues associated with treatment and research involving patients who are in a persistent vegetative or minimally conscious state. Concludes that patients in these states are at risk for therapeutic failures until physicians can more accurately determine which patients will benefit from treatment and accurately convey such information to families or surrogates. Quotes Principles VII and IX and Opinions 8.031, 8.0315, 9.065, 10.01, and 10.015. Tovino & Winslade, *A Primer on the Law and Ethics of Treatment, Research, and Public Policy in the Context of Severe Traumatic Brain Injury, 14 Ann. Health L. 1, 18, 38, 39, 40, 41 (2005).*

Journal 2004 Analyzes various issues relating to the role of mental health professionals in capital punishment in light of Albert Bandura's model of "mechanisms of moral disengagement." Concludes that facilitating participation of mental health professionals in executions creates conflicts with the humanistic norms of the profession. Quotes Preamble and Opinions 1.01, 1.02, 2.06, 2.067, 2.20, 2.21, 2.211, and 8.14. Judges, *The Role of Mental Health Professionals in Capital Punishment: An Exercise in Moral Disengagement, 41 Hous. L. Rev. 515, 562, 568, 569, 570, 571-72, 581, 586, 588, 598 (2004).*

Journal 2004 Examines the requirements of the Privacy Rule regarding use and disclosure of a patient's identifiable health information in the context of research. Concludes that the Rule's burdensome administrative requirements may discourage research and thus outweigh any benefits for research subject autonomy. Quotes Principle VIII and Opinions 5.051, 8.031, and 10.015. Tovino, *The Use and Disclosure of Protected Health Information for Research Under the HIPAA Privacy Rule: Unrealized Patient Autonomy and Burdensome Government Regulation, 49 S. D. L. Rev. 447, 496, 502 (2004).*

Journal 2004 Addresses the problem of pediatric obesity and examines various treatment options, including gastric bypass. Concludes that, before surgery is undertaken, the best interests of the child must be prioritized, with consultative input from specialists who have no stake in the decision. Quotes 10.015. Wilde, *Bioethical and Legal Implications of Pediatric Gastric Bypass, 40 Willamette L. Rev. 575, 613 (2004).*

Journal 2003 Highlights the legal and ethical concerns surrounding use of noncompetition clauses. Concludes that physicians should carefully evaluate these clauses given their likely enforceability. Quotes Opinions 9.02, 9.06, 10.01, and 10.015. Loeser, *The Legal, Ethical, and Practical Implications of Noncompetition Clauses: What Physicians Should Know Before They Sign,* 31 J. L. Med. & Ethics 283, 286, 287, 290 (2003).

Journal 2002 Examines sports-related concussions among football players. Considers the responsibilities of team physicians. Concludes that litigation will increase without treatment guidelines for concussion management. References Opinion 10.015. Hecht, *Legal and Ethical Aspects of Sports-Related Concussions: The Merril Hoge Story,* 12 Seton Hall J. Sport L. 17, 42-43 (2002).

10.016   The previous Opinion 10.016, "Pediatric Decision-Making," issued June 2008, was replaced by the current Opinion 10.016, "Pediatric Decision-Making."

10.016 Pediatric Decision-Making

Medical decision making for pediatric patients should be based on the child's best interest, which is determined by weighing many factors, including effectiveness of appropriate medical therapies, the patient's psychological and emotional welfare, and the family situation. When there is legitimate inability to reach consensus about what is in the best interest of the child, the wishes of the parents should generally receive preference.

Physicians treating pediatric patients generally must obtain informed consent from a parent or a legal guardian. Certain classes of children, such as emancipated or mature minors, may provide consent to their own medical care. Physicians should give pediatric patients the opportunity to participate in decision making at a developmentally appropriate level. The physician should seek the patient's assent, or agreement, by explaining the medical condition, its clinical implications, and the treatment plan in ways that take into account the child's cognitive and emotional maturity and social circumstances. The physician should provide a supportive environment and encourage reluctant parents to discuss their child's health status with the patient, in private themselves or with the physician. For HIV-infected children in particular, the physician should be sensitive to the fact that disclosure of health status can have implications for the child's relationships with biological relatives, household members, and peers; adherence to a complex medical regimen; and participation in behaviors that put the child or others at risk. Physicians should also be sensitive that disclosure of HIV and other conditions (eg, some inherited conditions) can also have implications for family members other than the child. If the patient does not or cannot assent, physicians should still explain the plan of care and tell him or her what to expect, without deception. In the case of an adolescent patient who has decision making capacity, the physician should encourage the patient's active participation in decision-making. The use of force such as with using physical restraints to carry out a medical intervention in adolescent patients who do not assent should be a last resort.

Parents and physicians may disagree about the course of action that best serves the pediatric patient's interests, including how much to tell the child about his or her health status, when and how to do so, and who should lead the discussion. When disagreements occur, institutional policies for timely conflict resolution should be followed, including consultation with an ethics committee, pastoral service, or other counseling resource. If a health care facility does not have policies for resolving conflicts in a timely manner, physicians should encourage their development. Physicians should treat reversible life-threatening conditions regardless of any persistent disagreement. Resolution of disagreements in the courts should be pursued only as a last resort. (IV, VIII)

Issued June 2011 based on the report "Amendment to E-10.016, 'Pediatric Decision-Making,'" adopted November 2010.

10.017 Gifts From Patients

Gifts that patients offer to physicians are often an expression of appreciation and gratitude or a reflection of cultural tradition, and can enhance the patient-physician relationship.

Some gifts signal psychological needs that require the physician's attention. Some patients may attempt to influence care or to secure preferential treatment through the offering of gifts or cash. Acceptance of such gifts is likely to damage the integrity of the patient-physician relationship. Physicians should make clear that gifts given to secure preferential treatment compromise their obligation to provide services in a fair manner.

There are no definitive rules to determine when a physician should or should not accept a gift. No fixed value determines the appropriateness or inappropriateness of a gift from a patient; however, the gift's value relative to the patient's or the physician's means should not be disproportionately or inappropriately large. One criterion is whether the physician would be comfortable if acceptance of the gift were known to colleagues or the public.

Physicians should be cautious if patients discuss gifts in the context of a will. Such discussions must not influence the patient's medical care.

If, after a patient's death, a physician should learn that he or she has been bequeathed a gift, the physician should consider declining the gift if the physician believes that its acceptance would present a significant hardship (financial or emotional) to the family.

The interaction of these various factors is complex and requires the physician to consider them sensitively. (I, II)

Issued December 2003 based on the report "Gifts From Patients," adopted June 2003.

Journal 2008 Argues that organ donation from a patient to his or her physician is unethical. Concludes that this practice would be exploitative to the patient and undermine public trust in the medical profession. Cites Opinions 8.14, 10.017, and 10.018. Steinberg & Pomfret, *A Novel Boundary Issue: Should a Patient Be an Organ Donor for Their Physician? 34 J. Med. Ethics 772,* 772 (2008).

10.018 Physician Participation in Soliciting Contributions From Patients

Donations play an important role in supporting and improving a community's health care. Physicians are encouraged to participate in fundraising and other solicitation activities while protecting the integrity of the patient-physician relationship, including patient privacy and confidentiality, and ensuring that all donations are fully voluntary. In particular:

(1) Appropriate means of soliciting contributions include making information available in a reception area and speaking at fundraising events. Physicians should avoid directly soliciting their own patients, especially at the time of a clinical encounter. They should reinforce the trust that is the foundation of the patient-physician relationship by being clear that patients' welfare is the primary priority and that patients need not contribute in order to continue receiving the same quality of care.

(2) The greater the separation between the request and the clinical encounter, the more acceptable the solicitation is likely to be.

(3) When physicians participate in solicitation efforts as members of the general community, they should seek to minimize perceptions of overlap with their professional roles.

(4) Physicians in institutions that rely on fundraising personnel for donation requests should work to protect privacy and confidentiality of patient information. In particular physicians should ensure that any patient information used for solicitation activities reveals only basic demographic data, not personal health information. When the medical service delivered or the diagnosis is identifiable by the nature of the physician's practice or the physician's specialty, permission from the patient should be obtained prior to divulging any information to third parties.

(5) When patients initiate requests to contribute, physicians should refer them to appropriate sources of information or fundraising personnel.

Issued December 2004 based on the report "Physician Participation in Soliciting Contributions From Patients," adopted June 2004.

Journal 2008 Argues that organ donation from a patient to his or her physician is unethical. Concludes that this practice would be exploitative to the patient and undermine public trust in the medical profession. Cites Opinions 8.14, 10.017, and 10.018. Steinberg & Pomfret, *A Novel Boundary Issue: Should a Patient Be an Organ Donor for Their Physician?* 34 J. Med. Ethics 772, 772 (2008).

Journal 2006 Examines the practice by physicians of billing a malpractice surcharge. Concludes that such practice is unethical and constitutes a breach of fiduciary duty. Quotes Opinions 10.015 and 10.018. Peterson, *The Malpractice Surcharge: A Simple Answer to Rising Malpractice Rates or a Greater Threat to Quality Patient Care?* 27 J. Legal Med. 87, 96, 97-98 (2006).

10.02 Patient Responsibilities

It has long been recognized that successful medical care requires an ongoing collaborative effort between patients and physicians. Physician and patient are bound in a partnership that requires both individuals to take an active role in the healing process. Such a partnership does not imply that both partners have identical responsibilities or equal power. While physicians have the responsibility to provide health care services to patients to the best of their ability, patients have the responsibility to communicate openly, to participate in decisions about the diagnostic and treatment recommendations, and to comply with the agreed-upon treatment program.

Like patients' rights, patients' responsibilities are derived from the principle of autonomy. The principle of patient autonomy holds that an individual's physical, emotional, and psychological integrity should be respected and upheld.

This principle also recognizes the human capacity to self-govern and choose a course of action from among different alternative options. Autonomous, competent patients assert some control over the decisions which direct their health care. With that exercise of self-governance and free choice comes a number of responsibilities.

(1) Good communication is essential to a successful patient-physician relationship. To the extent possible, patients have a responsibility to be truthful and to express their concerns clearly to their physicians.

(2) Patients have a responsibility to provide a complete medical history, to the extent possible, including information about past illnesses, medications, hospitalizations, family history of illness, and other matters relating to present health.

(3) Patients have a responsibility to request information or clarification about their health status or treatment when they do not fully understand what has been described.

(4) Once patients and physicians agree upon the goals of therapy and a treatment plan, patients have a responsibility to cooperate with that treatment plan and to keep their agreed-upon appointments. Compliance with physician instructions is often essential to public and individual safety. Patients also have a responsibility to disclose whether previously agreed-upon treatments are being followed and to indicate when they would like to reconsider the treatment plan.

(5) Patients generally have a responsibility to meet their financial obligations with regard to medical care or to discuss financial hardships with their physicians. Patients should be cognizant of the costs associated with using a limited resource like health care and try to use medical resources judiciously.

(6) Patients should discuss end-of-life decisions with their physicians and make their wishes known. Such a discussion might also include writing an advance directive.

(7) Patients should be committed to health maintenance through health-enhancing behavior. Illness can often be prevented by a healthy lifestyle, and patients should take personal responsibility when they are able to avert the development of disease.

(8) Patients should also have an active interest in the effects of their conduct on others and refrain from behavior that unreasonably places the health of others at risk. Patients should inquire as to the means and likelihood of infectious disease transmission and act upon that information which can best prevent further transmission.

(9) Participation in medical education is to the mutual benefit of patients and the health care system. Patients are encouraged to participate in medical education by accepting care, under appropriate supervision, from medical students, residents, and other trainees. Consistent with the process of informed consent, the patient or the patient's surrogate decision maker is always free to refuse care from any member of the health care team.

(10) Patients should discuss organ donation with their physicians and, if donation is desired, make applicable provisions. Patients who are part of an organ allocation system and await needed transplant should not try to go

outside of or manipulate the system. A fair system of allocation should be answered with public trust and an awareness of limited resources.

(11) Patients should not initiate or participate in fraudulent health care and should report illegal or unethical behavior by physicians and other providers to the appropriate medical societies, licensing boards, or law enforcement authorities. (I, IV, VI)

Issued June 1994 based on the report "Patient Responsibilities," adopted June 1993. Updated June 1998, December 2000, and June 2001.

Journal 2011 Examines the protection of a woman's autonomy in the context of reproductive choices including abortion. Argues that, when faced with such choices, women are not currently provided with balanced and comprehensive information necessary to promote autonomy. Concludes that the law should recognize the complexity involved in reproductive choices and provide an appropriate framework for women to make such choices in their own best interests. Cites Opinions 10.01 and 10.02. Laufer-Ukeles, *Reproductive Choices and Informed Consent: Fetal Interests, Women's Identity, and Relational Autonomy*, 37 Am. J. L. & Med. 567, 575 (2011).

Journal 2011 Examines the use of antibiotic prophylaxis for Lyme disease to prevent anaplasmosis from deer tick bites in patients in the upper Midwest. Concludes single-dose antibiotic prophylaxis is an appropriate response to bites, although an alternative recommendation of more aggressive antibiotic therapy following a bite may also be appropriate if patient is informed and such treatment is consistent with patient goals and values. References Opinions 10.01 and 10.02. Maloney, *The Management of Ixodes scapularis Bites in the Upper Midwest*, 110 World Med. J. 78, 80 (2011).

Journal 2011 Reviews the use and current regulation of medical marijuana to alleviate pain in terminally ill patients. Focusing on patient autonomy, concludes that patients should have access to medical marijuana in controlled doses under controlled conditions. Quotes Principle III and Opinions 10.01, 10.015, and 10.02. References Principle VIII. Pfeifer, *Smoking Gun: The Moral and Legal Struggle for Medical Marijuana*, 27 Touro L. Rev. 339, 340-41, 345-346 (2011).

Journal 2009 Explores the jurisprudential foundation of the fiduciary duty physicians owe their patients and discusses the failure of physicians to disclose to patients errors and other emergent medical risks. Concludes law should recognize the physician's duty to disclose such risks by enforcing a cause of action for breach of that duty. Quotes Principles III and VIII and Opinions 8.12, 10.015, and 10.02. References Opinion 8.12. Hafemeister, *Lean on Me: A Physician's Fiduciary Duty to Disclose an Emergent Medical Risk to the Patient*, 86 Wash. U. L. Rev. 1167, 1172-1173, 1178, 1182, 1185, 1188, 1209 (2009).

Journal 2002 Reviews how changes in the health care delivery system underscore the importance of information in patient empowerment. Concludes that patients should use information to take charge of their health care. Quotes Principle V and Opinion 10.02. Cites Opinion 10.01. Kane, *Information Is the Key to Patient Empowerment*, 11 Annals Health L. 25, 29-30, 44 (2002).

Journal 2002 Discusses state regulation of health information and the Federal Health Privacy Rule, noting that it provides inadequate protection. Concludes state laws can bridge gaps in protection. Quotes Opinion 10.02. Pritts, *Altered States: State Health Privacy Laws and the Impact of the Federal Health Privacy Rules*, 2 Yale J. Health Pol'y, L. & Ethics 327, 351 (2002).

Journal 1999 Discusses the need for physicians to advocate on behalf of patients' rights in the context of health care delivery. Evaluates the nature and scope of the physician's role as advocate, noting that physicians cannot be expected to engage in attorney-like advocacy. Quotes Principles IV and VI, Fundamental Elements (2), (4), and (6) [now Opinion 10.01], Patient Responsibilities 5 [now Opinion 10.02], and Opinions 2.03, 2.07, 2.09, 2.16, 2.19, 3.06, 4.01, 4.04, 6.01, 7.02, 8.02, 8.03, 8.13, 8.132, 9.06, 9.07, and 9.131. Cites Opinions 5.05, 5.09, 7.01, 8.135, and 9.02. Sage, *Physicians as Advocates*, 35 Hous. L. Rev. 1529, 1537, 1541, 1542, 1552-53, 1554, 1556, 1557, 1559, 1561-62, 1564, 1571, 1574, 1576, 1580 (1999).

Journal 1994 Discusses notions of quality in health care, asking who is responsible to define quality, who is responsible to deliver it, and who is responsible for quality of care when it is unsatisfactory. Concludes that significant economic changes will require a reallocation of these responsibilities among patients, providers, and payers. References Patient Responsibilities (1), (4), and (5) [now Opinion 10.02]. Morreim, *Redefining Quality by Reassigning Responsibility*, 20 Am. J. Law & Med. 79, 103 (1994).

10.03 Patient-Physician Relationship in the Context of Work-Related and Independent Medical Examinations

When a physician is responsible for performing an isolated assessment of an individual's health or disability for an employer, business, or insurer, a limited patient-physician relationship should be considered to exist. Both "industry-employed physicians" (IEPs), who are employed by businesses or insurance companies for the purpose of conducting medical examinations, and "independent medical examiners" (IMEs), who are independent contractors providing medical examinations within the realm of their specialty, may perform such medical examinations.

Despite their ties to a third party, the responsibilities of IEPs and IMEs are in some basic respects very similar to those of other physicians. IEPs and IMEs have the same obligations as physicians in other contexts to:

(1) Evaluate objectively the patient's health or disability. In order to maintain objectivity, IEPs and IMEs should not be influenced by the preferences of the patient-employee, employer, or insurance company when making a diagnosis during a work-related or independent medical examination.

(2) Maintain patient confidentiality as outlined by Opinion 5.09, "Confidentiality: Industry-Employed Physicians and Independent Medical Examiners."

(3) Disclose fully potential or perceived conflicts of interest. The physician should inform the patient about the terms of the agreement between himself or herself and the third party as well as the fact that he or she is acting as an agent of that entity. This should be done at the outset of the examination, before health information is gathered from the patient-employee. Before the physician proceeds with the exam, he or she should ensure to the extent possible that the patient understands the physician's unaltered ethical obligations, as well as the differences that exist between the physician's role in this context and the physician's traditional fiduciary role.

IEPs and IMEs are responsible for administering an objective medical evaluation but not for monitoring patients' health over time, treating patients, or fulfilling many other duties traditionally held by physicians. Consequently, a limited patient-physician relationship should be considered to exist during isolated assessments of an individual's health or disability for an employer, business, or insurer.

The physician has a responsibility to inform the patient about important health information or abnormalities that he or she discovers during the course of the examination. In addition, the physician should ensure to the extent possible that the patient understands the problem or diagnosis. Furthermore, when appropriate, the physician should suggest that the patient seek care from a qualified physician and, if requested, provide reasonable assistance in securing follow-up care. (I)

Issued December 1999 based on the report "Patient-Physician Relationship in the Context of Work-Related and Independent Medical Examinations," adopted June 1999.

Alaska 2010 Workers' compensation claimant appealed summary judgment in medical malpractice action against physician who performed independent medical examination. The court quoted Opinion 10.03 in holding that the claimant did not present any evidence the physician failed to abide by ethical standards. The court concluded in part that the claims were dependent upon claimant establishing a physician-patient relationship with the physician and affirmed the lower court's ruling. *Smith v. Radecki, 238 P.3d 111, 116.*

Ariz. 2003 Employee appealed summary judgment and dismissal in malpractice action against a radiologist and x-ray company for failure to inform her of medical results that could have led to an earlier diagnosis of lung cancer. Employee was referred by her employer to the radiologist for a chest x-ray. The radiologist did not inform the employee of abnormalities noted in his report. Quoting Opinion 10.03, the appellate court held the physician had a duty to directly inform the employee of the results. The x-ray company was not liable, however, since the radiologist was an independent contractor. *Stanley v. McCarver, 204 Ariz. 339, 63 P.3d 1076, 1081.*

N.J. 2001 Deceased patient's wife filed a medical malpractice action against a physician who conducted pre-employment screening. The physician failed to inform the deceased about a condition he discovered during the physical. The New Jersey Supreme Court reversed the lower courts and held that a physician under contract with a third party to perform pre-employment physicals has a nondelegable duty to inform the patient of any potentially serious medical conditions. The court quoted Opinion 10.03, expressing the view that, although this may not be a traditional physician-patient relationship, the physician still has a responsibility to inform the patient. *Reed v. Bojarski, 166 N.J.89, 764 A.2d 433, 444.*

N.Y. 2009 Plaintiff in a personal injury action sued the physician designated by the defendant in that action to conduct an independent medical examination of plaintiff. Plaintiff claimed he was injured during the examination by the physician. The court relied on Opinion 10.03 in distinguishing the relationship between a physician performing an independent medical examination on a person and an examination undertaken in a traditional physician-patient relationship. The court held that the duty owed to the examinee is to perform the examination in a manner so as not to cause physical harm to the examinee. The court found that plaintiff's claim was governed by the statute of limitations for professional malpractice actions. *Bazakos v. Lewis, 12 N.Y.3d 631, 911 N.E.2d 847, 850, 883 N.Y.S.2d 785.*

N.Y. App. 2008 Plaintiff in personal injury action brought suit against physician hired by alleged tortfeasor to conduct statutory medical examination to recover for injuries sustained during examination. The court quoted Opinion 10.03 in determining that a limited patient-physician relationship exists between the physician and the examinee in such a case. The court held that, despite precedent dictating otherwise, there was no physician-patient relationship in this case and that the statute of limitations for negligence should apply, rather than the statute of limitations for medical malpractice actions. *Bazakos v. Lewis, 56 A.D.3d 15, 864 N.Y.S.2d 505, 512, n. 3, rev'd, 12 N.Y.3d 631, 911 N.E.2d 847, 883 N.Y.S.2d 785.*

10.05 Potential Patients

(1) Physicians must keep their professional obligations to provide care to patients in accord with their prerogative to choose whether to enter into a patient-physician relationship.

(2) The following instances identify the limits on physicians' prerogative:

    (a) Physicians should respond to the best of their ability in cases of medical emergency (Opinion 8.11, "Neglect of Patient").

    (b) Physicians cannot refuse to care for patients based on race, gender, sexual orientation, gender identity, or any other criteria that would constitute invidious discrimination (Opinion 9.12, "Patient-Physician Relationship: Respect for Law and Human Rights"), nor can they discriminate against patients with infectious diseases (Opinion 2.23, "HIV Testing")

    (c) Physicians may not refuse to care for patients when operating under a contractual arrangement that requires them to treat (Opinion 10.015, "The Patient-Physician Relationship"). Exceptions to this requirement may exist when patient care is ultimately compromised by the contractual arrangement.

(3) In situations not covered above, it may be ethically permissible for physicians to decline a potential patient when:
   (a) The treatment request is beyond the physician's current competence.
   (b) The treatment request is known to be scientifically invalid, has no medical indication, and offers no possible benefit to the patient (Opinion 8.20, "Invalid Medical Treatment").
   (c) A specific treatment sought by an individual is incompatible with the physician's personal, religious, or moral beliefs.

(4) Physicians, as professionals and members of society, should work to assure access to adequate health care* (Opinion 10.01, "Fundamental Elements of the Patient-Physician Relationship"). Accordingly, physicians have an obligation to share in providing charity care (Opinion 9.065, "Caring for the Poor") but not to the degree that would seriously compromise the care provided to existing patients. When deciding whether to take on a new patient, physicians should consider the individual's need for medical service along with the needs of their current patients. Greater medical necessity of a service engenders a stronger obligation to treat. (I, VI, VIII, IX)

Issued December 2000 based on the report "Potential Patients, Ethical Considerations," adopted June 2000. Updated December 2003. Updated June 2008 based on the report "Modification of Ethics Policy to Ensure Inclusion for Transgender Physicians, Medical Students, and Patients;" adopted November 2007.

*Considerations in determining an adequate level of health care are outlined in Opinion 2.095, "The Provision of Adequate Health Care."

Journal 2011 Discusses advancements in modern reproductive technologies and the need for legislation to regulate these technologies. Concludes that regulating these technologies may violate modern views of personal autonomy and therefore should focus on the safety of the technologies and not be used to "protect" women from their ability to freely contract. Quotes Opinions 2.18 and 10.05. Neal, *Protecting Women: Preserving Autonomy in the Commodification of Motherhood,* 17 Wm. & Mary J. Women & L. 611, 630, 635 (2011).

Journal 2010 Discusses issues arising from the enactment of legislation by North Dakota involving a minor's reproductive rights. Explores ethical principles that govern physician's actions within the context of reproductive health. Concludes that, while a patient's expectation of confidentiality with a physician is critical, competing values come into play when the patient is a minor and parental involvement may be important. Provides practical guidance to address issues in this context. Quotes Opinions 2.01, 2.015, 5.055, 8.08, 8.115, 9.12, 10.01, 10.015, and 10.05. Cites Opinion 5.05, 5.055, 8.08, 8.11, 8.115, 9.12, and 10.05. Haas, *"Doctor, I'm Pregnant and Fifteen—I Can't Tell My Parents—Please Help Me": Minor Consent, Reproductive Rights, and Ethical Principles for Physicians,* 86 N.D. L. Rev. 63, 70, 73, 75-78, 82, 84, 86-88, (2010).

Journal 2009 Discusses the right of health care professionals to refuse to provide health care services to lesbian, gay, or bisexual (LGB) individuals, because of moral or religious objections, and its impact on access to health care services, including assisted reproduction and elder health care services, for such patients. Concludes physicians should adhere to professional ethical standards to promote LGB patients' autonomy and equal access to care. Quotes Opinion Preamble. Cites Opinion 10.05. Reibman, *The Patient Wanted the Doctor to Treat Her in the Closet, but the Janitor Wouldn't Open the Door: Healthcare Provider Rights of Refusal Versus LGB Rights to Reproductive and Elder Healthcare,* 28 Temp. J. Sci. Tech. & Envtl. L. 65, 90-91 (2009).

Journal 2006 Explores the legal and ethical issues surrounding concierge medicine. Concludes that concierge medicine is best restricted to a small class of wealthy individuals. Quotes Principle IX and Opinion 8.055. Cites Principle VI and Opinions 8.055, 8.11, 8.115, 9.065, and 10.05. Carnahan, *Law, Medicine, and Wealth: Does Concierge Medicine Promote Health Care Choice, or Is It a Barrier to Access?* 17 Stan. L. & Pol'y Rev. 121, 149-50, 151, 152, 153-54 (2006).

A P P E N D I X

American Medical Association

Relevant Bylaws

1.00   Membership

1.10   Categories. Categories of membership in the American Medical Association (AMA) are Active Constituent, Active Direct, Affiliate, Honorary, and International.

1.11   Active Membership.

1.111   Active Constituent. Constituent associations are recognized medical associations of states, commonwealths, districts, territories, or possessions of the United States of America. Active constituent members are members of constituent associations who are entitled to exercise the rights of membership in their constituent associations, including the right to vote and hold office, as determined by their respective constituent associations and who meet one of the following requirements:
a. Possess the United States degree of doctor of medicine (MD) or doctor of osteopathic medicine (DO), or a recognized international equivalent.
b. Are medical students in educational programs provided by a college of medicine or osteopathic medicine accredited by the Liaison Committee on Medical Education or the American Osteopathic Association leading to the MD or DO degree. This includes those students who are on an approved sabbatical, provided that the student will be in good standing upon returning from the sabbatical.

1.1111   Admission. Active constituent members are admitted to membership upon certification by the constituent association to the AMA, provided there is no disapproval by the Council on Ethical and Judicial Affairs.

1.112   Active Direct. Active direct members are those who apply for membership in the AMA directly. Applicants residing in states where the constituent association requires all of its members to be members of the AMA are not eligible for this category of membership unless the applicant is serving full time in the Federal Services that have been granted representation in the House of Delegates. Active direct members must meet one of the following requirements:

a. Possess the United States degree of doctor of medicine (MD) or doctor of osteopathic medicine (DO), or a recognized international equivalent.

b. Medical students in educational programs provided by a college of medicine or osteopathic medicine accredited by the Liaison Committee on Medical Education or the American Osteopathic Association leading to the MD or DO degree. This includes those students who are on an approved sabbatical, provided that the student will be in good standing upon returning from the sabbatical.

1.1121 Admission. Active direct members are admitted to membership upon application to the AMA, provided that there is no disapproval by the Council on Ethical and Judicial Affairs.

1.11211 Notice. The AMA shall notify each constituent association of the name and address of those applicants for active direct membership residing within its jurisdiction.

1.11212 Objections. Objections to applicants for active direct membership must be received by the Executive Vice President of the AMA within 45 days of receipt by the constituent association of the notice of the application for such membership. All objections will immediately be referred to the Council on Ethical and Judicial Affairs for prompt disposition pursuant to the rules of the Council on Ethical and Judicial Affairs.

1.113 Council on Ethical and Judicial Affairs Review. The Council on Ethical and Judicial Affairs may consider information pertaining to the character, ethics, professional status, and professional activities of the applicant for membership. The Council shall provide by rule for an appropriate hearing procedure to be provided to the applicant.

1.114 Rights and Privileges. Active members are entitled to receive the *Journal of the American Medical Association*, *American Medical News*, and such other publications as the Board of Trustees may authorize.

1.115 Dues and Assessments. Active members are liable for such dues and assessments as are determined and fixed by the House of Delegates.

1.1151 Active Constituent Members. Active constituent members shall pay their annual dues to the constituent associations for transmittal to the AMA, except as may be otherwise arranged by the Board of Trustees.

1.1152 Active Direct Members. Active direct members shall pay their annual dues directly to the AMA.

1.1153 Exemptions. On request, active members may be exempt from the payment of dues on January 1 following their sixty-fifth birthday, provided they are fully retired from the practice of medicine. Additionally, the Board of Trustees may exempt members from payment of dues to alleviate financial hardship or because of retirement from medical practice due to medical disability. The Board of Trustees shall establish appropriate standards and procedures for granting all dues exemptions. Members who were exempt from payment of dues based on age and retirement under Bylaw provisions applicable in prior years shall be entitled to maintain their dues-exempt status in all subsequent years. Dues exemptions for financial hardship or medical disability shall be reviewed annually.

1.1154 Delinquency. Active members are delinquent if their dues and assessments are not received by the date determined by the House of Delegates, and shall forfeit their membership in the AMA if such delinquent dues and assessments are not received by the AMA within 30 days after a notification to the delinquent member has been made on or following the delinquency date.

1.12 Affiliate Members. Persons who belong to one of the following classes are eligible to become affiliate members of the AMA:
a. Physicians in foreign countries who have attained distinction in medicine and who are members of their national medical society or such other medical organization as will verify their professional credentials.
b. American physicians located in foreign countries or in territories or possessions of the United States who are engaged in medical missionary, educational, or philanthropic endeavors.
c. Dentists who hold the degree of DMD or DDS who are members of the American Dental Association and their state and local dental societies.
d. Pharmacists who are active members of the American Pharmaceutical Association.
e. Teachers of medicine or of the sciences allied to medicine who are citizens of the United States and are ineligible for active membership.
f. Individuals engaged in scientific endeavors allied to medicine and others who have attained distinction in their fields of endeavor who are not eligible for other categories of membership.

1.121 Admission. Membership is conferred by majority vote of the House of Delegates following nomination by the Council on Ethical and Judicial Affairs. Nominations for d, e, and f must also be approved by the appropriate constituent association. The election of affiliate members shall take place at a time recommended by the Committee on Rules and Credentials and approved by the House of Delegates.

1.122 **Rights and Privileges.** Affiliate members may attend AMA meetings but may not vote or hold office, and they are not eligible to receive publications of the AMA except by subscription.

1.123 **Dues and Assessments.** Affiliate members are not subject to dues or assessments.

1.13 **Honorary Members.** Physicians of foreign countries who have achieved preeminence in the profession of medicine and who attend a meeting of the House of Delegates are eligible to become honorary members of the AMA.

1.131 **Admission.** Membership is conferred by majority vote of the House of Delegates following nomination by the Board of Trustees. The election of honorary members shall take place at a time recommended by the Committee on Rules and Credentials and approved by the House of Delegates.

1.132 **Rights and Privileges.** Honorary members may attend AMA meetings but may not vote or hold office, and they are not eligible to receive publications of the AMA except by subscription.

1.133 **Dues and Assessments.** Honorary members are not subject to dues or assessments.

1.14 **International Members.** Physicians who have graduated from medical schools located outside the United States and its territories and are ineligible for Active Constituent or Active Direct membership and who can fulfill and document the following requirements:
a. Graduation from a medical school listed in the World Health Organization Directory.
b. Possession of a valid license in good standing in the country of graduation or practice location documented by one of the following:
   (i) verification that the applicant is an international member of a national medical specialty society seated in the House of Delegates that has a procedure to verify the applicant's educational credentials;
   (ii) certification from the national medical association in the country of practice attesting to the applicant's valid authorization to practice medicine without limitation; or
   (iii) certification from the registry or licensing authority of the country of practice attesting to the applicant's valid license in good standing.

1.141 **Admission.** International members are admitted to membership by providing a completed application accompanied by the required documentation. The Council on Ethical and Judicial Affairs shall provide by rule for an appropriate hearing procedure to be provided to the applicant should denial of membership be based on information pertaining to the applicant's character, ethical conduct, or professional status.

1.142 Rights and Privileges. International members are entitled to receive the English edition of the Journal of the American Medical Association and such other benefits as the Board of Trustees may authorize. International members may attend AMA meetings, but may not vote or hold office.

1.143 Dues and Assessments. International members shall be subject to dues as established by the Board of Trustees, but they shall not be subject to assessments.

1.20 Maintenance of Membership. A member may hold only one category of membership in the AMA at any one time. Membership may be retained as long as the member complies with the provisions of the Constitution and Bylaws and Principles of Medical Ethics of the AMA.

1.30 Transfer of Membership. Members of the AMA, except members serving full time in the Federal Services, who move to a jurisdiction in which the constituent association requires that all members of the constituent association be members of the AMA, must apply for membership in the constituent association within one year after moving into the jurisdiction to continue membership in the AMA. Unless membership in the constituent association has been granted within 2 years after application, membership in the AMA shall cease.

1.40 Termination of Membership. Upon official notification to the AMA that an active constituent member is not in good standing in a constituent association, such member shall cease to be a member of the AMA, subject to the member's right of appeal as provided in Bylaw 6.54.

1.50 Discrimination. Membership in any category of the AMA or in any of its constituent associations shall not be denied or abridged because of sex, color, creed, race, religion, disability, ethnic origin, national origin, sexual orientation, gender identity, age, or for any other reason unrelated to character, competence, ethics, professional status, or professional activities.

1.60 Discipline. The Council on Ethical and Judicial Affairs, after due notice and hearing may censure, suspend, expel, or place on probation any member of the AMA for an infraction of the Constitution or these Bylaws, for a violation of the Principles of Medical Ethics, or for unethical or illegal conduct.

2.00 House of Delegates

2.6172 Opinions and Reports of the Council on Ethical and Judicial Affairs. The Council on Ethical and Judicial Affairs issues opinions and reports. Opinions will be considered informational and filed. Motions are in order to extract an opinion, and request that the Council reconsider or withdraw the opinion. Reports may be adopted, not adopted, or referred, and may be amended for clarification only with the concurrence of the Council.

6.00 Councils

6.01 Responsibilities.

6.011 Information and Recommendations. All Councils have a continuing duty to provide information and to submit recommendations to the House of Delegates, through the Board of Trustees, on matters relating to the areas of responsibility assigned to them under the provisions of these Bylaws.

6.0111 Method of Reporting. Councils, except the Council on Ethical and Judicial Affairs and the Council on Legislation shall submit their reports to the House of Delegates through the Board of Trustees. The Board of Trustees may make such nonbinding recommendations regarding the reports to the Councils as it deems appropriate, prior to transmitting the reports to the House of Delegates without delay or modification by the Board. The Board may also submit written recommendations regarding the reports to the House of Delegates.

6.0112 Method of Referral. Referrals from the House of Delegates to a Council shall be made through the Board of Trustees. The Board may, in addition, refer the matter to such other councils as it deems appropriate.

6.012 Strategic Planning. All Councils have a responsibility to participate in the strategic planning process with the Board of Trustees, other Councils, and other organizational units as may be appropriate.

6.013 Communications and Working Relationships. All Councils have a responsibility to communicate and develop working relationships with the Board of Trustees, other Councils, the Sections, organizations represented within the House of Delegates, and other organizational units as may be appropriate.

6.02 **Rules and Regulations.** Each Council shall select a Chair and Vice Chair or Chair-Elect and may adopt such rules and regulations as it deems necessary and appropriate for the conduct of its affairs, subject to approval by the Board of Trustees.

6.50 **Council on Ethical and Judicial Affairs.**

6.51 **Authority.** The Council on Ethical and Judicial Affairs is the judicial authority of the AMA, and its decision shall be final.

6.52 **Functions.**

6.521 To interpret the Principles of Medical Ethics of the AMA through the issuance of Opinions;

6.522 To interpret the Constitution, Bylaws, and rules of the AMA;

6.523 To investigate general ethical conditions and all matters pertaining to the relations of physicians to one another or to the public, and make recommendations to the House of Delegates or the constituent associations through the issuance of Reports or Opinions;

6.524 To receive appeals filed by applicants who allege that they, because of sex, color, creed, race, religion, disability, ethnic origin, national origin, sexual orientation, gender identity, age, or for any other reason unrelated to character or competence have been unfairly denied membership in a constituent association and/or component society, to determine the facts in the case, and to report the findings to the House of Delegates. If the Council determines that the allegations are indeed true, it shall admonish, censure, or in the event of repeated violations, recommend to the House of Delegates that the constituent association and/or component society involved be declared to be no longer a constituent association and/or component society member of the AMA;

6.525 To request that the President appoint investigating juries to which it may refer complaints or evidence of unethical conduct which in its judgment are of greater than local concern. Such investigative juries, if probable cause for action be shown, shall submit formal charges to the President, who shall appoint a prosecutor to prosecute such charges against the accused before the Council on Ethical and Judicial Affairs in the name and on behalf of the AMA. The Council may acquit, admonish, suspend, expel, or place on probation the accused; and

6.526 To approve applications and nominate candidates for affiliate membership as otherwise provided for in Bylaw 1.12.

6.53 **Original Jurisdiction.** The Council on Ethical and Judicial Affairs shall have original jurisdiction in:

6.531 All questions involving membership as provided in Bylaws 1.111, 1.112, 1.12, 1.14, and 1.60.

6.532 All controversies arising under this Constitution and Bylaws and under the Principles of Medical Ethics to which the AMA is a party.

6.533 Controversies between two or more state associations or their members and between a constituent association and a component society or societies of another state association or associations or their members.

6.54 **Appellate Jurisdiction.** The Council on Ethical and Judicial Affairs shall have appellate jurisdiction in questions of law and procedure but not of fact in all cases which arise:

a. Between a constituent association and one or more of its component societies.
b. Between component societies of the same constituent association.
c. Between a member or members and the component society to which the member or members belong following an appeal to the member's constituent association.
d. Between a member and the component society or the constituent association to which the member belongs regarding disciplinary action taken against the member by the society or association.
e. Between members of different component societies of the same constituent association following a decision by the constituent association.

6.541 **Appeal Mechanisms.** Notice of appeal shall be filed with the Council on Ethical and Judicial Affairs within 30 days of the date of the decision by the component society or the constituent association and the appeal shall be perfected within 60 days thereof; provided, however, that the Council on Ethical and Judicial Affairs, for what it considers good and sufficient cause, may grant an additional 30 days for perfecting the appeal.

6.55 **Membership.**

6.551 Nine active members of the AMA, one of whom shall be a resident/ fellow physician and one of whom shall be a medical student. Members elected to the Council on Ethical and Judicial Affairs shall resign all other positions held by them in the AMA upon their election to the Council. No member, while serving on the Council on Ethical and Judicial Affairs, shall be a delegate or an alternate delegate to the House of Delegates, or an Officer of the AMA, or serve on any other council, committee, or as representative to or Governing Council member of an AMA Section.

6.552 **Limit on Medical Student Participation.** The medical student member of the Council shall have the right to participate fully in the work of the Council, including the right to make motions and vote on policy issues, elections, appointments, or nominations conducted by the Council, except that in disciplinary matters and in matters relating to membership the medical student member shall participate only if a medical student is the subject of the disciplinary matter or is the applicant for membership.

6.56 **Nomination and Election.** The members of the Council shall be elected by the House of Delegates on nomination by the President-Elect who assumes the office of President at the conclusion of the meeting. State associations, national medical specialty societies, Sections, and other organizations represented in the House of Delegates, and members of the Board of Trustees may submit the names and qualifications of candidates for consideration by the President-Elect.

6.57 **Term.**

6.571 The medical student member of the Council shall be elected for a term of 2 years. If the medical student member ceases to be enrolled in an educational program at any time prior to the expiration of the term for which the medical student member was elected, the service of such medical student member on the Council shall thereupon terminate, and the position shall be declared vacant.

6.572 The resident/fellow physician member of the Council shall be elected for a term of 3 years provided that if the resident/fellow physician member ceases to be a resident/fellow physician at any time prior to the expiration of the term for which elected, the service of such resident/ fellow physician member on the Council shall thereupon terminate, and the position shall be declared vacant.

6.573 All other members of the Council shall be elected for a term of 7 years, so arranged that at each Annual Meeting the term of one member shall expire.

6.58 **Tenure.** Members of the Council may serve only one term, except that the resident/fellow physician member and the medical student member shall be eligible to serve for 2 terms. A member elected to serve an unexpired term shall not be regarded as having served a term unless such member has served at least half of the term.

6.59 **Vacancies.**

6.591 **Members other than the Resident/Fellow Physician Member.** Any vacancy among the members of the Council other than the resident/fellow physician member shall be filled at the next meeting of the House of Delegates. The new member shall be elected by the House of Delegates, on nomination by the President, for the remainder of the unexpired term.

6.592 Resident/Fellow Physician Member. If the resident/fellow physician member of the Council ceases to complete the term for which elected, the remainder of the term shall be deemed to have expired. The successor shall be elected by the House of Delegates at the next Annual Meeting, on nomination by the President, for a 3-year term.

Glossary of Terms

Council on Ethical and Judicial Affairs Opinions: Interpretations of the Principles of Medical Ethics on matters of (1) ethical principles or (2) social policy which involves issues of morality in the practice of medicine. Opinions establish standards of honorable conduct for physicians and cannot be amended by the House of Delegates. The Council may be requested by the House of Delegates to reconsider an opinion, but it is not required to do so. Unless withdrawn by the Council on Ethical and Judicial Affairs, Opinions of the AMA are published as Current Ethical Opinions in the AMA Policy Compendium and in the AMA Code of Medical Ethics.

Council on Ethical and Judicial Affairs Reports: Reports of the Council on Ethical and Judicial Affairs may be prepared in response to a resolution or on an issue of importance to physicians and may include recommendations for action by the House of Delegates. Recommendations in reports of the Council may be adopted, not adopted, or referred by the House of Delegates but cannot be amended without the concurrence of the Council. If adopted, the recommendations are included in the Policy Compendium.

Preface to the Rules of the Council on Ethical and Judicial Affairs

Professionalism generally is defined according to three key elements: the expertise that is acquired by a professional through specialized training; the commitment to providing services of value to others; and self-regulation, which often leads to the establishment of a code of conduct. These characteristics, which engender public trust, clearly pertain to the medical profession and have been embodied in many of the activities of the American Medical Association since it was established in 1847.

The Council on Ethical and Judicial Affairs, and its predecessors, have been instrumental in defining the elements of medical professional integrity by establishing standards of ethical conduct and by encouraging physicians to uphold these standards. The Council's work also includes the review of physician misconduct on the basis of our AMA's Principles of Medical Ethics and possible action against membership in the Association. These activities help fulfill the responsibility a profession holds in preserving professional integrity by establishing, as well as enforcing, standards of conduct. By conferring membership only upon those physicians who uphold the values of medical ethics and professionalism, the AMA assumes a leading role in demonstrating that the medical profession considers self-regulation a paramount responsibility.

General Rules of the Council on Ethical and Judicial Affairs

Rule I. Administration

A. **Meetings.** The Council on Ethical and Judicial Affairs will meet during the Annual and Interim Meetings of the American Medical Association. Other meetings of the Council may be called, on reasonable notice, by the Chair of the Council; or they shall be called, on reasonable notice, by the Executive Vice President of the American Medical Association on the written request of at least five members of the Council.

B. **Chair and Vice-Chair.** At the reorganization meeting of the Council which shall be held during each Annual Meeting of the AMA after election of members to the Council, the Council on Ethical and Judicial Affairs shall elect a chair and a vice-chair from among its members except that the resident physician and medical student members of the Council shall not be eligible to serve as chair or vice-chair. The chair and the vice-chair shall retain the right to vote on all matters. No member of the Council shall serve more than two consecutive years as chair or two consecutive years as vice-chair.

The chair and vice-chair to be so elected shall be elected on separate, secret ballots. The balloting and voting for chair shall be completed and a chair elected before the balloting and voting for the vice-chair begins. A majority vote of the entire Council shall be required to so elect either a chair or a vice-chair, with balloting and voting to be repeated, if necessary, until a member is elected to each position.

In the event that the position of chair becomes permanently vacant for any reason during the term of the then currently serving chair, the then currently serving vice-chair shall immediately assume the position of chair for the remainder of the term. A new vice-chair shall then be elected by secret ballot at the ensuing meeting of the Council to serve the remainder of the immediately preceding vice-chair's term. A majority vote of the entire Council, as then constituted, shall be required to so elect a vice-chair, with balloting and voting to be repeated, if necessary, until a member is elected vice-chair. The serving of the balance of a term as chair or vice-chair due to such a vacancy shall not be counted in determining whether a member of the Council has served more than two consecutive years as chair or two consecutive years as vice-chair.

In the event that the position of vice-chair becomes permanently vacant for any reason during the term of the then currently serving vice-chair, a new vice-chair shall be elected by secret ballot at the ensuing meeting of the Council to serve the remainder of the immediately preceding vice-chair's term. A majority vote of the entire Council, as then constituted, shall be required to so elect a vice-chair, with balloting and voting to be repeated, if necessary, until a member is elected vice-chair. The serving of the balance of a term as vice-chair due to such a vacancy shall not be counted in determining whether a member of the Council has served more than two consecutive years as vice-chair.

C. **Student Members**. The medical student member of the Council shall participate as a regular member in the interpretation of the Principles of Medical Ethics of the American Medical Association, the interpretation of the Constitution, Bylaws, and rules of the Association, and the investigation of general ethical conditions and all matters pertaining to the relations of physicians to one another or to the public. The medical student member of the Council shall have the right to participate in disciplinary matters and in matters relating to membership only if a medical student is the subject of the disciplinary matter or is the applicant for membership.

D. **Quorum.** A majority of the members of the Council on Ethical and Judicial Affairs eligible to vote on a matter shall constitute a quorum and shall be required to adopt any action.

E. **Confidentiality.** All matters under consideration for adoption by the Council shall be treated as confidential until adopted by the Council.

Rule II. Applications for Membership

A. **Active Membership**. Applications for membership in the American Medical Association will be considered by the Council on Ethical and Judicial Affairs at any meeting upon presentation of the applications by the Executive Vice President of the Association.

B. **Affiliate Membership**. Applications for affiliate membership submitted by (1) physicians in foreign countries who have attained distinction in medicine and who are members of the national medical society or such other organization as will verify their professional credentials, (2) American physicians located in foreign countries or possessions of the United States and engaged in medical missionary, educational, or philanthropic endeavors, (3) dentists who hold the degree of DDS or DMD, who are members of the American Dental Association and their state and local dental societies, (4) pharmacists who are active members of the American Pharmaceutical Association, (5) teachers of medicine or of the sciences allied to medicine who are citizens of the United States and are ineligible for active or associate membership, or (6) individuals engaged in scientific endeavors allied to medicine and others who have attained distinction in their fields of endeavor who are not otherwise eligible for membership, may be considered at any meeting of the Council on presentation of the applications by the Executive Vice President of the Association. The Council will consider and approve only those applications which are accompanied by a statement of a responsible and qualified individual attesting to the requirements set forth above. (Employees of the AMA or any AMA affiliate or subsidiary may be eligible affiliate members under subsection (6). They must have five years of employment at the AMA, affiliate, or subsidiary and their distinction in their field of endeavor must be certified by an AMA Senior Vice President, or if the employee is a Senior Vice President, the Executive Vice President.)

C. **Refusal of Approval.** An applicant for membership in the American Medical Association whose application has not been approved by the Council on Ethical and Judicial Affairs will be promptly notified of such fact.

Rule III. Physicians Denied Membership in Component or Constituent Associations

Pursuant to 6.4024 of the Bylaws, any physician whose application for member-ship in a component and/or constituent association has allegedly been denied unfairly because of color, creed, race, religion, ethnic origin, national origin, or sex may appeal to the Council on Ethical and Judicial Affairs. The Council shall determine the facts in the case and report the findings to the House of Delegates. If the Council determines that the allegations are indeed true, it shall admonish, censure or, in the event of repeated violations, recommend to the House of Delegates that the state association involved be declared to be no longer a constituent member of the American Medical Association. Proceedings for such determination shall be initiated by a written statement. Such statement shall: (1) identify the parties to the case, (2) show that the appellant has exhausted remedies made available by the constitution and bylaws of the component society and the state association, and (3) include a concise factual resume of the case in sufficient detail to enable the Council to ascertain the facts. The appellant should also furnish such other information as may be requested by or helpful to the Council in determining the facts.

Rule IV. Original Controversies

Original proceedings before the Council on Ethical and Judicial Affairs shall be initiated by a written statement. Such statement shall include information (1) identifying the parties to the controversy, including membership affilia-tions, if applicable, and (2) explaining the nature of the controversy, setting forth the provisions of the Constitution, Bylaws, Rules, or Principles of Medical Ethics concerned.

Rule V. Appeals

Appellate proceedings before the Council on Ethical and Judicial Affairs shall be perfected by a written statement of appeal. Such statement shall include information (1) identifying the parties to the case and indicating membership affiliations when appropriate, (2) showing that the appellant has exhausted remedies made available by the constitution and bylaws of the component society and the state association, and (3) describing the error of law or procedure which is believed to have occurred during the proceedings. The statement shall also include a concise, factual resume of the case. Appellant shall submit with the statement the charges, complaints, findings, opinions, and decisions previously entered in the case.

Rule VI. Interpretation of the Constitution, Bylaws, Rules, and Principles of Medical Ethics of the American Medical Association

A. **Requests for Interpretation.** Requests for interpretation of the Constitution, Bylaws, Rules, or Principles of Medical Ethics of the Association shall be in writing and shall describe the matter to be interpreted in sufficient detail to enable the members of the Council on Ethical and Judicial Affairs to evaluate the request in all its aspects.

B. **Interpretations Initiated by the Council.** The Council on Ethical and Judicial Affairs on its own motion, may render an opinion concerning the interpretation or application of the Constitution, Bylaws, Rules, or Principles of Medical Ethics of the Association and may, on its own motion, consider and decide the constitutionality and validity of all rules and regulations adopted by Councils and Committees of the Association pursuant to the Bylaws of the Association.

C. **Discretionary Power.** The Council on Ethical and Judicial Affairs may, in its own discretion, refuse to consider requests for interpretation of the Principles of Medical Ethics which in the opinion of the Council should be resolved by a component society or a state association. Requests for interpretation of the Principles of Medical Ethics which are not of national interest and relate to the observance of local customs and ideals may be readdressed to the component society or constituent association primarily responsible for knowledge of the requirements of such local customs and recognized ideals.

Rule VII. Jurisdiction

The Council on Ethical and Judicial Affairs may, on its own motion or on the motion of any party, determine the question of jurisdiction at any stage of the proceedings.

Rules for Review of Membership

1. Per AMA Bylaws B-1.111, B-1.121, B-1.131, B-1.151, B-1.611, and B-1.62, the Council on Ethical and Judicial Affairs may review information pertaining to the character, ethics, professional status, and professional activities of current members and applicants for AMA membership whenever evidence of improper conduct is brought to the Council's attention. Any misrepresentation in renewing or applying for AMA membership shall constitute cause for Council review.

2. The Council may seek such additional evidence as it deems appropriate. All persons connected with the review process and with any proceedings under these rules, other than the member or applicant being reviewed, shall take reasonable precautions to keep the proceedings confidential, consistent with AMA policies on due process in peer review. Such confidentiality is subject to the need to notify others in order to conduct the review, the notice requirements of these rules, and the reporting requirements of the Federal Health Care Quality Improvement Act.

Notice of possible disciplinary sanction or denial
3. If the Council finds reasonable cause to institute disciplinary proceedings, then prior to the final determination of whether to impose sanctions the member or applicant shall be offered a full hearing, at which there shall be no presumption that disciplinary action is warranted. The Council shall send notice of the basis for consideration of disciplinary sanction against or denial of AMA membership, along with a copy of these rules. The notice will state that the member or applicant may present to the Council additional information pertinent to the review. The AMA will use reasonable efforts to effect notification by registered or certified mail or by a commercial delivery service, at the last address known to the AMA.

4. Once the Council has determined such reasonable cause, it shall retain jurisdiction, notwithstanding any attempt by the member to resign or the applicant to withdraw the application, until the matter is fully resolved.

5. The member or applicant shall have thirty (30) days following the sending of the notice offering a hearing in which to file a written response and request a hearing.

6. Failure of the member or applicant to submit a written request for a plenary hearing shall waive the right to such hearing. Failure of the member or

applicant to keep the AMA apprised of his or her contact information or to be reasonably available for a hearing shall also be deemed a waiver of the right to such a hearing, notwithstanding a specific request for the hearing. The Council may then continue, dismiss, or decide the matter at its discretion, based upon the available evidence.

7. If the member or applicant submits a written request for a hearing, the Council shall notify the physician of the date and time of the hearing and the manner in which it will proceed, along with a copy of these rules.

Hearing procedure

8. The Council shall not be bound by technical rules of evidence usually employed in legal proceedings and may review any information deemed reliable and relevant. The Council generally will not consider evidence that purportedly contradicts the findings of a medical licensing board, a court, or a governmental agency that has made an adjudication relevant to the professional fitness of the member or applicant.

9. The member or applicant may opt to participate in the hearing in person or by teleconference and may be accompanied by legal counsel. Either party may retain a court reporter or stenographer to record the hearing at his, her, or its own expense.

10. The member or applicant may present witnesses or documentary evidence to the Council.

11. Members of the Council and its legal counsel may pose questions to the member or applicant, and to any witness.

12. Any significant misstatements in connection with a disciplinary proceeding may, within the Council's discretion, be grounds for discipline.

13. The Council may consider any mitigating or aggravating evidence, including the member or applicant's participation in rehabilitation or remedial activities.

Decision

14. The Council may issue appropriate sanctions, including denial of membership to an applicant or expulsion, probation, or suspension of a member.

15. Denial of membership to an applicant or expulsion of a member is imposed only when the Council determines that the physician under review has seriously violated the Principles of Medical Ethics and that it would discredit the AMA to have that physician as a member.

16. Probation stems from a determination that a physician may obtain or retain AMA membership, but only so long as the physician behaves ethically and submits written reports to the Council attesting to that conduct.

The period of probation is generally coincident with a probationary period imposed by the state authority.

17. Suspension is a conditional or temporary revocation of membership rights. It may be imposed when a member has violated the Principles of Medical Ethics but the violation is not so serious as to justify expulsion and the member is not on probation with a state authority. When the member is able to demonstrate to the Council that he or she will conform to the Principles of Medical Ethics, the suspension will be lifted.

18. For a less serious violation of the Principles of Medical Ethics, the Council may admonish, reprimand, or censure a member or applicant. Admonishment is less severe and censure is more severe than a reprimand. With such decisions, the applicant would be accepted for and a current member would retain his or her AMA membership.

19. As a nondisciplinary action, the Council may monitor a member or applicant. Monitoring will be for a defined period of time and may include requiring the member or applicant to provide periodic status reports. The Council will make a determination of membership status at the conclusion of the monitoring period. If the Council determines that disciplinary sanctions may be appropriate, the member or applicant will be notified of the possibility of such sanctions and offered a subsequent hearing.

20. The Council shall, within thirty (30) days after the hearing, notify the member or applicant of its decision.

21. Copies of the decision will be sent to any state medical societies and specialty medical societies that have representation in the AMA House of Delegates and in which, according to the records of the AMA, the member or applicant has membership.

22. The Council's decisions are effective on the sending of its decision to the member or applicant and are final.

23. If the Council expels a member or denies an application, the member or applicant may reapply to the AMA one year after the date of the decision.

24. If a lawsuit is brought in connection with any proceeding under these rules, the courts of Illinois shall have exclusive venue over such action, and the applicable law in such action shall be the law of Illinois (without regard to choice of law provisions).

Rules of the Council on Ethical and Judicial Affairs in Original Jurisdiction Cases

Preamble

6.4025 of the Bylaws provides that the Council on Ethical and Judicial Affairs may request the President of the Association to appoint investigating juries to which the Council may refer complaints or evidences of unethical conduct which, in its judgment, are of greater than local concern.

The following Rules of Procedure, respecting notice of charges, and the conduct of hearings before the Council on Ethical and Judicial Affairs are based upon this section of the Bylaws.

Investigating Jury

At the request of the Council on Ethical and Judicial Affairs, the President has appointed an investigating jury. Complaints or evidence of unethical conduct of greater than local concern will be submitted to this jury by the Council.

Institution of Proceedings

If after investigation a probable cause for action is shown, the investigating jury shall submit a statement of charges to the President. The President shall submit to the Council on Ethical and Judicial Affairs the statement of charges presented to him or her by the investigating jury for prosecution in the name and on behalf of the American Medical Association.

Statement of Charges

The statement of charges shall allege in writing an infraction of the AMA's Constitution or Bylaws or a violation of the Principles of Medical Ethics of the AMA. Exhibits may be attached.

Notice

A copy of the statement of charges shall be sent to the respondent physician by personal delivery or by registered or certified mail.

Answer

The respondent physician shall have thirty (30) days after personal delivery or mailing of the notice of statement of charges to file a written answer. If the respondent physician fails to file a written answer, the allegations shall be considered to be admitted.

Proceedings

The Chair of the Council on Ethical and Judicial Affairs shall designate one or more members of the Council to conduct a hearing on the statement of charges. This member or these members shall be known as the Hearing Officer.

Hearings shall be held at such reasonable time and place, designated by the Hearing Officer, as may be consistent with the nature of the proceedings and the convenience of the parties. The parties shall receive not less than fifteen (15) days of notice of the hearing.

The General Counsel of the American Medical Association or his or her designee shall prosecute the charges against the respondent physician. Attendance at hearings may be limited to the members of the Council on Ethical and Judicial Affairs, the staff, witnesses, if any, the parties, and counsel who may speak in their behalf.

The Hearing Officer or his or her counsel may question the parties and their witnesses. The Hearing Officer shall not be bound by technical rules of evidence usually employed in legal proceedings but may accept any evidence deemed appropriate and pertinent.

Should any party to the controversy fail to appear at the hearing, the Hearing Officer may, in his or her discretion, continue, dismiss, or proceed with the hearing?

Findings and Conclusions

At the conclusion of the hearing, the Hearing Officer shall render a report in writing containing findings and conclusions and recommendations, if any. This report, together with a transcript of the proceedings, shall be submitted to the Council on Ethical and Judicial Affairs. A copy of the report shall be mailed to all parties of record.

Written Objections

Any party to the proceedings may submit written objections to the report to the Council on Ethical and Judicial Affairs. These objections must be submitted within twenty-one (21) days after the report has been submitted by the Hearing Officer to the Council on Ethical and Judicial Affairs.

Oral Argument

In addition to written objections, any party may request an opportunity to present oral arguments on its objections to the report of the Hearing Officer before the Council on Ethical and Judicial Affairs. This request must be made within twenty-one (21) days after the report has been submitted to the Council. The granting of oral arguments shall be discretionary with the Council. If granted, the parties shall be notified by the Council of the place and date for such oral argument; all parties shall be given opportunity to be heard, and the time allotted to argument may be limited by the Council with due regard to the magnitude and complexities of the issues involved.

If any party fails to appear, the Council may continue or proceed with the oral argument.

Final Decision

The Council on Ethical and Judicial Affairs, including the member or members who serve as the Hearing Officer, shall render a final decision. A copy of that decision shall be mailed or otherwise served upon all parties.

Disciplinary Action

The Council on Ethical and Judicial Affairs shall have the authority to acquit, admonish, censure, or place on probation the accused physician or suspend or expel him or her from AMA membership as the facts may justify. This action shall be in accordance with the authority vested in the Council by 1.60, 6.401, and 6.402 of the Bylaws.

Transcript

A written transcript shall be made of the proceedings and of the oral argument before the Council on Ethical and Judicial Affairs.

If any party to the controversy requests a copy of the transcript, it shall be made available to the party at the party's expense.

Filing of Copies

Ten (10) copies of all pleadings and exhibits shall be submitted to AMA Headquarters to the Chair of the Council on Ethical and Judicial Affairs. One copy of each document shall be submitted at the same time to each of the other parties to the controversy.

Table of Cases

A Woman's Choice-East Side Women's Clinic v. Newman, 305 F.3d 684 (7th Cir. 2002) [8.08].

Abdur'Rahman v. Bredesen, 2004 WL 2246227 (Tenn. App. 2004) [2.06].

Acuna v. Turkish, 192 N.J. 399, 930 A.2d 416 (2007) [8.08].

Agee v. Grunert, 349 F. Supp.2d 838 (D. Vt. 2004) [9.031].

Aiken v. Business and Indus. Health Group, Inc., 886 F. Supp. 1565 (D. Kan. 1995) [I].

Allen v. Smith, 368 S.E.2d 924 (W. Va. 1988) [IV].

Amaral v. Saint Cloud Hospital, 598 N.W.2d 379 (Minn. 1999) [V].

American Medical Ass'n v. FTC, 638 F.2d 443, (2nd Cir. 1980), aff'd, 455 US 676 (1982) [5.02, 8.05].

American Medical Ass'n v. United States, 130 F.2d 233 (D.C. Cir. 1942), aff'd, 317 US 519 (1943) [8.05].

American Optometric Ass'n v. F.T.C., 626 F.2d 896 (D.C. Cir. 1980) [5.02].

Ancier v. State Dept. of Health, 140 Wash. App. 564, 166 P.3d 829 (2007) [5.026, 5.027].

Anderson v. Bd. of Trustees of Caro Community Hosp., 10 Mich. App. 348, 159 N.W.2d 347 (1968) [II; 9.031].

Anderson v. Florence, 288 Minn. 351, 181 N.W.2d 873 (1970) [II; 8.12].

Arizona State Bd. of Medical Examiners v. Clark, 97 Ariz. 205, 398 P.2d 908 (1965) [III, VII; 3.01, 8.11, 9.06].

Arlen v. State, 61 Ohio St. 2d 168, 399 N.E.2d 1251 (1980) [II, III; 8.06, 9.04].

Arroyo v. United States, 656 F.3d 663, 678 (7th Cir. 2011) [8.12].

Awwad v. Capital Region Otolaryngology Head & Neck Group, 2007 N.Y. Misc. LEXIS 8593 [9.02].

Axtell Clinic v. Cranston, No. 56,745 (Kan. Ct. App. June 20, 1985) (LEXIS, States Library, Kan. file) [6.02, 6.03, 9.02].

Balian v. Board of Licensure in Medicine, 722 A.2d 364 (Me. 1999) [7.01, 7.02].

Bates v. State Bar of Ariz., 433 US 350 (1977) [5.02].

Bay Ridge Diagnostic Laboratory, Inc. v. Dumpson, 400 F. Supp. 1104 (E.D.N.Y. 1975) [8.03, 8.032, 8.06, 9.06].

Bazakos v. Lewis, 12 N.Y.3d 631, 911 N.E.2d 847, 883 N.Y.S.2d 785 (2009) [10.03].

Bazakos v. Lewis, 56 A.D.3d 15, 864 N.Y.S.2d 505 (2008), rev'd, 12 N.Y.3d 631, 911 N.E.2d 847, 883 N.Y.S.2d 785 (2009) [10.03].

Baze v. Rees, 553 U.S. 35,64 (2008) (Alito, J., concurring) [2.06].

Belin v. Dingle, 127 Md. App. 68, 732 A.2d 301 (1999) [8.16].

Berger v. Sonneland, 101 Wash. App. 141, 1 P.3d 1187 (2000) [IV].

Bernstein v. Alameda-Contra Costa Medical Ass'n, 139 Cal. App. 2d 241, 293 P.2d 862 (1st Dist. 1956) [II; 9.04, 9.07].

Best v. Taylor Machine Works, 179 Ill. 2d 367, 689 N.E. 2d 1057 (Ill. 1997) [IV; 5.05].

Biddle v. Warren General Hospital, 86 Ohio St. 3d 395, 715 N.E. 2d 518 (1999) [IV; 5.05].

Bloomington Urological Associates v. Scaglia, 292 Ill. App. 3d, 793, 686 N.E. 2d 389 (4th Dist. 1997) [8.11].

Boike v. McLaren Health Care Corp., 2007 WL 1932029 (Mich. App. 2007) [II].

Boman v. Southeast Medical Services Group, 1998 WL 1182063 (Mass. Super. 1998) [6.02, 8.032].

Bouvia v. Superior Court, 179 Cal. App. 3d 1127, 225 Cal. Rptr. 297 (2d Dist. 1986) [2.20].

Bowman v. Beghin, 713 N.E.2d 913 (Ind. App. 1999) [8.08].

Brandt v. Medical Defense Assoc., 856 S.W.2d 667 (Mo. 1993) [IV; 5.05].

Bratt v. International Business Mach. Corp., 392 Mass. 508, 467 N.E.2d 126 (1984) [IV; 5.05, 5.09].

Brophy v. New England Sinai Hosp., Inc., 398 Mass. 417, 497 N.E.2d 626 (1986) [2.20].

Brown v. Bi-Lo, Inc, 354 S.C. 436, 581 S.E.2d 836 (2003) [IV].

Brown v. Warren, 858 So.2d 168 (Miss. App. 2003) [8.03, 8.05].

Bryant v. Hilst, 136 F.R.D. 487 (D. Kan. 1991) [IV; 5.05].

Bryson v. Tillinghast, 749 P.2d 110 (Okla. 1988) [IV; 5.05].

Cahill v. Rosa, 89 N.Y.2d 14, 24, 674 N.E.2d 274 651 N.Y.S.2d 344 (1996) [9.131].

Cal. Att'y Op. N. 98-104, 1998 WL 744399 [8.09].

Calhoun v. WHA Medical Clinic, PLLC, 178 N.C. App. 585, 632 S.E.2d 563 (2006) [9.02].

Calvert v. Sharp, 748 F.2d 861, 863 (4th Cir. 1984), cert. denied, 471 US 1132 (1985) [VI].

Carson v. Fine, 123 Wash. 2d 206, 867 P.2d 610 (1994) [9.07].

Carter-Shields v. Alton Health Institute, 317 Ill. App. 3d 260, 739 N.E.2d 569 (5th Dist. 2000) vacated 201 Ill. 2d 441, 777 N.E.2d 948 (2002) [9.02, 9.06].

Casperson v. N.E. Wis. Ctr. for Surgery & Rehab of Hand, Ltd., 2007 WL 1191782 (Wis. App. 2007) [8.115, 10.01].

Castillo-Plaza v. Green, 655 So. 2d 197 (Fla. App. 1995) [II, IV; 5.05, 5.06, 5.08].

Cent. Ind. Podiatry, P.C. v. Krueger, 882 N.E.2d 723 (Ind. 2008) [9.02].

Chiropractic Coop. Ass'n v. AMA, 617 F. Supp. 264 (E.D. Mich. 1985), aff'd in part and rev'd in part, 867 F.2d 270 (6th Cir. 1989) [VI; 3.01, 3.04].

Chiropractic Coop. Ass'n v. AMA, 867 F.2d 270 (6th Cir. 1989) [VI; 3.01, 3.05, 3.04].

Chiropractic Coop. Ass'n v. AMA, 1986-2 Trade Cas. (CCH) & 67, 294 (E.D. Mich. 1986), aff'd in part and rev'd in part, 867 F.2d 270 (6th Cir. 1989) [VI; 3.01, 3.04].

Clayton v. Harkey, 826 So.2d 1283 (Miss. 2002) [8.03, 8.05].

Cleveland Hair Clinic, Inc. v. Puig, 968 F. Supp. 1227 (N.D. Ill. 1996) [7.03, 9.02].

Colby v. Schwartz, 78 Cal. App. 3d 885, 144 Cal. Rptr. 624 (2d Dist. 1978) [VI; 8.11, 9.06].

Community Hosp. Group Inc. v. More, 183 N.J. 36, 869 A.2d 884 (2005) [9.02].

Community Hosp. Group Inc. v. More, 365 N.J. Super. 84, 838 A.2d 472 (2003) [9.02].

Compassion in Dying v. Washington, 79 F. 3d 790 (9th Cir. 1996), replacing, 49 F.3d 586 (9th Cir. 1995) [2.20, 2.21, 2.211].

Compassion in Dying v. Washington, 49 F.3d 586 (9th Cir. 1995), replaced, 79 F. 3d 790 (9th Cir. 1996) [2.211].

Conley v. Warren, 797 So. 2d 881 (Miss. 2001) [8.03, 8.05].

Cooey v. Strickland, 589 F.3d 210 (6th Cir. 2009) [2.06].

Cooey v. Strickland, 479 F.3d 412 (6th Cir. 2007) [2.06].

Corbett v. D'Alessandro, 487 So. 2d 368 (Fla. App. 1986) [IV; 2.20].

Corey v. Skelton, 834 So.2d 681 (Miss. 2003) [8.03, 8.05].

Cornfeld v. State Board of Physicians, 174 Md. App. 456, 921 A.2d 893 (2007) [II].

Couture v. Couture, 48 Ohio App. 3d 208, 549 N.E.2d 571 (1989) [2.20].

Crescenzo v. Crane, 350 N.J. Super. 531, 796 A.2d 283 (2002) [IV].

Crist v. Moffatt, 326 N.C. 326, 333, 389 S.E.2d 41 (1990) [IV; 5.05].

Cruzan v. Director, Missouri Department of Health, 497 US 261 (1990) [2.20].

Cruzan v. Harmon, 760 S.W.2d 408 (Mo. 1988), aff'd, 497 US 261 (1990) [2.20].

Culbertson v. Mernitz, 602 N.E. 2d 98 (Ind. 1992) [8.08].

D.A.B v. Brown, 570 N.W. 2d 168 (Minn. App. 1997) [8.06].

Dade County Medical Ass'n v. Samartino, 213 So. 2d 627 (Fla. App. 1968) [5.02].

Darke v. Estate of Isner, 2004 WL 1325635 (Mass. Super. 2004) [8.13].

DeGrella v. Elston, 858 S.W.2d 698 (Ky. 1993) [2.20].

Delio v. Westchester County Medical Center, 134 Misc. 2d 206, 510 N.Y.S.2d 415 (Sup. Ct. 1986), rev'd, 129 A.D.2d 1, 516 N.Y.S.2d 677 (1987) [2.20].

Dingle v. Belin, 358 Md. 354, 749 A.2d 157 (2000) [8.16].

Doe v. Roe, 93 Misc. 2d 201, 400 N.Y.S.2d 668 (Sup. Ct. 1977) [IV; 5.05].

Dominy v. Shumpert, 235 Ga. App. 500, 510 S.E.2d 81 (1998) [8.031].

Downey v. Weston, 451 Pa. 259, 301 A.2d 635 (1973) [IV; 5.05].

Dr. K. v. State Bd. of Physician Quality Assur., 98 Md. App. 103, 632 A.2d 453 (1993), cert. denied, 334 Md. 18, 637 A.2d 1191 (1994), and cert. denied, 115 S. Ct. 75, 130 L. Ed. 29 (1994) [II].

D'Souza v. State Med. Bd. of Ohio, 2009 WL 5108774 (Ohio 2009) [I, II, IV, VIII].

Dupree v. Malpractice Research, Inc., 179 Mich. App. 254, 445 N.W.2d 498 (1989) [6.01].

Duquette v. Superior Court, 161 Ariz. 269, 778 P.2d 634 (Ariz. App. 1989) [IV; 5.05].

Eli Lilly & Co. v. Marshall, 850 S.W.2d 155 (Tex. 1993) [V].

Emerich v. Philadelphia Center for Human Development, Inc., 554 Pa. 209, 720 A.2d 1032 (1999) [5.05].

Estate of Behringer v. Medical Ctr., 249 N.J. Super. 597, 592 A.2d 1251, 1268 (1991) [IV; 5.05, 9.13, 9.131].

Estate of Finkle, 90 Misc. 2d 550, 395 N.Y.S.2d 343 (Surr. Ct. 1977) [IV; 5.05, 7.04].

Estates of Morgan v. Fairfield Family Counseling Center, 77 Ohio St. 3d 284, 303, 673 N.E.2d 1311 (1997) [IV; 5.05].

Falcon v. Alaska Pub. Offices Comm'n, 570 P.2d 469 (Alaska 1977) [IV; 5.05].

Falcone v. Middlesex County Medical Soc'y, 62 N.J. Super. 184, 162 A.2d 324 (1960), aff'd, 34 N.J. 582, 170 A.2d 791 (1961) [VI; 3.01].

Falksen v. Sec. of the Dept. of Health and Human Services, 2004 WL 785056 (Fed. Cl. 2004) [9.07].

Faya v. Almaraz, 329 Md. 435, 620 A.2d 327 (1993) [9.13, 9.131].

Ferguson v. City of Charleston, 532 US 67, 121 S. Ct. 1281 (2001) [5.05].

Finucan v. Maryland State Board of Physicians Quality Assurance, 151 Md. App. 399, 827 A.2d 176 (2003) [8.14].

Fineman v. New Jersey Dept. of Human Servs., 272 N.J. Super. 606, 640 A.2d 1161 (App. Div. 1994), cert. denied, 138 N.J. 267, 649 A.2d 1287 (1994) [VI].

Forziati v. Board of Registration in Medicine, 333 Mass. 125, 128 N.E.2d 789 (1955) [II; 6.02].

Fosmire v. Nicoleau, 75 N.Y.2d 218, 551 N.E.2d 77, 551 N.Y.S.2d 876 (1990) [2.20].

Freeman v. Duluth Clinic, 334 N.W.2d 626 (Minn. 1983) [9.02].

Gadson v. Newman, 807 F. Supp. 1412 (C.D. Ill. 1992) [8.032].

Garby v. George Washington University Hosp., 886 A.2d 510 (D.C. App. 2005) [IV].

Geisberger v. Willuhn, 72 Ill. App. 3d 435, 390 N.E.2d 945 (2d Dist. 1979) [IV; 5.05].

Gladieux v. Ohio State Medical Board, 1999 WL 770959 (Ohio App. 1999) [I, IV].

Goad v. Virginia Board of Medicine, 40 Va. App. 621, 580 S.E.2d 494 (2003) [3.08, 9.05].

Gomez v. Chua Medical Corp., 510 N.E.2d 191 (Ind. App. 1987) [9.02].

Gonzales v. Oregon, 126 S. Ct. 904 (2006) [2.211].

Grabowski v. Quigley, 454 Pa. Super. 27, 684 A.2d 610 (1996) [8.16].

Greenberg v. Miami Children's Hospital Research Institute, Inc., 264 F. Supp. 2d 1064 (S.D. Fla. 2003) [2.08].

Greisman v. Newcomb Hosp., 40 N.J. 389, 192 A.2d 817 (1963) [3.01].

Gromis v. Medical Board, 8 Cal. App. 4th 589, 10 Cal. Rptr. 2d 452 (1st Dist. 1992), reh'g denied, 1992 Cal. App. LEXIS 1047, and review denied, 1992 Cal. LEXIS 5101 [8.14].

Grossman v. Columbine Medical Group, Inc., 1999 WL 1024015 (Colo. App. 1999) [10.01].

Group Health Coop. v. King County Medical Soc'y, 39 Wash. 2d 586, 237 P.2d 737 (1951) [VI; 8.04, 8.05, 9.06].

Hadix v. Caruso, 461 F.Supp. 2d 574 (W.D. Mich. 2006) [2.067].

Hague v. Williams, 37 N.J. 328, 181 A.2d 345 (1962) [IV; 5.05].

Hammonds v. Aetna Casualty & Sur. Co., 243 F. Supp. 793 (N.D. Ohio 1965) [IV; 5.08].

Harlan v. Lewis, 141 F.R.D. 107 (E.D. Ark. 1992) [5.05].

Health Sys. Agency v. Virginia State Bd. of Medicine, 424 F.Supp. 267 (E.D. Va. 1976) [5.02].

Heller v. Norcal Mutual Ins. Co., 8 Cal. 4th 30, 876 P.2d 999, 32 Cal. Rptr. 2d 200 (1994), cert. denied, 115 S. Ct. 669, 130 L. Ed. 2d 602 (1994) [5.05].

Hellman v. Board of Registration in Medicine, 404 Mass. 800, 537 N.E.2d 150 (1989) [IV].

Hiser v. Randolph, 126 Ariz. 608, 617 P.2d 774 (Ct. App. 1980) [VI; 8.11].

Hodder v. U.S., 328 F. Supp. 2d 335 (E.D.N.Y. 2004) [3.041].

Homer v. Long, 90 Md. App. 1, 3 n.1, 599 A.2d 1193 (1992) [8.14].

Hopkins v. Sec. of Dept. of Health and Human Services, 2007 WL 2454038 (Fed. Cl. 2007) [9.07].

Horn v. New York Times, 186 Misc. 2d 469, 719 N.Y.S. 2d 471 (Sup. Ct. 2000) [IV; 5.05, 5.09].

Horne v. Patton, 291 Ala. 701, 287 So. 2d 824 (1973) [IV; 5.05].

Hull v. Tate, No. 46443 (Okla. Ct. App. Apr. 16, 1974) (LEXIS States library, Okla. file), rev'd, No. 46443 (Okla. Sup. Ct. Oct. 29, 1974) (LEXIS, States library, Okla. file) [8.16].

Idbeis v. Wichita Surgical Specialists, 279 Kan. 755, 112 P.2d 81 (2005) [9.02].

In re AB, 196 Misc. 2d 940, 768 N.Y.S. 2d 256 (Sup. Ct. 2003) [2.20, 2.215].

In re Baska, 281 Ga. 676, 641 S.E.2d 533 (2007) [8.14].

In re Capt. Wool, Inc., 1995 US Dist. LEXIS 20128 (E.D. Va. 1995) [8.032].

In re Conroy, 190 N.J. Super. 453, 464 A.2d 303 (1983), rev'd, 98 N.J. 321, 486 A.2d 1209 (1985) [2.17, 2.20].

In re Culbertson's Estate, 57 Misc. 2d 391, 292 N.Y.S.2d 806 (Surr. Ct. 1968) [7.01, 7.02, 7.03, 7.05].

In re Doe, 16 Phila. 229, 1987 Phila. Cty. Rptr. LEXIS 30 (1987) [2.20].

In re Doe, 411 Mass. 512, 583 N.E.2d 1263 (1992) [2.20].

In re Drabick, 200 Cal. App. 3d 185, 245 Cal. Rptr. 840 (6th Dist. 1988) [2.20].

In re Eli Lilly & Co., 142 F.R.D. 454 (S.D. Ind. 1992) [V].

In re Estate of Longeway, 133 Ill.2d 33, 549 N.E.2d 292 (1989) [2.20].

In re Farrell, 108 N.J. 335, 529 A.2d 404 (1987) [2.20].

In re Fiori, 438 Pa. Super. 610, 652 A.2d 1350 (1995), app. granted, 655 A.2d 989 (Pa. 1995) [2.20].

In re Gardner, 534 A.2d 947 (Me. 1987) [2.20].

In re Grant, 109 Wash. 2d 545, 747 P.2d 445 (1987) [2.20].

In re Jobes, 108 N.J. 394, 529 A.2d 434 (1987) [2.20].

In re Lawrance, 579 N.E.2d 32 (Ind. 1991) [2.20].

In re Lifschutz, 2 Cal. 3d 415, 467 P.2d 557, 85 Cal. Rptr. 829 (1970) [IV; 5.05].

In re Managed Care Litigation, 150 F. Supp. 2d 1330 (S.D. Fla. 2001) [8.053].

In re Milton S. Hershey Medical Ctr., 407 Pa. Super. 565, 595 A.2d 1290, 1295 (1991) [9.131].

In re Odeh, 431 B.R. 807, 814 (N.D. Ill. 2010) [7.01, 8.03].

In re Peter, 108 N.J. 365, 529 A.2d 419 (1987) [2.20].

In re Prange, 166 Ill. App.3d 1091, 520 N.E.2d 946, vacated, 121 Ill. 2d 570, 527 N.E.2d 303 (1988) [2.20].

In re R.C., 775 P.2d 27 (Colo. 1989) [2.04, 2.05].

In re Rules Adoption, 224 N.J. Super. 252, 540 A.2d 212 (1988) [IV; 5.05].

In re Subpoena N. 22., Appeal of A.B., 709 A.2d 385 (Pa. Super. 1998) [5.05].

In re Vioxx Products Liability Litigation, 230 F.R.D. 473 (E.D. La. 2005) [5.05].

In re Woolley, 2005 WL 2077475 (Minn. App. 2005) [10.015].

Isles Wellness, Inc. v. Progressive N. Ins. Co., 703 N.W.2d 513 (Minn. 2005) [VI].

Jasty v. Wright Medical Technology, Inc., 528 F.3d 28 (1st Cir. 2008) [8.0501].

Johnson v. Blue Cross/Blue Shield, 677 F. Supp. 1112 (D.N.M. 1987) [VI; 3.01, 3.04].

Jones v. Fakehany, 261 Cal. App. 2d 298, 67 Cal. Rptr. 810 (2d Dist. 1968) [5.02, 5.05, 6.08].

K.A.C. v. Benson, 1993 Minn. App. LEXIS 1201 (Minn. 1993) [9.13, 9.131].

Kaiser Foundation Health Plan, Inc. v. Zingale, 99 Cal. App. 4th 1018, 121 Cal. Rptr. 2d 741 (2002) [8.135].

Kamelgard v. Macura, 585 F.3d 334 (7th Cir. 2009) [9.031].

Karlin v. Weinberg, 148 N.J. Super. 243, 372 A.2d 616 (1977), aff'd, 77 N.J. 408, 390 A.2d 1161 (1978) [9.02].

Karlin v. Weinberg, 77 N.J. 408, 390 A.2d 1161 (1978) [9.02].

Kartell v. Blue Shield of Mass., Inc., 749 F.2d 922 (1st Cir. 1984), cert. denied, 471 US 1029 (1985) [8.05].

Kelley v. Sec. of Dept. of Health and Human Services, 2005 WL 1125671 (Fed. Cl. 2005) [9.07].

Ketchup v. Howard, 247 Ga. App. 54, 543 S.E.2d 371 (2000) [8.08, 10.01].

Kirk v. Jefferson County Medical Soc'y, 577 S.W.2d 419 (Ky. App. 1978) [I, III].

Koefoot v. American College of Surgeons, 652 F. Supp. 882 (N.D. Ill. 1986) [3.01].

Korper v. Weinstein, 57 Mass. App. 433, 783 N.E.2d 877 (2003) [8.14].

Krischer v. McIver, 697 So. 2d 97 (Fla. 1997) [2.211].

Kunkel v. Walton, 179 Ill. 2d 519, 689 N.E. 2d 1047 (1997) [IV].

Kurdek v. West Orange Bd. of Educ., 222 N.J. Super. 218, 536 A.2d 332 (1987) [IV; 5.05].

L.W. v. L.E. Phillips Career Dev. Ctr., 167 Wis. 2d 53, 482 N.W.2d 60 (1992) [2.20].

Lemon v. Stewart, 111 Md. App. 511, 523, 682 A.2d 1177 (Md. App. 1996) [9.131].

Lisa M. v. Henry Mays Newhall Memorial Hosp. 12 Cal. 4th 291, 907 P.2d 358, 48 Cal. Rptr. 510 (1995) [8.14].

Littleton v. Good Samaritan Hospital, 39 Ohio St. 3d 86, 529 N.E.2d 449 (1988) [IV; 5.05].

Loudon v. Mhyre, 110 Wash. 2d 675, 756 P.2d 138 (1988) [IV; 5.05].

Loui v. Board of Medical Examiners, 78 Haw. 21, 889 P.2d 705 (1995) [Preamble].

Lurch v. United States, 719 F.2d 333 (10th Cir. 1983), cert. denied, 466 US 927 (1984) [8.03, 8.05].

Magan Medical Clinic v. California State Bd. of Medical Examiners, 249 Cal. App. 2d 124, 57 Cal. Rptr. 256 (2d Dist. 1967) [8.03, 8.032, 8.06].

Manion v. N.P.W. Medical Center of N.E. Pa., Inc., 676 F.Supp. 585 (M.D. Pa. 1987) [IV; 5.05, 5.06, 5.07].

Marsingill v. O'Malley, 58 P.3d 495 (Alaska 2002) [8.08].

Martin v. Baehler, 1993 Del. Super. LEXIS 199 (1993) [IV].

Maryland Att'y Gen. Op., 62 Op. Att'y Gen. 157 (1977) [IV; 2.02, 5.05].

Maryland Att'y Gen. Op. No. 89-022 (1989) [IV].

Maryland Att'y Gen. Op. No. 88-046, 73 Op. Att'y Gen. 162 (1988) [2.20].

Maryland Att'y Gen. Op. No. 86-030, 71 Op. Att'y. Gen. 407 (1986) [IV].

Matter of Lyle A., 14 Misc. 3d 842, 830 N.Y.S.2d 486 (2006) [8.08, 8.081, 8.11, 10.01].

Matthies v. Mastromonaco, 160 N.J. 26, 733 A.2d 456 (1999) [8.08].

Maxey v. United States, 1989 US Dist. LEXIS 5827 (W.D. Ark. 1989) [VI].

McConnell v. Beverly Enterprises-Connecticut, Inc., 209 Conn. 692, 553 A.2d 596 (1989) [2.20].

McCormick v. England, 328 S.C. 627, 494 S.E. 2d 431 (Ct. App. 1997) [IV].

McHugh v. Audet, 72 F.Supp. 394 (M.D. Pa. 1947) [9.07].

McIntosh v. Milano, 168 N.J. Super. 466, 403 A.2d 500 (1979) [Preamble; I, IV; 5.05].

McMurray v. Johnson, 481 So. 2d 887 (Ala. 1985) [8.16].

McNiel v. Cooper, 241 S.W. 3d 886 (Tenn. App. 2007) [7.02].

Memphis Planned Parenthood v. Sundquist, 175 F.2d 456 (6th Cir. 1999) [2.015].

Mich. Att'y Gen. Opinion No. 5229, 1977-78 Att'y. Gen. Op. 234 (1977) [8.03, 8.032].

Mich. Att'y Gen. Opinion No. 5024, 1977-78 Att'y. Gen. Op. 299 (1978) [5.02].

Midtown Medical Group, Inc. v. State Farm Mutual Automobile Insurance Co., 220 Ariz. 341, 206 P.3d 790 (Ariz. App. 2009) [VI].

Miller v. Meeks, 762 So. 2d 302 (Miss. 2000) [8.03, 8.05].

Miller v. Rupf, 2004 WL 2092015 (Cal. App. 2004) [II, V].

Missouri Att'y Gen. Op. N. 6 (July 8, 1982) (LEXIS, States Library, Mo. file) [8.06].

Mitchell v. Villien, 19 So. 3d 557 (La. App. 2009) [5.05].

Modi v. West Virginia Board of Medicine, 465 S.E.2d 230 (W. Va. 1995) [8.08].

Mohanty v. St. John Heart Clinic, S.C., 225 Ill.2d 52, 866 N.E.2d 85 (2006) [8.115, 9.02, 9.06, 10.01].

Monroe v. United States, 2008 U.S. Dist. LEXIS 22455 (N.D. Ill. 2008) [8.03, 8.05].

Montefiore Hosp. & Medical Center v. NLRB, 621 F.2d 510 (2d Cir. 1980) [VI].

Monturi v. Englewood Hosp., 246 N.J. Super. 547, 588 A.2d 408 (1991) [8.16].

Moore v. Rees, 2007 WL 1035013 (E.D. Ky. 2007) [2.06].

Morrison v. Abramovice, 206 Cal. App. 3d 304, 309, 253 Cal. Rptr. 530, 533 (1988) [2.20].

Moses v. McWilliams, 379 Pa. Super. 150, 549 A.2d 950 (1988), appeal denied, 521 Pa. 630, 558 A.2d 532 (1989) [IV; 5.05, 5.07].

Ms. B. v. Montgomery County Emergency Service, Inc., 799 F. Supp. 534 (E.D. Pa. 1992) cert. denied, 114 S.Ct. 174 (1993) [5.05].

Munn v. Montana Board of Medical Examiners, 329 Mont. 401, 124 P.3d 1123 (2005) [8.14].

Murfreesboro Med. Clinic v. Udom, 166 S.W.3d 674 (Tenn. 2005) [9.02, 9.06].

N.X. v. Cabrini Medical Center, 97 N.Y.2d 247, 765 N.E.2d 844, 739 N.Y.S.2d 348 (2002) [8.14].

Nash v. Wennar, 645 F.Supp. 238 (D. Vt. 1986) [I, IV; 8.05].

Neade v. Portes, 303 Ill. App. 3d 799, 710 N.E. 2d 418 (2d Dist. 1999) [8.132].

Nieto v. Kapoor, 268 F.3d 1208 (10th Cir. 2001) [I, IV].

Noble v. Sartori, 1989 Ky. App. LEXIS 67 (1989) [VI; 8.11].

North Carolina Department of Corrections v. North Carolina Medical Board, 363 N.C. 189, 675 S.E.2d 641 (2009) [2.06].

Oak Orchard Cmty. Health Ctr. v. Blasco, 8 Misc. 3d 927, 800 N.Y.S.2d. 277 (Sup. Ct. 2005) [9.02].

Ohio Att'y Gen. Op. No. 99-044, 1999 WL 692 623 [8.03, 8.11, 8.13].

Ohio Urology, Inc. v. Poll, 72 Ohio. App. 446, 594 N.E.2d 1027 (1991) [VI; 6.11, 9.02, 9.06].

Ojeda v. Sharp Cabrillo Hosp., 8 Cal. App. 4th 1, 10 Cal. Rptr. 2d 230 (1992) [6.01].

Otto v. Melman, 2009 WL 4348827 (N.Y. Sup. 2009) [8.062].

Painter v. Abels, 998 P.2d 931 (Wyo. 2000) [2.07].

People v. Anyakora, 162 Misc. 2d 47, 616 N.Y.S.2d 149 (Sup. Ct. 1993) [VI].

People v. Griffin, 242 A.D.2d 70, 671 N.Y.S. 2d 34 (1998) [8.14].

People v. Kevorkian, 248 Mich. App. 373, 639 N.W.2d 291 (2001) [2.20, 2.21, 2.211].

People v. Stritzinger, 137 Cal. App. 3d 126, 186 Cal. Rptr. 750 (2d Dist. 1982), rev'd 34 Cal. 3d 505, 668 P.2d 738, 194 Cal. Rptr. 431 (1983) [IV; 2.02, 5.05].

Perna v. Pirozzi, 182 N.J. Super 510, 442 A.2d 1016 (1982), rev'd, 92 N.J. 446, 457 A.2d 431 (1983) [8.16].

Perna v. Pirozzi, 92 N.J. 446, 457 A.2d 431 (1983) [8.16].

Perreira v. State, 768 P.2d 1198 (Colo. 1989) [IV; 5.05].

Petrillo v. Syntex Laboratories, Inc., 148 Ill. App. 3d 581, 499 N.E.2d 952 (1st Dist. 1986), cert. denied, 483 US 1007 (1987) [II, IV; 5.05, 5.06, 5.07, 5.08].

Phelps v. DeMello, 2007 WL 1063567 (E.D. Mo. 2007) [II].

Phoenix Orthopaedic Surgeons, Ltd. v. Peairs, 164 Ariz. 54, 790 P.2d 752 (Ct. App. 1989) [9.02].

Pierce v. Ortho Pharmaceutical Corp., 84 N.J. 58, 417 A.2d 505 (1980) [2.07].

Pierson v. Med. Health Ctrs., 2004 WL 1416265 (N.J. Super. 2004) [9.02].

Planned Parenthood League of Massachusetts, Inc. v. Attorney General, 424 Mass. 586, 677 N.E.2d 101, 107 (1997) [2.015].

Planned Parenthood of Central New Jersey v. Farmer, 165 N.J. 609, 762 A.2d 620 (2000) [2.015].

Planned Parenthood of Middle Tennessee v. Sundquist, 1998 WL 467110 (Tenn. App. 1998) [10.01].

Planned Parenthood v. Miller, 63 F.3d 1452 (8th Cir. 1995) [2.015].

Plastic Surgical Servs. of New England, P.C. v. Hall, 1993 WL 818637 (Mass. Super. 1993) [8.115].

Polo v. Gotchel, 225 N.J. Super. 429, 542 A.2d 947 (1987) [6.01].

Pons v. Ohio State Medical Bd., 66 Ohio St. 3d 619, 614 N.E.2d 748 (1993) [I, II, IV; 8.14].

Prairie Eye Center v. Butler, 329 Ill. App. 3d 293, 768 N.E.2d 414 (4th Dist. 2002) [9.02].

Prestrud v. Blanco, 2006 WL 1633707 (Wash. App. 2006) [8.14].

Pryzbowski v. US Health Care, Inc., 64 F. Supp. 2d 361 (D.N.J. 1999) [8.13].

Pullman v. Gormley, 13 Misc.3d 1234(A), 831 N.Y.S.2d 356, 2006 WL 3232182 (2006) [7.03, 7.04].

Quilico v. Kaplan, 749 F.2d 480 (7th Cir. 1984) [8.03, 8.05].

Rasmussen v. Fleming, 154 Ariz. 200, 741 P.2d 667 (Ct. App. 1986), aff'd in part and rev'd in part, 154 Ariz. 207, 741 P.2d 674 (1987) [2.20].

Rasmussen v. Fleming, 154 Ariz. 207, 741 P.2d 674 (1987) [2.20].

Reed v. Bojarski, 166 N.J.89, 764 A.2d 433 (2001) [10.03].

Reinninger v. Prestige Fabricators, Inc., 523 S.E. 2d 720 (N.C. App. 1999) [5.05].

Ritt v. Ritt, 98 N.J. Super. 590, 238 A.2d 196 (1967), rev'd, 52 N.J. 177, 244 A.2d 497 (1968) [IV; 5.05].

Rocca v. Southern Hills Counseling Center, Inc., 671 N.E. 2d 913 (Ind. App. 1996) [IV; 5.05].

Roe v. Wade, 410 US 113 (1973) [2.01].

Salerian v. Maryland State Board of Physicians, 176 Md. App. 231, 932 A.2d 1225 (2007) [IV; 5.05].

Salt River Project v. Industrial Comm'n, 1992 Ariz. App. LEXIS 323, 129 Ariz. Adv. Rep. 39 (1992) [IV].

Sampson v. State, 31 P.3d 88 (Alaska 2001) [2.211].

San Juan-Torregosa v. Garcia, 80 S.W.3d 539 (Tenn. App. 2002) [2.20].

Schaal v. Fender, 2007 WL 2461642 (D. Colo. 2007) [7.01].

Schechter v. Ohio State Med. Bd., 2005 WL 1869733 (Ohio App. 2005) [I, II, IV].

Scripps Clinic v. Superior Court, 108 Cal. App.4th 917, 134 Cal. Rptr. 2d 101 (2003) [VI, VIII].

Selkin v. State Board for Professional Medical Conduct, 63 F. Supp. 2d 397 (S.D.N.Y. 1999) [8.14].

Shankman v. Coastal Psychiatric Assoc., 258 Ga. 294, 368 S.E.2d 753 (1988) [9.02].

Singleton v. Norris, 319 F.3d 1018 (8th Cir. 2003) [2.06].

Singleton v. State, 437 S.E.2d 53 (S.C. 1993) [2.06].

Smith v. Radecki, 238 P.3d 111, 116 (Alaska 2010) [10.03].

Somoza v. St. Vincent's Hosp. & Medical Ctr. of New York, 192 A.D.2d 429, 596 N.Y.S.2d 789 (1993) [9.12].

Sorensen v. Barbuto, 143 P.3d 295 (Utah App. 2006) [5.05, 5.059].

South Carolina Att'y Gen. Op. 1978 S.C. AG LEXIS 806 [7.01, 7.02, 7.03].

Sperry Rand Corp. v. Hill, 356 F.2d 181 (1st Cir.), cert. denied, 384 US 973 (1966) [5.02].

Spock v. Pocket Books, Inc., 48 Misc. 2d 812, 266 N.Y.S.2d 77 (Sup. Ct. 1965) [II; 5.02].

Springdale Diagnostic Clinic v. Northwest Physicians, 2003 Ark. App. LEXIS 697 (2003) [7.03].

Stanley v. McCarver, 204 Ariz. 339, 63 P.3d 1076 (2003) [10.03].

State ex. rel. Kitzmiller v. Henning, 437 S.E.2d 452 (W.Va. 1993) [IV; 5.05].

State ex. rel. Stufflebam v. Appelquist, 694 S.W.2d 882 (Mo. App. 1985) overuled by State ex. rel. Woytus v. Ryan, 776 S.W.2d 389 (Mo. 1989) [IV; 5.05].

State ex. rel. Woytus v. Ryan, 776 S.W.2d 389 (Mo. 1989) [IV; 5.05].

State v. Agacki, 226 Wis. 2d 349, 595 N.W. 2d 31 (1999) [5.05].

State v. AMA, 1981-2 Trade Cas. (CCH) & 64,195 (1981) [V, VI; 3.04, 3.07].

State v. Johnson, 968 S.W.2d 123 (Mo. 1998) [IV].

State v. Naramore, 25 Kan. App. 2d 302, 965 P.2d 211 (1998) [2.20, 2.22].

State v. Perry, 610 So. 2d 746 (La. 1992) [2.06].

State v. Wood, 323 Wis. 2d 321, 780 N.W.2d 63, 82-83 (2010) [2.065, 2.19].

St. Clair Medical, P.C. v. Borgiel, 270 Mich. App. 260, 715 N.W.2d 914 (2006) [9.02].

Steele v. Hamilton County Cmty. Mental Health Bd., 90 Ohio St. 3d 176, 736 N.E.2d 10 (2000) [I].

Steeves v. United States, 294 F. Supp. 446 (D.S.C. 1968) [V; 8.04].

Steinberg v. Jensen, 186 Wis. 2d 237, 519 N.W.2d 753 (Ct. App. 1994), rev'd, 194 Wis. 2d 440, 534 N.W.2d 361 (1995) [IV; 5.05].

Steinberg v. Jensen, 194 Wis. 2d 440, 534 N.W.2d 361 (1995) [IV; 5.05].

Stempler v. Speidell, 100 N.J. 368, 495 A.2d 857 (1985), cert. denied, 483 US 1007 (1987) [IV; 5.05].

Stewart v. Midani, 525 F. Supp. 843 (N.D. Ga. 1981) [VI].

Stevens v. Sec. of Dept. of Health and Human Services, 2006 WL 659525 (Fed. Cl. 2006) [9.07].

Stidham v. Clark, 74 S.W.3d 719 (Ky. 2002) [5.05].

Stigliano v. Connaught Labs., Inc., 140 N.J. 305, 658 A.2d 715 (1995) [9.07].

Stone v. Secretary of the Department of Health and Human Services, 2010 WL 3790297, 8 (Fed. Cl. 2010) [9.07].

Sullivan v. Washington, 768 So. 2d 881 (Miss. 2000) [8.03, 8.05].

Swafford v. Harris, 967 S.W.2d 319 (Tenn. 1998) [6.01, 9.07].

Tarasoff v. Regents of Univ. of Cal., 17 Cal.3d 425, 551 P.2d 334, 131 Cal. Rptr. 14 (1976) [IV; 5.05].

Taylor v. Albert Einstein Medical Ctr., 723 A.2d 1027 (Pa. Super. 1998) [8.12, 8.16].

Thompson v. Astrue, 2008 WL 2444532 (W.D. Pa. 2008) [3.041].

Thompson v. Sun City Community Hosp., Inc., 141 Ariz. 597, 688 P.2d 605 (1984) [VI].

Total Care Physicians v. O'Hara, 2002 Del. Super. LEXIS 493 (2002) [7.01, 7.03].

Treister v. American Academy of Orthopaedic Surgeons, 78 Ill. App. 3d 746, 396 N.E.2d 1225 (1st Dist. 1979) [9.05].

Trevino v. Ortega, 41 Tex. Sup. 907, 969 S.W.2d 950 (1998) [7.05].

US v. Best, 59 M.J. 886 (Army Crim. App. 2004) [8.03, 10.015].

United States v. Ilayayev, 800 F. Supp. 2d 417, 435 (E.D.N.Y. 2011) [2.20].

United States v. Neufeld, 908 F. Supp. 491 (S.D. Ohio 1995) [3.04].

United States v. Weston, 134 F. Supp. 2d 115 (D.D.C. 2001) [2.06].

Utah Att'y Gen. Op. No. 77-294 (Feb. 15, 1978) [IV; 5.05].

Va. Att'y Gen. Op., 1994 Va. AG LEXIS 12 (1994) [2.06].

Va. Att'y Gen. Op., 1990 Va. AG LEXIS 63 (1990) [2.20].

Vacco v. Quill, 117 S. Ct. 2293, 138 L. Ed. 2d 834 (US 1997) [2.20, 2.211].

Valley Medical Specialists v. Farber, 194 Ariz. 363, 982 P.2d 1277 (1999) [9.02, 9.06].

Vassiliades v. Garfinckel's, Brooks Bros., 492 A.2d 580 (D.C. App. 1985) [IV; 5.05].

Vine Street Clinic v. Healthlink, Inc., 353 Ill. App. 3d 929, 819 N.E.2d 363 (4th Dist. 2004) [6.02].

Washington v. Glucksberg, 117 S. Ct. 2258, 138 L. Ed. 2d 772 (US 1997) [2.211].

Webb v. Jarvis, 575 N.E.2d 992 (Ind. 1991) [Preamble].

Weinberg v. Board of Registration in Medicare, 443 Mass. 679, 824 N.E.2d 38 (2005) [8.14].

Weiss v. Cigna Healthcare, Inc., 972 F. Supp. 748 (S.D.N.Y. 1997) [8.13].

Weiss v. Sec. of the Dept. of Health and Human Services, 2003 U.S. Claims LEXIS 359 (Fed. Cl. 2003) [9.07].

Weiss v. York Hosp., 745 F.2d 786 (3d Cir. 1984), cert. denied, 470 US 1060 (1985) [3.01].

Wenninger v. Muesing, 307 Minn. 405, 240 N.W.2d 333 (1976) [IV; 5.05].

Wilk v. American Medical Association, 895 F.2d 352 (7th Cir. 1990) [3.01].

Wilk v. American Medical Association, 671 F.Supp. 1465 (N.D. Ill. 1987), aff'd, 895 F.2d 352 (7th Cir. 1990) [3.01].

Wilk v. American Medical Association, 735 F.2d 217 (7th Cir. 1983), cert. denied, 467 US 1210 (1984) [3.01].

Wilk v. American Medical Association, 719 F.2d 207 (7th Cir. 1983), Cert. denied, 467 US 1210 (1984) [3.01].

Wisconsin Att'y Gen. Op. 10-87 (Mar. 16, 1987), (LEXIS, States library, Wis. file) [IV; 2.02, 5.05].

Wood v. Upjohn Co., No. 6093-1-II (Wash. Ct. App. Sept. 4, 1984) (LEXIS, States library, Wash. file) [VI].

Woods v. Commonwealth, 142 S.W.3d 24 (Ky. 2004) [2.20].

Wright v. Wasudev, 1994 Tenn. App. LEXIS 657 (1994) [IV; 5.05].

Yates v. El-Deiry, 160 Ill. App. 3d 198, 513 N.E.2d 519 (3d Dist. 1987) [IV; 5.05].

Table of Articles

Aarons, *Medicine and Its Alternatives: Health Care Priorities in the Caribbean,* 29 Hastings Center Rep. 23, 25 (July-Aug. 1999) [3.01].

Abemayor, *United We Stand, Divided We Fall,* 135 Arch. Otolaryngol. Head Neck Surg. 432, 432, 433 (2009) [9.012, 10.015].

Abernethy, *The Methodology of Death: Reexamining the Deterrence Rationale,* 27 Colum. Hum. Rts. L. Rev. 379, 410-11 (1996) [2.06].

Abrams, *The Vulnerable President and the Twenty-Fifth Amendment, With Observations on Guidelines, a Health Commission, and the Role of the President's Physician,* 30 Wake Forest L. Rev. 453, 466, 471 (1995) [5.04, 5.05, 8.03].

Acker, *When the Cheering Stopped: An Overview and Analysis of New York's Death Penalty Legislation,* 17 Pace L. Rev. 41, 221-22 (1996) [2.06].

Acosta, *The Texas Communicable Disease Prevention and Control Act: Are We Offering Enough Protection to Those Who Need It Most?* 36 Hous. L. Rev. 1819, 1822, 1830, 1831 (1999) [IV; 10.01].

Adams, *Live Organ Donors and Informed Consent: A Difficult Minuet,* 8 J. Legal Med. 555 (1987) [2.16].

Aden, *End of Life Decision Making: The Right to Die? You Can Go Your Own Way: Exploring the Relationship Between Personal and Political Autonomy in Gonzales v. Oregon,* 15 Temp. Pol. & Civ. Rts. L. Rev. 323, 329 (2006) [2.211].

Agich, *Rationing and Professional Autonomy,* 18 Law Med. & Health Care 77, 79, 82 (1990) [IV, VI].

Agnello, *Advocating for a Change in the Massachusetts HIV Statute: Putting an End to Physician Uncertainty,* 2 J. Trial App. Advoc. 105, 107 (1997) [IV].

Agrawal, *Chicago Hope Meets the Chicago School,* 96 Mich. L. Rev. 1793, 1804 (1998) [8.13].

Agrawal, *Resuscitating Professionalism: Self-regulation in the Medical Marketplace,* 66 Mo. L. Rev. 341, 354, 355, 360, 361, 378, 388 (2001) [2.03, 2.09, 2.095, 8.02, 8.021, 8.032, 8.051, 8.13, 9.04].

Ahronheim, *Service by Health Care Providers in a Public Health Emergency: The Physician's Duty and the Law,* 12 J. Health Care L. & Pol'y 195 (2009) [VI; 2.23, 9.06, 9.067, 9.12, 9.131].

Albert, *Cruzan v. Director, Missouri Department of Health: Too Much Ado,* 12 J. Legal Med. 331, 338, 343 (1991) [2.20].

Allen, *The Foreseeability of Transference: Extending Employer Liability Under Washington Law for Therapist Sexual Exploitation of Patients,* 78 Wash. L. Rev. 525, 531 (2003) [8.14].

Allenby, Arkin, Barrett, Borenstein, Gaudet, Kittrie, Lin, Lucas, Marchant, O'Meara, & Silberman, *International Governance of Autonomous Military Robots,* 12 Colum. Sci. & Tech. L. Rev. 272, 291 (2011) [Preamble; I, VI].

American Bar Association Task Force on Mental Disability and the Death Penalty (Igasaki, et al), *Recommendation and Report on the Death Penalty and Persons With Mental Disabilities,* 30 Mental & Physical Disability L. Rep. 668, 676 (2006) [2.06].

Anderson, *A Medical-Legal Dilemma: When Can "Inappropriate" Nutrition and Hydration Be Removed in Indiana?* 67 Ind. L. J. 479, 480 (1992) [2.20].

Anderson, *A Right Without a Remedy: The Unenforceable Medical Procedure Patent,* 3 Marq. Intell. Prop. L. Rev. 117, 132, 140 (1999) [9.08, 9.09].

Anderson, *Distinguishing Patentable Process Claims From Unpatentable Laws of Nature in the Medical Technology Field,* 59 Ala. L. Rev. 1203 (2008) [9.08].

Andrews, *Harnessing the Benefits of Biobanks,* 33 J. L. Med. & Ethics 22, 25 (2005) [2.08].

Andrews, *The Gene Patent Dilemma: Balancing Commercial Incentives With Health Needs,* 2 Hous. J. Health L. & Pol'y 65, 74, 104 (2002) [2.08, 9.095].

Andrews, *Two Perspectives: Rights of Donors: Who Owns Your Body? A Patient's Perspective on Washington University v. Catalona,* 34 J. L. Med. & Ethics 398, 404 (2006) [2.08].

Andrews & Jaeger, *Confidentiality of Genetic Information in the Workplace*, XVII Am. J. Law & Med. 75, 78 (1991) [5.05].

Annas, *Toxic Tinkering—Lethal-Injection Execution and the Constitution*, 359 New Engl. J. Med. 1512 (2009) [2.06].

Annas, Glantz, & Mariner, *The Right of Privacy Protects the Doctor-Patient Relationship*, 263 JAMA 858, 861 (1990) [2.20].

Antommaria, *Conscientious Objection in Clinical Practice: Notice, Informed Consent, Referral, and Emergency Treatment*, 9 Ave Maria L. Rev. 81, 98 (2010) [8.115].

Antommaria, *How Can I Give Her IV Antibiotics at Home When I Have Three Other Children to Care For? Using Dispute System Design to Address Patient Provider Conflicts in Health Care*, 29 Hamline J. Pub. L. & Pol'y 273 (2008) [8.115].

Appelbaum, Jorgenson, & Sutherland, *Sexual Relationships Between Physicians and Patients*, 154 Arch. Intern. Med. 2561, 2561 (1994) [8.14].

Aral, Mosher, & Cates, *Self-reported Pelvic Inflammatory Disease in the United States, 1988*, 266 JAMA 2570, 2573 (1991) [9.121].

Ares, *An Uncommon Skin Condition Illustrates the Need for Caution When Prescribing for Friends*, 20 J. Am. Acad. of Nurse Prac. 389, 390 (2008) [8.115, 8.19].

Ariens, *"Playing Chicken": An Instant History of the Battle Over Exceptions to Client Confidences*, 33 J. Legal Prof. 239 (2009) [IV].

Ashburn, Wilson, & Eisenstein, *Human Tissue Research in the Genomic Era of Medicine*, 160 Arch. Intern. Med. 3377, 3378 (2000) [2.132].

Avraham, *Private Regulation*, 34 Harv. J. L. & Pub. Pol'y 543, 614-15 (2011) [III].

Awad, *Attorney-Client Sexual Relations*, 22 J. Legal. Prof. 131, 190 (1998) [8.14].

Bagley, *Patent First, Ask Questions Later: Morality and Biotechnology in Patent Law*, 45 Wm. & Mary L. Rev. 469, 500 (2003) [9.095].

Bahnassi, *Keeping Doctors Out of the Interrogation Room: A New Ethical Obligation That Requires the Backing of the Law*, 19 Health Matrix 447 (2009) [Preamble; 2.06, 2.067, 2.068].

Bailey, *The Legal, Financial, and Ethical Implications of Online Medical Consultations*, 16 J. Tech. L. & Pol'y 53, 95 (2011) [10.015].

Baker, *Bioethics and History*, 27 J. Med. & Phil. 447, 455, 469 (2002) [2.20, 6.02, 6.03, 8.032, 8.06].

Baker, *In Defense of Bioethics*, 37 J. of Law, Med. and Ethics 83, 87 (2009) [3.01].

Baker & Emanuel, *The Efficacy of Professional Ethics: The AMA Code of Ethics in Historical and Current Perspective*, 30 Hastings Center Rep. S13, S14 (July/Aug. 2000) [I].

Balint, *Issues of Privacy and Confidentiality in the New Genetics*, 9 Alb. L. J. Sci. & Tech. 27, 32 (1998) [IV].

Banks, *Legal and Ethical Safeguards: Protection of Society's Most Vulnerable Participants in a Commercialized Organ Transplantation System*, XXI Am. J. Law & Med. 45, 77, 79, 95-96, 103-04 (1995) [2.15, 2.167].

Bard, *The Diagnosis Is Anencephaly and the Parents Ask About Organ Donation: Now What? A Guide for Hospital Counsel and Ethics Committees*, 21 W. New Eng. L. Rev. 49, 62 (1999) [2.162].

Barnes, Rango, Burke, & Chiarello, *The HIV-Infected Health Care Professional: Employment Policies and Public Health*, 18 Law Med. & Health Care 311, 314, 315 (1990) [9.131].

Baron, *Why Withdrawal of Life-Support for PVS Patients Is Not a Family Decision*, 19 Law Med. & Health Care 73 (1991) [2.20].

Baron, Bergstresser, Brock, Cole, Dorfman, Johnson, Schnipper, Vorenberg, & Wanzer, *A Model State Act to Authorize and Regulate Physician-Assisted Suicide*, 33 Harv. J. Legis. 1, 2, 7 (1996) [2.20, 2.211].

Barua, *"Synthetic Sanity": A Way Around the Eighth Amendment?* 44 Crim. Law Bulletin 561 (2008) [2.06].

Basanta, *"No-Hire" Clauses in Healthcare Sector Contracts: Their Use and Enforceability*, 39 J. Health L. 451, 453 (2006) [9.02].

Bassel, *Order at the End of Life: Establishing a Clear and Fair Mechanism for the Resolution of Futility Disputes*, 63 Vand. L. Rev. 491, 494, 523 (2010) [2.17, 2.20].

Battin, *Physician-Assisted Dying and the Slippery Slope: The Challenge of Empirical Evidence*, 45 Willamette L. Rev. 91 (2008) [2.21, 2.211].

Baum, *"To Comfort Always": Physician Participation in Executions*, 5 N. Y. U. J. Legis. & Pub. Pol'y 47, 56-57 (2001) [2.06].

Beane, *AIDS Crisis and the Health Care Community: Public Concerns Triggering Questionable Private Rights of Action for Emotional Harms and Legislative Response*, 45 Mercer L. Rev. 633, 669 (1994) [9.13, 9.131].

Beard, *The Impact of Changes in Health Care Provider Reimbursement Systems on the Recovery of Damages for Medical Expenses in Personal Injury Suits*, 21 Am. J. Trial Advoc. 453, 484 (1998) [6.11].

Beckwith & Peppin, *Physician Value Neutrality: A Critique*, 28 J. L. Med. & Ethics 67, 72-73 (2000) [2.01, 2.02, 8.032, 8.05, 8.08, 8.132].

Befort, *Pre-Employment Screening and Investigation: Navigating Between a Rock and a Hard Place*, 14 Hofstra Lab. L. J. 365, 391 (1997) [2.132].

Begg, *Revoking the Lawyers' License to Discriminate in New York: The Demise of a Traditional Professional Prerogative*, 7 Geo. J. Legal Ethics 275, 298, 299 (1993) [VI; 9.12, 9.131].

Bell, *Non–Heart Beating Organ Donation: Old Procurement Strategy—New Ethical Problems*, 29 J. Med. Ethics 176, 181 (2003) [2.155, 2.162].

Bellacosa, *The Fusion of Medicine and Law for In Extremis Health and Medical Decisions: Does It Produce Energy and Light or Just Cosmic Debris?* 18 Bull. Am. Acad. Psychiatry Law 5, 9 (1990) [2.20].

Belville, *Most Covenants Not to Compete Against Physicians are No Longer Enforceable in Tennessee*, 7 Transactions 419, 434 (2006) [9.02].

Benesch, *Disability Discrimination in the Health Care Workplace*, 9 Trends in Health Care, Law & Ethics 45, 46 (Summer 1994) [9.131].

Bennett, *Inclusion of Women in Clinical Trials—Policies for Population Subgroups*, 329 New Eng. J. Med. 288, 289 (1993) [9.122].

Bennett, *When Is Medical Treatment Futile?* 9 Issues in Law & Med. 35, 39 (1993) [2.22].

Benson, *The Social Control of Human Biomedical Research: An Overview and Review of the Literature*, 29 Soc. Sci. Med. 1 (1989) [2.07].

Berg, *Ethics and E-Medicine*, 46 St. Louis U. L. J. 61, 66 (2002) [8.062, 8.063].

Berg, *Grave Secrets: Legal and Ethical Analysis of Postmortem Confidentiality*, 34 Conn. L. Rev. 81, 87, 117 (2001) [5.051, 7.02].

Berg, *Of Elephants and Embryos: A Proposed Framework for Legal Personhood*, 59 Hastings L. J. 369, 377-78 (2007) [2.162].

Berg, *Understanding Waiver*, 40 Hous. L. Rev. 281, 329 (2003) [8.08].

Berger, *Lethal Injection and the Problem of Constitutional Remedies*, 27 Yale L. & Pol'y Rev. 259 (2009) [Preamble; 1.02, 2.06].

Berger, *Patient Confidentiality in a High Tech World*, 5 J. Pharmacy & L., 139, 141 (1996) [5.05].

Berger & Rosner, *Ethical Challenges Posed by Dementia and Driving*, 11 J. Clinical Ethics 304, 307, 308 (2000) [2.24].

Berger & Rosner, *The Ethics of Practice Guidelines*, 156 Arch. Intern. Med. 2051, 2053, 2056 (1996) [8.13].

Bergin, *Book Review: Law and Ethics in Biomedical Research: Regulation, Conflict of Interest, and Liability*, 23 Windsor Rev. Legal & Soc. Issues 117, 122 (2007) [2.07].

Berlan & Bravender, *Confidentiality, Consent and Caring for the Adolescent Patient*, 21 Current Opinion Pediatrics 450, 455 (2009) [5.055].

Bernat, *Quality of Neurological Care: Balancing Cost Control and Ethics*, 54 Arch. Neurol. 1341, 1343, 1345 (1997) [8.032, 8.13].

Bernstein, *Out of the Frying Pan and Into the Fire: The Expert Witness Problem in Toxic Tort Litigation*, 10 Rev. Litigation 117, 143 (1990) [9.07].

Bernstein & Seybert, *Everyone Pays the Price When Healthcare Providers Waive Patients' Co-insurance Obligations*, 21 Health Law. 20 (Dec. 2008) [6.12, 6.13].

Berrol, *Considerations for Management of the Persistent Vegetative State*, 67 Arch. Phys. Med. Rehabil. 283 (1986) [2.20].

Bertram, *How Current Informed Consent Protocols Flunk the Sham Surgery Test: A New Frontier in Medicine and Ethics*, 14 Quinnipiac Health L. J. 131, 133, 161-162 (2010) [2.07, 2.076].

Bessler, *Revisiting Beccaria's Vision: The Enlightenment, America's Death Penalty, and the Abolition Movement*, 4 NW J. L. & Soc. Pol'y 195 (2009) [2.06].

Bethard, *Physician Self-referral: Beyond Stark II*, 43 Brandeis L. J. 465, 468 (2005) [8.032].

Black & Sade, *Lethal Injection and Physicians: State Law vs Medical Ethics*, 298 JAMA 2779, 2780, 2781 (2007) [2.06, 2.211, 9.02].

Blair, *Lifting the Genealogical Veil: The Blueprint for Legislative Reform of the Disclosure of Health-Related Information in Adoption*, 70 No. Carolina L. Rev. 681, 692 (1992) [IV].

Blanchard, *"Medical Necessity" Determinations—A Continuing Healthcare Policy Problem*, 37 J. Health L. 599, 620 (2004) [8.05].

Blecker, *Killing Them Softly: Meditations on a Painful Punishment of Death*, 35 Fordham Urb. L. J. 969 (2008) [2.06].

Bobinski, *Autonomy and Privacy: Protecting Patients From Their Physicians*, 55 U. Pitt. L. Rev. 291, 302, 313 (1994) [8.03, 8.15, 9.13].

Bobinski, *Patients and Providers in the Courts: Fractures in the Americans with Disabilities Act*, 61 Alb. L. Rev. 785, 790, 806 (1998) [9.131].

Bobinski & Epps, *Women, Poverty, Access to Health Care, and the Perils of Symbolic Reform*, 5 J. Gender, Race & Just. 233, 238 (2002) [9.122].

Boden, *Compassion Inaction: Why President Bush's Faith-Based Initiatives Violate the Establishment Clause*, 29 Seattle U. L. Rev. 991, 1023 (2006) [II, VIII].

Bodenheimer & Grumbach, *Capitation or Decapitation: Keeping Your Head in Changing Times*, 276 JAMA 1025, 1031 (1996) [8.13].

Boire, *Neurocops: The Politics of Prohibition and the Future of Enforcing Social Policy From Inside the Body*, 19 J. L. & Health 215, 237 (2005) [8.08].

Bond, *Diverse and Perverse Incentives in Managed Care: Where Will the Pendulum Stop?* 1 Widener L. Symp. J. 141, 151, 154 (1996) [8.13].

Bonnie, *Mentally Ill Prisoners on Death Row: Unsolved Puzzles for Courts and Legislatures*, 54 Cath. U. L. Rev. 1169, 1175 (2005) [2.06].

Bonnie, Wright, & Dineen, *Legal Authority to Preserve Organs in Cases of Uncontrolled Cardiac Death: Preserving Family Choice*, 36 J. L. Med. & Ethics 741 (2008) [2.157, 8.181].

Booker, *Physicians, Malpractice, and State Lines: A Guide to Personal Jurisdiction in Medical Malpractice Lawsuits*, 20 J. Legal Med. 385, 394 (1999) [5.02].

Boozang, *Death Wish: Resuscitating Self-determination for the Critically Ill*, 35 Ariz. L. Rev. 23, 24, 28, 52 (1993) [2.22, 8.08].

Boozang, *Is the Alternative Medicine? Managed Care Apparently Thinks So*, 32 Conn. L. Rev. 567, 606 (2000) [II].

Bopp & Coleson, *The Constitutional Case Against Permitting Physician-Assisted Suicide for Competent Adults With Terminal Conditions*, 11 Issues in Law & Med. 239, 250 (1995) [2.211].

Bordone, *Fitting the Ethics to the Forum: A Proposal for Process-Enabling Ethical Codes*, 21 Ohio St. J. on Disp. Resol. 1, 35 (2005) [2.035].

Bostick, Sade, & McMahon, *Report of the Council on Ethical and Judicial Affairs: Physician Pay-for-Performance Programs*, 3 Ind. Health L. Rev. 429, 430, 431, 432-33, 434, 435, 436 (2006) [I, V, VIII, IX; 2.035, 2.095, 6.01, 8.021, 8.03, 8.0501, 8.053, 8.054, 8.121].

Bostick, Sade, McMahon, & Benjamin, *Report of the American Medical Association Council on Ethical and Judicial Affairs: Withholding Information From Patients: Rethinking the Propriety of "Therapeutic Privilege,"* 17 J. Clinical Ethics 302, 303 (Winter 2006) [8.08, 8.081, 8.121, 10.015].

Botkin, *Prenatal Diagnosis and the Selection of Children*, 30 Fla. St. U. L. Rev. 265, 289 (2003) [2.12].

Boumil, Freitas, & Freitas, *Multidisciplinary Representation of Patients: The Potential for Ethical Issues and Professional Duty Conflicts in the Medical-Legal Partnership Model*, 13 J. Health Care L. & Pol'y 107, 124 (2010) [8.0501].

Bourne, *Medical Malpractice: Should Courts Force Doctors to Confess Their Own Negligence to Their Patients?* 61 Ark. L. Rev. 621 (2009) [8.12].

Bovbjerg & Tancredi, *Liability Reform Should Make Patients Safer: "Avoidable Classes of Events" are a Key Improvement*, 33 J. L. Med. & Ethics 478, 482 (2005) [8.12].

Bowser, *Eliminating Racial and Ethnic Disparities in Medical Care*, 30 Brief 24, 25 (Summer 2001) [9.121].

Bowser, *Racial Profiling in Health Care: An Institutional Analysis of Medical Treatment Disparities*, 7 Mich. J. Race & L. 79, 119 (2001) [9.121].

Boyle, *Managed Care in Mental Health: A Cure, or a Cure Worse Than the Disease?* 40 St. Louis U. L. J. 437, 448 (1996) [8.13].

Brann, *Utah's Medical Malpractice Prelitigation Panel: Exploring State Constitutional Arguments Against a Nonbinding Inadmissible Procedure*, 2000 Utah L. Rev. 359, 399-400 (2000) [9.122].

Brennan, *Ensuring Adequate Health Care for the Sick: The Challenge of the Acquired Immunodeficiency Syndrome as an Occupational Disease*, 1988 Duke L. J. 29 (1988) [VI].

Brennan, *Torture of Guantanamo Detainees With the Complicity of Medical Health Personnel: The Case for Accountability and Providing a Forum for Redress for These International Wrongs*, 45 U.S.F. L. Rev. 1005, 1045 (2011) [2.067, 2.068].

Brennan, *Transmission of the Human Immunodeficiency Virus in the Health Care Setting— Time for Action*, 324 New Eng. J. Med. 1504, 1505, 1506 (1991) [9.131].

Brock, *Voluntary Active Euthanasia*, 22 Hastings Center Rep. 10 (March/April 1992) [2.20, 2.21].

Brody, *Ethical Questions Raised by the Persistent Vegetative Patient*, 18 Hastings Center Rep. 33 (Feb./ March 1988) [2.20].

Brody, *New Perspectives on Emergency Room Research*, 27 Hastings Center Rep. 7, 9 (Jan./Feb. 1997) [2.07].

Brody, *Special Ethical Issues in the Management of PVS Patients*, 20 Law Med. & Health Care 104, 109 (1992) [2.20, 2.22].

Brody, *The Physician as Professional and the Physician as Honest Businessman*, 119 Arch. Otolaryngol. Head Neck Surg. 495, 496 (1993) [6.11].

Brody & Avery, *Medicine's Duty to Treat Pandemic Illness: Solidarity and Vulnerability*, 39 Hastings Center Report 40, 44 (2009) [10.01, 10.015].

Brooks, Smith, & Anderson, *Medical Apartheid: An American Perspective*, 266 JAMA 2746, 2748 (1991) [9.121].

Brown-Cranstoun, *Kringen v. Boslough and Saint Vincent Hospital: A New Trend for Healthcare Professionals Who Treat Victims of Domestic Violence?* 33 J. Health L. 629, 649, 650 (2000) [2.02].

Brownrigg, *Mother Still Knows Best: Cancer-Related Gene Mutations, Familial Privacy, and a Physician's Duty to Warn*, 26 Fordham Urb. L. J. 247 (1999) [IV].

Bruening, Andrew, & Smith, *Concurrent Care: An Ethical Issue for Family Physicians*, 36 J. Fam. Practice 606, 607 (1993) [Preamble].

Brunetti, Weiss, Studenski, & Clipp, *Cardiopulmonary Resuscitation Policies and Practices: A Statewide Nursing Home Study*, 150 Arch. Intern. Med. 121, 122 (1990) [2.20, 2.22].

Bruns & Wolman, *Morality of the Privacy of Genetic Information: Possible Improvements of Procedures*, 19 Med. Law 127, 129 (2000) [2.132].

Brunsden, *Hepatitis C in Prisons: Evolving Toward Decency Through Adequate Medical Care and Public Health Reform*, 54 UCLA L. Rev. 465, 500 (2006) [Preamble; VII, VIII, IX; 10.015].

Buchanan, *Medical Ethics at the Millennium: A Brief Retrospective*, 26 Colo. Law. 141, 142, 143, 144, 145 (1997) [5.05, 5.057, 7.01, 8.115, 8.12, 8.13, 9.12, 9.131, 10.01].

Buckles, *Electronic Formulary Management and Medicaid: Maximizing Economic Efficiency and Quality of Care in the Age of Electronic Prescribing*, 11 U. Fla. J. L. & Pub. Pol'y 179, 182-83 (2000) [8.135].

Buhai, *Emotional Conflicts: Impaired Dispassionate Representation of Family Members*, 21 Geo. J. Legal Ethics 1159 (2008) [8.19].

Bulleit & Krause, *Kickbacks, Courtesies, or Cost-Effectiveness? Application of the Medicare Antikickback Law to the Marketing and Promotional Practices of Drug and Medical Device Manufacturers*, 54 Food & Drug L. J. 279, 296 (1999) [8.061].

Burman, *Lawyers and Domestic Violence: Raising the Standard of Practice*, 9 Mich. J. Gender & L. 207, 254 (2003) [5.05].

Burman, *Wyoming Attorneys' Pro Bono "Obligation,"* 5 Wyo. L. Rev. 421, 428 (2005) [9.065].

Burnette & Morning, *HIPAA and Ex Parte Interviews—The Beginning of the End?* 1 J. Health & Life Sci. L. 73 (2008) [IV, VIII; 5.05, 10.01].

Burris, *Dental Discrimination Against the HIV-Infected: Empirical Data, Law and Public Policy*, 13 Yale J. On Reg. 1, 41 (1996) [9.131].

Butler, *Baze v. Rees: Lethal Injection as a Constitutional Method of Execution*, 86 Denv. U. L. Rev. 509 (2009) [2.06].

Calabro: *Breaking the Shield of the Learned Intermediary Doctrine: Placing the Blame Where it Belongs*, 25 Cardozo L. Rev. 2241, 2262, 2263 (2004) [8.061].

Campbell: *Sell, Singleton, and Forcible Medication— Running Roughshod Over Liberty*, 35 U. Tol. L. Rev. 691, 716 (2004) [2.06].

Canning, *Privileged Communications in Ohio and What's New on the Horizon: Ohio House Bill 52 Accountant-Client Privilege,* 31 Akron L. Rev. 505, 550 (1998) [IV].

Cantor, *Discarding Substituted Judgment and Best Interests: Toward a Constructive Preference Standard for Dying, Previously Competent Patients Without Advance Instructions,* 48 Rutgers L. Rev. 1193, 1234, 1247 (1996) [2.17].

Cantor, *My Annotated Living Will,* 18 Law Med. & Health Care 114 (1990) [2.20].

Cantor, *Of Pills and Needles: Involuntarily Medicating the Psychotic Inmate When Execution Looms,* 2 Ind. Health L. Rev. 119, 154, 156, 164 (2005) [2.06].

Cantor, *On Hastening Death Without Violating Legal and Moral Prohibitions,* 37 Loy. U. Chi. L. J. 407, 427 (2006) [2.21].

Cantor, *On Kamisar, Killing, and the Future of Physician-Assisted Death,* 102 Mich. L. Rev. 1793, 1825 (2004) [2.215].

Cantor, *The Bane of Surrogate Decision-Making: Defining the Best Interests of Never-Competent Persons,* 26 J. Legal Med. 155, 160 (2005) [2.20].

Cantor, *The Permanently Unconscious Patient, Non-Feeding and Euthanasia,* XV Am. J. Law & Med. 381 (1989) [2.20].

Cantor, *The Relation Between Autonomy-Based Rights and Profoundly Mentally Disabled Persons,* 13 Annals Health L. 37, 70 (2004) [2.20].

Cantor & Baum, *The Limits of Conscientious Objection—May Pharmacists Refuse to Fill Prescriptions for Emergency Contraception?* 351 New Eng. J. Med. 2008, 2012 (2004) [2.01].

Cantor & Thomas, *The Legal Bounds of Physician Conduct Hastening Death,* 48 Buff. L. Rev. 83, 110, 131, 158 (2000) [2.21, 2.211, 2.18, 2.20].

Caplan, Cooper, Garcia-Prats, & Brody, *Diffusion of Innovative Approaches to Managing Hypoplastic Left Heart Syndrome,* 150 Arch. Pediatr. Adolesc. Med. 487, 490 (1996) [2.162].

Capron, *Ethics: Public and Private,* 24 Hastings Center Rep. 26, 27 (Nov./Dec. 1994) [2.162].

Cardi, *A Pluralistic Analysis of the Therapist/Physician Duty to Warn Third Parties,* 44 Wake Forest L. Rev. 877 (2009) [5.05].

Carlson, *Organ Donation Recovery and Improvement Act: How Congress Missed an Opportunity to Say "Yes" to Financial Incentives for Organ Donation,* 23 J. Contemp. Health L. & Pol'y 136, 145 (2006) [2.151].

Carnahan, *Concierge Medicine: Legal and Ethical Issues,* 35 J. L. Med. & Ethics 211, 212-13 (2007) [8.05, 8.055, 8.115, 9.06, 9.065].

Carnahan, *Law, Medicine, and Wealth: Does Concierge Medicine Promote Health Care Choice, or Is It a Barrier to Access?* 17 Stan. L. & Pol'y Rev. 121, 149-50, 151, 152, 153-54 (2006) [VI, IX; 8.055, 8.11, 8.115, 9.065, 10.05].

Carr, *Contracts—Murfreesboro Medical Clinic, P.A. v. Udom: Physician Noncompete Agreements Go Under the Knife: The Tennessee Supreme Court Rejects Physician Noncompete Agreements,* 36 U. Mem. L. Rev. 1115, 1128, 1131 (2006) [9.02, 9.06].

Carrese, *Refusal of Care: Patients' Well-being and Physicians' Ethical Obligations,* 296 JAMA 691, 692, 693 (2006) [IV; 10.01].

Carter, *Health Information Privacy: Can Congress Protect Confidential Medical Information in the "Information Age"?* 25 Wm. Mitchell L. Rev. 223, 236, 273 (1999) [5.05, 7.02, 7.05].

Casagrande, *Children Not Meant to Be: Protecting the Interests of the Child When Abortion Results in Live Birth,* 6 Quinnipiac Health L. J. 19, 44, 45, 47-48 (2002) [Preamble; I, III; 2.035, 2.20, 2.215].

Casarez, *Public Forums, Selective Subsidies, and Shifting Standards of Viewpoint Discrimination,* 64 Alb. L. Rev. 501, 558 (2000) [8.08].

Casell, *Lengthening the Stem: Allowing Federally Funded Researchers to Derive Human Pluripotent Stem Cells From Embryos,* 34 U. Mich. J. L. Ref. 547, 563 (2001) [2.141].

Castronova, *Operation Cyber Chase and Other Agency Efforts to Control Internet Drug Trafficking,* 27 J. Legal Med. 207, 219 (2006) [5.026].

Caveney, *Going, Going, Gone . . . The Opportunities and Legal Pitfalls of Online Surgical Auctions,* 103 W. Va. L. Rev. 591, 607 (2001) [9.12].

Cerminara, *Dealing With Dying: How Insurers Can Help Patients Seeking Last-Chance Therapies (Even When the Answer Is "NO"),* 15 Health Matrix 285, 293-94 (2005) [2.07].

Cerminara, *Musings on the Need to Convince Some People With Disabilities That End-of-Life Decision-Making Advocates Are Not Out to Get Them*, 37 Loy. U. Chi. L. J. 343, 347 (2006) [2.03, 2.035, 2.17, 2.22].

Cerminara, *Protecting Participants in and Beneficiaries of ERISA-Governed Managed Health Care Plans*, 29 U. Mem. L. Rev. 317, 324 (1999) [2.20, 2.225].

Cerminara, *The Class Action Suit As a Method of Patient Empowerment in the Managed Care Setting*, 24 Am. J. Law & Med. 7, 16, 17, 23 (1998) [8.13, 8.132].

Cerminara, Pizzetti, & Photangtham, *Schiavo Revisited? The Struggle for Autonomy at the End of Life in Italy*, 12 Marq. Elder's Advisor 295, 308 (2011) [2.20].

Chamberlain, *Looking for a "Good Death": The Elderly Terminally Ill's Right to Die by Physician-Assisted Suicide*, 17 Elder L. J. 61 (2009) [2.211].

Chand, *Deconstructing Gonzales v. Oregon: When Political Agendas Yield to Rudimentary Notions of Federalism and Statutory Interpretation*, 50 How. L. J. 229, 239-40 (2006) [2.211].

Chen, *Organ Allocation and the States: Can the States Restrict Broader Organ Sharing?* 49 Duke L. J. 261, 273 (1999) [2.16].

Chen, Mueller, Prasad, Greinwald, Manaligod, Muilenburg, Verhoeven, Van Camp, & Smith, *Presymptomatic Diagnosis of Nonsyndromic Hearing Loss by Genotyping*, 124 Arch. Otolaryngol. Head Neck Surg. 20, 23 (1998) [2.12].

Chervenak & McCullough, *The Ethics of Direct and Indirect Referral for Termination of Pregnancy*, 199 Am. J. Obstet. Gynecol. 232.e1, 232.e1 (2008) [10.01].

Cherry, *Polymorphic Medical Ontologies: Fashioning Concepts of Disease*, 25 J. Med. & Phil. 519, 532 (2000) [2.03].

Childress, *Ethics, Public Policy, and Human Fetal Tissue Transplantation Research*, 1 Kennedy Inst. Ethics J. 93, 116 (June 1991) [2.10].

Childress, *The Failure to Give: Reducing Barriers to Organ Donation*, 11 Kennedy Inst. Ethics J. 1, 13, 14 (2001) [2.155].

Chopko, *Responsible Public Policy at the End of Life*, 75 U. Det. Mercy L. Rev. 557, 573 (1998) [2.211].

Chouhan & Draper, *Modified Mandated Choice for Organ Procurement*, 29 J. Med. Ethics 157, 162 (2003) [2.155].

Chow, *Health Courts: An Extreme Makeover of Medical Malpractice With Potentially Fatal Complications*, 7 Yale J. Health Pol'y L. & Ethics 387, 399 (2007) [9.07].

Christensen & Orlowski, *Iatrogenic Cardiopulmonary Arrests in DNR Patients*, 11 J. Clinical Ethics 14, 15, 20 (2000) [2.22].

Chudoba, *Conscience in America: The Slippery Slope of Mixing Morality With Medicine*, 36 Sw. U. L. Rev. 85, 86, 103, 104, 105 (2007) [Preamble; V, VI, VIII].

Cibas, Alexander, Benson, Patricio de Agustín, Doherty, Faquin, Middleton, Miller, Raab, White, & Mandel, *Indications for Thyroid FNA and Pre-FNA Requirements: A Synopsis of the National Cancer Institute Thyroid Fine-Needle Aspiration State of the Science Conference*, 36 Diagnostic Cytopathology 390, 394 (2008) [8.08].

Clark, *Autonomy and Death*, 71 Tul. L. Rev. 45, 89 (1996) [2.21, 2.211].

Clark, *Confidential Communications in a Professional Context: Attorney, Physician, and Social Worker*, 24 J. Legal Prof. 79, 92 (2000) [5.05].

Clark, *Medical Ethics at Guantanamo Bay and Abu Ghraib: The Problem of Dual Loyalty*, 34 J. L. Med. & Ethics 570, 573 (2006) [2.067].

Clark, *Medication Errors in Family Practice, in Hospitals and After Discharge From the Hospital: An Ethical Analysis*, 32 J. L. Med & Ethics 349, 354 (2004) [10.01].

Clark, *Oregon's Death with Dignity Act and Alleged Patient Euthanasia After Hurricane Katrina—The Government's Role*, 18 Health Lawyer 1, 8 (2006) [2.211].

Clayton, *The Web of Relations: Thinking About Physicians and Patients*, 6 Yale J. Health Pol'y, L. & Ethics 465, 473 (2006) [8.061].

Clemmens, *Creating Human Embryos for Research: A Scientist's Perspective on Managing the Legal and Ethical Issues*, 2 Ind. Health L. Rev. 95, 99 (2005) [2.14].

Closen, *HIV-AIDS, Infected Surgeons and Dentists, and the Medical Profession's Betrayal of Its Responsibility to Patients*, 41 N. Y. L. Sch. L. Rev. 57, 65, 71-72, 129 (1996) [9.131].

Cohen, *An Examination of the Right of Hospitals to Engage in Economic Credentialing*, 77 Temp. L. Rev. 705, 741 (2004) [8.032].

Cohen, *Holistic Health Care: Including Alternative and Complementary Medicine in Insurance and Regulatory Schemes*, 38 Ariz. L. Rev. 83, 92 (1996) [3.01].

Cohen, *The Open Door: Will the Right to Die Survive Washington v. Glucksberg and Vacco v. Quill?* 16 In Pub. Interest 79, 94 (1998) [2.20, 2.211].

Cohen, *Toward a Bioethics of Compassion*, 28 Ind. L. Rev. 667, 673, 681-82, 683 (1995) [2.01, 2.211, 8.18].

Cohen-Almagor, *A Critique of Callahan's Utilitarian Approach to Resource Allocation in Health Care*, 17 Issues L. & Med. 247, 261 (2002) [2.037].

Cohen & Cohen, *Required Reconsideration of "Do-Not-Resuscitate" Orders in the Operating Room and Certain Other Treatment Settings*, 20 Law Med. & Health Care 354, 356 (1992) [2.22].

Cohn, Berger, Holzman, Lockhart, Reuben, Robertson, & Selbst, *Guidelines for Expert Witness Testimony in Medical Liability Cases*, 94 Pediatrics 755, 756 (1994) [9.07].

Cohen, Dicecco, & Levin, *Failure to Communicate: When It Comes to Hospital Patient Care, Communication Between Doctor and Nurse Should Be Seamless. If It's Not, Patients Suffer. Here's How to Find Out if a Miscommunication Is at the Core of Your Client's Case*, 46 Trial 38, 40-41 (May 2010) [3.02, 9.045].

Coker, Smith, Bethea, King, & McKeown, *Physical Health Consequences of Physical and Psychological Intimate Partner Violence*, 9 Arch. Fam. Med. 451, 456, 457 (2000) [2.02].

Cole, *Authentic Democracy: Endowing Citizens With a Human Right in Their Genetic Information*, 33 Hofstra L. Rev. 1241, 1251 (2005) [IV].

Cole, *Beyond Unconstitutional Conditions: Charting Spheres of Neutrality in Government-Funded Speech*, 67 N. Y. U. L. Rev. 675, 744 (1992) [8.08].

Coleman, *Beyond the Call of Duty: Compelling Health Care Professionals to Work During an Influenza Pandemic*, 94 Iowa L. Rev. 1 (2008) [9.067, 9.131].

Coleman, *Brother, Can You Spare a Liver? Five Ways to Increase Organ Donation*, 31 Val. U. L. Rev. 1, 30, 31 (1996) [2.06].

Coleman, *Privilege and Confidentiality in 12-Step Self-Help Programs*, 26 J. Legal Med. 435, 441 (2005) [5.05].

Coleman & Rosoff, *The Case for Legal Regulation of Physicians' Off-Label Prescribing*, 86 Notre Dame L. Rev. 649, 679 (2011) [10.01, 10.015].

Coleson, *The Glucksberg & Quill Amicus Curiae Briefs: Verbatim Arguments Opposing Assisted Suicide*, 13 Issues in Law & Med. 3, 67 (1997) [2.211].

Collett, *Protecting Our Daughters: The Need for the Vermont Parental Notification Law*, 26 Vt. L. Rev. 101, 106-07 (2001) [2.015].

Colletti, Mulholland, & Sonnad, *Perceived Obstacles to Career Success for Women in Academic Surgery*, 135 Arch. Surg. 972, 976 (2000) [9.035].

Collins, *Conscience Clauses and Oral Contraceptives: Conscientious Objection or Calculated Obstruction?* 15 Ann. Health L. 37, 54 (2006) [I, II, III, IV, V, VI, VII, VIII, IX].

Comment, *A Right to Die: Can a Massachusetts Physician Withdraw Artificial Nutrition and Hydration From a Persistently Vegetative Patient Following Cruzan v. Director, Missouri Department of Health?* 26 New Eng. L. Rev. 199, 216, 220 (1991) [2.20].

Comment, *AIDSphobia: Forcing Courts to Face New Areas of Compensation for Fear of a Deadly Disease*, 39 Vill. L. Rev. 241, 277 (1994) [9.13, 9.131].

Comment, *Alliances for the Future: Cultivating a Cooperative Environment for Biotech Success*, 11 Berkeley Tech. L. J. 311, 344 (1996) [8.031].

Comment, *An Illinois Physician-Assisted Suicide Act: A Merciful End to a Terminally Ill Criminal Tradition*, 28 Loy. U. Chi. L. J. 763, 775 (1997) [2.20].

Comment, *Artificial Nutrition and the Terminally Ill: How Should Washington Decide?* 61 Wash. L. Rev. 419 (1986) [2.20].

Comment, *Beyond Autonomy: Judicial Restraint and the Legal Limits Necessary to Uphold the Hippocratic Tradition and Preserve the Ethical Integrity of the Medical Profession*, 9 J. Contemp. Health L. & Pol'y 451, 467, 468 (1993) [2.20, 10.01].

Comment, *Curing the Health Care Industry: Government Response to Medicare Fraud and Abuse*, 5 J. Contemp. Health L. & Pol'y 175 (1989) [8.03].

Comment, *Dangerous Relations: Doctors and Extracorporeal Embryos, The Need For New Limits to Medical Inquiry*, 7 J. Contemp. Health L. & Pol'y 307, 309 (1991) [2.10, 2.14].

Comment, *Ethical Considerations in Resuscitation*, 268 JAMA 2282, 2283, 2287 (1992) [2.20, 2.22].

Comment, *From the Land of Lincoln a Healing Rule: Proposed Texas Rule of Civil Procedure Prohibiting Ex Parte Contact Between Defense Counsel and a Plaintiff's Treating Physician*, 25 Tex. Tech L. Rev. 1081, 1081, 1082 (1994) [II, IV; 5.05].

Comment, *Hold on Courts: May a Comatose Patient Be Denied Food and Water*, 31 St. Louis Univ. L. J. 749 (1987) [2.20].

Comment, *Medical Use of Marijuana: Legal and Ethical Conflicts in the Patient-Physician Relationship*, 30 U. Rich. L. Rev. 249, 268-69 (1996) [2.17].

Comment, *Noncompetition Clauses in Physician Employment Contracts in Oregon*, 76 Or. L. Rev. 195, 204-06 (1997) [Preamble; 6.11, 9.02, 9.06].

Comment, *Nonconsensual HIV Testing in the Health Care Setting: The Case for Extending the Occupational Protections of California Proposition 96 to Health Care Workers*, 26 Loy. L.A. L. Rev. 1251, 1269 (1993) [VI; 9.131].

Comment, *One Step Forward, Two Steps Back: A Constitutional and Critical Look at Ohio's New Living Will Statute*, 54 Ohio St. L. J. 445, 447, 460, 470 (1993) [2.20].

Comment, *Physician Assisted Suicide and the Right to Die With Assistance*, 105 Harvard L. Rev. 2021, 2027, 2035 (1992) [2.20].

Comment, *Physician-Assisted Suicide: Should Texas Be Different?* 33 Hous. L. Rev. 1475, 1480, 1488 (1997) [2.21, 2.211].

Comment, *Physician Gag Clauses—The Hypocrisy of the Hippocratic Oath*, 21 So. Ill. U. L. J. 313, 318, 320 (1997) [8.13].

Comment, *Physician Retaliation: Can the Physician-Patient Relationship Be Protected?* 94 Dickinson L. Rev. 965, 986 (1990) [9.131].

Comment, *Protecting Children Exposed to Domestic Violence in Contested Custody and Visitation Litigation*, 6 B.U. Pub. Int. L. J. 501, 502, 505 (1997) [2.02].

Comment, *Regulating Physician Investment and Referral Behavior in the Competitive Health Care Marketplace of the '90s—An Argument for Decentralization*, 65 Wash. L. Rev. 657, 658 (1990) [8.03].

Comment, *Right to Die: Oklahoma's Position on Nutrition and Hydration: Confusing or Unconstitutional?* 43 Okla. L. Rev. 143, 151 (1990) [2.20].

Comment, *Shielding the Plaintiff and Physician: The Prohibition of Ex Parte Contacts With a Plaintiff's Treating Physician*, 13 Campbell L. Rev. 233, 243, 248 (1991) [IV; 5.06].

Comment, *Statutory Immunity for Volunteer Physicians: A Vehicle for Reaffirmation of the Doctor's Beneficent Duties—Absent the Rights Talk*, 1 Widener L. Symp. J. 425, 448, 449 (1996) [9.065, 10.01].

Comment, *Surrogate Health Care Decision Making: The Pennsylvania Supreme Court Recognizes the Right of an Individual in a Permanent Vegetative State to Refuse Life-Sustaining Measures through a Surrogate Decision Maker*, 35 Duq. L. Rev. 849, 859-60 (1997) [2.20].

Comment, *Taking Tarasoff Where No One Has Gone Before: Looking at Duty to Warn Under the AIDS Crisis*, 15 St. Louis U. Pub. L. Rev. 471, 499 (1996) [2.23, 5.057].

Comment, *The Hospice Movement: A Renewed View of the Death Process*, 4 J. Contemp. Health L. & Pol'y 295 (1988) [2.20].

Comment, *The Living Will: Preservation of the Right-to-Die Demands Clarity and Consistency*, 95 Dickinson L. Rev. 209, 217 (1990) [2.20].

Comment, *The Right to Refuse Life Sustaining Medical Treatment and the Nonterminally Ill Patient: An Analysis of Abridgment and Anarchy*, 17 Pepperdine L. Rev. 461, 462 (1990) [2.20].

Comment, *The Role of the Family in Medical Decision Making for Incompetent Adult Patients: A Historical Perspective and Case Analysis*, 48 Univ. Pittsburgh L. Rev. 539 (1987) [2.20].

Comment, *Tort Reform to Ensure the Inclusion of Fertile Women in Early Phases of Commercial Drug Research*, 3 U. Chi. L. Sch. Roundtable 355, 359 (1996) [9.035].

Comment, *Who's in Charge: The Doctor or the Dollar? Assessing the Relative Liability of Third Party Payors and Doctors After Wickline and Wilson*, 18 J. Contemp. L. 285, 301, 302 (1992) [2.03].

Comment, *Withholding Lifesaving Treatment From Defective Newborns: An Equal Protection Analysis,* 29 St. Louis Univ. L. J. 853 (1985) [2.17].

Conde, *Embryo Donation: The Government Adopts a Cause,* 13 Wm. & Mary J. Women & L. 273, 288 (2006) [2.141].

Coombs, *The Medical Malpractice Myth,* 27 J. Legal Med. 243, 249-50 (2006) [8.12].

Cooper, *Restrictive Covenants,* 248 JAMA 3091 (1982) [9.02].

Cooper & Harper, *Life After Death: The Authority of Estate Fiduciaries to Dispose of Decendents' Reproductive Matter,* 26 Touro L. Rev. 649, 658 (2010) [2.04].

Coppolo, *Not Just a Minimum Income Policy for Physicians: The Need for Good Faith and Fair Dealing in Physician Deselection Disputes,* 48 Wm. and Mary L. Rev. 677, 686 (2006) [8.13].

Corcoran, Hodge, & Rutkow, *A Hidden Epidemic: Assessing the Legal Environment Underlying Mental and Behavioral Health Conditions in Emergencies,* 4 St. Louis U. J. Health L. & Pol'y 33, 68 (2010) [10.01].

Costantino, *Second Generation Organizational Conflict Management Systems Design: A Practitioner's Perspective on Emerging Issues,* 14 Harv. Negot. L. Rev. 81 (2009) [I, II, V, VIII].

Cotter, *Increasing Consent for Organ Donation: Mandated Choice, Individual Autonomy, and Informed Consent,* 21 Health Matrix 599, 606,607 (2011) [2.155].

Crabtree, Pelletier, Gleason, Pruett, & Sawyer, *Gender-Dependent Differences in Outcome After the Treatment of Infection in Hospitalized Patients,* 282 JAMA 2143, 2148 (1999) [9.122].

Crain, *The Transformation of the Professional Workforce,* 79 Chi.-Kent L. Rev. 543, 582 (2004) [9.025].

Cramton & Knowles, *Professional Secrecy and Its Exceptions: Spaulding v. Zimmerman Revisited,* 83 Minn. L. Rev. 63, 98 (1998) [5.09].

Crane, *The Problem of Physician Self-referral Under the Medicare and Medicaid Antikickback Statute: The Hanlester Network Case and the Safe Harbor Regulation,* 268 JAMA 85, 89, 90 (1992) [8.032].

Cranford, *Neurologic Syndromes and Prolonged Survival: When Can Artificial Nutrition and Hydration Be Foregone?* 19 Law Med. & Health Care 13, 14, 16, 17 (1991) [2.20].

Crespi, *Overcoming the Legal Obstacles to the Creation of a Futures Market in Bodily Organs,* 55 Ohio St. L. J. 1, 74 (1994) [2.15].

Crossley, *Infants With Anencephaly, the ADA, and the Child Abuse Amendments,* 11 Issues in Law & Med. 379, 385, 409 (1996) [2.162, 2.17].

Crossley, *Infected Judgment: Legal Responses to Physician Bias,* 48 Vill. L. Rev. 195, 239, 297 (2003) [9.121, 9.122].

Crossley, *Of Diagnoses and Discrimination: Discriminatory Nontreatment of Infants With HIV Infection,* 93 Columbia L. Rev. 1581, 1620, 1621 (1993) [2.09, 2.17, 2.20, 2.22, 4.04, 8.03].

Cultice, *Medical Futility: When Is Enough, Enough?* 27 J. Health & Hosp. Law 225, 230, 256 (1994) [2.03, 2.035, 2.095, 2.17, 2.19, 2.20, 2.22].

Cuzmanes & Orlando, *Automation of Medical Records: The Electronic Superhighway and Its Ramifications for Health Care Providers,* 6 J. Pharmacy & L. 19, 27 (1997) [IV].

Daar, *Accessing Reproductive Technologies: Invisible Barriers, Indelible Harms,* 23 Berkeley J. Gender L. & Just.18 (2008) [9.12].

Daar, *A Clash at the Bedside: Patient Autonomy v. a Physician's Professional Conscience,* 44 Hastings L. J. 1241, 1257, 1268, 1286 (1993) [2.20, 2.22].

Daar, *Medical Futility and Implications for Physician Autonomy,* XXI Am. J. Law & Med. 221, 234 (1995) [2.035].

Dahm, *Medical Futility and the Texas Medical Futility Statute: A Model to Follow or One to Avoid?* 20 Health Law 25 (2008) [2.035, 2.037, 2.20].

Dahm, *Using DNA Profile as the Unique Patient Identifier in the Community Health Information Network: Legal Implications,* 15 J. Marshall J. Computer & Info. L. 227, 266, 275 (1997) [5.05].

Dalton, *Domestic Violence, Domestic Torts and Divorce: Constraints and Possibilities,* 31 New. Eng. L. Rev. 319, 354 (1997) [2.02].

D'Amico, Krasna, Krasna, & Sade, *No Heroic Measures: How Soon Is Too Soon to Stop?* 87 Ann. Thorac. Surg. 11, 17 (2009) [8.081].

Daniels, *Duty to Treat or Right to Refuse?* 21 Hastings Center Rep. 36, 37, 42 (March/April 1991) [VI; 9.131].

Danino, *Dodging the Issue of Physician Assisted Suicide: The Supreme Court's Likely Response in Gonzales v. Oregon*, 10 Mich. St. U. J. Med. & L. 299, 305 (2006) [2.211].

Daugherty, *"Synthetic Sanity": The Ethics and Legality of Using Psychotropic Medications to Render Death Row Inmates Competent for Execution*, 17 J. Contemp. H. L. & Pol'y 715, 730 (2001) [2.06].

Davis & Grimaldi, *Sexual Confusion: Attorney-Client Sex and the Need for a Clear Ethical Rule*, 7 Notre Dame J. Law, Ethics, & Pub. Pol. 57, 61 (1993) [8.14].

Davison, Reisman, Pellegrino, Larson, Dermody, & Hutchison, *Perioperative Guidelines for Elective Surgery in the Human Immunodeficiency Virus–Positive Patient*, 121 Plastic and Reconstructive Surgery 1831, 1838 (2008) [II; 9.131].

Deady, *Cyberadvice: The Ethical Implications of Giving Professional Advice Over the Internet*, 14 Geo. J. Legal Ethics 891, 905 (2001) [10.01].

Deftos, *Genomic Torts: The Law of the Future— The Duty of Physicians to Disclose the Presence of a Genetic Disease to the Relatives of Their Patients With the Disease*, 32 USF. L. Rev. 105, 130 (1997) [10.01].

Dehlendorf & Wolfe, *Physicians Disciplined for Sex-Related Offenses*, 279 JAMA 1883 (1998) [8.14].

DeLair, *Ethical, Moral, Economic and Legal Barriers to Assisted Reproductive Technologies Employed by Gay Men and Lesbian Women*, 4 DePaul J. Health Care L. 147, 150 (2000) [VI].

Dellinger & Vickery, *When Staff Object to Participating in Care*, 28 J. Health & Hospital Law 269, 272, 276 (1995) [I, VI; 1.02, 2.035, 9.055].

Delmonico, Arnold, Scheper-Hughes, Siminoff, Kahn, & Youngner, *Ethical Incentives—Not Payment—for Organ Donation*, 346 New Eng. J. Med. 2002, 2005 (2002) [2.155].

Demaine, *"Playing Doctor" With the Patient's Spouse: Alternative Conceptions of Health Professional Liability*, 14 Va. J. Soc. Pol'y & L. 308, 325, 330-31, 331-32 (2007) [Preamble; I, II, VIII; 8.145, 9.04, 9.123, 10.015].

DeMarco & McKinnon, *Life After BRCA1/2 Testing: Family Communication and Support Issues*, 27 Breast Disease 127, 127 (2007) [2.131].

DeMitchell, *Immorality, Teacher Private Conduct, and Adverse Notoriety: A Needed Recalculation of Nexus?* 40 J. L & Educ. 327, 336 (2011) [1.01].

DeMuro, *A Review of Key Legal Requirements Affecting Ambulatory Surgical Centers*, 11 Health Law. 1, 7 (1999) [8.032].

DeNatale & Parrish, *Health Care Workers' Ability to Recover in Tort for Transmission or Fear of Transmission of HIV From a Patient*, 36 Santa Clara L. Rev. 751, 782-83, 787 (1996) [IV; 9.131].

Denbo, *What Your Genes Know Affects Them: Should Patient Confidentiality Prevent Disclosure of Genetic Test Results to a Patient's Biological Relatives?* 43 Am. Bus. L. J. 561, 572, 577 (2006) [IV; 5.05].

Dennis, *Promotion of Devices: An Extension of FDA Drug Regulation or a New Frontier?* 48 Food & Drug L. J. 87 (1993) [8.061].

Denno, *Getting to Death: Are Executions Constitutional?* 82 Iowa L. Rev. 319, 385-86 (1997) [2.06].

Denno, *The Lethal Injection Quandary: How Medicine Has Dismantled Death*, 76 Fordham L. Rev. 49, 80-81 (2007) [2.06].

Denno, *When Legislatures Delegate Death: The Troubling Paradox Behind State Uses of Electrocution and Lethal Injection and What It Says About Us*, 63 Ohio St. L. J. 63, 112-13 (2002) [2.06].

Dent, *Civil Rights for Whom? Gay Rights Versus Religious Freedom*, 95 Ky. L. J. 553, 569 (2007) [9.12].

Devettere, *The Imprecise Language of Euthanasia and Causing Death*, 1 J. Clinical Ethics 268, 268 (1990) [2.20].

DeVita, *Honestly, Do We Need a Policy on Truth?* 11 Kennedy Inst. Ethics J. 157, 158 (2001) [II; 8.12, 10.01].

Dickey, *Euthanasia: A Concept Whose Time Has Come?* 8 Issues in Law & Med. 521, 523, 524 (1993) [2.17, 2.20].

DiFonzo, *The End of the Red Queen's Race: Medical Marijuana in the New Century*, 27 Quinnipiac L. Rev. 673 (2009) [VIII; 2.17].

Dillon, *Contingent Fees and Medical-Legal Consulting Services: Economical or Unethical?* 11 J. Legal Med. 93, 101, 111 (1990) [6.01, 6.05, 9.07].

Dixon, *Conant v. McCaffrey: Physicians, Marijuana, and the First Amendment*, 70 U. Colo. L. Rev. 975, 977 (1999) [2.17].

Doherty & Freed, *User Fees in Health Care*, 39 Md. B.J. 5, 9 (April 2006) [4.01, 8.055].

Dolin, *A Defense of Embryonic Stem Cell Research*, 84 Ind. L. J. 1203 (2009) [2.20].

Dolin, *A Healer or an Executioner? The Proper Role of a Psychiatrist in a Criminal Justice System*, 17 J. L. & Health 169, 206, 213-14 (2003) [2.06, 8.08].

D'Orazio, *Half of the Family Tree: A Call for Access to a Full Genetic History for Children Born by Artificial Insemination*, 2 J. Health & Biomedical L. 249, 256 (2006) [2.05].

Dore, *Aid in Dying: Not Legal in Idaho; Not About Choice*, 53 The Advocate 18 (Sept. 2010) [2.211].

Dore, *Physician-Assisted Suicide: A Recipe for Elder Abuse and the Illusion of Personal Choice*, 36 Vt. B. J. 53, 53 (Winter 2011) [2.211].

Dowell, *The Corporate Practice of Medicine Prohibition: A Dinosaur Awaiting Extinction*, 27 J. Health & Hospital Law 369, 370 (1994) [VI].

Doyal, *Human Need and the Right of Patients to Privacy*, 14 J. Contemp. Health L. & Pol'y 1, 3 (1997) [IV].

Draper, *Preventive Law by Corporate Professional Team Players: Liability and Responsibility in the Work of Company Doctors*, 15 J. Contemp. Health L. & Pol'y. 525, 564 (1999) [2.132].

Dresser, *Pharmaceutical Company Gifts: From Voluntary Standards to Legal Demands*, 36 Hastings Center Rep. 8, 9 (May/June 2006) [8.061].

Dresser, *Relitigating Life and Death*, 51 Ohio St. L. J. 425, 436 (1990) [2.20].

Dresser, *Wanted: Single, White Male for Medical Research*, 22 Hastings Center Rep. 24, 28 (Jan./Feb. 1992) [9.122].

DuBois, *Non–Heart-Beating Organ Donation: A Defense of the Required Determination of Death*, 27 J. Law Med. & Ethics 126, 128 (1999) [2.06, 2.162].

Duncan & Lubin, *The Use and Abuse of History in Compassion in Dying*, 20 Harv. J. L. & Pub. Pol'y 175, 183 (1996) [2.211].

Duncan, Luginbill, Richardson, & Wilson, *Using Tort Law to Secure Patient Dignity*, 40 Trial 42, 46 (Oct. 2004) [8.087].

Dunn, George, Churchill, & Spindler, *Ethics in Sports Medicine*, 35 Am. J. of Sports Med. 840, 841, 842 (2007) [3.06].

Durst, *Cutting Through Pennsylvania's Medical Informed Consent Statute: A Reasonable Interpretation Abolishing the Surgical Requirement*, 104 Dick. L. Rev. 197, 225 (1999) [8.08].

Dworkin, *Getting What We Should From Doctors: Rethinking Patient Autonomy and the Doctor-Patient Relationship*, 13 Health Matrix 235, 240 (2003) [8.08].

Eaton & Reid, *Mirror, Mirror on the Wall: Evaluating Fair Market Value for Manufacturer-Physician Consulting Arrangements*, 65 Food & Drug L. J. 141, 147 (2010) [8.061].

Ebert, *Attorneys, Tell Your Clients to Say They're Sorry: Apologies in the Health Care Industry*, 5 Ind. Health L. Rev. 337 (2008) [8.08, 8.12, 10.01, 10.015].

Economou, *What About Families? A Different Perspective on Physician Assisted Suicide in California*, 7 Whittier J. Child & Fam. Advoc. 253 (2008) [2.211].

Egan, Parsi, & Ramirez, *Comparing Ethics Education in Medicine and Law: Combining the Best of Both Worlds*, 13 Annals Health L. 303, 316, 323 (2004) [Preamble; 9.11].

Ehrlich, *Grounded in the Reality of Their Lives: Listening to Teens Who Make the Abortion Decision Without Involving Their Parents*, 18 Berkeley Women's L. J. 61, 72, 84-85, 175-76 (2003) [2.015].

Ehrlich, *Journey Through the Courts: Minors, Abortion and the Quest for Reproductive Fairness*, 10 Yale J. L. & Feminism 1, 19 (1998) [2.015].

Ehrlich, *Minors as Medical Decision Makers: The Pretextual Reasoning of the Court in the Abortion Cases*, 7 Mich. J. Gender & L. 65, 91 (2000) [2.015].

Ehrlich, *Shifting Boundaries: Abortion, Criminal Culpability and the Indeterminate Legal Status of Adolescents*, 18 Wis. Women's L. J. 77, 105 (2003) [2.015].

Eisenstat, *An Analysis of the Rationality of Mandatory Testing for the HIV Antibody: Balancing the Governmental Public Health Interests With the Individual's Privacy Interest*, 52 Univ. Pittsburgh L. Rev. 327, 347 (1991) [9.131].

Eitel, Hegeman, & Evans, *Medicine on Trial: Physicians' Attitudes About Expert Medical Witnesses*, 18 J. Legal Med. 345, 355, 358 (1997) [II, VI; 9.07].

Elliott, *The Charity Care Crisis—Where Does the Money Go?* 8 J. Health Care Compliance 11, 13 (September/October 2006) [9.065].

Elsas, *A Clinical Approach to Legal and Ethical Problems in Human Genetics*, 39 Emory L. J. 811, 816, 820 (1990) [5.05].

Eltis, *Predicating Dignity on Autonomy? The Need for Further Inquiry Into the Ethics of Tagging and Tracking Dementia Patients With GPS Technology*, 13 Elder L. J. 387, 403 (2005) [I].

Emanuel, *Do Physicians Have an Obligation to Treat Patients With AIDS?* 318 New Eng. J. Med. 1686 (1988) [9.12].

Emanuel, *Justice and Managed Care: Four Principles for the Just Allocation of Health Care Resources*, 30 Hastings Center Rep. 8, 16 (May/June 2000) [8.032].

Emanuel & Goldman, *Protecting Patient Welfare in Managed Care: Six Safeguards*, 23 J. Health Pol. Pol'y & L. 635, 641 (1998) [8.061].

Emanuel, Barry, Stoeckle, Ettelson, & Emanuel, *Advance Directives for Medical Care—A Case for Greater Use*, 324 New Eng. J. Med. 889 (1991) [2.20].

Emanuel, Emanuel, Stoeckle, Hummel, & Barry, *Advance Directives: Stability of Patients' Treatment Choices*, 154 Arch. Intern. Med. 209, 217 (1994) [2.20].

Emanuel, von Gunten, & Ferris, *Advance Care Planning*, 9 Arch. Fam. Med. 1181, 1181 (2000) [2.225].

Engelhardt, Jr, *Giving, Selling, and Having Taken: Conflicting Views of Organ Transfer*, 1 Ind. Health L. Rev. 29, 33-34 (2004) [2.15, 2.151].

Erwin, *Analyzing the Disruptive Physician: How State and Federal Courts Should Handle Whistleblower Cases Brought by Disruptive Physicians*, 44 Duq. L. Rev. 275, 276 (2006) [9.045].

Etzioni, *Organ Donation: A Communitarian Approach*, 13 Kennedy Inst. Ethics J. 1, 3, 4, 16 (March 2003) [2.15, 2.155].

Ewart, *Use of the Drug Pavulon in Lethal Injections: Cruel and Unusual?* 14 Wm. & Mary Bill of Rts. J. 1159, 1182 (2006) [2.06].

Fahrenkrog, *A Comparison of International Regulation of Preimplantation Genetic Diagnosis and a Regulatory Suggestion for the United States*, 15 Transnat'l L. & Contemp. Probs. 757, 759 (2006) [2.12].

Falit, *Ancillary Service and Self-referral Arrangements in the Medical and Legal Professions: Do Current Ethical, Legislative, and Regulatory Policies Adequately Serve the Interests of Patients and Clients?* 58 S. C. L. Rev. 371, 373-74 (2006) [8.032].

Falk & Cary, *Death-Defying Feats: State Constitutional Challenges to New York's Death Penalty*, 4 J. L. & Pol'y 161, 233, 234 (1995) [2.06].

Fallek, *The Pain Relief Promotion Act: Will It Spell Death to "Death With Dignity" or Is It Unconstitutional?* 27 Fordham Urb. L. J. 1739, 1755 (2000) [2.20].

Farber, Davis, Weiner, Jordan, Boyer, & Ubel, *Physicians' Attitudes About Involvement in Lethal Injection for Capital Punishment*, 160 Arch. Intern. Med. 2912, 2912 (2000) [2.06].

Farber, Jordan, Silverstein, Collier, Weiner, & Boyer, *Primary Care Physicians' Decisions About Discharging Patients From Their Practices*, 23 J. of General Internal Med. 283, 283 (2008) [10.015].

Farber, Novack, & O'Brien, *Love, Boundaries, and the Physician-Patient Relationship*, 157 Arch. Intern. Med. 2291, 2292, 2293, 2294 (1997) [8.14].

Farley, *The Medicare Antifraud Statute and Safe Harbor Regulations: Suggestions for Change*, 81 Georgetown L. J. 167, 184 (1992) [8.032].

Farrow, *The Anti-Patient Psychology of Health Courts: Prescriptions From a Lawyer-Physician*, 36 Am. J. L. & Med. 188, 219 (2010) [9.07].

Fedder, *To Know or Not to Know: Legal Perspectives on Genetic Privacy and Disclosure of an Individual's Genetic Profile*, 21 J. Legal Med. 557, 563 (2000) [2.139].

Feldhammer, *Medical Torture: End of Life Decision-Making in the United Kingdom and United States*, 14 Cardozo J. Int'l & Comp. L. 511, 514-15, 532 (2006) [2.037, 9.115].

Fentiman, *Patient Advocacy and Termination From Managed Care Organizations: Do State Laws Protecting Health Care Professional Advocacy Make Any Difference?* 82 Neb. L. Rev. 508, 515-16, 517-18 (2003) [8.054, 8.13, 10.01].

Ferguson, *Ethical Postures of Futility and California's Uniform Health Care Decisions Act*, 75 S. Cal. L. Rev. 1217, 1252-53 (2002) [2.037].

Fernandez, *Is AIDS Different?* 61 Alb. L. Rev. 1053 (1998) [2.23].

Fichter, *The Law of Doctoring: A Study of the Codification of Medical Professionalism*, 19 Health Matrix 317 (2009) [II, III, IV, V, VI, VII, VIII].

Field, *New Ethical Relationships Under Health Care's New Structure: The Need for a New Paradigm*, 43 Vill. L. Rev. 467, 468 (1998) [I].

Field, *Overview: Computerized Medical Records Create New Legal and Business Confidentiality Problems*, 11 HealthSpan 3, 4 (1994) [5.05].

Field, *Testing for AIDS: Uses and Abuses*, XVI Am. J. Law & Med. 34, 50 (1990) [9.131].

Fiestal, *A Solomonic Decision: What Will Be the Fate of Frozen Preembryos?* 6 Cardozo Women's L. J. 103, 110 (1999) [2.141].

Fine, *Exploitation of the Elite: A Case for Physician Unionization*, 45 St. Louis L. J. 207, 207 (2001) [I].

Fink, *Time to Stop Dialyzing the Dead (and Treating Other Patients Too Aggressively, Too), Dialysis & Transplantation* May 2009, 1, 1 [2.035].

Finks, *Lethal Injection: An Uneasy Alliance of Law and Medicine*, 4 J. Legal Med. 383 (1983) [2.06].

Fischer, Alpert, Stoeckle, & Emanuel, *Can Goals of Care Be Used to Predict Intervention Preferences in an Advance Directive?* 157 Arch. Intern. Med. 801, 807 (1997) [2.20, 2.21].

FitzGibbon, *The Failure of the Freedom-Based and Utilitarian Arguments for Assisted Suicide*, 42 Am. J. Juris. 211, 252 (1997) [2.211].

FitzGibbon & Lai, *The Model Physician-Assisted Suicide Act and the Jurisprudence of Death*, 13 Issues in Law & Med. 173, 203-04 (1997) [2.211].

Flamholz, *A Penny for Your Organs: Revising New York's Policy on Offering Financial Incentives for Organ Donation*, 14 J. L. & Pol'y 329, 330, 374 (2006) [2.151, 2.16].

Fleming, *Healthcare Access: Conflicts of Interest Presented by Managed Care ICU Bedside Rationing and Their Impact on Minorities and Women*, 5 Geo. J. Gender & L. 663, 667 (2004) [2.035].

Flick, *The Due Process of Dying*, 79 Cal. L. Rev. 1121, 1152 (1991) [2.22].

Forell & Sortun, *The Tort of Betrayal of Trust*, 42 U. Mich. J. L. Reform, 557 (2009) [VIII].

Forrester, *AIDS: The Responsibility to Care*, 34 Vill. L. Rev. 799, 811 (1989) [VI; 9.131].

Forster, *The Legal and Ethical Debate Surrounding the Storage and Destruction of Frozen Human Embryos: A Reaction to the Mass Disposal in Britain and the Lack of Law in the United States*, 76 Wash. U. L.Q. 759, 766-67, 770 (1998) [2.141].

Freedman, *Health Professions, Codes, and the Right to Refuse to Treat HIV-Infectious Patients*, 18 Hastings Center Rep. 20 (Supp.) (April/May 1988) [VI; 8.11, 9.12].

Freedman & Halpern, *The Erosion of Ethics and Morality in Medicine: Physician Participation in Legal Executions in the United States*, 41 N. Y. L. Sch. L. Rev. 169, 174 (1996) [2.06].

Freeman, *Dealing With Doctors*, 13 S. C. Law 11, 11 (July/Aug. 2001) [5.05].

Freiman, *The Abandonment of the Antiquated Corporate Practice of Medicine Doctrine: Injecting a Dose of Efficiency Into the Modern Health Care Environment*, 47 Emory L. J. 697, 712 (1998) [VI].

Friedland, *HIV Confidentiality and the Right to Warn—The Health Care Provider's Dilemma*, 80 Mass. L. Rev. 3, 4 (March 1995) [IV; 5.05, 10.01].

Friedland, *Managed Care and the Expanding Scope of Primary Care Physicians' Duties: A Proposal to Redefine Explicitly the Standard of Care*, 26 J. Law Med. & Ethics 100, 104 (1998) [I].

Friedland, *Physician-Patient Confidentiality: Time to Re-Examine a Venerable Concept in Light of Contemporary Society and Advances in Medicine*, 15 J. Legal Med. 249, 257, 264, 276 (1994) [I, IV; 5.05].

Frishman, *Wisconsin Act 110: When an Infant Survives an Abortion*, 20 Wis. Women's L. J. 101, 117 (2005) [2.01].

Frye, *The International Bill of Gender Rights vs. the Cider House Rules: Transgenders Struggle With the Courts Over What Clothing They Are Allowed to Wear on the Job, Which Restroom They Are Allowed to Use on the Job, Their Right to Marry, and the Very Definition of Their Sex*, 7 Wm. & Mary J. Women & L. 133, 149 (2000) [2.132, 2.135, 2.137, 5.08, 5.09].

Frye & Meiselman, *Same-Sex Marriages Have Existed Legally in the United States for a Long Time Now*, 64 Alb. L. Rev. 1031, 1053 (2001) [2.132, 2.135, 2.137, 5.08, 5.09].

Fry-Revere, Ray, & Reher, *Death: A New Legal Perspective*, 27 J. Contemp. Health L. & Pol'y 1, 11, 50, 53 (2010) [2.157, 10.01].

Furman, *Genetic Test Results and the Duty to Disclose: Can Medical Researchers Control Liability?* 23 Seattle Univ. L. R. 391, 408-09 (1999) [2.07].

Furrow, *Doctor's Dirty Little Secrets: The Dark Side of Medical Privacy*, 37 Washburn L. Rev. 283, 290 (1998) [9.131].

Furrow, *Incentivizing Medical Practice: What (if Anything) Happens to Professionalism?* 1 Widener L. Symp. J. 1, 9 (1996) [2.03].

Gabos, *The Perils of Singleton v. Norris: Ethics and Beyond*, 32 Am. J. L. & Med. 117, 118, 125-26, 127 (2006) [I, III, VIII; 2.06].

Gaitan, *Challenges Facing Society in the Implementation of the Death Penalty*, 35 Fordham Urb. L. J. 763 (2008) [2.06].

Gamble & Stone, *U.S. Policy on Health Inequities: The Interplay of Politics and Research*, 31 J. Health Pol. Pol'y & L. 93, 105-06 (2006) [9.121].

Garfield, *Bridging a Gap in Human Rights Law: Prisoner of War Abuse as "War Tort,"* 37 Geo. J. Int'l L. 725, 743 (2006) [2.068].

Garrett & Garis, *Leveling the Playing Field in the Pharmacy Benefit Management Industry*, 42 Val. U. L. Rev. 33, 64 (2007) [8.06].

Garris, *The Case for Patenting Medical Procedures*, XXII Am. J. Law & Med. 85, 93, 94-95 (1996) [9.08, 9.09, 9.095].

Gatter, *A Prisoner's Constitutional Right to Medical Information: Doctrinally Flawed and a Threat to State Informed Consent Law*, 45 Wake Forest L. Rev. 1025, 1062 (2010) [8.08].

Gatter, *Protecting Patient-Doctor Discourse: Informed Consent and Deliberative Autonomy*, 78 Or. L. Rev. 941, 956 (1999) [Preamble; 8.03].

Gauthier, *Active Voluntary Euthanasia, Terminal Sedation, and Assisted Suicide*, 12 J. Clinical Ethics 43, 43-44, 49 (2001) [2.20, 2.21].

Geckeler, *The Clinton-Obama Approach to Medical Malpractice Reform: Reviving the Most Meaningful Features of Alternative Dispute Resolution*, 8 Pepp. Disp. Resol. L. J. 171, 193 (2007) [8.12, 8.082].

Geiger, *The Ailing Labor Rights of Medical Residents: Curable Ill or a Lost Cause?* 8 U. Pa. J. Lab. & Emp. L. 523, 538 (2006) [9.025].

Gelein, *Are Online Consultations a Prescription for Trouble? The Uncharted Waters of Cybermedicine*, 66 Brook. L. Rev. 209, 239 (2000) [10.01].

Gellman, *Prescribing Privacy: The Uncertain Role of the Physician in the Protection of Patient Privacy*, 62 No. Carolina L. Rev. 255 (1984) [5.03, 5.04, 5.06, 5.07, 5.08, 5.09].

Gerbert, Bleecker, Miyasaki, & Maguire, *Possible Health Care Professional-to-Patient HIV Transmission: Dentists' Reactions to a Centers for Disease Control Report*, 265 JAMA 1845, 1846, 1847 (1991) [9.131].

Gerbert, Maguire, Bleecker, Coates, & McPhee, *Primary Care Physicians and AIDS: Attitudinal and Structural Barriers to Care*, 266 JAMA 2837, 2838 (1991) [9.131].

Gibbs, *State Regulation of Pharmaceutical Clinical Trials*, 59 Food & Drug L. J. 265, 279 (2004) [8.0315].

Gibbs, Nsiah-Jefferson, McHugh, Trivedi, & Prothrow-Stith, *Reducing Racial and Ethnic Health Disparities: Exploring an Outcome-Oriented Agenda for Research and Policy*, 31 J. Health Pol. Pol'y & L. 185, 216 (2006) [9.121].

Gilbert, *Emerging Issues in Global AIDS Policy: Preserving Privacy*, 25 Whittier L. Rev. 273, 276 (2003) [7.025].

Gilmore, *Employment Protection for Lesbians and Gay Men*, 6 L. & Sex. 83, 95 (1996) [9.03].

Gimbel & Zaremski, *Medical Restrictive Covenants in Illinois: At the Crossroads of Carter-Shields and Prairie Eye Center*, 12 Annals Health L. 1, 12 (2003) [9.02].

Ginsberg, *Informed Consent: No Longer Just What the Doctor Ordered? The "Contributions" of Medical Associations and Courts to a More Patient Friendly Doctrine*, 15 Mich. St. J. Med. & Law 17, 23, 24, 25, 26, 46 (2011) [2.065, 8.08, 10.01, 10.015].

Gitter, *Ownership of Human Tissue: A Proposal for Federal Recognition of Human Research Participants' Property Rights in Their Biological Material*, 61 Wash. & Lee L. Rev. 257, 334 (2004) [2.08].

Gittler & Rennart, *HIV Infection Among Women and Children and Antidiscrimination Laws: An Overview*, 77 Iowa L. Rev. 1313, 1363 (1992) [VII; 9.131].

Glass & Waring, *The Physician/Investigator's Obligation to Patients Participating in Research: The Case of Placebo Controlled Trials*, 33 J. L. Med. & Ethics, 575, 576 (2005) [2.07].

Glynn, *Multidisciplinary Representation of Children: Conflicts Over Disclosures of Client Communications*, 27 J. Marshall L. Rev. 617, 625, 626, 630-32, 637, 639, 643 (1994) [III, IV; 1.02, 2.02, 5.05, 10.01].

Glynn, *Turning to State Legislatures to Legalize Physician-Assisted Suicide for Seriously Ill, Non-Terminal Patients After Vacco v. Quill and Washington v. Glucksberg*, 6 J. L. & Pol'y. 329, 345 (1997) [2.211].

Godoy, *Where Is Biotechnology Taking the Law? An Overview of Assisted Reproductive Technology, Research on Frozen Embryos and Human Cloning*, 19 J. Juv. L. 357, 363 (1998) [2.141].

Gold, *Physicians' "Right of Conscience"—Beyond Politics*, 38 (1) J. L. Med & Ethics, 138 (2010) [VII].

Goldberg, *Sex and the Attorney-Client Relationship: An Argument for a Prophylactic Rule*, 26 Akron L. Rev. 45 (1992) [8.14].

Goldman, *Revising Iowa's Life-Sustaining Procedures Act: Creating a Practical Guide to Living Wills in Iowa*, 76 Iowa L. Rev. 1137, 1149 (1992) [2.20].

Goldstone, *Symposium: "Torture and the War on Terror": Combating Terrorism: Zero Tolerance for Torture*, 37 Case W. Res. J. Int'l L. 343, 346 (2006) [2.067].

Gomez, *Silencing the Hired Guns: Ensuring Honesty in Medical Expert Testimony Through State Legislation*, 26 J. Legal Med. 385, 399 (2005) [II].

Gordon, *Is There an Accuser in the House? Evaluating Statements Made to Physicians and Other Medical Personnel in the Wake of Crawford v. Washington and Davis v. Washington*, 38 N. M. L. Rev. 529 (2009) [2.02, 9.07].

Gorman, *Empirical Studies of the Legal Profession: What Do We Know About Lawyers' Lives? Explaining the Spread of Law Firm In-House Counsel Positions: A Response to Professor Chambliss.* 84 N. C. L. Rev. 1577, 1585 [VIII].

Gorsuch, *The Legalization of Assisted Suicide and the Law of Unintended Consequences: A Review of the Dutch and Oregon Experiments and Leading Utilitarian Arguments for Legal Change*, 2004 Wis. L. Rev. 1347, 1379 (2004) [2.211].

Gorsuch, *The Right to Assisted Suicide and Euthanasia*, 23 Harv. J. L. & Pub. Pol'y 599, 653, 707 (2000) [2.20, 2.21, 2.211].

Gostin, *Deciding Life and Death in the Courtroom: From Quinlan to Cruzan, Glucksberg, and Vacco—A Brief History and Analysis of Constitutional Protection of the Right to Die*, 278 JAMA 1523, 1525, 1528 (1997) [2.211].

Gostin, *Drawing a Line Between Killing and Letting Die: The Law, and Law Reform, on Medically Assisted Dying*, 21 J. Law Med. & Ethics 94, 98 (1993) [2.20].

Gostin, *Ethics, the Constitution, and the Dying Process: The Case of Theresa Marie Schiavo*, 293 JAMA 2403, 2405 (2005) [2.20].

Gostin, *Physician-Assisted Suicide: A Legitimate Medical Practice?* 295 JAMA 1941, 1942 (2006) [2.211].

Gottlieb, *Executions and Torture: The Consequences of Overriding Professional Ethics*, 6 Yale J. Health Pol'y, L. & Ethics 351, 366, 367 (2006) [2.06].

Grabois, *The Liability of Psychotherapists for Breach of Confidentiality*, 12 J. Law & Health 39, 53-54 (1998) [5.05, 5.06, 5.07, 5.08, 5.09].

Gray, *Trust and Trustworthy Care in the Managed Care Era*, 16 Health Affairs 34, 38, 47-48 (1997) [8.03].

Graybill, *Assisting Minors Seeking Abortions in Judicial Bypass Proceedings: A Guardian Ad Litem Is No Substitute for an Attorney*, 55 Vand. L. Rev. 581, 583 (2002) [2.015].

Greely, *Direct Financial Incentives in Managed Care: Unanswered Questions*, 6 Health Matrix 53, 81 (1996) [8.13].

Greely, *Neuroscience and Criminal Justice: Not Responsibility but Treatment*, 56 U. Kan. L. Rev. 1103 (2008) [2.065].

Green, *NHGRI's Intramural Ethics Experiment*, 7 Kennedy Inst. of Ethics J. 181, 185, 188 (1997) [2.138].

Green, *Physician-Assisted Suicide and Euthanasia: Safeguarding Against the "Slippery Slope"—The Netherlands Versus the United States*, 13 Ind. Int'l & Comp. L. Rev. 639, 662 (2003) [2.21, 2.211].

Green & Thomas, *DNA: Five Distinguishing Features for Policy Analysis*, 11 Harv. J. L. & Tech. 571, 582-83 (1998) [2.138].

Green, Haggerty, & Hale, *Community-Based Plan for Treating Human Immunodeficiency Virus–Infected Individuals Sponsored by Local Medical Societies and an Acquired Immunodeficiency Syndrome Service Organization*, 151 Arch. Intern. Med. 2061, 2064 (1991) [9.131].

Greenfield, *Greenberg v. Miami Children's Hospital: Unjust Enrichment and the Patenting of Human Genetic Material*, 15 Ann. Health L. 213, 248 (2006) [2.08].

Greenstein, *Against Professionalism*, 22 Geo. J. Legal Ethics 327 (2009) [Preamble; VII].

Greer, *Legal Injection: The Supreme Court Enters the Lethal Injection Debate: Hill v. McDonough, 126 S. Ct. 2096 (2006)*, 30 Harv. J. L. & Pub. Pol'y 767, 774 (2007) [2.06].

Gregg, *The Supreme Court and the Purposes of Medicine*, 354 New Eng. J. Med. 993, 994 (2006) [2.211].

Grewal, Sofair, Guevara, & Manthous, *Medicaid Patients' Access to Subspecialty Care in Connecticut*, 75 Connecticut Med. 489, 490 (2011) [2.095, 9.065].

Grimm, *Informed Consent for All! No Exceptions*, 37 N.M. L. Rev. 39, 39, 61 (2007) [I, VIII; 2.08, 8.08, 8.082].

Groner, *The Hippocratic Paradox: The Role of the Medical Profession in Capital Punishment in the United States*, 35 Fordham Urb. L. J. 883 (2008) [2.06].

Gross, *Wagging the Watchdog: Law and the Emergence of Bioethical Norms*, 21 Med. & L. 687, 702 (2002) [2.20].

Guanzon, *Health Care Law*, 41 U. Rich. L. Rev. 179, 199 (2006) [3.03, 3.08, 5.01, 5.015, 5.02, 5.04, 5.055, 6.02, 6.021, 6.03, 6.04, 7.03, 7.04, 7.05, 8.054, 8.08, 8.081, 8.085, 8.115, 8.12, 8.14, 8.145, 8.19, 9.045].

Guise, *Expansion of the Scope of Disclosure Required Under the Informed Consent Doctrine: Moore v. The Regents of the University of California*, 28 San Diego L. Rev. 455, 462 (1991) [Preamble].

Gunz & Jennings, *A Proactive Proposal for Self-regulation of the Actuarial Profession: A Means of Avoiding the Audit Profession's Post-Enron Regulatory Fate*, 48 Am. Bus. L.J. 641, 654 (2011) [VIII].

Gutheil, Jorgenson, & Sutherland, *Prohibiting Lawyer-Client Sex*, 20 Bull. Am. Acad. Psychiatry Law 365 (1992) [8.14].

Haas, *"Doctor, I'm Pregnant and Fifteen—I Can't Tell My Parents—Please Help Me": Minor Consent, Reproductive Rights, and Ethical Principles for Physicians*, 86 N.D. L. Rev. 63, 70, 73, 75-78, 82, 84, 86-88, (2010) [2.01, 2.015, 5.05, 5.055, 8.08, 8.11, 8.115, 9.12, 10.01, 10.015, 10.05].

Haas, *Who Will Make Room for the Intersexed?* 30 Am. J. L. & Med. 41, 63 (2004) [8.08].

Hackett, *Smoke-Free State Psychiatric Facility Grounds: Is Legislation Necessary and Appropriate to Remove Tobacco From These Treatment Settings?* 53 N. Y. L. Sch. L. Rev. 99 (2009) [I, III].

Hackler & Hiller, *Family Consent to Orders Not to Resuscitate: Reconsidering Hospital Policy*, 264 JAMA 1281, 1282 (1990) [2.17].

Haddon, *Baby Doe Cases: Compromise and Moral Dilemma*, 34 Emory L. J. 545 (1985) [2.20].

Hafemeister, *End-of-Life Decision Making, Therapeutic Jurisprudence, and Preventive Law: Hierarchical v. Consensus-Based Decision-Making Model*, 41 Ariz. L. Rev. 329 (1999) [2.20].

Hafemeister, *If All You Have Is a Hammer: Society's Ineffective Response to Intimate Partner Violence*, 60 Cath. U. L. Rev. 919, 962 (2011) [5.05].

Hafemeister, *Lean on Me: A Physician's Fiduciary Duty to Disclose an Emergent Medical Risk to the Patient*, 86 Wash. U. L. Rev. 1167 (2009) [III, VIII; 8.12, 10.015, 10.02].

Hafemeister, *The Fiduciary Obligation of Physicians to "Just Say No" if an "Informed" Patient Demands Services That Are Not Medically Indicated*, 39 Seton Hall L. Rev. 335 (2009) [Preamble; I, VIII; 2.035, 8.03, 10.015].

Hafemeister & Bryan, *Beware Those Bearing Gifts: Physicians' Fiduciary Duty to Avoid Pharmaceutical Marketing*, 57 U. Kan. L. Rev. 491 (2009) [8.061].

Halberstam, *Commercial Speech, Professional Speech, and the Constitutional Status of Social Institutions*, 147 U. Pa. L. Rev. 771, 857 (1999) [III].

Halevy, *AIDS, Surgery, and the Americans with Disabilities Act*, 135 Arch. Surg. 51, 52, 53 (2000) [9.13, 9.131].

Halevy & Brody, *Acquired Immunodeficiency Syndrome and the Americans with Disabilities Act: A Legal Duty to Treat*, 96 Am. J. Med. 282, 283, 284 (1994) [VI; 9.12, 9.131].

Halevy & Mcguire, *The History, Successes and Controversies of the Texas "Futility" Policy*, 43 Houston Lawyer 38, 39 (2006) [2.037].

Hall, *A Theory of Economic Informed Consent*, 31 Ga. L. Rev. 511, 521, 524-25 (1997) [8.13].

Hall, *Bargaining With Hippocrates: Managed Care and the Doctor-Patient Relationship*, 54 S. C. L. Rev. 689, 696, 735 (2003) [VII; 8.03].

Hall, *Confidentiality as an Organizational Ethics Issue*, 10 J. Clinical Ethics 230, 232 (1999) [5.05].

Hall, *Law, Medicine, and Trust*, 55 Stan. L. Rev. 463, 471 (2002) [II; 8.12].

Hall, *Paying for What You Get and Getting What You Pay For: Legal Responses to Consumer-Driven Health Care*, 69 Law & Contemp. Prob. 159, 165 (2006) [8.055, 9.065].

Hall, *Rationing Health Care at the Bedside*, 69 N. Y. U. L. Rev. 693, 704 (1994) [2.03].

Hall, *The Promise and Peril of Direct-to-Consumer Prescription Drug Promotion on the Internet*, 7 DePaul J. Health Care L. 1, 35 (2003) [5.015].

Hall, *Third-Party Payor Conflicts of Interest in Managed Care: A Proposal for Regulation Based on the Model Rules of Professional Conduct*, 29 Seton Hall L. Rev. 95, 96, 107, 108, 109, 110, 111, 112, 134, 135, 136 (1998) [Preamble; 2.07, 2.08, 2.132, 4.04, 5.01, 8.03, 8.13, 9.06, 10.01].

Hall & Boswell, *Ethics, Law, and Pain Management as a Patient Right*, 12 Pain Physician 499, 500 (2009) [I, II, IV, VIII].

Hall & Schneider, *The Professional Ethics of Billing and Collections*, 300 JAMA 1806, 1807 (2008) [6.08, 6.12].

Hall & Schneider, *When Patients Say No (to Save Money): An Essay on the Tectonics of Health Law*, 41 Conn. L. Rev. 743 (2009) [I].

Hall & Sobotka, *Inconsistent Government Policies: Why FDA Off-Label Regulation Cannot Survive First Amendment Review Under Greater New Orleans*, 62 Food Drug L. J. 1, 31 (2007) [5.015].

Halldorson, Bakthavatsalam, Fix, Reyes, & Perkins, *D-MELD, a Simple Predictor of Post Liver Transplant Mortality for Optimization of Donor/Recipient Matching*, 9 Am. J. of Transplantation 318, 324 (2009) [2.03].

Halpern, Ubel, & Caplan, *Solid-Organ Transplantation in HIV-Infected Patients*, 347 New Eng. J. Med. 284, 287 (2002) [2.16, 9.131].

Hamilton, *Religious Institutions, the No-Harm Doctrine, and the Public Good*, 2004 B.Y.U. L. Rev. 1099, 1175, 1176 (2004) [Preamble].

Hamilton, Edwards, Boehnlein, & Hamilton, *The Doctor-Patient Relationship and Assisted Suicide: A Contribution From Dynamic Psychiatry*, 19 Am. J. Forensic Psychiatry 59, 60 (1998) [2.211].

Hammes & Webster, *Professional Ethics and Managed Care in Dermatology*, 132 Arch. Dermatol. 1070, 1072, 1073 (1996) [8.13].

Hanlon, Weiss, & Rees, *British Community Pharmacists' Views of Physician-Assisted Suicide (PAS)*, 26 J. Med. Ethics 363, 367, 369 (2000) [2.211].

Hanson, *Informed Consent and the Scope of a Physician's Duty of Disclosure*, 77 N.D. L. Rev. 71, 89, 91 (2001) [8.13].

Harbinson, *Crawford v. Washington and Davis v. Washington's Originalism: Historical Arguments Showing Child Abuse Victims' Statements to Physicians Are Nontestimonial and Admissible as an Exception to the Confrontation Clause*, 58 Mercer L. Rev. 569, 617 (2007) [VIII].

Hardaway, Peterson, & Mann, *The Right to Die and the Ninth Amendment: Compassion and Dying After Glucksberg and Vacco*, 7 Geo. Mason L. Rev. 313, 342 (1999) [2.211].

Harmon, *Back From Wonderland: A Linguistic Approach to Duties Arising From Threats of Physical Violence*, 37 Cap. U. L. Rev. 27 (2008) [5.05].

Haroun & Morris, *Weaving a Tangled Web: The Deceptions of Psychiatrists*, 10 J. Contemp. Leg. Issues 227, 235 (1999) [II, III].

Harris, *The Regulation of Managed Care: Conquering Individualism and Cynicism in America*, 6 Va. J. Soc. Pol'y. & L. 315, 329 (1999) [2.16].

Harris & Foran, *The Ethics of Middle-Class Access to Legal Services and What We Can Learn From the Medical Profession's Shift to a Corporate Paradigm*, 70 Fordham L. Rev. 775, 817, 821, 822, 823, 824 (2001) [VI; 2.03, 2.09, 8.02, 8.021, 8.03, 8.05, 8.051, 8.054, 8.13, 8.132].

Hartman, *Face Value: Challenges of Transplant Technology*, 31 Am. J. L. & Med. 7, 25, 31 (2005) [2.15].

Hartog, *The Psychological Impact of AIDS on Real Property and a Real Estate Broker's Duty to Disclose*, 36 Ariz. L. Rev. 757, 772 (1994) [9.13, 9.131].

Harvey, *Confidentiality: A Measured Response to the Failure of Privacy*, 140 Univ. Pa. L. Rev. 2385, 2454 (1992) [8.08].

Hashimoto, *The Future Role of Managed Care and Capitation in Workers' Compensation*, XXII Am. J. Law & Med. 233, 258, 259 (1996) [8.13].

Hasko, *Persuasion in the Court: Nonlegal Materials in US Supreme Court Opinions*, 94 Law Libr. J. 427, 444, 453 (2002) [2.20, 2.211].

Haut, *Divorce and the Disposition of Frozen Embryos*, 28 Hofstra L. Rev. 493, 519 (1999) [2.141].

Hawkins, *Doctors as Bankers: Evidence From Fertility Markets*, 84 Tul. L. Rev. 841, 848, 874 (2010) [2.055, 6.08].

Healey & Dowling, *Controlling Conflicts of Interest in the Doctor-Patient Relationship: Lessons From Moore v. Regents of the University of California*, 42 Mercer L. Rev. 989, 997, 998 (1991) [2.19, 8.032, 8.06].

Hecht, *Legal and Ethical Aspects of Sports-Related Concussions: The Merril Hoge Story*, 12 Seton Hall J. Sport L. 17, 42-43 (2002) [10.015].

Heilman, *Contemplating "Cruel and Unusual": A Critical Analysis of Baze v. Rees in the Context of the Supreme Court's Eighth Amendment "Proportionality" Jurisprudence*, 58 Am. U. L. Rev. 633 (2009) [2.06].

Heimer, *Responsibility in Health Care: Spanning the Boundary Between Law and Medicine*, 41 Wake Forest L. Rev. 465, 498 (2006) [Preamble; VII, IX].

Helft, Siegler, & Lantos, *The Rise and Fall of the Futility Movement*, 343 New Eng. J. Med. 293, 294 (2000) [2.037].

Hellman, *Money Talks But It Isn't Speech*, 95 Minn. L. Rev. 953, 1002 (2011) [10.01].

Hellman, *Prosecuting Doctors for Trusting Patients*, 16 Geo. Mason L. Rev. 701 (2009) [8.14].

Henderson & Cassady, *Drug Deals in 2006: Cutting Edge Legal and Regulatory Issues in the Pharmaceutical Industry*, 15 Ann. Health L. 107, 131-32 (2006) [8.061].

Hensl, *Restored to Health to Be Put to Death: Reconciling the Legal and Ethical Dilemmas of Medicating to Execute in Singleton v. Norris*, 49 Vill. L. Rev. 291, 324 (2004) [2.06, 2.065].

Hermer, *Paradigms Revised: Intersex Children, Bioethics & the Law*, 11 Annals Health L. 195, 221 (2002) [10.01].

Hermer, *The Scapegoat: EMTALA and Emergency Department Overcrowding*, 14 J. L. & Pol'y 695, 713-14 (2006) [IX; 9.065].

Heyman, *Military Medical Ethics*, 395 New Eng. J. Med. 2728, 2729 (2009) [2.068].

Hillerich, Ellerin, & Frieder, *Selecting and Presenting a Failure to Diagnose Breast Cancer Case*, 20 Am. J. Trial Advoc. 253, 271 (1996-97) [5.05, 5.06].

Hilliard, *The Politics of Palliative Care and the Ethical Boundaries of Medicine: Gonzales v. Oregon as a Cautionary Tale*, 35 J. L. Med. & Ethics 158, 170 (2007) [2.211].

Hinkie, *Free Speech and Rule 3.6: How the Object of Attorney Speech Affects the Right to Make Public Criticism*, 20 Geo. J. Legal Ethics 695, 695 (2007) [IV].

Hirshfeld, *Defining Full and Fair Disclosure in Managed Care Contracts*, 60 The Citation 67 (1990) [8.03, 8.032, 8.132].

Hirshfeld, *Economic Considerations in Treatment Decisions and the Standard of Care in Medical Malpractice Litigation*, 264 JAMA 2004, 2007 (1990) [2.03, 2.09].

Hirshfeld, *Should Ethical and Legal Standards for Physicians Be Changed to Accommodate New Models for Rationing Health Care?* 140 Univ. Pa. L. Rev. 1809, 1816 (1992) [2.03, 2.09, 4.04].

Hirshfeld, *Should Third Party Payors of Health Care Services Disclose Cost Control Mechanisms to Potential Beneficiaries?* 14 Seton Hall Legis. J. 115 (1990) [2.03, 2.09, 2.19, 4.04, 4.06, 8.03, 8.032].

Hirshfeld & Thomason, *Medical Necessity Determinations: The Need for a New Legal Structure*, 6 Health Matrix 3, 8-9 (1996) [I, II, III, IV, V, VI, VII; 2.03].

Ho, *Lessons From Laboratory Corp. of America Holdings v. Metabolite Laboratories, Inc.*, 23 Santa Clara Computer & High Tech. L. J. 463, 482 (2007) [9.095].

Ho, *Patents, Patients, and Public Policy: An Incomplete Intersection at 35 USC § 287(c)*, 33 U.C. Davis L. Rev. 601, 603, 623, 624, 625, 631 (2000) [V; 8.03, 9.08, 9.09, 10.01].

Hodges, Tolle, Stocking, & Cassel, *Tube Feeding: Internists' Attitudes Regarding Ethical Obligations*, 154 Arch. Intern. Med. 1013, 1020 (1994) [2.20].

Hoffmann, *Physicians Who Break the Law*, 53 St. Louis U. L. J. 1049 (2009) [1.02].

Hoffman, *Preplacement Examinations and Job-Relatedness: How to Enhance Privacy and Diminish Discrimination in the Workplace*, 49 U. Kan. L. Rev. 517, 534, 535, 556, 565 (2001) [2.132, 2.139].

Hoffman, *The Use of Placebos in Clinical Trials: Responsible Research or Unethical Practice?* 33 Conn. L. Rev. 449, 454-55, 496 (2001) [2.075].

Hoge, *APA Resource Document: I. The Professional Responsibilities of Psychiatrists in Evolving Health Care Systems*, 24 Bull. Am. Acad. Psychiatry Law 393, 405 (1996) [2.095, 8.13, 8.132].

Hoge, *APA Resource Document: II. Regulatory Guidelines for Protecting the Interests of Psychiatric Patients in Emerging Health Care Systems*, 24 Bull. Am. Acad. Psychiatry Law 407, 412, 418 (1996) [8.13].

Hoge, *Proposed Federal Legislation Jeopardizes Patient Privacy*, 23 Bull. Am. Acad. Psychiatry Law 495, 498, 500 (1995) [IV; 5.07].

Holland, *Should Parents Be Permitted to Authorize Genetic Testing for Their Children?* 31 Fam. L. Q. 321, 346-47 (1997) [2.132].

Holliday, *Traditional Medicines in Modern Societies: An Exploration of Integrationist Options Through East Asian Experience*, 28 J. Med. & Phil. 373, 387 (2003) [Preamble; V].

Holman & Jacoby, *Managing Medical Bills on the Brink of Bankruptcy*, 10 Yale J. Health Pol'y, L. & Ethics 239, 255 (2010) [6.08].

Horan & Grant, *The Legal Aspects of Withdrawing Nourishment*, 5 J. Legal Med. 595 (1984) [2.20].

Horner & Minifie, *Research Ethics III: Publication Practices and Authorship, Conflicts of Interest, and Research Misconduct*, 54 J. Speech, Language Hearing Res. S346, S351, S352 (2011) [VIII; 8.031].

Horstman, *Commuting Death Sentences of the Insane: A Solution for a Better, More Compassionate Society*, 36 USF.L. Rev. 823, 848 (2002) [2.06].

Hsu, *Legal Issues Concerning Retail Clinics*, 20 Health Law 13 (June 2008) [Preamble].

Huberfeld, *Be Not Afraid of Change: Time to Eliminate the Corporate Practice of Medicine Doctrine*, 14 Health Matrix 243, 256 (2004) [VI].

Huddle, *Medical Professionalism and Medical Education Should Not Involve Commitments to Political Advocacy*, 86 Acad. Med. 378, 379 (2011) [IX].

Hughes, *The Oregon Death with Dignity Act: Relief of Suffering at the End of Medicine's Ability to Heal*, 95 Geo. L. J. 207, 219 (2006) [2.211].

Hughes, *The Tri-chemical Cocktail: Serene Brutality*, 72 Alb. L. Rev. 527 (2009) [2.06].

Hughes, *The Uniform Mediation Act: To the Spoiled Go the Privileges*, 85 Marq. L. Rev. 9, 26 (2001) [5.05].

Hunter, *Justice Blackmun, Abortion, and the Myth of Medical Independence*, 72 Brooklyn L. Rev. 147, 190-91 (2006) [IV; 5.05].

Hunter, *Managed Process, Due Care: Structures of Accountability in Health Care*, 6 Yale J. Health Pol'y L. & Ethics 93, 107, 113 (2006) [8.05, 8.13].

Hurley, *Cashing in on the Transplant List: An Argument Against Offering Valuable Compensation for the Donation of Organs*, 4 J. High Tech. L. 117, 130 (2004) [2.151].

Hutchinson, *Marsingill v. O'Malley: The Duty to Disclose Becomes the Duty to Divine*, 25 Alaska L. Rev. 241 (2008) [8.08].

Hyams, *Expert Psychiatric Evidence in Sexual Misconduct Cases Before State Medical Boards*, XVIII Am. J. Law & Med. 171, 173, 174 (1992) [8.14].

Hyams, Shapiro, & Brennan, *Medical Practice Guidelines in Malpractice Litigation: An Early Retrospective*, 21 J. Health Pol. Pol'y & L. 289, 298 (1996) [8.16].

Hyman, *Getting the Haves to Come Out Behind: Fixing the Distributive Injustices of American Health Care*, 69 Law & Contemp. Probs. 265, 268-69 (2006) [6.01].

Hyman & Silver, *Just What the Patient Ordered: The Case for Result-Based Compensation Arrangements*, 29 J. L. Med. & Ethics 170, 170 (2001) [6.01].

Hyman & Silver, *The Poor State of Health Care Quality in the U.S.: Is Malpractice Liability Part of the Problem or Part of the Solution?* 90 Cornell L. Rev. 893, 926, 965 (2005) [6.01, 8.12].

Hyman & Silver, *You Get What You Pay For: Result-Based Compensation for Health Care*, 58 Wash. & Lee L. Rev. 1427, 1459, 1460, 1461, 1481-82 (2001) [6.01, 9.121, 9.122].

Iffy, Varadi, Portuondo, & Ende, *Collection of Fetal Blood for Stem Cell Research and Therapy*, 25 Med. & L. 553, 555 (2006) [2.165].

Iheukwumere, *Doctor, Are You Experienced? The Relevance of Disclosure of Physician Experience to a Valid Informed Consent*, 18 J. Contemp. Health L. & Pol'y 373, 376-77 (2002) [II; 8.12].

Iheukwumere, *HIV-Positive Medical Practitioners: Legal and Ethical Obligations to Disclose*, 71 St. John's L. Rev. 715, 732-34 (1997) [9.13, 9.131].

Ikemoto, *The Fuzzy Logic of Race and Gender in the Mismeasure of Asian American Women's Health Needs*, 65 U. Cin. L. Rev. 799, 800, 804, 810 (1997) [9.121, 9.122].

Ile, *Should Physicians Treat Patients Who Seek Second Opinions?* 266 JAMA 273, 274 (1991) [6.11, 9.02, 9.06, 9.12].

Isaacman & Miller, *Neonatal HIV Seroprevalence Studies*, 14 J. Legal Med. 413, 428 (1993) [2.07].

Iserson, Heine, Larkin, Moskop, Baruch, & Aswegan, *Fight or Flight: The Ethics of Emergency Physician Disaster Response*, 51 Annals of Emergency Med. 345, 346-47 (2008) [Preamble; 2.25, 9.067, 9.131].

Jacobi, *Patients at a Loss: Protecting Health Care Consumers Through Data Driven Quality Assurance*, 45 U. Kan. L. Rev. 705, 720, 721, 759 (1997) [2.03, 2.09, 8.13].

Jacobs & Goodman, *Splitting Fees or Splitting Hairs? Fee Splitting and Health Care—The Florida Experience*, 8 Annals Health L. 239, 244 (1999) [6.02].

Jacoby, *Show Me the Money: Making Markets in Forbidden Exchange: The Debt Financing of Parenthood*, 72 Law & Contemp. Prob. 147 (2009) [6.01].

Javitt, Stanley, & Hudson, *Direct-to-Consumer Genetic Tests, Government Oversight, and the First Amendment: What the Government Can (and Can't) Do to Protect the Public's Health*, 57 Okla. L. Rev. 251, 280 (2004) [5.015].

Jecker, *Genetic Testing and the Social Responsibility of Private Health Insurance Companies*, 21 J. Law Med. & Ethics 109, 112 (1993) [2.132].

Jecker, *Privacy Beliefs and the Violent Family: Extending the Ethical Argument for Physician Intervention*, 269 JAMA 776, 778, 779 (1993) [IV; 5.05, 8.14, 9.131].

Jecker & Schneiderman, *An Ethical Analysis of the Use of "Futility" in the 1992 American Heart Association Guidelines for Cardiopulmonary Resuscitation and Emergency Cardiac Care*, 153 Arch. Intern. Med. 2195, 2197 (1993) [2.22].

Jensen, *Organ Procurement: Various Legal Systems and Their Effectiveness*, 22 Hous. J. Int'l L. 555, 578 (2000) [2.15].

Jerdee, *Breaking Through the Silence: Minnesota's Pregnancy Presumption and the Right to Refuse Medical Treatment*, 84 Minn. L. Rev. 971, 980 (2000) [2.20].

Jesson & Knapp, *My Lawyer Told Me to Say I'm Sorry: Lawyers, Doctors, and Medical Apologies*, 35 Wm. Mitchell L. Rev. 1410 (2009). [8.121].

Johns, *Multidisciplinary Practice and Ethics Part II— Lawyers, Doctors, and Confidentiality*, 6 NAELA J. 55, 57-65, 68 (2010) [IV; 2.02, 2.23, 2.24, 5.05].

Johnson, *ERISA Doctor in the House? The Duty to Disclose Physician Incentives to Limit Health Care*, 82 Minn. L. Rev. 1631, 1639, 1649, 1655 (1998) [8.13, 8.132].

Johnson, *Habit and Discernment in Abortion Practice: The Partial-Birth Abortion Ban Act of 2003 as Morals Legislation*, 36 Rutgers L. J. 549, 582 (2005) [2.211].

Johnson, *Harm to the "Fabric of Society" as a Basis for Regulating Otherwise Harmless Conduct: Notes on a Theme From Ravin v. State*, 27 Seattle U. L. Rev. 41, 55 (2003) [2.211].

Johnson, *HIV Testing of Health Care Workers: Conflict Between the Common Law and the Centers for Disease Control*, 42 Am. Univ. L. Rev. 479, 518 (1993) [9.131].

Johnson, *"I Will Not Divulge": How to Resolve the "Mass of Legal Confusion" Surrounding the Physician-Patient Relationship in West Virginia*, 110 W. Va. L. Rev. 1231 (2008) [IV; 5.05].

Johnson, *Judicial Review of Disciplinary Action for Sexual Misconduct in the Practice of Medicine*, 270 JAMA 1596 (1993) [8.14].

Johnson, *Keeping a Critical Eye on Chiropractic*, 31 J. of Manipulative and Physiological Therapeutics 559, 559 (2008) [1.01, 1.02, 3.01, 5.02].

Johnson, *Minnesota's "Crack Baby" Law: Weapon of War or Link in a Chain?* 8 Law & Ineq. 485, 494, 495, 496 (1990) [8.08].

Johnson, *Polluting Medical Judgment? False Assumptions in the Pursuit of False Claims Regarding Off-Label Prescribing*, 9 Minn. J. L. Sci. & Tech. 61 (2009) [8.06].

Johnson, *The Death-Prolonging Procedures Act and Refusal of Treatment in Missouri*, 30 St. Louis Univ. L. J. 805 (1986) [2.19].

Johnson, Gibbons, Goldner, Wiener, & Eton, *Legal and Institutional Policy Responses to Medical Futility*, 30 J. Health & Hosp. L. 21, 26, 31, 35, 36 (1997) [2.035, 2.22].

Johnson, Grasso, & Maslowski, *Conflicts Between Ethics and Law for Military Mental Health Providers*, 175 Mil. Med. 548, 549 (2010) [1.02].

Jones, *Battered Spouses' Damage Actions Against Non-Reporting Physicians*, 45 DePaul L. Rev. 191 (1996) [2.02].

Jones, *Kentucky Tort Liability for Failure to Report Family Violence*, 26 N. Ky. L. Rev. 43, 58 (1999) [2.02].

Jones, *Primum Non Nocere: The Expanding "Honest Services" Mail Fraud Statute and the Physician-Patient Fiduciary Relationship*, 51 Vand. L. Rev. 139, 161, 164 (1998) [2.03, 8.03, 8.06].

Jones & McCullough, *What to Do When a Patient's International Medical Care Goes South*, 46 J. of Vascular Surgery 1077, 1078 (2007) [VI].

Joralemon, *Shifting Ethics: Debating the Incentive Question in Organ Transplantation*, 27 J. Med. Ethics 30, 31, 34 (2001) [2.15].

Jordan, *Financial Conflicts of Interest in Human Subjects Research: Proposals for a More Effective Regulatory Scheme*, 60 Wash. & Lee L. Rev. 15, 23 (2003) [9.095].

Jost, *Confronting Conflict: Addressing Institutional Conflicts of Interest in Academic Medical Centers*, 36 Am. J. L. & Med. 326, 336 (2010) [8.061].

Jost, *Health Law and Administrative Law: A Marriage Most Convenient*, 49 St. Louis U. L. J. 1, 20 (2004) [8.14].

Jost & Davies, *The Empire Strikes Back: A Critique of the Backlash Against Fraud and Abuse Enforcement*, 51 Ala. L. Rev. 239, 240 (1999) [II].

Joynt, *Neurology*, 263 JAMA 2660 (1990) [2.161].

Jozefowicz, *The Case Against Having Professional Privilege in the Physician-Patient Relationship*, 16 Med. & L. 385, 386-87, 391 (1997) [Preamble; IV; 5.05].

Judge, *Issues Surrounding the Patenting of Medical Procedures*, 13 Santa Clara Computer & High Tech. L. J. 181, 202-03 (1997) [9.08, 9.095].

Judges, *The Role of Mental Health Professionals in Capital Punishment: An Exercise in Moral Disengagement*, 41 Hous. L. Rev. 515, 562, 568, 569, 570, 571-72, 581, 586, 588, 598 (2004) [Preamble; 1.01, 1.02, 2.06, 2.067, 2.20, 2.21, 2.211, 8.14].

Jung, Lurie, & Wolfe, *U.S. Physicians Disciplined for Criminal Activity*, 16 Health Matrix 335, 335 (2006) [II, III].

Jurevic, *Disparate Impact Under Title VI: Discrimination, by Any Other Name, Will Still Have the Same Impact*, 15 St. Louis U. Pub. L. Rev. 237, 253 (1996) [2.03].

Jurevic, *When Technology and Health Care Collide: Issues With Electronic Medical Records and Electronic Mail*, 66 UMKC L. Rev. 809, 819-20 (1998) [5.05, 5.07].

Kachalia, Choudhry, & Studdert, *Physician Responses to the Malpractice Crisis: From Defense to Offense*, 33 J. L. Med. & Ethics 416, 419, 421, 424 (2005) [VIII; 9.025, 10.015].

Kallmyer, *A Chimera in Every Sense: Standard of Care for Physicians Practicing Complementary and Alternative Medicine*, 2 Ind. Health L. Rev. 225, 229, 231 (2005) [10.01, 10.02].

Kalt, *Death, Ethics, and the State*, 23 Harv. J. L. & Pub. Pol'y 487, 537, 539 (2000) [2.211].

Kamisar, *On the Meaning and Impact of the Physician-Assisted Suicide Cases*, 82 Minn. L. Rev. 895, 909, 918 (1998) [2.211].

Kamisar, *When Is There A Constitutional "Right to Die?" When Is There No Constitutional "Right to Live?"*, 25 Georgia L. Rev. 1203, 1207, 1208, 1222 (1991) [2.20].

Kane, *Driving Into the Sunset: A Proposal for Mandatory Reporting to the DMV by Physicians Treating Unsafe Elderly Drivers*, 25 U. Haw. L. Rev. 59, 59, 61, 62, 67, 69, 82, 83 (2002) [1.02, 2.24, 5.05, 10.01].

Kane, *Information Is the Key to Patient Empowerment*, 11 Annals Health L. 25, 29-30, 44 (2002) [V; 10.01, 10.02].

Kao & Linden, *Direct-to-Consumer Advertising and the Internet: Informational Privacy, Product Liability and Organizational Responsibility*, 46 St. Louis U. L. J. 157, 170 (2002) [5.015].

Kapp, *Drug Companies, Dollars, and the Shaping of American Medical Practice*, 29 S. Ill. U. L. J. 237, 249 (2005) [8.061].

Kapp, *Legal Standards for the Medical Diagnosis and Treatment of Dementia*, 23 J. Legal Med. 359, 382 (2002) [2.24].

Kapp, *Conscripted Physician Services and the Public's Health*, 39 J.L. Med. & Ethics 414 (2011) [2.09, 9.06, 10.015].

Kapp, *Patient Autonomy in the Age of Consumer-Driven Health Care: Informed Consent and Informed Choice*, 2 J. Health & Biomedical L. 1, 5 (2006) [10.01].

Kapp, *Physicians' Legal Duties Regarding the Use of Genetic Tests to Predict and Diagnose Alzheimer Disease*, 21 J. Legal Med. 445, 456-57, 465-66 (2000) [2.132, 2.139, 8.032].

Kapp, *Placebo Therapy and the Law: Prescribe With Care*, 8 Am. J. Law & Med. 371 (1983) [8.08, 8.12].

Kaserman, *Fifty Years of Organ Transplants: The Successes and the Failures*, 23 Issues L. & Med. 45, 60 (2007) [2.151].

Kass & Lund, *Physician-Assisted Suicide, Medical Ethics and the Future of the Medical Profession*, 35 Duq. L. Rev. 395, 404 (1996) [2.211].

Kassel, *Counterpoint . . . Defense Counsel's Ex Parte Communication With Plaintiff's Doctors: A Bad One-Sided Deal*, 9 S.C. Law. 42, 43 (Sept./Oct. 1997) [IV; 5.05].

Kassirer, *Managing Care Should We Adopt a New Ethic?* 339 New Eng. J. Med. 397 (1998) [8.13].

Katner, *Confidentiality and Juvenile Mental Health Records in Dependency Proceedings*, 12 Wm. & Mary Bill of Rts. J. 511, 529 (2004) [IV].

Katner, *The Ethical Dilemma Awaiting Counsel Who Represent Adolescents with HIV/AIDS: Criminal Law and Tort Suits Pressure Counsel to Breach the Confidentiality of the Clients' Medical Status*, 70 Tul. L. Rev. 2311, 2341 (1996) [5.05].

Katz, *Informed Consent—Must It Remain a Fairy Tale?* 10 J. Contemp. Health L. & Pol'y 69, 80 (1994) [8.08].

Katz, *The Pregnant Child's Right to Self-determination*, 62 Alb. L. Rev. 1119, 1142 (1999) [2.015].

Kaufman, *The Demise of Medical Malpractice Screening Panels and Alternative Solutions Based on Trust and Honesty*, 28 J. Legal Med. 247, 250 (2007) [10.015].

Keim, *Physicians for Professional Sports Teams: Health Care Under the Pressure of Economic and Commercial Interests*, 9 Seton Hall. J. Sport L. 196, 218-19 (1999) [3.06].

Kelley, *The Meanings of Professional Life: Teaching Across the Health Professions*, 27 J. Med. & Phil. 475, 485, 490, 491 (2002) [2.161, 8.13].

Kelly, *The "Right to Die" in America: The Ninth Circuit's Decision in Compassion in Dying v. The State of Washington*, 29 J. Health & Hosp. L. 246, 255 (1996) [2.211].

Kelly & Robinson, *Disclosure of Membership in the Lesbian, Gay, Bisexual, and Transgender Community by Individuals With Communication Impairments: A Preliminary Web-Based Survey*, 20 Am. J. Speech-Language Pathology 86, 90 (2011) [VI].

Kenworthy, *The Austrian Psychotherapy Act: No Legal Duty to Warn*, 11 Ind. Int'l & Comp. L. Rev. 469, 480-81, 485, 490, 496 (2001) [2.23, 5.05, 5.06].

Kerr, Hays, Mittman, Siu, Leake, & Brook, *Primary Care Physicians' Satisfaction With Quality of Care in California Capitated Medical Groups*, 278 JAMA 308, 312 (1997) [8.13].

Kesselheim & Mello, *Medical-Process Patents—Monopolizing the Delivery of Health Care*, 355 New Eng. J. Med. 2036, 2036 (2006) [9.095].

Keyes, *The Choice of Participation by Physicians in Capital Punishment*, 22 Whittier L. Rev. 809, 810-11, 838 (2001) [2.06].

Khan, *Taking Ownership of Legal Outcomes: An Argument Against Dissociation Paradigm and Analytical Gaming*, 55 St. Louis U. L.J. 887 (2011) [1.02].

Khan & Lea, *Paging King Solomon: Towards Allowing Organ Donation From Anencephalic Infants*, 6 Ind. Health L. Rev. 17 (2009) [2.147, 2.162].

Khanna, Silverman, & Schwartz, *Disclosure of Operating Practices by Managed-Care Organizations to Consumers of Healthcare: Obligations of Informed Consent*, 9 J. Clinical Ethics 291, 293, 296 (1998) [8.13].

Kibler, *Administrative Law*, 38 U. Rich. L. Rev. 39, 47 (2003) [8.181].

Kimbler, *Psychotic Journeys of the Green Mile*, 22 T.M. Cooley L. Rev. 27, 48 (2005) [2.06].

King, *The Standard of Care for Residents and Other Medical School Graduates in Training*, 55 Am. U. L. Rev. 683, 727 (2006) [8.16].

Kinney, *Hospital Peer Review of Physicians: Does Statutory Immunity Increase Risk of Unwarranted Professional Injury?* 13 Mich. St. U. J. Med. & L. 57 (2009) [9.045].

Kinney, *Procedural Protections for Patients in Capitated Health Plans*, XXII Am. J. Law & Med. 301, 319-20 (1996) [8.13].

Kinney, *Tapping and Resolving Consumer Concerns About Health Care*, 26 Am. J. Law & Med. 335, 337, 375 (2000) [VI; 8.13, 9.065].

Kinney, *The Corporate Transformation of Medical Specialty Care: The Exemplary Case of Neonatology*, 36 J. L. Med. & Ethics 790 (2008) [9.02].

Kinney & Clark, *Provisions for Health and Health Care in the Constitutions of the Countries of the World*, 37 Cornell Int'l L. J. 285, 289 (2004) [2.095].

Kinney, McCabe, Gilbert, & Shisler, *Altered Standards of Care for Health Care Providers in the Pandemic Influenza*, 6 Ind. Health L. Rev. 1 (2009) [9.067].

Kinney & Sage, *Resolving Medical Malpractice Claims in the Medicare Program: Can It Be Done?* 12 Conn. Ins. L. J. 77, 105 (2006) [8.082].

Kinney & Selby, *History and Jurisprudence of the Physician-Patient Relationship in Indiana*, 30 Ind. L. Rev. 263, 269, 272, 276 (1997) [2.20, 8.08, 9.06, 9.12].

Kirschenbaum & Kuhlik, *Federal and State Laws Affecting Discounts, Rebates, and Other Marketing Practices for Drugs and Devices*, 47 Food & Drug L. J. 533, 560 (1992) [8.06, 8.061].

Klein, *An Analysis of the Death Penalty Jurisprudence of the October 2007 Supreme Court Term*, 25 Touro L. Rev. 625 (2009) [2.06].

Klein, *Death Penalty and Right to Counsel Decisions in the October 2005 Term*, 22 Touro L. Rev. 1003, 1012 (2007) [2.06].

Kleinman, *Health Care in Crisis: A Proposed Role for the Individual Physician as Advocate*, 265 JAMA 1991 (1991) [9.121].

Klimkina, *Are Noncompete Contracts Between Physicians Bad Medicine? Advocating in the Affirmative by Drawing a Public Policy Parallel to the Legal Profession*, 98 Ky. L. J. 131, 147-148 (2010) [9.02, 9.06].

Klocke, *Prescription Records for Sale: Privacy and Free Speech Issues Arising From the Sale of De-identified Medical Data*, 44 Idaho L. Rev. 511 (2008) [5.05].

Knaplund, *Postmortem Conception and a Father's Last Will*, 46 Ariz. L. Rev. 91, 96 (2004) [2.04].

Kolder & Julian, *Teaching About Sexual Minorities: An Iowa Experience*, 1 Proc. Obstetrics Gynecology 1 (April 2010, Article 10) [VI].

Koniak, *The Law Between the Bar and the State*, 70 No. Carolina L. Rev. 1389, 1396 (1992) [1.02].

Koons, *Physician Employee Non-Compete Agreements on the Examining Table: The Need to Better Protect Patients' and the Public's Interests in Indiana*, 6 Ind. Health L. Rev. 253 (2009) [IV, VI, VII; 5.02, 8.041, 8.115, 9.02, 9.06, 9.065, 9.067, 9.09, 10.01, 10.015].

Kramer, Gruenberg, & Fidler, *Psychiatrists' Attitudes Toward Physician-Assisted Suicide: A Survey*, 19 Am. J. Forensic Psychiatry 81, 87, 90 (1998) [2.06, 2.20].

Krause, *"Promises to Keep": Health Care Providers and the Civil False Claims Act*, 23 Cardozo L. Rev. 1363, 1365 (2002) [I, II, IV].

Krause, *The Brief Life of the Gag Clause: Why Antigag Clause Legislation Isn't Enough*, 67 Tenn. L. Rev. 1, 4, 43 (1999) [8.13].

Kreitzberg & Richter, *But Can It Be Fixed? A Look at Constitutional Challenges to Lethal Injection Executions*, 47 Santa Clara L. Rev. 445, 448, 449, 499, 502 (2007) [2.06].

Krishnan, Diette, Skinner, Clark, Steinwachs, & Wu, *Race and Sex Differences in Consistency of Care With National Asthma Guidelines in Managed Care Organizations*, 161 Arch. Intern. Med. 1660, 1660 (2001) [9.122].

Krumm, *Genetic Discrimination: Why Congress Must Ban Genetic Testing in the Workplace*, 23 J. Legal Med. 491, 506 (2002) [2.20].

Kruse, *A Call for New Perspectives for Living Wills (You Might Like It Here)*, 37 Real Prop., Prob. & Tr. J. 545, 550 (2002) [2.035].

Kumar & Kinney, *Indiana Lawmakers Face National Health Policy Issues*, 25 Indiana L. Rev. 1271, 1275, 1276 (1992) [2.20].

Kurfirst, *The Duty to Disclose HMO Physician Incentives*, 13 (3) Health Law 18, 18, 22 (2001) [8.132].

Kurtz, *The Law of Informed Consent: From "Doctor Is Right" to "Patient Has Rights,"* 50 Syracuse L. Rev. 1243, 1245 (2000) [8.08].

Kutzko, Boyer, Thoman, & Scott, *HIPAA in Real Time: Practical Implications of the Federal Privacy Rule*, 51 Drake L. Rev. 403, 408 (2003) [5.05, 5.055, 5.057, 5.06, 5.07, 5.075, 5.08, 5.09].

Kwiecinski, *Limiting Conflicts of Interest Arising From Physician Investment in Specialty Hospitals*, 88 Marq. L. Rev. 413, 414, 428 (2004) [8.032].

Kwiecinski, *To Be or Not to Be, Should Doctors Decide? Ethical and Legal Aspects of Medical Futility Policies,* 7 Marq. Elder's Advisor 313, 323-24 (2006) [2.037].

Labowitz, *Beyond Tarasoff: AIDS and the Obligation to Breach Confidentiality,* 9 St. Louis Univ. Pub. L. Rev. 495, 514 (1990) [2.23].

Lafferty, *Statutory and Ethical Barriers in the Patenting of Medical and Surgical Procedures,* 29 J. Marshall L. Rev. 891, 912 (1996) [9.08].

Landis, *The Team Physician: An Analysis of the Causes of Action, Conflicts, Defenses and Improvements,* 1 DePaul J. Sports L. & Contemp. Probs. 139, 144 (2003) [I, II].

Landfair, *Transforming Physicians Into Business Savvy Entrepreneurs: Patient Surcharges Charge Onto the Scene of Physician Reimbursement,* 43 Duq. L. Rev. 257, 268, 269 (2005) [IX; 6.12].

Langston, *Ethical Treatment of Military Detainees,* 370 Lancet 1999, 1999 (2007) [2.067, 2.068].

Langwell & Moser, *Strategies for Medicare Health Plans Serving Racial and Ethnic Minorities,* 23 Health Care Financing Rev. 131, 134, 146 (2002) [9.121].

Lapertosa, *End of Life Decision Making: The Right to Die? Preventing the "Right to Refuse" From Becoming a License to Kill: Adopting a Constitutional Minimum Standard for Approving Withdrawal of Life Support for Legally Incompetent Patients,* 15 Temp. Pol. & Civ. Rts. L. Rev. 483, 488 (2006) [2.211].

Larson, *Prescription for Death: A Second Opinion,* 44 DePaul L. Rev. 461, 472 (1995) [2.21, 2.211].

Larson, *Tales of Death: Storytelling in the Physician-Assisted Suicide Litigation,* 39 Washburn L. J. 159, 177 (2000) [2.211].

Lasken, *The Incoherent Right to Die,* 4 NAELA J. 167 (2008) [2.20].

Laufer-Ukeles, *Reproductive Choices and Informed Consent: Fetal Interests, Women's Identity, and Relational Autonomy,* 37 Am. J. L. & Med. 567, 575 (2011) [10.01, 10.02].

Laurie, *Challenging Medical-Legal Norms: The Role of Autonomy, Confidentiality, and Privacy in Protecting Individual and Familial Group Rights in Genetic Information,* 22 J. Legal Med. 1, 24 (2001) [IV; 10.01].

Law, *Silent No More: Physicians' Legal and Ethical Obligations to Patients Seeking Abortions,* 21 N. Y. U. Rev. L. & Soc. Change 279, 289, 290, 300 (1994) [3.04, 8.04].

Lazzarini, *An Analysis of Ethical Issues in Prescribing and Dispensing Syringes to Injection Drug Users,* 11 Health Matrix 85, 107, 119 (2001) [III; 1.02, 5.05].

LeBlanc, *Abandoning Patients and Clients: Where Medicine Can Learn From Law,* 1 Charleston L. Rev. 237, 237-38, 256 (2007) [Preamble; 8.115].

LeBlang, *Obligations of HIV-Infected Health Professionals to Inform Patients of Their Serological Status: Evolving Theories of Liability,* 27 J. Marshall L. Rev. 317, 318 (1994) [9.131].

LeDoux, *Interspousal Liability and the Wrongful Transmission of HIV-AIDS: An Argument for Broadening Legal Avenues for the Injured Spouse and Further Expanding Children's Rights to Sue Their Parents,* 34 New Eng. L. Rev. 392, 411 (2000) [9.131].

Lee, *35 USC §287(c)—The Physician Immunity Statute,* 79 J. Pat. & Trademark Off. Soc'y 701, 702-04 (1997) [9.095].

Leflar, *Advance Health Care Directives Under Arkansas Law,* 1994 Ark. L. Notes 37, 42. [2.20].

LeGros & Pinkall, *The New JCAHO Patient Safety Standards and the Disclosure of Unanticipated Outcomes,* 35 J. Health L. 189, 203 (2002) [8.12].

Lemmens & Miller, *The Human Subjects Trade: Ethical and Legal Issues Surrounding Recruitment Incentives,* 31 J. L. Med. & Ethics 398, 407 (2003) [6.03, 8.031].

Lenrow, *The Treating Physician as Researcher: Is Assuming This Dual Role a Violation of the Nuremberg Code?* 25 Temp. J. Sci. Tech. & Envtl. L. 15, 42-43 (2006) [8.115, 10.015].

Leppert, *Doreika v. Blotner: Affirming Ketchup Against Judicial Mustard,* 60 Mercer L. Rev. 807 (2009) [8.08, 8.15].

Lerman, *Second Opinion: Inconsistent Deference to Medical Ethics in Death Penalty Jurisprudence,* 95 Geo. L. J. 1941, 1945, 1974-75, 1976, 1977 (2007) [I; 2.06, 4.01, 5.02, 7.05].

Leubsdorf, *Against Lawyer Retaining Liens,* 72 Fordham L. Rev. 849, 864, 865 (2004) [7.02, 8.10].

Levine, *Medicalization of Psychoactive Substance Use and the Doctor-Patient Relationship,* 69 Milbank Quarterly 623, 624 (1991) [III].

Levitt & Ryan, *Not Competent to Be Executed: Dilemmas Faced by Psychiatrists and Attorneys*, 23 Am. J. Forensic Psych. 39, 47 (July 2002) [2.06].

Levy, *Because Judges Went to Law School, Not Medical School: Restrictive Covenants in the Practices of Law and Medicine*, 30 J. Health & Hosp. L. 89, 92, 101 (1997) [9.02].

Levy, *Collective Bargaining in the Elite Professions—Doctors' Application of the Labor Law Model to Negotiations With Health Plan Providers*, 13 U. Fla. J. L. & Pub. Pol'y 269, 277 (2002) [II].

Levy, *Conflict of Duty: Capital Punishment Regulations and AMA Medical Ethics*, 26 J. Legal Med. 261, 268, 269, 270, 273 (2005) [2.01, 2.06, 2.21].

Levy, *Gonzales v. Oregon and Physician-Assisted Suicide: Ethical and Policy Issues*, 42 Tulsa L. Rev. 699, 699 (2007) [2.211].

Liang & Mackey, *Confronting Conflict: Addressing Institutional Conflicts of Interest in Academic Medical Centers*, 36 Am. J. L. & Med. 136, 149 (2010) [8.061].

Liang & Ren, *Medical Liability Insurance and Damage Caps: Getting Beyond Band Aids to Substantive Systems Treatment to Improve Quality and Safety in Healthcare*, 30 Am. J. L. & Med. 501, 534 (2004) [8.12].

Liddle, *Gene Patents: The Controversy and the Law in the Wake of Myriad*, 44 Suffolk U. L. Rev. 683, 686 (2011) [9.095].

Lieberman & Derse, *HIV-Positive Health Care Workers and the Obligation to Disclose: Do Patients Have a Right to Know?* 13 J. Legal Med. 333, 353, 354, (1992) [8.03, 8.032, 9.131].

Linder & Meyers, *"Don't Let Me Die in Prison"—Palliative Care for Prison Inmates*, 298 JAMA 894, 898 (2007) [5.059].

Liner, *Physician Deselection: The Dynamics of a New Threat to the Physician-Patient Relationship*, 23 Am. J. Law & Med. 511, 513, 527 (1997) [I, III; 8.05, 8.13].

Lininger, *From Park Place to Community Chest: Rethinking Lawyers' Monopoly*, 101 Nw. U. L. Rev. 1343, 1349 (2007) [9.065, 10.01].

Lipschitz, *Psychiatry and Consent for Physician-Assisted Suicide*, 19 Am. J. Forensic Psychiatry 91, 103, 104 (1998) [2.06, 2.211].

Lipsky, *Dealing With the NFL's Concussion Problems of Yesterday, Today, and Tomorrow*, 18 Fordham Intell. Prop. Media & Ent. L. J. 959 (2008) [3.06].

Liu & Sato, *Patent Protection of Medical Methods—Focusing on Ethical Issues*, 20 Pac. Rim. L. & Pol'y J. 125, 135 (2011) [V].

Livingston, *When Libido Subverts Credo: Regulation of Attorney-Client Sexual Relations*, 62 Fordham L. Rev. 5, 55 (1993) [8.14].

Lloyd, *Primum Non Nocere: Singleton v. Norris and the Ethical Dilemma of Medicating the Condemned*, 58 Ark. L. Rev. 225, 232, 233 (2005) [VIII; 1.02, 2.06].

Lockhart, *The Safest Care Is to Deny Care: Implications of Corporate Health Insurance, Inc. v. Texas Department of Insurance on HMO Liability in Texas*, 41 S. Tex. L. Rev. 621, 628, 634 (2000) [8.13].

Loeser, *The Legal, Ethical, and Practical Implications of Noncompetition Clauses: What Physicians Should Know Before They Sign*, 31 J. L. Med. & Ethics 283, 286, 287, 290 (2003) [9.02, 9.06, 10.01, 10.015].

Loftus, Paddock, & Guernsey, *Patient-Psychotherapist Privilege: Access to Clinical Records in the Tangled Web of Repressed Memory Litigation*, 30 U. Rich L. Rev. 109, 127 (1996) [IV; 5.05].

Lonchyna, *To Resuscitate or Not . . . In the Operating Room: The Need for Hospital Policies for Surgeons Regarding DNR Orders*, 6 Annals Health L. 209, 215, 217 (1997) [2.22, 8.08].

Loue, *Access to Health Care and the Undocumented Alien*, 13 J. Legal Med. 271, 291 (1992) [VI, VII].

Loue, *Intimate Partner Violence: Bridging the Gap Between Law and Science*, 21 J. Legal Med. 1, 18 (2000) [2.02].

Lubet, *Expert Witnesses: Ethics and Professionalism*, 12 Geo. J. Legal Ethics 465, 466 (1999) [IV].

Luetkemeyer, *Who's Guarding the Henhouse and What Are They Doing With the Eggs (and Sperm)? A Call for Increased Regulation of Gamete Donation and Long-Term Tracking of Donor Gametes*, 3 St. Louis U. J. Health L. & Pol'y 397, 414 (2010) [VIII].

Luna, *Sovereignty and Suspicion*, 48 Duke L. J. 787, 884 (1999) [2.132].

Lund, *The President as Client and the Ethics of the President's Lawyers*, 61 L. & Contemp. Probs. 65, 68 (1998) [IV].

Lundmark, *Surgery by an Unauthorized Surgeon as a Battery*, 10 J. L. & Health 287, 293 (1996) [8.16].

Lunstroth, *Voluntary Self-regulation of Complementary and Alternative Medicine Practitioners*, 70 Alb. L. Rev. 209, 243 (2006) [8.06, 8.062].

Lyons, *In Incognito—The Principle of Double Effect in American Constitutional Law*, 57 Fla. L. Rev. 469, 474 (2005) [2.20].

MacDonald, *Organ Donation: The Time Has Come to Refocus the Ethical Spotlight*, 8 Stan. L. & Pol'y Rev. 177, 179, 185 (1997) [2.155].

Mack & Sade, *Relations Between Cardiothoracic Surgeons and Industry*, 87 Ann. Thorac. Surg. 1334, 1335 (2009) [8.061].

Madison, *ERISA and Liability for Provision of Medical Information*, 84 N. C. L. Rev. 471, 540 (2006) [8.053, 8.135].

Madow, *Forbidden Spectacle: Executions, the Public and the Press in Nineteenth Century New York*, 43 Buff. L. Rev. 461, 475 (1995) [2.06].

Maerz, *Death of the Challenge to Lethal Injection? Missouri's Protocol Deemed Constitutional Yet Again*, 75 Mo. L. Rev. 1323, 1340-41 (2010) [2.06].

Mahoney, *The Market for Human Tissue*, 86 Va. L. Rev. 163, 179 (2000) [2.15].

Mahowald, *Aren't We All Eugenicists? Commentary on Paul Lombardo's "Taking Eugenics Seriously,"* 30 Fla. St. U. L. Rev. 219, 234 (2003) [2.12].

Maizlin, Barnard, Gourlayz, & Brown, *Economic and Ethical Impact of Extrarenal Findings on Potential Living Kidney Donor Assessment with Computed Tomography Angiography*, 20 Transplant Int'l. 338, 341 (2007) [VIII].

Makar, *Domestic Violence: Why the Florida Legislature Must Do More to Protect the "Silent" Victims*, 72 Fla. Bar J. 10, 16 (Nov. 1998) [2.02].

Malinowski, *Capitation, Advances in Medical Technology, and the Advent of a New Era in Medical Ethics*, XXII Am. J. Law & Med. 331, 337 (1996) [2.09].

Malinowski, *Conflicts of Interest in Clinical Research: Legal and Ethical Issues: Institutional Conflicts and Responsibilities in an Age of Academic-Industry Alliances*, 8 Wid. L. Symp. J. 47, 70 (2001) [8.031].

Malinowski, *Dealing With the Realities of Race and Ethnicity: A Bioethics-Centered Argument in Favor of Race-Based Genetics Research*, 45 Hous. L. Rev. 1415 (2009) [8.08].

Malinowski, *Law, Policy, and Market Implications of Genetic Profiling in Drug Development*, 2 Hous. J. Health L. & Pol'y 31, 51 (2002) [8.031].

Malloy, *Physician Restrictive Covenants: The Neglect of Incumbent Patient Interests*, 41 Wake Forest L. Rev. 189, 207-08, 217, 218 (2006) [6.11, 8.11, 8.115, 9.02, 9.06].

Malone, *Medical Authority and Infanticide*, 1 J. Law & Health 77 (1985-86) [2.17].

Maloney, *The Management of Ixodes scapularis Bites in the Upper Midwest*, 110 World Med. J. 78, 80 (2011) [10.01, 10.02].

Mancino, *New GCM Suggests Rules for Ventures Between Nonprofit Hospitals and Doctors*, 76 J. Taxation 164, 167 (1992) [8.032].

Manian, *The Irrational Woman: Informed Consent and Abortion Decision-Making*, 16 Duke J. Gender L. & Pol'y 223 (2009) [8.08].

Manthous, *Counterpoint: Is It Ethical to Order "Do Not Resuscitate" Without Patient Consent?* 132 Chest 751, 753 (2007) [2.035].

Mareiniss, *A Comparison of Cruzan and Schiavo: The Burden of Proof, Due Process, and Autonomy in the Persistently Vegetative Patient*, 26 J. Legal Med. 233, 248, 250 (2005) [2.035, 2.20].

Marks, *Doctors as Pawns? Law and Medical Ethics at Guantanamo Bay*, 37 Seton Hall L. Rev. 711, 725 (2007) [2.068].

Mars, *The Corporate Practice of Medicine: A Call for Action*, 7 Health Matrix 241, 267 (1997) [VI].

Marsh, *Sacrificing Patients for Profits: Physician Incentives to Limit Care and ERISA Fiduciary Duty*, 77 Wash. U. L. Q. 1323, 1332 (1999) [8.03].

Marshall, O'Keefe, Fisher, Caruso, & Surdukowski, *Patients' Fear of Contracting the Acquired Immune Deficiency Syndrome From Physicians*, 150 Arch. Intern. Med. 1501, 1505 (1990) [9.131].

Martens, *Necessity of Adapting Psychiatric Treatment to Relevant Ethical Guidelines*, 20 Med. Law 393, 394 (2001) [VII].

Martin, *Hugs and Drugs: Research Ethics, Conflict of Interest, and Why the FDA's Attempt to Preempt Pharma Failure-to-Warn Claims Is a Dangerous Prescription,* 6 Ave Maria L. Rev. 587 (2008) [10.015].

Martin, *Legal Malpractice: Negligent Referral as a Cause of Action,* 29 Cumb. L. Rev. 679, 686 (1999) [8.132].

Martin, *Patentability of Methods of Medical Treatment: A Comparative Study,* 82 J. Pat. & Trademark Off. Soc'y 381, 383-84, 388, 423 (2000) [9.08, 9.09, 9.095].

Martin, *Tessie Hutchinson and the American System of Capital Punishment,* 59 Md. L. Rev. 553, 565 (2000) [2.06].

Martin, *Who Will Take the Keys From Grandpa?* 21 T.M. Cooley L. Rev. 257, 263, 264 (2004) [2.24].

Martin & Bjerknes, *The Legal and Ethical Implications of Gag Clauses in Physician Contracts,* XXII Am. J. Law & Med. 433, 465-66 (1996) [Preamble; II, V, VI; 10.01].

Martin, Kurtzberg, & Hesse, *Umbilical Cord Blood: A Guide for Primary Care Physicians,* 84 Am. Fam. Physician 661 (2011) [2.165].

Martin & Lagod, *The Human Preembryo, the Progenitors, and the State: Toward a Dynamic Theory of Status, Rights, and Research Policy,* 5 High Tech. L. J. 257, 304 (1990) [2.141].

Marzen, *Out, Out Brief Candle: Constitutionally Prescribed Suicide for the Terminally Ill,* 21 Hastings Const. L.Q. 799, 821 (1994) [2.06, 2.211].

Mason, *Ignoring It Will Not Make It Go Away: Guidelines for Statutory Regulation of Physician-Assisted Death,* 45 New Eng. L. Rev. 139, 142 (2010) [2.211].

Mayer, *Bergman v. Chin: Why an Elder Abuse Case Is a Stride in the Direction of Civil Culpability for Physicians Who Undertreat Patients Suffering From Terminal Pain,* 37 New Eng. L. Rev. 313, 340 (2003) [2.20].

Mayo, *Sex, Marriage, Medicine, and Law: "What Hope of Harmony?"* 42 Washburn L. J. 269, 271 (2003) [2.162].

McAbee, *Improper Expert Medical Testimony: Existing and Proposed Mechanisms of Oversight,* 19 J. Legal Med. 257, 265 (1998) [6.01, 8.04, 9.07].

McAneeley, *Physician-Assisted Suicide: Expanding the Laboratory to the State of Hawai'i,* 29 Hawaii L. Rev. 269, 294 (2006) [2.211].

McCarthy, *Conversations About Medical Marijuana Between Physicians and Their Patients,* 25 J. Legal Med. 333, 343 (2004) [2.17].

McClellan, *Health Disparities, Health Care Reform, Morality, and the Law: "Keep Your Government Hands Off of My Medicare,"* 82 Temp. L. Rev 1141, 1151, 1154-55 (2010) [2.03].

McClimans, *Elective Twin Reductions: Evidence and Ethics,* 24 Bioethics 295, 297 (2010) [I].

McConnell, *Confidentiality and the Law,* 20 J. Med. Ethics 47, 47 (1994) [IV; 10.01].

McConnell, *Quality Control: The Implications of Negative Genetic Selection and Pre-Birth Genetic Enhancement,* 15 UCLA Women's L. J. 47, 61 (2006) [2.11].

McConnell, *The Right to Die and the Jurisprudence of Tradition,* 1997 Utah L. Rev. 665, 703-04 (1997) [2.211].

McCormick, *Pharmaceutical Manufacturer's Duty to Warn of Adverse Drug Interactions,* 66 Def. Couns. J. 59, 61 (1999) [9.032].

McCullough, *A Basic Concept in the Clinical Ethics of Managed Care: Physicians and Institutions as Economically Disciplined Moral Co-Fiduciaries of Populations of Patients,* 24 J. Med. Phil. 77, 82-83, 87, 89, 91, 96 (1999) [8.13].

McEntire, *Compensating Post-Conception Prenatal Medical Malpractice While Respecting Life: A Recommendation to North Carolina Legislators,* 29 Campbell L. Rev. 761, 763 (2007) [10.01].

McFarlane, *Mandatory Reporting of Domestic Violence: An Inappropriate Response for New York Health Care Professionals,* 17 Buff. Pub. Int. L. J. 1, 29 (1998) [2.02].

McGonnigal, *This Is Who Will Die When Doctors Are Allowed to Kill Their Patients,* 31 J. Marshall L. Rev. 95, 103 (1997) [2.211].

McGrath, *Raising the "Civilized Minimum" of Pain Amelioration for Prisoners to Avoid Cruel and Unusual Punishment,* 54 Rutgers L. Rev. 649, 657, 660 (2002) [V; 2.20].

McGuire, *AIDS and the Sexual Offender: The Epidemic Now Poses New Threats to the Victim and the Criminal Justice System,* 96 Dickinson L. Rev. 95, 109, 110 (1991) [5.05].

McGuire & Bruce, *Keeping Children's Secrets: Confidentiality in the Physician-Patient Relationship,* 8 Hous. J. Health L. & Pol'y 315 (2008) [5.055].

McIntyre, *Loosening Criteria for Withholding Prehospital Cardiopulmonary Resuscitation*, 153 Arch. Intern. Med. 2189, 2190 (1993) [2.22].

McKinney, Winslade, & Stone, *Offender Organ Transplants: Law, Ethics, Economics, and Health Policy*, 9 Hous. J. Health L. & Pol'y 39 (2008) [VIII].

McKnight & Bollis, *Foregoing Life-Sustaining Treatment for Adult Developmentally Disabled, Public Wards: A Proposed Statute*, XVIII Am. J. Law & Med. 203, 206, 220, 227 (1992) [2.20].

McLaughlin, *Pandora's Box: Can HIPAA Still Protect Patient Privacy Under a National Health Care Information Network?* 42 Gonz. L. Rev. 29, 42 (2006) [5.07].

McLean & Richards, *Managed Care Liability for Breach of Fiduciary Duty After Pegram v. Herdrich: The End of ERISA Preemption for State Law Liability for Medical Care Decision Making*, 53 Fla. L. Rev. 1, 38 (2001) [8.06].

McMullen, *Equitable Allocation of Human Organs: An Examination of the New Federal Regulations*, 20 J. Legal Med. 405, 412 (1999) [2.03].

McNaughton & McNaughton, *Divided Loyalty: The Dilemma of the Treating Physician Advocate*, 22 Okla. City U. L. Rev. 1051, 1052, 1054, 1056, 1058, 1059, 1062 (1997) [5.05, 5.07, 5.08, 7.02, 8.02, 8.03, 9.07].

McNoble, *The Cruzan Decision—A Surgeon's Perspective*, 20 Memphis State Univ. L. Rev. 569, 581, 600, 601 (1990) [2.20].

McQuire, Majumder, & Cheney, *The Ethical Health Lawyer*, 33 J. L. Med. & Ethics 603, 604 (2005) [9.11].

Mechanic, *The Functions and Limitations of Trust in the Provision of Medical Care*, 23 J. Health Pol. Pol'y & Law 661, 667 (1998) [6.02, 8.03].

Meerschaert, *Physicians' Duty to Participate in Pandemic Care*, 300 JAMA 284, 284 (2008) [2.25, 9.067].

Mehlman, *Dishonest Medical Mistakes*, 59 Vand. L. Rev. 1137, 1144 (2006) [VIII; 8.03].

Mehlman, *How Will We Regulate Genetic Enhancement?* 34 Wake Forest L. Rev. 671, 693-94, 695 (1999) [2.11, 2.138, 9.065].

Mehlman, *Medical Advocates: A Call for a New Profession*, 1 Widener L. Symp. J. 299, 314 (1996) [2.03].

Mehlman, *Rationing Expensive Lifesaving Medical Treatments*, 1985 Wisconsin L. Rev. 239, 250, 260 (1985) [2.03].

Mehlman, *The Law of Above Averages: Leveling the New Genetic Enhancement Playing Field*, 85 Iowa L. Rev. 517, 527-28, 559 (2000) [2.11, 2.12].

Mehlman, *The Patient-Physician Relationship in an Era of Scarce Resources: Is There a Duty to Treat?* 25 Conn. L. Rev. 349 (1993) [2.09].

Mehlman & Massey, *The Patient-Physician Relationship and the Allocation of Scarce Resources: A Law and Economics Approach*, 4 Kennedy Inst. Ethics J. 291, 292 (1994) [2.09, 2.095].

Mehta, *Why Self-regulation Does Not Work: Resolving Prescription Corruption Caused by Excessive Gift-Giving by Pharmaceutical Manufacturers*, 63 Food & Drug L. J. 799 (2008) [8.061].

Meisel, *A Retrospective on Cruzan*, 20 Law Med. & Health Care 340, 345 (1992) [2.20].

Meisel, *Barriers to Forgoing Nutrition and Hydration in Nursing Homes*, XXI Am. J. Law & Med. 335, 353-54 (1995) [2.20].

Meisel, *Legal Myths About Terminating Life Support*, 151 Arch. Intern. Med. 1497, 1499 (1991) [2.20].

Meisel, *Lessons From Cruzan*, 1 J. Clinical Ethics 245, 248 (1990) [2.20].

Meisel, *The Legal Consensus About Forgoing Life-Sustaining Treatment: Its Status and Its Prospects*, 2 Kennedy Inst. Ethics J. 309, 325 (1992) [2.20].

Melvin, *An Unacceptable Exception: The Ramifications of Physician Immunity From Medical Procedure Patent Infringement Liability*, 91 Minn. L. Rev. 1088, 1090 (2007) [9.095].

Menikoff, *Organ Swapping*, 29 Hastings Center Rep. 28, 32 (Nov./Dec. 1999) [2.15].

Merkatz, *Women in Clinical Trials: An Introduction*, 48 Food & Drug L. J. 161, 163 (1993) [9.122].

Meruelo, *The Need to Understand Why Patients Sue and a Proposal for a Specific Model of Mediation*, 29 J. Legal Med. 285 (2008) [10.015].

Merz, *Psychosocial Risks of Storing and Using Human Tissues in Research*, 8 Risk: Health Safety & Env't 235, 236 (1997) [2.132].

Merz, Sankar, & Yoo, *Hospital Consent for Disclosure of Medical Records*, 26 J. Law Med. & Ethics 241, 248 (1998) [IV; 5.05].

Messerly & Warwick, *Nowhere to Turn: A Glance at the Facts Behind the Supposed Need for Tort "Reform,"* 28 Hamline L. Rev. 489, 506 (2005) [I, II, III, IV, V, VI, VII, VIII, IX].

Michalos, *Medical Ethics and the Executing Process in the United States of America,* 16 Med. & Law 125, 131, 133 (1997) [2.06].

Michels & Rothman, *Update on Unethical Use of Placebos in Randomised Trials,* 17 Bioethics 188, 200 (2003) [2.075].

Mikel, *Drivers' Licenses and Age Limits: Imposition of Driving Restrictions on Elderly Drivers,* 9 Marq. Elder's Advisor 359 (2008) [5.05].

Mikk, *Making the Plaintiff's Bar Earn Its Keep: Rethinking the Hospital Incident Report,* 53 N. Y. L. Sch. L. Rev. 133 (2009) [8.121].

Milani, *Better Off Dead Than Disabled? Should Courts Recognize a Wrongful Living Cause of Action When Doctors Fail to Honor Patients' Advance Directives?* 54 Wash. & Lee L. Rev. 149, 151-52 (1997) [2.22].

Miles, *Medical Ethics and the Interrogation of Guantanamo 063,* 7 Am. J. Bioethic, 5, 9 (April 2007) [2.068].

Miles, *Medical Futility,* 20 Law Med. & Health Care 310, 311, 313 (1992) [2.20, 2.21, 2.22].

Miles, *On a New Charter to Defend Medical Professionalism: Whose Profession Is It Anyway?* 32 Hastings Center Rep. 46, 47 (May/June 2002) [2.06].

Miles, *What Are We Teaching About Indigent Patients?* 268 JAMA 2561, 2562 (1992) [9.131].

Miles & Freedman, *Medical Ethics and Torture: Revising the Declaration of Tokyo,* 373 Lancet 344, 344-45 (2009) [2.068].

Miller, *A Death by Any Other Name: The Federal Government's Inconsistent Treatment of Drugs Used in Lethal Injections and Physician-Assisted Suicide,* 17 J. L. & Health 217, 234-35 (2003) [2.06, 2.211].

Miller, *Managed Care Regulation: In the Laboratory of the States,* 278 JAMA 1102, 1104, 1108-09 (1997) [8.13].

Miller, *Norms and Interests,* 32 Hofstra L. Rev. 637, 650, 670 (2003) [II, VIII].

Miller, *Trusting Doctors: Tricky Business When It Comes to Clinical Research,* 81 B. U. L. Rev. 423, 427-28 (2001) [IV; 8.032].

Miller & Sage, *Disclosing Physician Financial Incentives,* 281 JAMA 1424, 1425 (1999) [8.032, 8.13, 8.132].

Miller-Rice, *The "Insane" Contradiction of Singleton v. Norris: Forced Medication in a Death Row Inmate's Medical Interest Which Happens to Facilitate His Execution,* 22 U. Ark. Little Rock L. Rev. 659, 673 (2001) [2.06].

Minor, *Identity Cards and Databases in Health Care: The Need for Federal Privacy Protections,* 28 Colum. J. L. & Soc. Probs. 253, 279 (1995) [5.05].

Minsker, *Prosecutorial Misconduct in Death Penalty Cases,* 45 Cal. W. L. Rev. 373 (2009) [2.06].

Mishu, Schaffner, Horan, Wood, Hutcheson, & McNabb, *A Surgeon With AIDS: Lack of Evidence of Transmission to Patients,* 264 JAMA 467 (1990) [9.131].

Misocky, *The Patients' Bill of Rights: Managed Care Under Siege,* 15 J. Contemp. Health L. & Pol'y 57, 73 (1998) [8.13].

Mitchell, *My Father, John Locke, and Assisted Suicide: The Real Constitutional Right,* 3 Ind. Health L. Rev. 45, 60 (2006) [2.211].

Mitchell, *Physician-Assisted Suicide: A Survey of the Issues Surrounding Legalization,* 74 N.D. L. Rev. 341, 349 (1998) [2.20, 2.211, 8.08].

Mitchell, *The Ethics of Passer-by Diagnosis,* 371 Lancet 85, 87 (2008) [VI].

Mitchell & Scott, *Evidence on Complex Structures of Physician Joint Ventures,* 9 Yale J. Regulation 489, 503 (1992) [8.032].

Mitchell & Scott, *New Evidence of the Prevalence and Scope of Physician Joint Ventures,* 268 JAMA 80, 84 (1992) [8.032].

Mitchell & Scott, *Physician Ownership of Physical Therapy Services: Effects on Charges, Utilization, Profits, and Service Characteristics,* 268 JAMA 2055, 2058 (1992) [8.032].

Mitchell & Sunshine, *Consequences of Physicians' Ownership of Health Care Facilities—Joint Ventures in Radiation Therapy,* 327 New Eng. J. Med. 1497, 1500 (1992) [8.032].

Mitten, *Team Physicians and Competitive Athletes: Allocating Legal Responsibility for Athletic Injuries,* 55 U. Pitt. L. Rev. 129, 140 (1993) [3.06].

Mitter, *Deputizing Internet Service Providers: How the Government Avoids Fourth Amendment Protections*, 67 N.Y.U. Ann. Surv. Am. L. 235, 273 (2011) [5.05].

Modlin, *Forensic Psychiatry and Malpractice*, 18 Bull. Am. Acad. Psychiatry Law 153, 161 (1990) [II, IV].

Molen, *Recognizing the Larger Sacrifice: Easing the Burdens Borne by Living Organ Donors Through Federal Tax Deductions*, 21 BYU J. Pub. L. 459, 463 (2007) [2.155].

Moore, *Mr. Prinzo's Breakthrough and the Limits of Confidentiality*, 51 St. Louis L. J. 1059, 1064 (2007) [IV].

Moore, *Physician-Assisted Suicide: Does "The End" Justify the Means?* 40 Ariz. L. Rev. 1471, 1472, 1481-82, 1491 (1998) [2.20, 2.211].

Moore, *What Doctors Can Learn From Lawyers About Conflicts of Interest*, 81 B. U. L. Rev. 445, 447, 449-50 (2001) [Preamble; IV; 2.07, 8.03, 8.031, 10.01].

Moore, Pichert, Hickson, Federspiel, & Blackford, *Rethinking Peer Review: Detecting and Addressing Medical Malpractice Claims Risk*, 59 Vand. L. Rev. 1175, 1144 (2006) [4.07, 9.10].

Morawetz, *Confidentiality and Common Sense: Insights From Philosophy*, 48 San Diego L. Rev. 357, 373 (2011) [5.05].

Morgan & Sutherland, *Last Rights? Confronting Physician-Assisted Suicide in Law and Society: Legal Liturgies on Physician-Assisted Suicide*, 26 Stetson L. Rev. 481, 484 (1996) [2.20, 2.21, 2.211].

Morgan, Marks, & Harty-Golder, *The Issue of Personal Choice: The Competent Incurable Patient and the Right to Commit Suicide?* 57 Mo. L. Rev. 1, 44, 45 (1992) [2.21, 2.211].

Morley, *Increasing the Supply of Organs for Transplantation Through Paired Organ Exchanges*, 21 Yale L. & Pol'y Rev. 221, 255 (2003) [2.15].

Morreim, *Am I My Brother's Warden? Responding to the Unethical or Incompetent Colleague*, 23 Hastings Center Rep. 19, 23 (May/June 1993) [II; 8.14, 9.031].

Morreim, *Blessed Be the Tie That Binds? Antitrust Perils of Physician Investment and Self-referral*, 14 J. Legal Med. 359, 367, 374, 377, 394, 409 (1993) [8.032].

Morreim, *Diverse and Perverse Incentives of Managed Care: Bringing Patients Into Alignment*, 1 Widener L. Symp. J. 89, 129 (1996) [8.13].

Morreim, *Economic Disclosure and Economic Advocacy: New Duties in the Medical Standard of Care*, 12 J. Legal Med. 275, 306 (1991) [8.08, 8.12].

Morreim, *Patient-Funded Research: Paying the Piper or Protecting the Patient?* 13 IRB 1, 2 (May/June 1991) [8.031].

Morreim, *Physician Investment and Self-referral: Philosophical Analysis of a Contentious Debate*, 15 J. Med. & Phil. 425, 428, 429, 430, 431 (1990) [8.032].

Morreim, *Redefining Quality by Reassigning Responsibility*, 20 Am. J. Law & Med. 79, 103 (1994) [10.02].

Morris, *Dissing Disclosure: Just What the Doctor Ordered*, 44 Ariz. L. Rev. 313, 344, 349, 362, 363, 366 (2002) [VII; 8.03, 8.053, 8.054, 8.08].

Morrison & Allokotte, *Duty First: Towards Patient-Centered Care and Limitations on the Right to Refuse for Moral, Religious or Ethical Reasons*, 9 Ave Maria L. Rev. 141, 168 (2010) [10.015].

Morrow, *Insuring Fairness: The Popular Creation of Genetic Antidiscrimination*, 98 Geo. L. J. 215 (2009) [IV].

Morse, *Whistleblowers and Tax Enforcement: Using Inside Information to Close the "Tax Gap,"* 24 Akron Tax J. 1 (2009) [IV].

Moses, *Understanding Legal Responses to Technological Change: The Example of In Vitro Fertilization*, 6 Minn. J. L. Sci. & Tech. 505, 543, 615 (2005) [2.055, 2.141].

Moskowitz, *Saving Granny From the Wolf: Elder Abuse and Neglect—The Legal Framework*, 31 Conn. L. Rev. 77, 116, 120, 121, 122 (1998) [2.02, 5.05].

Mossinghoff, *Remedies Under Patents on Medical and Surgical Procedures*, 78 J. Pat. & Trademark Off. Soc'y 789, 790 (1996) [9.095].

Mossman, *Is Prosecution "Medically Appropriate"?* 31 New Eng. J. on Crim. & Civ. Confinement 15, 53-54, 59 (2005) [III; 2.06].

Mossman, *Critique of Pure Risk Assessment or, Kant Meets Tarasoff*, 75 U. Cin. L. Rev. 523, 579 (2006) [Preamble; III, IV, VIII; 5.05].

Mossman & Steinberg, *Promoting, Prescribing, and Pushing Pills: Understanding the Lessons of Anti-Psychotic Drug Litigation*, 13 Mich. St. U. J. Med. & L. 263 (2009) [8.061].

Mottor, Morales and Taylor: *The Future of Lethal Injection*, 6 Appalachian J. L. 287, 300-01 (2007) [2.06].

Mowery, *A Patient's Right of Privacy in Computerized Pharmacy Records*, 66 U. Cin. L. Rev. 697, 717 (1998) [5.05].

Mullins, *The Need for Guidance in Decision Making for Terminally Ill Incompetents: Is the Ohio Legislature in a "Persistent Vegetative State?"* 17 Ohio No. Univ. L. Rev. 827, 844 (1991) [2.20].

Muñoz, *Privacy at the Cost of Public Safety: Reevaluating Mental Health Laws in the Wake of the Virginia Tech Shootings*, 18 S. Cal. Interdisc. L. J. 161 (2008) [IV].

Munoz, Nichols, Okata, Pitt, & Seager, *The Two Faces of Gag Provisions: Patients and Physicians in a Bind*, 17 Yale L. & Pol'y Rev. 249, 258 (1998) [II].

Murphy, *Expert Witnesses at Trial: Where Are the Ethics?* 14 Geo. J. Legal Ethics 217, 231-32 (2000) [I, II, III, V; 1.02, 6.01, 9.07].

Murphy, Stee, McEvoy, & Oshiro, *Journal Reporting of Medical Errors*, 131 Chest 890, 892 (2007) [8.12].

Myers, Sonenshein, & Hofstein, *To Regulate or Not to Regulate Attorney-Client Sex? The Ethical Question in Pennsylvania*, 69 Temp. L. Rev. 741, 780 (1996) [II].

Naccasha, *The Permissibility of Routine AIDS Testing in the Health Care Context*, 5 Notre Dame J. L. Ethics & Pub. Pol'y, 223, 241 (1990) [VI; 9.131].

Naiser, *Physician Noncompetition Agreements in Kentucky: The Past Discounting of Public Interests and a Proposed Solution*, 47 U. Louisville L. Rev. 195 (2008) [VIII; 9.02].

Nandi, *Ethical Aspects of Clinical Practice*, 135 Arch. Surg. 22, 23 (2000) [Preamble].

Napoli, *The Doctrine of Informed Consent and Women: The Achievement of Equal Value and Equal Exercise of Autonomy*, 4 J. Gender & L. 335, 336 (1996) [9.122].

Nash, *Considering the Scope of Advisal Duties Under Padilla*, 33 Cardozo L. Rev. 549, 550 (2011) [8.12].

National Council on Disability, *Assisted Suicide: A Disability Perspective*, 14 Issues L. & Med. 273, 292 (1998) [2.20].

Neal, *Protecting Women: Preserving Autonomy in the Commodification of Motherhood*, 17 Wm. & Mary J. Women & L. 611, 630, 635 (2011) [2.18, 10.05].

Needell, *Legal Ethics in Medicine: Are Medical Ethics Different From Legal Ethics?* 14 St. Thomas L. Rev. 31, 35, 50 (2001) [II; 5.02].

Nelson, *AETNA v. DAVILA/CIGNA v. CALAD: A Missed Opportunity*, 31 Wm. Mitchell L. Rev. 843, 847, 849, 850, 880 (2005) [VIII; 8.054, 8.13, 8.135, 9.123, 10.01, 10.015].

Nelson & Ashby, *Rethinking the Ethics of Physician Participation in Lethal Injection Execution*, 41 Hastings Center Rep., 28, 29, 35 (May-June 2011) [2.06].

Nelson, Becker, & Morrisey, *Medical Liability and Health Care Reform*, 21 Health Matrix 443, 510 (2011) [8.12].

Nelson, Swanson, & Buckley, *Lebron v. Gottlieb Memorial Hospital: Capping Medical Practice Reform in Illinois*, 20 Annals Health L. 1, 7, 11 (Winter 2011) [9.10, 10.015].

Nelson & Cranford, *Legal Advice, Moral Paralysis and the Death of Samuel Linares*, 17 Law Med. & Health Care 316 (1989) [2.20].

Newdick, *Public Health Ethics and Clinical Freedom*, 14 J. Contemp. Health L. & Pol'y 335, 336, 339, 356, 359, 361 (1998) [8.13].

Newman, *Baby Doe, Congress and the States: Challenging the Federal Treatment Standard for Impaired Infants*, XV Am. J. Law and Med. 1 (1989) [2.17].

Nidich, *Zinermon v. Burch and Voluntary Admissions to Public Hospitals: A Common Sense Proposal for Compromise*, 25 N. Ky. L. Rev. 699, 710 (1998) [I, III].

Noah, *A Drug by Any Other Name. . . ? Paradoxes in Dietary Supplement Risk Regulation*, 17 Stan. L. & Pol'y Rev. 165, 192 (2006) [8.063].

Noah, *Adverse Drug Reactions: Harnessing Experimental Data to Promote Patient Welfare*, 49 Cath. U. L. Rev. 449, 477, 497-98 (2000) [V; 5.05, 9.032].

Noah, *Bioethical Malpractice: Risk and Responsibility in Human Research*, 7 J. Health Care L. & Pol'y 175, 183, 235 (2004) [2.071, 2.075, 8.0315].

Noah, *Comfortably Numb: Medicalizing (and Mitigating) Pain-and-Suffering Damages*, 42 U. Mich. J. L. Reform 431 (2009) [2.20].

Noah, *Death of a Salesman: To What Extent Can the FDA Regulate the Promotional Statements of Pharmaceutical Sales Representatives?* 47 Food & Drug L. J. 309, 316 (1992) [8.061].

Noah, *Informed Consent and the Elusive Dichotomy Between Standard and Experimental Therapy*, 28 Am. J. L. & Med. 361, 394, 395 (2002) [2.07, 9.032].

Noah, *Medicine's Epistemology: Mapping the Haphazard Diffusion of Knowledge in the Biomedical Community*, 44 Ariz. L. Rev. 373, 404, 447, 448 (2002) [V; 9.08, 9.095].

Noah, *Pigeonholing Illness: Medical Diagnosis as a Legal Construct*, 50 Hastings L. J. 241, 301, 302 (1999) [II; 9.07].

Noah, *The Participation of Underrepresented Minorities in Clinical Research*, 29 Am. J. Law & Med. 221, 223 (2003) [9.121].

Noah, *Triage in the Nation's Medicine Cabinet: The Puzzling Scarcity of Vaccines and Other Drugs*, 54 S. C. L. Rev. 741, 755 (2003) [2.16].

Noah & Brushwood, *Adverse Drug Reactions in Elderly Patients: Alternative Approaches to Postmarket Surveillance*, 33 J. Health L. 383, 400, 445 (2000) [V; 9.032].

Nodzenski, *HIV-Infected Health Care Professionals and Informed Consent*, 2 S. Cal. Interdisciplinary L. J. 299, 327 (1993) [9.13].

Noonan, *Patenting Medical Technology*, 11 J. Legal Med. 263, 268 (1990) [9.09].

Northern, *Procreative Torts: Enhancing the Common-Law Protection for Reproductive Autonomy*, 1998 U. Ill. L. Rev. 489, 525 (1998) [8.08].

Note, *A Case Study of New Textualism in State Courts: Doe v. Marselle and the Confidentiality of HIV-Related Information*, 30 Conn. L. Rev. 295, 297 (1997) [5.05].

Note, *Administrative Agencies Get Their Way Over Constitutional Rights in Rust v. Sullivan*, 28 Willamette L. Rev. 173, 193 (1991) [8.08].

Note, *Aid-in-Dying: Should We Decriminalize Physician-Assisted Suicide and Physician-Committed Euthanasia?* XVIII Am. J. Law & Med. 369, 370 (1992) [2.211].

Note, *AIDS: Establishing a Physician's Duty to Warn*, 21 Rutgers L. J. 645, 652 (1990) [5.05].

Note, *Constitutional Aspects of Physician-Assisted Suicide After Lee v. Oregon*, XXIII Am. J. Law & Med. 69 (1997) [2.211].

Note, *Constitutional Law—Judicial Deference— Supreme Court Will Defer to "Reasonable" Abortion Restrictions*, 14 Univ. Ark. Little Rock 557, 573 (1992) [8.08].

Note, *Contingent Expert Witness Fees: Access and Legitimacy*, 64 So. Cal. L. Rev. 1363, 1374, 1382 (1991) [8.04].

Note, *Covenants Not to Compete and Liquidated Damages Clauses: Diagnosis and Treatment for Physicians*, 46 S. C. L. Rev. 505, 514 (1995) [9.02, 9.06].

Note, *Cruzan v. Director, Missouri Department of Health: To Die or Not to Die: That Is the Question— But Who Decides?* 51 Louisiana L. Rev. 1307, 1327, 1333 (1991) [2.20].

Note, *Denial of Coverage for "Experimental" Medical Procedures: The Problem of De Novo Review Under ERISA*, 79 Kentucky L. J. 801, 824 (1990-91) [2.03, 2.09].

Note, *Ethics and AIDS: A Summary of the Law and a Critical Analysis of the Individual Physician's Ethical Duty to Treat*, XVI Am. J. Law & Med. 249, 262 (1990) [VI].

Note, *Exercising the Right to Die: North Carolina's Amended Natural Death Act and the 1991 Health Care Power of Attorney Act*, 70 No. Carolina L. Rev. 2108, 2116 (1992) [2.20].

Note, *Healer-Patient Privilege: Extending the Physician-Patient Privilege to Alternative Health Practitioners in California*, 48 Hastings L. J. 633, 657 (1997) [5.05].

Note, *Health Care Proxies: New York's Attempt to Resolve the Right to Die Dilemma*, 57 Brooklyn L. Rev. 145, 168 (1991) [2.20].

Note, *HIV and Dentistry*, 29 Val. U. L. Rev. 297, 317 (1994) [9.131].

Note, *HMO Exclusion of Chiropractors*, 66 So. Cal. L. Rev. 807, 823 (1993) [3.04].

Note, *I Have a Conscience, Too: The Plight of Medical Personnel Confronting the Right to Die*, 65 Notre Dame L. Rev. 699, 706 (1990) [2.20].

Note, *Informed Choice: Physicians' Duty to Disclose Nonreadily Available Alternatives, 43 Case W. Res. L. Rev. 491, 491, 498-99, 508, 509 (1993) [I, II, III, IV, V; 8.08].*

Note, *Leading Cases—Public Employee Speech, 120 Harv. L. Rev. 125, 282 (2006) [II].*

Note, *Patenting Medical Procedures: A Search for a Compromise Between Ethics and Economics, 18 Cardozo L. Rev. 1527, 1544, 1547, 1554 (1997) [9.08, 9.09, 9.095].*

Note, *Perry v. Louisiana: Medical Ethics on Death Row—Is Judicial Intervention Warranted? 4 Georgetown J. Legal Ethics 707, 714 (1991) [2.06].*

Note, *Physician-Patient Sexual Contact: The Battle Between the State and the Medical Profession, 50 Wash. & Lee L. Rev. 1725, 1725-26, 1734, 1752 (1993) [8.14].*

Note, *Physicians, Bound and Gagged: Federal Attempts to Combat Managed Care's Use of Gag Clauses, 21 Seton Hall Legis. J. 567, 601-02 (1997) [II, V; 8.13, 10.01].*

Note, *Preventing Patient Dumping: Sharpening the COBRA's Fangs, 61 N. Y. U. L. Rev. 1186 (1986) [VI; 8.11].*

Note, *Professional Ethics Codes in Court: Redefining the Social Contract Between the Public and the Professions, 25 Georgia L. Rev. 1327, 1335, 1351 (1991) [II; 2.19].*

Note, *Redefining the Right to Die in Illinois, 15 So. Ill. Univ. L. J. 1261, 1273 (1991) [2.20].*

Note, *Restricting Ex Parte Interviews With Nonparty Treating Physicians: Crist v. Moffatt, 69 No. Carolina L. Rev. 1381, 1391, 1392 (1991) [5.50].*

Note, *Rust on the Constitution: Politics and Gag Rules, 37 How. L. J. 83, 96 (1993) [8.08].*

Note, *Sexual Conduct Within the Physician-Patient Relationship: A Statutory Framework for Disciplining This Breach of Fiduciary Duty, 1 Widener L. Symp. J. 501, 507 (1996) [II; 8.14].*

Note, *Something Worth Writing Home About: Clear and Convincing Evidence, Living Wills, and Cruzan v. Director, Missouri Department of Health, 22 Univ. Toledo L. Rev. 871, 879 (1991) [2.20].*

Note, *State Natural Death Acts: Illusory Protection of Individuals' Life-Sustaining Treatment Decisions, 29 Harvard J. Legis. 175, 186, 194, 195, 201 (1992) [2.20, 2.22].*

Note, *Stop Gagging Physicians! 7 Health Matrix 187, 193, 200, 208-09 (1997) [8.13].*

Note, *The Americans with Disabilities Act: Magic Bullet or Band-Aid for Patients and Health Care Workers Infected With the Human Immunodeficiency Virus? 57 Brooklyn L. Rev. 1277, 1279, 1305 (1992) [9.131].*

Note, *The Economic Wisdom of Regulating Pharmaceutical "Freebies," 1991 Duke L. J. 206, 216, 233, 234 (1991) [8.061, 8.08].*

Note, *The Informed-Consent Policy of the International Conference on Harmonization of Technical Requirements for Registrations of Pharmaceuticals for Human Use: Knowledge Is the Best Medicine, 30 Cornell Int'l L. J. 203, 209 (1997) [2.07].*

Note, *The New Patent Infringement Liability Exception for Medical Procedures, 23 J. Legis. 265, 268 (1997) [9.095].*

Note, *The Ohio Physician-Patient Privilege: Modified, Revised, and Defined, 49 Ohio St. L. J. 1147 (1989) [II, IV; 5.05].*

Note, *The Policy Against Federal Funding for Abortions Extends Into the Realm of Free Speech After Rust v. Sullivan, 19 Pepperdine L. Rev. 637, 681 (1992) [8.08].*

Note, *Torts: Defining the Duty Imposed on Physicians by the Doctrine of Informed Consent, 22 Wm. Mitchell L. Rev. 149, 160 (1996) [9.13].*

Note, *Toward a More Perfect Union: A Federal Cause of Action for Physician Aid-in-Dying, 27 U. Mich. J. L. Ref. 521, 538 (1994) [I, III; 2.06].*

Note, *Who Decides if There Is Triumph in the Ultimate Agony? Constitutional Theory and the Emerging Right to Die With Dignity, 37 Wm. & Mary L. Rev. 827, 829 (1996) [2.20, 2.211].*

Novy, Ritter, & McNeill, *A Primer of Ethical Issues Involving Opioid Therapy for Chronic Nonmalignant Pain in a Multidisciplinary Setting, 10 Pain Med. 356, 360 (2009) [8.083].*

Noyes, *Higher Penalties for Failing to Pay Child Support: A Look at Medical License Revocation, 19 J. Legal Med. 127, 138 (1998) [5.05, 9.02, 9.06].*

Nugent, *Patenting Medical Devices: The Economic Implications of Ethically Motivated Reform, 17 Ann. Health L. 135 (2008) [9.08].*

Nunziato, *Preventing Prescription Drug Overdose in the Twenty-First Century: Is the Controlled Substances Act Enough?* 38 Hofstra L. Rev. 1261, 1277 (2010) [10.015].

Obade, *Whisper Down the Lane: AIDS, Privacy, and the Hospital Grapevine,* 2 J. Clinical Ethics 133, 133 (1991) [5.05].

Oberheu, Jones, & Sade, *A Surgeon Operates on His Son: Wisdom or Hubris?* 84 Ann. Thorac. Surg. 723, 725, 726 (2007) [VI; 8.19].

Oberman, *Mothers and Doctors' Orders: Unmasking the Doctor's Fiduciary Role in Maternal-Fetal Conflicts,* 94 Nw. U. L. Rev. 451, 456, 462, 493 (2000) [8.08, 8.13, 10.01].

Oberman, *Panel Discussion American Association of Law Schools Panel: Panel on the Use of Patients for Teaching Purposes Without Their Knowledge or Consent,* 8 J. Health Care L. & Pol'y 210, 210 (2005) [8.08].

O'Brien, *The Momentum of Posthumous Conception: A Model Act,* 25 J. Contemp. Health L. & Pol'y 332 (2009) [2.04].

Oddi, *Reverse Informed Consent: The Unreasonably Dangerous Patient,* 46 Vand. L. Rev. 1417, 1449, 1463, 1465, 1479 (1993) [IV, VI; 8.11, 9.131].

Offit, Groeger, Turner, Wadsworth, & Weiser, *The "Duty to Warn" a Patient's Family Members About Hereditary Disease Risks,* 292 JAMA 1469, 1471 (2004) [2.131].

Offit, Sagi, & Hurley, *Preimplantation Genetic Diagnosis for Cancer Syndromes: A New Challenge for Preventive Medicine,* 296 JAMA 2727, 2727 (2006) [2.12].

Ogbogu, Fleischer, Brodell, Bhalla, Draelos, & Feldman, *Physicians' and Patients' Perspectives on Office-Based Dispensing: The Central Role of the Physician-Patient Relationship,* 137 Arch. Dermatol. 151, 151 (2001) [8.06].

Oken, *Curing Healthcare Providers' Failure to Administer Opioids in the Treatment of Severe Pain,* 23 Cardozo L. Rev. 1917, 1925-26, 1952, 1954 (2002) [2.20, 2.21, 2.211].

Oleson, *Swilling Hemlock: The Legal Ethics of Defending a Client Who Wishes to Volunteer for Execution,* 63 Wash. & Lee L. Rev. 147, 277, 325 (2006) [2.20, 2.211].

Olson, *Physician Specialty Advertising: The Tendency to Deceive?* 11 J. Legal Med. 351, 354 (1990) [5.02].

O'Neill, *Surrogate Health Care Decisions for Adults in Illinois—Answers to the Legal Questions That Health Care Providers Face on a Daily Basis,* 29 Loy. Univ. Chi. L. J. 411, 445, 448 (1998) [2.035, 2.22, 8.11].

Oppenheim, *Physicians as Experts Against Their Own Patients? What Happened to the Privilege?* 63 Def. Couns. J. 254, 257, 261 (1996) [IV; 5.05].

Orenstein, *Apology Excepted: Incorporating a Feminist Analysis Into Evidence Policy Where You Would Least Expect It,* 28 S.W. U. L. Rev. 221, 264 (1999) [I, II].

Orentlicher, *Advance Medical Directives,* 263 JAMA 2365 (1990) [2.20].

Orentlicher, *Cloning and the Preservation of Family Integrity,* 59 La. L. Rev. 1019, 1022 (1999) [2.147].

Orentlicher, *Denying Treatment to the Noncompliant Patient,* 265 JAMA 1579, 1581 (1991) [VI; 9.12].

Orentlicher, *Health Care Reform and the Patient-Physician Relationship,* 5 Health Matrix 141, 143, 148 (1995) [5.05, 10.01].

Orentlicher, *HIV-Infected Surgeons: Behringer v. Medical Center,* 266 JAMA 1134, 1136 (1991) [8.032, 9.131].

Orentlicher, *Paying Physicians More to Do Less: Financial Incentives to Limit Care,* 30 U. Rich. L. Rev. 155, 167 (1996) [8.13].

Orentlicher, *The Illusion of Patient Choice in End-of-Life Decisions,* 267 JAMA 2101, 2102 (1992) [2.20, 2.22, 9.121].

Orentlicher, *The Influence of a Professional Organization on Physician Behavior,* 57 Alb. L. Rev. 583, 592, 593, 594, 595, 596 (1994) [1.01, 1.02, 8.061, 9.04, 9.131].

Orentlicher, *The Legalization of Physician Assisted Suicide: A Very Modest Revolution,* 38 B. C. L. Rev. 443, 459-60 (1997) [2.211].

Ornish, Mills, & Ornish, *Prearraignment Forensic Evaluations: Toward a New Policy,* 24 Bull. Am. Acad. Psychiatry Law 453, 454, 469 (1996) [Preamble; IV; 5.05].

Orr & Bishop, *Why Psychiatrists Should Not Participate in Euthanasia and Physician-Assisted Suicide,* 19 Am. J. Forensic Psychiatry 35, 36 (1998) [2.211].

Orr & Hook, *Stem Cell Research: Magical Promise v. Moral Peril,* 2 Yale J. Health Pol'y, Law & Ethics 189, 197 (2001) [2.30].

Orr, Johnston, Ashwal, & Bailey, *Should Children With Severe Cognitive Impairment Receive Solid Organ Transplants?* 11 J. Clinical Ethics 219, 222-23, 228 (2000) [2.16].

O'Shaughnessy, *The Worst of Both Worlds? Parental Involvement Requirements and the Privacy Rights of Mature Minors*, 57 Ohio St. L. J. 1731, 1764-65 (1996) [2.015].

O'Sullivan & Borcherding, *Informed Consent for Medication in Persons With Mental Retardation and Mental Illness*, 12 Health Matrix 63, 75, 86, 87, 88 (2002) [Preamble; I, III, IV, VIII, IX; 8.08].

O'Toole, *HIV-Specific Crime Legislation: Targeting an Epidemic for Criminal Prosecution*, 10 J. L. & Health 183, 195, 199 (1995) [2.23].

Overgaard, *Balancing the Interests of Researchers and Donors in the Commercial Scientific Research Marketplace*, 74 Brook. L. Rev. 1473 (2009) [2.08].

Packer, *Embryonic Stem Cells, Intellectual Property, and Patents: Ethical Concerns*, 37 Hofstra L. Rev. 487 (2008) [8.031].

Packer, *Ethics and Medical Patents*, 117 Arch. Ophthalmol. 824, 825 (1999) [9.08].

Packer, Parke II, & Pellegrino, *Should Ophthalmologists Teach Surgery to Optometrists?* 126 Arch. Ophthalmol. 1458, 1458 (2008) [3.03].

Paltrow, *The War on Drugs and the War on Abortion: Some Initial Thoughts on the Connections, Intersections and the Effects*, 28 S.U. L. Rev. 201, 219 (2001) [10.01].

Paradise & Andrews, *Tales From the Crypt: Scientific, Ethical, and Legal Considerations for Biohistorical Analysis of Deceased Historical Figures*, 26 Temp. J. Sci. Tech. & Envtl. L. 223, 287-88 (2007) [Preamble; 2.079, 2.08, 2.105, 5.05, 5.051, 5.075, 8.03, 8.031, 9.095, 9.10].

Park, *Physician-Assisted Suicide: State Legislation Teetering at the Pinnacle of a Slippery Slope*, 7 Wm. & Mary Bill Rts. J. 277, 292, 293 (1998) [2.211].

Parker, *Corporate Practice of Medicine: Last Stand or Final Downfall?* 29 J. Health & Hosp. L. 160, 167, 173 (1996) [VI].

Parmet, *The Supreme Court Confronts HIV: Reflections on Bragdon v. Abbott*, 26 J. Law Med. & Ethics 225 (1998) [9.131].

Partlett, *Misuse of Genetic Information: The Common Law and Professionals' Liability*, 42 Washburn L. J. 489, 503 (2003) [2.132].

Pasquale, *The Three Faces of Retainer Care: Crafting a Tailored Regulatory Response*, 7 Yale J. Health Pol'y L. & Ethics 39, 74 (2007) [8.055].

Paterson, *Can We Mandate Compassion?* 41 Hastings Center Rep. 20, 21 (Mar.-Apr. 2011) [I].

Patterson, *Conflicts of Interest in Scientific Expert Testimony*, 40 Wm. & Mary L. Rev. 1313, 1330, 1332, 1335, 1371 (1999) [8.061, 9.07].

Patterson, *Planning for Health Care Using Living Wills and Durable Powers of Attorney: A Guide for the South Carolina Attorney*, 42 So. Carolina L. Rev. 525, 535, 541, 547, 548 (1991) [2.20].

Patton, *A Call for Common Sense: Organ Donation and the Executed Prisoner*, 3 Va. J. Soc. Pol'y & L. 387, 404, 405, 407-10 (1996) [VII; 2.06, 2.162].

Pearlman, Cain, Patrick, Appelbaum-Maizel, Starks, Jecker, & Uhlmann, *Insights Pertaining to Patient Assessments of States Worse Than Death*, 4 J. Clinical Ethics 33, 40 (1993) [2.20, 2.21].

Pearlmutter, *Physician Apologies and General Admissions of Fault: Amending the Federal Rules of Evidence*, 72 Ohio St. L. J. 687, 713) (2011) [8.12].

Pearson, Kahn, Harrison, Rubenstein, Rogers, Brook, & Keeler, *Differences in Quality of Care for Hospitalized Elderly Men and Women*, 268 JAMA 1883 (1992) [9.122].

Peccarelli, *A Moral Dilemma: The Role of Judicial Intervention in Withholding or Withdrawing Nutrition and Hydration*, 23 John Marshall L. Rev. 537, 539, 540, 541 (1990) [Preamble; I, II, III, IV, V, VI, VII; 2.20].

Pegalis, *A Proposal to Use Common Ground That Exists Between the Medical and Legal Professions to Promote a Culture of Safety*, 51 N. Y. L. Sch. L. Rev. 1057, 1070, 1073 (2006) [8.12, 10.015].

Peltier & Guisti, *Commerce and Care: The Irreconcilable Tension Between Selling and Caring*, 39 McGeorge L. Rev. 785 (2008) [8.054].

Pena, *Reevaluating Privacy and Disability Laws in the Wake of the Virginia Tech Tragedy: Considerations for Administrators and Lawmakers*, 87 N. C. L. Rev. 305 (2008) [5.05].

Perales, *Rethinking the Prohibition of Death Row Prisoners as Organ Donors: A Possible Lifeline to Those on Organ Donor Waiting Lists*, 34 St. Mary's L. J. 687, 721, 725 (2003) [VII; 2.06].

Perdue & Binion, *A License to Kill: The Unintended (?) Consequence of Milo on Kramer*, 41 S. Tex. L. Rev. 293, 309 (2000) [8.12].

Pereira & Pearson, *Patient Attitudes Toward Physician Financial Incentives*, 161 Arch. Intern. Med. 1313, 1316, 1317 (2001) [8.132].

Pergament, *Internet Psychotherapy: Current Status and Future Regulation*, 8 Health Matrix 233, 253 (1998) [9.12].

Perkin & Resnik, *The Agony of Agonal Respiration: Is the Last Gasp Necessary?* 28 J. Med. Ethics 164, 169 (2002) [2.211].

Persels, *Forcing the Issue of Physician-Assisted Suicide: Impact of the Kevorkian Case on the Euthanasia Debate*, 14 J. Legal Med. 93, 115 (1993) [2.06, 2.20].

Peschel, *Revisiting the Compromise of 35 USC § 287(c)*, 16 Tex. Intell. Prop. L. J. 299 (2008) [V; 9.08].

Pessagno, *Prometheus and Bilski: Pushing the Bounds of Patentable Subject Matter in Medical Diagnostic Techniques With the Machine-or-Transformation Test*, 36 Am. J. L. & Med. 619, 620 (2010) [9.08].

Peterson, *The Malpractice Surcharge: A Simple Answer to Rising Malpractice Rates or a Greater Threat to Quality Patient Care?* 27 J. Legal Med. 87, 96, 97-98 (2006) [10.015, 10.018].

Petrila, *Ethics, Money, and the Problem of Coercion in Managed Behavioral Health Care*, 40 St. Louis U. L. J. 359, 377 (1996) [2.03, 4.04].

Pfeifer, *Smoking Gun: The Moral and Legal Struggle for Medical Marijuana*, 27 Touro L. Rev. 339, 340-41, 345-346 (2011) [III, VIII; 10.01, 10.015, 10.02].

Phan, *Physician Unionization: The Impact on the Medical Profession*, 20 J. Legal Med. 115, 136, 137 (1999) [9.025].

Philip, Conant, & Heilig, *Participation of Health Care Personnel in Torture and Interrogation*, 353 New Eng. J. Med. 1634, 1634 (2005) [1.02].

Pierucci, Kirby, & Leuthner, *End-of-Life Care for Neonates and Infants: The Experience and Effects of a Palliative Care Consultation Service*, 108 Pediatrics 653, 659 (2001) [2.215].

Pittman, *Any Willing Provider Laws and ERISA's Saving Clause: A New Solution for an Old Problem*, 64 Tenn. L. Rev. 409, 416 (1997) [8.13].

Pittman, *Physician-Assisted Suicide in the Dark Ward: The Intersection of the Thirteenth Amendment and Health Care Treatments Having Disproportionate Impacts on Disfavored Groups*, 28 Seton Hall L. Rev. 774, 784 (1998) [2.211].

Plambeck, *Divided Loyalties: Legal and Bioethical Considerations of Physician–Pregnant Patient Confidentiality and Prenatal Drug Abuse*, 23 J. Legal Med. 1, 8, 25 (2002) [IV; 10.01].

Polsky, *Winning Medicine: Professional Sports Team Doctors' Conflicts of Interest*, 14 J. Contemp. Health L. & Pol'y 503, 505 (1998) [VI].

Pope, *Multi-Institutional Healthcare Ethics Committees: The Procedurally Fair Internal Dispute Resolution Mechanism*, 31 Campbell L. Rev. 257 (2009) [9.11, 9.115].

Pope, *Surrogate Selection: An Increasingly Viable, but Limited, Solution to Intractable Futility Disputes*, 3 St. Louis U. J. Health L. & Pol'y 183, 207, 208, 211-214, 224, 228 (2010) [2.20, 8.081].

Pope, *The Maladaptation of Miranda to Advance Directives: A Critique of the Implementation of the Patient Self-Determination Act*, 9 Health Matrix 139, 178 (1999) [2.20].

Porter, *Physician Advertising—What Is Legal? What Is Ethical? What Is Acceptable?* 80 Ohio State Med. J. 437 (1984) [5.02].

Portman & Romanow, *Concierge Medicine: Legal Issues, Ethical Dilemmas, and Policy Challenges*, 1 J. Health & Life Sci. L. 1 (2008) [II, VI; 8.055].

Poser, *Unlabeled Drug Samples and the Learned Intermediary: The Case for Drug Company Liability Without Preemption*, 62 Food Drug L. J. 653, 667 (2007) [8.061].

Post, *Subsidized Speech*, 106 Yale L. J. 151, 173 (1996) [8.08].

Post, Blustein, Gordon, & Dubler, *Pain: Ethics, Culture, and Informed Consent to Relief*, 24 J. Law Med. & Ethics 348, 349, 356 (1996) [2.20].

Potter, *Failure to Disclose HMO Incentives and the Breach of Fiduciary Duty: Is a New Cause of Action Against Physicians the Best Solution?* 34 USF L. Rev. 733, 753 (2000) [8.132].

Povenmire, *Do Parents Have the Legal Authority to Consent to the Surgical Amputation of Normal, Healthy Tissue From Their Infant Children? The Practice of Circumcision in the United States*, 7 Am. U. J. Gender Soc. Pol. & L. 87, 96 (1999) [IV].

Prasse, *Hippocrates Would Roll Over in His Grave: An Examination of Why Internet Health Care Programs Should Obtain Informed Consent From Their Users*, 42 Creighton L. Rev. 733 (2009) [IV].

Pratt, *Too Many Physicians: Physician-Assisted Suicide After Glucksberg/Quill,* 9 Alb. L. J. Sci. & Tech. 161, 208 (1999) [2.20, 2.21, 2.211].

Prentice, *Clinical Trial Results, Physicians, and Insider Trading,* 20 J. Legal Med. 195, 221 (1999) [8.032].

Preston, *Baby Spice: Lost Between Feminine and Feminist,* 9 Am. U. J. Gender Soc. Pol'y & L. 541, 590 (2001) [9.122].

Price, *Between Scylla and Charybdis: Charting a Course to Reconcile the Duty of Confidentiality and the Duty to Warn in the AIDS Context,* 94 Dickinson L. Rev. 435, 477 (1990) [2.23].

Pritts, *Altered States: State Health Privacy Laws and the Impact of the Federal Health Privacy Rules,* 2 Yale J. Health Pol'y, L. & Ethics 327, 351 (2002) [10.02].

Pronovost & Williams, *Telemedicine and End-of-Life Care: What's Wrong With This Picture?* 12 J. Clinical Ethics 64, 68 (2001) [2.20].

Puglise, *"Calling Dr. Love": The Physician-Patient Sexual Relationship as Grounds for Medical Malpractice—Society Pays While the Doctor and Patient Play,* 14 J. L. & Health 321, 324-25, 349 (2000) [8.14].

Pugno, *Hospital Privileges for Family Physicians: Rights, Rationale, and Resources,* 17 J. Fam. Practice 77 (1983) [9.05].

Quick, *Contract Law: Physician, Meet Thy Covenant: Noncompete Agreements in the Medical Profession,* 86 Mich. Bar J. 22, 23 (2007) [9.02].

Quill & Cassel, *Nonabandonment: A Central Obligation for Physicians,* 10 Trends in Health Care, Law & Ethics 25, 27 (Winter/Spring 1995) [8.11].

Quill, Cassel, & Meier, *Care of the Hopelessly Ill: Proposed Clinical Criteria for Physician-Assisted Suicide,* 327 New Eng. J. Med. 1380, 1381 (1992) [2.20].

Quinn, *The Best Interests of Incompetent Patients: The Capacity for Interpersonal Relationships as a Standard for Decisionmaking,* 76 Cal. L. Rev. 897 (1988) [2.20].

Rabeneck, McCullough, & Wray, *Ethically Justified, Clinically Comprehensive Guidelines for Percutaneous Endoscopic Gastrostomy Tube Placement,* 349 Lancet 496, 497, 498 (1997) [2.17].

Radelet, *Capital Punishment in Colorado: 1859-1972,* 74 U. Colo. L. Rev. 885, 940 (2003) [2.06].

Radnor, *How to Prepare for and Take a Doctor's Deposition,* 22 Prac. Litigator 40, 52 (May 2011) [6.01].

Rai, Siegler, & Lantos, *The Physician as a Health Care Proxy,* 29 Hastings Center Rep. 14, 19 (Sep./Oct. 1999) [2.03].

Rajkumar, *A Human Rights Approach to Routine Provider-Initiated HIV Testing,* 7 Yale J. Health Pol'y L. & Ethics 319, 371 (2007) [2.23].

Rand, *An Interdisciplinary Search for Help Through Social Work's Empowerment Approach,* 13 Clinical L. Rev. 459, 477 (2006) [VII].

Ratcliffe, *The Ethics of Genetic Patenting and the Subsequent Implications on the Future of Health Care,* 27 Touro L. Rev. 435, 438-39, 449 (2011) [2.079, 2.105].

Raz, Campbell, Guindi, Holcraft, Déry, & Cukier, *Placebos in Clinical Practice: Comparing Attitudes, Beliefs, and Patterns of Use Between Academic Psychiatrists and Nonpsychiatrists,* 56 Can. J. Psychiatry 199 (2011) [8.083].

Reardon, *American Medical Association Perspective on Physician Assisted Suicide,* 75 U. Det. Mercy L. Rev. 515 (1998) [2.211].

Rediger, *Living in a World With HIV: Balancing Privacy, Privilege and the Right to Know Between Patients and Health Care Professionals,* 21 Hamline J. Pub. L. & Pol'y 443, 456-57, 461, 472 (2000) [2.23, 9.13, 9.131].

Reed, *Cybermedicine: Defying and Redefining Patient Standards of Care,* 37 Ind. L. Rev. 845, 850, 859, 862 (2004) [5.027].

Reese & Burry, *Evaluating Maryland's Response to Drug-Exposed Babies,* 10 Psychol. Pub. Pol'y & L. 343, 353 (2004) [10.01].

Regan, *Regulating the Business of Medicine: Models for Integrating Ethics and Managed Care,* 30 Colum. J. L. & Soc. Probs. 635, 651, 656, 657 (1997) [Preamble; I, II, III, IV, V; 8.13].

Reibman, *The Patient Wanted the Doctor to Treat Her in the Closet, but the Janitor Wouldn't Open the Door: Healthcare Provider Rights of Refusal Versus LGB Rights to Reproductive and Elder Healthcare,* 28 Temp. J. Sci. Tech. & Envtl. L. 65 (2009) [Preamble; 10.05].

Reisman, *Physicians and Surgeons as Inventors: Reconciling Medical Process Patents and Medical Ethics,* 10 High Tech. L. J. 355, 356, 368-70, 385 (1995) [VII; 9.08, 9.09, 9.095].

Reiss, *Commentary on Payment and Reimbursement Issues Affecting the Marketing of Drugs, Medical Devices, and Biologics, With Emphasis on the Anti-Kickback Statute and Stark II*, 52 Food & Drug L. J. 99, 107 (1997) [8.061].

Relman, *"Self-referral"—What's at Stake?* 327 New Eng. J. Med. 1522, 1524 (1992) [8.032].

Resnik, *DNA Patents and Human Dignity*, 29 J. L. Med. & Ethics 152, 158, 159 (2001) [2.105].

Reuland, *Health Maintenance Organizations and Physician Financial Incentive Plans: Should Physician Disclosure be Mandatory?* 27 Iowa J. Corp. L. 293, 312 (2002) [8.13].

Reutenauer, *Medical Malpractice Liability in the Era of Genetic Susceptibility Testing*, 19 QLR 539, 571 (2000) [10.01].

Reza, *Religion and the Public Defender*, 26 Fordham Urb. L. J. 1051, 1062, 1063 (1999) [VI; 8.11, 9.06, 9.12].

Rheinstein, *MedWatch: The FDA Medical Products Reporting Program*, 48 Am. Fam. Physician 636, 636 (1993) [9.032].

Rice, *The Superior Orders Defense in Legal Ethics: Sending the Wrong Message to Young Lawyers*, 32 Wake Forest L. Rev. 887, 908-09 (1997) [9.055].

Rich, *A Prescription for the Pain: The Emerging Standard of Care for Pain Management*, 26 Wm. Mitchell L. Rev. 1, 35-36, 85 (2000) [V; 2.20, 9.011].

Rich, *Advance Directives: The Next Generation*, 19 J. Legal Med. 63, 79 (1998) [2.20].

Rich, *Prognostication in Clinical Medicine: Prophecy or Professional Responsibility?* 23 J. Legal Med. 297, 299, 318, 327 (2002) [IV; 8.12, 10.01].

Rich, *The Assault on Privacy on Healthcare Decision Making*, 68 Denver L. Rev. 1, 10 (1991) [2.20].

Richards, *Reconciling Data Privacy and the First Amendment*, 52 UCLA L. Rev. 1149, 1195 (2005) [5.05].

Richards & Wolf, *Medical Confidentiality and Disclosure of Paternity*, 48 S. D. L. Rev. 409, 411, 412, 413 (2003) [I, II, IV, V; 1.02, 5.05, 5.055, 10.01].

Rickard & Fehn, *Recent Developments in Regulation of Pharmaceutical Marketing Practices*, 19 Health Lawyer 16, 17 (Dec. 2006) [8.061].

Rie, *The Limits of a Wish*, 21 Hastings Center Rep. 24 (July/August 1991) [2.20].

Risley, *Ethical and Legal Issues in the Individual's Right to Die*, 20 Ohio N. U. L. Rev. 597, 605 (1993) [2.20].

Rivo & Satcher, *Improving Access to Health Care Through Physician Workforce Reform*, 270 JAMA 1074, 1075 (1993) [9.121].

Roach, *Paradox and Pandora's Box: The Tragedy of Current Right-to-Die Jurisprudence*, 25 Univ. Mich. J. Law Reform 133, 137, 158 (1991) [2.20].

Robbins, *Open Your Mouth and Say "Ideology": Physicians and the First Amendment*, 12 U. Pa. J. Const. L. 155 (2009) [8.08].

Roberts, *Rust v. Sullivan and the Control of Knowledge*, 61 Geo. Wash. L. Rev. 587, 641 (1993) [8.08].

Roberts, Roberts, Warner, Solomon, Hardee, & McCarty, *Internal Medicine, Psychiatry, and Emergency Medicine Residents' Views of Assisted Death Practices*, 157 Arch. Intern. Med. 1603, 1609 (1997) [2.211].

Robertson, *Dilemma in Danville*, 11 Hastings Center Rep. 5 (Oct. 1981) [2.17].

Robertson, *Prior Agreements for Disposition of Frozen Embryos*, 51 Ohio St. L. J. 407, 419 (1990) [2.141].

Robertson, *Procreative Liberty and Harm to Offspring in Assisted Reproduction*, 30 Am. J. L. & Med. 7, 22 (2004) [9.131].

Robertson, *Seeking a Seat at the Table: Has Law Left Environmental Ethics Behind as It Embraces Bioethics?* 32 Wm. & Mary Envtl. L. & Pol'y Rev. 273 (2008) [I, II, III, IV, V, VI, VII, VIII, IX].

Robertson, *The Dead Donor Rule*, 29 Hastings Center Rep. 6, 13 (Nov./Dec. 1999) [2.162].

Rode, *End-of-Life Decision Making for Patients in Persistent Vegetative States: A Comparative Analysis*, 30 Hastings Int'l & Comp. L. Rev. 477, 499, 500 (2007) [2.035, 2.037, 2.20].

Rodes, *On Law and Chastity*, 76 Notre Dame L. Rev. 643, 675 (2001) [8.14].

Rodriguez, *Suing Health Care Providers for Saving Lives: Liability for Providing Unwanted Life-Sustaining Treatment*, 20 J. Legal Med. 1, 62 (1999) [2.20].

Rodwin, *Reforming Pharmaceutical Industry-Physician Financial Relationships: Lessons From the United States, France, and Japan*, 39 J. L. Med. & Ethics 662, 664 (2011) [8.061].

Rodwin, *Strains in the Fiduciary Metaphor: Divided Physician Loyalties and Obligations in a Changing Health Care System*, XXI Am. J. Law & Med. 241, 246, 250 (1995) [Preamble; 8.032].

Rodwin & Okamoto, *Physicians' Conflicts of Interest in Japan and the United States: Lessons for the United States*, 25 J. Health Pol. Pol'y & L. 343, 355, 358 (2000) [8.032, 8.061].

Roko, *Executioner Identities: Toward Recognizing a Right to Know Who Is Hiding Beneath the Hood*, 75 Fordham L. Rev. 2791, 2799 (2007) [2.06].

Rooksby, *Ethics Education in Medical Schools: Problems, Practices, and Possibilities*, 10 Quinnipiac Health L. J. 181, 205 (2007) [Preamble].

Rosato, *The Ultimate Test of Autonomy: Should Minors Have a Right to Make Decisions Regarding Life-Sustaining Treatment?* 49 Rutgers L. Rev. 1, 80-81, 82 (1996) [2.20].

Rosato, *Using Bioethics Discourse to Determine When Parents Should Make Health Care Decisions for Their Children: Is Deference Justified?* 73 Temp. L. Rev. 1, 40, 44 (2000) [2.20].

Rose, *Financial Conflicts of Interest: How Are We Managing?* 8 Wid. L. Symp. J. 1, 24 (2001) [8.03, 8.031].

Rosenfeld, *Assisted Suicide, Depression, and the Right to Die*, 6 Psychol. Pub. Pol'y & L. 467, 469 (2000) [2.21, 2.211].

Rosner, Cassell, Friedland, Landolt, Loeb, Numann, Ora, Risemberg, & Sordillo, *Ethical Considerations of Reproductive Technologies*, 87 N.Y. State J. Med. 398 (1987) [2.04, 2.05, 2.14, 2.18].

Rosoff, *Breach of Fiduciary Duty Lawsuits Against MCOs*, 22 J. Legal Med. 55, 65 (2001) [8.0132].

Rosoff, *The Changing Face of Pharmacy Benefits Management: Information Technology Pursues a Grand Mission*, 42 St. Louis U. L. J. 1, 25-26 (1998) [5.05].

Rosoff & Coleman, *The Case for Legal Regulation of Physicians' Off-Label Prescribing*, 86 Notre Dame L. Rev. 649, 675 (2011) [I, V].

Ross, Lackner, Lurie, Gross, Wolfe, & Krumholz, *Pharmaceutical Company Payments to Physicians: Early Experiences With Disclosure Laws in Vermont and Minnesota*, 297 JAMA 1216, 1216 (2007) [8.061].

Roth & Levin, *Dilemma of Tarasoff: Must Physicians Protect the Public or Their Patients?* 11 Law Med. & Health Care 104 (1983) [IV].

Rothenberg, *Gestational Surrogacy and the Health Care Provider: Put Part of the IVF Genie Back Into the Bottle*, 18 Law Med. & Health Care 345, 346 (1990) [2.18].

Rothenberg, *Who Cares? The Evolution of the Legal Duty to Provide Emergency Care*, 26 Houston L. Rev. 21 (1989) [VI].

Rothstein, *Is Deidentification Sufficient to Protect Health Privacy in Research?* 10 Am. J. Bioethics 3, 5 (Sept. 2010) [IV; 5.05, 7.025].

Rothstein, *Should Health Care Providers Get Treatment Priority in an Influenza Pandemic?* 38 J. L. Med. & Ethics 412, 413, 415 (2010) [2.03, 9.067].

Rothstein, *The Role of IRBs in Research Involving Commercial Biobanks*, 30 J. Law Med. & Ethics 105, 106, 108 (2002) [8.031].

Rothstein, *Worst Case Bioethics: Death, Disaster, and Public Health*, 31 J. Legal Med. 331, 333 (2010) [8.02].

Rothstein & Hoffman, *Genetic Testing, Genetic Medicine, and Managed Care*, 34 Wake Forest L. Rev. 849, 883 (1999) [2.23].

Rothstein, Gelb, & Craig, *Protecting Genetic Privacy by Permitting Employer Access Only to Job-Related Employee Medical Information: Analysis of a Unique Minnesota Law*, 24 Am. J. Law & Med. 399, 400 (1998) [2.132].

Rothstein & Talbott, *Compelled Disclosure of Health Information: Protecting Against the Greatest Potential Threat to Privacy*, 295 JAMA 2882, 2883 (2006) [IV; 5.05].

Rothstein & Talbott, *Job Security and Income Replacement for Individuals in Quarantine: The Need for Legislation*, 10 J. Health Care L. & Pol'y 239, 239-40 (2007) [2.25].

Rowland, *Communicating Past the Conflict: Solving the Medical Futility Controversy With Process-Based Approaches*, 14 U. Miami Int'l & Comp. L. Rev. 271, 278-79 (2006) [2.03, 2.035].

Rozenek, *Whose Conscience Is It Anyway? The State's Role in Conscience Clause Creation and the Denial of Contraception*, 40 Suffolk U. L. Rev. 215, 220 (2006) [VIII].

Rubenstein, *First, Do No Harm: Health Professionals and Guantanamo*, 37 Seton Hall L. Rev. 733, 738 (2007) [2.067].

Rubenstein, Pross, Davidoff, & Iacopino, *Coercive US Interrogation Policies: A Challenge to Medical Ethics*, 294 JAMA 1544 (2005) [1.02, 2.067].

Ruebner & Reis, *Hippocrates to HIPAA: A Foundation for a Federal Physician-Patient Privilege*, 77 Temp. L. Rev. 505, 572 (2004) [5.05].

Ruger, *Health, Capability, and Justice: Toward a New Paradigm of Health Ethics, Policy and Law*, 15 Cornell J. L. & Pub. Pol'y 403, 425, 465 (2006) [2.22, 8.13].

Rugg, *An Old Solution to a New Problem: Physician Unions Take the Edge Off Managed Care*, 34 Colum. J. L. & Soc. Probs. 1, 41 (2000) [VI, VII; 10.01].

Rundle, *The Physician's Immunity Statute: A Botched Operation or a Model Procedure?* 34 J. Corp. L. 943 (2009) [9.08, 9.09].

Rupprecht, *Compelling Choice: Forcibly Medicating Death Row Inmates to Determine Whether They Wish to Pursue Collateral Relief*, 114 Penn St. L. Rev. 333 (2009) [2.06].

Russano, *Is Boutique Medicine a New Threat to American Health Care or a Logical Way of Revitalizing the Doctor-Patient Relationship?* 17 Wash. U.J. L. & Pol'y 313, 331, 332 (2005) [VII, IX; 8.055].

Rutkow, *Dying to Live: The Effect of the Patient Self-Determination Act on Hospice Care*, 7 N. Y. U. J. Legis. & Pub. Pol'y 393, 413, 430 (2004) [2.035, 2.22].

Sabo, *Limiting a Surrogate's Authority to Terminate Life-Support for an Incompetent Adult*, 79 N. C. L. Rev. 1815, 1815 (2001) [2.20].

Sade, *Broadcast of Surgical Procedures as a Teaching Instrument in Cardiothoracic Surgery*, 86 Ann. Thorac. Surg. 357, 359 (2008) [VIII; 8.121].

Sadoff, *Ethical Obligations for the Psychiatrist: Confidentiality, Privilege, and Privacy in Psychiatric Treatment*, 29 Loy. L.A. L. Rev. 1709, 1710, 1711 (1996) [IV; 5.05].

Safriet, *Closing the Gap Between Can and May in Health-Care Providers' Scopes of Practice: A Primer for Policymakers*, 19 Yale J. on Reg. 301, 311 (2002) [I, II].

Sage, *Managed Care's Crimea: Medical Necessity, Therapeutic Benefit, and the Goals of Administrative Process in Health Insurance*, 53 Duke L. J. 597, 634 (2003) [10.01].

Sage, *Pay for Performance: Will It Work In Theory?* 3 Ind. Health L. Rev. 305, 308-09 (2006) [6.01].

Sage, *Physicians as Advocates*, 35 Hous. L. Rev. 1529, 1537, 1541, 1542, 1552-53, 1554, 1556, 1557, 1559, 1561-62, 1564, 1571, 1574, 1576, 1580 (1999) [IV, VI; Elements (2), (4), (6); 2.03, 2.07, 2.09, 2.16, 2.19, 3.06, 4.01, 4.04, 6.01, 7.02, 8.02, 8.03, 8.13, 8.132, 9.06, 9.07, 9.131, 10.01, 10.02].

Sage, *Regulating Through Information: Disclosure Laws and American Health Care*, 99 Colum. L. Rev. 1701, 1753, 1758, 1760 (1999) [8.032, 8.051, 8.13].

Sage, *Some Principles Require Principals: Why Banning "Conflicts of Interest" Won't Solve Incentive Problems in Biomedical Research*, 85 Tex. L. Rev. 1413, 1458 (2007) [6.02].

Sage & Kalyan, *Horses or Unicorns: Can Paying for Performance Make Quality Competition Routine?* 31 J. Health Pol. Pol'y & L. 531, 531-32, 554 (2006) [6.01, 8.056].

Sage, Zivin, & Chase, *Bridging the Relational-Regulatory Gap*, 59 Vand. L. Rev. 1263, 1284 (2006) [8.12].

Sanematsu, *Taking a Broader View of Treatment Disputes Beyond Managed Care: Are Recent Legislative Efforts the Cure?* 48 UCLA L. Rev. 1245, 1258, 1284 (2001) [2.035, 2.037, 2.17, 2.22].

Sangree, *Control of Childbearing by HIV-Positive Women: Some Responses to Emerging Legal Policies*, 41 Buff. L. Rev. 309, 362 (1993) [8.08].

Santayana, *The Michigan Legislature Persists in Prohibiting Assisted Suicide*, 77 U. Det. Mercy L. Rev. 875, 886 (2000) [2.211].

Sargent, *Treating the Condemned to Death*, 16 Hastings Center Rep. 5 (Dec. 1986) [I; 2.06].

Sarnoff, *Patent Eligible Medical and Biotechnology Inventions After Bilski, Prometheus, and Myriad*, 19 Tex. Intell. Prop. L. J. 393, 407 (2011) [9.08].

Saver, *In Tepid Defense of Population Health: Physicians and Antibiotic Resistance*, 34 Am. J. L. & Med. 431(2008) [VII, VIII; 2.03, 2.09, 10.015].

Saver, *Squandering the Gain: Gainsharing and the Continuing Dilemma of Physician Financial Incentives*, 98 Nw. U. L. Rev. 145, 219, 221, 222 (2003) [2.03, 2.09, 4.04, 8.03, 8.13].

Sawicki, *Character, Competence, and the Principles of Medical Discipline*, 13 J. Health Care L. & Pol'y 285, 291 (2010) [10.015].

Sawicki, *Doctors, Discipline, and the Death Penalty: Professional Implications of Safe Harbor Policies*, 27 Yale L. & Pol'y Rev. 107 (2008) [2.06].

Sawyer, *The Death Penalty Is Dead Wrong: Jus Cogens Norms and the Evolving Standard of Decency*, 22 Penn. St. Int'l L. Rev. 459, 477 (2004) [2.06].

Schawbel, *Are You Taking Any Prescription Medication? A Case Comment on Weld v. CVS Pharmacy, Inc.*, 35 New Eng. L. Rev. 909, 957 (2001) [5.05].

Schiff, *The Lawyer's Role in Restoring Adolescents' Abortion Rights*, 44 Fed. Law. 60, 62 (May 1997) [2.015].

Schlesinger, Gray, & Perreira, *Medical Professionalism Under Managed Care: The Pros and Cons of Utilization Review*, 16 Health Affairs 106, 119, 120, 124 (1997) [8.13, 9.031].

Schmid, *Protecting the Physician in HIV Misdiagnosis Cases*, 46 Duke L. J. 431, 458 (1996) [IV].

Schmidt, *Professional Courtesy Discounts Under Siege—Part II*, 29 Colo. Law. 59, 62 (Jan. 2000) [6.12, 6.13].

Schneider, *Adverse Impact of Predisposition Testing on Major Life Activities: Lessons From BRCA1/2 Testing*, 3 J. Health Care L. & Pol'y 365, 380 (2000) [2.132].

Schneider, *After Autonomy*, 41 Wake Forest L. Rev. 411, 429-30 (2006) [8.13].

Schneiderman, Teetzel, & Kalmanson, *Who Decides Who Decides? When Disagreement Occurs Between the Physician and the Patient's Appointed Proxy About the Patient's Decision-Making Capacity*, 155 Arch. Intern. Med. 793, 796 (1995) [2.20].

Schnibbe, *Recent Legislative Developments in Utah Law: Family Law*, 1996 Utah L. Rev. 1335, 1394 (1996) [8.08].

Schoenholtz, Freedman, & Halpern, *The Legal Abuse of Physicians in Deaths in the United States: The Erosion of Ethics and Morality in Medicine*, 42 Wayne L. Rev. 1505, 1542 (1996) [2.06].

Schuler, *Knock Out? Supreme Court Deals a Blow to Non-Competes for Docs, but This Fight Is Not Over.* 41 Tenn. B.J. 16, 19 (Dec. 2005) [9.02, 9.06].

Schulkin, *Hormone Therapy, Dilemmas, Medical Decisions*, 36 J. L. Med. & Ethics 73 (2008) [8.061].

Schwartz, *Doubtful Duty: Physicians' Legal Obligation to Treat During an Epidemic*, 60 Stan. L. Rev. 657, 662, 663 (2007) [VII; 2.25, 9.067, 9.131].

Schwartz, *Privacy and the Economics of Personal Health Care Information*, 76 Tex. L. Rev. 1, 59 (1997) [5.07].

Schwartz, *The Ethical Health Lawyer: When Doing the Right Thing Means Breaking the Law—What Is the Role of the Health Lawyer?* 34 J. L. Med. & Ethics 624, 625, 626 (2006) [VIII; 1.02].

Schwartz & Gibson, *Defining the Role of the Physician: Medical Education, Tradition, and the Legal Process*, 18 Houston L. Rev. 779 (1981) [IV].

Schwartz, Silverman, Hulka, & Appel, *Marketing Pharmaceutical Products in the Twenty-First Century: An Analysis of the Continued Viability of Traditional Principles of Law in the Age of Direct-to-Consumer Advertising*, 32 Harv. J. L. & Pub. Pol'y 333 (2009) [5.015].

Sciarrino, *Ferguson v. City of Charleston: "The Doctor Will See You Now, Be Sure to Bring Your Privacy Rights in With You!"* 12 Temp. Pol. & Civ. Rts. L. Rev. 197, 213, 215, 220, 221, 222 (2002) [Preamble; VIII, IX; 2.136, 5.05, 10.01].

Scordato, *Understanding the Absence of a Duty to Reasonably Rescue in American Tort Law*, 82 Tul. L. Rev. 1447 (2008) [VI].

Scott, *Cybermedicine and Virtual Pharmacies*, 103 W. Va. L. Rev. 407, 441, 451 (2001) [5.05, 6.02, 6.03].

Scott, *Doctors as Advocates, Lawyers as Healers*, 29 Hamline J. Pub. L. Pol'y, 331 (2008) [I, II, VIII; 8.12, 10.01, 10.015].

Scott, *Is Too Much Privacy Bad for Your Health? An Introduction to the Law, Ethics, and HIPAA Rule on Medical Privacy*, 17 Ga. St. U. L. Rev. 481, 494 (2000) [10.01].

Searl, *Ward v. Summa Health System*, 37 Ohio N.U. L. Rev. 879, 887-888 (2011) [8.12].

Sears, *HIV Discrimination in Health Care Services in Los Angeles County: The Results of Three Testing Studies*, 15 Wash. & Lee J. Civil Rts. & Soc. Just. 85 (2008) [9.131].

Seng, *Legal and Regulatory Barriers to Adequate Pain Control for Elders in Long-Term Care Facilities*, 6 N.Y. City L. Rev. 95, 97 (2003) [2.20].

Severyn, *Jacobson v. Massachusetts: Impact on Informed Consent and Vaccine Policy*, 5 J. Pharmacy & L. 249, 253, 274 (1996) [8.08, 10.01].

Sewall, *Pushing Execution Over the Constitutional Line: Forcible Medication of Condemned Inmates and the Eighth and Fourteenth Amendments, 51 B.C. L. Rev. 1279, 1301 (2010)* [2.06].

Shaivitz, *Medicate-to-Execute: Current Trends in Death Penalty Jurisprudence and the Perils of Dual Loyalty, 7 J. Health Care L. & Pol'y 149, 167, 168 (2004)* [2.06].

Shapiro, *On the Possibility of "Progress" in Managing Biomedical Technologies: Markets, Lotteries, and Rational Moral Standards in Organ Transplantation, 31 Cap. U. L. Rev. 13, 29 (2003)* [2.16].

Shea, *Hurricane Katrina and the Legal and Bioethical Implications of Involuntary Euthanasia as a Component of Disaster Management in Extreme Emergency Situations, 19 Annals Health L. 133, 137-138 (2010)* [2.20, 2.21].

Shepherd, *Face to Face: A Call for Radical Responsibility in Place of Compassion, 77 St. John's L. Rev. 445, 472 (2003)* [VI].

Shepherd, *HIV, the ADA, and the Duty to Treat, 37 Hous. L. Rev. 1055, 1061, 1083-84 (2000)* [Preamble; VI; 9.131].

Shepherd, *In Respect of People Living in a Permanent Vegetative State—And Allowing Them to Die, 16 Health Matrix 631, 671 (2006)* [2.20].

Shepherd, *Sophie's Choices: Medical and Legal Responses to Suffering, 72 Notre Dame L. Rev. 103, 106, 133 (1996)* [VI; 2.162].

Shewmon, *Active Voluntary Euthanasia: A Needless Pandora's Box, 3 Issues in Law and Med. 219 (1987)* [2.06, 8.11, 9.06].

Shimm & Spece, *Conflict of Interest and Informed Consent in Industry-Sponsored Clinical Trials, 12 J. Legal Med. 477, 481, 507, 510 (1991)* [8.031].

Shin, *Redressing Wounds: Finding a Legal Framework to Remedy Racial Disparities in Medical Care, 90 Cal. L. Rev. 2047, 2056, 2057, 2100 (2002)* [9.121].

Shiner, *Medical Futility: A Futile Concept? 53 Wash. & Lee L. Rev. 803, 834 (1996)* [10.01].

Shorr, *AIDS, Judaism, and the Limits of the Secular Society, 20 Second Opinion 23, 24, 27 (1995)* [5.05, 9.131].

Shultz, *From Informed Consent to Patient Choice: A New Protected Interest, 95 Yale L. J. 219 (1985)* [II, IV; 6.02, 8.03, 8.032].

Siegal & Bonnie, *Closing the Organ Gap: A Reciprocity-Based Social Contract Approach, 34 J. L. Med. & Ethics 415, 415 (2006)* [2.155].

Sierles, Brodkey, Cleary, McCurdy, Mintz, Frank, Lynn, Chao, Morgenstern, Shore, & Woodard, *Medical Students' Exposure to and Attitudes About Drug Company Interactions: A National Survey, 294 JAMA 1034, 1035 (2005)* [8.061].

Sigman, Kraut, & La Puma, *Disclosure of a Diagnosis to Children and Adolescents When Parents Object, 147 Am. J. Diseases Children 764, 766 (1993)* [II].

Silver, *From Baby Doe to Grandpa Doe: The Impact of the Federal Age Discrimination Act on the Hidden Rationing of Medical Care, 37 Catholic Univ. L. Rev. 993 (1988)* [2.03].

Silver, *Love, Hate, and Other Emotional Interference in the Lawyer/Client Relationship, 6 Clinical L. Rev. 259, 266 (1999)* [8.14].

Silverstein & Speitel, *"Honey, I Have No Idea": Court Readiness to Handle Petitions to Waive Parental Consent for Abortion, 88 Iowa L. Rev. 75, 116, 117 (2002)* [2.015].

Simon, *Treatment Boundary Violations: Clinical, Ethical, and Legal Considerations, 20 Bull. Am. Acad. Psychiatry Law 269, 282 (1992)* [6.07].

Singleton, *Privacy Versus the First Amendment: A Skeptical Approach, 11 Fordham Intell. Prop. Media & Ent. L. J. 97, 122 (2000)* [5.05].

Sirmon & Kreisberg, *The Invisible Patient, 334 New Eng. J. Med. 908, 910, 911 (1996)* [8.12].

Skiver & Hickey, *AIDS: Legal Issues 1992, 19 Ohio No. Univ. L. Rev. 839, 860 (1993)* [5.05].

Sklansky, *Neonatal Euthanasia: Moral Considerations and Criminal Liability, 27 J. Med. Ethics 5, 8, 9 (2001)* [2.215].

Skobeloff, Spivey, St. Clair, & Schoffstall, *The Influence of Age and Sex on Asthma Admissions, 268 JAMA 3437, 3439, 3440 (1992)* [9.122].

Sladden & Graydon, *Liability for Medical Malpractice—Recent New Zealand Developments, 28 Med. & L. 301 (2009)* [8.12].

Smetanka, *Who Will Protect the "Disruptive" Dialysis Patient? 32 Am. J. L. & Med. 53, 89 (2006)* [Preamble].

Smith, *Euphemistic Codes and Tell-Tale Hearts: Humane Assistance in End-of-Life Cases, 10 Health Matrix 175, 177 (2000)* [2.22].

Smith, *Ignorance Is Not Bliss: Why a Ban on Human Cloning Is Unacceptable,* 9 Health Matrix 311, 330, 331 (1999) [2.162].

Smith, *Legal Recognition of Neocortical Death,* 71 Cornell L. Rev. 850 (1986) [2.20].

Smith, *Murder, She Wrote or Was It Merely Selective Nontreatment?* 8 J. Contemp. Health L. & Pol'y 49, 53 (1992) [2.17, 2.20].

Smith, *Our Hearts Were Once Young and Gay: Health Care Rationing and the Elderly,* 8 U. Fla. J. L. & Pub. Pol'y 1, 21 (1996) [2.09].

Smith, *Rethinking Prison Sex: Self-expression and Safety,* 15 Colum. J. Gender & L. 185, 202 (2006) [3.08, 8.14, 8.145, 10.015].

Smith, *The Elderly and Health Care Rationing,* 7 Pierce L. Rev. 171 (2009) [2.09].

Sneed, May, & Stencel, *Physicians' Reliance on Specialists, Therapists, and Vendors When Prescribing Therapies and Durable Medical Equipment for Children With Special Health Care Needs,* 107 Pediatrics 1283, 1287, 1288, 1289 (2001) [8.06, 9.132].

Snyder, *Artificial Feeding and the Right to Die: The Legal Issues,* 9 J. Legal Med. 349 (1988) [2.20].

Solomon & Asaro, *Community-Based Health Care: A Legal and Policy Analysis,* 24 Fordham Urb. L. J. 235, 276-77 (1997) [9.065, 10.01].

Solove, *Digital Dossiers and the Dissipation of Fourth Amendment Privacy,* 75 S. Cal. L. Rev. 1083, 1155 (2002) [5.05].

Sonderling, *POLST: A Cure for the Common Advance Directive—It's Just What the Doctor Ordered,* 33 Nova L. Rev. 451 (2009) [2.225].

Sontag, *Are Clinical Ethics Consultants in Danger? An Analysis of the Potential Legal Liability of Individual Clinical Ethicists,* 151 U. Pa. L. Rev. 667, 679 (2002) [9.11].

Spece, *Medical Tourism: Protecting Patients From Conflicts of Interest in Broker's Fees Paid by Foreign Providers,* 6 J. Health & Biomedical L. 1, 3, 19 (2010) [6.02, 6.021].

Spece & Marchalonis, *Sound Constitutional Analysis, Moral Principle, and Wise Policy Judgment Require a Clear and Convincing Evidence Standard of Proof in Physician Disciplinary Proceedings,* 3 Ind. Health L. Rev. 107, 109 (2006) [9.05].

Spector, *Managed Healthcare Liability Issues,* 32 Cumb. L. Rev. 311, 335-36 (2002) [8.132].

Spellman, *Encouragement Is Not Enough: The Benefits of Instituting a Mandated Choice Organ Procurement System,* 56 Syracuse L. Rev. 353, 371 (2006) [2.155].

Sperling, *Breaking Through the Silence: Illegality of Performing Resuscitation Procedures on the "Newly-Dead,"* 13 Ann. Health L. 393, 394, 396, 401, 425 (2004) [8.181].

Spielberg, *On Call and Online: Sociohistorical, Legal, and Ethical Implications of E-mail for the Patient-Physician Relationship,* 280 JAMA 1353, 1356 (1998) [5.04, 5.05, 5.057, 5.07, 5.075, 5.08].

Spielberg, *Online Without a Net: Physician-Patient Communication by Electronic Mail,* 25 Am. J. Law & Med. 267, 284-85 (1999) [5.04, 5.05, 5.06, 5.07].

Spielman, *After the Gag Episode: Physician Communication in Managed Care Organizations,* 22 Seton Hall Legis. J. 437, 453, 461, 463 (1998) [8.13].

Spielman, *Managed Care Regulation and the Physician-Advocate,* 47 Drake L. Rev. 713, 717, 719 (1999) [8.13].

Spielman, *Professionalism in Forensic Bioethics,* 30 J. L. Med. & Ethics 420, 425, 427, 436 (2002) [9.07].

Spreng, *Pharmacists and the "Duty" to Dispense Emergency Contraceptives,* 23 Issues L. & Med. 215 (2008) [9.12].

Sprung, *Changing Attitudes and Practices in Forgoing Life-Sustaining Treatments,* 263 JAMA 2211, 2213 (1990) [2.20].

Staihar, *The State's Unqualified Interest in Preserving Life: A Critique of the Formulations of Life's Sanctity in Washington v. Glucksberg,* 34 Idaho L. Rev. 401, 415 (1998) [2.211].

Stamatakis, *Beyond Advance Directives: Personal Autonomy and the Right to Refuse Life-Sustaining Medical Treatment,* 47 N. H. B. J. 20, 29-30 (2007) [2.035, 2.037, 2.20, 2.225, 8.08, 8.081, 8.082, 9.11, 9.115, 10.015].

Stark, *Bio-Ethics and Physician Liability: The Liability Effects of Developing Pain Management Standards,* 14 St. Thomas L. Rev. 601, 631 (2002) [2.21, 2.211].

Stein & Savulescu, *Welfare Versus Autonomy in Human Subjects Research,* 38 Fla. St. U. L. Rev. 303, 332 (2011) [8.08].

Steinberg & Pomfret, *A Novel Boundary Issue: Should a Patient Be an Organ Donor for Their Physician?* 34 J. Med. Ethics 772, 772 (2008) [8.14, 10.017, 10.018].

Steinbrook, *Physician-Industry Relations—Will Fewer Gifts Make a Difference? 360 New Eng. J. Med. 557 (2009)* [8.061].

Steinbrook & Lo, *Artificial Feeding—Solid Ground, Not a Slippery Slope, 318 New Eng. J. Med. 286 (1988)* [2.20].

Steinbuch, *Placing Profits Above Hippocrates: The Hypocrisy of General Service Hospitals, 31 U. Ark. Little Rock L. Rev. 505 (2009)* [9.02].

Stinneford, *Incapacitation Through Maiming: Chemical Castration, The Eighth Amendment, and the Denial of Human Dignity, 3 U. St. Thomas L. J. 559, 576 (2006)* [2.065].

Stith, *The Semblance of Autonomy: Treatment of Persons With Disabilities Under the Uniform Health-Care Decisions Act, 22 Issues L. & Med. 39, 63-64 (2006)* [8.13].

Stoever, *Stories Absent From the Courtroom: Responding to Domestic Violence in the Context of HIV and AIDS, 87 N. C. L. Rev. 1157 (2009)* [2.02].

Stone & Winslade, *Physician-Assisted Suicide and Euthanasia in the United States: Legal and Ethical Observations, 16 J. Legal Med. 481, 483, 490, 497, 498, 499 (1995)* [III, IV, VI; 2.20, 2.21, 8.11, 9.12].

Stonefield, *Lawyer Discrimination Against Clients: Outright Rejection—No; Limitations on Issues and Arguments—Yes, 20 W. New Eng. L. Rev. 103, 112 (1998)* [9.12].

Storey, *Does Ethics Make Good Law? A Case Study, 19 Cardozo Arts & Ent. L. J. 467, 470 (2001)* [1.02].

Strasser, *The Futility of Futility? On Life, Death, and Reasoned Public Policy, 57 Md. L. Rev. 505, 523, 552, 553 (1998)* [2.22].

Strong, *Consent to Sperm Retrieval and Insemination After Death or Persistent Vegetative State, 14 J. L. & Health 243, 248 (2000)* [2.22].

Studdert, Mello, & Brennan, *Financial Conflicts of Interest in Physicians' Relationships with the Pharmaceutical Industry—Self-regulation in the Shadow of Federal Prosecution, 351 New Eng. J. Med. 1891, 1900 (2004)* [8.061].

Sugarman & Yarashus, *Admissibility of Managed Care Financial Incentives in Medical Malpractice Cases, 34 Tort & Ins. L. J. 735, 743, 746, 759 (1999)* [8.13, 8.132].

Sullivan, *Naked Fitzies and Iron Cages: Individual Values, Professional Virtues, and the Struggle for Public Space, 78 Tul. L. Rev. 1687, 1702, 1703 (2004)* [V; 5.05].

Sullivan & Reynolds, *Where Law and Bioethics Meet . . . and Where They Don't, 75 U. Det. Mercy L. Rev. 607, 612 (1998)* [8.08, 8.115].

Sulmasy, Geller, Faden, & Levine, *The Quality of Mercy: Caring for Patients With "Do Not Resuscitate" Orders, 267 JAMA 682 (1992)* [2.22].

Sulmasy & Pellegrino, *The Rule of Double Effect: Clearing Up the Double Talk 159 Arch. Intern. Med. 545, 550 (1999)* [2.20].

Summerhill & Chandler, *Company Representatives in the Operating & Treatment Room: How to Navigate the Ever-Expanding Theories of Liability for Medical Device & Pharmaceutical Companies, 12 DePaul J. Health Care L. 253 (2009)* [Preamble; 2.06, 2.067, 2.068].

Sundram, *In Harm's Way: Research Subjects Who Are Decisionally Impaired, 1 J. Health Care L. & Pol'y 36, 43-44 (1998)* [2.07].

Susman, *Your Karma Ran Over My Dogma: Bikram Yoga and the (Im)Possibilities of Copyrighting Yoga, 25 Loy. L.A. Ent. L. Rev. 245, 272 (2005)* [9.095].

Suter, *A Brave New World of Designer Babies? 22 Berkeley Tech. L. J. 897, 936-37 (2007)* [2.137].

Suter, *Disentangling Privacy From Property: Toward a Deeper Understanding of Genetic Privacy, 72 Geo. Wash. L. Rev. 737, 787 (2004)* [IV; 5.05].

Suzuki, *When Something Is Not Quite Right: Considerations for Advising a Client to Seek Mental Health Treatment, 6 Hastings Race & Poverty L. J. 209 (2009)* [IV].

Swanson, *The Right to Know: An Approach to Gun Licenses and Public Access to Government Records, 56 UCLA L. Rev. 1579 (2009)* [5.05].

Swartz, *"Conscience Clauses" or "Unconscionable Clauses": Personal Beliefs Versus Professional Responsibilities, 6 Yale J. Health Pol'y, L. & Ethics 269, 317, 347 (2006)* [2.20, 8.032].

Svoboda, Van Howe, & Dwyer, *Informed Consent for Neonatal Circumcision: An Ethical and Legal Conundrum, 17 J. Contemp. Health L. & Pol'y 61, 67, 73, 82 (2000)* [8.08, 8.03, 9.011].

Swedlow, Johnson, Smithline, & Milstein, *Increased Costs and Rates of Use in the California Workers' Compensation System as a Result of Self-referral by Physicians,* 327 New Eng. J. Med. 1502 (1992) [8.032].

Szczygiel, *Beyond Informed Consent,* 21 Ohio N. U. L. Rev. 171, 217, 218, 220, 225, 226, 256 (1994) [Preamble; I, II, III, IV, V, VI; 1.01, 1.02, 8.08, 10.01].

Tabler, *Should Physicians Apologize for Medical Errors?* 19 Health Lawyer 23, 23 (Jan. 2007) [I, II, III, IV; 8.12].

Tabor, *The Battle for Hospital Privileges,* 251 JAMA 1602 (1984) [9.05].

Tadd & Bayer, *Commentary: Medical Decision Making Based on Chronological Age—Cause for Concern,* 11 J. Clinical Ethics 328, 330 (2000) [2.035].

Talesh, *Breaking the Learned Helplessness of Patients: Why MCOs Should be Required to Disclose Financial Incentives,* 26 Law & Psychol. Rev. 49, 60-61, 63 (2002) [2.03, 8.13].

Tames, Cotter, Melendez, Scudder, & Colvin, *Medical-Legal Partnership: Evolution or Revolution,* 45 Clearinghouse Rev. 124, 127 (2011) [9.065].

Tapocsi, *Three Steps to Death: The Use of the Drug Pavulon in the Lethal Injection Protocol Utilized Today Violates the Eighth Amendment's Protection Against Cruel and Unusual Punishment,* 35 Ohio N.U. L. Rev. 425 (2009) [2.06].

Tarantino, *Withdrawal of Life Support: Conflict Among Patient Wishes, Family, Physicians, Courts and Statutes, and the Law,* 42 Buff. L. Rev. 623, 638, 639, 646 (1994) [2.20].

Taslitz, *A Feminist Fourth Amendment? Consent, Care, Privacy, and Social Meaning in Ferguson v. City of Charleston,* 9 Duke J. Gender L. & Pol'y 1, 18, 19 (2002) [II, IV; 10.01].

Tasse, *The Return of Results of Deceased Research Participants,* 39 J. L. Med. & Ethics 621, 624-625 (2011) [5.051].

Taub, *Withholding Treatment From Defective Newborns,* 10 Law Med. & Health Care 4 (Feb. 1982) [2.17].

Tenery, *Interactions Between Physicians and the Health Care Technology Industry,* 283 JAMA 391, 393 (2000) [8.061, 9.011].

Teninbaum, *How Medical Apology Programs Harm Patients,* 15 Chap. L. Rev. 307, 310 (2011) [8.12].

Terry, *An eHealth Diptych: The Impact of Privacy Regulation on Medical Error and Malpractice Litigation,* 27 Am. J. L. & Med. 361, 402 (2001) [IV].

Terry, *Physicians and Patients Who "Friend" or "Tweet": Constructing a Legal Framework for Social Networking in a Highly Regulated Domain,* 43 Ind. L. Rev. 285, 314-16, 319, 334-36, 338 (2010) [5.026, 5.027, 5.045, 5.046, 5.05, 5.059, 5.0591, 8.14, 9.031, 9.08, 9.12, 9.123].

Terry, *Prescriptions sans Frontières (or How I Stopped Worrying About Viagra on the Web but Grew Concerned About the Future of Healthcare Delivery),* 4 Yale J. Health Pol'y L. & Ethics 183, 240, 244, 251 (2004) [5.026, 5.027].

Terry, *Under-Regulated Health Care Phenomena in a Flat World: Medical Tourism and Outsourcing,* 29 W. New Eng. L. Rev. 421, 441 (2007) [7.05].

Terzian, *Direct-to-Consumer Prescription Drug Advertising,* 25 Am. J. Law & Med. 149, 165 (1999) [II, III].

Testa, *Sentenced to Life? An Analysis of the United States Supreme Court's Decision in Washington v. Glucksberg,* 22 Nova L. Rev. 821, 839 (1998) [2.211].

Thomasma, *When Physicians Choose to Participate in the Death of Their Patients: Ethics and Physician-Assisted Suicide,* 24 J. Law Med. & Ethics 183, 184, 195 (1996) [2.211].

Thompson, *Understanding Financial Conflicts of Interest,* 329 New Eng. J. Med. 573 (1993) [8.032].

Tironi, *Pharmaceutical Pricing: A Review of Proposals to Improve Access and Affordability of Prescription Drugs,* 19 Ann. Health L. 311, 360 (2010) [8.061].

Todres, *Toward Healing and Restoration for All: Reframing Medical Malpractice Reform,* 39 Conn. L. Rev. 667, 728-29 (2006) [8.12].

Toll, *For My Doctor's Eyes Only: Ferguson v. City of Charleston,* 33 Loy. U. Chi. L. J. 267, 305 (2001) [5.05].

Tovino, *The Use and Disclosure of Protected Health Information for Research Under the HIPAA Privacy Rule: Unrealized Patient Autonomy and Burdensome Government Regulation,* 49 S. D. L. Rev. 447, 496, 502 (2004) [VIII; 5.051, 8.031, 10.015].

Tovino & Winslade, *A Primer on the Law and Ethics of Treatment, Research, and Public Policy in the Context of Severe Traumatic Brain Injury,* 14 Ann. Health L. 1, 18, 38, 39, 40, 41 (2005) [VII, IX; 8.031, 8.0315, 9.065, 10.01, 10.015].

Trehan, *Fear of Prescribing: How the DEA Is Infringing on Patients' Right to Palliative Care*, 61 U. Miami L. Rev. 961, 975 (2007) [2.20].

Trew, *Regulating Life and Death: The Modification and Commodification of Nature*, 29 U. Tol. L. Rev. 271, 292 (1998) [2.162].

Tribbensee, *Privacy and Confidentiality: Balancing Student Rights and Campus Safety*, 34 J.C. & U. L. 393 (2008) [5.05].

Trunkey, Cahn, Lenfesty, & Mullins, *Management of the Geriatric Trauma Patient at Risk of Death: Therapy Withdrawal Decision Making*, 135 Arch. Surg. 34, 35 (2000) [2.037].

Truog, *Brain Death—Too Flawed to Endure, Too Ingrained to Abandon*, 35 J. L. Med. & Ethics 273, 280 (2007) [2.162].

Truog, *Futility in Pediatrics: From Case to Policy*, 11 J. Clinical Ethics 136, 139, 141 (2000) [2.037].

Truog & Brennan, *Participation of Physicians in Capital Punishment*, 329 New Eng. J. Med. 1346 (1993) [2.06].

Tsai, *Cheaper and Better: The Congressional Administrative Simplification Mandate Facilitates the Transition to Electronic Medical Records*, 19 J. Legal Med. 549, 570, 581 (1998) [IV; 5.07, 5.075, 8.061].

Turkington, *Medical Record Confidentiality Law, Scientific Research, and Data Collection in the Information Age*, 25 J. Law Med. & Ethics 113, 126 (1997) [IV].

Turner, *Going After the "Hired Guns": Is Improper Expert Witness Testimony Unprofessional Conduct or the Negligent Practice of Medicine?* 33 Pepp. L. Rev. 275, 304 (2006) [9.07].

Tyler, *Allies Not Adversaries: Teaching Collaboration to the Next Generation of Doctors and Lawyers to Address Social Inequality*, 11 J. Health Care L. & Pol'y 249 (2008) [9.065].

Underwood & Cadle, *Genetics, Genetic Testing, and the Specter of Discrimination: A Discussion Using Hypothetical Cases*, 85 Ky. L. J. 665, 684 (1996-97) [2.12].

Urofsky, *Do Go Gentle Into That Good Night: Thoughts on Death, Suicide, Morality and the Law*, 59 Ark. L. Rev. 819, 832 (2007) [2.211].

Urofsky, *Justifying Assisted Suicide: Comments on the Ongoing Debate*, 14 Notre Dame J. L. Ethics & Pub. Pol'y 893, 918, 923 (2000) [2.06, 2.211].

Urofsky, *Leaving the Door Ajar: The Supreme Court and Assisted Suicide*, 32 U. Rich. L. Rev. 313, 336 (1998) [2.211].

Van Der Goes, *Opportunity Lost: Why and How to Improve the HHS-Proposed Legislation Governing Law Enforcement Access to Medical Records*, 147 U. Pa. L. Rev. 1009, 1063 (1999) [IV].

Vanderstappen, *Internet Pharmacies and the Specter of the Dormant Commerce Clause*, 22 Wash. U. J. L. & Pol'y 619, 628 (2006) [5.026].

Vars, *Illusory Consent: When an Incapacitated Patient Agrees to Treatment*, 87 Or. L. Rev. 353 (2008) [8.08].

Veatch, *Abandoning Informed Consent*, 25 Hastings Center Rep. 5, 6 (March/April 1995) [8.08].

Veatch, *Doctor Does Not Know Best: Why in the New Century Physicians Must Stop Trying to Benefit Patients*, 25 J. Med. & Phil. 701, 710, 711 (2000) [II; 8.08].

Veatch, *Why Liberals Should Accept Financial Incentives for Organ Procurement*, 13 Kennedy Inst. Ethics J. 19, 34 (March 2003) [2.15].

Velikonia, *The Costs of Multiple Gestation Pregnancies in Assisted Reproduction*, 32 Harv. J. L. & Gender 463 (2009) [2.055].

Virmani, Schneiderman, & Kaplan, *Relationship of Advance Directives to Physician-Patient Communication*, 154 Arch. Intern. Med. 909, 913 (1994) [2.20].

Vital, *Mandatory Reporting Statutes and the Violence Against Women Act: An Analytical Comparison*, 10 Geo. Mason U. Civ. Rts. L. J. 171, 189 (2000) [2.02].

Volkert, *Telemedicine: Rx for the Future of Health Care*, 6 Mich. Telecomm. & Tech. L. Rev. 147, 214, 225 (2000) [5.05, 5.07].

Vukadinovich, *Minors' Rights to Consent to Treatment: Navigating the Complexity of State Laws*, 37 J. Health L. 667, 689-90 (2004) [2.015].

Wagner, Kane, & Kallman, *Suicide Killing of Human Life as a Human Right*, 6 Liberty U. L. Rev. 27, 38 (2011) [2.211].

Walker, *Protecting the Public: The Impact of the Americans with Disabilities Act on Licensure Considerations Involving Mentally Impaired Medical and Legal Professionals*, 25 J. Legal Med. 441, 454 (2004) [9.031].

Wallace, *Incompetency for Execution: The Supreme Court Challenges the Ethical Standards of the Mental Health Professions*, 8 J. Legal Med. 265 (1987) [2.06].

Waller & Fulton, *The Electronic Chart: Keeping It Confidential and Secure*, 26 J. Health & Hosp. L. 104, 105 (April 1993) [IV; 5.07].

Walters, *Life-Sustaining Medical Decisions Involving Children: Father Knows Best*, 15 T. M. Cooley L. Rev. 115, 128, 138, 151 (1998) [2.20].

Walters & Ashwal, *Organ Prolongation in Anencephalic Infants: Ethical and Medical Issues*, 18 Hastings Center Rep. 19 (Oct./Nov. 1988) [2.20].

Walzer, *Impaired Physicians: An Overview and Update of the Legal Issues*, 11 J. Legal Med. 131, 174, 192 (1990) [IV; 4.07].

Wampler, *To Be or Not to Be in Tennessee: Deciding Surrogate Issues*, 34 U. Mem. L. Rev. 333, 365 (2004) [2.035, 8.081, 8.115].

Wang, *Race as Proxy: Situational Racism and Self-fulfilling Stereotypes*, 53 DePaul L. Rev. 1013, 1082-83 (2004) [9.121].

Wann, Nassef, Jeffrey, Messer, Wilke, Duerinckx, Blankenship, Rosenberg, & Dembo, *Ethical Considerations in CT Angiography*, 23 Int. J. Cardiovasc. Imaging 379, 384 (2007) [V].

Wanzer, Federman, Adelstein, Cassel, Cassem, Cranford, Hook, Lo, Moertel, Safar, Stone, & Van Eys, *The Physician's Responsibility Toward Hopelessly Ill Patients: A Second Look*, 320 New Eng. J. Med. 844 (1989) [2.20].

Warren, *Pennsylvania Medical Informed Consent Law: A Call to Protect Patient Autonomy Rights by Abandoning the Battery Approach*, 38 Duq. L. Rev. 917, 925 (2000) [IV; 8.08, 10.01].

Washko, *Should Ethics Play a Special Role in Patent Law?* 19 Geo. J. Legal Ethics 1027, 1029 (2006) [9.095].

Washlick & Welch, *Physician-Vendor Marketing and Financial Relationships Under Attack*, 2 J. Health & Life Sci. L. 151 (2008) [8.061].

Watson, *Medicaid Physician Participation: Patients, Poverty, and Physician Self-interest*, XXI Am. J. Law & Med. 191, 218 (1995) [VI].

Watson, *Race, Ethnicity and Quality of Care: Inequalities and Incentives*, 27 Am. J. L. & Med. 203, 206 (2001) [9.121].

Wazana, *Physicians and the Pharmaceutical Industry: Is a Gift Ever Just a Gift?* 283 JAMA 373, 380 (2000) [8.061].

Wear, Coles, Szczygiel, McEvoy, & Pegels, *Patenting Medical and Surgical Techniques: An Ethical-Legal Analysis*, 23 J. Med. Phil. 75, 76, 87 (1998) [9.08, 9.095].

Weeks, *Loopholes: Opportunity, Responsibility, or Liability?* 35 J. L. Med. & Ethics 320, 322 (2007) [8.09].

Weiner & Wettstein, *Confidentiality of Patient-Related Information*, 112 Arch. Ophthalmology 1032, 1033 (1994) [IV; 10.01].

Weinstock, Leong & Silva, *Competence to Be Executed: an Ethical Analysis Post Panetti*, 28 Behav. Sci. Law 690, 691 (2010) [2.06].

Weinstock, Leong, & Silva, *Opinions by AAPL Forensic Psychiatrists on Controversial Ethical Guidelines: A Survey*, 19 Bull. Am. Acad. Psychiatry Law 237, 238 (1991) [1.02, 5.09].

Weir & Gostin, *Decisions to Abate Life-Sustaining Treatment for Nonautonomous Patients: Ethical Standards and Legal Liability for Physicians After Cruzan*, 264 JAMA 1846, 1849, 1850 (1990) [2.20].

Weissbrodt & Wilson, *Piercing the Confidentiality Veil: Physician Testimony in International Criminal Trials Against Perpetrators of Torture*, 15 Minn. J. Int'l L. 43, 68, 68-69 (2006) [IV; 5.05].

Weisser, *Abolishing the Pharmacist's Veto: An Argument in Support of a Wrongful Conception Cause of Action Against Pharmacists Who Refuse to Provide Emergency Contraception*, 80 S. Cal. L. Rev. 865, 881-81 (2007) [8.08].

Wentz, Osteen, & Gannon, *Continuing Medical Education: Unabated Debate*, 268 JAMA 1118 (1992) [8.061, 9.011].

Wentz, Osteen, & Gannon, *Refocusing Support and Direction*, 266 JAMA 953 (1991) [8.061, 9.011].

Wertheimer, *Ockham's Scalpel: A Return to a Reasonableness Standard*, 43 Vill. L. Rev. 321, 327 (1998) [8.13].

Wertheimer, *Of Apples and Trees: Adoption and Informed Consent*, 25 QLR 601, 618 (2007) [8.082].

Westfall, McCabe, & Nicholas, *Personal Use of Drug Samples by Physicians and Office Staff*, 278 JAMA 141, 142 (1997) [8.061].

White, *Health Care Professionals and Treatment of HIV-Positive Patients*, 20 J. Legal Med. 67, 86 (1999) [VI; 2.23, 9.131].

White & Zimbelman, *Abandoning Informed Consent: An Idea Whose Time Has Not Yet Come*, 23 J. Med. Phil. 477, 496 (1998) [Preamble].

Widmer, *South Dakota Should Follow Public Policy and Switch to the Preponderance Standard for Medical License Revocation After In Re the Medical License of Dr. Reuben Setliff, M.D.*, 48 S. D. L. Rev. 388, 396-97, 402 (2003) [II, III, IV; 1.02, 9.07].

Wilcox, *Enforcing Lawyer Non-Competition Agreements While Maintaining the Profession: The Role of Conflict of Interest Principles*, 84 Minn. L. Rev. 915, 966 (2000) [9.02].

Wilde, *Air Force Women's Access to Abortion Services and the Erosion of 10 USC § 1093*, 9 Wm. & Mary J. Women & L. 351, 371 (2003) [8.08, 10.01].

Wilde, *Bioethical and Legal Implications of Pediatric Gastric Bypass*, 40 Willamette L. Rev. 575, 613 (2004) [10.015].

Wilde, *The Liability of Alaska Mental Health Providers for Mandated Treatment*, 20 Alaska L. Rev. 271, 276 (2003) [10.01].

Williams, *Fluconomics: Preserving Our Hospital Infrastructure During and After a Pandemic*, 7 Yale J. Health Pol'y L. & Ethics 99, 115 (2007) [2.25, 9.067].

Williams, *Managing Physician Financial Conflicts of Interest in Clinical Trials Conducted in the Private Practice Setting*, 59 Food & Drug L. J. 45, 67 (2004) [8.061].

Williams, *The Trouble With Texting: The Future of Searches Under the Automobile Exception After Arizona v. Gant*, 4 Charleston L. Rev. 919, 929 (2010) [5.05].

Williams & Rucker, *Understanding and Addressing Racial Disparities in Health Care*, 21 Health Care Fin. Rev. 75, 88 (2000) [9.122].

Wilson, *Dwindling Community Involvement: A Sign of Professional Failure to Thrive?* 162 Arch. Pediatr. Adolesc. Med. 695, 695 (2008) [VII].

Wilson, *"Unauthorized Practice": Regulating the Use of Anesthetized, Recently Deceased, and Conscious Patients in Medical Teaching*, 44 Idaho L. Rev. 423 (2008) [8.087].

Wiltbank, *Informed Consent and Physician Inexperience: A Prescription for Liability?* 42 Willamette L. Rev. 563, 570 (2006) [8.16].

Windsor, *Disposition of Cryopreserved Preembryos After Divorce*, 88 Iowa L. Rev. 1001, 1026 (2003) [2.141].

Winn, *Confidentiality in Cyberspace: The HIPAA Privacy Rules and the Common Law*, 33 Rutgers L. J. 617, 622 (2002) [5.05].

Winslade & McKinney, *The Ethical Health Lawyer: To Tell or Not to Tell: Disclosing Medical Error*, 34 J. L. Med. & Ethics 813, 814 (2006) [8.12].

Wiseman, *Pro Bono Publico: The Growing Need for Expert Aid*, 60 S. C. L. Rev. 493 (2008) [9.07].

Woan, *Buy Me a Pound of Flesh: China's Sale of Death Row Organs on the Black Market and What Americans Can Learn From It*, 47 Santa Clara L. Rev. 413, 439 (2007) [2.151].

Wolf, *Health Care Reform and the Future of Physician Ethics*, 24 Hastings Center Rep. 28, 32, 40 (March/ April 1994) [2.03, 2.09, 4.04, 5.01, 8.03, 9.121, 9.122].

Wolf, *Toward a Systemic Theory of Informed Consent in Managed Care*, 35 Hous. L. Rev. 1631, 1641, 1658, 1661, 1662, 1679 (1999) [2.03, 8.03, 8.032, 8.051, 8.13, 8.132].

Wolf & Kahn, *Genetic Testing and the Future of Disability Insurance: Ethics, Law & Policy*, 35 J. L. Med. & Ethics 6, 23 (2007) [2.138].

Wolf, Kahn, & Wagner, *Using Preimplantation Genetic Diagnosis to Create a Stem Cell Donor: Issues, Guidelines & Limits*, 31 J. L. Med. & Ethics 327, 329, 339 (2003) [2.12].

Wolfson, *A Quality of Mercy: The Struggle of the AIDS-Afflicted to Use Marijuana as Medicine*, 22 T. Jefferson L. Rev. 1, 24 (1999) [2.17].

Wong, *A Matter of Life and Death: A Very Personal Discourse*, 1 Geo. J. L. & Pub. Pol'y 339, 350 (2003) [2.211].

Wong, *Lethal Injection Protocols: The Failure of Litigation to Stop Suffering and the Case for Legislative Reform*, 25 Temp. J. Sci. Tech. & Envtl. L. 263, 282 (2006) [2.06].

Wong, *Whose Life Is It Anyway?* 5 Cardozo Pub. L. Pol'y & Ethics J. 233, 271-72 (2006) [2.035, 2.211].

Wood, *Protective Privilege Versus Public Peril: How Illinois Has Failed to Balance Patient Confidentiality With the Mental Health Professional's Duty to Protect the Public*, 29 N. Ill. U. L. Rev. 571 (2009) [Preamble; 5.05].

Woodward, *Medical Record Confidentiality and Data Collection: Current Dilemmas*, 25 J. Law Med. & Ethics 88, 90, 95 (1997) [5.07].

Wusthoff, *Medical Mistakes and Disclosure: The Role of the Medical Student*, 286 JAMA 1080, 1080 (2001) [8.12].

Wyatt, *Buy Out or Get Out: Why Covenants Not to Compete in Surgeon Employment Contracts Are Truly Bad Medicine*, 45 Washburn L. J. 715, 720 (2006) [9.02, 9.06].

Wynia, *Breaching Confidentiality to Protect the Public: Evolving Standards of Medical Confidentiality for Military Detainees*, 7 Am. J. Bioethics, 1, 2 (Aug. 2007) [III; 1.02, 5.05].

Xenakis, *How Should We Respond? Seton Hall University School of Law Guantanamo Teach-In*, 37 Seton Hall L. Rev. 703, 709 (2007) [II].

Yang & Gorman, *What's Yours Is Mine: Protection and Security in a Digital World*, 36 Md. B.J. 24, 28-29 (Nov./Dec. 2003) [5.05].

Young, *Telemedicine: Patient Privacy Rights of Electronic Medical Records*, 66 UMKC L. Rev. 921, 926 (1998) [IV; 5.05].

Zer-Gutman, *Revising the Ethical Rules of Attorney-Client Confidentiality: Towards a New Discretionary Rule*, 45 Loy. L. Rev. 669, 683-84, 699, 709, 718 (1999) [IV; 5.05, 5.07].

Ziegler, Mosier, Buenaver, & Okuyemi, *How Much Information About Adverse Effects of Medication Do Patients Want From Physicians?* 161 Arch. Intern. Med. 706, 710 (2001) [10.01].

Zoellner, *Medical Repatriation: Examining the Legal and Ethical Implications of an Emerging Practice*, 32 Wash. U. J. L. & Pol'y 515, 530-532 (2010) [Preamble; I, II, III, IV, V, VI, VII, VIII, IX].

Zonana, *Physicians Must Honor Refusal of Treatment to Restore Competency by Non-Dangerous Inmates on Death Row*, 38 J. L. Med. & Ethics 764, 766 (Winter 2010) [2.06].

Zwirn, *Professionalism, Mental Disability, and the Death Penalty*, 41 N. Y. L Sch. L. Rev. 163, 165 (1996) [2.06].

Index to Opinions

Indexed here are Opinions of the AMA Council on Ethical and Judicial Affairs. Opinions are cited by opinion number, (eg, advertising and managed care organizations, 5.01). Also cited here are Principles of Medical Ethics, found on page xvii (eg, Principle IX).

Ability to pay, *See* Financial incentives and interests
Abnormalities, genetic counseling, 2.12
Abortion, 2.01
    fetal tissue transplantation, medical applications of, 2.161
    genetic counseling, 2.12
    mandatory parental consent, 2.015
Abuse, *See* Violence and abuse
Abuse, health care fraud and, 9.132
Access to care, *See also* Health disparities; 10.05, Principle IX
    allocating limited medical resources, 2.03
    denial, in allocating limited medical resources, 2.03
    efforts to increase organ donation, 2.151, 2.155
    fetal umbilical cord donations, public vs. private blood banking, 2.165
    financial barriers to health care access, 9.0651
    gender disparities in health care, 9.122
    health disparities, 9.121, 9.122
    managed care appeals, 8.13
    managed care restrictions, bedside rationing, 8.13
    medical directors' ethical obligations, 8.021
    patenting medical procedures to limit availability, 9.095
    patient's right to continuity of care, 10.01
    pay-for-performance programs, 8.056
    provision of adequate care, 2.095, 8.021, 10.01
    racial and ethnic health care disparities, 9.121
    retainer practices providing care and urgent care to patients in need, 8.055
Accident prevention, *See also* Patient safety
    impaired drivers, 2.24
Accreditation, 9.01
    fertility labs, 2.055
    industry development of accredited educational programs (guideline 7), 8.061
Acquired immunodeficiency syndrome, *See* headings beginning with HIV
Adequate health care, provision of, 2.095, 8.021, 10.01
Admission fee, 4.01
Adolescents, *See also* Children
    mandatory parental consent for abortion, 2.015
    minors' confidential care, 5.055
Adoption
    genetic testing of children, 2.138
    surrogate mothers and, 2.18

Advance directives, 2.225
    do-not-resuscitate orders, 2.22
    optimal use of orders not-to-intervene and, 2.225
    patient responsibilities in end-of-life decisions, 10.02
    surrogate decision making, 8.081
    withholding/withdrawing life-sustaining treatment, 2.20
Adverse drug or device events, 9.032
Adverse event reporting, 9.032
Advertising and publicity, 5.01-5.027
    claims of exclusive or unique skills or remedies, 5.02
    creating false expectations, 5.015, 5.02
    direct-to-consumer diagnostic imaging tests, 8.045
    managed care organizations and, 5.01
    physician publicity and, 5.02
    prescription drugs, direct-to-consumer, 5.015
    records disclosure to data collection companies, 5.075
    truthful, 5.02
Advisory services, *See* Consultation, medical
Advocacy for change in law and policy, 9.025
Advocacy, patient, *See* Patient advocacy
Age, allocation (rationing) of limited medical resources, 2.03
Aging, medical futility in end-of-life care, 2.037
AIDS, *See* headings beginning with HIV
Alcohol and Alcoholism
    minors' confidential care, 5.055
    reporting impaired, incompetent or unethical colleagues, 9.0305, 9.031
    substance abuse, 8.15
Allied health professionals, 3.03, *See also* Health personnel
    surgical comanagement, 8.043
Allocation of limited medical resources, 2.03
Allocation of resources, *See* Access to care; Health care delivery
Allow visitors extended hours (AVEH) orders, 2.225
American Medical Association, *See* Council on Ethical and Judicial Affairs; Principles of Medical Ethics
Amniocentesis, 2.12
Anatomical gifts, *See* Transplantation
Anencephalic neonates as organ donors, 2.162
Animals, xenotransplantation, 2.169

Anonymous donor, artificial insemination by, 2.05
Antitrust violations, physician unions, strikes, collective action, 9.025
Appointment charges, 8.01
Appointments, 10.02
    missed, 8.01
Artificial insemination, *See also* Reproductive medicine
    by anonymous donor, 2.05
    by known donor, 2.04
    surrogate mothers, 2.18
Artificial life support, *See* Life-sustaining treatment
Assessments, compulsory, 4.02
Assisted reproductive technology, *See also* Reproductive medicine
    ethical conduct in, 2.055
Assisted suicide, 2.211
Athletes, *See* Sports medicine
Attendees, *See* Meetings
Attorney-physician relation: confidentiality, 5.06
Automobile drivers, impaired, 2.24
Autopsy, postmortem medical information, 5.051
Availability of information to other physicians: records of physicians, 7.01
Availability of medical procedures, use of patents and other means to limit, 9.095
AVEH (allow visitors extended hours) orders, 2.225

Barriers, financial, to health care access, 9.0651
Basic benefits package, *See* Insurance, health
Behavior
    disruptive, 9.045
    healthy, 10.02
    unethical, 9.031
Benefits, insurance, *See* Insurance, health
Best interests analysis, *See* Decision making
Biased behavior, *See* Discrimination
Billing, *See also* Fees and charges
    housestaff and student services, 4.03
    laboratory, 6.09
Biological weapons, 2.078
Biomedical research, *See also* Research
    conflicts of interest, 8.031
    embryonic stem cells, 2.146
    guidelines to prevent malevolent use of, 2.078
Biotechnology
    commercial use of human tissue, 2.08
    continuing medical education sponsorship by industry, 9.0115
Blood, fetal umbilical cord donations, public vs. private blood banking, 2.165
Blood-borne pathogens, artificial insemination, 2.04, 2.05
Bodily restraints, *See* Patient safety
Bone marrow, fetal umbilical cord blood banking, 2.165
"Boutique medicine,", *See* Retainer practices
Breach of electronic health information, 5.10
Breaches of confidentiality, *See* Confidentiality
Broadcast media, *See* Media relations
Business, *See* Economics

Cadaveric organ donation, *See also* Transplantation
    encouraging study of motivation, 2.151
Cannulation, 2.157
Capital punishment, 2.06
    lethal injection, 2.06
    mental competence of condemned prisoners, 2.06
    physician actions not constituting participation in executions, 2.06
    relieving suffering of condemned persons, 2.06
    treating mentally incompetent condemned prisoners, 2.06
    witnessing an execution, 2.06
Capitation
    conflicts of interest, 8.051
    determining rates, 8.051
    negotiating discounts for specialty care, 8.052
    stop-loss plans to prevent catastrophic expenses, 8.051, 8.054
Cardiac death, organ donation after, 2.157
Cardiopulmonary resuscitation, do-not-resuscitate orders, 2.22
Care, futile, 2.035
Care, levels of, and economic incentives, 4.04
Caring for the poor, 9.065
Carrier screening, *See also* Genetics
    ethical issues in, 2.137
Change in law and policy, advocacy for, 9.025
Chaperones during physical exams, 8.21
Character, physician, Principle II
Charges, *See also* Fees and charges
    completion of insurance form, 6.07
    interest and finance, 6.08
    missed appointments, 8.01
Charity care, *See* Indigent care
Chemical weapons, 2.078
Child abuse, *See* Violence and abuse
Children
    clinical investigation guidelines, 2.07
    cloning to produce, 2.147
    filming patients for education of health professionals, 5.046
    genetic testing, 2.138
    genetically identical, 2.145
    medical record retention, 7.05
    minors' confidential care, 5.055
    organ transplantation from living donors, 2.15
    pediatric decision making, 10.016
    physician treatment of family members, 8.19
    xenotransplantation, 2.169
Chiropractic, 3.01, 3.04, 3.041
Choice, free, 9.06
    patient neglect, 8.11
    physician, Principle VI
Chorionic villus sampling, 2.12
Civil rights and professional responsibility, 9.03
Clinical encounter, patient privacy and outside observers to, 5.0591
Clinical investigations, *See* Research
Clinical practice, placebo use in, 8.083
Clinical settings, industry representatives in, 8.047

Clinical skills, medical students performing
  procedures on fellow students, 3.09
Clinical test results, general guidelines for
  reporting, 8.095
Clinical trials, *See also* Research
  clinical investigation guidelines, 2.07
  managing conflicts of interest in the conduct
    of, 8.0315
  subject selection for, 2.071
  use of placebo controls in, 2.075
Cloning
  to produce children, 2.147
Colleagues, *See* Physician colleagues
Collections, *See* Fees and charges
Collective action, 9.025
Collections, *See* Fees and charges
Comanagement, surgical, ethical implications
  of, 8.043
Comfort care, *See* Pain and pain control;
  Terminally ill patients
Commercial interests, *See* Financial incentives
  and interests
Commercial use of human tissue, 2.08
Communicable diseases, *See* Infectious diseases;
  Public health
Communication
  clinical test result reporting guidelines, 8.095
  disrespect, derogatory conduct in patient-
    physician relationship, 9.123
  electronic mail, 5.026
  informing families of patient's death, 8.18
  patient responsibilities, 10.02
  political, with patients and their families, 9.012
  professionalism in using social media, 9.124
  racial and ethnic health care disparities, 9.121
  referral services by telecommunication, 5.025
  understanding cultural or ethnic
    characteristics, 9.121
Communications media, *See also* Media relations
  standards of professional responsibility, 5.04
Community fundraising
  contribution solicitation from patients, 10.018
  non-health-related products sold in physicians'
    offices, 8.062
Community participation, Principle VII
Compassion, Principle I
Competence, medical, Principle I
Competence, mental, *See* Mental competence
Competition, *See also* Financial incentives
  and interests
  covenants not-to-compete for physicians-in-
    training, 9.021
  factors in, 6.11
Compulsory assessments, 4.02
Computed tomography, direct-to-consumer
  diagnostic imaging tests, 8.045
Computers, *See also* Internet
  authorized personnel and access, 5.07
  breaches of electronic health information, 5.10
  confidentiality, security safeguards, 5.07
  data erasure, 5.07
Concierge practices, 8.055

Condemned prisoners, *See* Capital punishment
Conferences and meetings, See
  Education; Meetings
Confidential care for minors, 5.055
Confidentiality, Principle IV, 5.05-5.09, *See also*
  Medical records
  abrogation of, in abortion for legal minors, 2.015
  artificial insemination by anonymous
    donor, 2.05
  attorney-physician relation, 5.06
  breaches of electronic health information, 5.10
  carrier screening of genetic disorders, 2.137
  chaperones during physical examinations, 8.21
  clinical investigation guidelines, 2.07
  clinical test result reporting guidelines, 8.095
  communications media, professional
    responsibility, standards, 5.04
  computer records, databases, 5.07
  contribution solicitation from patients, 10.018
  court-ordered disclosure, 5.05
  criminal justice system and genetic
    information, 2.136
  disclosing information to patients'
    attorneys, 5.06
  disclosure of records to data collection
    companies, 5.075
  DNA databank safeguards, 2.079
  document destruction when discarding old
    medical records, 7.05
  electronic mail, 5.026
  ethics committees, 9.11
  ethics consultations, 9.115
  familial risk disclosures in genetic testing, 2.131
  filming patients for education of health
    professionals, 5.046
  filming patients in health care settings, 5.045
  full disclosure of information by patients, 5.05
  fundamental elements of patient-physician
    relationship, 10.01
  genetic testing of children, 2.138
  HIV testing, 2.23
  impaired drivers, 2.24
  industry-employed physicians and independent
    medical examiners, 5.09, 10.03
  industry representatives in clinical
    settings, 8.047
  information disclosed by patients, 5.05
  information on specific patients released to the
    media, 5.04
  insurance company representatives and, 5.08
  lawsuits involving, 5.05
  mandatory parental consent for abortion, 2.015
  medical record access by non-treating medical
    staff, 7.025
  medical record disposal, 7.05
  medical students performing procedures on
    fellow students, 3.09
  minors' care, 5.055
  online sites with patient-specific
    information, 5.027
  patient privacy and outside observers, 5.0591
  patient threats and physician precautions, 5.05

patients' attorneys, 5.06
physician disruptive behavior, 9.045
physician records, 7.02
postmortem medical information, 5.051
potential breaches, in electronic mail, 5.026
public health interventions, quarantine,
    isolation, 2.25
radio frequency ID devices, 2.40
record access by nontreating medical staff, 7.025
records disclosure to data collection
    companies, 5.075
release of medical records, 7.02
reporting impaired, incompetent or unethical
    physicians, 9.0305, 9.031
required disclosure of confidential
    information, 5.05
safeguards in genomic research, 2.079
social media use by physicians, 9.124
supervisor-trainee disputes, 9.055
work-related and independent
    examinations, 10.03
Conflict of interest
abortion and fetal tissue transplantation, 2.161
biomedical research, 8.031
capitation, 8.051
clinical investigation guidelines, 2.07
clinical trials, 8.0315
contingent physician fees, 6.01
continuing medical education sponsorship by
    industry, 9.0115
death determination, organ donors, 2.16
direct-to-consumer diagnostic imaging
    tests, 8.045
disclosure in biomedical research, 8.031
disclosure in clinical trials, 8.0315
disclosure, physician ownership of health
    facilities, 8.0321
disclosures by CME faculty, 9.011
disclosures when health-related products are
    sold in physicians' offices, 8.063
financial gain in genomic research, 2.079
financial incentives and medical practice, 8.054
guidelines, 8.03
health product endorsements, efficacy, 8.063
health-related online sites, 5.027
industry gifts to physicians (guidelines), 8.061
industry-employed physicians and independent
    medical examiners, 10.03
lawsuits involving, 8.03
managed care financial incentives, 8.13
managing conflicts of interest in the conduct of
    clinical trials, 8.0315
non-health-related products sold in physicians'
    offices, 8.062
organ donors and recipients, 2.15
organ transplant team members, in cases of
    cardiac death, 2.157
patient referral and disclosure of
    limitations, 8.132
physician contractual relationships, 8.05, 8.0501
physician employment by nonphysician
    supervisee, 3.05

physician markups, commissions or profits
    involving laboratory services, 8.09
physician ownership of health facilities, 8.0321
physician ownership of pharmacies, 8.06
physician self-referral (financial interest in
    facilities outside their practices), 8.0321
professionalism and contractual
    relations, 8.0501
self-referrals, 8.0321
treating second-opinion patients, 8.041
Consent, informed, See Informed consent
Consent, parental, See Parents
Consent, presumed, See Transplantation
Consultation, medical, Principle V, 8.04
advisory or referral services by
    telecommunication, 5.025
allied health professionals, 3.03
ethics clarifications, 9.115
second opinions, 8.041
token, and industry payment, 8.061
Consultations, ethics, 9.115
Consumers, See also Advertising and publicity;
    Drugs and Devices
diagnostic imaging tests, direct to, 8.045
direct advertisements of prescription
    drugs, 5.015
health-related online sites, 5.027
managed care benefits package
    formulation, 8.13
managed care plan selection, 8.13
Contact lenses, 8.06
Contingent physician fees, 6.01
Continuing medical education, See Education,
    medical, continuing
Contraception, minors' confidential care, 5.055
Contracts
capitation, 8.051
clinical trials and management of conflicts of
    interest, 8.0315
employee/employment, 8.05
gestational surrogacy, 2.18
health plan restrictions on disclosure ("gag
    clauses"), 8.053
lawsuits and, 8.05, 9.02, 9.06
noncompetition covenants for physicians in
    training, 9.021
physician contractual relationships, 8.05, 8.0501
physician-hospital, 4.06
physician income and benefits
    arrangements, 8.05
physician refusals to provide care, 10.05
prior evaluation of health plan financial
    incentives, 8.054
respect for law and human rights in patient-
    physician relationships, 9.12
restrictive covenants, 9.02, 9.06
retainer practices, distinguishing special
    services and amenities from reimbursable
    medical services, 8.055
surrogate mothers, 2.18
terms compromising professional judgment,
    integrity, 8.0501

Contributions, *See also* Donations
   from patients, physician participation in
      soliciting, 10.018
Copayment, *See* Fees and charges;
      Insurance, health
Costs, See also Financial incentives and interests
   awareness, 2.09
   prescription drugs in health care plans, 8.135
   managed care, 8.13
   medical record transfer, 7.04
   quality and, 2.09
Council on Ethical and Judicial Affairs, AMA
   disciplinary actions, 1.01
   physician discipline, 9.04
Counseling, genetic, *See* Genetic counseling
Court-initiated medical treatments in criminal
      cases, 2.065
Courtesy, professional, 6.13
Courts, *See* Law
Covenants not-to-compete for physicians-in-
      training, 9.021
CPR, *See* Cardiopulmonary resuscitation
Crime
   court-initiated treatments in criminal
      cases, 2.065
   justice system and genetic information, 2.136
   physician illegal conduct, 9.04
Criminal cases, court-initiated medical treatments
   in, 2.065
Criminal justice system, genetic information
   and, 2.136
Cultural characteristics, *See* Ethnic groups

Data collection
   employee statistical information with identities
      deleted, 5.09
   error reporting systems, 8.121
   records disclosure for marketing purposes, 5.075
Databases
   confidentiality, 5.07
   DNA, 2.079
   genetic, and criminal justice system, 2.136
   living organ donor outcomes, 2.15
Death, *See also* Suicide; Terminally ill patients
   certification, physician actions not constituting
      participation in executions, 2.06
   determination of, anencephalic neonates as
      organ donors, 2.162
   determination, organ donors, 2.16
   information release to the media, 5.04
   informing families of, 8.18
   medical futility in end-of-life care, 2.037
   organ donation after cardiac death, 2.157
   palliative care for dying patients, 2.20
   postmortem medical information, 5.051
   presumed consent and mandated choice for
      organs from deceased donors, 2.155
   procedures on newly deceased patients for
      training purposes, 8.181
Death, cardiac, organ donation after, 2.157
Death certification, physician actions not
   constituting participation in executions, 2.06

Death row, *See* Capital punishment
Deceased donors, presumed consent and mandated
      choice for organs from, 2.155
Deceased patients, performing procedures on the
      newly deceased for training purposes, 8.181
Deception, *See also* Fraud and abuse; Principle II
Decision making, *See also* Informed consent;
      Surrogate decision makers
   abortion, and motivation to donate fetal
      tissue, 2.161
   acceptable mechanisms in allocating limited
      resources, 2.03
   advance directives, 2.225
   allocation (rationing) of limited medical
      resources, 2.03
   best-interest principle, 8.081
   conflicts in determining futility in end-of-life
      care, 2.037
   discussions in advance by patient with surrogate
      decision makers, 8.081
   do-not-resuscitate orders, 2.22
   end-of-life decisions, 10.02
   excluding resident physicians from a patient's
      care, 8.088
   financial incentives and medical practice, 8.054
   frozen pre-embryos, 2.141
   fundamental elements of patient-physician
      relationship, 10.01
   gender disparities in health care, 9.122
   informed consent and, 8.08
   life support withdrawal, in organ donation after
      cardiac death, 2.157
   managed care benefits package
      formulation, 8.13
   mandatory parental consent for abortion, 2.015
   medical futility in end-of-life care, 2.037
   medical need, 2.03
   medical need, xenotransplantation, 2.169
   medical students' involvement in patient
      care, 8.087
   minors' confidential care, 5.055
   orders not to intervene, 2.225
   organ transplantation from living donors, 2.15
   patient responsibilities, autonomy, 10.02
   pediatric, 10.016
   quality of life, 2.17
   sedation to unconsciousness at end of life, 2.201
   seriously ill newborns, 2.215
   substituted judgment and best interests
      analysis, 2.20, 8.081
   surrogate, 8.081
   surrogate, in organ donation after cardiac
      death, 2.157
   valid treatment alternatives, 8.20
   withdrawal of consent by potential organ
      donors, 2.15
   withholding information from patients, 8.082
   withholding/withdrawing life-sustaining
      treatment, 2.20
Definitions, *See* Terminology
Delinquent accounts, *See* Fees and charges
Delivery of health care, *See* Health care delivery

Denial of treatment, *See* Treatment denial

Departure from a group, records of physicians upon retirement or, 7.03

Derogatory conduct and disrespect in the patient-physician relationship, 9.123

Designated organ donation, *See* Transplantation

Detail visits, *See* Drugs and devices

Detainees, *See* Prisoners

Developing countries, infrastructure development in international research, 2.077

Devices, medical, *See* Drugs and devices

Diagnosis, *See also* Genetic testing

    clinical test result reporting guidelines, 8.095

    court-initiated treatments in criminal cases, 2.065

    direct-to-consumer imaging tests, 8.045

    excessive or unnecessary testing while waiving copayments, 6.12

    information on specific patients released to the media, 5.04

    informing patients of changes, 8.12

    laboratory services, 8.09

    multiplex genetic testing, 2.139

    physician advisory or referral services by telecommunication, 5.025

    surgical or diagnostic instrument patents, 9.09

    timely reporting of test results, 8.095

Diagnostic imaging tests, direct-to-consumer, 8.045

Diagnostic or surgical instrument, patent for, 9.09

Dignity, Principle I, 10.01

Direct-to-consumer advertising, *See also* Advertising; Consumers

    advertisements of prescription drugs, 5.015

    diagnostic imaging tests, 8.045

Directed organ donation, *See* Transplantation

Disabilities

    evaluation, 5.09, 10.03

    quality of life, 2.17

    seriously disabled newborns, 2.17

Disaster preparedness and response, physician obligation in, 9.067

Disciplinary actions

    assisted reproductive technology, unethical conduct, 2.055

    censure, suspension or expulsion from medical society membership, 1.01

    due process, 9.05

    illegal, unethical conduct, 9.04

Discipline and medicine, 9.04

Disclosure in health care plan contracts, restrictions on, 8.053

Disclosure of familial risk in genetic testing, 2.131

Disclosure of information and records, *See* Confidentiality; Medical records

Disclosure of interests, *See* Conflict of interest

Disclosure of limitations: referral of patients, 8.132

Disclosure of risks, *See* Informed consent

Discounts for specialty care, 8.052

Discrimination

    carrier screening of genetic disorders, 2.137

    civil rights, equal opportunity, in professional activities, organizations, 9.03

declining to accept patients, 9.12

disrespect, derogatory conduct, prejudice in patient-physician relationship, 9.123

eliminating biased behavior by health personnel, 9.121

employers' genetic testing as basis for hiring, 2.132

gender, 9.035

gender disparities in health care, 9.122

HIV-infected patients, 9.131

multiplex genetic testing, 2.139

physician refusals to provide care, 10.05

racial and ethnic health care disparities, 9.121

respect for law and human rights in patient-physician relationships, 9.12

Disparities, *See* Health disparities

Dispensing drugs and devices, *See* Drugs and devices

Disputes between medical supervisors and trainees, 9.055

Disrespect and derogatory conduct in the patient-physician relationship, 9.123

Disruptive behavior, physicians with, 9.045

DNA

    criminal justice system and genetic information, 2.136

    databanks in genomic research, safeguards, 2.079

    gene replacement, 2.13

    recombinant, 2.13

    sequences, 2.105

    viral delivery systems (gene therapy, genetic engineering), 2.11, 2.13

DND (do not defibrillate) orders, 2.225

DNI (do not intubate) orders, 2.225

DNLH (do not leave home) orders, 2.225

DNR (do not resuscitate) orders, 2.22

DNT (do not treat) orders, 2.225

DNTransfer (do not transfer) orders, 2.225

Do-not-defibrillate (DNF) orders, 2.225

Do-not-intubate (DNI) orders, 2.225

Do-not-leave-home (DNLH) orders, 2.225

Do-not-resuscitate orders, 2.22

Do-not-transfer (DNTransfer) orders, 2.225

Do-not-treat (DNT) orders, 2.225

Domestic partners, surrogate decision making, 8.081

Domestic violence, *See* Violence and abuse

Donations, contribution solicitation from patients, 10.018

Donors, *See also* Organ donation and organ donors; Reproductive medicine; Transplantation

    deceased, presumed consent and mandated choice for organs from, 2.155

    gamete providers, 2.141, 2.145

    living, transplantation of organs from, 2.15

Drivers, impaired, 2.24

Drug abuse, 8.15; *See also* Substance abuse

    minors' confidential care, 5.055

    reporting impaired, incompetent or unethical colleagues, 9.0305, 9.031

Drug formularies, 8.135

Drug industry
    assistance programs, 8.135
    clinical trials and management of conflicts of
        interest, 8.0315
    continuing medical education sponsors,
        9.011, 9.0115
    direct and indirect subsidies to meeting/
        conference attendees, 8.061
    gifts tied to prescribing practices, 8.061
    gifts to physicians (guidelines), 8.061
Drug samples, free, for physicians' personal or
    family member use (guideline 1), 8.061
Drugs and devices
    adverse event reporting, 9.032
    adverse reactions in expedited partner therapy
        (STDs), 8.07
    clinical investigation guidelines, 2.07
    compensation from or financial interest in drug
        firms, 8.06
    continuing medical education sponsorship by
        industry, 9.0115
    controlled substance prescriptions for physician
        family members, 8.19
    cost containment, cost-effectiveness, 8.135
    direct and indirect subsidies to meeting/
        conference attendees (guideline 5), 8.061
    direct-to-consumer advertisements, 5.015
    dispensing within physicians' office practices, 8.06
    experimental treatment, investigational therapy
        continuation, 2.071
    fee splitting, 6.02
    free samples (guideline 1), 8.061
    incentives to promote cost-effectiveness, 8.135
    industry gifts tied to prescribing practices
        (guideline 7), 8.061
    industry gifts to physicians (guidelines), 8.061
    industry representatives in clinical
        settings 8.047
    patent for surgical or diagnostic instruments, 9.09
    patient freedom of choice in filling
        prescriptions, 8.06
    patient's right to written copies of
        prescriptions, 8.06
    pharmaceutical benefit management, 8.135
    pharmacy and therapeutics committees, 8.135
    physician ownership of pharmacies, 8.06
    physician self-treatment, treatment of
        immediate family members, 8.19
    physician-assisted suicide, 2.211
    placebo use, 8.083
    prescribing and dispensing, 8.06
    prescription changes, 8.135
    provision from physician's office in cases of
        patient hardship, 8.063
    reporting adverse events, 9.032
    sedation to unconsciousness at end of life, 2.201
Due process, 9.05
    determining adequate health care, 2.095
    medical futility in end-of-life care, 2.037
    fairness, safeguards, 9.05
    peer review, 9.10
Dying, See Death

E-mail, See Electronic mail
Economic competition, 6.11
Economic incentives and levels of care, 4.04
Economic issues, See Conflict of interest; Cost;
    Fees and charges; Financial incentives
    and interests
Education, medical, Principle V
    ethical research principles, 2.078
    gender discrimination, 9.035
    industry scholarship and special funds for
        medical trainees (guideline 6), 8.061
    medical students' involvement in patient
        care, 8.087
    medical students performing procedures on
        fellow students, 3.09
    patient participation in, 10.02
    postmortem medical information disclosed for
        educational purposes, 5.051
    procedures on newly deceased patients for
        training purposes, 8.181
    sexual harassment and exploitation between
        medical supervisors and trainees, 3.08
    signing bonuses to attract graduates of US
        medical schools, 9.037
    supervisor-trainee disputes, 9.055
    violence and abuse detection, treatment, 2.02
Education, medical, continuing, Principle V
    credit, 9.011
    financial relationships with industry, 9.0115
    genetic information, 2.131
    independence of, 9.0115
    industry development of accredited programs
        (guideline 7), 8.061
    industry gifts, travel expenses and
        honoraria for faculty at meetings
        (guideline 5), 8.061
    industry input in development of conferences,
        meetings, lectures (guideline 7), 8.061
    industry promotional activities, 9.011
    industry sponsorship, 9.0115
    industry subsidies for (guideline 4), 8.061
    industry scholarships, funds for medical trainees
        attending educational conferences,
        (guideline 6), 8.061
    keeping current with best practices,
        competence, 9.14
    non-CME, primarily promotional
        activities, 9.011
    physician obligations, 9.011
    sponsors, 9.011
    token vs. actual consulting in industry
        compensation for meeting-related
        expenses (guideline 5), 8.061
    unfair profits, excessive fees, 9.011
    value of, 9.011
Education, medical, graduate
    adequate rest, "moonlighting" by
        residents, 8.088
    noncompetition covenants for physicians in
        training, 9.021
    resident physicians' involvement in patient
        care, 8.088

signing bonuses for attracting US graduates, 9.037
supervisor-trainee disputes, 9.055
Elder abuse, *See* Violence and abuse
Electronic health information, breach of, 5.10
Electronic mail, 5.026
Electronic medical records, *See* Medical records
E-mail, *See* Electronic mail
Embryos, *See also* Reproductive medicine
destruction, 2.146
frozen pre-embryos, 2.141
moral status, 2.146
pre-embryo splitting, 2.145
stem cell research, 2.146
transplantation, 2.14
Emergency situations, waiver of informed consent
for research in, 8.085
Emergency treatment, Principle VI
informed consent waiver for research in
emergency situations, 8.085
nurses acting contrary to physicians' orders, 3.02
patient neglect, 8.11
physician self-treatment, treatment of
immediate family members, 8.19
physicians' obligations in disaster preparedness
and response, 9.067
potential patients, 10.05
waiver of informed consent for research, 8.085
Employers, genetic testing by, 2.132
Employment
gender discrimination, 9.035
genetic testing by employers, 2.132
industry-employed physicians, independent
medical examiners, and confidentiality,
5.09, 10.03
physician, by nonphysician supervisee, 3.05
physician contractual relationships, 8.05
physician-hospital contractual relations, 4.06
sexual harassment and hostile work
environment, 3.08
workers' compensation, 10.03
EMRs, *See* Medical records
End-of-life care, *See* Terminally ill persons
Engineering, genetic, *See* Genetic engineering
Environmental exposure, genetic susceptibility to
injury in the workplace, 2.132
Epidemics, *See* Disaster preparedness and response;
Public health
Equal opportunity, *See* Discrimination
Equal opportunity, *See* Health care delivery;
Health disparities
Equipment, *See* Drugs and devices
Error and harm, ethical responsibility to study and
prevent, 8.121
Errors, medical, *See* Medical errors; Patient safety
"Ethical" (term), 1.01
Ethical conduct, 1.01
Ethical conduct in assisted reproductive
technology, 2.055
Ethical considerations in international
research, 2.077
Ethical guidelines for physicians in administrative
or other nonclinical roles, 8.02

Ethical implications of surgical
comanagement, 8.043
Ethical implications of xenotransplantation, 2.169
Ethical issues in carrier screening of genetic
disorders, 2.137
Ethical obligations of medical directors, 8.021
Ethical responsibility to study and prevent error
and harm, 8.121
Ethics committees, 9.11
disputes in surrogate decision making, 8.081
ethics consultations, 9.115
in health care institutions, 9.11
medical futility in end-of-life care, 2.037
pediatric decision making, disagreements, 10.016
surrogate decision making, 8.081
treatment decisions for seriously ill
newborns, 2.215
withholding/withdrawing life-sustaining
treatment, 2.20
Ethics consultations, 9.115
Ethics, medical
medical society disciplinary proceedings, 9.04
Principles of Medical Ethics, page xvii
relationship to law, 1.02
reporting unethical physicians, 9.031
Ethnic discrimination, *See* Discrimination
Ethnic groups
declining patients on basis of race, color,
religion, national origin, 9.12
increasing diversity in medical profession, 9.121
racial and ethnic health care disparities, 9.121
understanding cultural or ethnic
characteristics, 9.121
Eugenics, 2.11
cloning, 2.147
genetic counseling and testing, 2.12
Euthanasia, 2.21
physician-assisted suicide, 2.20, 2.211
Evaluations, medical, 5.09, 10.03
Evidence-based medicine, pay-for-performance
programs, 8.056
Executions, *See* Capital punishment
Existential suffering, *See* Terminal care
Expedited partner therapy, 8.07
Experimental treatments, *See* Research
Experiments, *See* Research
Experiments, unethical, information from, 2.30
Expert testimony, 9.07
attorney-physician confidentiality, 5.06
determining competence to stand trial (capital
punishment), 2.06
Eyeglasses, 8.06

Faculty, medical, *See also* Education, medical;
Education, medical, continuing
CME conflict of interest disclosures, 9.011
continuing medical education, 9.011
disputes between trainees and, 9.055
gender discrimination and tenure, 9.035
honoraria and reasonable compensation
for services at conferences/meetings
(guideline 5), 8.061

industry gifts, travel expenses and honoraria for, at educational meetings (guideline 5), 8.061
objective presentations, 9.011
physicians teaching allied health professionals, 3.03
promotional activity at CME events, 9.011
resident physicians' involvement in patient care, 8.088
schools of chiropractic, 3.041
sexual harassment and exploitation between medical supervisors and trainees, 3.08
supervisor-trainee disputes, 9.055
tenure decisions, 9.035
Familial risk, disclosure of, in genetic testing, 2.131
Family, *See also* Parents
burdens of care and quality of life, 2.17
disputes in withholding/withdrawing treatment, 2.20
genetic testing of children, 2.138
genetically identical children, 2.145
impact of cloning to produce children, 2.147
informing families of patient's death, 8.18
physician self-treatment, treatment of immediate family members, 8.19
private fetal umbilical cord blood banking, 2.165
risk disclosures, notification, in genetic testing, 2.131
sexual/romantic relations between physicians and key third parties, 8.145
sibling tissue donations (tissue harvesting), 2.145
surrogate decision makers, 2.20, 8.081
withholding/withdrawing life-sustaining treatment, 2.20
Family members, physician treatment of, 8.19
Family violence, *See* Violence and abuse
FCCO (full comfort care only) orders, 2.225
FDA, *See* Food and Drug Administration
Fee, admission, 4.01
Fee splitting, 6.02
Fee splitting: referrals to health care facilities, 6.03
Fees and charges, 6.01-6.13
acquisition or processing charges for laboratory services, 8.09
basis for determining reasonableness, 6.05
co-payment forgiveness, waiver, 6.12, 6.13
collection policies, 6.08
competition, 6.11
contingent, 6.01
copayment forgiveness or waiver, 6.12
copying medical records, 7.02, 7.04
customary, 6.05
delinquent accounts, 6.08, 7.01, 7.02
excessive or unnecessary testing while waiving copayments, 6.12
fee splitting, 6.02, 6.03, 8.043
fee-splitting, referrals to health facilities, 6.03
finance charges, 6.08
financial incentives to patients for referrals, 6.021
finder's fees, 6.03
guarantees of successful outcomes, 6.01

hospital admissions, 4.01
housestaff and student services billing, 4.03
illegal or excessive, 6.05
insurance claim form completion, 6.07
interest, finance charges (delinquent accounts), 6.08
laboratory bills, 6.09
laboratory services, 8.09
lien laws, 8.10
managed care fee withholds, 8.13
medical record copying, 7.02
medical record transfer costs, 7.04
medical service fees, 6.05
Medicare assignment, 6.05
missed, cancelled appointments, 8.01
multiple physicians, separate billing, 6.10
patient record-related, 7.02
personally rendered services, 6.10
professional courtesy, 6.13
reasonable, 6.05
referrals to companies selling medical products, 6.02
retainer practices, distinguishing special services and amenities from reimbursable medical services, 8.055
separate bills by each physician, 6.10
splitting, 6.02, 8.043
splitting, for referrals to health facilities, 6.03
surgical assistants, 6.10
surgical comanagement and fee-splitting, 8.043
unnecessary medical services, 2.19
withholding records because of unpaid bills, 7.01, 7.02
Fees, contingent, 6.01
Fees for medical services, 6.05
Fellow students, medical students performing procedures on, 3.09
Fertility laboratories, 2.055
Fertilization in vitro, *See also* Reproductive medicine
advance agreements for disposition of frozen pre-embryos, 2.141
frozen pre-embryos, 2.141
human ova maintenance in research, 2.14
pre-embryo splitting, 2.145
Fetal research guidelines, 2.10
Fetal tissue transplantation, medical applications of, 2.161
Fetoscopy, prenatal genetic testing, 2.12
Fetus, dead, 2.10
Filming patients for the education of health professionals, 5.046
Filming patients in health care settings, 5.045
Finance charges, *See* Fees and charges
Financial barriers to health care access, 9.0651
Financial gain, *See* Conflict of interest
Financial incentives and interests
ability to pay and allocation (rationing) of limited medical resources, 2.03
biomedical research conflicts of interest, 8.031
bracketed system of widely varied bonuses and penalties, 8.054

cadaveric organ donation financial incentives, motivation, 2.151

clinical trials and management of conflicts of interest, 8.0315

commercial use of human tissue, 2.08

competition, 6.11

conflicts of interest under capitation, 8.051

continuing medical education sponsors, 9.011, 9.0115

cost containment and prescription drugs, 8.135

costs and quality of care, 2.09

determining capitation rates, 8.051

direct-to-consumer diagnostic imaging tests, 8.045

disclosure of financial interests and sponsorship in health-related online sites, 5.027

drug and device prescribing and dispensing, 8.06

drug formularies, 8.135

exclusive distributorships of health-related products, 8.063

factors in evaluation of health plan financial incentives, 8.054

fetal tissue transplantation and financial remuneration, 2.161

filming patients for education of health professionals, 5.046

financial barriers to health care access, 9.0651

financial gain in filming patients in health care settings, 5.045

financial incentives and medical practice, 8.054

financial incentives or administrative conditions compromising professionalism, 8.0501, 8.054, 8.056

financial incentives to patients for referrals, 6.021

health fraud and abuse, 9.132

health-related online sites, 5.027

health-related products sold in physicians' offices, 8.063

incentives applied across broad physician groups, 8.054

incentives based on longer time periods preferable, 8.054

incentives based on quality and patient satisfaction, 8.054

incentives calculated on continuum of utilization preferable to trigger points, 8.054

incentives that promote efficiency, 8.054

industry representatives in clinical settings, 8.047

interest and finance charges, 6.08

larger patient pools preferable to reduce financial risks, 8.054

lien laws, 8.10

living organ donor compensation, 2.15

managed care financial incentives, 8.13

medical staff privileging decisions, 4.07

non-health-related products sold in physicians' offices, 8.062

noncompetition covenants for physicians in training, 9.021

patenting human genes, 2.105

patient financial obligations, 10.02

patient's inability to pay for care, 10.01

pay-for-performance programs, 8.056

physician conflict of interest guidelines, 8.03

physician contractual relationships, 8.05, 8.0501

physician ownership of health facilities and conflicts of interest, 8.0321

physician self-referral (financial interest in facilities outside their practices), 8.0321

physician-hospital contractual relations, 4.06

physician-owned laboratory services, 8.09

professionalism and contractual relations, 8.0501

provision of health products free or at cost, 8.063

quality considerations above cost considerations, 2.09

records disclosure to data collection companies, 5.075

referrals to companies selling medical products, 6.02

regulation in health facility accreditation, 9.01

restrictive covenants, 9.02

risk and case-mix adjustment in pay for performance, 8.056

Finder's fees, 6.03

"First come, first served," *See* Health care delivery

Food and Drug Administration
    direct-to-consumer advertisements of prescription drugs, 5.015
    drug or device adverse event reporting, 9.032
    experimental treatment, investigational therapy continuation, 2.071

Forgiveness or waiver of insurance copayments, 6.12

Fraud and abuse
    advertising and publicity, 5.02
    clinical investigation guidelines, 2.07
    co-payment forgiveness, waiver, 6.12, 6.13
    excessive or unnecessary testing while waiving copayments, 6.12
    excessive testing, 6.12
    forgiveness or waiver of insurance copayments, 6.12
    nonscientific practitioners, 3.01
    patient responsibilities in preventing, reporting, 10.02
    preventing, 9.132
    reporting, Principle II
    surgeon substitution without patient knowledge, 8.16
    unnecessary testing by clinics, 6.12

Free choice, Principle VI, 9.06
    medical student involvement in care, 8.087
    patient neglect, 8.11
    physician, Principle VI
    physician acceptance and declining of patients, 3.01
    potential patients, 10.05
    prescription filling, 8.06

Free drug samples for physicians' personal or family member use (guideline 1), 8.061

Free market conditions, *See* Competition
Freedom of choice, *See* Free choice
Frozen pre-embryos, 2.141, 2.145
Frozen semen, *See* Reproductive medicine
Full-comfort-care-only (FCCO) orders, 2.225
Fundamental elements of the patient-physician
    relationship, 10.01
Fundraising
    contribution solicitation from patients, 10.018
    non-health-related products sold in physicians'
        offices, 8.062
Futile care, 2.035
    do-not-resuscitate orders, 2.22
    end-of-life care, 2.037
    institutional policies on, 2.037
    organ transplantation from living donors, 2.15
    patient demands and reasons for treatment
        denial, 2.035

"Gag" clauses, 8.053
Gamete providers, 2.141, 2.145
Gender
    discrimination in the medical profession, 9.035
    disparities in health care, 9.122
    preference, artificial insemination, 2.04, 2.05
    sex-linked inherited diseases, 2.04, 2.05
Gene patenting, 2.105
Gene pool, 2.147
Gene replacement, 2.13
Gene splicing, 2.13
Gene therapy, 2.11, 2.13
Gene transfer, 2.13
Genes, human, patenting, 2.105
Genetic counseling, 2.12, 2.131
    artificial insemination by known donor, 2.04
    carrier screening, 2.137, 2.138
    children, 2.138
    familial risk disclosures in genetic testing, 2.131
    physicians' moral values and judgment, 2.12
    pre-embryo analysis, 2.12
    prenatal testing, counseling, 2.12
    private fetal umbilical cord blood banking, 2.165
    screening donors in artificial insemination,
        2.04, 2.05
    sex-linked disease, and artificial insemination,
        2.04, 2.05
Genetic disorders, ethical issues in carrier
    screening, 2.137
Genetic engineering, 2.13
Genetic information and the criminal justice
    system, 2.136
Genetic information, insurance companies
    and, 2.135
Genetic manipulation, *See* Gene therapy
Genetic selection, 2.12
Genetic testing, 2.13-2.139
    artificial insemination, 2.04, 2.05
    by employers, 2.132
    carrier screening, 2.137, 2.138
    children, 2.138
    criminal justice system and genetic
        information, 2.136

    disclosure of familial risk in, 2.131
    insurance companies, 2.135
    multiplex, 2.139
    prenatal, 2.12
    worker susceptibility to injury, 2.132
Genetics, 2.079-2.147
    carrier screening, 2.137
    cloning to produce children, 2.147
    criminal justice system and genetic
        information, 2.136
    deceased victims' information, 2.136
    destruction of samples, 2.136
    DNA databank safeguards in genomic
        research, 2.079
    engineering, 2.13
    eugenics, 2.11
    gene therapy, 2.11
    identical children, 2.145
    implications of germline therapy, 2.11
    in vitro fertilization, human ova maintenance
        in research, 2.14
    information and insurance companies, 2.135
    patenting human genes, 2.105
    predisposition to disease, 2.135
    stem cell research, 2.146
    susceptibility to injury in the workplace, 2.132
Genomic research, 2.079
    privacy safeguards for samples, protecting
        individual identity, 2.079
    safeguards for specific communities in
        studies, 2.079
    safeguards in use of DNA databanks in, 2.079
Germline modification, 2.13
Germline therapy, 2.11
Gestational surrogacy contracts, 2.18
Ghost surgery, *See* Surgery
Gifts from patients, 10.017
Gifts to physicians
    bequests, 10.017
    by patients, 10.017
    from industry, 8.061
    guidelines, 8.061
Goodwill, 7.04
Graduates of US medical schools, signing bonuses
    to attract, 9.037
Group practice
    contractual relationships, 8.05
    records at retirement, departure, 7.03
    Guidelines, ethical
    conflicts of interest, 8.03
    fetal research, 2.10
    gifts to physicians, 8.061
    organ transplantation, 2.16
    reporting clinical test results, 8.095
    preventing malevolent use of biomedical
        research, 2.078

Harassment, sexual, *See* Sexual misconduct
Harm, *See also* Medical errors; Patient safety
    breaches of minors' confidential care, 5.055
    cadaveric organ donation financial incentives,
        motivation, 2.151

cloning to produce children, 2.147
euthanasia, 2.21
HIV-infected physicians, 9.131
infectious disease transmission by physicians, 9.13
organ transplantation from living donors, 2.15
patient threats and disclosure of confidential information, 5.05
physician-assisted suicide, 2.20, 2.211
postmortem medical information, 5.051
preventing malevolent use of biomedical research, 2.078
studying and preventing, 8.121
Harm and error, ethical responsibility to study and prevent, 8.121
Health and wellness, physician, 9.0305
Health care access, See Access to care
Health care, adequate, 2.095, 8.021, 10.01
Health care delivery
access to care, 10.05
allocation (rationing) of limited medical resources, 2.03
competition, 6.11
costs, 2.09
equal opportunity in allocating limited resources, 2.03
evaluation of procedures in determinations of adequate health care, 2.095
"first come, first served," 2.03
foreign infrastructure development in international research, 2.077
medical need and prioritizing of patients, 2.03
minimal threshold approach, 2.03
patient's right to continuity of care, and adequate care, 10.01
provision of adequate care, 2.095, 8.021, 10.01
reforms, 9.025
three-tiered system, 2.03
unnecessary medical services, 2.19
weighted formula in allocating limited resources, 2.03
Health care disparities, See Health disparities
Health care fraud and abuse, See Fraud and abuse
Health care institutions, ethics committees in, 9.11
Health care plans, See Insurance, health; Managed care
Health care, privacy in the context of, 5.059
Health care proxy, 8.081
Health care settings, filming patients in, 5.045
Health disparities, See also Access to care; Discrimination
allocation (rationing) of limited medical resources, 2.03
basic benefits package, provision of adequate health care, 2.095
clinical trial subject selection, 2.071
fetal umbilical cord donations, public vs. private blood banking, 2.165
gender bias, 9.122
racial and ethnic, 9.121
Health education
direct-to-consumer advertisements of prescription drugs, 5.015

filming patients in health care settings, 5.045
Health facilities, See Hospitals and health facilities; Laboratories
Health insurance, See Insurance, health
Health maintenance organizations, See Managed care
Health personnel
allied health professionals, 3.03
physician immunization for vaccine-preventable diseases, 9.133
public and occupational health protective measures taken by, 2.25
referral of patients to limited practitioners, 3.04
substitution of services by allied health professionals, 3.03
surgical comanagement, 8.043
Health plans, See Insurance, health; Managed care
Health policy
allocation (rationing) of limited medical resources, 2.03
change advocacy, 9.025
evaluation of procedures in determinations of adequate health care, 2.095
financial barriers to health care access, 9.0651
health costs, 2.09
managed care restrictions, 8.13
social and economic issues, 2.09
Health products, 8.063
Health professionals, See Allied health professionals; Health personnel; Interprofessional relations; Nurses; Physicians
Health-related online sites, 5.027
Health-related products, sale of, from physicians' offices, 8.063
Health resource allocation, See Access to care; Adequate health care; Health care delivery; Transplantation
Health worker safety, See Occupational health
Health workers, See Health personnel
Healthy behaviors (patient responsibilities), 10.02
Hearings, See Due process
Heart disease, organ donation after cardiac death, 2.157
Hematopoietic stem cells, See Stem cells
Hereditary diseases, See Genetic counseling; Genetic testing
Heredity, See Genetics
History of medicine, unethical experiment results, information, 2.30
History-taking, See Medical records
HIV-infected patients and physicians, 9.131
HIV testing, 2.23
Homosexuality
artificial insemination for couples, 2.05
declining patients on basis of sexual orientation, 9.12
Honesty, Principle II; see also Conflict of interest
health care fraud and abuse, 9.132
patient information, 8.12
Honoraria, 8.061
Hospice care, 2.211
Hospital medical staff, See Medical staff

Hospital-physician contractual relations, 4.06

Hospital relations, 4.01-4.07

Hospitals and health facilities, 4.01-4.07; *See also* Ethics committees; Medical staff
accreditation standards, 9.01
admission fees charged by physicians, 4.01
biomedical research conflicts of interest, 8.031
do-not-resuscitate orders, policies, 2.22
economic regulation in accreditation, 9.01
ethics committees, 9.11
ethics consultations, 9.115
fee-splitting, referrals to, 6.03
housestaff and student services billing, 4.03
noncompetition covenants for physicians in training, 9.021
physician contractual relations, 4.06
physician ownership and conflicts of interest, 8.0321
physician self-referral (financial interest in facilities outside their practices), 8.0321
record access by nontreating medical staff, 7.025
referrals, fee splitting, 6.03
review committees for biomedical conflict of interest, 8.031
utilization committees and peer review, 9.10
Housestaff and student services, billing for, 4.03

Human cloning, *See* Cloning

Human dignity, Principle I, 10.10

Human gene pool, 2.147

Human genes, patenting, 2.105

Human Genome Project, 2.132

Human rights, Principle I
respect for, in patient-physician relationships, 9.12
torture, 2.067

Human subjects, *See* Research subjects

Human tissue, *See also* Stem cells
commercial use, 2.08
DNA databanks, genomic research, 2.079
fetal tissue transplantation, 2.161

Humans, radio frequency ID devices in, 2.40

IAC (inquire about comfort) orders, 2.225

Identification devices, radio frequency ID, 2.40

Illegal conduct, 1.02

Imaging, direct-to-consumer diagnostic tests, 8.045

Immediate family members, physician treatment of, 8.19

Immunization
medical record retention, 7.05
protective measures taken by physicians and other health personnel, 2.25, 9.133

Impaired drivers, 2.24

Impaired physicians
reporting impaired, incompetent or unethical colleagues, 9.0305, 9.031
substance abuse, 8.15
supervisor-trainee disputes, 9.055

Implants, radio frequency ID devices, 2.40

In vitro fertilization, 2.14, *See also* Reproductive medicine

advance agreements for disposition of frozen pre-embryos, 2.141
frozen pre-embryos, 2.141
human ova maintenance in research, 2.14
pre-embryo splitting, 2.145

Incentives, economic, See Financial incentives and interests

Incompetence, mental, *See* Mental competence

Incompetent physicians, Principle II, 9.031

Independent medical examiners and examinations, 5.09, 10.03

Indigent care, 9.065, 10.05
caring for the poor, 9.065
fundamental elements of patient-physician relationship, 10.01
physician obligations, 10.05

Industry, *See* Drug industry; Drugs and devices; Industry gifts to physicians

Industry-employed physicians and independent medical examiners: confidentiality, 5.09

Industry gifts to physicians, 8.061
development of conferences, meetings, lectures by companies (guideline 7), 8.061
direct subsidies to conference attendees (guideline 4), 8.061
educational materials (guideline 1), 8.061
faculty honoraria and reasonable reimbursement for CME meeting-related expenses, (guideline 5), 8.061
legitimate conferences (guideline 3), 8.061
meals at conferences (guideline 5), 8.061
modest hospitality at conferences and meetings (guideline 5), 8.061
scholarships, funding for medical trainees to attend carefully selected educational conferences (guideline 6), 8.061
subsidies for travel, lodging and personal expenses of meeting attendees (guideline 5), 8.061
token advisory or consulting services (guideline 5), 8.061

Industry representatives in clinical settings, 8.047

Infants
anencephalic neonates as organ donors, 2.162
fetal umbilical cord blood banking, 2.165
seriously disabled, 2.17
treatment decisions for seriously ill newborns, 2.215

Infection control, disease transmission by physicians, 9.13

Infectious diseases
artificial insemination, 2.04, 2.05
patient responsibilities, 10.02
physician refusals to provide care, 10.05
physician immunization, 9.133
physicians with, precautions, 9.13
public health interventions, quarantine, isolation, 2.25
screening donors in artificial insemination, 2.04, 2.05
xenotransplantation risks, 2.169

Information and patients: records of physicians, 7.02

Information availability, Principle V

Information, availability of records of physicians to other physicians, 7.01

Information, electronic, breach of, 5.10

Information from unethical experiments, 2.30

Information, genetic, and insurance companies, 2.135

Information, genetic, and the criminal justice system, 2.136

Information, medical, postmortem, 5.051

Information, patient, 8.12

Information, withholding from patients, 8.082

Informed consent, 8.08

    abortion and fetal tissue transplantation, 2.161

    advance directives, 2.225

    artificial insemination by anonymous donor, 2.05

    artificial insemination by known donor, 2.04

    assisted reproductive technology, 2.055

    carrier screening of genetic disorders, 2.137

    children in clinical investigations, 2.07

    clinical investigation guidelines, 2.07

    cloning for biomedical research, 2.146

    cloning to produce children, 2.147

    commercial use of human tissue, 2.08

    communicating information in more than one session, 8.08

    computerized patient records and medical information, 5.07

    court-initiated treatments in criminal cases, 2.065

    criminal justice system and genetic information, 2.136

    direct-to-consumer ads for prescription drugs, 5.015

    direct-to-consumer diagnostic imaging tests, 8.045

    disclosure obligations of physicians, 8.08

    disclosure of patient information to insurance company representatives, 5.08

    disclosure of patient records to data collection companies for marketing purposes, 5.075

    distinguishing between investigators and clinicians, 8.0315

    DNA databank safeguards in genomic research, 2.079

    do-not-resuscitate orders, 2.22

    ethics consultations, 9.115

    expedited partner therapy (STDs), 8.07

    fetal research guidelines, 2.10

    fetal umbilical cord blood banking, 2.165

    filming patients for education of health professionals, 5.046

    filming patients in health care settings, 5.045

    filming patients in health care settings, 5.045

    gene therapy, 2.11

    genetic counseling and testing, 2.12

    genetic engineering, 2.13

    genetic testing by employers, 2.132

    HIV testing, 2.23

    international research, 2.077

    lawsuits involving, 8.08

    managed care full disclosure, 8.13

    mandatory parental consent for abortion, 2.015

    medical students performing procedures on fellow students, 3.09

    medical students' involvement in patient care, 8.087

    mentally incompetent persons in clinical investigations, 2.07

    minors' confidential care, 5.055

    orders not to intervene, 2.225

    organ donation after cardiac death, 2.157

    organ donation by children and incompetent adults, 2.15

    organ donors and recipients, 2.16

    organ transplantation from living donors, 2.15

    organ transplantation guidelines, 2.16

    patient decision making, 8.08

    patient restraint, 8.17

    peers as patients, 8.191

    physician obligations to patients, 8.08

    physician participation in clinical trials and conflict of interest, 8.0315

    physician self-treatment, treatment of immediate family members, 8.19

    placebo controls in clinical trials, 2.075

    placebo use, 8.083

    presumed consent and mandated choice for organs from deceased donors, 2.155

    radio frequency ID devices, 2.40

    reporting violence and abuse, 2.02

    resident physicians' involvement in patient care, 8.088

    routine HIV testing, 2.23

    sedation to unconsciousness at end of life, 2.201

    stem cell recipients, 2.146

    surgeon substitution without patient knowledge, 8.16

    surgical comanagement, 8.043

    surgical "placebo" controls, 2.076

    treatment decisions for seriously ill newborns, 2.215

    waiver for research in emergency situations, 8.085

    withholding information from patients, 8.082

    xenotransplantation, 2.169

Informing families of a patient's death, 8.18

Inherited diseases, See Genetic counseling; Genetic testing; Genetics

Inquire about comfort (IAC) orders, 2.225

Insemination, artificial, See Artificial insemination; Reproductive medicine

Institutional review boards, See also Ethics committees

    filming patients in health care settings, 5.045

    international research criteria, 2.077

    placebo controls in clinical trials, 2.075

Institutionalized persons, clinical investigation guidelines, 2.07

Instruments, surgical or diagnostic, patent for, 9.09

Insurance companies, See Insurance, health; Managed care

Insurance, health, *See also* Managed care
basic benefits package, provision of adequate
    health care, 2.095
    bracketed incentive system with widely varied
        bonuses and penalties, 8.054
    claim form completion charges, 6.07
    co-payment forgiveness, waiver, 6.12, 6.13
    company representatives and
        confidentiality, 5.08
    contract restrictions on disclosure ("gag
        clauses"), 8.053
    contractual relationships, 8.05
    cost containment and prescription drugs, 8.135
    coverage decisions by medical directors, 8.021
    forgiveness or waiver of insurance
        copayments, 6.12
    form completion charges, 6.07
    fraud and abuse, 9.132
    genetic information, 2.135
    incentives based on quality and patient
        satisfaction, 8.054
    incentives that promote efficiency, 8.054
    larger patient pools preferable to reduce
        financial risks, 8.054
    managed care appellate mechanisms, 8.13
    managed care benefits package
        formulation, 8.13
    managed care restrictions, allocations, 8.13
    medical directors' ethical obligations, 8.021
    patient advocacy, 10.01
    patient referral and disclosure of
        limitations, 8.132
    physician incentives applied across broad
        physician groups, 8.054
    physician incentives based on longer time
        periods preferable, 8.054
    physician incentives calculated on continuum
        of utilization preferable to trigger
        points, 8.054
    retainer practices, distinguishing special
        services and amenities from reimbursable
        medical services, 8.055
Intelligence gathering, *See* Interrogations
Interest charges, *See* Fees and charges
Interest charges and finance charges, 6.08
International health
    guidelines on cloning to produce children, 2.147
International medical graduates, 9.037
International research, 2.077
    ethical considerations in, 2.077
    preventing malevolent use of biomedical
        research, 2.078
Internet, *See also* Computers
    health-related online sites, 5.027
    patient-specific information, 5.027
    physician Web sites and sales of health- and
        non-health-related products, 8.062; 8.063
    social media use by physicians, 9.124
Interpersonal violence, *See* Violence and abuse
Interprofessional relations, 3.00-3.09
    allied health professionals, 3.03
    chiropractic, 3.041

    nonscientific practitioners, 3.01
    nurses, 3.02
    physician employment by nonphysician
        supervisee, 3.05
    referral of patients, 3.04
    sexual harassment and exploitation between
        medical supervisors and trainees, 3.08
Interrogation, physician participation in, 2.068
Invalid medical treatment, 8.20, 10.05
Investigation, clinical, 2.07
Investigational therapies, *See* Research
Investments, *See* Conflict of interest
Involvement in patient care, medical
    student, 8.087
Involvement in patient care, resident
    physicians, 8.088
Isolation and quarantine as public health
    interventions, 2.25

Journals, medical
    gender discrimination in medical
        publishing, 9.035
    physician obligation to share knowledge, skills,
        new procedures, 9.08
    unethical experiment results, information, 2.30
Judicial Council, AMA, *See* Council on Ethical
    and Judicial Affairs, AMA

Key third parties, sexual or romantic relations
    between physicians and, 8.145
Knowledge, scientific, *See* Scientific knowledge
Known donor, artificial insemination by, 2.04

Laboratory services, 8.09
    billing for actual charges, 6.09
    clinical test result reporting guidelines, 8.095
    fee-splitting, referrals to, 6.03
    fertility labs, 2.055
    ownership, operation and supervision by
        nonphysicians, 8.09
    physician acquisition or processing charges, 8.09
    physician markups, commissions or profits, 8.09
Language
    barriers in racial and ethnic health care
        disparities, 9.121
    derogatory, in patient-physician
        relationship, 9.123
Law, *See also* Contracts
    abortion, 2.01
    abuse reporting, 2.02
    advance agreements for disposition of frozen
        pre-embryos, 2.141
    advocacy for change in, 9.025
    artificial insemination by known donor, 2.04
    assisted reproductive technology, 2.055
    capital punishment, 2.06
    change advocacy, 9.025
    changing, Principle III
    cloning to produce children, 2.147
    court-initiated treatments in criminal
        cases, 2.065
    court-ordered care, 10.015

criminal justice system and genetic
information, 2.136
deceased victims' genetic information, 2.136
direct-to-consumer advertisements of
prescription drugs, 5.015
enforcement, interrogations, 2.068
equal standing of cloned children, 2.147
expedited partner therapy (STDs), 8.07
fetal research, 2.10
genetic testing of children, 2.138
gestational surrogacy contracts, 2.18
illegal conduct compared with unethical
conduct, 1.02
immunity from punitive action in studying and
preventing error and harm, 8.121
impaired drivers, 2.24
invalid treatment, 8.20, 10.05
liens, 8.10
mandatory parental consent for abortion, 2.015
mandatory reporting of violence and
abuse, 2.02
medical record retention, disposal, 7.05
medical records retention, 7.05
medical testimony, 9.07
nonscientific practitioners, 3.01
patient access to medical records, 7.02
patients' attorney-physician relationship,
confidentiality, 5.06
pediatric decision making,
disagreements, 10.016
physician illegal conduct, 9.04
physician participation in interrogation, 2.068
physician political activity, 9.012
physician records, 7.02
physician respect for, Principle III
physician testimony, 5.06
presumed consent and mandated choice for
organs from deceased donors, 2.155
relationship to ethics, 1.02
reporting impaired drivers, 2.24
reporting unethical physicians, 9.031
reporting violence and abuse, 2.02
required disclosure of confidential
information, 5.05
respect for, in patient-physician
relationships, 9.12
routine forgiveness or waiver of insurance
copayments, 6.12
statute of limitations and medical record
retention, 7.05
studying and preventing error and harm, 8.121
surgical or diagnostic instrument patents, 9.09
surrogate decision making, 8.081
surrogate mothers, 2.18
unjust, 1.02
Lawyers, See Attorneys
Legal issues, See Law
Lethal injections, See also Capital punishment
euthanasia, 2.21
physician participation in executions, 2.06
Levels of care and economic incentives, 4.04
Liability, See Law; Professional liability

Licensure
false medical testimony, 9.07
nonscientific practitioners, 3.01
reporting unethical physicians, 9.031
substitution of services by allied health
professionals, 3.03
Lien laws, 8.10
Lifesaving skills, 8.181
Life support, See Life-sustaining treatment
Life-sustaining treatment
decisions for seriously ill newborns, 2.215
substituted judgment and best interests analysis,
2.20, 8.081
withdrawal, and organ donation after cardiac
death, 2.157
withdrawal, and quality of life
considerations, 2.17
withholding/withdrawing, 2.20
Lifesaving skills, 8.181
Limitations, disclosure of: referral of patients, 8.132
Limited medical resources, allocation of, 2.03
Limited practitioners, See Health personnel
Limiting medical procedures, use of patents and
other means, 9.095
Living donors, See also Transplantation
transplantation of organs from, 2.15
Living wills, 8.081
Lodging at conferences, See Meetings

Malevolent use of biomedical research, 2.078
Malpractice, See Professional liability
Managed care, 8.13
advertising, 5.01
appeals, 8.13
benefits package formulation, 8.13
bracketed incentive system with widely varied
bonuses and penalties, 8.054
capitation, 8.051, 8.052
conflicts of interest under capitation, 8.051
contracts, 8.05, 8.053
cost containment and prescription drugs, 8.135
fee withholds, 8.13
freedom of choice and, 9.06
gatekeepers, 8.13
health maintenance organizations, 5.01
incentives based on quality and patient
satisfaction, 8.054
incentives that promote efficiency, 8.054
larger patient pools preferable to reduce
financial risks, 8.054
medical directors' ethical obligations, 8.021
patient referral and disclosure of
limitations, 8.132
physician incentives applied across broad
physician groups, 8.054
physician incentives based on longer time
periods preferable, 8.054
physician incentives calculated on continuum
of utilization preferable to trigger
points, 8.054
physician obligation to disclose treatment
options, alternatives, 8.13

physician rosters, 5.01

restrictions on disclosures ("gag" clauses), 8.053

Managing conflicts of interest in the conduct of clinical trials, 8.0315

Mandated choice for organs from deceased donors, 2.155

Mandatory parental consent to abortion, 2.015

Marketing

records disclosure to data collection companies, 5.075

referrals to companies selling medical products, 6.02

Media relations, 5.04-5.046, *See also* Advertising

clinical investigation guidelines, 2.07

communications media, professional responsibility, standards, 5.04

filming patients in health care settings, 5.045

medical news reports, 2.07

patient consent to information release, 5.04

physician advisory or referral services by telecommunication, 5.025

public solicitation for directed organ donation, 2.152

Mediation, ethics consultations, 9.115

Medicaid, medical record retention, 7.05

Medical applications of fetal tissue transplantation, 2.161

Medical care, charges, services provided by multiple physicians, 6.10

Medical centers, *See* Hospitals and health facilities

Medical devices, *See* Drugs and devices

Medical directors, 8.021

Medical education, *See* Education, medical; Education, medical, continuing; Education, medical, graduate

Medical errors, *See also* Patient safety

informing patients of, 8.12

reporting systems, 8.121

resident physicians' involvement in patient care, 8.088

studying and preventing, 8.121

supervisor-trainee disputes, 9.055

Medical examinations, independent, 10.03

Medical examiners, independent: confidentiality, 5.09

Medical futility, *See* Futile care

Medical history of patient, *See also* Medical records

patient responsibilities, 10.02

Medical information postmortem, 5.051

Medical licensure, *See* Licensure

Medical malpractice, *See* Professional liability

Medical need, *See* Decision making

Medical practice, 8.01-8.21

expedited partner therapy (STDs), 8.07

financial incentives and, 8.054

invalid treatment, 8.20, 10.05

managed care, 8.13

medical directors' ethical obligations, 8.021

medical necessity, situations engendering stronger obligation to treat, 10.05

medical need and prioritizing of patients, 2.03

new procedures, 9.08

patenting medical procedures to limit availability, 9.095

patient transfers when converting to a retainer practice, 8.055

peers as patients, 8.191

physician disciplinary measures, 9.04

physician self-treatment, treatment of immediate family members, 8.19

physicians in management positions or other nonclinical roles, 8.02

placebo use, 8.083

restrictive covenants, 9.02

retainer practices, 8.055

risk and case-mix adjustment in pay for performance, 8.056

second opinions, 8.041

sexual misconduct, 8.14

unlicensed individuals, 3.01

Medical offices and practices, *See* Practice management; Practice sale

Medical procedures

clinical investigation guidelines, 2.07

evaluation of, in determinations of adequate health care, 2.095

medical students performing procedures on fellow students, 3.09

new, and physician obligation to share knowledge, 9.08

newly deceased patients for training purposes, 8.181

use of patents and other means to limit availability, 9.095

Medical profession, gender discrimination in, 9.035

Medical records, 7.01-7.05

access by non-treating medical staff, 7.025

advance directives, advisory documents, 2.225

artificial insemination, anonymous donor's medical history, 2.05

availability of information to other physicians, 7.01

breaches of electronic health information, 5.10

children's, 7.05

computerized, and confidentiality, 5.07

confidentiality, 7.02

copying charges, 7.02, 7.04

criminal justice system and genetic information release, 2.136

departure from group, 7.03

destruction to preserve confidentiality, 7.05

detecting breaches of confidentiality, 7.025

disclosure of patient information to insurance company representatives, 5.08

disclosure to data collection companies for marketing purposes, 5.075

disposal, 7.05

do-not-resuscitate orders, 2.22

electronic, 7.025

filming patients for education of health professionals, 5.046

forwarding, 7.01, 7.03

fundamental elements of patient-physician relationship, 10.01

genetic information and insurance companies, 2.135
genetic testing of children, 2.138
group practice departure, 7.03
immunizations, 7.05
information and patients, 7.02
Medicare and Medicaid patients, 7.05
monitoring user access, 7.025
new treating physicians, 7.01
non-physician custodians, 7.04
nontreating medical staff access, 7.025
old, and document destruction, 7.05
orders not to intervene, 2.225
patient access, 7.02
patient authorization for release, 7.01
patient opportunity to claim, 7.05
patient's right to written copies of prescriptions, 8.06
physician retirement or departure from a group, 7.03
physicians' notes, 7.02
postmortem medical information, 5.051
practice sale and, 7.04
prescriptions for drugs and devices in, 8.06
providing records of former patients, 7.01
record access by nontreating medical staff, 7.025
retention, 7.03, 7.05
statute of limitations and malpractice claims, 7.05
transfer of, with sale of practice, 7.04
user access, 7.025
withholding, for unpaid bills, 7.01, 7.02
Medical resources, See Access to care; Adequate health care; Health care delivery; Transplantation
Medical schools, US, signing bonuses to attract graduates of, 9.037
Medical services, fees for, 6.05
Medical services, unnecessary, 2.19
Medical societies, See Societies, medical
Medical staff, 4.05
actions by, 4.05
compulsory vs. self-imposed assessments, 4.02
core responsibilities, 4.05
do-not-resuscitate orders, policies, 2.22
due process, 9.05
economic incentives and levels of care, 4.04
ethics committee representation, 9.11
governing board interaction, 4.05
non-treating, access to records, 7.025
organized, 4.05
peer review, 9.10
physician disruptive behavior, 9.045
physician-hospital contractual relations and financial arrangements, 4.06
privileges, 4.07
record access by nontreating medical staff, 7.025
responsibilities, 4.05
supervisor-trainee disputes, 9.055
wasteful or unnecessary hospital care, 4.04
Medical students, See Students, medical

Medical supervisors, See also Faculty, medical
disputes between trainees and, 9.055
sexual harassment and exploitation between trainees and, 3.08
Medical testimony, 9.07
Medical trainees, See Education, medical; Education, medical, graduate; Resident physicians; Students, medical
Medical treatment, invalid, 8.20, 10.05
Medical treatment, life-sustaining, See Life-sustaining treatment
Medical treatments, court-initiated, in criminal cases, 2.065
Medical witness testimony, 9.07
attorney-physician confidentiality, 5.06
determining competence to stand trial, 2.06
Medicare
assignment, and illegal or excessive fees, 6.05
illegal, excessive fees, 6.05
medical record retention, 7.05
Medications, See Drugs and devices
Medicine and discipline, 9.04
Medicine, practice of, and financial incentives, 8.054
Medicolegal issues, See Law
Meetings
continuing medical education, 9.011
direct subsidies to attendees, 8.061
honoraria and reasonable compensation for services of faculty and consultants, 8.061
industry gifts, travel expenses and honoraria for faculty at, 8.061
industry subsidies of travel-related expenses, (guideline 5), 8.061
industry travel subsidies for trainees to attend, 8.061
legitimate conferences (guideline 3), 8.061
Mental competence
condemned prisoners, 2.06
do-not-resuscitate orders, 2.22
euthanasia, 2.21
filming patients for education of health professionals, 5.046
incompetent persons, clinical investigation guidelines, 2.07
minors' confidential care, 5.055
organ transplantation from living donors, 2.15
withholding/withdrawing life-sustaining treatment, 2.20
xenotransplantation, 2.169
Mental health records, 7.02
Military intelligence, interrogations, 2.068
Minimal threshold, See Health care delivery
Minority groups, See Discrimination; Ethnic groups; Health disparities
Minors, See Adolescents; Children
Moral principles, 1.01
embryonic stem cell research, 2.146
Mothers, surrogate, See Pregnancy
Motion pictures
filming patients for education of health professionals, 5.046

filming patients in health care
settings, 5.045
Motivation in cadaveric organ donation, 2.151
Motor vehicle drivers, *See* Automobile drivers
Multiple physicians, services provided by, 6.10
Multiplex genetic testing, 2.139

National security, interrogations, 2.068
Nazi experiments, 2.30
NBD (no blood draws) orders, 2.225
Need, medical, *See* Decision making
Neglect of patient, 8.11
Negotiating discounts for specialty care, 8.052
Neonates, *See* Infants
New medical procedures, 9.08
Newborns, *See* Infants
Newly deceased patients, *See* Death
News, medical, *See* Media relations; Research
NFT (no feeding tube) orders, 2.225
NIL (no intravenous lines) orders, 2.225
No blood draws (NBD) orders, 2.225
No feeding tube (NFT) orders, 2.225
No intravenous lines (NIL) orders, 2.225
No vital signs (NVS) orders, 2.225
Nonclinical roles, ethical guidelines for physicians
in, 8.02
Noncompetition clauses
covenants not-to-compete for physicians-in-
training, 9.021
Non-health-related goods, sale of, from physicians'
offices, 8.062
Nonphysician supervisee, physician employment
by, 3.05
Nonscientific practitioners, 3.01
Nonscientific treatment
invalid treatment, 8.20, 10.05
Non-treating medical staff, access by, to records of
physicians, 7.025
Notes, physicians', *See* Medical records
Novel vectors, 2.13
Nurses, 3.02, 3.03
questioning physicians' orders, 3.02
NVS (no vital signs) orders, 2.225

Occupational health
genetic testing by employers, 2.132
immunization for vaccine-preventable
diseases, 9.133
protective measures taken by physicians and
other health personnel, 2.25, 9.133
work-related and independent examinations,
5.09, 10.03
Online sites, *See* Internet
Oocyte donors, 2.146, 2.147
Optimal use of orders not-to-intervene and
advance directives, 2.225
Orders, *See* Physicians' orders
Organ swaps, *See* Transplantation
Organ donation and organ donors, *See*
also Transplantation
after cardiac death, 2.157
anencephalic neonates as organ donors, 2.162

cadaveric organ donation financial incentives,
motivation, 2.151
condemned prisoners, 2.06
dead fetus tissue, organs, 2.10
directed (designated) fetal tissue transplantation
prohibited, 2.161
directed (designated) organ donations, 2.15, 2.152
distribution of organs, 2.15, 2.151
donated organs as national rather than regional
resource, 2.16
donor advocate team separate from organ
recipient's care, 2.15
donor evaluation by advocate team, 2.15, 2.152
efforts to increase organ donation, 2.151, 2.155
fetal tissue, and financial remuneration, 2.161
fetal tissue, medical applications of, 2.161
geographical priorities and, 2.16
guidelines, 2.16
living donors, 2.15
living organ donor compensation, 2.15
organ swaps (paired donation), 2.15
patient responsibilities, 10.02
presumed consent and mandated choice for
organs from deceased donors, 2.155
psychosocial evaluation of donors, 2.15, 2.152
public solicitation for directed organ
donation, 2.152
purchase of donated organs, 2.151
single waiting lists, 2.16
tissue harvesting from genetically identical
children, 2.145
withdrawal decisions by potential donors, 2.15
xenotransplantation, 2.169
Organized medical staff, *See* Medical staff
Outcome measures, medical futility in end-of-life
care, 2.037
Outside observers to the clinical encounter and
patient privacy, 5.0591
Ova donors, frozen pre-embryos, 2.141, 2.145
Ova, human, 2.14

Pain and pain control
euthanasia prohibition, 2.21
full-comfort-care-only (FCCO) orders, 2.225
hastening patient death, 2.20
organ donation after cardiac death, 2.157
physician-assisted suicide, 2.20, 2.211
sedation to unconsciousness at end of life, 2.201
surrogate decision making, 8.081
treatment decisions for seriously ill
newborns, 2.215
Palliative care, *See* Pain and pain control;
Terminally ill patients
Parents
gamete providers, in vitro fertilization,
2.141, 2.145
genetic testing of children, 2.138
involvement, and minors' confidential
care, 5.055
mandatory parental consent for abortion, 2.015
minors' confidential care, 5.055
pediatric decision making, 10.016

rights, artificial insemination, 2.05
sexual/romantic relations between physicians
and key third parties, 8.145
treatment decisions for seriously ill
newborns, 2.215
Partner therapy, expedited, 8.07
Patents
human genes, 2.105
limiting availability of medical procedures, 9.095
surgical or diagnostic instruments, 9.09
Patient advocacy
collective action and, 9.025
fundamental elements of patient-physician
relationship, 10.01
managed care restrictions, 8.13
physician obligations, 10.015
Patient care, medical student involvement
in, 8.087
Patient care, resident physicians' involvement
in, 8.088
Patient-centered care, quality improvement, 9.14
Patient consent, See Decision making;
Informed consent
Patient decision making, See Decision making
Patient education, See also Informed consent
expedited partner therapy (STDs), 8.07
filming patients in health care settings, 5.045
health products sold in or given at physicians'
offices, 8.063
Patient information, 8.12
Patient, neglect of, 8.11
Patient-physician relationship, Principle VIII;
10.01-10.05;See also Confidentiality
assisted suicide, 2.20, 2.211
best interests of patient paramount, 10.015
breaches of electronic health information, 5.10
capitation agreements affecting, 8.051
care by physicians providing second
opinions, 8.041
clinical investigation guidelines, 2.07
communication by electronic mail, 5.026
conditions creating the existence of, 10.015
confidential nature of, and required disclosure
of confidential information, 5.05
confidentiality and required disclosures of
confidential information, 5.05
conflict of interest guidelines, 8.03
contract restrictions on disclosure ("gag
clauses"), 8.053
contribution solicitation from patients, 10.018
declining patients on basis of race, color,
religion, national origin, sexual
orientation, gender identity, 9.12
direct-to-consumer diagnostic imaging
tests, 8.045
disclosure, physician ownership of health
facilities (physician self-referral
possibilities), 8.0321
discrimination on ethnic, religious, sexual
orientation, gender identity or other
basis, 9.12
disrespect and derogatory conduct in, 9.123

economic gain as subordinate to patient
interests, 8.03
euthanasia prohibition, 2.21
expedited partner therapy (STDs), 8.07
financial incentives and medical practice, 8.054
financial incentives in patient
recruitment, 6.021
first duty is to individual patient, 8.054
free choice in, 9.06
fundamental elements, 10.01
health-related products sold in physicians'
offices, 8.063
HIV-infected patients, 9.131
information on specific patients released to the
media, 5.04
informing families of patient's death, 8.18
informing patients about health plan financial
incentives, 8.054
informing patients of mistakes, 8.12
insurance company representatives and
confidentiality, 5.08
limited, industry-employed physicians and
independent medical examiners, 10.03
managed care, 8.13
medical necessity, situations engendering
stronger obligation to treat, 10.05
medical testimony and physician obligation to
individual patients, 9.07
neglect of patient, 8.11
organ transplantation guidelines, 2.16
patient gifts to physicians, 10.017
patient notification of physician's departure
from a group, 7.03
patient notification of physician departure from
group, 7.03
patient privacy protections, 5.059
patient responsibilities, 10.02
patient transfers when converting to a retainer
practice, 8.055
patient's right to continuity of care, and
adequate care, 10.01
patients harmed by an error, 8.121
pediatric decision making, 10.016
peers as patients, 8.191
physician records, 7.02
physician refusals to provide care, 10.05
physician responsibility to patient is paramount,
Principle VIII
physician self-treatment, treatment of
immediate family members, 8.19
placebo use, 8.083
political communications with patients and
their families, 9.012
potential patients, 10.05
public health interventions, quarantine,
isolation, 2.25
records disclosure to data collection
companies, 5.075
respect for law and human rights, 9.12
retainer practices, 8.055
role of treating physician in allocating limited
medical resources, 2.03

sexual misconduct, 8.14

sexual/romantic relations between physicians and key third parties, 8.145

social media use and professional boundaries, 9.124

surgeon substitution without patient knowledge, 8.16

termination of, continuity of care, timely notification, 8.115

trust in, 10.015

unrealistic expectations and false promises based on outcome, 6.01

withholding information from patients, 8.082

Patient privacy and outside observers to the clinical encounter, 5.0591

Patient responsibilities, 10.02

Patient rights, fundamental elements of patient-physician relationship, 10.01

Patient safety

abortion procedures and fetal tissue transplantation, 2.161

direct-to-consumer advertisements of prescription drugs, 5.015

drug or device adverse event reporting, 9.032

error reporting systems, 8.121

expedited partner therapy (STDs), 8.07

gene therapies, 2.11

guidelines, organ donors and recipients, 2.16

hospital medical staff responsibilities, 4.05

impaired physicians, 9.0305, 9.031

implications of germline therapy, 2.11

informed consent waiver for research in emergency situations, 8.085

informing patients of mistakes, 8.12

living organ donor outcomes, 2.15

organ transplantation from living donors, 2.15

patients harmed by an error, 8.121

pay-for-performance programs, 8.056

placebo controls in clinical trials, 2.075

quality improvement, 9.14

radio frequency ID devices, 2.40

resident physicians' involvement in patient care, 8.088

restraints, 8.17

studying and preventing error and harm, 8.121

transplantation procedures by competent physicians in adequate facilities, 2.16

Patient transfer

do not transfer orders, 2.225

medical futility in end-of-life care, 2.037

Patient's death, informing families, 8.18

Patients, See also Advance directives; Confidentiality; Decision making; Informed consent; Patient advocacy; Patient-physician relationship; Patient safety; Patients' rights; Quality of life, autonomy and privacy in context of health care, 5.059

autonomy of, 10.02

chaperones during physical examinations, 8.21

clinical trial subject selection, 2.071

commercial use of, profits from human tissue, 2.08

compliance with treatment plans, 10.02

cooperation with treatment, 10.02

criminal justice system and genetic information, 2.136

deceased patient's bequest to a physician, 10.017

deception of, by nonscientific practitioners, 3.01

demands for treatments, 2.035

do-not-resuscitate orders, 2.22

filming, for the education of health professionals, 5.046

filming, in health care settings, 5.045

financial incentives to, for referrals, 6.021

financial obligations, 10.02

free choice of physicians, 9.06

freedom of choice in filling prescriptions, 8.06

genetic information and insurance companies, 2.135

gifts to physicians, 10.017

healthy lifestyle commitment, 10.02

HIV-infected, 9.131

impaired drivers, 2.24

informed consent, 8.08

informing families of death, 8.18

international research, 2.077

involuntary restraints, 8.17

keeping appointments, 10.02

managed care benefits package formulation, 8.13

managed care plan selection, 8.13

minors' autonomy, confidential care, 5.055

missed, cancelled appointments, 8.01

newly deceased, procedures performed on, for training purposes, 8.181

notification of physician's departure from a group, 7.03

opportunity to claim medical records, 7.05

physician responsibility to, is paramount, Principle VIII

physician-assisted suicide, 2.20, 2.211

placebo controls in clinical trials, 2.075

potential, 10.05

public health interventions, quarantine, isolation, 2.25

quality of life, 2.17

radio frequency ID devices, 2.40

research subjects in clinical investigations, 2.07

responsibilities of, 10.02

restraints, 8.17

right to courtesy, respect, dignity, responsiveness and timely attention, 10.01

soliciting contributions from, 10.018

testimonials, 5.02

withdrawing consent for filming, 5.045

withholding information from, 8.082

withholding/withdrawing life-sustaining treatment, 2.20

Patients, mentally incompetent, See Mental competence

Patients who are peers, 8.191

Patients, referral of, See Referrals

Patients' records, See Medical records

Patients' rights, respect for, Principle IV

Pay-for-performance programs, 8.056
Payment, *See* Fees and charges; Financial
    incentives and interests
Pediatric care, *See* Children
Pediatric decision making, 10.016
Peer review, 9.10
    allocation policies for limited medical
        resources, 2.03
    forms and types of, 9.10
    quality monitoring, 9.14
Peers as patients, 8.191
Performance improvement, *See* Quality of care
Perfusion
    cold preservation fluid, for organ donation after
        cardiac death, 2.157
    without consent to organ donation, 2.157
Personal injury, physician testimony, 5.06
Pharmaceutical benefit management, 8.135
Pharmacy, *See also* Drugs and devices
    drug and device prescribing and
        dispensing, 8.06
    physician ownership of pharmacies, 8.06
Pharmacy and therapeutics committees, 8.135
Physical abuse, *See* Violence and abuse
Physical examination
    chaperones during, 8.21
    gowns, privacy for undressing, draping, 8.21
    work-related and independent
        examinations, 10.03
Physical restraints, 8.17
Physician advisory or referral services by
    telecommunication, 5.025
Physician assistants, allied health
    professionals, 3.03
Physician-assisted suicide, 2.20, 2.211
Physician-attorney relation: confidentiality, 5.06
Physician colleagues
    disruptive behavior, 9.045
    knowledge and skill sharing, 9.08, 9.095
    peers as patients, 8.191
    physicians as patients, 8.191, 9.0305
    professional courtesy, 6.13
    records of physicians: availability of information
        to other physicians, 7.01
    reporting deficiencies, Principle II
    reporting impairment, incompetence, unethical
        behavior, 9.0305, 9.031
    respect for rights of, Principle IV
    surgical comanagement, 8.043
Physician conflict of interest, *See* Conflict
    of interest
Physician employment by nonphysician
    supervisee, 3.05
Physician fees, *See* Fees and charges
Physician health and wellness, 9.0305
Physician-hospital contractual relations, 4.06
Physician obligation in disaster preparedness and
    response, 9.067
Physician ownership of health facilities, services,
    See Financial incentives and interests;
    Hospitals and health facilities; Referrals;
    Self-referral

Physician participation in interrogation, 2.068
Physician participation in soliciting contributions
    from patients, 10.018
Physician-patient relationship, *See* Patient-
    physician relationship; Patients
Physician pay-for-performance programs, 8.056
Physician records, *See* Confidentiality;
    Medical records
Physicians
    administrative or other nonclinical roles, 8.02
    advertising and publicity, 5.02
    censure, suspension or expulsion from medical
        society membership, 1.01
    change advocacy for laws and health
        policy, 9.025
    civil rights in professional activities,
        organizations, 9.03
    clinical trial participation and conflict of
        interest, 8.0315
    conflict of interest guidelines, 8.03
    deceased patient's bequests, 10.017
    disaster preparedness and response
        obligations, 9.067
    disciplinary measures, 9.04
    disruptive behavior, 9.045
    due process, 9.05
    employed by hospitals, 4.06
    employment by nonphysician supervisee, 3.05
    financial interests in imaging facilities, 8.045
    financial interests subordinate to patient
        interests, 8.03
    free drug samples for personal or family member
        use (guideline 1), 8.061
    freedom of choice in service, associations, and
        environment, Principle VI
    gender discrimination, 9.035
    gifts to, from industry, 8.061
    health and wellness, 9.0305
    health facility ownership and conflicts of
        interest, 8.0321
    HIV-infected, 9.131
    hospital contractual relations and financial
        arrangements, 4.06
    illegal conduct, 1.02
    immunization for vaccine-preventable
        diseases, 9.133
    impaired, 9.0305
    increasing diversity in medical profession, 9.121
    industry-employed and independent medical
        examiners, 10.03
    infectious disease precautions, 9.13
    management positions or other nonclinical
        roles, 8.02
    medical directors' ethical obligations, 8.021
    medical testimony, 9.07
    moral values and judgment in genetic
        counseling, 2.12
    multiple, services provided by, 6.10
    need for a personal physician of their
        own, 9.0305
    obligation to share knowledge, skills, new
        procedures, 9.08

patient free choice of, 9.06
patient gifts, 10.017
peer review, 9.10
peers as patients, 8.191
persecution of, when they treat torture
    victims, 2.067
personal moral decisions (capital
    punishment), 2.06
personal, religious, moral beliefs of, and refusal
    to provide a specific treatment, 10.05
political communications with patients and
    their families, 9.012
professional courtesy, 6.13
public and occupational health protective
    measures taken by, 2.25
reporting deficiencies in character or
    competence, Principle II
reporting impaired, incompetent or unethical
    colleagues, 9.0305, 9.031
respect for colleagues' rights, Principle IV
self-treatment, treatment of immediate family
    members, 8.19
sexual harassment and exploitation between
    medical supervisors and trainees, 3.08
sexual misconduct, 8.14
sexual or romantic relationships with former
    patients, 8.14
sexual/romantic relations between key third
    parties and, 8.145
social media use and boundaries between
    private and professional areas, 9.124
substance abuse, 8.15
surgical comanagement, 8.043
unions, strikes, collective action, 9.025
Physicians and infectious diseases, 9.13
Physicians in training, covenants
    not-to-compete, 9.021
Physicians' obligations in preventing, identifying
    and treating violence and abuse, 2.02
Physicians' offices, See Practice management
Physicians' orders
    do-not-resuscitate, 2.22
    not-to-intervene and advance directives,
        optimal use of, 2.225
Physician's political communications with patients
    and their families, 9.012
Physician's role following breach of electronic
    health information, 5.10
Physicians' self-referral, 8.0321
Physicians with disruptive behavior, 9.045
Placebo controls in clinical trials, 2.075
"Placebo" controls, surgical, 2.076
Placebo use in clinical practice, 8.083
Policy change and policy making, See
    Health policy
Political activity
    change advocacy for laws and health
        policy, 9.025
    communications with patients and their
        families, 9.012
Poor, See Poverty
Postmortem medical information, 5.051

Postmortem procedures, 8.181
Potential patients, 10.05
Poverty, See also Indigent care
    caring for the poor, 9.065
    clinical trial subject selection, 2.071
    fundamental elements of patient-physician
        relationship, 10.01
Practice management, 8.01-8.21; See also
    Contracts; Fees and charges; Medical records
    contribution solicitation from patients, 10.018
    eliminating biased behavior by health
        personnel, 9.121
    exclusive distributorships of health-related
        products, 8.063
    lien laws, 8.10
    non-health-related products sold in physicians'
        offices, 8.062
    practice sale and physician records, 7.04
    retainer practices, 8.055
    sale of health-related products from physicians'
        offices, 8.063
Practice matters, See Medical practice;
    Practice management
Practice of medicine, See Licensure;
    Medical practice
Practice sales, medical records transfer, 7.04
Practitioners, nonscientific, 3.01
Pre-embryos, See also Reproductive medicine
    frozen, 2.141
    splitting, 2.145
Pregnancy
    abortion, 2.01
    fetal research guidelines, informed consent, 2.10
    fetal tissue transplantation, medical
        applications of, 2.161
    fetal umbilical cord blood banking, 2.165
    gene transfer in utero, 2.13
    mandatory parental consent for abortion, 2.015
    minors' confidential care, 5.055
    prenatal genetic testing, counseling, 2.12
    safety in abortion procedures, 2.161
    surrogate mothers, 2.18
Pregnancy termination, See Abortion
Prenatal testing, See Pregnancy
Prescribing and prescription drugs, See Drugs
    and device
Presumed consent and mandated choice for organs
    from deceased donors, 2.155
Principles of Medical Ethics, page xvii
Prisoners
    coercive interrogations, 2.068
    condemned, capital punishment, 2.06
    interrogation strategies, 2.068
    physical and mental assessments, 2.068
    physician participation in interrogation, 2.068
    torture, 2.067
Privacy, Principle IV; see also Confidentiality
    chaperones during physical examinations, 8.21
    confidentiality of information disclosed by
        patients, 5.05
    electronic mail, 5.026
    expedited partner therapy (STDs), 8.07

filming patients for education of health
    professionals, 5.046
filming patients in health care settings, 5.045
in the context of health care, 5.059
industry representatives in clinical
    settings, 8.047
online sites with patient-specific
    information, 5.027
outside observers, 5.0591
patient autonomy and, 5.059
potential breaches, in electronic mail, 5.026
protection of patients, 5.059
social media use by physicians, 9.124
Privileges, *See* Medical staff
PRN orders, *See* Pro re nata orders
Pro re nata orders, 8.17
Procedures, medical, *See* Medical procedures
Professional courtesy, 6.13
Professional liability
    breach of confidentiality cases, 5.05
    conflict of interest lawsuits, 8.03
    contingent physician fees, 6.01
    drug and device prescribing and
        dispensing, 8.06
    HIV-infected physicians, 9.131
    informed consent and, 8.08
    informing patients of mistakes, 8.12
    medical records retention, statute of
        limitations, 7.05
    medical testimony, 9.07
    patient neglect lawsuits, 8.11
    reporting impaired drivers, 2.24
    statute of limitations and medical records
        retention, 7.05
    studying and preventing error and harm, 8.121
    surgeon substitution without patient
        knowledge, 8.16
    workers' compensation lawsuits, 10.03
Professional rights and responsibilities, 9.01-9.14
    civil rights and, 9.03
    communications media, 5.04
Professional standards, *See* Standards
Professionalism and contractual relations, 8.0501
Prognosis, information on specific patients released
    to the media, 5.04
Provision of adequate health care, 2.095
Proxy decision making, *See* Surrogate
    decision makers
Psychological abuse, *See* Violence and abuse
Psychosocial evaluation and support
    euthanasia, 0-2.21
    existential suffering, 2.201
    organ donors, 2.15, 2.152
    terminal patients contemplating suicide, 2.211
    treatment decisions for seriously ill
        newborns, 2.215
Public health, *See also* Infectious diseases
    community improvement, Principle VII
    drug or device adverse event reporting, 9.032
    epidemics and public health interventions, 2.25
    expedited partner therapy (STDs), 8.07
    HIV-infected physicians, 9.131

HIV testing, 2.23
impaired drivers, 2.24
infectious disease transmission by
    physicians, 9.13
interventions, quarantine, isolation, 2.25
patient responsibilities, 10.02
physicians' obligations in disaster preparedness
    and response, 9.067
physician immunization for vaccine-preventable
    diseases, 9.133
prevention of violence and abuse, 2.02
routine HIV testing, 2.23
third-party notification of HIV status, 2.23
Public solicitation for directed donation of organs
    for transplantation, 2.152
Publicity, *See* Advertising and publicity
Publishing, *See* Journals, medical

Quality of care
    conflicts of interest under capitation, 8.051
    contractual terms compromising professional
        judgment, integrity, 8.0501, 8.054, 8.056
    cost considerations subordinate to, 2.09
    economic incentives and levels of care, 4.04
    ethics committees, 9.11
    evaluation of health plan financial
        incentives, 8.054
    evaluation of procedures in determinations of
        adequate health care, 2.095
    hospital medical staff responsibilities, 4.05
    improvement of, 9.14
    laboratory services ownership, operation and
        supervision by nonphysicians, 8.09
    managed care financial incentives, 8.13
    managed care restrictions, 8.13
    monitoring, 9.14
    pay-for-performance programs, 8.056
    performance improvement, 9.14
    physician employment by nonphysician
        supervisee, 3.05
    physician health and wellness, 9.0305
    physician refusals to provide care, 10.05
    racial and ethnic health care disparities, 9.121
    reporting impaired, incompetent or unethical
        physicians, 9.0305, 9.031
    retainer practices, 8.055
    standard of care in medical testimony, 9.07
    supervisor-trainee disputes, 9.055
Quality of life, 2.17
    allocation (rationing) of limited medical
        resources, 2.03
    seriously disabled newborns, 2.17
    surrogate decision making, 8.081
    treatment decisions for seriously ill
        newborns, 2.215
Quality, 9.14
Quarantine and isolation as public health
    interventions, 2.25

Racial and ethnic health care disparities, 9.121
Racial discrimination, *See* Discrimination
Racial groups, *See* Ethnic groups

Radio frequency ID devices, 2.40
Rationing, *See* Access to care; Health care delivery
Records, *See* Confidentiality; Medical records
Records of physicians, *See* Medical records
Referral of patients, *See* Referrals
Referral services by telecommunication, 5.025
Referrals, 3.04; see also Consultation, medical
    chiropractic, 3.041
    consultation, 8.04
    direct-to-consumer diagnostic imaging
      tests, 8.045
    disclosure of health plan limitations, 8.132
    fee splitting, 6.02
    fee splitting, 6.02, 6.03
    financial incentives to patients for, 6.021
    managed care, 8.13
    negotiating discounts for specialty care, 8.052
    not billable, 6.10
    outside health plan coverage, 8.132
    physician ownership of health facilities and
      conflicts of interest, 8.0321
    physician self-referral (financial interest in
      facilities outside their practices), 8.0321
    physician services by telecommunication, 5.025
    research studies, 6.03
    surgical co-management, 8.043
    to health facilities, 6.03
    to specialists, limited practitioners, other health
      professionals, 3.04
Reforms, *See* Health care delivery; Health
    policy; Law
Refusal of CPR, *See* Do-not-resuscitate orders
Refusal to treat, *See* Treatment denial
Reimbursement, *See* Fees and charges; Financial
    incentives and interests; Insurance, health;
    Managed care
Relation of law and ethics, 1.02
Religion
    ethics committees in religiously affiliated
      facilities, 9.11
    physician's personal, religious, moral beliefs
      and refusal to provide a specific
      treatment, 10.05
Religious discrimination, *See also* Discrimination
    civil rights, professional responsibility, 9.03
    declining patients on basis of, 9.12
Reporting adverse drug or device events, 9.032
Reporting clinical test results: general
    guidelines, 8.095
Reporting (notification) obligations
    deficiencies in physician character or
      competence, Principle II
    impaired drivers, 2.24
    impaired, incompetent or unethical colleagues,
      9.0305, 9.031
    patient responsibilities in preventing,
      reporting, 10.02
Reproductive medicine
    advance agreements for disposition of frozen
      pre-embryos, 2.141
    artificial insemination by anonymous
      donor, 2.05

    artificial insemination by known donor, 2.04
    assisted reproductive technology, 2.055
    cloning, 2.147
    compensation of donors, 2.05
    death of donors of frozen semen, 2.04
    frozen pre-embryos, 2.141
    identical siblings, 2.145
    immortal cell lines, 2.146
    in vitro fertilization, 2.14
    parental rights in artificial insemination, 2.05
    pre-embryo analysis, 2.12
    pre-embryo splitting, 2.145
    reporting unethical practices, 2.05
    sale of pre-embryos, 2.145
    semen donor's death, 2.04
    stem cells, human, 2.146
    surrogate mothers, 2.18
Reproductive technology, assisted, 2.055
Research
    advancement of scientific knowledge,
      Principle V
    cadaveric organ donation financial incentives,
      motivation, 2.151
    clinical investigation guidelines, 2.07
    clinical trials and management of conflicts of
      interest, 8.0315
    commercial use of human tissue, 2.08
    conflicts of interest, 2.079, 8.031, 8.0315
    delay or obstruction of results by clinical trial
      sponsors, 8.0315
    disclosure of company ties, potential conflicts of
      interest, 8.031
    DNA databank safeguards in genomic
      research, 2.079
    embryonic stem cells, 2.146
    experimental treatment, investigational therapy
      continuation, 2.071
    fair market value of physician compensation for
      clinical trials, 8.0315
    fee splitting, finder's fees, 6.03
    fetal, guidelines, 2.10
    fetal umbilical cord blood collection, 2.165
    funding medical care for complications
      associated with clinical trials, 8.0315
    gender discrimination, 9.035
    gender disparities in health care, 9.122
    genetic engineering, 2.13
    immortal cell lines, 2.146
    in vitro fertilization, human ova
      maintenance, 2.14
    industry travel subsidies for genuine research
      purposes (guideline 5), 8.061
    industry-sponsored, in CME, 9.011
    informed consent waiver for, in emergency
      situations, 8.085
    institutional responsibility for ethical
      conduct, 2.07
    international, 2.077
    malevolent use of, 2.078
    medical news reports, 2.07
    Nazi experiments, 2.30
    new procedures, 9.08

news, publicity about, 2.07
patenting human genes, 2.105
payments for referring patients for
    studies, 6.03
placebo controls in clinical trials, 2.075
postmortem medical information, 5.051
presumed consent and mandated choice for
    organs from deceased donors, 2.155
preventing exploitation in foreign
    countries, 2.077
preventing malevolent use of biomedical
    research, 2.078
publication, 8.031, 8.0315, 9.08
racial and ethnic health care disparities, 9.121
radio frequency ID devices, 2.40
referrals for studies, 6.03
responsibilities of institutions conducting
    clinical investigations, 2.07
restrictions on dissemination of results, 2.078
scientific knowledge secondary to concern for
    research subjects, 2.07
studying and preventing error and harm, 8.121
surgical "placebo" controls, 2.076
termination of studies with placebo
    controls, 2.075
time length of studies with placebo
    controls, 2.075
training in ethical principles, 2.078
treating patients and also conducting
    research, 8.0315
Tuskegee study, 2.30
unethical experiment results, information, 2.30
withholding new medical knowledge, 9.08
xenotransplantation, 2.169
Research subjects
clinical investigation guidelines, 2.07
commercial use of, profits from human
    tissue, 2.08
financial gain in genomic research, 2.079
international research, 2.077
safeguards for communities and individuals in
    genomic research, 2.079
selection for clinical trials, 2.071
unethical experiment results, information, 2.30
xenotransplantation, 2.169
Resident physicians, See also Education,
    medical, graduate
adequate rest, "moonlighting," 8.088
due process, 9.05
industry scholarship and special funds
    (guideline 6), 8.061
industry travel subsidies directly given to,
    (guideline 6), 8.061
industry-sponsored conferences, symposia
    designed specifically for medical trainees
    (guideline 6), 8.061
informing families of patient's death, 8.18
involvement in patient care, 8.088
noncompetition covenants, 9.021
peers as patients, 8.191
sexual harassment and exploitation between
    medical supervisors and trainees, 3.08

signing bonuses for attracting US
    graduates, 9.037
supervisor-trainee disputes, 9.055
surgeon substitution, 8.16
Resource allocation, See Health care delivery
Resources, limited, allocation of, 2.03
Respect for law and human rights: patient-
    physician relationship, 9.12
Respect (patient-physician relationship
    disrespect, derogatory conduct, 9.123
    right to courtesy, respect, dignity,
        responsiveness and timely attention, 10.01
Responsibilities, patient, 10.02
Responsibility, professional, civil rights and, 9.03
Responsibility, professional :communications
    media standards, 5.04
Restraints, use of, 8.17
Restrictions on disclosure in health care plan
    contracts, 8.053
Restrictive covenants, 9.02
    excessiveness in duration or geographic
        scope, 9.02
    noncompetition covenants for physicians in
        training, 9.021
Retainer practices, 8.055
Retention of medical records, See Medical records
Retirement, 7.03
RFID, See Radio frequency ID devices
Risk disclosure, See Informed consent
Romantic relations between physicians and key
    third parties, 8.145

Safeguards in use of DNA databanks in genomic
    research, 2.079
Sale of a medical practice, 7.04
Sale of health-related products from physicians'
    offices, 8.063
Sale of non-health-related goods from physicians'
    offices, 8.062
Scarce resources, See Access to care;
    Adequate health care; Health care
    delivery; Transplantation
Scientific investigations, See Research
Schools, medical, See Education, medical
Scientific knowledge, Principle V
    obligation to share knowledge, skills, new
        procedures, 9.08
    patenting medical procedures to limit
        availability, 9.095
Screening, direct-to-consumer diagnostic imaging
    tests, 8.045
Screening, genetic, See Genetic testing
Second opinions, 8.041
Security, computer
    breaches of electronic health information, 5.10
    patient records and medical information, 5.07
Sedation, See Drugs
Sedation to unconsciousness in end-of-life
    care, 2.201
Self-referral, 8.0321, 8.06
Self-treatment or treatment of immediate family
    members, 8.19

Semen, frozen, 2.04, 2.05
Seriously ill newborns, treatment decisions
    for, 2.215
Services provided by multiple physicians, 6.10
Sex selection, *See* Gender preference
Sexual abuse, *See* Violence and abuse
Sexual harassment
    exploitation and, between medical supervisors
        and trainees, 3.08
    gender discrimination, 9.035
Sexual misconduct, 8.14, 8.145
Sexual orientation, discrimination based on, 9.03,
    9.12, 10.05
Sexual relationships, key third parties, 8.145
Sexually transmitted diseases
    expedited partner therapy, 8.07
    minors' confidential care, 5.055
    third-party notification of HIV status, 2.23
Siblings, *See* Family
Signing bonuses to attract graduates of US medical
    schools, 9.037
Social events, modest vs. lavish, industry
    subsidies at conferences and meetings
    (guideline 5), 8.061
Social media, 9.124
Social policy issues, 2.01-2.40
    morality and, 1.01
Social worth in allocation (rationing) of limited
    medical resources, 2.03
Societies, medical
    civil rights in professional activities,
        organizations, 9.03
    due process, 9.05
    false medical testimony, 9.07
    member censure, suspension, expulsion, 1.01
    peer review, 9.10
    physician discipline, expulsion, 9.04
    reporting unethical physicians, 9.031
    specialty organization determination of valid
        treatments, 2.065
    Socioeconomic conditions, *See* Access to
        care; Discrimination; Health disparities;
        Indigent care; Poverty
Solicitation of the public for directed donation of
    organs for transplantation, 2.152
Soliciting contributions from patients, 10.018
Somatic cell donors, 2.146, 2.147
Somatic cell nuclear transfer technology,
    2.146, 2.147
Somatic cell therapy, 2.11
Specialty care
    negotiating discounts, 8.052
    patient referral and disclosure of health plan
        limitations, 8.132
Sperm donors, 2.04, 2.05
    compensation, 2.05
    frozen pre-embryos, 2.141, 2.145
Splitting pre-embryos, 2.145
Sports medicine, 3.06
Spouse abuse, *See* Violence and abuse
Staff privileges, 4.07
Standards, professional, Principle II

State executions, *See* Capital punishment
State law, *See* Law
Stem cells, 2.146
    donors and recipients, 2.146
    embryonic, 2.146
    fetal umbilical cord blood banking, 2.165
    immortal cell lines, 2.146
    research with, 2.146
Stop-loss plans, 8.051, 8.054
Strikes, 9.025
Student services, billing for, 4.03
Students, medical
    due process, 9.05
    industry scholarship and special funds for
        educational meeting attendees
        (guideline 6), 8.061
    informing families of patient's death, 8.18
    involvement in patient care, 8.087
    peers as patients, 8.191
    performing procedures on fellow
        students, 3.09
    sexual harassment and exploitation between
        medical supervisors and trainees, 3.08
    signing bonuses to attract graduates of US
        medical schools, 9.037
    supervisor-trainee disputes, 9.055
Subject selection for clinical trials, *See*
    Research subjects
Subsidies by industry, *See* Meetings
Substance abuse
    physician impairment, 8.15
    reporting impaired, incompetent or unethical
        colleagues, 9.0305, 9.031
Substituted judgment, *See* Decision making;
    Surrogate decision makers
Substitution of surgeon without patient's
    knowledge or consent, 8.16
Suffering, existential, *See* Terminal care
Suicide, physician-assisted, 2.20, 2.211
Supervisee, nonphysician, physician employment
    by, 3.05
Supervisors, medical
    disputes between trainees and, 9.055
    sexual harassment and exploitation between
        trainees and, 3.08
Surgeon, substitution of, without patient's
    knowledge or consent, 8.16
Surgery
    assistants, 8.16
    comanagement and self-referral
        restrictions, 8.043
    multiple physicians providing services, 6.10
    "placebo" controls, 2.076
    second opinions, 8.041
    self-referral restrictions, 8.043
    studies involving minor modifications of
        procedures, 2.076
    studies of new surgical procedures, 2.076
    surgeon substitution without patient
        knowledge, 8.16
    surgical or diagnostic instrument patents, 9.09
Surgical "placebo" controls, 2.076

Surgical comanagement, ethical implications of, 8.043
Surgical or diagnostic instruments, patent for, 9.09
Surrogate decision makers, 8.081
  discussions in advance by patient with, 8.081
  do-not-resuscitate orders, 2.22
  filming patients for education of health professionals, 5.046
  filming patients in health care settings, 5.045
  medical students' involvement in patient care, 8.087
  organ donation after cardiac death, 2.157
  substituted judgment, 8.081
  withholding/withdrawing life-sustaining treatment, 2.20
Surrogate mothers, 2.18

Team physicians, See Sports medicine
Technology, assisted reproductive, 2.055
Teenagers, See Adolescents
Telecommunication, See also Internet
  diagnosis by, 5.025
  electronic mail, 5.026
  health-related online sites, 5.027
  physician advisory or referral services, 5.025
Telephone, physician advisory or referral services, 5.025
Terminally ill patients
  advance directives, 2.225
  do-not-resuscitate orders, 2.22
  end-of-life decisions, 10.02
  euthanasia, 2.21
  existential suffering, 2.201
  intentionally causing death, 2.201
  medical futility in end-of-life care, 2.037
  orders not to intervene, 2.225
  organ transplant team members excluded from decision making, in cases of cardiac death, 2.157
  physician-assisted suicide, 2.20, 2.211
  sedation to unconsciousness, 2.201
  xenotransplantation, 2.169
Termination of physician-patient relationship, 8.115
Terminology, 1.01
  capital punishment, physician participation, 2.06
  conditions creating the existence of patient-physician relationship, 10.015
  criteria determining "genuine research purposes" (guideline 5), 8.061
  defining "carefully selected educational conferences" (guideline 6), 8.061
  definition of legitimate industry conferences and meetings (guideline 3), 8.061
  detainees, 2.068
  ethical conduct, 1.01
  "futility," as concept, 2.035
  interrogations, 2.068
  medical futility in end-of-life care, 2.037
  sexual harassment, 3.08
  surgical "placebo" controls, 2.076

  torture, 2.067
  unethical conduct, 1.01
Test results, See Diagnosis
Testimonials, patient, 5.02
Testimony, 5.06, 9.07
  physician actions not constituting participation in executions, 2.06
Tests, diagnostic, See Diagnosis
"Therapeutic privilege," 8.082
Third parties, sexual or romantic relations between physicians and, 8.145
Three-tiered allocation system, See Health care delivery
Tissue harvesting, 2.145
Tissue, human, See Human tissue
Token advisory or consulting services, See Consultation, medical
Tomography, computed, direct-to-consumer diagnostic imaging tests, 8.045
Torture, 2.067
Touring, See Travel
Trainees and training, See Education, medical; Education, medical, graduate; Resident physicians; Students, medical
Transfer, See Patient transfer
Transplantation, 2.16
  allocation guidelines on organ recipients, 2.16
  anencephalic neonates as organ donors, 2.162
  assistance to sustain organ perfusion in anencephalic neonates, 2.162
  cadaveric organ donation financial incentives, motivation, 2.151
  dead fetus tissue, organs, 2.10
  directed (designated) fetal tissue transplantation prohibited, 2.161
  directed (designated) organ donations, 2.15, 2.152
  distribution of organs, 2.15, 2.151
  donated organs as national rather than regional resource, 2.16
  donor advocate team separate from organ recipient's care, 2.15
  donor evaluation by advocate team, 2.15, 2.152
  efforts to increase organ donation, 2.151, 2.155
  fetal tissue, and financial remuneration, 2.161
  fetal tissue, medical applications of, 2.161
  fetal umbilical cord, 2.165
  geographical priorities and, 2.16
  guidelines, 2.16
  in vitro fertilization, 2.14
  living donors, 2.15
  living organ donor compensation, 2.15
  organ donation after cardiac death, 2.157
  organ donation and patient responsibilities, 10.02
  organ donation by condemned prisoners, 2.06
  organ recipient selection, 2.16
  organ swaps (paired donation), 2.15
  presumed consent and mandated choice for organs from deceased donors, 2.155
  procedures by competent physicians in adequate facilities, 2.16

psychosocial evaluation of donors, 2.15, 2.152

public solicitation for directed organ donation, 2.152

purchase of donated organs, 2.151

single waiting lists for organ recipients, 2.16

tissue harvesting from genetically identical children, 2.145

withdrawal decisions by potential donors, 2.15

xenotransplantation, 2.169

Transsexual identity, declining patients on basis of, 9.12

Travel subsidies, prizes and industry gifts to physicians, 8.061

Treatment decisions for seriously ill newborns, 2.215

Treatment denial

allocating limited medical resources, 2.03

discrimination and, 9.12

futile care, 2.035

HIV-infected patients, 2.23, 9.131

medical futility in end-of-life care, 2.037

potential patients, 10.05

physician's personal, religious, moral beliefs and refusal to provide a specific treatment, 10.05

Tuskegee Study, 2.30

Ultrasonography, prenatal genetic testing, 2.12

Umbilical cord blood banking, 2.165

Uncompensated care, See Indigent care

Unconsciousness, sedation to, in end-of-life care, 2.201

Unethical conduct, 1.01, 9.031, 9.04

Unethical experiments, information from, 2.30

Unionization, 9.025

Unnecessary medical services, 2.19

Unscientific practitioners, See Nonscientific practitioners

Unscientific procedures, See Nonscientific treatment

US Food and Drug Administration, See Food and Drug Administration

Utilization committees, See Peer review

Utilization review, physician self-referral (financial interest in facilities outside their practices), 8.0321

Vaccination, See Immunization

Vegetative state, See Life-sustaining treatment

Vehicle drivers, See Automobile drivers

Victims, See Torture; Violence and abuse

Violence and abuse

community and health resources, 2.02

mandatory reporting, 2.02

patient threats and disclosure of confidential information, 5.05

physician training, 2.02

physicians' obligations in preventing, identifying and treating, 2.02

societal misconceptions, 2.02

Viral delivery systems (gene therapy), 2.11, 2.13

Volunteering, caring for the poor, 9.065

Waiting lists, See Transplantation

Waiver of co-payment, See Fees and charges

Waiver of informed consent for research in emergency situations, 8.085

War, biological and chemical weapons, 2.078

Web sites, See also Internet

health-related, 5.027

sales of health- and non-health-related products, 8.062, 8.063

Weighted formula, See Health care delivery

Wellness, physician, 9.0305

Withdrawing/withholding treatment, See Life-sustaining treatment; Treatment denial

Withholding information from patients, 8.082

Women, See also Abortion; Gender; Pregnancy

fetal research guidelines, 2.10

gender discrimination, 9.035

gender disparities in health care, 9.122

sexual harassment in medicine, 9.035

single, artificial insemination by anonymous donor, 2.05

surrogate mothers, 2.18

Work, See Employment

Work-related and independent medical examinations, 5.09, 10.03

Worker health, See Occupational health

Workers' compensation

contingent physician fees, 6.01

industry-employed physicians, independent medical examiners, and confidentiality, 5.09

physician testimony, 5.06

work-related and independent examinations, 10.03

Workplace issues, See Employment

World health, See Developing countries; International health; International research

Xenotransplantation, 2.169